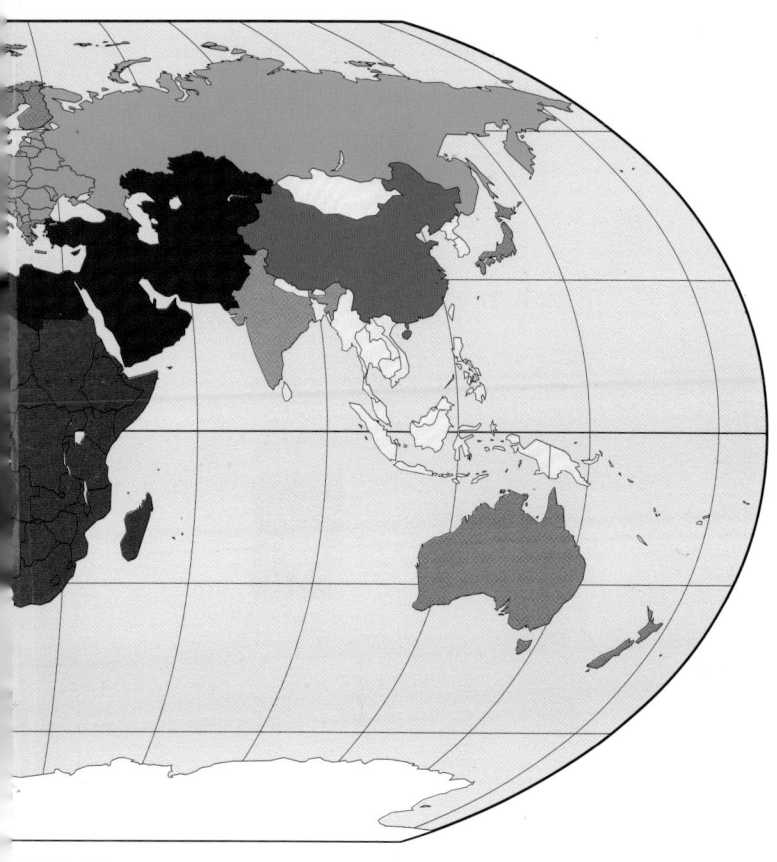

OUPINGS

- Other Asia and Islands (OAI)
  Otros países asiáticos e insulares (OPAI)
  Autres pays d'Asie et îles (APAI)

- Sub-Saharan Africa (SSA)
  Africa al Sur del Sahara (ASS)
  Afrique sub-saharienne (ASS)

- Latin America and the Caribbean (LAC)
  América Latina y el Caribe (ALC)
  Amérique latine et Caraïbes (ALC)

- Middle Eastern Crescent (MEC)
  Arco del Oriente Medio (AOM)
  Croissant moyen-oriental (CMO)

GLOBAL BURDEN OF DISEASE AND INJURY SERIES
VOLUME II

GLOBAL HEALTH STATISTICS

A Compendium of Incidence, Prevalence and Mortality Estimates for Over 200 Conditions

CHRISTOPHER J. L. MURRAY
HARVARD UNIVERSITY
BOSTON, MA, USA

ALAN D. LOPEZ
WORLD HEALTH ORGANIZATION
GENEVA, SWITZERLAND

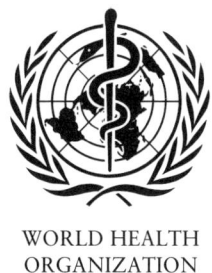

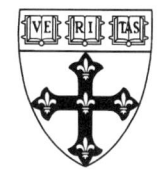

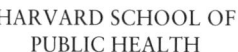

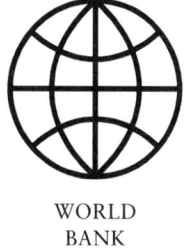

WORLD HEALTH
ORGANIZATION

HARVARD SCHOOL OF
PUBLIC HEALTH

WORLD
BANK

PUBLISHED BY THE HARVARD SCHOOL OF PUBLIC HEALTH ON BEHALF OF
THE WORLD HEALTH ORGANIZATION AND THE WORLD BANK
DISTRIBUTED BY HARVARD UNIVERSITY PRESS

Library of Congress Cataloging-in-Publication (CIP) Data

Murray, Christopher J.L.
  Global health statistics : a compendium of incidence, prevalence,
and mortality estimates for over 200 conditions / Christopher J.L.
Murray, Alan D. Lopez.
      p. cm. -- (Global burden of disease and injury series : 2)
  "Harvard School of Public Health."
  Includes bibliographical references and index.
  Introd. also in Spanish and French.
  ISBN 0-674-35449-4
  1. Medical statistics. I. Lopez, Alan D. II. World Health
Organization. III. World Bank. IV. Harvard School of Public
Health. V. Title VI. Series.
  [DNLM: 1. Epidemiology--tables. 2. Public Health--statistics.
3. Health Status Indicators--tables.   WA 16 M981g 1996]
RA407. M87   1996
614.4'2--dc20
DNLM/DLC
for Library of Congress   96-26652
                                                    CIP

Printed in the United States of America

For Brian Abel-Smith, Richard Peto, Sam Preston, Lado Ruzicka and Edward O. Wilson who guided and encouraged us in our careers; and for Agnes and Lene, our infinitely patient and supporting wives.

TABLE OF CONTENTS

LIST OF TABLES

FOREWORD TO
THE *GLOBAL BURDEN OF DISEASE AND INJURY SERIES*

RALPH H. HENDERSON

The collection and use of timely and reliable health information in support of health policies and programmes have been actively promoted by the World Health Organization since its foundation. Valid health statistics are required at all levels of the health system, ranging from data for health services support at the local community level, through to national statistics and information used to monitor the effectiveness of national health strategies. Equally, regional and global data are required to monitor global epidemics and to continuously assess the effectiveness of global public health approaches to disease and injury prevention and control, as coordinated by WHO technical programmes. Despite the clear need for epidemiological data, reliable and comprehensive health statistics are not available in many Member States of WHO, and, indeed, in many countries the ascertainment of disease levels, patterns and trends is still very uncertain.

In recent years, monitoring systems, community-level research and disease registers have improved in both scope and coverage. Simultaneously, research on the epidemiological transition has increased our understanding of how the cause structure of mortality changes as overall mortality rates decline. As a consequence, estimates and projections of various epidemiological parameters, such as incidence, prevalence and mortality, can now be made at the global and regional level for many diseases and injuries. The Global Burden of Disease Study has now provided the public health community with a set of consistent estimates of disease and injury rates in 1990. The Study has also attempted to provide a comparative index of the burden of each disease or injury, namely the number of Disability-Adjusted Life Years (DALYs) lost as a result of either premature death or years lived with disability.

The findings published in the *Global Burden of Disease and Injury Series* provide a unique and comprehensive assessment of the health of populations as the world enters the third millennium. We also expect that the methods described in the various volumes in the series will stimulate

Member States to improve the functioning and usefulness of their own health information systems. Nonetheless, it must be borne in mind that the results from an undertaking as ambitious as the Global Burden of Disease Study can only be approximate. The reliability of the data for certain diseases, and for some regions, is extremely poor, with only scattered information available in some cases. To extrapolate from these sources to global estimates is clearly very hazardous, and could well result in errors of estimation. The methods that were used for some diseases (e.g. cancer) are not necessarily those applied by other scientists or institutions (e.g. the International Agency for Research on Cancer) and hence the results obtained may differ, sometimes considerably, from theirs. Moreover, the concept of the DALY as used in this Study is still under development, and further work is needed to assess the relevance of the social values that have been incorporated in the calculation of DALYs, as well as their applicability in different sociocultural settings. In this regard, WHO and its various partners are continuing their efforts to investigate burden-of-disease measurements and their use in health policy decision-making.

Dr Ralph H. Henderson is Assistant Director-General of the World Health Organization.

Foreword to
The *Global Burden of*
Disease and Injury Series

Dean T. Jamison

Rational evaluation of policies for health improvement requires four basic types of information: a detailed, reliable assessment of epidemiological conditions and the burden of disease; an inventory of the availability and disposition of resources for health (i.e. a system of what has become known as national health accounts); an assessment of the institutional and policy environment; and information on the cost-effectiveness of available technologies and strategies for health improvement. The *Global Burden of Disease and Injury Series* provides, on a global and regional level, a detailed and internally consistent approach to meeting the first of these information needs, that concerning epidemiological conditions and disease burden. It fully utilizes what information exists while, at the same time, pointing to great variation—across conditions and across countries—in data quality. In the *Global Burden of Disease and Injury Series*, Christopher Murray, Alan Lopez and literally scores of their collaborators from around the world present us with a *tour de force*: its (initial) 10 volumes summarize epidemiological knowledge about all major conditions and most risk factors; they generate assessments of numbers of deaths by cause that are consistent with the total numbers of deaths by age, sex and region provided by demographers; they provide methodologies for and assessments of aggregate disease burden that combine—into the Disability-Adjusted Life Year or DALY measure—burden from premature mortality with that from living with disability; and they use historical trends in main determinants to project mortality and disease burden forward to 2020. Publication of the *Global Burden of Disease and Injury Series* marks the transition to a new era of health outcome accounting—an era for which these volumes establish vastly higher standards for rigour, comprehensiveness and internal consistency. I firmly predict that by the turn of the century the official reporting of health outcomes in dozens of countries and globally will embody the approach and standards described in this series.

The *Global Burden of Disease and Injury Series* culminates an evolutionary process that began in the late 1980s. Close and effective collaboration between the World Bank and the World Health Organization initiated, supported and contributed substantively to that process.

BACKGROUND

Work leading to the *Global Burden of Disease and Injury Series* proceeded in three distinct phases beginning in 1988. Intellectual antecedents go back much further (see Murray 1996, or Morrow and Bryant 1995); perhaps the most relevant are Ghana's systematic assessment of national health problems (Ghana Health Assessment Project Team 1981) and the introduction of the QALY (quality-adjusted life year)—see, for example Zeckhauser and Shepard (1976). My comments here focus on the three phases leading directly to the *Global Burden of Disease and Injury Series*.

Phase 1 constituted an input to a four-year long "Health Sector Priorities Review" initiated in 1988 by the World Bank; its purpose was to assess "...the significance to public health of individual diseases (or related clusters of diseases)...and what is now known about the cost and effectiveness of relevant interventions for their control" (Jamison et al. 1993, p. 3; that volume provides the results of the review). Dr Christopher Murray of Harvard University introduced the DALY as a common measure of effectiveness for the review to use across interventions dealing with diverse diseases, and Dr Alan Lopez of the World Health Organization prepared estimates of child death by cause that were consistent with death totals provided by demographers at the World Bank (Lopez 1993). At the same time, and in close coordination, a World Bank effort was preparing consistent estimates for adult (ages 15–59) mortality by cause for much of the developing world (Feachem et al. 1992). Ensuring this consistency was a major advance and is a precondition for systematic attempts to measure disease burden. (Estimates of numbers of deaths by cause that are not constrained to sum to a demographically-derived total seem inevitably to result in substantial overestimates of deaths due to each cause.) Phase I of this effort, then, introduced the DALY and established important consistency standards to guide estimation of numbers of deaths by cause.

Phase 2 constituted the first attempt to provide a comprehensive set of estimates not only of numbers of deaths by cause but also of total disease burden including burden from disability. This effort was commissioned as background for the World Bank's *World Development Report 1993: Investing in Health*; it was co-sponsored by the World Bank and the World Health Organization; and it was undertaken under the general guidance of a committee chaired by Dr JP Jardel (then Assistant Director-General of WHO). The actual work was conceptualized, managed and integrated by Drs Murray and Lopez and involved extensive efforts by a large number of individuals, most of whom were on the WHO staff. First publication of the estimates of 1990 disease burden appeared in Appendix B of *Investing in Health* (World Bank 1993); the World Health Organization subsequently published a volume containing a full account of the methods used and a somewhat revized and far more extensive presentation of the results (Murray and Lopez 1994).

Preparation and publication of the *Global Burden of Disease and Injury Series* constitutes Phase 3 of this sequence of efforts. As in the earlier phases, the *Global Burden of Disease and Injury Series* was undertaken to inform a policy analysis—in this case an assessment of priorities for health research and development in developing countries being guided by WHO's Ad Hoc Committee on Health Research Relating to Future Intervention Options. The Committee sought updated estimates of disease burden for 1990, projections to 2020 and an extension of the methods to allow assessment of burden attributable to selected risk factors (volume 9 of the *Global Burden of Disease and Injury Series*). The committee's report (Ad Hoc Committee 1996) and the *Global Burden of Disease and Injury Series* appear as companion documents.

Chapters summarizing results from the *Global Burden of Disease and Injury Series* appear in volume I, *The Global Burden of Disease;* underlying epidemiological statistics for over 200 conditions appear in volume II, *Global Health Statistics.* The next six volumes of the *Series* provide, for the first time, chapters detailing the data on each condition or cluster of conditions. These condition-specific chapters were extremely difficult to prepare under the constraints of time, consistency and comprehensiveness imposed by Murray and Lopez. (As co-author of the chapter on intestinal helminthiases I am well aware of the difficulties involved!) Yet the results, individually and collectively, enrich greatly the summaries that were hitherto published. The selection of subjects for the individual volumes—reproductive health, infectious diseases, non-communicable diseases, neurological and psychiatric disorders, injury and malnutrition—will make individual volumes of value to specialist communities. Volume IX reports on the burden due to selected risk factors. The tenth and final volume for the initial series—additional volumes are in the planning stage—reports country-specific analyses (the first of which, for Mexico, had been published previously by Lozano et al. 1994), describes applications of the analyses and introduces alternative methodological approaches.

Will there be a fourth phase? I am sure there will. Reporting of the disease-specific and risk factor analysis in the *Global Burden of Disease and Injury Series* will provoke constructive and perhaps substantial criticism and improvements; country-specific assessments will multiply (over 20 are now under way) and they, too, will modify and enrich current estimates. Country and global estimates for times in the past will most likely be prepared; estimates of years of life lost for the Unites States in 1900 have already been made (Jamison 1995). Methodologies will be criticized and, I would predict, constructively revised. Unfinished elements of the agenda discussed in the next section will be completed. Phase 4, perhaps centred on the estimation of global and regional disease burden for 1995 and including a look at the past, will take us well beyond where we now are.

THE AGENDA

Disease burden (or numbers of deaths by cause) can be partitioned in three separate ways for different age, sex and regional groupings (Murray et al. 1994). One partition is by *risk factor*—genetic, behavioural, environmental and physiological. The second is by *disease*. The third is by consequence—*premature mortality* at different ages and different *types of disability* (e.g. sensory, cognitive functioning, pain, affective state, etc.).

Disaggregation by risk factor helps guide policy concerning primary and secondary prevention, including development of new preventive measures. Disaggregation by disease helps guide policy concerning cure, secondary prevention and palliation; and disaggregation by consequence helps guide policies for rehabilitation.

Work on the disease burden assessment agenda began with assessments of mortality and burden by disease; the *Global Burden of Disease and Injury Series* advances the agenda in that domain by revising and adding great detail on disease burden estimates. Additionally the *Global Burden of Disease and Injury Series* makes a major advance by assessing burden due to selected major risk factors (Volume 9); this extends usefulness of the work to the domain of prevention policy.

There remains, however, an important unfinished agenda. The disease burden associated with different types of disability remains to be assessed; perhaps part of the reason for neglect of rehabilitation in most discussion of health policy is the lack of even approximate information on burden due to disability or on the DALY gains per unit cost of rehabilitative intervention.

A related agenda item—relevant to planning for curative and, particularly, rehabilitative intervention—is to present disease burden estimates from a current prevalence perspective. The dominant perspective of work so far undertaken, including in the *Global Burden of Disease and Injury Series*, is that of adding up over time the burden that will result from all conditions incident in a given year (here 1990); this well serves the development of primary prevention policy and of treatment policy for diseases of short duration. The prevalence perspective complements the incidence one by assessing how much burden is being experienced during a particular year by chronic conditions or by disabilities; those conditions or disabilities will often have been generated some time in the past. From an incidence perspective, disability in this year from, say, an injury occurring a decade ago would generate DALY loss in the year of incidence; but to guide investment in rehabilitation we need to know how much disability exists today, i.e., we need a prevalence perspective. Murray and Lopez in *The Global Burden of Disease* and in *Global Health Statistics* provide the basic estimates of prevalence of different disabilities and first glimpses of the prevalence perspective.

A final major agenda item is to establish for each condition and in the aggregate how much of the potential current burden is in fact being averted by existing interventions and how much of the remaining burden persists because of lack of any intervention, lack of cost-effective interventions, or because of inefficiency of the system.

USES OF DALYs AND DISEASE BURDEN MEASUREMENT

DALYs have six major uses to underpin health policy. Five of these relate to measurement of the burden of disease; the final one concerns judging the relative priority of interventions in terms of cost-effectiveness.

Assessing performance. A country-specific (or regional) assessment of the burden of disease provides a performance indicator that can be used over time to judge progress or across countries or regions to judge relative performance. These comparisons can be either quite aggregated (in terms of DALYs lost per thousand population) or finely disaggregated to allow focused assessment of where relative performance is good and where it is not. The *Global Burden of Disease and Injury Series* with its burden assessments for eight regions in 1990—and with the increasing number of country-specific assessments that it will report—will provide, I predict, the benchmark for all subsequent work. The most natural comparison is to the development of National Income and Product Accounts (NIPAs) by Simon Kuznets and others in the 1930s, which culminated in 1939 with a complete NIPA for the United Kingdom prepared by James Meade and Richard Stone at the request of the UK Treasury. NIPAs have, in the subsequent decades, transformed the empirical underpinnings of economic policy analysis. One of the leading proponents of major changes in NIPAs has put it this way:

> The national income and product accounts for the United States (NIPAs), and kindred accounts in other nations, have been among the major contributions to economic knowledge over the past half century....Several generations of economists and practitioners have now been able to tie theoretical constructs of income, output, investment, consumption, and savings to the actual numbers of these remarkable accounts with all their fine detail and soundly meshed interrelations. (Eisner 1989)

My own expectation is that this series will, over a decade or two, initiate a transformation of health policy analysis analogous to that initiated for economic policy by the introduction of NIPAs in the late 1930s. Today most health policy work concerns only cost, finance, process and access; burden of disease (and risk factor) assessments should soon allow full incorporation of performance measures in policy analysis.

Generating a forum for informed debate of values and priorities. The assessment of disease burden in a country-specific context in practice involves participation of a broad range of national disease specialists, epidemiologists and, often, policy makers. Debating the appropriate values for, say, disability weights or for years of life lost at different ages helps clarify values and objectives for national health policy. Discussing the inter-relations among diseases and their risk factors in the light of local conditions sharpens consideration of priorities. And the entire process brings technically informed participants to the table where policy is discussed. The preparation of a well-defined product generates a process with much value of its own.

Identifying national control priorities. Many countries now identify a relatively short list of interventions, the full implementation of which becomes an explicit priority for national political and administrative attention. Examples include interventions to control tuberculosis, poliomyelitis, HIV infection, smoking and specific micronutrient deficiencies. Because political attention and administrative capacity are in relatively fixed and short supply, the benefits from using those resources will be maximized if they are directed to interventions that are both cost-effective and aimed at problems associated with a high burden. Thus, national assessments of disease burden are instrumental for establishing this short list of control priorities.

Allocating training time for clinical and public health practitioners. Medical schools offer a fixed number of instructional hours; training programmes for other levels and types of practitioners are likewise limited. A major instrument for implementing policy priorities is to allocate this fixed time resource well—again that means allocation of time to training in interventions where disease burden is high and cost-effective interventions exist.

Allocating research and development resources. Whenever a fixed effort will have a benefit proportional not to the size of the effort but rather to the size of the problem being addressed, estimates of disease burden become essential for formulation of policy. This is the case with political attention and with time in the medical school curriculum; and it is likewise true for the allocation of research and development resources. Developing a vaccine for a broad range of viral pneumonias, for example, would have perhaps hundreds of times the impact of a vaccine against disease from Hanta virus infection. Thus information on disease or risk factor burden is one (of several) vital inputs to inform research and development resource allocation. Indeed, as previously noted, this series—with its disease burden assessments for 1990, its projections to 2020 and its initial assessment of burden due to risk factors—was commissioned to inform a WHO Committee charged with assessing health research and development priorities for developing countries (Ad Hoc Committee 1996).

The Committee sought not only to know the burden by condition, but also to partition the burden remaining for each condition into several distinct parts reflecting the importance of the reasons for the remaining disease burden. This division into four parts was undertaken for several conditions; a major agenda item for future analysis is to undertake such a partitioning systematically for all conditions so that there could be reasonably approximate answers to such questions as "How much of the remaining disease burden cannot be addressed without major biomedical advances?" or, "How much of the remaining disease burden could be averted by utilizing existing interventions more efficiently?" Arguably most of the spectacular gains in human health of the past century have resulted from advances in knowledge (although improvements in income and education have also played a role). If so, improving research and development policy in health may be more important than improving policy in health systems or finance; improved assessments and projections of disease burden will be critical to that undertaking.

Allocating resources across health interventions. Here disease burden assessment often plays a minor role; the task is to shift resources to interventions which, at the margin, will generate the greatest reduction in DALY loss. When there are major fixed costs in mounting an intervention—as is the case with political and managerial attention for national control priorities—burden estimates are indeed required to optimize resource allocation. But, typically, much progress can be made with only an understanding of how the DALYs gained from an intervention vary with the level of expenditure on it; such assessments are the stuff of cost-effectiveness analysis. The DALY as a common measure of effectiveness allows comparison of cost-effectiveness across interventions addressing all conditions; such an initial effort was undertaken for the World Bank's "Health Sector Priorities Review" (Jamison et al. 1993) in the late 1980s using a forerunner to the DALY utilized in this series.

* * *

The *Global Burden of Disease and Injury Series* contains the only available internally consistent, comprehensive and comparable assessments of causes of death, incidence and prevalence of disease and injury, measures and projections of disease burden, and measures of risk factor burden. In that sense the authors' contributions represent a landmark achievement and provide an invaluable resource for policy analysts and scholars. This effort dramatically raises the standard by which future reporting of health conditions will be judged. Yet, the very need for the ad hoc assessments that the volumes in this series report, points to important gaps in the international system for gathering, analysing and distributing policy-relevant data on the health of populations. Without information on how levels and trends in key indicators in their own countries compare with other countries, national decision-makers will lack benchmarks for judging performance. Likewise students of health systems will lack the empirical basis for forming outcome-based judgements on which policies work—and which do not. I hope, then, that one follow-on to the *Global*

Burden of Disease and Injury Series will be the institutionalization of continued efforts to generate and analyse internationally comparable data on health outcomes.

Dean T. Jamison is Professor of Public Health and of Education at the University of California, Los Angeles, and Economic Adviser to the Human Development Department of the World Bank. He recently served as Chairman of the World Health Organization's Ad Hoc Committee on Health Research Relating to Future Intervention Options.

REFERENCES

Ad Hoc Committee on Health Research Relating to Future Intervention Options (1996) *Investing in health research and development.* World Health Organization. Geneva (Document TDR/Gen/96.1).

Eisner R (1989) *The total incomes system of accounts.* Chicago, University of Chicago Press.

Feachem RGA et al., eds. (1992) *The health of adults in the developing world.* New York, Oxford University Press for the World Bank.

Ghana Health Assessment Project Team (1981) A quantitative method of assessing the health impact of different diseases in less developed countries. *International journal of epidemiology*, 10: 73–80.

Goerdt A et al. (1996) Disability: definition and measurement issues. In: Murray CJL and Lopez AD, eds., *The global burden of disease: a comprehensive assessment of mortality and disability from diseases, injuries, and risk factors in 1990 and projected to 2020.* Cambridge, Harvard University Press.

Jamison DT et al., eds. (1993) *Disease control priorities in developing countries.* New York, Oxford University Press for the World Bank.

Jamison JC (1995) The mortal burden: disability adjusted life years lost to premature mortality in the United States in 1900. Economic history paper, MIT Department of Economics.

Lopez AD (1993) Causes of death in industrial and developing countries: estimates for 1985–1990. In: Jamison DT et al., eds. *Disease control priorities in developing countries.* New York, Oxford University Press for the World Bank, 35–50.

Lozano R et al. (1994) *El peso de la enfermedad en México: un doble reto.* [The national burden of disease in México: a double challenge.] Mexico, Mexican Health Foundation, (Documentos para el análisis y la convergencia, No. 3).

Morrow RH, Bryant JH (1995) Health policy approaches to measuring and valuing human life: conceptual and ethical issues. *American journal of public health*, 85(10): 1356–1360.

Murray CJL (1996) Rethinking DALYs. In: Murray CJL and Lopez AD, eds., *The global burden of disease: a comprehensive assessment of mortality and disability from diseases, injuries, and risk factors in 1990 and projected to 2020.* Cambridge, Harvard University Press.

Murray CJL and Lopez AD, eds. (1994) *Global comparative assessments in the health sector: disease burden, expenditures and intervention packages.* Geneva, World Health Organization.

Murray CJL, Lopez AD, Jamison DT (1994) The global burden of disease in 1990: summary results, sensitivity analysis and future directions. *Bulletin of the World Health Organization*, 72(3):495–509.

World Bank (1993) *World development report 1993: investing in health.* New York, Oxford University Press for the World Bank.

World Health Organization. *World health statistics annual*, various years. Geneva, WHO.

Zeckhauser R, Shepard D (1976) Where now for saving lives? *Law and contemporary problems*, 40:5–45.

Foreword

Richard Peto

Until the twentieth century, human mortality was caused primarily by infections, malnutrition, and trauma. About half of all persons in Europe and elsewhere died in infancy or childbirth, and few survived long enough to be at much risk from the noncommunicable diseases of middle and old age. During this century, however, there has been a great change in this pattern, dubbed the "epidemiological transition." First, especially in developed countries, childhood death rates have decreased substantially and are continuing to decrease. These decreases notwithstanding, 1990 death rates indicate that one in every six persons in developing countries dies before reaching middle age.

Most of these early deaths are caused by injuries or communicable diseases, while most deaths at later ages are caused by noncommunicable diseases. The increasing relative importance of causes such as cancer or cardiovascular disease is attributed not to any general increase in the age-specific death-rates of noncommunicable diseases, but rather to a general decrease in deaths from other causes. Worldwide, HIV and tobacco are the only large causes of death whose effects are increasing rapidly. Apart from these two factors (and the temporary effects of wars and famines), life expectancy is increasing. Indeed, life expectancy in developing countries today is greater than was the life expectancy in any developed country at the start of this century.

Vast problems remain, however, particularly in infancy and childhood. In 1990, during which there were 140 million births, there were 50 million deaths, of which thirteen million were of children aged between 0 and 4 years. These numbers indicate the complementary needs for better family planning and better child survival. The analyses presented in this volume show more specifically where large improvements might be possible: 2.5 million deaths before age five years were due to conditions arising in the perinatal period, most of which could have been avoided. Another seven million deaths before age five were attributable to diarrhoea, respiratory infections, malaria, measles, or tetanus; most of these, too, were avoidable.

Over the past twenty years, remarkable progress has been made toward describing the patterns of disease and the trends in mortality. Until the 1970s, no clear assessment of the relative importance of different diseases as causes of either death or disability was available. It was therefore difficult to devise appropriately balanced strategies for disease control. Since then, numerical estimates have been devised and improved, helping to engender appropriate emphasis on the more pressing needs: selective primary care; child survival and safe motherhood; vaccination; breast-feeding and other methods of prevention and treatment of diarrhoeal and respiratory diseases; tuberculosis control; and the control of avoidable causes of cardiovascular diseases.

It is easy to underestimate the extraordinary importance and power of purely descriptive statistics. For in the long term, they have an enormous influence on major public policies, special disease control programmes, and research agendas. And, in recent years, Murray and Lopez have produced the best descriptive statistics in the world, particularly for mortality.

The authors have consulted widely and, in so doing, have produced estimates that are more consistent and plausible than any others. Their large picture is unlikely to be altered by future evidence, even though later data may better inform the details. For example, later analyses may reveal the heterogeneity that undoubtedly occurs within each of the eight world regions for which data are evaluated here. But the present volume attempts to provide a broad picture for the entire population of the world. In so doing, it presents much of substantial importance and of substantial novelty. From these estimates, several trustworthy conclusions have already emerged—such as the great relative importance of mental health—that will withstand any doubts concerning data or methodology.

Murray and Lopez also present estimates of the trends in disease. These trends appear to be plausible, but so too might other estimates based on different data, assumptions and methods. John Kenneth Galbraith has said that economists fall into two classes, those who cannot predict the future and those who know they cannot predict the future; and the same may be true of epidemiologists. Because of the sheer uncertainty in an exercise of projection, some of the future trends presented here will prove to be incorrect. For those disease trends for which knowledge is particularly reliable—such as the increasing mortality from tobacco use or HIV and the decreasing mortality in infancy and childhood—the future projections presented here are of substantial interest.

Analysis of the present and the recent past, however, is the core of this work. The estimates of the global burden of disease in 1990 are for most practical purposes good enough to be trusted and their wide availability is welcomed.

Richard Peto is a Fellow of The Royal Society. He is Professor of Medical Statistics and Epidemiology at the University of Oxford.

Acknowledgements

An undertaking such as this book is simply not possible without the support and contribution of many individuals and institutions throughout the world. A large number of scientists, both within the World Health Organization and elsewhere, provided epidemiological data, research reports, and other information on specific diseases and injuries, which greatly facilitated the preparation of regional estimates published in this book. Many, but not all of those involved have authored chapters on their particular disease that appear in other volumes of the *Global Burden of Disease and Injury Series*. The cooperation of several scientific organizations, government research institutes and non-governmental organizations in providing datasets and advice on their reliability is also gratefully acknowledged.

We wish to acknowledge particularly the dedication, long days and long nights, and truly extraordinary contribution made by Steven Goodreau, Caroline Cook, Joshua Salomon, Robert Ashley, William Whang, Arnab Acharya, Xinjian Qiao, Rafael Lozano, Bonifasiyo Ssennyamantono, Emmanuela Gakidou, Catherine Michaud, Prasanta Mahapatra and Kenji Shibuya at the Burden of Disease Unit, Harvard Center for Population and Development Studies. We are particularly grateful to Rafael Lozano and Catherine Michaud, for the Spanish and French translations, respectively, of the Introduction and Explanatory Notes. Special thanks go to Sonia Contreras, Joaquin Pereira, and S. Venkatesh for proofreading the manuscript.

A special acknowledgement is due to Dean Jamison who inspired all of this.

This work would not have been possible without the financial support of the Edna McConnell Clark Foundation, the Rockefeller Foundation, and the World Bank. We wish to specifically acknowledge the collegial environment and financial support provided by the WHO Ad Hoc Committee on Health Research Relating to Future Intervention Options, chaired by Dean Jamison. Although the preparation of the *Global Burden of Disease and Injury Series* began prior to the Committee's establishment, these books describe in some detail the analytical basis of the Committee's Report, and are thus complementary to it.

While these individuals and institutions played a substantial role in the preparation of this book, they are not responsible for the estimates reported herein. Rather, these numbers represent the outcome of a long series of discussions with scientists, and we alone assume responsibility for their accuracy and plausibility.

CJLM

ADL

INTRODUCTION

Objective, comparable and reliable information on the nature, extent and distribution of diseases and health problems is an essential input into health policy formulation, evaluation, monitoring, and research into the determinants of health. The reality, however, is that despite decades of efforts by countries, supported by international organizations, particularly the World Health Organization, reliable regional and global information on health status is still not widely available. In order to meet the urgent data needs of global health policy formulation, the World Bank and the World Health Organization commissioned the Global Burden of Disease Study (GBD) in 1992 to provide an objective comparable assessment of health status, based on what was then known about the occurrence of disease and injury throughout the world. The results of this study were widely used in the *World Development Report 1993: Investing in Health* (World Bank 1993). A more detailed but nevertheless abbreviated presentation of methods and results was published in a series of articles in the *Bulletin of WHO*, and subsequently reprinted in a book published by the World Health Organization in 1994 (Murray 1994, Murray and Lopez 1994a, Murray and Lopez 1994b, Murray and Lopez 1994c, Murray et al. 1994). The *Global Burden of Disease and Injury Series*, to which this volume belongs, is intended to provide full details of the methods, materials and results for each disease and injury included in the Global Burden of Disease Study, and on the applications of the methods at the national and sub-national level.

The Global Burden of Disease Study was designed in part to address three major limitations of available information on the magnitude of health problems. First, too often health information is provided to decision makers by disease advocates. This link between advocacy and epidemiological estimation can raise doubts about the objectivity of the conclusions. In particular, advocates, often unintentionally, tend to overestimate the magnitude of their specific health concerns. Decoupling advocacy from the process of generating epidemiological assessments is an essential step towards more plausible and useful estimates. Second, international datasets which are based on similar diagnostic and reporting procedures are almost exclusively focused on mortality and fail to incorporate comparable information on non-fatal health outcomes. The absence of plausible information on disability and other indicators of morbidity has contributed to the continued neglect of these problems in national and international health policy debate. Despite the enormous gap in knowledge about the epidemiology of many non-fatal health outcomes, a second major goal of the GBD study was to generate plausible estimates of the incidence, prevalence and duration for a number of important diseases and injuries. Third, a common metric, the Disability-Adjusted Life Year or DALY, has been used to aggregate and summarize the data and information on mortality and non-fatal health outcomes and thus permit comparisons of the impact of various health-related conditions. As DALYs can also be used in cost-effectiveness analyses, they greatly facilitate the joint assessment of the magnitude of health problems with the array of interventions—and their costs—that are available to address these problems. With such a common metric, the combination of burden of disease results and the cost-effectiveness analysis of available interventions can be, and has been, used to identify a set of priority interventions, such as the essential packages described in the *World Development Report* 1993.

The more specific objectives of the Global Burden of Disease Study were four-fold. The first of these was to develop internally consistent estimates of mortality by age, sex and region for more than 100 important causes of death. A second goal was to develop internally consistent estimates of incidence, prevalence, case-fatality and mortality by age, sex and region for the major sequelae of more than 100 leading causes of ill-health. Recognizing the important role of certain exposures in the etiology of disease and injury, a third objective was to estimate the amount of premature mortality and disability attributable to selected risk factors such as air pollution, unsafe sex, hypertension, alcohol and tobacco. The fourth objective was to provide a set of projections of the burden of disease by age, sex, region and cause up until the year 2020.

The purpose of this volume is to facilitate access to the detailed estimates of incidence, prevalence, duration and death which have been prepared for the Global Burden of Disease Study. Designed primarily as a convenient reference source for global epidemiological estimates, much of the volume is dedicated to the tabular presentation of results. Following this brief introduction describing the methods used to prepare the estimates, the remainder of the volume includes a series of tables containing basic demographic information for each of the eight geographical regions used in the *World Development Report 1993*, followed by a much larger number of tables which provide estimates of incidence, prevalence, average age of onset, average duration, deaths in 1990 and projected deaths in 2000 for various diseases and sequelae. The discussion which follows briefly outlines the GBD classification system, the basic demography of each of the eight regions, the cause of death estimation procedures, and the methods used to estimate incidence, prevalence, case-fatality and duration for major sequelae. Readers interested in more detail about the methods and assumptions concerning the empirical basis and estimation process for each disease are referred to the relevant volume(s) in the series.

GBD CLASSIFICATION SYSTEM

For the Global Burden of Disease Study, a so-called 'tree' structure of diseases and injuries has been used. This is presented in Table I. At the first level of disaggregation, overall mortality is divided into three broad cause groups: Group I, consisting of communicable diseases, maternal causes, conditions arising in the perinatal period and nutritional deficiencies[1]; Group II, encompassing the noncommunicable diseases; and Group III, comprizing all injuries. Group I causes of death, the pre-transitional causes, consist of the cluster of conditions that typically decline at a faster pace than all-cause mortality during the process of the epidemiological transition. As a result, in low mortality populations, these causes account for only a small proportion of deaths. Conversely, the noncommunicable diseases clustered in Group II are the most important health problems in populations that have undergone the epidemiological transition. While it is true that mortality rates from some noncommunicable conditions such as stomach cancer may decline faster than all-cause mortality, these conditions have been maintained in Group II along with other cancers, since death rates from cancer as a whole appear to be relatively constant throughout the transition. Finally, injuries are separately classified into Group III, in part because their etiology is very different from that of most diseases, but also because there is no generalized pattern of change in injury mortality that accompanies the epidemiological transition.

Each Group has then been divided into several major sub-categories of disease and injury that are mutually exclusive and exhaustive. These sub-categories are identified with capital letters in Table I. Specifically, Group I has been divided into infectious and parasitic causes, respiratory infections, maternal causes, conditions arising during the perinatal period and nutritional deficiencies. Noncommunicable causes (Group II) have been divided into 14 categories (see Table I). Group III (Injuries) has been divided into two major sub-categories, unintentional injuries (IIIA) and intentional injuries (IIIB).

A third level of disaggregation is used to identify more specific causes of death within each of these second-level categories. For example, within the category infectious and parasitic diseases (IA), specific causes such as tuberculosis (IA1), HIV (IA3) and diarrhoea (IA4) have been identified. Finally, for some diseases such as sexually transmitted diseases (IA2), a fourth level of disaggregation is provided, in this case syphilis (IA2a), gonorrhoea (IA2b) and chlamydia (IA2c). The set of disaggregated causes was selected on the basis of three criteria: the probable magnitude of the disease or injury as a cause of death or disability as evaluated at the beginning of the study; health conditions for which considerable health

Table I   Global Burden of Disease Study classification system for diseases and injuries

Title of GBD cause	ICD-9 Code	ICD-9 BTL Code	ICD-10 Code
I. Communicable, maternal, perinatal and nutritional conditions	001-139, 243, 260-269, 280-285,320-322, 381-382, 614-616, 460-465, 466, 480-487, 614-616, 630-676, 760-779	01-07, 19, 200, 220, 240, 310-312, 320-322, 371-373, 38-41, 45	A00-B99, G00, N70-N73, J00-J06, J10-J18, J20-J22, H65-H66, O00-O99, P00-P06, E00-E02, E40-E46, E50, D50
A. Infectious and parasitic diseases	001-139,320-322, 614-616	01-07, 220, 371-373	A00-B99, G00, N70-N73
1. Tuberculosis	010-018, 137	02, 077	A15-A19, B90
2. Sexually transmitted diseases excluding HIV	090-099, 614-616	06, 371-373	A50-A64, N70-N73
a. Syphilis	090-097	060	A50-A53
b. Chlamydia	i	ii	A55-A56
c. Gonorrhoea	098	061	A54
3. HIV	i		B20-B24
4. Diarrhoeal diseases	001, 002, 004, 006-009	01 minus 013	A01-A04, A06-A09
5. Childhood-cluster diseases	032, 033, 037, 045, 050, 055, 056, 138	033, 034, 037, 040-043, 078	A33-37, A80, B05, B91
a. Pertussis	033	034	A37
b. Poliomyelitis	045, 138	040, 078	A80, B91
c. Diphtheria	032	033	A36
d. Measles	055	042	B05
e. Tetanus	037, 771.3	037[iii]	A33-A35
6. Bacterial meningitis and meningococcaemia	036, 320-322	036, 220[iv]	A39, G00
7. Hepatitis B and hepatitis C	070.2-070.9	046[v]	B16-B19
8. Malaria	084	052	B50-B54
9. Tropical-cluster diseases	085, 086, 120, 125	053, 054, 072, 074	B55-B57, B65, B73-B74
a. Trypanosomiasis	086.3, 086.4, 086.5, 086.9[vi]	054[ii]	B56
b. Chagas disease	086.0, 086.1, 086.2, 086.9[vi]	054[vii]	B57
c. Schistosomiasis	120	072	B65
d. Leishmaniasis	085	053	B55
e. Lymphatic filariasis	125.0, 125.1	ii	B74.0-B74.2
f. Onchocerciasis	125.3	ii	B73
10. Leprosy	030	032	A30
11. Dengue	061	ii	A90-A91
12. Japanese encephalitis	062.0	ii	A83.0
13. Trachoma	076	048	A71
14. Intestinal nematode infections	126-129	ii	
a. Ascariasis	127.0	ii	B77
b. Trichuriasis	127.3	ii	B79
c. Ancylostomiasis and necatoriasis	126	ii	B76
B. Respiratory infections	460-466, 480-487, 381-382	310-312, 320-322, 240	J00-J06, J10-J18, J20-J22, H65-H66
1. Lower respiratory infections	466, 480-487	320-322	J10-J18, J20-J22
2. Upper respiratory infections	460-465	310-312	J00-J06
3. Otitis media	381-382	240	H65-H66
C. Maternal conditions	630-676	38-41	O00-O99
1. Maternal haemorrhage	640, 641, 666	390	O44-O46, O67, O72
2. Maternal sepsis	670	ii	O85-O86
3. Hypertensive disorders of pregnancy	642	ii	O10-O16
4. Obstructed labour	660	393	O64-O66
5. Abortion	630-639	38	O00-O08
D. Conditions arising during the perinatal period	760-779	45	P00-P06
1. Low birth weight	764-765	452	P05-P07
2. Birth asphyxia and birth trauma	767-770	453-454	P03, P10-P15, P20-P29

Table I   (continued)

Title of GBD cause	ICD-9 Code	ICD-9 BTL Code	ICD-10 Code
E. Nutritional deficiencies	243, 260-269, 280-285	19, 200[viii]	E00-E02, E40-E46, E50, D50
1. Protein-energy malnutrition	260-263	190-192	E40-E46
2. Iodine deficiency	243	ii	E00-E02
3. Vitamin A deficiency	264	ii	E50
4. Iron-deficiency anaemia	280	200[viii]	D50
II. Noncommunicable diseases	140-242, 244-259, 270-279, 286-319, 323-380, 383-459, 467-479, 488-613, 617-629, 680-759	08-18, 20-37, 42-44. [minus 200, 220, 240, 310-312, 320-322, 371-373]	C00-C97, D00-D48, D55-D80, E03-E07, E10-E16, E20-E34, E51-E89, F00-F99, G03-G99, H00-H61, H68-H95, I00-I99, J30-J99, K20-K99, N00-N64, N75-N99, L00-L99, M00-M99, Q00-Q99, K00-K99
A. Malignant neoplasms	140-209	08-14	C00-C97
1. Mouth and oropharynx cancers	140-149	08	C00-C14
2. Oesophagus cancer	150	090	C15
3. Stomach cancer	151	091	C16
4. Colon and rectum cancers	153, 154	093, 094	C18-C21
5. Liver cancer	155	095	C22
6. Pancreas cancer	157	096	C25
7. Trachea, bronchus and lung cancers	162	101	C33-C34
8. Melanoma and other skin cancers	172-173	111, 112	C43-C44
9. Breast cancer	174	113	C50
10. Cervix uteri cancer	180	120	C53
11. Corpus uteri cancer	179, 182	122	C54-C55
12. Ovary cancer	183	123	C56
13. Prostate cancer	185	124	C61
14. Bladder cancer	188	126	C67
15. Lymphomas and multiple myeloma	200-202	14 [minus 141]	C81-C90, C96
16. Leukaemia	204-208	141	C91-C95
B. Other neoplasms	210-239	15, 16, 17	D00-D48
C. Diabetes mellitus	250	181	E10-E14
D. Endocrine disorders	240-242, 244-246, 251-259, 270-279, 281-289	18, 20 [minus 200[ix]]	D55-D80, E03-E07, E15-E16, E20-E34, E51-E89
E. Neuro-psychiatric conditions	290-319, 323-359	21-22 [minus 220]	F00-F99, G03-G99
1. Unipolar major depression	i	ii	F32-F33
2. Bipolar disorder	296	212	F30-F31
3. Schizophrenia	295	211	F20-F29
4. Epilepsy	345	225	G40-G41
5. Alcohol use	291, 303, 305.0	215x	F10
6. Dementia and other degenerative and hereditary CNS disorders	330, 331, 290	222, 210[xi]	F01, F03, G30-G31
7. Parkinson disease	332	221	G20-G21
8. Multiple sclerosis	340	223	G35
9. Drug use	304, 305.2-305.9	216[xii]	F11-F16, F18-F19
10. Post-traumatic stress disorder	i	ii	xvii
11. Obsessive-compulsive disorders	300.3	ii	F42
12. Panic disorder	300.2	ii	F40.0, F41.0
F. Sense organ diseases	360-380, 383-389	23, 24 [minus 240]	H00-H61, H68-H95
1. Glaucoma	365	230	H40
2. Cataracts	366	231	H25-H26
G. Cardiovascular diseases	390-459	25-30	I00-I99
1. Rheumatic heart disease	390-398	25	I01-I09
2. Ischaemic heart disease	410-414, Proportion of: 428, 427.1, 427.4, 427.5, 440.9, 429.0-429.2, 429.9[xiii]	27 xiv	I20-I25 xv
3. Cerebrovascular disease	430-438	29	I60-I69
4. Inflammatory heart diseases	420, 421, 422, 425, Proportion of 428[xvi]	ii	I30-I33, I38, I40, I42

Table I (continued)

Title of GBD cause	ICD-9 Code	ICD-9 BTL Code	ICD-10 Code
H. Respiratory diseases	470-478, 490-519	31-32 [minus 310-312, 320-322]	J30-J99
1. Chronic obstructive pulmonary disease	490-492, 495-496	ii	J40-J44
2. Asthma	493	ii	J45-J46
I. Digestive diseases	530-579	34	K20-K99
1. Peptic ulcer	531-533	341	K25-K27
2. Cirrhosis of the liver	571	347	K70, K74
3. Appendicitis	540-543	342	K35-K37
J. Genito-urinary diseases	580-611, 617-629	35-37 [minus 371-373]	N00-N64, N75-N99
1. Nephritis and nephrosis	580-589	350	N00-N19
2. Benign prostatic hypertrophy	600	360	N40
K. Skin diseases	680-709	42	L00-L99
L. Musculo-skeletal diseases	710-759	43	M00-M99
1. Rheumatoid arthritis	714	430	M05-M06
2. Osteoarthritis	715	ii	M15-M19
M. Congenital anomalies	740-759	44	Q00-Q99
1. Abdominal wall defect	i	ii	xvii
2. Anencephaly	740.0	ii	Q00
3. Anorectal atresia	751.2	ii	Q42
4. Cleft lip	749.1	ii	Q36
5. Cleft palate	749.0	ii	Q35,Q37
6. Oesophageal atresia	750.3	ii	Q39.0-Q39.1
7. Renal agenesis	753.0	ii	Q60
8. Down syndrome	758.0	ii	Q90
9. Congenital heart anomalies	745-747	442	Q20-Q28
10 Spina bifida	741	ii	Q05
N. Oral conditions	520-529	33	K00-K14
1. Dental caries	521.0	ii	K02
2. Periodontal disease	523	ii	K05
3. Edentulism	i	ii	xvii
III. Injuries	E800-999	E47-E56	V01-Y98
A. Unintentional injuries	E800-921, 923-949	E47-E51, E520-E523, E53	V01-X59, Y40-Y98
1. Road traffic accidents	E810-819, 826-829, 928-929	E471,E472	V01-V89
2. Poisonings	E850-869	E48	X40-X49
3. Falls	E880-888	E50	W00-W19
4. Fires	E890-899	E51	X00-X09
5. Drownings	E910	E521	W65-W74
6. Other unintentional injuries	E800-E807, E820-825, E830-E848, E870-E879, E900-E909, E911-E921, E923-E949	E470, E473-E474, E49, E520, E522-E523, E53	V90-V99, W20-W64, W75-W99, X10-X39, X50-X59
B. Intentional injuries	E922, 950-979, 990-999	E524, E54-E55, E561	X60-Y09,Y35-Y36
1. Self-inflicted injuries	E950-959	E54	X60-X84
2. Violence	E922, 960-969	E55	X85-Y09
3. War	E990-999	E561	Y35-Y36

NOTES

1. "Symptoms, signs and ill-defined conditions" (Chapter XVI in ICD-9 and R00-R99 in ICD-10) is included in Group I for persons aged under 5 years and in Group II for persons aged 5 years and over, and distributed proportionally to all causes below the Group level.
2. Cause E560 of ICD-9 BTL code (E980-E989 of ICD-9, Y10-Y34 in ICD-10) is distributed proportionally to all injury causes below the Group level.

i No ICD-9 code is available.
ii No ICD-9 BTL code is available.
iii There is no BTL code for neonatal tetanus.
iv BTL 220 includes unspecified causes of meningitis which can be excluded when 4-digit ICD-9 data are available.
v BTL 046 includes hepatitis A which should not be part of this category.
vi 086.9 in SSA is African trypanosomiasis and 086.9 in LAC is Chagas disease.
vii 054 in SSA is African trypanosomiasis and 054 in LAC is Chagas disease.

ix Some of BTL 200, anaemias other than from iron deficiency, should be included here.
x BTL 215 does not include deaths from ICD-9 detailed codes 303 and 305.0.
xi BTL 210 includes ICD-9 detailed codes 330-336 which should not be part of this category.
xii BTL 216 does not include ICD-9 detailed codes 305.2-305.9 which should be included here.
xiii The proportion of these ill-defined cardiovascular codes that should be included with ischaemic heart disease depends on the proportion of cardiovascular deaths that were originally coded to 410-414. See Murray and Lopez (1996b) for a detailed analysis and recommended correction methods.
xiv See Murray and Lopez (1996b) for an equation to approximate ischaemic heart disease mortality using BTL data.
xv No algorithm has been developed yet for ICD-10 data to correct for miscoding of ischaemic heart disease deaths.
xvi 2.5% of deaths at ages 30-44, 5% of deaths at ages 45-59, and 10% of deaths at ages 60+.
xvii No ICD-10 code is available.

services are provided such as appendicitis; and conditions which are a focus of current health policy debate.

Since the category of signs, symptoms and ill-defined conditions—Chapter XVI in the Ninth Revision of the International Classification of Diseases, Injuries and Causes of Death (ICD-9) (Chapter XVIII in the Tenth Revision of the ICD)—has no public health relevance in terms of interventions, it was not used as one of the major causes in our classification system. Deaths assigned to this category, as well as certain other codes used for ill-defined diagnoses, were reassigned to specific causes of death. From the perspective of generating information in order to inform the choice of alternative health policies and strategies, the assignment of deaths to an ill-defined category is uninformative and potentially misleading. Each person who dies does so from some specific underlying cause and the best possible estimate of the magnitude of each such cause is required for policy formation.[2]

Table I lists the four digit ICD-9 codes corresponding to each cause of death in our classification tree. The Ninth Revision of the ICD was used as the basis for developing the cause of disease and injury list since this was the Revision of the ICD in use in 1990, the base year for the GBD study. As ICD-10 is being progressively implemented by countries during the 1990s, the corresponding codes in the Tenth Revision are also included for future reference.

For each disease or injury, one or more sequelae have also been evaluated. For example, for diabetes mellitus, we have included diabetic foot ulcers, amputations, neuropathy and blindness from retinopathy, in addition to diabetes itself. For convenience, each sequela has also been assigned a code, namely the disease code followed by a dash and a number. For example, diabetic foot is coded as IIC-2. Not all sequelae are evaluated in this volume, due to space considerations. This is particularly true of the large number of sequelae arising from each of the causes listed under Group III (Injuries). Death estimates for 1990 and projections for 2000 are presented for each disease or injury only, and are not disaggregated by sequelae. To facilitate the presentation of tables, deaths have been included in the same table as the primary presentation of the disease or injury, or that of the most important outcome. This is an arbitrary but necessary choice in order to reduce the number of tables published for each disease and its sequelae.

REGIONS

The GBD analysis was carried out for eight geographical regions specifically developed by the World Bank for the *World Development Report 1993*. These regions, and their abbreviations, are as follows: the Established Market Economies (EME), the Formerly Socialist Economies of Europe (FSE), Latin America and the Caribbean (LAC), China (CHN), India (IND), Other Asia and Islands (OAI), Middle Eastern Crescent (MEC) (which includes North Africa, the Middle East, Pakistan and the Central Asian republics of the Former Soviet Union), and sub-Saharan Africa (SSA). The assignment of countries by the World Bank to each region is shown in Table II. The criteria used to define these regions included the level of socio-economic development, epidemiological homogeneity and geographic contiguity. The colour map included in this volume illustrates the location and composition of each region.

REGIONAL DEMOGRAPHIC ESTIMATES

The starting point for global, regional or national estimation of the burden of disease is a reliable assessment of the size and distribution of population and deaths, by age and sex. Through the combined efforts of many individuals, organizations and governments, much is known about the basic demography of each region in the world. Unquestionably, the database for estimating child mortality levels in all regions is more developed than for adult mortality (United Nations 1992; Hill and Yazbeck 1994). Indeed, there is considerable controversy among demographers over levels of adult mortality in some developing regions without good vital registration systems, where mortality is estimated indirectly from census and survey data (Timaeus 1991). For example, estimates of adult mortality by age and sex from the World Bank and the United Nations Population Division can differ by as much as 50 percent, but in general the uncertainties are less extreme than this. Demographic estimates of deaths and population in 1990, by age and sex, were developed specifically for the *World Development Report 1993*. We have continued to use them in the Global Burden of Disease Study to ensure comparability with other publications where burden of disease results have been included. Tables 1–9 provide the 1990 estimates of population and deaths by 5-year age group and sex for each of the 8 regions, and for the world. In addition, aggregate population and death figures for the five broad age groups used for preparing the epidemiological assessments in this study are also provided.[3]

ESTIMATING CAUSES OF DEATH

This section provides a very brief overview of the various data sources available for estimating cause-of-death patterns and the methods used to derive cause-of-death estimates based on this information. Much more detailed information on the methods and approaches followed to derive estimates of all epidemiological parameters reported in this book, as well as for making projections of mortality, can be found in *The Global Burden of Disease*, the first volume of the *Global Burden of Disease and Injury Series*.

Sources of Data

In order to estimate cause-of-death patterns, four broad types of sources of information on mortality can be used: vital registration systems, sample death registration systems, epidemiological assessments and cause-of-death models. Table III summarizes the availability of reliable vital registration data by age and region in 1990. Only EME and FSE have complete vital registration systems; for the developing regions, other sources including sample registration systems, population laboratories, epidemiological estimates and models were used to supplement information from vital registration.

While routine death registration is not widely available in India and China, there exist functioning sample registration systems that can be used as a basis for estimating mortality by cause. Thus, in China, the Chinese Academy of Preventive Medicine operates what is known as the Disease Surveillance Points (DSP) system. Established in the early 1980s, this system monitors vital events in a representative sample of 10 million people in rural and vital events in urban areas of China. Each surveillance point maintains a team, including a physician, which investigates every reported death to assign a cause of death using medical records and interviews with family members of the deceased.

India, like China, does not have complete vital registration and reliable cause-of-death attribution. Two systems, however, provide information that can be used to estimate cause-of-death patterns. In urban areas, medically certified deaths which occur in hospitals are tabulated and published each year by the Registrar-General. While in most States the quality of data generated by this system is quite poor, in Maharashtra State the coverage of medical certification of causes of death is estimated to be greater than 80 percent (Government of India, Registrar-General 1992a). This information has been used as the basis for estimating urban cause-of-death patterns in India. In rural areas of India, a 'verbal autopsy' sample registration system based on Primary Health Centres (PHC) and their catchment areas has been in operation since 1965. Known as the Survey of Causes of Death (Rural), SCD(R), the system currently includes over 1300 PHCs (Government of India, Registrar-General 1992b) and provides useful information on broad causes of mortality in rural areas. Since the cause of death is assigned by "lay" (non-medical) personnel, the returns from this system are only likely to be useful for estimating broad cause-of-death groups, and not for specific categories of disease or injury.

Even though no sample registration system is available for much of the population in sub-Saharan Africa, small scale population laboratories such as those operating in Niakhar (Senegal), Keneba (The Gambia), Navrongo (Ghana), Machakos (Kenya), and Morogoro, Hai and Dar es

Table II States or territories included in the Global Burden of Disease Study, by demographic region

Demographically developed regions		Demographically developing regions
Established market economies (EME)	Formerly socialist economies of Europe (FSE)	India (IND)
		China (CHN)
		Other Asia and islands (OAI)
Andorra	Albania	
Australia	Belarus	
Austria	Bosnia and Herzegovina	American Samoa
Belgium	Bulgaria	Bangladesh
Bermuda	Croatia	Bhutan
Canada	Czech Republic	Brunei Darussalam
Channel Islands	Estonia	Cambodia
Denmark	Hungary	Cook Islands
Faeroe Islands	Latvia	Federated States of Micronesia
Finland	Lithuania	Fiji
France	Macedonia,The Former Yugoslav	French Polynesia
Germany	Republic of	Guam
Gibraltar	Moldova	Hong Kong
Greece	Poland	Indonesia
Greenland	Romania	Johnston Island
Holy See	Russian Federation	Kiribati
Iceland	Slovakia	Korea, Democratic People's Republic of
Ireland	Slovenia	Korea, Republic of
Isle of Man	Ukraine	Lao People's Democratic Republic
Italy	Yugoslavia	Macao
Japan		Malaysia
Liechtenstein		Maldives
Luxembourg		Marshall Islands
Monaco		Mauritius
Netherlands		Midway Island
New Zealand		Mongolia
Norway		Myanmar
Portugal		Nauru
San Marino		Nepal
Spain		New Caledonia
St. Pierre and Miquelon		Niue
Sweden		Northern Mariana Islands
Switzerland		Palau
United Kingdom		Papua New Guinea
United States		Philippines
		Pitcairn Island
		Reunion
		Seychelles
		Singapore
		Solomon Islands
		Sri Lanka
		Taiwan
		Thailand
		Tokelau Island
		Tonga
		Tuvalu
		Vanuatu
		Viet Nam
		Wake Island
		Wallis and Futuna Islands
		Western Samoa

Table II (continued)

Demographically developing regions, continued

Sub-Saharan Africa (SSA)	Latin America and the Caribbean (LAC)	Middle Eastern crescent (MEC)
Angola	Anguilla	Afghanistan
Ascension	Antigua and Barbuda	Algeria
Benin	Argentina	Armenia
Botswana	Aruba	Azerbaijan
Burkina Faso	Bahamas	Bahrain
Burundi	Barbados	Cyprus
Cameroon	Belize	Egypt
Cape Verde	Bolivia	Former Spanish Sahara
Central African Republic	Brazil	Georgia
Chad	British Virgin Islands	Iran, Islamic Republic of
Comoros	Cayman Islands	Iraq
Congo	Chile	Israel
Côte d'Ivoire	Colombia	Jordan
Djibouti	Costa Rica	Kazakhstan
Equatorial Guinea	Cuba	Kuwait
Eritrea	Dominica	Kyrgyzstan
Ethiopia	Dominican Republic	Lebanon
Gabon	Ecuador	Libyan Arab Jamahiriya
Gambia	El Salvador	Malta
Ghana	French Guiana	Morocco
Guinea	Grenada	Oman
Guinea-Bissau	Guadeloupe	Pakistan
Kenya	Guatemala	Qatar
Lesotho	Guyana	Saudi Arabia
Liberia	Haiti	Syrian Arab Republic
Madagascar	Honduras	Tajikistan
Malawi	Jamaica	Tunisia
Mali	Martinique	Turkey
Mauritania	Mexico	Turkmenistan
Mayotte	Montserrat	United Arab Emirates
Mozambique	Netherlands Antilles	Uzbekistan
Namibia	Nicaragua	West Bank and Gaza Strip
Niger	Panama	Yemen
Nigeria	Paraguay	
Rwanda	Peru	
São Tomé and Principe	Puerto Rico	
Senegal	St. Kitts and Nevis	
Sierra Leone	St. Lucia	
Somalia	St. Vincent and the Grenadines	
South Africa	Suriname	
St. Helena	Trindad and Tobago	
Sudan	Turks and Caicos Islands	
Swaziland	Uruguay	
Tanzania	U.S. Virgin Islands	
Togo	Venezuela	
Tristan da Cunha		
Uganda		
Zaire		
Zambia		
Zimbabwe		

Table III   Sources used to estimate mortality by cause for
each region in 1990.

	Vital registration (% coverage)			Sample registration	
	Under 5 years	5 years and over	TOTAL	Urban	Rural
EME	99	99	99		
FSE	99	99	99		
IND				ICD	SCD(R)
CHN				DSP	DSP
OAI	2	14	10		
SSA	<1	2	1		
LAC	28	47	43		
MEC	12	27	22		

Salaam (Tanzania) provide some limited verbal autopsy information on
causes of death. While these reporting systems are helpful in delineating
local patterns of causes of death, their usefulness in estimating regional
patterns of causes of death is limited.

For several specific conditions, epidemiologists have developed estimates of cause-specific mortality based on the natural history of a given
disease. Incidence and/or prevalence rates estimated from specific surveys
are combined with information on case-fatality rates for treated and
untreated cases to yield approximate death rates. For some causes of
death, such as acute respiratory infection, diarrhoea and malaria, surveys
have been undertaken to more directly measure cause-specific mortality,
often with limited success (for more details, see the relevant chapters in
volumes of the *Global Burden of Disease and Injury Series*). The major
limitation of epidemiological estimates is that they tend to over-estimate
the burden of a particular disease. When epidemiological estimates for
major causes of death are summed, the total number of deaths estimated
in this way often exceeds (sometimes considerably) the number of deaths
from all causes based on demographic analyses. The tendency of epidemiological estimates to over-estimate disease levels arises from several
sources of bias. First, many deaths are multi-causal, yet each death in
epidemiological assessments is often fully attributed to each of several
causes. Second, when there is uncertainty as to incidence, prevalence or
case-fatality rates, analysts tend to err on the side of higher rates despite
frequent claims to the contrary. Third, because epidemiological assessments are usually undertaken without consideration of other causes of
death, authors of epidemiological assessments are often unaware of the
comparative magnitude of their claims on mortality. Epidemiological
assessments of the magnitude of health problems can be very informative
but, when considered independently of other causes of death and disability, they can be misleading.

Where no vital registration, sample registration or epidemiological
estimates are available, cause-of-death models may be helpful to estimate

patterns. Indirect techniques to estimate cause-of-death structure were first developed by Preston (1976) who modelled the relationship between total mortality and cause-specific mortality for twelve broad groups of causes, based on an analysis of historical vital registration data for developed nations and a few developing countries. In particular, cause-specific mortality was postulated to be a linear function of all-cause mortality. Preston's work has formed the basis of nearly all subsequent approaches to estimating cause-of-death patterns in regions without vital registration. Typically, these refinements have involved estimating equations for specific age groups, incorporating more recent data or examining more detailed causes (Hakulinen et al. 1986, Hull et al. 1981, Lopez and Hull 1983, Murray et al. 1992).

Previous attempts to use these models to estimate cause-of-death patterns in regions or countries without reliable data on mortality patterns have been hampered by a number of concerns, including the diversity of cause-of-death patterns by age and sex, the limited range of reliable observations on cause of death structure at high mortality levels, the analytical complications created by the use of Chapter XVI of the ICD-9 (Signs, Symptoms and Ill-Defined Conditions) and the true functional form of the relationship between cause-specific mortality and all-cause mortality. We have endeavoured to address each of these limitations in the models developed for this study—details of the database and methods used are given in Murray and Lopez (1996b). In view of the requirements of the GBD study to estimate cause-of-death patterns by age and sex for several broad age groups, cause-of-death models were developed separately for males and females for each of the seven age groups: 0–4 years, 5–14, 15–29, 30–44, 45–59, 60–69, and 70 years and over.[4]

Methods

The sequential procedure for estimating age-, sex- and cause-specific mortality rates for each region can be summarized as follows: (1) first estimates were prepared largely from vital registration and sample registration data; (2) estimates for selected cause-groups, such as malignant neoplasms and asthma, were then corrected using specific methods; (3) cause-specific mortality rates for selected causes were adjusted based on epidemiological analyses; and (4) final adjustments were made to ensure that the sum of cause-specific mortality rates was identical to total age-specific mortality as estimated from demographic methods. The application of each of these steps differed by region; in the following description some of these differences are highlighted—see Murray and Lopez (1996a) for a more complete description.

For EME and FSE, first estimates were derived solely from vital registration data (covering virtually all deaths in both regions). For China, first estimates were calculated using Disease Surveillance Points data from 1991 on 52 734 deaths in a population of 10 million, adjusted to match the total deaths in each age and sex group in China. For India, first estimates were derived from the ICD-9 Medical Certification of Causes of Death database inflated to match the estimated number of urban deaths in each age and sex group (based on the returns of the Indian Sample Registration Scheme). Estimates of mortality by cause in rural areas were based on the Survey of Causes of Death (Rural) results for 1991–1993, inflated to match the estimated rural deaths for the entire country.

In the four remaining regions, LAC, OAI, MEC and SSA, some vital registration data were available, but the majority of deaths are not captured by existing systems (see Table III). Moreover, those deaths that are recorded cannot be considered as representative of mortality conditions for the entire region. Each of these regions can be divided into a registration area, for which vital registration data are available, and a residual area. To develop plausible estimates of mortality by cause in the residual areas, a two-step procedure was followed. First, a new Lorenz-curve method based on the geographical inequality of death distribution was developed; this yielded estimates of age- and sex-specific mortality rates from all causes combined in the residual areas—see Murray and Lopez (1996b) for more details. Second, for the registration areas, the percentage distribution of recorded deaths in each age group assigned to Groups I, II and III was compared with the percentage predicted by the cause-of-death models. The number of standard deviations above or below the predicted value for each Group is a measure of how much the registration areas in the region deviate from the cause-of-death patterns reflected in the models. To estimate the disaggregation of all-cause mortality into Groups I, II and III in the residual areas, we have assumed that the pattern of deviation of the cause-of-death structure as compared to the cause-of-death models is similar to that of the registration areas. In other words, if the registration areas in LAC yield a percentage of all-cause mortality from Group I diseases that is 2.3 standard deviations higher than expected, then we have assumed that the residual areas also have a percentage of all-cause mortality due to Group I that is 2.3 standard deviations higher than predicted.

In SSA, a slightly different method was used because registration data were available only for South Africa.[5] The region was divided into two components: Southern Africa, including South Africa, Botswana, Namibia, Mozambique, Zimbabwe, Swaziland, Zambia and Malawi; and Northern Africa, which included all other countries in SSA. The Lorenz-curve method was then used to estimate the pattern for Southern Africa based on the vital registration data from South Africa. For the remainder of SSA, the mortality pattern was based on the difference between the regional estimates and the estimates for the Southern African subregion. The distribution of deaths across Groups I, II and III for registered deaths in South Africa was within one standard deviation of that predicted by the models. For the remaining SSA subregion, we have applied the same pattern of deviation as suggested by the registration areas of South Africa.

To estimate mortality from the more detailed causes within each Group in the residual areas, we have assumed that in LAC, MEC, SSA and OAI the proportionate distribution for a given age-sex group is the same as in the registration areas. The alternative would have been to use the small cause regression models as discussed above. We feel, however, that it is preferable to base the estimation of more detailed cause-of-death patterns on local data than on the patterns implied by vital registration data from industrialized countries.

For a number of categories of diseases, such as malignant neoplasms, cardiovascular diseases, neuro-psychiatric conditions and chronic respiratory conditions, a standard series of corrections was also applied. These are described in detail in Murray and Lopez (1996b).

Based on the detailed epidemiological reviews undertaken for many conditions, estimates were also generated for many diseases in all developing regions by disease experts. These epidemiological assessments were used to adjust first-round mortality estimates for selected causes. Because of the greater concentration on infectious disease epidemiology in most developing countries, epidemiologically-based estimates of mortality exist for many more diseases in Group I than in Group II. As epidemiological assessments tend to yield rates which are higher than those based on vital registration, this tends to bias the final results towards Group I diseases and away from Group II diseases. For the detailed basis of each epidemiological assessment, the reader is referred to the relevant chapter(s) in the appropriate volume(s) of the *Global Burden of Disease and Injury Series*.

Because of the sporadic but intense nature of war-related injuries, the epidemiological estimates of war deaths have been incorporated in a slightly different manner. In brief, we have chosen to consider war deaths as deaths which are additional to those estimated from the basic demographic analyses used to determine the number of deaths in each age-sex group in each region. Thus, the epidemiological estimates of war deaths have not been subject to the final adjustment algorithm described below.

In accordance with the principles of the ICD, in the primary tabulations (Murray and Lopez 1996b) for the GBD study, each death has been assigned to a single underlying cause. For example, deaths from hepatoma due to chronic hepatitis B infection are assigned to hepatoma in the primary tabulations. Likewise, following ICD conventions, deaths from tuberculosis in HIV positives are assigned to HIV in the primary tabulations. In this volume, most of the tables show the number of deaths assigned to a cause in the primary tabulation; however, some tables, such as for tuberculosis/HIV, show the number of deaths associated with the joint condition. The technical notes accompanying the tables indicate clearly the type of mortality shown.

After correcting many causes based on epidemiological assessments, the sum of cause-specific mortality often exceeded total mortality for a number of age groups in several regions. In some cases, the sum of Group-specific causes of death exceeded the total mortality for that Group in a given age group—a common problem for Group I in the adult age groups. To force the sum of cause-specific deaths to equal deaths from all causes in any given age-sex group, two additional adjustment algorithms were applied, one for neonatal causes and one for all other age groups.

In most regions, 80–90 percent of neonatal deaths are due to a limited number of causes: congenital syphilis, neonatal tetanus, conditions arising during the perinatal period and congenital anomalies. We first estimated the number of neonatal deaths in each region based on the findings of major demographic research projects such as the Demographic and Health Surveys Project, and then required that the sum of deaths from congenital syphilis, neonatal tetanus, conditions arising during the perinatal period and congenital anomalies expected during the neonatal period equal 85 percent of estimated neonatal deaths. Where epidemiologically-based estimates of deaths from these four causes expected in the first month of life exceeded 85 percent of estimated neonatal deaths, these causes were proportionately reduced.

The extent of overestimation of mortality in each of the fourteen age-sex groups, and in each region, was evaluated by comparing the number of standard deviations above or below the proportionate mortality for a Group, as predicted by the cause-of-death models, with the number of standard deviations above or below in the first estimates. To adjust for overestimation based on the epidemiological approach, we have arbitrarily chosen the following algorithm. If first estimates for Group I or Group II based on vital registration or sample registration data were already more than 2.5 standard deviations above or below the expected value, we did not allow epidemiological assessments to increase the degree of deviation. If the first assessment for Group I was less than 2.5 standard deviations greater than expected, or Group II was more than 2.5 standard deviations below the expected value, then the results from epidemiological assessments were permitted to change the proportion in either Group by 2 standard deviations. If a change of 2 standard deviations would increase the percentage of deaths due to Group I to be more than 2.5 standard deviations above the mean, or decrease the percentage of deaths due to Group II to be more than 2.5 standard deviations below the mean, the percentage of deaths due to Group I was set equal to a value 2.5 standard deviations above the mean and the percentage of deaths due to Group II was set equal to 2.5 standard deviations below the mean.

INCIDENCE, PREVALENCE, CASE-FATALITY AND DURATION

For the Global Burden of Disease Study, estimates were required of the incidence, prevalence, remission, duration, case-fatality and mortality for each disease or injury and its sequelae. Valid community-based epidemiological studies that could be used to derive these estimates do not exist for several of these epidemiological parameters in some regions. In order to identify all useful sources of data and information, and to supplement empirical data with informed judgement, the estimates presented in this volume were obtained in close collaboration with a large number of experts familiar with specific diseases or injuries, and are the result of an iterative process spanning more than four years (1992–1996). The following steps summarize the actual mechanism used to generate estimates for each disease and its sequelae.

1. Disease experts, or groups of experts in some cases, were identified for each of the more than 100 conditions in the Global Burden of Disease Study. Study participants were drawn from the World Health Organization, the International Agency for Research on Cancer, the World Bank, the United States Centers for Disease Control, and academic institutions in several countries including the United States, the United Kingdom, France, Mexico, New Zealand, India, Sri Lanka, China and South Africa.

2. First-round estimates of incidence, remission, case-fatality, prevalence, duration and death were made by experts on the basis of published and unpublished studies. Where no data for a region were available, experts were encouraged to make informed estimates. Frequently, age-patterns of incidence or remission were based on the assumption that regions have similar epidemiological profiles. In the worst case scenario, when no information was available at all, the preliminary estimates were based on data and information from other regions.

3. These estimates were critically reviewed and the internal consistency of estimates of incidence, remission, case-fatality rates, duration and prevalence was ascertained using DisMod.[6] These checks identified major inconsistencies with many estimates. Disease experts were then invited to revise their estimates in consultation with the authors, in order to make them internally consistent.

4. Revised estimates were used to produce preliminary results. These estimates were extensively reviewed by a group of international health experts at a meeting hosted by the World Health Organization in Geneva, from 8–11 December 1992. Subsequent revisions were again subject to internal consistency validation and the modified estimates formed the basis of the results published in the *World Development Report 1993: Investing in Health.*

5. As part of the follow-up to the *WDR 1993*, disease experts were asked to write detailed chapters on the data and methods used to generate the estimates. These authors had the opportunity during this process to go through three more iterations of estimating incidence, prevalence, duration, case-fatality, remission and death incorporating the widespread discussion and review of the results published in 1993 and 1994. Each of these revisions has been reviewed for internal consistency. In many cases, we have revised estimates in collaboration with the disease experts to ensure internal consistency. For certain clusters of conditions, such as the neuro-psychiatric disorders, specific international seminars were convened to review the epidemiological estimates.

PROJECTING CAUSES OF DEATH 1990–2020

Strategies and policies to support health promotion and disease prevention must have a forward-looking perspective. To meet this need, we have also included in this volume projections of mortality for each cause to the year 2000. The projection method developed for the Global Burden of Disease Study is fully described elsewhere (Murray and Lopez 1996a). Briefly, the approach used was to develop a statistical or econometric model to predict different scenarios of cause-specific mortality based on a very restricted number of independent variables. This approach may be overly simplistic but it generates plausible predictions based largely on empirical observations across a wide range of countries over many decades. Rather than projecting total mortality and then decomposing it into component causes based on a set of relationships between total mortality and cause-specific mortality, we have chosen to model clusters of causes independently. Our projections of total mortality for each age and sex group are calculated as the sum of the projections for each of the causes. Causes of death have been divided into nine clusters of causes: all Group I diseases, cancers, cardiovascular diseases, digestive diseases, chronic respiratory diseases, other Group II diseases, road traffic accidents, other unintentional injuries and intentional injuries. These nine causes sum up to total mortality within each age and sex group. We have chosen these particular clusters of causes because mortality trends in countries with good vital registration data over the past 40 years suggest that the more specific causes within each cluster have been following a similar time trend. There are some obvious exceptions, such as the rise of tuberculosis in EME over the past 5–10 years, and the HIV epidemic, for which separate methods have been used. In general, however, these nine clusters of causes appear to capture reasonably well the range of different trends in specific causes.

Four independent variables were chosen for inclusion in the predictive model: income per capita, human capital, smoking intensity and time. Income per capita, measured in international dollars, which are adjusted for differences in purchasing power not reflected in official exchange rates, was used as a general proxy for many aspects of economic development. The average number of years of schooling of the population, a measure of education and human capital formation, was used to capture this key determinant of health status and the ability of the population to make use of available health knowledge and interventions. One dominant determinant of adult health status that is not well captured by income or education is cumulative exposure to smoking, since cigarette smoking is a principal cause of several major diseases. Smoking prevalence rates from surveys are not a reliable measure of the impact of smoking since other factors, including duration, type, amount and mode of smoking, are critical determinants of cumulative past exposure. Based on the approach developed by Peto and Lopez, we have taken estimated lung cancer rates minus non-smoker lung cancer rates for each age and sex group to estimate a smoking intensity parameter (see Peto et al. 1994 for further details on this method[7]). Smoking intensity is then used as one of the independent variables in the predictive equations for cancer, cardiovascular disease and chronic respiratory disease. The fourth independent variable used in the projections is time itself. Thus, secular trends in mortality not explained by income, education or smoking may be due to changes in technology or knowledge which we crudely capture using time as a variable. In addition, as discussed below, independent projections of the HIV epidemic were added to the basic projections generated from the predictive model.

For each of the nine clusters of causes of death, for each of seven age groups and for each sex, various functional forms of the regression equations were evaluated. The final equation used was based on the smallest set of independent variables that had reasonable predictive power as measured by the proportion of variance explained. In addition, if the parameter estimate for a variable had the opposite sign of what was expected and the coefficient was not significant at the 1% level, this variable was dropped from the equation. Projections for more detailed causes were based on regression equations relating the mortality rate from a detailed cause to the mortality rate for one of the nine clusters of causes.

Given a set of equations relating mortality rates by age, sex and cause to income per capita, human capital, smoking intensity and time, projections of each of these independent variables were required in order to project mortality by cause. For each independent variable, pessimistic, baseline and optimistic scenarios were generated. However, due to lack of space, only the baseline scenario results are presented in this volume. Projections of income per capita for each region were based on World Bank economic forecasts and plausible assumptions about long-term per capita income growth. Human capital has been projected based on the median growth rate in human capital recorded over the period 1950–1990 for each region. In addition, we assume that as levels of human capital grow, the growth rate declines. To project smoking intensity to the year 2020, we examined the relationship between cigarettes consumed per adult in the United Kingdom from 1900–1990 and smoking intensity estimates in the United Kingdom for a similar period. To project smoking intensity, it is assumed that the time course of the smoking epidemic in the United Kingdom will be repeated in each region. Using estimates of cigarette consumption per capita for males and females for each region, we have used the relationship in the United Kingdom to estimate smoking intensity thirty years after a given level of cigarette consumption per capita has been reached. This figure was used as the projected value of smoking intensity for each region in 2020. For the intervening years, we assumed that current values of the smoking intensity variable will increase, or decrease, in a linear fashion towards the projected value in 2020.

As mentioned earlier, the past experience of countries with good vital registration data, as embodied in the predictive equations described above, does not adequately capture the path of the HIV epidemic. To estimate the possible impact of the HIV epidemic in each region between 1990 and 2020, we have prepared independent projections of HIV incidence and HIV mortality in each year for each age, sex and region. These projections agree closely with those of the former WHO Global Programme on AIDS (GPA) for the phase of the epidemic during which incidence is rising. For the phase of the epidemic when incidence is declining, the GPA projection model assumes that incidence falls to zero very quickly in all regions, so that by the year 2020, there would be essentially little or no HIV incidence. This appears to us to be too optimistic a scenario. Our baseline projections are based on the assumption that incidence numbers will decline to an equilibrium value that is one-half of peak incidence. As no region, except for EME, is near the point where incidence is half of peak incidence, we do not know at what incidence level the HIV epidemic will stabilize in each region. To estimate mortality from HIV, we have used the same assumptions as included in the GPA projection model concerning the distribution of time required for progression from HIV to AIDS, and the distribution of deaths from AIDS over time. These projections are likely to be quite pessimistic, particularly for regions such as India and OAI, where the GPA assumed that the epidemic will follow a much more accelerated time course as compared, for example, to SSA.

ORGANIZATION OF TABLES

Table IV provides a complete listing of all diseases and injuries, and of the sequelae of each disease and injury included in the Global Burden of Disease Study. Due to limitations of space, not all these sequelae can be presented in this volume. The right hand column of Table IV indicates which sequelae have been included. For each of the sequelae, there are three pages of tables containing identical sets of estimates for each of the eight geographical regions used for the *WDR 1993*, plus a summary table giving aggregate estimates for the world. The data on the various epidemiological indicators included in the tables represent the basic epidemiological information required to compute DALYs for each disease or injury. The actual DALY estimates are not shown in the tables but are given in summary form in *The Global Burden of Disease*, the first volume of the *Global Burden of Disease and Injury Series*, and are reported in more detail in the specific disease or injury chapters in subsequent volumes.

The epidemiological indicators included in the tables are intended to reflect the essential information that health planners and other public health workers might require in order to formulate, implement and evaluate appropriate strategies for the prevention and treatment of disease and injury. Thus, the tables present data on the 1990 burden of disease and injury in the region, how this burden is distributed across different age groups and between males and females, how rapidly the condition is increasing (or decreasing), whether or not the condition

Table IV Cause groups, diseases and injuries, and sequelae
included in the Global Burden of Disease Study
and the set of sequelae for which data are presented
in this volume

GBD Classification Code	Cause group, disease, injury, or sequela	Data presented in this volume (table number)
I	Communicable, maternal, perinatal, and nutritional conditions	
IA	Infectious and parasitic diseases	
IA1	Tuberculosis	
IA1-1	HIV sero-negative cases	10
IA1-2	HIV sero-positive cases	11
IA2	Sexually transmitted diseases excluding HIV	
IA2a	Syphilis	
IA2a-1	Congenital syphilis	12
IA2a-2	Low birth weight	13
IA2a-3	Primary	14
IA2a-4	Secondary	15
IA2a-5	Tertiary – cardiovascular	16
IA2a-6	Tertiary – gummas	17
IA2a-7	Tertiary – neurologic	18
IA2b	Chlamydia	
IA2b-1	Ophthalmia neonatorum	19
IA2b-2	Low birth weight	20
IA2b-3	Corneal scar – blindness	21
IA2b-4	Corneal scar – low vision	22
IA2b-5	Cervicitis	23
IA2b-6	Neonatal pneumonia	24
IA2b-7	Pelvic inflammatory disease	25
IA2b-8	Ectopic pregnancy	26
IA2b-9	Tubo-ovarian abscess	27
IA2b-10	Chronic pelvic pain	28
IA2b-11	Infertility	29
IA2b-12	Symptomatic urethritis	30
IA2b-13	Epididymitis	31
IA2b-14	Stricture	32
IA2c	Gonorrhoea	
IA2c-1	Ophthalmia neonatorum	33
IA2c-2	Low birth weight	34
IA2c-3	Corneal scar – blindness	35
IA2c-4	Corneal scar – low vision	36
IA2c-5	Cervicitis	37
IA2c-6	Pelvic inflammatory disease	38
IA2c-7	Ectopic pregnancy	39
IA2c-8	Tubo-ovarian abscess	40
IA2c-9	Chronic pelvic pain	41
IA2c-10	Infertility	42
IA2c-11	Symptomatic urethritis	43
IA2c-12	Epididymitis	44
IA2c-13	Stricture	45
IA3	HIV	
IA3-1	Cases	46
IA3-2	AIDS	47
IA4	Diarrhoeal diseases	
IA4-1	Episodes	48

Table IV   (continued)

GBD Classification Code	Cause group, disease, injury, or sequela	Data presented in this volume (table number)
IA5	Childhood-cluster diseases	
IA5a	Pertussis	
IA5a-1	Episodes	49
IA5a-2	Mental retardation	50
IA5b	Poliomyelitis	
IA5b-1	Lameness	51
IA5c	Diphtheria	
IA5c-1	Episodes	52
IA5c-2	Neurological complications	53
IA5c-3	Myocarditis	54
IA5d	Measles	
IA5d-1	Episodes	55
IA5e	Tetanus	
IA5e-1	Episodes	56
IA6	Bacterial meningitis and meningococcaemia	
IA6-1	All forms – episodes	57
IA6-2	Streptococcus pneumoniae – episodes	58
IA6-3	Haemophilus influenzae – episodes	59
IA6-4	Neisseria meningitidis – episodes	60
IA6-5	Meningococcaemia without meningitis – episodes	61
IA6-6	Deafness	62
IA6-7	Seizure disorder	63
IA6-8	Motor deficit	64
IA6-9	Mental retardation	65
IA7	Hepatitis B and hepatitis C	
IA7-1	Episodes	66
IA7-2	Cirrhosis of the liver – symptomatic cases	67
IA7-3	Hepatoma	68
IA8	Malaria	
IA8-1	Episodes	69
IA8-2	Anaemia	70
IA8-3	Neurological sequelae	71
IA9	Tropical-cluster diseases	
IA9a	Trypanosomiasis	
IA9a-1	Episodes	72
IA9b	Chagas disease	
IA9b-1	Infection	73
IA9b-2	Cardiomyopathy without congestive heart failure	74
IA9b-3	Cardiomyopathy with congestive heart failure	75
IA9b-4	Megaviscera	76
IA9c	Schistosomiasis	
IA9c-1	Infection	77
IA9d	Leishmaniasis	
IA9d-1	Visceral	78
IA9d-2	Cutaneous	79
IA9e	Lymphatic filariasis	
IA9e-1	Hydrocele > 15 cm	80
IA9e-2	Bancroftian lymphoedema	81
IA9e-3	Brugian lymphoedema	82
IA9f	Onchocerciasis	
IA9f-1	Blindness	83

Table IV (continued)

GBD Classification Code	Cause group, disease, injury, or sequela	Data presented in this volume (table number)
IA9f-2	Itching	84
IA9f-3	Low vision	85
IA10	Leprosy	
IA10-1	Cases	86
IA10-2	Disabling leprosy	87
IA11	Dengue	
IA11-1	Dengue haemorrhagic fever	88
IA12	Japanese encephalitis	
IA12-1	Episodes	89
IA12-2	Cognitive impairment	90
IA12-3	Neurological sequelae	91
IA13	Trachoma	
IA13-1	Blindness	92
IA13-2	Low vision	93
IA14	Intestinal nematode infections	
IA14a	Ascariasis	
IA14a-1	High intensity infection	94
IA14a-2	Cotemporaneous cognitive deficit	95
IA14a-3	Cognitive impairment	96
IA14a-4	Intestinal obstruction	97
IA14b	Trichuriasis	
IA14b-1	High intensity infection	98
IA14b-2	Cotemporaneous cognitive deficit	99
IA14b-3	Massive dysentery syndrome	100
IA14b-4	Cognitive impairment	101
IA14c	Ancylostomiasis and necatoriasis	
IA14c-1	High intensity infection	102
IA14c-2	Anaemia	103
IA14c-3	Cognitive impairment	104
IB	Respiratory infections	
IB1	Lower respiratory infections	
IB1-1	Episodes	105
IB1-2	Chronic sequelae	106
IB2	Upper respiratory infections	
IB2-1	Episodes	107
IB2-2	Pharyngitis	108
IB3	Otitis media	
IB3-1	Episodes	109
IB3-2	Deafness	110
IC	Maternal conditions	
IC1	Maternal haemorrhage	
IC1-1	Episodes	111
IC1-2	Sheehan syndrome	112
IC1-3	Severe anaemia	113
IC2	Maternal sepsis	
IC2-1	Episodes	114
IC2-2	Infertility	115
IC3	Hypertensive disorders of pregnancy	
IC3-1	Episodes	116
IC3-2	Neurological sequelae	117
IC4	Obstructed labour	
IC4-1	Episodes	118

Table IV (continued)

GBD Classification Code	Cause group, disease, injury, or sequela	Data presented in this volume (table number)
IC4-2	Stress incontinence	119
IC4-3	Rectovaginal fistula	120
IC5	Abortion	
IC5-1	Episodes	121
IC5-2	Infertility	122
ID	Conditions arising during the perinatal period	
ID1	Low birth weight	
ID1-1	All sequelae	123
ID2	Birth asphyxia and birth trauma	
ID2-1	All sequelae	124
IE	Nutritional deficiencies	
IE1	Protein-energy malnutrition	
IE1-1	Wasting	125
IE1-2	Stunting	126
IE1-3	Developmental disability	127
IE2	Iodine deficiency	
IE2-1	Goitre – grade 0	128
IE2-2	Goitre – grade 1	129
IE2-3	Goitre – grade 2	130
IE2-4	Mild developmental disability	131
IE2-5	Cretinoidism	132
IE2-6	Cretinism	133
IE3	Vitamin A deficiency	
IE3-1	Xerophthalmia	134
IE3-2	Corneal scar	135
IE4	Iron-deficiency anaemia	
IE4-1	All forms	136
IE4-2	Mild	137
IE4-3	Moderate	138
IE4-4	Severe	139
IE4-5	Very severe	140
IE4-6	Cognitive impairment	141
II	Noncommunicable diseases	
IIA	Malignant neoplasms	
IIA1	Mouth and oropharynx cancers	
IIA1-1	Cases	142
IIA2	Oesophagus cancer	
IIA2-1	Cases	143
IIA3	Stomach cancer	
IIA3-1	Cases	144
IIA4	Colon and rectum cancers	
IIA4-1	Cases	145
IIA5	Liver cancer	
IIA5-1	Cases	146
IIA6	Pancreas cancer	
IIA6-1	Cases	147
IIA7	Trachea, bronchus and lung cancers	
IIA7-1	Cases	148
IIA8	Melanoma and other skin cancers	
IIA8-1	Cases	149
IIA9	Breast cancer	
IIA9-1	Cases	150

Table IV (continued)

GBD Classification Code	Cause group, disease, injury, or sequela	Data presented in this volume (table number)
IIA10	Cervix uteri cancer	
IIA10-1	Cases	151
IIA11	Corpus uteri cancer	
IIA11-1	Cases	152
IIA12	Ovary cancer	
IIA12-1	Cases	153
IIA13	Prostate cancer	
IIA13-1	Cases	154
IIA14	Bladder cancer	
IIA14-1	Cases	155
IIA15	Lymphomas and multiple myeloma	
IIA15-1	Cases	156
IIA16	Leukaemia	
IIA16-1	Cases	157
IIB	Other neoplasms	
IIC	Diabetes mellitus	
IIC-1	Cases	158
IIC-2	Diabetic foot	159
IIC-3	Neuropathy	160
IIC-4	Retinopathy – blindness	161
IIC-5	Amputation	162
IID	Endocrine disorders	
IIE	Neuro-psychiatric conditions	
IIE1	Unipolar major depression	
IIE1-1	Depressive episodes	163
IIE2	Bipolar disorder	
IIE2-1	Cases	164
IIE3	Schizophrenia	
IIE3-1	Cases	165
IIE4	Epilepsy	
IIE4-1	Cases	166
IIE5	Alcohol use	
IIE5-1	Alcohol dependence syndrome	167
IIE6	Dementia and other degenerative and hereditary CNS disorders	
IIE6-1	Cases	168
IIE7	Parkinson disease	
IIE7-1	Cases	169
IIE8	Multiple sclerosis	
IIE8-1	Cases	170
IIE9	Drug use	
IIE9-1	Dysfunctional and harmful drug use	171
IIE10	Post-traumatic stress disorder	
IIE10-1	Cases	172
IIE11	Obsessive-compulsive disorders	
IIE11-1	Cases	173
IIE12	Panic disorder	
IIE12-1	Cases	174
IIF	Sense organ diseases	
IIF1	Glaucoma	
IIF1-1	Blindness	175
IIF2	Cataracts	
IIF2-1	Blindness	176

Table IV   (continued)

GBD Classification Code	Cause group, disease, injury, or sequela	Data presented in this volume (table number)
IIG	Cardiovascular diseases	
IIG1	Rheumatic heart disease	
IIG1-1	Congestive heart failure	177
IIG2	Ischaemic heart disease	
IIG2-1	Acute myocardial infarction	178
IIG2-2	Angina pectoris	179
IIG2-3	Congestive heart failure	180
IIG3	Cerebrovascular disease	
IIG3-1	First-ever stroke	181
IIG4	Inflammatory heart diseases	
IIG4-1	Myocarditis	182
IIG4-2	Pericarditis	183
IIG4-3	Endocarditis	184
IIG4-4	Cardiomyopathy	185
IIH	Respiratory diseases	
IIH1	Chronic obstructive pulmonary disease	
IIH1-1	Symptomatic cases	186
IIH2	Asthma	
IIH2-1	Cases	187
III	Digestive diseases	
III1	Peptic ulcer	
III1-1	Cases	188
III2	Cirrhosis of the liver	
III2-1	Symptomatic Cases	189
III3	Appendicitis	
III3-1	Episodes	190
IIJ	Genito-urinary diseases	
IIJ1	Nephritis and nephrosis	
IIJ1-1	Acute glomerulonephritis	191
IIJ1-2	End-stage renal disease	192
IIJ2	Benign prostatic hypertrophy	
IIJ2-1	Symptomatic cases	193
IIK	Skin diseases	
IIL	Musculo-skeletal diseases	
IIL1	Rheumatoid arthritis	
IIL1-1	Cases	194
IIL2	Osteoarthritis	
IIL2-1	Hip	195
IIL2-2	Knee	196
IIM	Congenital anomalies	
IIM1	Abdominal wall defect	
IIM1-1	Cases	197
IIM2	Anencephaly	
IIM2-1	Cases	198
IIM3	Anorectal atresia	
IIM3-1	Cases	199
IIM4	Cleft lip	
IIM4-1	Cases	200
IIM5	Cleft palate	
IIM5-1	Cases	201
IIM6	Oesophageal atresia	
IIM6-1	Cases	202

Table IV (continued)

GBD Classification Code	Cause group, disease, injury, or sequela	Data presented in this volume (table number)
IIM7	Renal agenesis	
IIM7-1	Cases	203
IIM8	Down syndrome	
IIM8-1	Cases	204
IIM9	Congenital heart anomalies	
IIM9-1	Cases	205
IIM10	Spina bifida	
IIM10-1	Cases	206
IIN	Oral conditions	
IIN1	Dental caries	
IIN1-1	Episodes	207
IIN2	Periodontal disease	
IIN2-1	Episodes	208
IIN3	Edentulism	
IIN3-1	Cases	209
III	Injuries	
IIIA	Unintentional injuries	
IIIA1	Road traffic accidents	
IIIA1-1	Episodes	210
IIIA1-2	Fractured skull – short term	
IIIA1-3	Fractured skull – long term	211
IIIA1-4	Fractured face bones	
IIIA1-5	Fractured vertebral column	
IIIA1-6	Injured spinal cord	212
IIIA1-7	Fractured rib or sternum	
IIIA1-8	Fractured pelvis	
IIIA1-9	Fractured clavicle, scapula, or humerus	
IIIA1-10	Fractured radius or ulna	
IIIA1-11	Fractured hand bones	
IIIA1-12	Fractured femur – short term	
IIIA1-13	Fractured femur – long term	213
IIIA1-14	Fractured patella, tibia, or fibula	
IIIA1-15	Fractured ankle	
IIIA1-16	Fractured foot bones	
IIIA1-17	Other dislocation	
IIIA1-18	Dislocated shoulder, elbow, or hip	
IIIA1-19	Sprains	
IIIA1-20	Intracranial injury – short term	214
IIIA1-21	Intracranial injury – long term	215
IIIA1-22	Internal injuries	
IIIA1-23	Open wound	
IIIA1-24	Injury to eyes	
IIIA1-25	Amputated thumb	
IIIA1-26	Amputated finger	
IIIA1-27	Amputated arm	
IIIA1-28	Amputated toe	
IIIA1-29	Amputated foot	
IIIA1-30	Amputated leg	
IIIA1-31	Crushing	
IIIA1-32	Burns < 20% – short term	
IIIA1-33	Burns < 20% – long term	
IIIA1-34	Burns > 20% and < 60% – short term	

Table IV　(continued)

GBD Classification Code	Cause group, disease, injury, or sequela	Data presented in this volume (table number)
IIIA1-35	Burns > 20% and < 60% – long term	
IIIA1-36	Burns > 60% – short term	
IIIA1-37	Burns > 60% – long term	
IIIA1-38	Injured nerves	
IIIA1-39	Poisoning	
IIIA1-40	Residual	
IIIA2	Poisonings	
IIIA2-1	Episodes	216
IIIA3	Falls	
IIIA3-1	Episodes	217
IIIA3-2	Fractured skull – short term	
IIIA3-3	Fractured skull – long term	218
IIIA3-4	Fractured face bones	
IIIA3-5	Fractured vertebral column	
IIIA3-6	Injured spinal cord	219
IIIA3-7	Fractured rib or sternum	
IIIA3-8	Fractured pelvis	
IIIA3-9	Fractured clavicle, scapula, or humerus	
IIIA3-10	Fractured radius or ulna	
IIIA3-11	Fractured hand bones	
IIIA3-12	Fractured femur – short term	220
IIIA3-13	Fractured femur – long term	221
IIIA3-14	Fractured patella, tibia, or fibula	
IIIA3-15	Fractured ankle	
IIIA3-16	Fractured foot bones	
IIIA3-17	Other dislocation	
IIIA3-18	Dislocated shoulder, elbow, or hip	
IIIA3-19	Sprains	
IIIA3-20	Intracranial injury – short term	
IIIA3-21	Intracranial injury – long term	222
IIIA3-22	Internal injuries	
IIIA3-23	Open wound	
IIIA3-24	Injury to eyes	
IIIA3-25	Amputated thumb	
IIIA3-26	Amputated finger	
IIIA3-27	Amputated arm	
IIIA3-28	Amputated toe	
IIIA3-29	Amputated foot	
IIIA3-30	Amputated leg	
IIIA3-31	Crushing	
IIIA3-32	Burns < 20% – short term	
IIIA3-33	Burns < 20% – long term	
IIIA3-34	Burns > 20% and < 60% – short term	
IIIA3-35	Burns > 20% and < 60% – long term	
IIIA3-36	Burns > 60% – short term	
IIIA3-37	Burns > 60% – long term	
IIIA3-38	Injured nerves	
IIIA3-39	Poisoning	
IIIA4-40	Residual	
IIIA4	Fires	
IIIA4-1	Episodes	223
IIIA4-2	Fractured skull – short term	

Table IV (continued)

GBD Classification Code	Cause group, disease, injury, or sequela	Data presented in this volume (table number)
IIIA4-3	Fractured skull – long term	
IIIA4-4	Fractured face bones	
IIIA4-5	Fractured vertebral column	
IIIA4-6	Injured spinal cord	224
IIIA4-7	Fractured rib or sternum	
IIIA4-8	Fractured pelvis	
IIIA4-9	Fractured clavicle, scapula, or humerus	
IIIA4-10	Fractured radius or ulna	
IIIA4-11	Fractured hand bones	
IIIA4-12	Fractured femur – short term	
IIIA4-13	Fractured femur – long term	
IIIA4-14	Fractured patella, tibia, or fibula	
IIIA4-15	Fractured ankle	
IIIA4-16	Fractured foot bones	
IIIA4-17	Other dislocation	
IIIA4-18	Dislocated shoulder, elbow, or hip	
IIIA4-19	Sprains	
IIIA4-20	Intracranial injury – short term	
IIIA4-21	Intracranial injury – long term	
IIIA4-22	Internal injuries	
IIIA4-23	Open wound	
IIIA4-24	Injury to eyes	
IIIA4-25	Amputated thumb	
IIIA4-26	Amputated finger	
IIIA4-27	Amputated arm	
IIIA4-28	Amputated toe	
IIIA4-29	Amputated foot	
IIIA4-30	Amputated leg	
IIIA4-31	Crushing	
IIIA4-32	Burns < 20% – short term	225
IIIA4-33	Burns < 20% – long term	226
IIIA4-34	Burns > 20% and < 60% – short term	227
IIIA4-35	Burns > 20% and < 60% – long term	228
IIIA4-36	Burns > 60% – short term	
IIIA4-37	Burns > 60% – long term	
IIIA4-38	Injured nerves	
IIIA4-39	Poisoning	
IIIA4-40	Residual	
IIIA5	Drownings	
IIIA5-1	Episodes	229
IIIA5-2	Quadriplegia	230
IIIA6	Other unintentional injuries	
IIIA6-1	Episodes	231
IIIA6-2	Fractured skull – short term	
IIIA6-3	Fractured skull – long term	
IIIA6-4	Fractured face bones	
IIIA6-5	Fractured vertebral column	
IIIA6-6	Injured spinal cord	232
IIIA6-7	Fractured rib or sternum	
IIIA6-8	Fractured pelvis	
IIIA6-9	Fractured clavicle, scapula, or humerus	
IIIA6-10	Fractured radius or ulna	

Table IV (continued)

GBD Classification Code	Cause group, disease, injury, or sequela	Data presented in this volume (table number)
IIIA6-11	Fractured hand bones	
IIIA6-12	Fractured femur – short term	
IIIA6-13	Fractured femur – long term	
IIIA6-14	Fractured patella, tibia, or fibula	
IIIA6-15	Fractured ankle	
IIIA6-16	Fractured foot bones	
IIIA6-17	Other dislocation	
IIIA6-18	Dislocated shoulder, elbow, or hip	
IIIA6-19	Sprains	
IIIA6-20	Intracranial injury – short term	
IIIA6-21	Intracranial injury – long term	233
IIIA6-22	Internal injuries	
IIIA6-23	Open wound	
IIIA6-24	Injury to eyes	
IIIA6-25	Amputated thumb	
IIIA6-26	Amputated finger	234
IIIA6-27	Amputated arm	
IIIA6-28	Amputated toe	
IIIA6-29	Amputated foot	
IIIA6-30	Amputated leg	
IIIA6-31	Crushing	
IIIA6-32	Burns < 20% – short term	
IIIA6-33	Burns < 20% – long term	235
IIIA6-34	Burns > 20% and < 60% – short term	
IIIA6-35	Burns > 20% and < 60% – long term	
IIIA6-36	Burns > 60% – short term	
IIIA6-37	Burns > 60% – long term	
IIIA6-38	Injured nerves	236
IIIA6-39	Poisoning	
IIIA6-40	Residual	
IIIB	Intentional injuries	
IIIB1	Self-inflicted injuries	
IIIB1-1	Episodes	237
IIIB1-2	Fractured skull – short term	
IIIB1-3	Fractured skull – long term	
IIIB1-4	Fractured face bones	
IIIB1-5	Fractured vertebral column	
IIIB1-6	Injured spinal cord	
IIIB1-7	Fractured rib or sternum	
IIIB1-8	Fractured pelvis	
IIIB1-9	Fractured clavicle, scapula, or humerus	
IIIB1-10	Fractured radius or ulna	
IIIB1-11	Fractured hand bones	
IIIB1-12	Fractured femur – short term	
IIIB1-13	Fractured femur – long term	
IIIB1-14	Fractured patella, tibia, or fibula	
IIIB1-15	Fractured ankle	
IIIB1-16	Fractured foot bones	
IIIB1-17	Other dislocation	
IIIB1-18	Dislocated shoulder, elbow, or hip	
IIIB1-19	Sprains	
IIIB1-20	Intracranial injury – short term	

Table IV   (continued)

GBD Classification Code	Cause group, disease, injury, or sequela	Data presented in this volume (table number)
IIIB1-21	Intracranial injury – long term	
IIIB1-22	Internal injuries	
IIIB1-23	Open wound	
IIIB1-24	Injury to eyes	
IIIB1-25	Amputated thumb	
IIIB1-26	Amputated finger	
IIIB1-27	Amputated arm	
IIIB1-28	Amputated toe	
IIIB1-29	Amputated foot	
IIIB1-30	Amputated leg	
IIIB1-31	Crushing	
IIIB1-32	Burns < 20% – short term	
IIIB1-33	Burns < 20% – long term	
IIIB1-34	Burns > 20% and < 60% – short term	
IIIB1-35	Burns > 20% and < 60% – long term	
IIIB1-36	Burns > 60% – short term	
IIIB1-37	Burns > 60% – long term	
IIIB1-38	Injured nerves	
IIIB1-39	Poisoning	
IIIB1-40	Residual	
IIIB2	Violence	
IIIB2-1	Episodes	238
IIIB2-2	Fractured skull – short term	
IIIB2-3	Fractured skull – long term	239
IIIB2-4	Fractured face bones	
IIIB2-5	Fractured vertebral column	
IIIB2-6	Injured spinal cord	240
IIIB2-7	Fractured rib or sternum	
IIIB2-8	Fractured pelvis	
IIIB2-9	Fractured clavicle, scapula, or humerus	
IIIB2-10	Fractured radius or ulna	
IIIB2-11	Fractured hand bones	
IIIB2-12	Fractured femur – short term	
IIIB2-13	Fractured femur – long term	
IIIB2-14	Fractured patella, tibia, or fibula	
IIIB2-15	Fractured ankle	
IIIB2-16	Fractured foot bones	
IIIB2-17	Other dislocation	
IIIB2-18	Dislocated shoulder, elbow, or hip	
IIIB2-19	Sprains	
IIIB2-20	Intracranial injury – short term	241
IIIB2-21	Intracranial injury – long term	242
IIIB2-22	Internal injuries	
IIIB2-23	Open wound	
IIIB2-24	Injury to eyes	
IIIB2-25	Amputated thumb	
IIIB2-26	Amputated finger	
IIIB2-27	Amputated arm	
IIIB2-28	Amputated toe	
IIIB2-29	Amputated foot	
IIIB2-30	Amputated leg	
IIIB2-31	Crushing	

Table IV   (continued)

GBD Classification Code		Cause group, disease, injury, or sequela	Data presented in this volume (table number)
IIIB2-32		Burns < 20% – short term	
IIIB2-33		Burns < 20% – long term	
IIIB2-34		Burns > 20% and < 60% – short term	
IIIB2-35		Burns > 20% and < 60% – long term	
IIIB2-36		Burns > 60% – short term	
IIIB2-37		Burns > 60% – long term	
IIIB2-38		Injured nerves	243
IIIB2-39		Poisoning	
IIIB2-40		Residual	
IIIB3	War		
IIIB3-1		Episodes	244
IIIB3-2		Fractured skull – short term	
IIIB3-3		Fractured skull – long term	
IIIB3-4		Fractured face bones	
IIIB3-5		Fractured vertebral column	
IIIB3-6		Injured spinal cord	
IIIB3-7		Fractured rib or sternum	
IIIB3-8		Fractured pelvis	
IIIB3-9		Fractured clavicle, scapula, or humerus	
IIIB3-10		Fractured radius or ulna	
IIIB3-11		Fractured hand bones	
IIIB3-12		Fractured femur – short term	
IIIB3-13		Fractured femur – long term	
IIIB3-14		Fractured patella, tibia, or fibula	
IIIB3-15		Fractured ankle	
IIIB3-16		Fractured foot bones	
IIIB3-17		Other dislocation	
IIIB3-18		Dislocated shoulder, elbow, or hip	
IIIB3-19		Sprains	
IIIB3-20		Intracranial injury – short term	
IIIB3-21		Intracranial injury – long term	245
IIIB3-22		Internal injuries	
IIIB3-23		Open wound	
IIIB3-24		Injury to eyes	
IIIB3-25		Amputated thumb	
IIIB3-26		Amputated finger	
IIIB3-27		Amputated arm	246
IIIB3-28		Amputated toe	
IIIB3-29		Amputated foot	247
IIIB3-30		Amputated leg	
IIIB3-31		Crushing	
IIIB3-32		Burns < 20% – short term	
IIIB3-33		Burns < 20% – long term	248
IIIB3-34		Burns > 20% and < 60% – short term	
IIIB3-35		Burns > 20% and < 60% – long term	
IIIB3-36		Burns > 60% – short term	
IIIB3-37		Burns > 60% – long term	
IIIB3-38		Injured nerves	249
IIIB3-39		Poisoning	
IIIB3-40		Residual	

occurs early or later in life, how long, on average, does the condition persist and how many people die from the condition in different population subgroups.

The format of the tables is as follows. At the top of the page, the abbreviated disease or injury short title is provided. Directly beneath the short disease or injury name is the name of the sequela. Three different terms are used repetitively to describe some sequelae: episodes, cases, and symptomatic cases. For diarrhoeal diseases, only one sequela is provided, namely episodes of diarrhoea itself. For consistency, all outcomes related to a disease, including the primary manifestation of the disease or injury, are called sequelae. When the term episodes is used, it indicates that we are providing estimates of incidence and prevalence of episodes of the disease or injury. For some chronic conditions, we provide estimates of the incidence or prevalence of individuals with the condition such as diabetes—this is indicated by using the term cases. Finally, for other chronic conditions, such as COPD or cirrhosis, we have given estimates of the incidence or prevalence of individuals with symptoms of the disease, labelled as symptomatic cases.

The following descriptions and definitions apply to all tables.

Reference year: all estimates refer to calendar year 1990, the base year for the Global Burden of Disease Study. The single exception is the projection of mortality which is shown for the year 2000.

Demographic variables: estimates are presented separately for males and females in view of their different risks of incurring disease and injury. Estimates are shown first for males in the top half of each table, and then for females in the bottom half of the table. Age is perhaps the most important variable in describing disease and injury patterns, since virtually all conditions reported in this book are strongly age-dependent. Estimates are presented for five broad age groups which roughly describe the phases of the life cycle during which disease and injury patterns are likely to be similar. Estimates are also presented for all ages combined, without any attempt at age-standardization. At the bottom of each table, estimates are provided for the total population of the region, including all age groups and for males and females combined.

Incidence: this indicator measures the occurrence of new cases of disease or injury in 1990. The estimated *number* of new cases (in thousands) is shown, along with the estimated incidence rate in the region, expressed as the number of new cases per 100 000 population per year in the respective age-sex group.

Prevalence: in addition to estimating the number of new cases, it is important to be able to estimate the amount of disease or injury which was actually present in each region in 1990, either due to new cases (incidence) in 1990, or from previous years. The estimated number (in thousands) of prevalent cases of disease or injury in 1990 is shown in the table, as is the point prevalence rate, expressed as the number of prevalent cases per 100 000 population.

Average age at onset: this parameter measures the average age (in years) at which new cases of disease or injury occurred in 1990, within each specific age group, and across all ages.

Average duration: an important input into the calculation of DALYs is the average duration of time (in years) that new cases can be expected to spend in a state of ill-health as a result of the disease or injury. These average durations of illness have been calculated for each specific age group, and for all ages combined (unweighted). Duration is measured as the time between occurrence of disease or injury and the absence of the condition, either through remission or death.

Deaths: estimated mortality from each cause and for two time periods is presented in four columns. First, the estimated number of deaths in 1990 (in thousands) within each age-sex group are shown, along with the corresponding age-sex-specific mortality rate for the region in 1990 (expressed per 100 000 population). Next, the *projected* number of deaths in the year 2000, and the *projected* mortality rate per 100 000 in the same year have been included in the extreme right-hand panels of each table. These projections have been made on the basis of the methods and assumptions described earlier and are included to provide a forward-looking perspective of the probable epidemiological profile of each region at the turn of the century.

Precision: Depending on the magnitude of the condition, many significant digits are shown in the tables for some estimates. The large number of significant digits should not convey a false sense of precision. In the era of computers, it is more practical to simply provide the reader with the results of various calculations and estimations rather than to round the figures to one or two significant digits. It is particularly problematic to round the results of this study to one or two significant digits because of the wide range in orders of magnitude of basic incidence and prevalence rates. In order to maintain consistency of units (e.g. per 100 000) across tables, the same number of significant digits for the more common sequelae is shown. In the tables, we have chosen to show the number of decimal places necessary so that for a given parameter at least two significant digits are shown.

DISCUSSION

There is a need, be it for global health policy debate, for monitoring the progress of health development, for research, or for many other public health purposes, to describe in some detail and with some confidence the health status of populations. This book is an attempt to meet that need. The estimates and projections presented here are deliberately ambitious and comprehensive: more than 200 conditions have been reviewed, estimates have been prepared for each sex separately, for five broad age groups and for the various major epidemiological indicators which are commonly used to describe health status. In this respect, the book provides a compendium of data, for major geographical regions of the world, which should help to inform the work of those concerned with improving public health.

Through the application of a sophisticated model of disease occurrence, prevalence, mortality and remission, the estimates presented here for each disease and injury are both internally consistent and consistent with what is known about their natural history. On the other hand, the *reliability* of the estimates is highly variable, and great caution is required when using them. By applying several different methods and approaches, we have tried to confirm the plausibility of estimates. However, no amount of methodological rigour can compensate for the extremely poor datasets and lack of epidemiological information which was commonly encountered in preparing the numbers. For large populations, including much of sub-Saharan Africa, India, other Asia and Islands and parts of Latin America and the Caribbean, very little is reliably known about the causes of mortality, or indeed about disease incidence, prevalence and duration. For these regions, no amount of epidemiological manipulation, extrapolation and estimation can change the fact that the epidemiological assessments reported here are imprecise. For other regions, more data are available and there is proportionately more confidence in the estimates, but even for the industrialized regions, diagnostic and other differences in coding practices among countries cast doubt on the reliability of estimates for specific conditions.

Rather than limiting this assessment to those regions or conditions for which reasonably reliable data were available for estimation, we have opted to prepare a truly global and, we believe, comprehensive assessment of health status in 1990 and beyond. We have done this fully cognizant of the substantial degree of uncertainty underlying many of the estimates. We are also aware that a global assessment of this kind, despite all expressed (and unexpressed) caveats, will most probably be used with a much greater degree of confidence than the underlying data justify. This is inevitable given the need for such an assessment. However, the availability of estimates must not detract from the urgent need to improve the epidemiological information systems which underly them, so that national health status monitoring and assessment can be more reliably performed and health development policies made more effective.

As a consequence of the strengthening of national health statistics systems, future global assessments will undoubtedly become more reliable and, thus, more useful. In the meantime, we hope that the estimates and projections presented here will be used, critically reviewed, and, in due course, updated on the basis of these reviews and critiques. Given the choice of partial, more confident, epidemiological assessments, or the uncertainty associated with the global estimates which are presented here, we have opted for the latter, taking some solace in Greenwood's (1948) remark that: "Making the best the enemy of the good is a sure way to hinder any statistical progress. The scientific purist who will wait for medical statistics until they are nosologically exact, is no wiser than Horace's rustic waiting for the river to flow away."

NOTES

1. In earlier versions of the Global Burden of Disease Study, the nutritional deficiencies, namely protein-energy malnutrition, vitamin A deficiency, iodine deficiency disorders and anaemias were included in Group II. These conditions clearly meet the criteria defining the pre-transitional cluster in Group I. However, they were not included in Group I in earlier versions of this study because of the difficulty in distinguishing some of these deaths from other nutritional and endocrine causes using the datasets available at that time. Considerably more effort has gone into the analysis of these conditions in this fifth and final version of the study, permitting the transfer of these causes to Group I.

2. Chapter XVI deaths have been proportionately reallocated under age 5 to all Group I causes and over age 5 to all Group II causes. Specific algorithms have been developed to deal with imprecise coding of cardiovascular deaths, such as those assigned to heart failure, and ill-defined intentional and unintentional injury deaths.

3. The numbers of deaths for some regions have been slightly modified from those reported in the *WDR 1993* to reflect the high level of war-related mortality around 1990 in some regions. In our opinion, the estimation methods underlying the 1990 demographic assessment did not adequately reflect this war-related mortality.

4. The cause-of-death models used in earlier versions of the Global Burden of Disease Study are not exactly the same as presented here for Version 5. Although the functional form of the two sets of models is similar, the specific results differ because of the addition of more recent information and refinements of the estimation procedures as described in Murray and Lopez (1996b).

5. The analysis of data for South Africa was based largely on the work of Stephen Hendrix, who generously allowed us access to his work prior to publication.

6. In order to ensure internal consistency among the epidemiological estimates presented in this volume, a computer programme, DISMOD, was developed that formalizes the relationship between incidence, remission, case-fatality and prevalence. Susceptibles in the population are assumed to contract a disease or disability at rate i and to die at a general mortality rate m. Cases of disease can either remit at rate r back to being susceptible, die from general causes at the same rate as the susceptibles m, or die from cause-specific mortality at rate f. DISMOD uses the finite difference method to solve the set of linear differential equations defined by these relationships.

7. Non-smoker lung cancer rates for all regions except China and OAI are assumed to be the same as non-smoker lung cancer rates recorded in the CPS-II follow-up survey in the US. For China and OAI, the non-smoker lung cancer rate in women is assumed to be substantially higher based on evidence from various epidemiological studies (Murray and Lopez 1996a).

INTRODUCCIÓN

La objetividad, comparabilidad y confiabilidad de la información sobre la magnitud y distribución de las enfermedades y de los problemas de salud es un punto de partida esencial en la formulación de las políticas de salud, evaluación, supervisión e incluso en la investigación de los determinantes de la salud. Sin embargo, a pesar de décadas de esfuerzos realizados por los países y del apoyo de organismos internacionales, como la Organización Mundial de la Salud, la confiabilidad de la información sobre el estado de salud regional y mundial no está suficientemente disponible.

Para encontrar rápidamente los datos necesarios para la formulación de las políticas de salud, el Banco Mundial y la Organización Mundial de la Salud encargaron el Estudio de la Carga Global de la Enfermedad (CGE) en 1992 para proporcionar una medición objetiva y comparable del estado de salud, y saber cual era entonces el conocimiento sobre la ocurrencia de las enfermedades y de las lesiones en todo el mundo. Los resultados de este estudio fueron ampliamente usados en el *Informe sobre el Desarrollo Mundial 1993: Invertir en Salud* (Banco Mundial, 1993). Una presentación más detallada, aunque todavía abreviada, de los métodos y resultados fue publicada en una serie de artículos en el Boletín de la OMS y posteriormente reimpresos en un libro publicado por la Organización Mundial de la Salud en 1994 (Murray 1994, Murray y Lopez 1994a, Murray y Lopez 1994b, Murray et al. 1994, Murray y Lopez 1994c). La *Serie sobre la Carga Global de la Enfermedad y Lesión*, que se inicia con este volumen, intenta presentar en detalle los métodos, materiales y resultados de cada enfermedad y lesión incluida en el Estudio de la Carga Global de la Enfermedad y las aplicaciones de éstos métodos tanto en el nivel nacional y como al interior de los países.

El Estudio de la Carga Global de la Enfermedad fue diseñado en parte para superar las tres principales limitaciones de la información disponible sobre la magnitud de los problemas de salud. En primer lugar, la información en salud es sumistrada frecuentemente a quienes toman decisiones, por personas implicadas con las enfermedades. El hecho de que estas mismas personas lleven a cabo las estimaciones epidemiológicas puede aumentar las dudas sobre la objetividad de las conclusiones. Más concretamente, sus preocupaciones específicas, les hacen sobrestimar la magnitud de las enfermedades de forma no intencionada. La separación de la «defensa» de los enfermos del proceso de generación de mediciones epidemiológicas es un paso esencial para conseguir estimaciones más plausibles y útiles.

En segundo lugar, los datos internacionales que están basados en diagnósticos y en procedimientos similares reportados están casi exclusivamente enfocados a mortalidad y les falta incorporar información comparable sobre resultados no fatales. La ausencia de información de buena calidad sobre discapacidad y otros resultados no fatales ha contribuido al continuo abandono de esos problemas en el debate nacional e internacional. A pesar de la enorme brecha en el conocimiento acerca de la epidemiología de muchos de los resultados no fatales, la segunda meta del Estudio de la CGE fue generar estimaciones creíbles sobre incidencia, prevalencia y duración de un número importante de enfermedades. En tercer lugar, una métrica comun, los años de vida ajustados por discapacidad o AVAD, han sido usados para agregar y resumir los datos y la información sobre mortalidad y resultados no fatales y así permitir las comparaciones del impacto de varias condiciones de salud. Los AVADs también pueden ser usados en el análisis de costo-efectividad, ya que en gran medida facilitan las mediciones conjuntas sobre la magnitud de los problemas de salud, las distintas series de intervenciones, disponibles para enfrentar estos problémas. Con una métrica común, la combinación de los resultados sobre la carga de la enfermedad y del análisis de costo-efectividad de las intervenciones disponibles, ha sido y puede ser usada para identificar un conjunto de intervenciones prioritarias en forma de paquetes esenciales descritos en el *Informe sobre el Desarrollo Mundial 1993*.

Los objetivos específicos del Estudio de la Carga de la Enfermedad fueron cuatro. El primero fue desarrollar estimaciones consistentes internamente de la mortalidad por edad, sexo y región para más de 100 causas de muerte. La segunda meta fue desarrollar estimaciones consistentes internamente de incidencia, prevalencia, letalidad y mortalidad por edad, sexo y región, de las principales secuelas de más de 100 causas de enfermedad, reconociendo el importante papel de ciertas exposiciones en la etiología de la enfermedad y de las lesiones. Un tercer objetivo fue estimar la cantidad de muertes prematuras y discapacidad atribuibles a ciertos factores de riesgo seleccionados, como la contaminación del aire, prácticas sexuales no seguras, hipertensión arterial, alcoholismo y tabaquismo. Finalmente, el cuarto objetivo fue proveer un conjunto de proyecciones sobre la carga de la enfermedad por edad, sexo, región y causa hasta el año 2020.

El propósito de este volumen es facilitar el acceso a estimaciones detalladas de incidencia, prevalencia, duración y muerte, que fueron preparadas para el estudio de la carga de la enfermedad. Fue diseñado primariamente como una referencia para estimaciones epidemiológicas a nivel mundial. Gran parte de este volumen esta dedicado a las presentaciones tabulares de los resultados. Después de esta breve introducción se describen los métodos usados para el cálculo las estimaciones, el resto del volumen contiene las tablas con la información demográfica básica para cada una de las ocho regiones geográficas usadas en el *Informe sobre el Desarrollo Mundial 1993,* seguida de un gran número de cuadros que proporcionan las estimaciones de incidencia, prevalencia, promedio de la edad de inicio, duración promedio, muertes en 1990 proyectadas al año 2000 para varias enfermedades y secuelas. La discusión posterior muestra brevemente el sistema de clasificación de la CGE, la demografía básica para cada una de las ocho regiones, los procedimientos empleados en las estimaciones de las causas de muerte y los métodos usados para estimar la incidencia, prevalencia, letalidad y duración de la secuela principal. Los lectores interesados en mas detalles acerca de los métodos y de los supuestos concernientes a las bases empíricas y procesos de estimación para cada una de las enfermedades pueden encontrarlos en otros los volúmenes relevantes en esta serie.

SISTEMA DE CLASIFICACIÓN DE LA CGE

Para el Estudio de la Carga Global de la Enfermedad, se ha usado una estructura de «árbol» para las enfermedades y lesiones. Esta se presenta en el cuadro I. En el primer nivel de desagregación, la mortalidad total se dividide en tres grandes grupos de causas: Grupo I, comprende en las enfermedades transmisibles, causas maternas, condiciones relacionadas con el periodo perinatal y deficiencias de la nutrición[1]; Grupo II, abarca las enfermedades no transmisibles y el Grupo III que agrupa todas las lesiones. Las causas de muerte del Grupo I, causas pretransicionales son en una agrupación de condiciones que típicamente estan disminuyendo a un ritmo mayor que todas las causas de muerte durante el proceso de transición epidemiológica. Como resultado, en las poblaciones de baja mortalidad, estas causas contribuyen con una baja proporción de muertes. Recíprocamente, las enfermedades del Grupo II son los problemas de salud más importantes en las poblaciones que han realizado la transición epidemiológica. Aún cuando es verdad que algunas tasas de mortalidad de condiciones no transmisibles como el cáncer de estómago puede descender más rápidamente que todas las causas de mortalidad en conjunto, estas enfermedades se han mantenido en el Grupo II junto con otros cánceres ya que las tasas de muerte por cáncer en total aparecen relativamente constantes a lo largo de la transición. Finalmente, las lesiones son separadas y clasificadas en el Grupo III, en parte porque su etiología es muy diferente de las otras enfermedades, pero tambien porque no hay patrones de cambio generalizables en la mortalidad por lesiones que acompañen la transición epidemiológica.

Cada grupo ha sido dividido en varias subcategorias de enfermedades y lesiones que son mutuamente excluyentes. Estas subcategorias son

Cuadro I Estudio de la Carga Global de la Enfermedad, sistema de clasificación de enfermedades

Título de las Causas de CGE	CIE 9a lista detallada	CIE 9a lista básica	CIE 10a lista
I. Condiciones transmisibles, maternas, perinatales y de la nutrición.	001–139, 243, 260–269, 280–285,320–322, 381–382, 614–616, 460–465, 466, 480–487, 614–616, 630–676, 760–779	01–07, 19, 200, 220, 240, 310–312, 320–322, 371–373, 38–41, 45.	A00–B99, G00, N70–N73, J00–J06, J10–J18, J20–J22, H65–H66, O00–O99, P00–P06, E00–E02, E40–E46, E50, D50
A. Enfermedades infecciosas y parasitarias	001–139,320–322, 614–616	01–07, 220, 371–373	A00–B99, G00, N70–N73
1. Tuberculosis	010–018, 137	02, 077	A15–A19, B90
2. Enfermedades de transmisión sexual excepto VIH	090–099, 614–616	06, 371–373	A50–A64, N70–N73
a. Sífilis	090–097	060	A50–A53
b. Clamidia	i	ii	A55–A56
c. Gorronea	098	061	A54
3. VIH	i	ii	B20–B24
4. Enfermedades diarreicas	001, 002, 004, 006–009	01 minus 013	A01–A04, A06–A09
5. Enfermedades de la infancia	032, 033, 037, 045, 050, 055, 056, 138	033, 034, 037, 040–043, 078	A33–37, A80, B05, B91
a. Tosferina	033	034	A37
b. Poliomielitis	045, 138	040, 078	A80, B91
c. Difteria	032	033	A36
d. Sarampión	055	042	B05
e. Tétanos	037, 771.3	037[iii]	A33–A35
6. Meningitis bacteriana y meningococcemia	036, 320–322	036, 220[iv]	A39, G00
7. Hepatitis B y hepatitis C	070.2–070.9	046[v]	B16–B19
8. Paludismo	084	052	B50–B54
9. Enfermedades tropicales	085, 086, 120, 125	053, 054, 072, 074	B55–B57, B65, B73–B74
a. Tripanosomiasis	086.3, 086.4, 086.5, 086.9[vi]	054[ii]	B56
b. Enfermedad de Chagas	086.0, 086.1, 086.2, 086.9[vi]	054[vii]	B57
c. Esquistosomiasis	120	072	B65
d. Leishmaniasis	085	053	B55
e. Filariasis linfática	125.0, 125.1	ii	B74.0–B74.2
f. Oncocercosis	125.3	ii	B73
10. Lepra	030	032	A30
11. Dengue	061	ii	A90–A91
12. Encefalitis japonesa	062.0	ii	A83.0
13. Tracoma	076	048	A71
14. Infecciones intestinales por nemátodos	126–129	ii	
a. Ascaridiasis	127.0	ii	B77
b. Tricocefalosis	127.3	ii	B79
c. Anquilostomiasis y necatoriasis	126	ii	B76
B. Infecciones respiratorias	460–466, 480–487, 381–382	310–312, 320–322, 240	J00–J06, J10–J18, J20–J22, H65–H66
1. Infecciones de las vías respiratorias inferiores	466, 480–487	320–322	J10–J18, J20–J22
2. Infecciones de las vías respiratorias superiores	460–465	310–312	J00–J06
3. Otitis media	381–382	240	H65–H66
C. Condiciones maternas	630–676	38–41	O00–O99
1. Hemorragia materna	640, 641, 666	390	O44–O46, O67, O72
2. Sepsis puerperal	670	ii	O85–O86
3. Trastornos hipertensivos del embarazo	642	ii	O10–O16
4. Parto obstruido	660	393	O64–O66
5. Aborto	630–639	38	O00–O08
D. Condiciones que aparecen durante el período perinatal	760–779	45	P00–P06
1. Bajo peso al nacer	764–765	452	P05–P07

Cuadro I (continuado)

Título de las Causas de CGE	CIE 9a lista detallada	CIE 9a lista básica	CIE 10a lista
2. Asfixia y trauma al nacer	767–770	453–454	P03, P10–P15, P20–P29
E. Deficiencias de la nutrición	243, 260–269, 280–285	19, 200[viii]	E00–E02, E40–E46, E50, D50
1. Desnutrición proteínico – calórica	260–263	190–192	E40–E46
2. Deficiencia de yodo	243	[ii]	E00–E02
3. Deficiencia de vitamina A	264	[ii]	E50
4. Anemia por deficiencia de hierro	280	200[viii]	D50
II. Enfermedades no transmisibles	140–242, 244–259, 270–279, 286–319, 323–380, 383–459, 467–479, 488–613, 617–629, 680–759	08–18, 20–37, 42–44. [menos 200, 220, 240, 310–312, 320–322, 371–373]	
A. Neoplasias malignas	140–209	08–14	C00–C97
1. Cánceres de boca y orofaringe	140–149	08	C00–C14
2. Cáncer de esófago	150	090	C15
3. Cáncer de estómago	151	091	C16
4. Cánceres de colon y recto	153, 154	093, 094	C18–C21
5. Cáncer de hígado	155	095	C22
6. Cáncer de páncreas	157	096	C25
7. Cánceres de tráquea, bronquios y pulmones	162	101	C33–C34
8. Melanoma y otros tumores de la piel	172–173	111, 112	C43–C44
9. Cáncer de mama	174	113	C50
10. Cáncer cervicouterino	180	120	C53
11. Cáncer de cuerpo de utero	179, 182	122	C54–C55
12. Cáncer de ovario	183	123	C56
13. Cáncer de próstata	185	124	C61
14. Cáncer de vesícula	188	126	C67
15. Linfomas y mieloma múltiple	200–202	14 [menos 141]	C81–C90, C96
16. Leucemia	204–208	141	C91–C95
B. Otras neoplasias	210–239	15, 16, 17	D00–D48
C. Diabetes mellitus	250	181	E10–E14
D. Trastornos endocrinos	240–242, 244–246, 251–259, 270–279, 281–289	18 20 [menos 200[ix]]	D55–D80, E03–E07, E15–E16, E20–E34, E51–E89
E. Condiciones neuropsiquiatricas	290–319, 323–359	21–22 [menos 220]	F00–F99, G03–G99
1. Depresión mayor unipolar	[i]	[ii]	F32–F33
2. Trastornos bipolar	296	212	F30–F31
3. Esquizofrenia	295	211	F20–F29
4. Epilesia	345	225	G40–G41
5. Uso de alcohol	291, 303, 305.0	215[x]	F10
6. Demencia y otros trastornos degenerativos y hereditarios del SNC	330, 331, 290	222, 210[xi]	F01, F03, G30–G31
7. Enfermedad de Parkinson	332	221	G20–G21
8. Esclerosis múltiple	340	223	G35
9. Uso de drogas	304, 305.2–305.9	216[xii]	F11–F16, F18–F19
10. Trastorno de estrés post-traumático	[i]	[ii]	[xvii]
11. Trastornos obsesivo-compulsivos	300.3	[ii]	F42
12. Trastorno de pánico	300.2	[ii]	F40.0, F41.0
F. Enfermedades de los órganos de los sentidos	360–380, 383–389	23, 24 [menos 240]	H00–H61, H68–H95
1. Glaucoma	365	230	H40
2. Cataratas	366	231	H25–H26
G. Enfermedades cardiovasculares	390–459	25–30	I00–I99
1. Cardiotapía reumática	390–398	25	I01–I09
2. Cardiotapía isquémica	410–414	27	I20–I25
	Proporción de: 428, 427.1, 427.4, 427.5, 440.9, 429.0 -429.2, 429.9[xiii]	[xiv]	[xv]

Cuadro I   (continuado)

Título de las Causas de CGE	CIE 9a lista detallada	CIE 9a lista básica	CIE 10a lista
3. Enfermedad cerebrovascular	430–438	29	I60–I69
4. Enfermerdades inflamatorias del corazón	420, 421, 422, 425 Proporción de 428[xvi]	ii	I30–I33, I38, I40, I42
H. Enfermedades respiratorias	470–478, 490–519	31–32 [minus 310–312, 320–322]	J30–J99
1. Enfermedad pulmonar obstructiva crónica	490–492, 495–496	ii	J40–J44
2. Asma	493	ii	J45–J46
I. Enfermedades digestivas	530–579	34	K20–K99
1. Ulcera péptica	531–533	341	K25–K27
2. Cirrosis hepática	571	347	K70, K74
3. Apendicitis	540–543	342	K35–K37
J. Enfermedades del aparato genitourinario	580–611, 617–629	35–37 [minus 371–373]	N00–N64, N75–N99
1. Nefritis y nefrosis	580–589	350	N00–N19
2. Hipertrofia prostática benigna	600	360	N40
K. Enfermedades de la piel	680–709	42	L00–L99
L. Enfermedades del sistema osteomuscular	710–759	43	M00–M99
1. Artritis reumatoide	714	430	M05–M06
2. Osteoartritis	715	ii	M15–M19
M. Anomalías congénitas	740–759	44	Q00–Q99
1. Defecto de la pared abdominal	i	ii	xvii
2. Anencefalia	740.0	ii	Q00
3. Atresia anorectal	751.2	ii	Q42
4. Labio leporino	749.1	ii	Q36
5. Paladar hendido	749.0	ii	Q35,Q37
6. Atresia esofágica	750.3	ii	Q39.0–Q39.1
7. Agenesia renal	753.0	ii	Q60
8. Síndrome de Down	758.0	ii	Q90
9. Anomalías congénitas del corazón	745–747	442	Q20–Q28
10. Espina bífida	741	ii	Q05
N. Afecciones de la cavidad bucal	520–529	33	K00–K14
1. Caries dentales	521.0	ii	K02
2. Enfermedad periodontal	523	ii	K05
3. Edentulismo	i	ii	xvii
III. Lesiones	E800–999	E47–E56	V01–Y98
A. Lesiones no intencionales	E800–921, 923–949	E47–E51, E520–E523, E53	V01–X59, Y40–Y98
1. Accidentes de tráfico	E810–819, 826–829, 928–929	E471,E472	V01–V89
2. Envenenamientos	E850–869	E48	X40–X49
3. Caídas	E880–888	E50	W00–W19
4. Fuegos	E890–899	E51	X00–X09
5. Ahogamientos	E910	E521	W65–W74
6. Otras lesiones no intencionales	E800–E807, E820–825, E830–E848, E870–E879, E900–E909, E911–E921, E923–E949	E470, E473–E474, E49, E520, E522–E523, E53	V90–V99, W20–W64, W75–W99, X10–X39, X50–X59
B. Lesiones intencionales	E922, 950–979, 990–999	E524, E54–E55, E561	X60–Y09,Y35–Y36
1. Lesiones autoinfligidas	E950–959	E54	X60–X84
2. Violencias	E922, 960–969	E55	X85–Y09
3. Guerra	E990–999	E561	Y35–Y36

Notas

1. «Senilidad y mal definidas» (Capítulo XVI de la 9a Clasificación Internacional de Enfermedades y R00–R99 en la 10a Clasificación Internacional de Enfermedades es incluida en el grupo I para personas menores de cinco años y en el grupo II para personas mayores de cinco años y distribuida proporcionalmente en todas las causas bajo los niveles del grupo.

2. La causa E560 (lista básica) de la 9a revisión de la Clasificación Internacional de Enfermedades, (E980–E989 lista detallada y Y10–Y34 de la 10a revisión) se distribuyeron preoporcionalmente en todas las causas de lesiones siguiendo los niveles del grupo.

i   «Senilidad y mal definidas» (Capítulo XVI de la 9a Clasificación Internacional de Enfermedades y R00–R99 en la 10a
    Clasificación Internacional de Enfermedades, es encluida en el grupo I para personas menores de cinco años y en el grupo
    II para personas mayores de cinco años y distribuida proporcionalmente en todas las causas bajo los niveles del grupo.
ii   No hay código disponible de la lista detallada de la CIE-9.
iii No hay código disponible de la lista básica de la CIE-9.
iv   El código 220 de la lista básica incluye causas inespecíficas de meningitis las cuales son excluidas cuando el cuarto dígito
    de la lista detallada esta disponible.
v   El código 46 de la lista básica incluye hepatitis A el cual no es parte de esta categoría.
vi   086.9 en ASS es tripanosomiasis africana y en ALC es enfermeded de Chagas.
vii 054 en ASS es tripanosomiasis africana y en ALC es enfermeded de Chagas.
viii El código 200 de la lista básica incluye otras anemias no ferroprivas que deben ser clasificadas en IID «Desordenes
    endócrinos.»
ix   Algunas anemias clasificadas con el código 200 de la lista básica deben ser incluidas aquí.
x   El código 215 de la lista básica no incluye muertes de los códigos 303 y 305.0 de la lista detallada.
xi   El código 210 de la lista básica incluye muertes de los códigos 330 a 336 los cuales no debieran ser parte de esta
    categoría en la lista detallada.
xii El código 216 de la lista básica no incluye los códigos 305.2 y 305.9 de la lista detallada los cuales deverian de estar
    incluidos aquí.
xiii La proporción de «códigos basura» de muertes cardiovasculares deberian ser incluidos en enfermedad isquémica del
    corazón dependiendo de la proportión de muertes cardiovasculares que originalmente había en los códigos 410 a 414.
    Favor de ver Murray y Lopez (1996a) para el análisis detallado y métodos recomendados para las correcciones.
xiv Ver Murray y Lopez (1996b) para una ecuación por aproximar la mortalidad por cardiotapía isquémica utilizando datos de
    la lista básica.
xv   No se ha desarrollado ningún algoritmo para la CIE 10a revisión por corregir por los muertes por cardiotapía isquémica en
    los códigos incorrecto.
xvi 2.5% 30–44, 5% 45–59 y 10% 60+.
xvii No hay código disponible en la CIE 10a revisión.

identificadas con letras mayúsculas en el Cuadro I. Específicamente, el Grupo I ha sido dividido en infecciones y parasitosis, infecciones respiratorias, causas maternas, condiciones perinatales y deficiencias nutricionales. Las enfermedades no transmisibles (Grupo II) han sido divididas en 14 categorias (ver Cuadro I). El Grupo III (las lesiones) han sido divididas en dos grandes subcategorias, lesiones no intencionales (IIIA) y lesiones intencionales (IIIB).

Un tercer nivel de desagregación es usado para identificar causas más específicas de muerte entre cada una de estas categorías del segundo nivel. Por ejemplo, entre las categorias de infecciones y parasitosis (IA), las causas específicas como la tuberculosis (IA1), VIH (IA3) y diarrea (IA4) han sido identificadas. Finalmente, para algunas enfermedades como las de transmisión sexual (IA2) existe un cuarto nivel de desagregación: en sífilis (IA2a), gonorrea (IA2b) y clamidia (IA2c). El conjunto de causas desagregadas fue seleccionado sobre la base de tres criterios: la probable magnitud de la enfermedad o de las lesiones como causa de muerte o discapacidad evaluada al principio del estudio; condiciones de salud para las cuales se proporcionan considerables servicios de salud, por ejemplo, apendicitis, y condiciones que son actualmente consideradas en los debates de salud pública como focos de atención.

La categoría de signos y síntomas mal definidos—Capítulo XVI de la Clasificación Internacional de Enfermedades, novena revisión (Capítulo XVIII de la décima revisión de la CIE)—no tiene relevancia en términos de intervenciones en salud pública, y no ha sido usada como una causa en nuestro sistema de clasificación. Las muertes asignadas a esta categoría, así como otros códigos usados para diagnósticos mal definidos, fueron reasignadas a causas de muerte específicas. Desde la perspectiva de generar datos para la elección de alternativas de políticas o estrategias de salud , la asignación de muertes a una categoría mal definida es inapropiada y potencialente engañosa. Cada persona que muere lo hace por alguna causa específica subyacente y se requiere la mejor estimación posible de la magnitud de cada una, para la formulación de políticas.[2]

El Cuadro I enlista los códigos de la CIE 9a revisión con cuatro dígitos correspondientes a cada causa de muerte en nuestra clasificación. La novena revisión de la CIE fue usada como base para el desarrollo de la lista de causas de enfermedad y lesiones, dado que estoba uigente en 1990, año base en el Estudio de la CGE. Como la 10a revisión de la CIE se distintos progresivamente implementará en los distintos países durante los la siguiente década se incluye también la correspondencia de códigos con la Décima revisión para futuras referencias.

Para cada enfermedad o lesión se han evaluado además una o más secuelas. Por ejemplo, para diabetes mellitus hemos incluido úlceras del pie diabético, amputaciones, neuropatía y ceguera por retinopatía en adición a la diabetes misma. Por conveniencia, cada secuela ha recibido un código compuesto por el mismo código de la enfermedad seguido de un guión y un número específico para cada secuela. Por ejemplo, el pie diabético es codificado como IIC-2. No todas las secuelas fueron evaluadas en este volumen debido a consideraciones de espacio. Esto es particularmente cierto para un gran número de secuelas provenientes de cada una de las causas listadas en el Grupo III (lesiones). Las muertes estimadas para 1990 y las proyecciones al año 2000 son presentadas solamente para cada enfermedad o lesión y no desagregadas por secuelas. Para facilitar la presentación de las tablas, se han incluido las muertes en la misma tabla junto a la presentación primaria de la enfermedad o el resultado más importante. Esto es arbitario pero necesario, pues permite reducir el número de tablas publicadas para cada enfermedad o secuela.

REGIONES

El análisis de la CGE fue llevado a cabo para ocho regiones geográficas específicamente desarrolladas por el Banco Mundial para el *Informe sobre el Desarrollo Mundial 1993*. Estas regiones y sus abreviaturas son las siguentes: Países con economía de mercado consolidada (PEMC), Países europeos antes socialistas (PEAS), América Latina y el Caribe (ALC), China (CHI), India (IND), Otros países asiáticos e insulares (OPAI), Arco del Oriente Medio (la cual incluye el Norte de Africa, el Oriente Medio, Pakistan y repúblicas de Asia Central de la antes Unión Sovietica) (AOM) y Africa al Sur del Sahara (ASS). La asignación de países realizada por el Banco Mundial a cada región se muestran en la cuadro II. El criterio usado para definir estas regiones incluyó el nivel de desarrollo socioeconómico, la homogeneidad epidemiológica y la contiguidad geográfica. El mapa en colores incluido en este volúmen ilustra la localización y composición de cada región.

ESTIMACIONES DEMOGRÁFICAS REGIONALES

El punto de partida para la estimación mundial, regional o nacional de la carga de la enfermedad es una medición confiable del tamaño y distribución de las poblaciones y muertes por edad y sexo. A través de la combinación de esfuerzos de muchos individuos, organizaciones y gobiernos se conoce bastante acerca de la demografía básica de cada región del mundo. Incuestionablemente, las bases de datos para estimar la mortalidad en la infancia en todas las regiones estan más desarrolladas que las relacionadas con la mortalidad en el adulto (Naciones Unidas 1992; Hill y Yazbeck 1994). Ciertamente, hay una considerable controversia entre los demógrafos sobre los niveles de mortalidad en adultos en algunas regiones en desarrollo donde no existe un buen registro de estadísticas vitales y donde la mortalidad es estimada indirectamente a partir de censos de población o encuestas (Timaeus 1991). Por ejemplo, las estimaciones de mortalidad en el adulto por edad y sexo del Banco Mundial y de la división de población de la Organización de las Naciones Unidas pueden diferir en más del 50%, pero en general el grado de incertidumbre es menor. Las estimaciones demográficas de muertes y población para 1990 por edad y sexo fueron desarrolladas específicamente para el *Informe sobre el Desarrollo Mundial 1993*. Hemos continuado usando el estudio de la Carga Global de la Enfermedad para asegurar comparabilidad con otras publicaciones donde los resultados de la carga de la Enfermedad han sido incluidos.

Los Cuadros 1 a 9 proporcionan las estimaciones de 1990 de población y muertes por grupos quinquenales por sexo, para cada una de las ocho regiones y para el total mundial. Adicionalmente se agregan figuras para la población y muertes en los cinco grandes grupos de edad usados para preparar las mediciones epidemiológicas.[3]

ESTIMACIÓN DE LAS CAUSAS DE MUERTE

Esta sección presenta una revisión muy breve de las diferentes fuentes de datos disponibles para la estimación de las causas de muerte, de los métodos usados para generar las estimaciones de causas de muerte basados en estos datos. Información mucho más detallada sobre los métodos y aproximaciones seguidas para generar estimaciones de todos los parámetros epidemiológicos reportados en este libro, así como para llevar cabo las proyecciones de mortalidad, pueden ser encontradas en *La Carga Global de la Enfermedad*, primer volumen de la *Serie sobre la Carga Global de la Enfermedad y Lesión*.

Fuentes de Datos

Para estimar los patrones de causas de muerte, cuatro fuentes de información pueden ser utilizados: registros de estadísticas vitales, muestras de los registros de defunciones, mediciones epidemiológicas y modelos para causas de muerte. El Cuadro III resume la disponibilidad de registros vitales confiables por edad y región en 1990. Solo los PEMC y los PEAS

Cuadro II   Países o territorios en el Estudio de la Carga Global de la Enfermedad, por región demográfica

Regiones demográficamente desarrolladas		Regiones en transición demográfica
Países con economía de mercado consolidada (PEMC)	Países europeos antes socialistas (PEAS)	India (IND)
		China (CHN)
Alemania	Albania	Otros países asiáticos e insulares (OPAI)
Andorra	Belarús	
Australia	Bosnia y Herzegovina	
Austria	Bulgaria	Bangladesh
Bélgica	Croacia	Bhután
Bermuda	Eslovaquia	Brunei Darussalam
Canadá	Eslovenia	Camboya
Dinamarca	Estonia	Corea, República de
España	Federación de Rusia	Corea, República Popular Democrática de
Estados Unidos	Hungría	Estados Federados de Micronesia
Finlandia	Letonia	Fiji
Francia	Lituania	Filipinas
Gibraltar	Macedonia, la ex República Yugoslava de	Grupo norte de las Islas Marianas
Grecia	Moldova	Guam
Groenlandia	Polonia	Hong Kong
Irlanda	República Checa	Indonesia
Isla de Man	Rumania	Isla de Wake
Islandia	Ucrania	Isla Johnston
Islas Anglonormandas	Yugoslavia	Isla Midway
Islas Feroé		Isla Pitcairn
Italia		Islas Cook
Japón		Islas Tokelau
Liechtenstein		Islas Marshall
Luxemburgo		Islas Salomón
Mónaco		Islas Wallis y Futuna
Noruega		Kiribati
Nueva Zelandia		Macao
Países Bajos		Malasia
Portugal		Maldivas
Reino Unido		Mauricio
Saint-Pierre-et-Miquelon		Mongolia
San Marino		Myanmar
Santa Sede		Nauru
Suecia		Nepal
Suiza		Niie
Suiza		Nueva Caledonia
		Palau
		Papua Nueva Guinea
		Polinesia Francesa
		Reunión República Democrática Popular de Laos
		Samoa Americana
		Samoa Occidental
		Seychelles
		Singapur
		Sri Lanka
		Tailandia
		Taiwan
		Tonga
		Tuvalu
		Vanuatu
		Viet Nam

Cuadro II   (continuado)

Regiones en transición demográfica, continuado

Africa al Sur del Sahara (ASS)	América Latina y el Caribe (ALC)	Arco del Oriente Medio (AOM)
Angola	Anguila	Afganistán
Ascención	Antigua y Barbuda	Arabia Saudita
Benin	Antillas Neerlandesas	Argelia
Botswana	Argentina	Armenia
Burkina Faso	Aruba	Azerbaiyán
Burundi	Bahamas	Bahrein
Cabo Verde	Barbados	Chipre
Camerún	Belice	Egipto
Chad	Bolivia	Emiratos Arabes Unidos
Comoras	Brasil	Georgia
Congo	Chile	Irán, República Isleamica del
Côte d'Ivoire	Colombia	Iraq
Djibouti	Costa Rica	Israel
Eritrea	Cuba	Jamahiriya Arabe Libia
Etiopía	Dominica	Jordania
Gabón	Ecuador	Kazajstán
Gambia	El Salvador	Kirguistán
Ghana	Granada	Kuwait
Guinea	Guadalupe	Líbano
Guinea Ecuatorial	Guatemala	Malta
Guinea-Bissau	Guayana Francesa	Marruecos
Kenya	Guyana	Omán
Lesotho	Haití	Pakistán
Liberia	Honduras	Qatar
Madagascar	Isla Vírgenes Británicas	República Arabe Siria
Malawi	Islas Caimán	Ribera Occidenta y Faja de Gaza
Malí	Islas Turcas y Caicos	Sahara Occidental
Mauritania	Islas Vírgenes (E.U.)	Tayikistán
Mozambique	Jamaica	Túnez
Namibia	Martinica	Turkmenistán
Níger	México	Turquía
Nigeria	Montserrat	Uzbekistán
República Centroafricana	Nicaragua	Yemen
Rwanda	Panamá	
Santo Tomé y Príncipe	Paraguay	
Senegal	Perú	
Sierra Leona	Puerto Rico	
Somalia	República Dominicana	
Sudáfrica	Saint Kitts y Nevis	
Sudán	San Vicentelas Granadinas	
Swazilandia	Santa Lucía	
Tanzaniá	Suriname	
Togo	Trinidad y Tabago	
Tristán da Cunha	Uruguay	
Uganda	Venezuela	
Zaire		
Zambia		
Zimbabwe		

Cuadro III   Disponibilidad de datos en registros vitales por
                  causas de muerte y por región, 1990.

	Registros vitales (% de cobertura)			Registros por muestreo	
	Menores de 5	**5+**	**Total**	**Urbano**	**Rural**
PEMC	99	99	99		
PEAS	99	99	99		
IND				ICD	SCD(R)
CHN				DSP	DSP
OPAI	2	14	10		
ASS	<1	2	1		
ALC	28	47	43		
AOM	12	27	22		

tienen sistemas de registros vitales completos; para las regiones en desarrollo otras fuentes fueron usadas, incluyendo muestras de registros vitales, comunidades laboratorio, estimaciones epidemiológicas y modelación , como suplemento de la información de registros vitales.

Aún cuando los registros de rutina no están ampliamente disponibles en India y China, están funcionando sistemas de registro de muestras de población que pueden ser usados como base para la estimación de la mortalidad por causas. En China, la Academia China de Medicina Preventiva opera con el conocido Sistema de Puntos de Vigilancia de Enfermedades (SPVE). Establecido a principios de los 80, este sistema supervisa una muestra representativa de 10 millones de personas en áreas rurales y urbanas de China. Cada punto de vigilancia mantiene un equipo, que incluye al médico. Dicho equipo investiga cada defunción reportada y le asigna una causa de muerte usando los registros médicos y entrevistas a miembros de la familia del fallecido.

La India, como China, no tiene un sistema completo y confiable de registros vitales para atribuir las causas de muerte. Sin embargo, dos sistemas que proporcionan información pueden ser usados para estimar patrones de causas de muerte. En áreas urbanas, la certificación médica de las muertes se realiza en hospitales y son tabuladas y publicadas cada año por el Registro General. Mientras en muchos estados la calidad de los datos generados es demasiado pobre, en el estado de Maharashtra la cobertura de la certificación médica de las causas de muerte es mayor del 80% (Oficina del Registro General 1992a). Esta información ha sido usada como base para la estimación de las causas de muerte urbanas. En las áreas rurales de la India, un sistema de muestreo de autopsias verbales basado en los Centros de Atención Primaria (CAP) y en sus áreas de influencia han estado en operación desde 1965.

Conocida como la encuesta de causas de muerte en el area rural (ECM-R), este sistema actualmente incluye información sobre 1300 CAPs (Oficina del Registro General 1992b) y proporciona información útil de amplios grupos de causas de muertes en areas rurales. Ya que la causa de muerte es asignada por un «lego», (personal no médico), este sistema solo es útil para estimar grupos amplios de causas de muerte y no para categorias específicas de enfermedad o lesiones.

Aunque ningún sistema de registro por muestreo esta disponible para una población amplia de Africa al Sur del Sahara, «a pequeña escala ciertas comunidades laboratorio» operan en Niakhar (Senegal), Keneba (Gambia), Navrongo (Ghana), Machakos (Kenia) y Morogoro, Hai y Dar es-Salaam (Tanzania) proporcionan información limitada sobre autopsias verbales sobre causas de muerte. Aún cuando este sistema de registro es útil para delinear los perfiles locales de causas de muerte, su utilidad en las estimaciones de perfiles regionales es limitada.

Para varias condiciones específicas, los epidemiólogos han desarrollado estimaciones de causas específicas de mortalidad basadas en la historia natural de una enfermedad dada. Las tasas estimadas de incidencia y/o prevalencia de encuestas específicas se combinan con información de tasas de letalidad para casos tratados y no tratados para producir tasas de mortalidad. Para algunas causas de muerte como la infección respiratoria aguda, la diarrea el paludismo se han desarrollado encuestas con el fin de realizar mediciones más directas de la mortalidad específica, a menudo con limitado éxito (para más detalles, ver los capítulos relevantes en la *Serie sobre la Carga Global de la Enfermedad y Lesión*). La mayor limitación de las estimaciones epidemiológicas es que tienden a sobreestimar la carga de cada enfermedad en particular. Cuando se suman las estimaciones epidemiológicas para cada una de las causas de muerte, el total número de muertes estimadas por esta vía generalmente excede (algunas veces considerablemente) al número de muertes para todas las causas que resultan del análisis demográfico. La tendencia de las estimaciones epidemiológicas a sobreestimar los niveles de morbilidad es ocasionada por de diferentes fuentes de sesgo. En primer lugar, aunque muchas defunciones son multicausales, los cálculos epidemiológicos atribuyen todavía frecuentement cada muerte a cada una sus muchas causas. En segundo lugar cuando existe incertudumbre sobre la incidencia, prevalencia o letalidad, los analistas tienden a elevar las tasas estimadas, a pesar de que se les reclame lo contrario. En tercer lugar, los cálculos epidemíologos se emprenden sin considerar las otras causas de muerte. De esta forma los autores de los cálculos son frecuentemente incosiententes de la magnitud comparativa de sus estimaciones de mortalidad. Las mediciones epidemiológicas de la magnitud de los problemas de salud pueden a portar mucha información, pero cuando son considerados independientemente de otras causas de muerte o discapacidad puede ser engañosas.

Donde no están disponibles los registros vitales o estimaciones epidemiológicas, la modelación de las causas de muerte puede resultar útil para estimar los perfiles. Preston (1976) inició el desarrollo de técnicas indirectas para estimar la proporción de causas de muerte, relacionando la mortalidad general con la mortalidad específica para doce grandes grupos de causas, basándose en el análisis histórico de registros vitales en naciones desarrolladas y en algunos países en desarrollo. Concretamente postulava que la mortalidad por causa específica es una función líneal de la mortalidad general. El trabajo de Preston ha sido la base de todas las aproximaciones subsecuentes para estimar los perfiles de causas de muerte en regiones sin registros vitales. Concretamente algunos refinamientos al trabajo original de Preston han involucrado ecuaciones para grupos específicos de edad, incorporando datos más recientes o examinando causas más detalladas (Hakulinen et al. 1986, Hull et al. 1981, Lopez y Hull 1983, Murray et al. 1993).

Algunos intentos previos de usar estos modelos para estimar perfiles de causas de muerte en regiones o países sin datos confiables han sido obstaculizados por buen número de problemas, incluyendo la diversidad de las causas de muerte por edad y sexo, el limitando margen de confiabilidad de las estimaciones de las causas de defunciónen en niveles de alta mortalidad, las complicaciones analíticas creadas por el uso del capítulo XVI de la 9a revisión de CIE (signos y síntomas mal definidos) y la forma real de relacionarse la mortalidad por causas específicas con la mortalidad general. Nos hemos esforzado en superar cada una de estas limitaciones en los modelos desarrollados para este estudio, los detalles de las bases de datos y métodos son presentados en Murray y Lopez (1996b). En vista de los requerimientos del Estudio de la CGE para estimar los perfiles de mortalidad para varios grupos de edad y sexo, los modelos fueron desarrollados separadamente para hombres y mujeres y para cada uno de los siete grupos de edad: 0–4 años, 5–14, 15–29, 30–44, 45–59, 60–69 y 70 y más.[4]

Métodos

El procedimiento secuencial para la estimación de tasas de mortalidad por edad, sexo y causa específica de muerte se describe a continuación: (1) primero las primeras estimaciones fueron preparadas a partir de los registros vitales y de las muestras de registros de datos; (2) las estimaciones para grupos de causas seleccionadas, como neoplasias malignas o asma fueron corregidas usando métodos específicos; (3) las tasas de mortalidad específica para causas seleccionadas fueron ajustadas basándose en análisis epidemiológico y (4) los ajustes finales fueron hechos para garantizar que la suma de la mortalidad por causas fuera idéntica a la mortalidad total de cada grupo de edad estimada por métodos demográficos. La aplicación de cada uno de estos pasos difiere por región; a continuación se destacan algunas de estas diferencias, para una completa descripción ver Murray y Lopez (1996b).

Para los PEMC y los PEAS, las primeras estimaciones fueron obstenidas solamente de los registros vitales (la cobertura es virtualmente total muertes en ambas regiones). Para China, las primeras estimaciones fueron calculadas usando los datos de los Puntos de Vigilancia de Enfermedades de 1991, 52 734 muertes en una población de 10 millones, ajustada y parada adaptada al total de muertes en cada sexo y grupo de edad. Para la India, las primeras estimaciones fueron derivadas de la base de datos de Certificación Médica de Causas de Muerte CIE 9a revisión expandidas para adapter la al número estimado de muertes urbanas en cada Grupo de edad y sexo (basada en los ingresos al esquema de Registro muestral de la India). Las estimaciones de mortalidad por causas en áreas rurales estuvieron basadas en los resultados de la encuesta de causas de muerte (rural) de 1991 a 1993; expandida para adaptada a las estimación rural de muerte para el país entero.

En las cuatro regiones restantes, ALC, OPAI, AOM y ASS, algunos registros vitales estaban disponibles, pero la mayoría de las muertes no están capturadas por los sistemas existentes (ver Cuadro III). Además muertes las registradas no fueron consideradas representativas de las condiciones de mortalidad para toda la región. Cada una de estas regiones pudo ser dividida dentro del área de registro, para la cual los registros vitales estan disponibles. Para desarrollar las posibles estimaciones de mortalidad por causa en las áreas residuales realizó el siguiente procedimiento. Primero, fue desarrollada una nueva curva de Lorenz basada con la desigualdad geográfica de la distribución de la muerte; así pudo estimarse la tasa específica de mortalidad por edad y sexo para todas las causas combinando en las áreas residuales, ver Murray y Lopez, (1996b) para más detalles. Segundo, para las areas con registros, el porcentaje de la distribución de las muertes registradas en cada grupo de edad asignada a los Grupos I, II y III fue comparada con el porcentaje predicho por los modelos de causas de muerte. El número de desviaciones estandar por arriba o abajo del valor predicho para cada grupo es una medida de cuanto se apartan las áreas con registros en la región de los perfiles de causas reflejados en los modelos. Para estimar la desagregación de todas las causas de mortalidad dentro de los Grupos I, II y III en las áreas residuales, hemos asumido que el perfil o la desviación de la estructura de causas de muerte de estas areas es similar a las areas con registro. En otras palabras, si los registros de las areas de ALC producen un porcentaje para todas las causas de muerte del Grupo I de 2.3 desviaciones estandar por arriba de lo esperado, entonces tenemos que asumir que las áreas residuales tienen tambien un porcentaje de todas las causas del Grupo I de 2.3 desviaciones estandar por arriba de lo esperado.

En ASS, se empleó un método ligeramente diferente porque los registros vitales solo estuvieron disponibles para Sudafrica.[5] La región fue dividida en dos componentes: el Sur de Africa, incluyendo Sudafrica, Botswana, Namibia, Mozambique, Zimbabwe, Swazilandia, Zambia y Malawi; y el Norte de Africa que incluye los otros países de Africa al Sur del Sahara. El método de la curva de Lorenz fue usado para estimar los perfiles del sur de Africa basados en los registros vitales de Sudafrica. Para el resto de los países africanos del sur del Sahara, los perfiles de mortalidad estuvieron basados en la diferencia entre las estimaciones regionales y las estimaciones para la subregión del Sur de Africa. La distribución de muertes entre los

Grupos I, II y III para las muertes registradas en Sudafrica estaban en centro del intervalo de tre una desviación estandar de los modelos predictivos. Para el área restante de ASS, aplicamos el mismo patrón de la desviación sugerida para las áreas con registro en el Sur de Africa.

Para estimar la mortalidad de causas más detalladas entre cada grupo en las áreas residuales, asumimos que en ALC, AOM, ASS y OPAI la distribución proporcional para un grupo de edad y sexo dado era el mismo que en las áreas de registro. La alternativa fue usar los pequeños modelos de regresión discutidos anteriormente. Sin embargo, creemos que es preferible basar la estimación de causas más detalladas en los datos locales que en los perfiles de los registros vitales de países industrializados.

Para un cierto número de enfermedades, como neoplasias malignas, enfermedades cardiovasculares, condiciones neuropsiquiatricas y enfermedades respiratorias crónicas, tambien se aplicaron series estandar. Estas están descritas en detalle en Murray y Lopez (1996b).

Basándose en revisiones epidemiológicas detalladas de algunas enfermedades, grupos de expertos generaron también estimaciones de estas enfermedades para todas las regiones en desarrollo. Estos cálculos epidemiológicos se utilizaron para quitar las estimaciones de mortalidad de causas relacionadas en una primera ronda. Debido a la gran concentración epidemiologica de las enfermedades infecciosas en paises mas desarrollados, existen estimaciones, epidemiológicas para más enfermadades del Grupo I que del Grupo II. Como las mediciones epidemiológicas tienden a producir tasa más altas que las basadas en registros vitales, existe una tendencia a sesgar los resultados finales hacia las enfermedades del Grupo I a costa de las del Grupo II. Para conocer detalladamente las bases de cada medición epidemiológica, el lector puede consultar los capítulos relevantes en el volumen correspondiente de la *Serie sobre la Carga Global de la Enfermedad y Lesión.*

Debido a la esporádica pero intensa naturaleza de las lesiones relacionadas con la guerra, las estimaciones epidemiológicas de muertes por guerra han sido incorporadas de una manera ligeramemente diferente. Brevemente, hemos decidido considerar las muertes de guerra como defunciones adicionales a las estimaciones demográficas básicas usadas para determinar el número de muertes en cada grupo de edad y sexo en cada región. De esta forma las estimaciones epidemiológicas de las muertes por la guerra no han sido sometidas a ajustes finales del algoritmo descrito anteriormente.

En concordancia con los principios de la CIE, en las tabulaciones primarias (Murray y Lopez 1996b) para el Estudio de la Carga Global de la Enfermedad, cada muerte ha sido asignada a una única causa subyacente. Por ejemplo, las muertes por hepatoma debido a hepatitis crónica posthepatititis tipo B son asignadas a hepatoma en la tabulación primaria. Asimismo siguiendo las convenciones de la CIE, muertes por tuberculosis con VIH positivos son asignadas a VIH en las tabulaciones primarias. En este volumen, muchas de las tablas muestran el número de muertes asignadas a cada causa en las tabulaciones primarias; sin embargo, algunas tablas, como la de tuberculosis/VIH muestra el número de muertes asociadas a ambas causa. Las notas técnicas que acompañan las tablas indican claramente el tipo de mortalidad que refieren.

Despúes de corregir muchas causas basadas en mediciones epidemiológicas, la suma de las causas específicas de mortalidad a menudo exceden el total de la mortalidad, para algunas grupos de edad en varias regiones. En algunos casos, la suma de las muertes de un grupo específico de causas exceden el total de la mortalidad para ese grupo en una edad dada; un problema común para el Grupo I en los adultos, por ejemplo. Para forzar que la suma de las muertes por causa específica sea igual a las muertes por todas las causas en un grupo de edad y sexo dados, dos algoritmos con ajustes adicionales fueron aplicados, uno para causas neonatales y otro para todos los otros grupos.

Estimamos primero el número de muertes neonatales en cada región, basándonos en las recomendaciones de los principales proyectos de investigación demográfica, como Proyecto de Encuestas de Demografía y Salud. Luego establecimos como requisito que la suma de muertes por sífilis congénita, tétanos neonatal, problemas que aparecen durante el período perinatal y anomalías congénitas esperadas debe ser igual al 85 porciento de las muertes neonatales. Cuando las estimaciones de defunciones basadas epidemiológicamente para estas cuatro causas esperadas en el primer mes de vida exceden el 85 porciento de las muertes neonatales estimadas, estas muertes deben ser proporcionalmente reducidas.

Se evaluó la extensión de la sobreestimación de la mortalidad en cada uno de los 14 grupos de edad y sexo en cada región, comparando el número de desviaciones estandar arriba o abajo de la mortalidad propor-cional para cada grupo pronosticado por el modelo de causas de muerte, con el número de desviaciones estandar arriba o abajo de las primeras estimaciones. Para ajustarla sobreestimación de la aproximación epidemiológica, hemos seleccionado arbitrariamente siguiente el algoritmo. Si las primeras estimaciones para el Grupo I o el Grupo II basadas en registros vitales o en muestras de datos de los registros fueron también más de 2.5 desviaciones estandar arriba o abajo del valor esperado, no permitimos mediciones epidemiológicas que aumenten el grado de desviación. Si la primera medición para el Grupo I era menor de 2.5 desviaciones estandar mayor de lo esperado, o el Grupo II estaba más de 2.5 desviaciones estandar por abajo de los valores esperados, entonces los resultados de las mediciones epidemiológicas fueron permitidos para cambiar la proporción en cada Grupo por dos desviaciones estandar. Si un cambio de dos desviaciones estandar incrementaran el porcentaje de muertes debidas al Grupo I para ser más que 2.5 desviaciones estandar encima de la media, o disminuyendo el porcentaje de muertes debidas al Grupo II para ser más de 2.5 desviaciones estandar abajo de la media, el porcentaje de muertes debidas al Grupo I es igual a un valor de 2.5 desviaciones estandar arriba de la media y el porcentaje de muertes debidas al Grupo II es igual a 2.5 desviaciones estandar abajo de la media.

INCIDENCIA, PREVALENCIA, LETALIDAD Y DURACIÓN

Para el Estudio de la Carga Global de la Enfermedad fueron requeridas estimaciones de incidencia, prevalencia, remisión, duración, letalidad y mortalidad de cada enfermedad o lesión y de sus secuelas. No existen estudios epidemiológicos válidos basados en la comunidad que pueden ser usados para derivar estimaciones para varios de estos parámetros epidemiológicos en algunas regiones. Para identificar todas las fuentes de datos e información útiles y suplementar datos empíricos con juicios informados, las estimaciones presentadas en este volumen fueron obtenidas en estrecha colaboración con un gran número de expertos familiarizados con las enfermedades específicas o lesiones y son el resultado de un proceso iterativo que abarcó cuatro años y medio (1992–1996). Los siguientes pasos resumen el mecanismo usado para generar estimaciones de cada enfermedad y sus secuelas.

1. Fueron identificados expertos en enfermedades, o grupos de expertos en algunos casos, para cada una de las más de 100 condiciones en el Estudio de la Carga Global de la Enfermedad. Los participantes del estudio fueron invitados de la Organización Mundial de la Salud, de la Agencia Internacional para la Investigación del Cáncer, del Banco Mundial, del Centro para el Control de la Enfermedades de los Estados Unidos y de instituciones académicas del Reino Unido, Francia, México, Nueva Zelanda, India, Sri Lanka, China y Sudafrica.

2. La primera ronda de estimaciones de incidencia, remisión, letalidad, prevalencia, duración y muertes fueron hechas por expertos sobre la base de estudios publicados y no publicados. Cuando los datos no estaban disponibles por región, los expertos fueron alentados a hacer estimaciones informadas. Frecuentemente, los perfiles de incidencia y remisión por edad están basados en los supuestos de las regiones que tienen perfiles similares. En el peor de los casos, cuando la información no estaba disponible, las estimaciones preliminares se basaron en los datos de otras regiones.

3. Estas estimaciones fueron críticamente revisadas y usando el DISMOD[6] fue determinada la consistencia interna de las estimaciones de inciden- cia, remisión, letalidad, duración y prevalencia. Estas verificaciones identificaron las inconsistencias en muchas de las estimaciones. Los expertos de las enfermedades fueron invitados a revisar sus estimacio- nes en comunicación con los autores para hacerlas consistentes inter- namente.

4. Las estimaciones revisadas fueron usadas para producir los resultados preliminares. Estas estimaciones fueron extensamente revisadas por un Grupo de expertos internacionales en una reunión auspiciada por la OMS en Ginebra del 8 al 11 de diciembre de 1992. Revisiones subsecuentes fueron también sujetas a validación de su consistencia interna y las estimaciones modificadas formaron la base de los resulta- dos publicados en el *Informe sobre el Desarrollo Mundial 1993: Invertir en Salud.*

5. Como parte del seguimiento del IDM 1993, los expertos de las enfermedades fueron invitados a escribir capítulos detallados con los métodos usados para generar los datos estimados. Estos autores tuvieron la oportunidad durante este proceso iterativo de realizar tres estimaciones de condiciones de la incidencia, prevalencia, duración, letalidad, remisión y muertes, incorporando la extensa discusión y revisión de los resultados publicados en 1993 y 1994. En cada una de estas revisiones ha sido evaluada su consistencia interna. En muchos casos, hemos revisado las estimaciones en colaboración con los expertos de las enfermedades para garantizar la consistencia interna. Para ciertos Grupos de condiciones, como las neuropsiquiátricas, fueron convocados seminarios internacionales para revisar las estimaciones epidemiológicas.

PROYECCIÓN DE CAUSAS DE MUERTE 1990–2020

Las estrategias y políticas dirigidas a la promoción de la salud y prevención de las enfermedades debe tener una perspectiva al futuro. Para cubrir esta necesidad, tambien hemos incluido en este volumen proyecciones de mortalidad para cada causa para el año 2000. El método desarrollado para las proyecciones del Estudio de la Carga Global de la Enfermedad está ampliamente descrito en otra parte (Murray y Lopez 1996a). Brevemente, el ampliament enfoque usado fue el desarrollo de un modelo estadístico econométrico para predecir diferentes escenarios para causas específicas de mortalidad basados en un número restringuido de variables independientes. Esta aproximación puede resultar muy simplista pero genera predicciones plausibles basadas en muchas observaciones empíricas en un amplio número de países durante varias décadas. En vez de proyectar la mortalidad total y luego descomponerla por causas específicas basándonos en la relación entre mortalidad general y mortalidad por causas específicas, hemos elegido el modelo de Grupos de causas independientes. Nuestras proyecciones de la mortalidad general para cada Grupo de edad y sexo se calculan sumardo las proyeciones de cada una de las causas. Las causas de muerte han sido divididas en nueve Grupos: el Grupo I completo, cánceres, enfermedades cardiovasculares, enfermedades digestivas, enfermedades respiratorias crónicas, otras del Grupo II, accidentes de tráfico, otras lesiones no intencionales y las lesiones intencionales. Estas nueve causas suman el total de la mortalidad entre cada Grupo de edad y sexo. Hemos elegido estos grupos en particular porque las tendencias de mortalidad en los países con buenos registros vitales en los últimos 40 años, sugieren que las causas más específicas dentro del cada uno de este grupos de causas siguen tendencias similares. Existen algunas excepciones obvias como la tuberculosis en los PEMC en los últimos 5 a 10 años y la epidemia de VIH, para los cuales se usaron métodos separados. Sin embargo en general, estos nueve grupos de causas parecen captar razonablemente bien las causas específicas.

Las cuatro variables independientes elegidas para ser incluidas en el modelo predictivo fueron: ingreso per capita, capital humano, intensidad de tabaquismo y tiempo. Se utilizó como medida representativa del desarrollo económico de los paises, el ingreso per-capita, medido en dolares internacionales ajustados según la paridad de poder de compra, lo cual no queda reflegarlo en las tasas oficiles de cambio. El promedio de años de escolaridad de la población, una medida de educación y formación de capital humano, fue usada para captar un determinante del estado de salud de la población y de su capacidad de hacer uno de sus conocimientos en salud y las intervenciones disponibles. Un determinante importante del estado de salud de los adultos que no es bien captado por el ingreso o la educación es la exposition acumulada al tabaquismo, ya que el tabaquismo es la principal causa de varias enfermedades. Las tasas de prevalencia de tabaquismo de las encuestas no son medidas confiables del impacto del tabaquismo ya que otros factores como la duración, tipo, cautidad y modo de fumar son determinantes críticos de la acumulación de la exposición ex pasado. Basados en la aproximación de Peto y Lopez, hemos estimado la tasa de cáncer pulmonar restando la tasa de cáncer pulmonar de los no fumadores en cada Grupo de edad y sexo para estimar un parámetro de intensidad del tabaquismo (ver Peto et al. 1994 para mayores detalles de este método[7]). Es así que, la intensidad del tabaquismo se usa como una de las variables independientes en las ecuaciones predictivas de cáncer, enfermedad cardiovascular y enfermedad respiratoria crónica. La cuarta variable independiente usada en la proyección es el tiempo. De esta forma las tendencias seculares de mortalidad no explicadas por ingreso, educación y tabaquismo pueden ser debidos a cambios en la tecnología o al conocimiento de las enfermedades el cual es captado de manera cruda usando el tiempo como una variable. Además, como se explica más adelante, que las proyecciones independientes de VIH fueron añadidas a las proyecciones básicas generadas por el modelo.

Para cada uno de los nueve grupos de causas de muerte y para cada uno de los siete grupos de edad y sexo, se evaluaron varias tipos de ecuaciones de regresión. La ecuación usada finalmente estuvo basada en un pequeño grupo de variables independientes que tenían un razonable valor predictivo medido por la proporción de la varianza explicada. Además, si los parámetros estimados para una variable tenían signo opuesto al esperado y el coeficiente no era significativo al nivel 1%, esta variable era retirada de la ecuación. Las proyecciones para causas más detalladas se basaron en ecuaciones de regresión que evaluaban tasa de mortalidad de causas más detalladas con la tasa de mortalidad de los nueve grupos de causas.

Para proyectar la mortalidad por causa se requerió un grupo de ecuaciones que relacionoban las tasas de mortalidad por edad, sexo y causa al ingreso per capita, capital humano, intensidad de tabaquismo y tiempo, a portir de proyecciones de cada una de estas variables independientes. Para cada variable fueron generados una línea basal, se escenario pesimista y otro optimista. Sin embargo, debido a la falta de espacio solo la línea basal se presenta este volumen. Las proyecciones del ingreso percapita para cada región se basaron en las predicciones económicas del Banco Mundial y en posibles supuestos acerca del crecimiento a largo plazo del ingreso per capita. El capital humano se proyectó basándose en la mediana de la tasa de crecimiento del capital humano registrado para el período de 1950–1990 en cada región. En las proyecciones de intensidad de tabaquismo al año 2020 examinamos la relación entre cigarros consumidos por adulto en el Reino Unido de 1900 a 1990 y las estimaciones de intensidad de tabaquismo en el Reino Unido para el período similar. En la proyección de intensidad de tabaquismo se asume que la evolución temporal de la epidemia de tabaquismo en el Reino Unido se repetirá en cada región (Lopez et al. 1994). Para realizar a estimaciones del consumo de cigarros per capita en hombres y mujeres de cada región hemos usado la relación del Reino Unido para, la intensidad del tabaquismo que ha sido alcanzada treinta años después de un nivel dado de consumo de cigarros per capita.

Este supuesto se usó para proyectar los valores de tabaquismo en cada región en el año 2020. Para los años futuros, hemos asumido que los valores actuales de la intensidad de tabaquismo pueden aumentar o disminuir en forma lineal hacia los valores proyectados al año 2020.

Como se mencionó anteriormente, cuando se incluía en las susodichas ecuaciones lo experimenta en el pasado de los paises con buenos registros de estadisticas viatales, no se capta adecuadamente la evolución de la epidemia de SIDA. Para estimar el posible impacto de la epidemia de VIH en cada región entre 1990 y el año 2020, hemos preparado proyecciones independientes de la incidencia y mortalidad por VIH para cada año y en cada grupo de edad, sexo y región. Estas proyecciones concuerdan estrechamente con las que temá el programa Mundial de SIDA de la OMS (PMS) en la fase epidémica en que la incidencia aumentaba. Para la fase en que la incidencia disminuye, el modelo de proyección del PMS asume que la incidencia cae rápidamente a cero en todas las regiones, de tal forma que para el año 2020 habría esencialmente una pequeña o nula incidencia. Esto nos parece también un escenario optimista. Nuestras proyecciones básicas se sustentan en el supuesto de que las cifras de incidencia iran declinando hacia un valor equilibrado que será la mitad del pico máximo de incidencia. No hay región, excepto la de los PEMC, en que la incidencia se acerque a la mitad de la cresta y no sabemos en qué nivel de la epidemia se estabilizará la incidencia de VIH en cada región. Para estimar la mortalidad de VIH hemos usado los mismos supuestos incluidos en las proyecciones del PMS cocernientes a la distribución del tiempo requerido para la progresión de VIH a SIDA y la distribución de muertes por SIDA en el tiempo. Estas proyecciones son pesimistas, particularmente para regiones como la India, OPAI y China donde el PMS asumió que la epidemia seguiría un curso mucho más acelerado que el de otras regiones como Africa al Sur del Sahara.

ORGANIZACIÓN DE LA TABLAS

El Cuadro IV proporciona un listado completo de todas las enfermedades y lesiones y cada una de las secuelas incluidas en el Estudio de la Carga Global de la Enfermedad. Debido a las limitaciones de espacio no todas las secuelas se pueden presentar en este volumen. En la columna del lado derecho del Cuadro IV se indica que secuela ha sido incluida. Por cada una de las secuelas, existen tres páginas de cuadros, que contienen grupos idénticos de estimaciones por cada una de las ocho regiones geográficas utilizadas para el *IDM1993*, más un cuadro resumen que proporciona las estimaciones agregadas para el mundo. Los datos sobre los indicadores epidemiológicos incluidos en los cuadros representan la información epidemiológica básica requerida para calcular los AVADs para cada enfermedad o lesión. Las estimaciones actuales de AVADs no se muestran en los cuadros, sin embargo, son presentadas en forma resumida en *La Carga Global de la Enfermedad*, el primer volumen de la *Serie sobre la Carga Global de la Enfermedad y Lesión*, y son reportadas con mas detalle en los capítulos de enfermedades y lesiones específicas, los cuales se encuentran en los volúmenes subsecuentes.

Los indicadores epidemiológicos incluidos en los cuadros tienen la función de reflejar la información esencial que los planificadores de salud y otros trabajadores en salud pública podrían requerir para poder formu-lar, implementar y evaluar estrategias apropiadas para la prevención y tratamiento de enfermedades y lesiones. Por lo tanto, los cuadros presentan datos útiles de 1990 sobre la carga de la enfermedad y lesion de cada región: cómo ésta carga se distribuye entre diferentes grupos de edad y entre hombres y mujeres, cómo cada condición está aumentando (o disminuyendo) rápidamente pues ocurre temprana o tardíamente en la vida, por cuánto tiempo en promedio la enfermedad persiste, y cuánta gente muere por la enfermedad en diferentes sub-grupos de población.

El formato de los cuadros es el siguiente. En la parte superior de la página se proporciona el título abreviado de la enfermedad o lesión. Abajo de la abreviatura de la enfermedad o lesión se encuentra el nombre de la secuela. Tres diferentes términos son utilizados repetitivamente para describir algunas secuelas: episodio, caso, y caso sintomático. Para las enfermedades diarreícas, solamente se registra una secuela, denominada episodios de diarrea. Por consistencia, todos los resultados relacionados con una enfermedad, incluyendo la manifestación primaria de la enfermedad o lesión, son nombrados secuelas. Cuando el término «episodios» es empleado, indica que estamos realizando estimaciones de incidencia y prevalencia de episodios de la enfermedad o lesión. Para algunas condiciones crónicas , proporcionomos estimaciones de la incidencia o prevalencia de individuos con la condición como en el caso de diabetes; esto es indicado por el uso del término casos. Finalmente, para otras condiciones crónicas como enfermedad pulmonar obstructiva crónica o cirrosis, ofrecemos estimaciones de la incidencia o prevalencia de individuos con síntomas de la enfermedad, etiquetados como casos sintomáticos.

La siguiente explicación se aplica a todas los cuadros.

Año de Referencia: todas las estimaciones se refieren al año 1990, año base para el Estudio Global de la Carga de la Enfermedad. La única excepción es la proyección, que muesta la de mortalidad para el año 2000.

Variables Demográficas: las estimaciones son presentadas separadamente para hombres y mujeres teniendo en aventa sus diferentes riesgos de presentar la enfermedad o lesión. En la primera mitad de cada cuadro se muestran las estimaciones para los hombres y en la segunda mitad del cuadro, las de las mujeres. La edad es probablemente la variable más importante al describir los patrones de la enfermedad o lesión, ya que virtualmente todas las condiciones reportadas en este libro dependen muy intensamente de la edad. Las estimaciones están presentadas por cinco grandes grupos de edad los cuales describen aproximadamente las fases del ciclo de vida donde los patrones de la enfermedad y lesión probablemente son similares. Las estimaciones se presentan también para todas las edades combinadas, sin ningún intento de estandarización por la edad. Al final de cada cuadro, se presentan las estimaciones para la población total de la región son provistas, incluyendo todos los grupos de edad, asi como hombres y mujeres combinados.

Incidencia: este indicador mide la ocurrencia de nuevos casos de enfermedad o lesión en 1990. El *número* de nuevos casos (en miles) es mostrado junto con la tasa de incidencia estimada en la región, expresada como el número de nuevos casos por 100 000 habitantes por año en el respectivo grupo de edad y sexo.

Prevalencia: Además de estimar el número de nuevos casos, es importante poder estimar la cantidad de enfermedad o lesión, que estuvo presente en cada región en 1990, ya sea debido a nuevos casos (incidencia) en 1990 o provenientes de años previos. El *número* estimado (en miles) de casos prevalentes de enfermedad o lesión en 1990 se muestra en la tabla, asi como la *tasa de prevalencia*, expresada en número de casos prevalentes por 100 000 habitantes.

Edad de inicio promedio: este parámetro mide la edad promedio (en años) de casos nuevos de la enfermedad o lesión ocurridos en 1990, en cada grupo de edad específico y en todas la edades.

Duración promedio: un dato importante dentro del cálculo de los AVADs es la duración promedio de tiempo (medido en años que se puede esperar para que los casos nuevos pasen de un estado de salud a un estado de enfermedad o lesión. Estas duraciones promedio de enfermedad han sido calculadas para cada grupo de edad específico y para todas las edades combinadas (no ponderadas). La duración es medida como el tiempo entre la ocurrencia de la enfermedad o lesión y la ausencia de dicha condición, ya sea a través de remisión o muerte.

Muertes: la mortalidad estimada por cada causa está presentada en cuatro columnas y en dos períodos de tiempo. Primeramente se muestra el número estimado de muertes en 1990 (en miles) dentro de cada grupo

Cuadro IV   Causas, enfermedades y lesiones y secuelas incluidas en el Estudio de la Carga Global de la Enfermedad y las secuelas para las cuales los datos son presentados en este volumen

CGE Código de Clasificación	Grupo de causas, enfermedad, lesión o secuela	Datos presentados en este volumen (Número de cuadro)
I	Conditiones transmisibles, maternas, perinatales de la nutrición	
IA	Enfermedades infecciosas y parasitarias	
IA1	Tuberculosis	
IA1-1	Casos sero-negative para VIH	10
IA1-2	Casos sero-positive par VIH	11
IA2	Enfermedades de transmisión sexual excepto VIH	
IA2a	Sífilis	
IA2a-1	Sífilis congénita	12
IA2a-2	Bajo peso al nacer	13
IA2a-3	Primaria	14
IA2a-4	Secundaria	15
IA2a-5	Terciaria – cardiovascular	16
IA2a-6	Terciaria – gomas	17
IA2a-7	Terciaria – neurosífilis	18
IA2b	Clamidia	
IA2b-1	Oftalmía neonatal	19
IA2b-2	Bajo peso al nacer	20
IA2b-3	Cicatriz de la córnea – ceguera	21
IA2b-4	Cicatriz de la córnea – disminución de la agudeza visual	22
IA2b-5	Cervicitis	23
IA2b-6	Neumonía neonatal	24
IA2b-7	Enfermedad inflamatoria pélvica	25
IA2b-8	Embarazo ectópico	26
IA2b-9	Absceso tuboovárico	27
IA2b-10	Dolor pélvico crónico	28
IA2b-11	Infertilidad	29
IA2b-12	Uretritis sintomática	30
IA2b-13	Epidedimitis	31
IA2b-14	Obstrucción ureteral	32
IA2c	Gonorrea	
IA2c-1	Oftalmía neonatal	33
IA2c-2	Bajo peso al nacer	34
IA2c-3	Cicatriz de la córnea – ceguera	35
IA2c-4	Cicatriz de la córnea – disminución de la agudeza visual	36
IA2c-5	Cervicitis	37
IA2c-6	Enfermedad inflamatoria pélvica	38
IA2c-7	Embarazo ectópico	39
IA2c-8	Absceso tuboovárico	40
IA2c-9	Dolor pélvico crónico	41
IA2c-10	Infertilidad	42
IA2c-11	Uretritis sintomática	43
IA2c-12	Epidedimitis	44
IA2c-13	Obstrucción ureteral	45
IA3	VIH	
IA3-1	Casos	46
IA3-2	SIDA	47
IA4	Enfermedades diarreicas	
IA4-1	Episodios	48

Cuadro IV   (continuado)

CGE Código de Clasificación	Grupo de causas, enfermedad, lesión o secuela	Datos presentados en este volumen (Número de cuadro)
IA5	Enfermedades de la infancia	
IA5a	Tosferina	
IA5a-1	Episodios	49
IA5a-2	Retraso mental	50
IA5b	Poliomielitis	
IA5b-1	Paralítica	51
IA5c	Difteria	
IA5c-1	Episodios	52
IA5c-2	Complicaciones neurológicas	53
IA5c-3	Miocarditis	54
IA5d	Sarampión	
IA5d-1	Episodios	55
IA5e	Tétanos	
IA5e-1	Episodios	56
IA6	Meninigitis bacteriana y meningococemia	
IA6-1	Todas las formas – episodios	57
IA6-2	Streptoccus pneumoniae – episodios	58
IA6-3	Haemophilus influenzae – episodios	59
IA6-4	Neisseria meningitidis – episodios	60
IA6-5	Meningococcemia sin meningitis – episodios	61
IA6-6	Sordera	62
IA6-7	Trastorno convulsivo	63
IA6-8	Déficit motriz	64
IA6-9	Retraso mental	65
IA7	Hepatitis B y hepatitis C	
IA7-1	Episodios	66
IA7-2	Cirrosis hepática – casos sintomáticos	67
IA7-3	Hepatoma	68
IA8	Paludismo	
IA8-1	Episodios	69
IA8-2	Anemia	70
IA8-3	Secuelas neurológicas	71
IA9	Enfermedades tropicales	
IA9a	Tripanosomiasis	
IA9a-1	Episodios	72
IA9b	Enfermedad de Chagas	
IA9b-1	Infección	73
IA9b-2	Cardiomiopatía sin insuficiencia cardiaca congestiva	74
IA9b-3	Cardiomiopatía con insuficiencia cardiaca congestiva	75
IA9b-4	Megavícera	76
IA9c	Esquistosomiasis	
IA9c-1	Infección	77
IA9d	Leishmaniasis	
IA9d-1	Visceral	78
IA9d-2	Cutánea	79
IA9e	Filariasis linfática	
IA9e-1	Hidrocele > 15 cm	80
IA9e-2	Linfedema bancroftiano	81
IA9e-3	Linfedema brugiano	82
IA9f	Oncocercosis	
IA9f-1	Ceguera	83

Cuadro IV   (continuado)

CGE Código de Clasificación	Grupo de causas, enfermedad, lesión o secuela	Datos presentados en este volumen (Número de cuadro)
IA9f-2	Prurito	84
IA9f-3	Disminución de la agudeza visual	85
IA10	Lepra	
IA10-1	Casos	86
IA10-2	Lepra discapacitante	87
IA11	Dengue	
IA11-1	Fiebre del dengue hemorrágico	88
IA12	Encefalitis japonesa	
IA12-1	Episodios	89
IA12-2	Deficiencia cognocitiva	90
IA12-3	Secuela neurológica	91
IA13	Tracoma	
IA13-1	Ceguera	92
IA13-2	Disminución de la agudeza visual	93
IA14	Infecciónes intestinales por nemátodos	
IA14a	Ascaridiasis	
IA14a-1	Infección de alta intensidad	94
IA14a-2	Deficit cognocitivo contemporaneo	95
IA14a-3	Deficiencia cognocitiva	96
IA14a-4	Obstruccíon intestinal	97
IA14b	Tricocefalosis	
IA14b-1	Infección de alta intensidad	98
IA14b-2	Deficit cognocitivo contemporaneo	99
IA14b-3	Síndrome masivo de dysenteria	100
IA14b-4	Deficiencia cognocitiva	101
IA14c	Anquilostomiasis y necatoriasis	
IA14c-1	Infección de alta intensidad	102
IA14c-2	Anemia	103
IA14c-3	Deficiencia cognocitiva	104
IB	Infecciones respiratorias	
IB1	Infecciones de las vías respiratorias inferiores	
IB1-1	Episodios	105
IB1-2	Secuelas crónicas	106
IB2	Infecciones de las vías respiratorias superiores	
IB2-1	Episodios	107
IB2-2	Faringuitis	108
IB3	Otitis media	
IB3-1	Episodios	109
IB3-2	Sordera	110
IC	Condiciones maternas	
IC1	Hemorragia materna	
IC1-1	Episodios	111
IC1-2	Sindrome de Sheehan	112
IC1-3	Anemia severa	113
IC2	Sepsis puerperal	
IC2-1	Episodios	114
IC2-2	Infertilidad	115
IC3	Trastornos hipertensivos del embarazo	
IC3-1	Episodios	116
IC3-2	Secuelas neurológicas	117
IC4	Parto obstruido	
IC4-1	Episodios	118

Cuadro IV (continuado)

CGE Código de Clasificación	Grupo de causas, enfermedad, lesíon o secuela	Datos presentados en este volumen (Número de cuadro)
IC4-2	Incontinencia por stress	119
IC4-3	Fístula rectovaginal	120
IC5	Aborto	
IC5-1	Episodios	121
IC5-2	Infertilidad	122
ID	Condiciones que aparecen durante el período perinatal	
ID1	Bajo peso al nacer	
ID1-1	Todas las secuelas	123
ID2	Asfixia y trauma al nacer	
ID2-1	Todas las secuelas	124
IE	Deficiencias de la nutrición	
IE1	Desnutrición proteínico-calórica	
IE1-1	Emaciación	125
IE1-2	Retraso de crecimiento	126
IE1-3	Discapacidad en el desarrollo	127
IE2	Deficiencia de yodo	
IE2-1	Bocio – grado 0	128
IE2-2	Bocio – grado 1	129
IE2-3	Bocio – grado 2	130
IE2-4	Discapacidad leve en el desarrollo	131
IE2-5	Cretinoidismo	132
IE2-6	Cretinismo	133
IE3	Deficiencia de vitamina A	
IE3-1	Xeroftalmia	134
IE3-2	Cicatriz de la córnea	135
IE4	Anemia por deficiencia de hierro	
IE4-1	Todas las formas	136
IE4-2	Leve	137
IE4-3	Moderada	138
IE4-4	Severa	139
IE4-5	Muy severa	140
IE4-6	Deficiencia cognocitivo	141
II	Enfermedades no transmisibles	
IIA	Neoplasias malignas	
IIA1	Cánceres de boca y orofaringue	
IIA1-1	Casos	142
IIA2	Cáncer de esófago	
IIA2-1	Casos	143
IIA3	Cáncer de estómago	
IIA3-1	Casos	144
IIA4	Cánceres de colon y recto	
IIA4-1	Casos	145
IIA5	Cáncer de higado	
IIA5-1	Casos	146
IIA6	Cáncer de páncreas	
IIA6-1	Casos	147
IIA7	Cánceres de traquea, bronquios y pulmones	
IIA7-1	Casos	148
IIA8	Melanoma y otros tumores de la piel	
IIA8-1	Casos	149
IIA9	Cáncer de mama	
IIA9-1	Casos	150

Cuadro IV (continuado)

CGE Código de Clasificación	Grupo de causas, enfermedad, lesión o secuela	Datos presentados en este volumen (Número de cuadro)
IIA10	Cáncer cervicouterino	
IIA10-1	Casos	151
IIA11	Cáncer de cuerpo de útero	
IIA11-1	Casos	152
IIA12	Cáncer de ovario	
IIA12-1	Casos	153
IIA13	Cáncer de próstata	
IIA13-1	Casos	154
IIA14	Cáncer de vesícula	
IIA14-1	Casos	155
IIA15	Linfomas y mieloma múltiple	
IIA15-1	Casos	156
IIA16	Leucemia	
IIA16-1	Casos	157
IIB	Otras neoplasias	
IIC	Diabetes mellitus	
IIC-1	Casos	158
IIC-2	Pie diabético	159
IIC-3	Neuropatía	160
IIC-4	Retinopatía-ceguera	161
IIC-5	Amputación	162
IID	Trastornos endocrinos	
IIE	Condiciones neuropsiquiatricas	
IIE1	Depresión mayor unipolar	
IIE1-1	Episodios depresivos	163
IIE2	Trastorno bipolar	
IIE2-1	Casos	164
IIE3	Esquizofrenia	
IIE3-1	Casos	165
IIE4	Epilepsia	
IIE4-1	Casos	166
IIE5	Uso de alcohol	
IIE5-1	Síndrome de dependencia del alcohol	167
IIE6	Demencia y otros trastornos degenerativos y hereditarios del SNC	
IIE6-1	Casos	168
IIE7	Enfermedad de Parkinson	
IIE7-1	Casos	169
IIE8	Esclerosis múltiple	
IIE8-1	casos	170
IIE9	Uso de drogas	
IIE9-1	Uso disfuncional y dañino de drogas	171
IIE10	Trastorno de estrés post-traumático	
IIE10-1	Casos	172
IIE11	Trastornos obsesivo-compulsivos	
IIE11-1	Casos	173
IIE12	Trastorno de pánico	
IIE12-1	Casos	174
IIF	Enfermedades de los órganos de los sentidos	
IIF1	Glaucoma	175
IIF1-1	Ceguera	
IIF2	Cataratas	176
IIF2-1	Ceguera	

Cuadro IV (continuado)

CGE Código de Clasificación	Grupo de causas, enfermedad, lesión o secuela	Datos presentados en este volumen (Número de cuadro)
IIG	Enfermedades cardiovasculares	
IIG1	Cardiopatía reumática	
IIG1-1	Insuficiencia cardíaca congestiva	177
IIG2	Cardiopatía isquémica	
IIG2-1	Infarto agudo del miocardio	178
IIG2-2	Angina de pecho	179
IIG2-3	Insuficiencia cardíaca congestiva	180
IIG3	Enfermedad cerebrovascular	
IIG3-1	Primer accidente cerebrovascular	181
IIG4	Enfermedades inflamatorias del corazón	
IIG4-1	Miocarditis	182
IIG4-2	Pericarditis	183
IIG4-3	Endocarditis	184
IIG4-4	Cardiomiopatia	185
IIH	Enfermedades respiratorias	
IIH1	Enfermedad pulmonar obstructiva crónica	
IIH1-1	Casos sintomáticos	186
IIH2	Asma	
IIH2-1	Casos	187
III	Enfermedades digestivas	
III1	Ulcera péptica	
III1-1	Casos	188
III2	Cirrosis hepática	
III2-1	Casos sintomáticos	189
III3	Apendicitis	
III3-1	Episodios	190
IIJ	Enfermedades del aparato genitourinario	
IIJ1	Nefritis y nefrosis	
IIJ1-1	Glomérulo nefritis aguda	191
IIJ1-2	Enfermedad renal terminal	192
IIJ2	Hipertrofia prostática benigna	
IIJ2-1	Casos sintomáticos	193
IIK	Enfermedades de la piel	
IIL	Enfermedades del sistema osteomuscular	
IIL1	Artritis reumatoide	
IIL1-1	Casos	194
IIL2	Osteoartritris	
IIL2-1	Cadera	195
IIL2-2	Rodilla	196
IIM	Anomalías congénitas	
IIM1	Defecto de la pared abdominal	
IIM1-1	Casos	197
IIM2	Anencefalia	
IIM2-1	Casos	198
IIM3	Atresia anorectal	
IIM3-1	Casos	199
IIM4	Labio leporino	
IIM4-1	Casos	200
IIM5	Paladar hendido	
IIM5-1	Casos	201
IIM6	Atresia esofágica	
IIM6-1	Casos	202

Cuadro IV   (continuado)

CGE Código de Clasificación	Grupo de causas, enfermedad, lesión o secuela	Datos presentados en este volumen (Número de cuadro)
IIM7	Agenesia renal	
IIM7-1	Casos	203
IIM8	Síndrome de Down	
IIM8-1	Casos	204
IIM9	Anomalías congénitas del corazón	
IIM9-1	Casos	205
IIM10	Espina bífida	
IIM10-1	Casos	206
IIN	Afecciones de la cavidad bucal	
IIN1	Caries dentales	
IIN1-1	Episodios	207
IIN2	Enfermedad periodontal	
IIN2-1	Episodios	208
IIN3	Edentulismo	
IIN3-1	Casos	209
III	Lesiones	
IIIA	Lesiones no intencionales	
IIIA1	Accidentes de tráfico	
IIIA1-1	Episodios	210
IIIA1-2	Fractura de cráneo – corta duración	
IIIA1-3	Fractura de cráneo – larga duración	211
IIIA1-4	Fractura de los huesos de la cara	
IIIA1-5	Fractura de la columna vertebral	
IIIA1-6	Lesión de la medula espinal	212
IIIA1-7	Fractura de costilla o esternón	
IIIA1-8	Fractura de pelvis	
IIIA1-9	Fractura de clavícula escápula o número	
IIIA1-10	Fractura de radio o cúbito	
IIIA1-11	Fractura de huesos de la mano	
IIIA1-12	Fractura de femur – corta duración	
IIIA1-13	Fractura de femur – larga duración	213
IIIA1-14	Fractura de patela, tibia o peroné	
IIIA1-15	Fractura de tobillo	
IIIA1-16	Fractura de huesos del pie	
IIIA1-17	Otra dislocación	
IIIA1-18	Dislocación de hombro, de codo o de cadera	
IIIA1-19	Esguinces	
IIIA1-20	Lesión intracraneal – corta duración	214
IIIA1-21	Lesión intracraneal – larga duración	215
IIIA1-22	Lesión interna	
IIIA1-23	Herida abierta	
IIIA1-24	Lesiones en los ojos	
IIIA1-25	Amputación de pulgar	
IIIA1-26	Amputación de dedo de la mano	
IIIA1-27	Amputación de brazo	
IIIA1-28	Amputación de dedo del pie	
IIIA1-29	Amputación del pie	
IIIA1-30	Amputación de la pierna	
IIIA1-31	Magulladuras	
IIIA1-32	Quemaduras < 20% – corta duración	
IIIA1-33	Quemaduras < 20% – larga duración	
IIIA1-34	Quemaduras > 20% y < 60% – corta duración	

Cuadro IV   (continuado)

CGE Código de Clasificación	Grupo de causas, enfermedad, lesión o secuela	Datos presentados en este volumen (Número de cuadro)
IIIA1-35	Quemaduras > 20% y < 60% – larga duración	
IIIA1-36	Quemaduras > 60% – corta duración	
IIIA1-37	Quemaduras > 60% – larga duración	
IIIA1-38	Traumatismo de nervios	
IIIA1-39	Envenenamiento	
IIIA1-40	Residual	
IIIA2	Envenenamientos	
IIIA2-1	Episodios	216
IIIA3	Caídas	
IIIA3-1	Episodios	217
IIIA3-2	Fractura de craneo – corta duración	
IIIA3-3	Fractura de craneo – larga duración	218
IIIA3-4	Fractura de los huesos de la cara	
IIIA3-5	Fractura de la columna vertebral	
IIIA3-6	Lesión de la medula espinal	219
IIIA3-7	Fractura de costilla o esternón	
IIIA3-8	Fractura de pelvis	
IIIA3-9	Fractura de clavícula, escápula o húmero	
IIIA3-10	Fractura de radio o cúbito	
IIIA3-11	Fractura de huesos de la mano	
IIIA3-12	Fractura de femur – corta duración	220
IIIA3-13	Fractura de femur – larga duración	221
IIIA3-14	Fractura de patela, tibia o peroné	
IIIA3-15	Fractura de tobillo	
IIIA3-16	Fractura de huesos del pie	
IIIA3-17	Otra dislocación	
IIIA3-18	Dislocación de hombro, de codo o de cadera	
IIIA3-19	Esguinces	
IIIA3-20	Lesión intracraneal – corta duración	
IIIA3-21	Lesión intracraneal – larga duración	222
IIIA3-22	Lesión interna	
IIIA3-23	Herida abierta	
IIIA3-24	Lesiones en los ojos	
IIIA3-25	Amputación de pulgar	
IIIA3-26	Amputación de dedo de la mano	
IIIA3-27	Amputación de brazo	
IIIA3-28	Amputación de dedo del pie	
IIIA3-29	Amputación del pie	
IIIA3-30	Amputación de la pierna	
IIIA3-31	Magulladuras	
IIIA3-32	Quemaduras < 20% – corta duración	
IIIA3-33	Quemaduras < 20% – larga duración	
IIIA3-34	Quemaduras > 20% y < 60% – corta duración	
IIIA3-35	Quemaduras > 20% y < 60% – larga duración	
IIIA3-36	Quemaduras > 60% – corta duración	
IIIA3-37	Quemaduras > 60% – larga duración	
IIIA3-38	Traumatismo de nervios	
IIIA3-39	Envenenamiento	
IIIA4-40	Residual	
IIIA4	Fuegos	
IIIA4-1	Episodios	223
IIIA4-2	Fractura de craneo – corta duración	

Cuadro IV   (continuado)

CGE Código de Clasificación	Grupo de causas, enfermedad, lesión o secuela	Datos presentados en este volumen (Número de cuadro)
IIIA4-3	Fractura de craneo – larga duración	
IIIA4-4	Fractura de los huesos de la cara	
IIIA4-5	Fractura de la columna vertebral	
IIIA4-6	Lesión de la medula espinal	224
IIIA4-7	Fractura de costilla o esternón	
IIIA4-8	Fractura de pelvis	
IIIA4-9	Fractura de clavícula, escápula o húmero	
IIIA4-10	Fractura de radio o cúbito	
IIIA4-11	Fractura de huesos de la mano	
IIIA4-12	Fractura de femur – corta duración	
IIIA4-13	Fractura de femur – larga duración	
IIIA4-14	Fractura de patela, tibia o peroné	
IIIA4-15	Fractura de tobillo	
IIIA4-16	Fractura de huesos del pie	
IIIA4-17	Otra dislocación	
IIIA4-18	Dislocación de hombro, de codo o de cadera	
IIIA4-19	Esguinces	
IIIA4-20	Lesión intracraneal – corta duración	
IIIA4-21	Lesión intracraneal – larga duración	
IIIA4-22	Lesión interna	
IIIA4-23	Herida abierta	
IIIA4-24	Lesiones en los ojos	
IIIA4-25	Amputación de pulgar	
IIIA4-26	Amputación de dedo de la mano	
IIIA4-27	Amputación de brazo	
IIIA4-28	Amputación de dedo del pie	
IIIA4-29	Amputación del pie	
IIIA4-30	Amputación de la pierna	
IIIA4-31	Magulladuras	
IIIA4-32	Quemaduras < 20% – corta duración	225
IIIA4-33	Quemaduras < 20% – larga duración	226
IIIA4-34	Quemaduras > 20% y < 60% – corta duración	227
IIIA4-35	Quemaduras > 20% y < 60% – larga duración	228
IIIA4-36	Quemaduras > 60% – corta duración	
IIIA4-37	Quemaduras > 60% – larga duración	
IIIA4-38	Traumatismo de nervios	
IIIA4-39	Envenenamiento	
IIIA4-40	Residual	
IIIA5	Ahogamientos	
IIIA5-1	Episodios	229
IIIA5-2	Cuadriplejia	230
IIIA6	Otras lesiones no intencionales	
IIIA6-1	Episodios	231
IIIA6-2	Fractura de craneo – corta duración	
IIIA6-3	Fractura de craneo – larga duración	
IIIA6-4	Fractura de los huesos de la cara	
IIIA6-5	Fractura de la columna vertebral	
IIIA6-6	Lesión de la medula espinal	232
IIIA6-7	Fractura de costilla o esternón	
IIIA6-8	Fractura de pelvis	
IIIA6-9	Fractura de clavícula, escápula o húmero	
IIIA6-10	Fractura de radio o cúbito	

Cuadro IV (continuado)

CGE Código de Clasificación	Grupo de causas, enfermedad, lesión o secuela	Datos presentados en este volumen (Número de cuadro)
IIIA6-11	Fractura de huesos de la mano	
IIIA6-12	Fractura de femur – corta duración	
IIIA6-13	Fractura de femur – larga duración	
IIIA6-14	Fractura de patela, tibia o peroné	
IIIA6-15	Fractura de tobillo	
IIIA6-16	Fractura de huesos del pie	
IIIA6-17	Otra dislocación	
IIIA6-18	Dislocación de hombro, de codo o de cadera	
IIIA6-19	Esguinces	
IIIA6-20	Lesión intracraneal – corta duración	
IIIA6-21	Lesión intracraneal – larga duración	233
IIIA6-22	Lesión interna	
IIIA6-23	Herida abierta	
IIIA6-24	Lesiones en los ojos	
IIIA6-25	Amputación de pulgar	
IIIA6-26	Amputación de dedo de la mano	234
IIIA6-27	Amputación de brazo	
IIIA6-28	Amputación de dedo del pie	
IIIA6-29	Amputación del pie	
IIIA6-30	Amputación de la pierna	
IIIA6-31	Magulladuras	
IIIA6-32	Quemaduras < 20% – corta duración	
IIIA6-33	Quemaduras < 20% – larga duración	235
IIIA6-34	Quemaduras > 20% y < 60% – corta duración	
IIIA6-35	Quemaduras > 20% y < 60% – larga duración duración	
IIIA6-36	Quemaduras > 60% – corta duración	
IIIA6-37	Quemaduras > 60% – larga duración	
IIIA6-38	Traumatismo de nervios	236
IIIA6-39	Envenenamiento	
IIIA6-40	Residual	
IIIB	Lesiones intencionales	
IIIB1	Lesiones autoinfligidas	
IIIB1-1	Episodios	237
IIIB1-2	Fractura de craneo – corta duración	
IIIB1-3	Fractura de craneo – larga duración	
IIIB1-4	Fractura de los huesos de la cara	
IIIB1-5	Fractura de la columna vertebral	
IIIB1-6	Lesión de la medula espinal	
IIIB1-7	Fractura de costilla o esternón	
IIIB1-8	Fractura de pelvis	
IIIB1-9	Fractura de clavícula, escápula o húmero	
IIIB1-10	Fractura de radio o cúbito	
IIIB1-11	Fractura de huesos de la mano	
IIIB1-12	Fractura de femur – corta duración	
IIIB1-13	Fractura de femur – larga duración	
IIIB1-14	Fractura de patela, tibia o peroné	
IIIB1-15	Fractura de tobillo	
IIIB1-16	Fractura de huesos del pie	
IIIB1-17	Otra dislocación	
IIIB1-18	Dislocación de hombro, de codo o de cadera	
IIIB1-19	Esguinces	
IIIB1-20	Lesión intracraneal – corta duración	

Cuadro IV (continuado)

CGE Código de Clasificación	Grupo de causas, enfermedad, lesión o secuela	Datos presentados en este volumen (Número de cuadro)
IIIB1-21	Lesión intracraneal – larga duración	
IIIB1-22	Lesión interna	
IIIB1-23	Herida abierta	
IIIB1-24	Lesiones en los ojos	
IIIB1-25	Amputación de pulgar	
IIIB1-26	Amputación de dedo de la mano	
IIIB1-27	Amputación de brazo	
IIIB1-28	Amputación de dedo del pie	
IIIB1-29	Amputación del pie	
IIIB1-30	Amputación de la pierna	
IIIB1-31	Magulladuras	
IIIB1-32	Quemaduras < 20% – corta duración	
IIIB1-33	Quemaduras < 20% – larga duración	
IIIB1-34	Quemaduras > 20% y < 60% – corta duración	
IIIB1-35	Quemaduras > 20% y < 60% – larga duración	
IIIB1-36	Quemaduras > 60% – corta duración	
IIIB1-37	Quemaduras > 60% – larga duración	
IIIB1-38	Traumatismo de nervios	
IIIB1-39	Envenenamiento	
IIIB1-40	Residual	
IIIB2	Violencias	
IIIB2-1	Episodios	238
IIIB2-2	Fractura de craneo – corta duración	
IIIB2-3	Fractura de craneo – larga duración	239
IIIB2-4	Fractura de los huesos de la cara	
IIIB2-5	Fractura de la columna vertebral	
IIIB2-6	Lesión de la medula espinal	240
IIIB2-7	Fractura de costilla o esternón	
IIIB2-8	Fractura de pelvis	
IIIB2-9	Fractura de clavícula, escápula o húmero	
IIIB2-10	Fractura de radio o cúbito	
IIIB2-11	Fractura de huesos de la mano	
IIIB2-12	Fractura de femur – corta duración	
IIIB2-13	Fractura de femur – larga duración	
IIIB2-14	Fractura de patela, tibia o peroné	
IIIB2-15	Fractura de tobillo	
IIIB2-16	Fractura de huesos del pie	
IIIB2-17	Otra dislocación	
IIIB2-18	Dislocación de hombro, de codo o de cadera	
IIIB2-19	Esguinces	
IIIB2-20	Lesión intracraneal – corta duración	241
IIIB2-21	Lesión intracraneal – larga duración	242
IIIB2-22	Lesión interna	
IIIB2-23	Herida abierta	
IIIB2-24	Lesiones en los ojos	
IIIB2-25	Amputación de pulgar	
IIIB2-26	Amputación de dedo de la mano	
IIIB2-27	Amputación de brazo	
IIIB2-28	Amputación de dedos del pie	
IIIB2-29	Amputación del pie	
IIIB2-30	Amputación de la pierna	
IIIB2-31	Magulladuras	

Cuadro IV (continuado)

CGE Código de Clasificación	Grupo de causas, enfermedad, lesión o secuela	Datos presentados en este volumen (Número de cuadro)
IIIB2-32	Quemaduras < 20% – corta duración	
IIIB2-33	Quemaduras < 20% – larga duración	
IIIB2-34	Quemaduras > 20% y < 60% – corta duración	
IIIB2-35	Quemaduras > 20% y < 60% – larga duración	
IIIB2-36	Quemaduras > 60% – corta duración	
IIIB2-37	Quemaduras > 60% – larga duración	
IIIB2-38	Traumatismo de nervios	243
IIIB2-39	Envenenamiento	
IIIB2-40	Residual	
IIIB3	Guerra	
IIIB3-1	Episodios	244
IIIB3-2	Fractura de craneo – corta duración	
IIIB3-3	Fractura de craneo – larga duración	
IIIB3-4	Fractura de los huesos de la cara	
IIIB3-5	Fractura de la columna vertebral	
IIIB3-6	Lesión de la medula espinal	
IIIB3-7	Fractura de costilla o esternón	
IIIB3-8	Fractura de pelvis	
IIIB3-9	Fractura de clavícula, escápula o húmero	
IIIB3-10	Fractura de radio o cúbito	
IIIB3-11	Fractura de huesos de la mano	
IIIB3-12	Fractura de femur – corta duración	
IIIB3-13	Fractura de femur – larga duración	
IIIB3-14	Fractura de patela, tibia o peroné	
IIIB3-15	Fractura de tobillo	
IIIB3-16	Fractura de huesos del pie	
IIIB3-17	Otra dislocación	
IIIB3-18	Dislocación de hombro, de codo o de cadera	
IIIB3-19	Esguinces	
IIIB3-20	Lesión intracraneal – corta duración	
IIIB3-21	Lesión intracraneal – larga duración	245
IIIB3-22	Lesión interna	
IIIB3-23	Herida abierta	
IIIB3-24	Lesiones en los ojos	
IIIB3-25	Amputación de pulgar	
IIIB3-26	Amputación de dedo de la mano	
IIIB3-27	Amputación de brazo	246
IIIB3-28	Amputación de dedo del pie	
IIIB3-29	Amputación del pie	247
IIIB3-30	Amputación de la pierna	
IIIB3-31	Magulladuras	
IIIB3-32	Quemaduras < 20% – corta duración	
IIIB3-33	Quemaduras < 20% – larga duración	248
IIIB3-34	Quemaduras > 20% y < 60% – corta duración	
IIIB3-35	Quemaduras > 20% y < 60% – larga duración	
IIIB3-36	Quemaduras > 60% – corta duración	
IIIB3-37	Quemaduras > 60% – larga duración	
IIIB3-38	Traumatismo de nervios	249
IIIB3-39	Envenenamiento	
IIIB3-40	Residual	

de edad y sexo, junto con la correspondiente tasa de mortalidad específica por grupo de edad y sexo de la región en 1990 (expresada por 100 000 habitantes). Posteriormente, el número proyectado de muertes para el año 2000 y la tasa de mortalidad proyectada por 100 000 habitantes en el mismo año, han sido incluidos en los paneles de la extrema derecha de cada tabla. Estas proyecciones han sido realizadas basándose en los métodos y supuestos descritos anteriormente y han sido incluidos para ofrecer una perspectiva futura del perfil epidemiológico probable de cada región a fines de siglo.

Precisión: dependiendo en la magnitud de la condición, algunas cifras significativas son mostradas en las tablas para algunas estimaciones. El gran número de dígitos significativos no debe llevar a un falso sentido de precisión. En la era de las computadoras es más práctico proporcionar al lector simplemente con los resultados de varios cálculos y estimaciones a redondear las tablas con uno o dos dígitos significativos. Es particularmente problemático redondear los resultados de este estudio con uno o dos dígitos debido a las amplias variaciones en la magnitud de incidencia básica y tasas de prevalencia. Para poder mantener la consistencia de las unidades (por ejemplo: por 100 000) en las tablas, nos vemos obligados a imprimir un número artificialmente elevado de dígitos significativos para las secuelas más comunes.

DISCUSIÓN

Existe una necesidad, ya sea para el debate de la política global de salud, para supercisar los progresos del desarrollo de la salud, para investigación, o para muchos otros propósitos en salud pública, de describir con detalle y con cierta certidumbre el estado de salud de los habitantes. Este libro es un intento por satisfacer esa necesidad. Las estimaciones y proyecciones aquí presentadas son deliberadamente ambiciosas y comprensivas: más de 200 condiciones de salud han sido revisadas, las estimaciones han sido preparadas separadamente por sexos, para cinco amplios grupos de edad, y por los más importantes indicadores epidemiológicos, que son comúnmente empleados para describir el estado de salud. En este sentido, el libro proporciona un compendio de datos, para amplias regiones geográficas del mundo, que debería servir de ayuda al trabajo de todas aguellas personas preocupadas por mejorar la salud pública.

Aplicando un modelo sofisticado sobre la ocurrencia de enfermedad, prevalencia, mortalidad, y remisión, las estimaciones aquí presentadas para cada enfermedad y lesión son consistentes internamente y consistentes con lo que se sabe de su historia natural. Por otro lado, la confiabilidad de las estimaciones es muy variable y se requiere gran precaución al emplearlas. Al aplicar varios diferentes métodos y enfoques, hemos tratado de confirmar la plausibilidad de las estimaciones. Sin embargo, ninguna aumento de rigor metodológico puede compensar los extremadamente es casos datos y la falta de información epidemiológica, la cual fue comúnmente encontrada durante la preparación de los números. En los casos de grandes poblaciones, incluyendo gran parte del Africa al Sur del Sahara, India, Otros países asiáticos e insulares y partes de América Latina y el Caribe, muy poco se sabe con certeza acerca de las causas de mortalidad o inclusive de la incidencia de enfermedad, prevalencia, y duración. Para estas regiones ninguna manipulación epidemiológica, extrapolación estimación o supocisión puedan cambiar el hecho de que las mediciones epidemiológicas aquí presentadas son imprecisas. Para otras regiones hay más datos disponibles y hay proporcionalmente más confianza en las estimaciones, pero aún para las regiones industrializadas, los diagnósticos y otras diferencias en la codificación entre países crean dudas sobre la precisión de las estimaciones para condiciones de salud específicas.

En vez de limitar los calculos a esas regiones o a enfermedades para las cuales había datos disponibles y razonablemente confiables para la estimación, hemos optado por preparar un cálculo realmente global y lo consideramos comprensivo del estado de salud en 1990 y más allá años despues de éste año. Estamos plenamente conscientes del grado substancial de incertidumbre subyacente en muchas de las estimaciones. También somos conscientes que una medición global de este tipo, a pesar de todas las advertencias ya expresadas (y las no expresadas), muy probablemente será empleada con un grado mucho mayor de confianza, que lo que los datos subyacentes justifican. Esto es innevitable dada la necesidad de este cálculo. Sin embargo, la disponibilidad de estimaciones no debe ir en detrimento de la urgente necesidad de mejorar los sistemas de información epidemiológico, premisa fundamental para que tanto la vigilancia del estado de salud como la evaluación puedan ser ejecutadas con mayor fiabilidad, y de esta forma las políticas de desarrollo de salud sean más efectivas.

Como consecuencia del fortalecimiento de los sistemas nacionales de estadísticas de salud, las evaluaciones globales futuras se llegavón a ser, indudablemente, más confiables y por lo tanto, más útiles. Mientras tanto, esperamos que las estimaciones y proyecciones aquí presentadas sean utilizadas, críticamente y en ciertos casos, actualizadas a través de estas revisiones y críticas. Ante la opción de elegir entre cálculos epidemiológicos parciales de mayor confianza o las estimaciones globales que aquí se presentan hemos optado por lo último, encontrando cierto conseulo en el comentario de Greenwood (1948): «Hacer lo mejor sea enemigo de lo bueno, es la forma más segura de impedir cualquier progreso estadístico». El científico purista que permanezca esperando hasta que las estadísticas médicas sean nosológicamente exactas no habrá superado la rustica espera de Horacio de que el rio fluya y desaparezca.

NOTAS

1. En versiones anteriores del Estudio de la Carga Global de la Enfermedad, las deficiencias de la nutrición, llamada malnutrición proteínico-calórica, deficiencia de vitamina A, alteraciones relacionadas con la deficiencia de yodo y las anemias fueron incluidas en el Grupo II. Estas condiciones claramente se identifican con los criterios definidos en el Grupo I como enfermedades

pretransicionales. Sin embargo, anteriormente no fueron incluidas en el Grupo I por la dificultad de distinguir algunas de estas muertes de otras causas nutricionales o endócrinas usando las bases de datos disponibles en aquel tiempo. La introducción de un esfuerzo mayor en el análisis de estas condiciones en la quinta y versión final del estudio, ha permitido la transferencia de estas causas al Grupo I.

2. El capítulo XVI ha sido proporcionalmente reasignado en los menores de cinco años a todas las causas del Grupo I y en los mayores de 5 años a todas las causas del Grupo II. Algoritmos específicos han sido desarrollados para distribuir la codificación imprecisa de las muertes cardiovasculares como aquellas asignadas a insuficiencia cardiaca y las muertes por lesiones no intencionales mal definidas.

3. Los números de defunciones para algunas regiones han sido ligeramente modificadas de lo reportado en el *IDM 1993* que refleja un alto nivel de muertes relacionadas con guerras alrededor de 1990 en algunas regiones. En nuestra opinión, los métodos de estimación que subyacen a las estimaciones de 1990 no reflejan adecuadamente la mortalidad relacionda con guerra.

4. Las causas de muerte usadas en el modelo en las versiones iniciales del Estudio de la Carga Global de la Enfermedad no son exactamente las mismas que se presentan aquí en la versión 5. Aunque la forma funcional de estos dos Grupos de modelos es similar, los resultados específicos difieren por la adición de información reciente y el refinamiento de los procedimientos de estimación descritos en Murray y Lopez (1996b).

5. El análisis de los datos de Sudafrica fue basado en un extenso trabajo de Stephen Hendrix, a quien se le agradece el acceso a su trabajo antes de ser publicado.

6. Para garantizar la consistencia interna entre las estimaciones epidemiológicas presentadas en este volumen, un programa de computadora, DisMod, fue desarrollado para formalizar la relación entre incidencia, remisión, letalidad y prevalencia. Los suceptibles en la población son asumidos para contraer una enfermedad o discapacidad a la tasa I y para morir a la tasa de mortalidad general m. Los casos de una enfermedad pueden remitir a la tasa r y regresar a ser suceptible, morir de una causa general a la misma tasa de los suceptibles m o morir de una causa específica de muerte a la tasa f. DisMod usa el método de la diferencia finita para resolver un Grupo de ecuaciones lineales diferenciales definidas por esta relación.

7. Las tasas de cáncer pulmonar de los no fumadores para todas las regiones excepto para China y OPAI se asumieron de las mismas tasas de cáncer de no fumadores registrados en la encuesta de seguimiento CPS-II de los Estados Unidos. Para China y OPAI la tasa de cáncer en mujeres se asumió que es sustancialmente más elevada basada en la evidencia de varios estudios epidemiológicos (Murray y Lopez 1996a).

Introduction

Une information objective, comparable, et fiable quant à la nature, l'étendue et la distribution des maladies et des problèmes de santé constitue un apport essentiel à la formulation et à l'évaluation des politiques de santé, y compris la recherche relative aux facteurs déterminants de la santé. En réalité, en dépit de l'effort soutenu par les pays au cours de plusieures décennies avec l'appui d'organisations internationales telles que l'Organisation Mondiale de la Santé, les renseignements fiables sur l'état de santé, régionaux ou globaux, restent limités. Pour répondre à l'urgent besoin d'obtenir les données nécessaires à la formulation de politiques globales de santé, la Banque Mondiale et l'Organisation Mondiale de la Santé ont commissioné l'Etude de la Charge Globale des Maladies (CGM) en 1992 dans le but de produire une évaluation objective et comparable de l'état de santé à partir des connaissances sur l'occurrence des maladies et des traumatismes qui étaient alors disponibles dans le monde. Les résultats de cette étude ont été largement utilisés dans le *Rapport sur le Développement dans le Monde 1993: Investir dans la Santé* (Banque Mondiale 1993). Une présentation plus détaillée, mais néanmoins abrégée, de la méthode et des résultats a été publiée dans une série d'articles du *Bulletin de l'OMS*, et par la suite réimprimée dans un livre publié par l'Organisation Mondiale de la Santé en 1994 (Murray 1994, Murray et Lopez 1994a, Murray et Lopez 1994b, Murray et al. 1994, Murray et Lopez 1994c). La *Série sur la Charge Globale des Maladies et Traumatismes*, dont ce volume fait partie, a pour but de fournir l'ensemble des détails relatifs aux méthodes, matériel, et résultats, pour chaque maladie et traumatisme inclus dans l'Etude de la Charge Globale des Maladies, ainsi que l'application des méthodes au niveau national et sub-national.

L'Etude de la Charge Globale des Maladies a été conçue en partie pour appréhender trois limitations majeures de l'information disponible quant à la magnitude des problèmes de santé. Tout d'abord, l'information sanitaire est trop souvent fournie aux décideurs par des avocats de maladies particulières. Ce lien entre plaidoyer et estimations épidémiologiques peut mettre en doute l'objectivité des conclusions. En particulier, les avocats ont tendance à surestimer la magnitude du problème de santé qui les préoccupe, souvent non intentionnellement. Le fait de séparer le plaidoyer de la démarche nécessaire à la génération d'évaluations épidémiologiques constitue une étape essentielle dans la préparation d'estimations plus utiles et plus plausibles. Deuxièmement, les banques de données internationales, établies à partir de procédures diagnostiques et de protocoles similaires, ont trait presqu'exclusivement à la mortalité et négligent de prendre en compte les données comparables relatives aux conséquences non-fatales sur l'état de santé. L'absence d'information plausible sur l'invalidité et autres issues non-fatales a contribué à perpétuer la négligence de ces problèmes dans les débats nationaux et internationaux des politiques de santé. En dépit de l'immense lacune en matière de données épidémiologiques concernant les issues non-fatales, le second but majeur de l'Etude de la Charge Globale des Maladies a été de générer des estimations plausibles de l'incidence, de la prévalence, et de la durée, de plusieures issues sanitaires non-fatales. Troisièmement, une métrique commune, l'Année de Vie Corrigée du Facteur d'Invalidité (AVCI), a été utilisée pour agréger et résumer les données et informations sur la mortalité et les issues de santé non-fatales. Cette approche a permis de comparer l'impact de différents états de santé. Le fait que les AVCI puissent également être utilisées pour l'analyse du coût-efficacité, facilite beaucoup l'évaluation conjointe de la magnitude des problèmes de santé, de la gamme des interventions disponibles, et de leurs coûts respectifs. Cette métrique commune, permettant de combiner les résultats relatifs à la charge des maladies aux analyses des interventions disponibles en terme de coût-efficacité, peut être et a été utilisée, pour identifier un ensemble d'interventions prioritaires, telles les prestations de services de santé essentiels décrites dans le *Rapport sur le Développement dans le Monde 1993*.

Les objectifs plus spécifiques de l'Etude de la Charge Globale des Maladies étaient quadruples. Le premier était de développer des estimations de la mortalité selon l'âge, le sexe et la région, qui aient une cohérence interne, pour plus de 100 causes importantes de décès. Le second objectif était de développer des estimations de l'incidence, de la prévalence, et du taux de létalité selon l'âge, le sexe et la région, pour les séquelles majeures de plus de 100 causes principales de mauvaise santé. Tenant compte du rôle important de certaines expositions dans l'étiologie des maladies et traumatismes, le troisième objectif était d'estimer la quantité de mortalité prématurée et d'invalidité pouvant être attribuée à des facteurs de risques choisis, tels que la pollution atmosphérique, les relations sexuelles dangereuses, l'hypertension, la consommation d'alcool et le tabagisme. Finalement, le quatrième objectif était de fournir un ensemble de projections de la charge des maladies selon l'âge, le sexe, la région, et la cause, à l'an 2020.

Le but de ce volume est de faciliter l'accès aux estimations détaillées de l'incidence, de la prévalence, de la durée, et du taux de létalité, qui ont été préparées pour l'Etude de la Charge Globale des Maladies. Ayant été conçue principalement comme source de référence pratique, une grande partie du volume est attribuée à la présentation tabulaire des résultats. Suivant cette brève introduction aux méthodes utilisées pour préparer les estimations, le reste du volume inclut une série de tableaux contenant des données démographiques de base pour chacune des huit régions utilisées dans le *Rapport sur le Développement dans le Monde 1993*, suivies d'un plus grand nombre de tableaux donnant des estimations de l'incidence, de la prévalence, et de la durée moyenne, des décès en 1990 et des décès projetés à l'an 2000 pour différentes maladies et séquelles. La discussion qui suit expose brièvement le système de classification de la Charge Globale des Maladies, la démographie de base de chacune des huit régions, les procédures d'estimation des causes de décès, et les méthodes utilisées pour estimer l'incidence, la prévalence, le taux de létalité, et la durée des séquelles majeures. Les lecteurs intéressés par plus de détails relatifs aux méthodes et assomptions des bases empiriques et le processus d'estimation pour chacune des maladies peuvent se référer au(x) volume(s) pertinent(s) dans la série.

SYSTÈME DE CLASSIFICATION DE LA CHARGE GLOBALE DES MALADIES

Pour l'Etude de la Charge Globale des Maladies, une structure «ramifiée» des maladies et traumatismes a été utilisée. Elle est présentée dans le Tableau I. Au premier niveau de ventilation, la mortalité générale est divisée en trois grands groupes de causes: le Groupe I inclut les maladies transmissibles, les causes maternelles, les conditions apparaissant dans la période périnatale, et les carences nutritionnelles.[1] Le Groupe II inclut les maladies non-transmissibles, et le Groupe III est limité aux traumatismes. Les causes de décès du Groupe I, les causes pré-transitionnelles, constituent la constellation des conditions qui typiquement diminuent plus rapidement que la mortalité générale au cours du processus de transition épidémiologique. Par conséquent, ces causes représentent seulement une petite proportion des décès chez les populations à faible taux de mortalité. Inversement, les maladies non-transmissibles, assemblées dans le Groupe II, constituent les problèmes de santé les plus importants chez les populations qui ont achevé la transition épidémiologique. Bien que certaines conditions non-transmissibles, telles que les cancers de l'estomac, puissent suivre un taux de déclin plus rapide que la mortalité due à l'ensemble des causes, elles ont néanmions été retenues dans le Groupe II avec d'autres cancers du fait que les décès dûs à l'ensemble des cancers semblent rester relativement constants au cours de la transition. Finalement, les traumatismes sont classés séparément dans le Groupe III, d'une part parce que leur étiologie est très différente de celle de la plupart des maladies, et d'autre part parce qu'aucune tendance n'a été observée au cours de la transition épidémiologique dans la mortalité due aux traumatismes.

Tableau I Système de classification des maladies et traumatismes de l'Etude de la Charge Globale des Maladies

Titre des causes CGM	Codes CIM-9	Codes BTL, CIM-9	Codes CIM-10
I. Affections transmissibles, périnatales, maternelles et nutritionelles	001–139, 243, 260–269, 280–285,320–322, 381–382, 614–616, 460–465, 466, 480–487, 614–616, 630–676, 760–779	01–07, 19, 200, 220, 240, 310–312, 320–322, 371–373, 38–41, 45.	A00–B99, G00, N70–N73, J00–J06, J10–J18, J20–J22, H65–H66, O00–O99, P00–P06, E00–E02, E40–E46, E50, D50
A. Maladies infectieuses et parasitaires	001–139,320–322, 614–616	01–07, 220, 371–373	A00–B99, G00, N70–N73
1. Tuberculose	010–018, 137	02, 077	A15–A19, B90
2. Maladies sexuellement transmissibles hormis le VIH	090–099, 614–616	06, 371–373	A50–A64, N70–N73
a. Syphilis	090–097	060	A50–A53
b. Chlamydiose	i	ii	A55–A56
c. Gonorrhée	098	061	A54
3. VIH	i		B20–B24
4. Maladies diarrhéiques	001, 002, 004, 006–009	01 minus 013	A01–A04, A06–A09
5. Maladies infantiles	032, 033, 037, 045, 050, 055, 056, 138	033, 034, 037, 040–043, 078	A33–37, A80, B05, B91
a. Coqueluche	033	034	A37
b. Poliomyélite	045, 138	040, 078	A80, B91
c. Diphtérie	032	033	A36
d. Rougeole	055	042	B05
e. Tétanos	037, 771.3	037iii	A33–A35
6. Méningite bactérienne et méningococcémie	036, 320–322	036, 220iv	A39, G00
7. Hépatite B et hépatite C	070.2–070.9	046v	B16–B19
8. Paludisme	084	052	B50–B54
9. Maladies tropicales	085, 086, 120, 125	053, 054, 072, 074	B55–B57, B65, B73–B74
a. Trypanosomiase	086.3, 086.4, i 086.5, 086.9v	054ii	B56
b. Maladie de Chagas	086.0, 086.1, 086.2, 086.9vi	054vii	B57
c. Schistosomiase	120	072	B65
d. Leishmaniose	085	053	B55
e. Filariose lymphatique	125.0, 125.1	ii	B74.0–B74.2
f. Onchocercose	125.3	ii	B73
10. Lèpre	030	032	A30
11. Dengue	061	ii	A90–A91
12. Encéphalite japonaise	062.0	ii	A83.0
13. Trachome	076	048	A71
14. Infections à nématodes intestinaux	126–129	ii	
a. Ascaridose	127.0	ii	B77
b. Tricocéphalose	127.3	ii	B79
c. Ankylostomiase et nécatoriose	126	ii	B76
B. Infections des voies respiratoires	460–466, 480–487, 381–382	310–312, 320–322, 240	J00–J06, J10–J18, J20–J22, H65–H66
1. Infections des voies respiratoires inférieures	466, 480–487	320–322	J10–J18, J20–J22
2. Infections des voies respiratoires supérieures	460–465	310–312	J00–J06
3. Otite moyenne	381–382	240	H65–H66
C. Affections maternelles	630–676	38–41	O00–O99
1. Hémorragie maternelle	640, 641, 666	390	O44–O46, O67, O72
2. Septicémie maternelle	670	ii	O85–O86
3. Troubles hypertensifs de la grossesse	642	ii	O10–O16
4. Dystocie d'obstacle	660	393	O64–O66
5. Avortement	630–639	38	O00–O08
D. Affections de la période périnatale	760–779	45	P00–P06
1. Poids insuffisant à la naissance	764–765	452	P05–P07
2. Asphyxie néonatale et traumatismes de l'accouchement	767–770	453–454	P03, P10–P15, P20–P29

Tableau I (suite)

Titre des causes CGM	Codes CIM-9	Codes BTL, CIM-9	Codes CIM-10
E. Carences nutritionnelles	243, 260–269, 280–285	19, 200[viii]	E00–E02, E40–E46, E50, D50
1. Malnutrition protéino-calorique	260–263	190–192	E40–E46
2. Déficience en iode	243	[ii]	E00–E02
3. Avitaminose A	264	[ii]	E50
4. Anémie ferriprive	280	200[viii]	D50
II. Maladies non-transmissibles	140–242, 244–259, 270–279, 286–319, 323–380, 383–459, 467–479, 488–613, 617–629, 680–759	08–18, 20–37, 42–44. [minus 200, 220, 240, 310–312, 320–322, 371–373.]	
A. Tumeurs malignes	140–209	08–14	C00–C97
1. Cancers de la bouche et de l'oropharynx	140–149	08	C00–C14
2. Cancer de l'oesophage	150	090	C15
3. Cancer de l'estomac	151	091	C16
4. Cancers du côlon et du rectum	153, 154	093, 094	C18–C21
5. Cancer du foie	155	095	C22
6. Cancer du pancréas	157	096	C25
7. Cancers de la trachée, des bronches et du poumon	162	101	C33–C34
8. Melanome et autres tumeurs cutanées	172–173	111, 112	C43–C44
9. Cancer du sein	174	113	C50
10. Cancer du col de l'utérus	180	120	C53
11. Cancer du corps de l'utérus	179, 182	122	C54–C55
12. Cancer de l'ovaire	183	123	C56
13. Cancer de la prostate	185	124	C61
14. Cancer de la vessie	188	126	C67
15. Lymphomes et myélome multiple	200–202	14 [minus 141]	C81–C90, C96
16. Leucémie	204–208	141	C91–C95
B. Autres néoplasmes	210–239	15, 16, 17	D00–D48
C. Diabète sucré	250	181	E10–E14
D. Troubles endocriniens	240–242, 244–246, 251–259, 270–279, 281–289	18, 20 [minus 200[ix]]	D55–D80, E03–E07, E15–E16, E20–E34, E51–E89
E. Affections neuro-psychiatriques	290–319, 323–359	21–22 [minus 220]	F00–F99, G03–G99
1. Dépression unipolaire majeure	[i]	[ii]	F32–F33
2. Trouble bipolaire	296	212	F30–F31
3. Schizophrénie	295	211	F20–F29
4. Epilepsie	345	225	G40–G41
5. Usage d'alcool	291, 303, 305.0	215[x]	F10
6. Démence et autres troubles dégénératifs et héréditaires du SNC	330, 331, 290	222, 210[xi]	F01, F03, G30–G31
7. Maladie de Parkinson	332	221	G20–G21
8. Sclérose en plaques	340	223	G35
9. Usage de drogues	304, 305.2–305.9	216[xii]	F11–F16, F18–F19
10. Troubles anxieux post-traumatiques	[i]	[ii]	[xvii]
11. Troubles obsessionnels et compulsifs	300.3	[ii]	F42
12. Trouble d'angoisse	300.2	[ii]	F40.0, F41.0
F. Maladies des organes des sens	360–380, 383–389	23, 24 [minus 240]	H00–H61, H68–H95
1. Glaucome	365	230	H40
2. Cataractes	366	231	H25–H26
G. Maladies cardio-vasculaires	390–459	25–30	I00–I99
1. Cardiopathie rhumatismale	390–398	25	I01–I09
2. Cardiopathie ischémique	410–414 Proportion de: 428, 427.1, 427.4, 427.5, 440.9, 429.0–429.2, 429.9[xiii] 430–438	27 [xiv]	I20–I25 [xv]
3. Maladie cérébrovasculaire		29	I60–I69
4. Maladies cardiaques inflammatoires	420, 421, 422, 425 Proportion de 428[xvi]	[ii]	I30–I33, I38, I40, I42

Tableau I (suite)

Titre des causes CGM	Codes CIM-9	Codes BTL, CIM-9	Codes CIM-10
H. Affections respiratoires	470–478, 490–519	31–32 [minus 310–312, 320–322]	J30–J99
1. Maladie pulmonaire obstructive chronique	490–492, 495–496	ii	J40–J44
2. Asthme	493	ii	J45–J46
I. Maladies de l'appareil digestif	530–579	34	K20–K99
1. Ulcère peptique	531–533	341	K25–K27
2. Cirrhose du foie	571	347	K70, K74
3. Appendicite	540–543	342	K35–K37
J. Maladies de l'appareil génito-urinaire	580–611, 617–629	35–37 [minus 371–373]	N00–N64, N75–N99
1. Néphrite et néphrose	580–589	350	N00–N19
2. Hypertrophie bénigne de la prostate	600	360	N40
K. Maladies de la peau	680–709	42	L00–L99
L. Maladies ostéo-musculaires	710–759	43	M00–M99
1. Arthrite rhumatoïde	714	430	M05–M06
2. Ostéoarthrite	715	ii	M15–M19
M. Anomalie congénitales	740–759	44	Q00–Q99
1. Anomalie de la paroi abdominale	i	ii	xvii
2. Anencéphalie	740.0	ii	Q00
3. Atrésie anorectale	751.2	ii	Q42
4. Bec de lièvre	749.1	ii	Q36
5. Fissure du palais	749.0	ii	Q35,Q37
6. Atrésie de l'oesophage	750.3	ii	Q39.0–Q39.1
7. Agénésie rénale	753.0	ii	Q60
8. Syndrome de Down	758.0	ii	Q90
9. Anomalies cardiaques congénitales	745–747	442	Q20–Q28
10 Spina bifida	741	ii	Q05
N. Affections de la cavité buccale	520–529	33	K00–K14
1. Caries dentaires	521.0	ii	K02
2. Maladie périodontale	523	ii	K05
3. Edentation	i	ii	xvii
III. Traumatismes	E800–999	E47–E56	V01–Y98
A. Traumatismes non-intentionnels	E800–921, 923–949	E47–E51, E520–E523, E53	V01–X59, Y40–Y98
1. Accidents de la voie publique	E810–819, 826–829, 928–929	E471,E472	V01–V89
2. Empoisonnements	E850–869	E48	X40–X49
3. Chutes	E880–888	E50	W00–W19
4. Incendies	E890–899	E51	X00–X09
5. Noyades	E910	E521	W65–W74
6. Autres traumatismes non-intentionnels	E800–E807, E820–825, E830–E848, E870–E879, E900–E909, E911–E921, E923–E949	E470, E473–E474, E49, E520, E522–E523, E53,	V90–V99, W20–W64, W75–W99, X10–X39, X50–X59
B. Traumatismes intentionnels	E922, 950–979, 990–999	E524, E54–E55, E561	X60–Y09,Y35–Y36
1. Traumatismes auto-infligés	E950–959	E54	X60–X84
2. Violence	E922, 960–969	E55	X85–Y09
3. Guerre	E990–999	E561	Y35–Y36

NOTES

1. «Symptômes, signes et états morbides mal définis» (Chapitre XVI de la CIM9 et R00–R99 de la CIM10) est inclus dans le Groupe I pour les personnes de moins de 5 ans et dans le Groupe II pour les personnes de 5 ans et plus, et sont distribués proportionellement à toutes les causes comprises à l'intérieur du Groupe.
2. Les cause E560 de la CIM9 code BTL (E980–E989 de la CIM 9, Y10–Y34 de la CIM10) sont redistribuées proportionellement à toutes les causes de traumatimes comprises à l'intérieur du Groupe.

i Il n'y a pas de code dans la CIM-9.
ii Il n'y a pas de code CIM-9 BTL.
iii Il n'y a pas de code BTL pour le tétanos néonatal.
iv BTL 220 inclut les causes non spécifées de méningites qui peuvent être exclues lorsqu'il y a un code CIM-9 à quatre chiffres.

ᵛ   BTL 046 inclut l'hépatite A qui ne devrait pas faire partie de cette catégorie.

ᵛⁱ 086.9 est la trypanosomiase Africaine en ASS et 086.9 est la maladie de Chagas en ALC.

ᵛⁱⁱ 054 est la trypanosomiase Africaine en ASS et 054 est la maladie de Chagas en ALC.

ᵛⁱⁱⁱ BTL 200 inclut les anémies autres que l'anémie ferriprive qui devraient être classées sous IID Troubles endocriniens.

ⁱˣ Une partie de BTL 200, les anémies autres que l'anémie ferriprive devraient être incluses ici.

ˣ   BTL 215 n'inclut pas les décès des codes détaillés 303 et 305.0 de la CIM-9.

ˣⁱ BTL 210 inclut les codes détaillés 330–336 qui de devraient pas faire partie de cette catégorie.

ˣⁱⁱ BTL 216 n'inclut pas les codes détaillés 305.2–305.9 qui devraient être inclus ici.

ˣⁱⁱⁱ La proportion de ces codes qui devrait être incluse dans les cardiopathies ischémiques dépend de la proportion des décès cardio-vasculaires qui sont codés comme 410–414 à l'origine. Veuillez vous référer à Murray et Lopez (1996b) pour une analyse détaillée et pour les méthodes de correction recommendées.

ˣⁱᵛ Voir Murray et Lopez (1996b) pour une équation qui permette d'approximer les cardiopathies ischémiques à partir des codes BTL.

ˣᵛ Aucun algorithme n'a été développé jusqu'ici pour corriger la codification des décès dus aux cardiopathies ischémiques mal codés définies dans la CIM-10.

ˣᵛⁱ 2.5% 30–44, 5% 45–59, 10% 60+.

ˣᵛⁱⁱ Il n'y a pas de code CIM-10.

Chacun des groupes a ensuite été divisé en plusieures sous-catégories majeures de maladies et traumatismes mutuellement exclusives et exhaustives. Ces sous-catégories sont identifiées par des lettres majuscules dans le Tableau I. Spécifiquement, le Groupe I a été sub-divisé en causes infectieuses et parasitaires, infections des voies respiratoires, causes maternelles, conditions apparaissant durant la période périnatale, et carences nutritionnelles. Les causes non-transmissibles (Groupe II) ont été divisées en 14 catégories (voir Tableau I). Le Groupe III (traumatismes) a été divisé en deux sous-catégories majeures, les traumatismes non-intentionnels (IIIA) et les traumatismes intentionnels (IIIB).

Un troisième niveau de ventilation a été utilisé pour identifier des causes de décès plus spécifiques à l'intérieur de chacune des catégories de second niveau. Par exemple, à l'intérieur de la catégorie IA (maladies infectieuses et parasitaires), des causes spécifiques telles la tuberculose (IA1), le VIH (IA3) et les maladies diarrhéiques (IA4) ont été identifiées. Finalement, pour certaines maladies telles que les maladies sexuellement transmissibles (IA2), un quatrième niveau de ventilation est donné: la syphilis (IA2a), la gonorrhée (IA2b), et la chlamydiose (IA2c). Cet ensemble de causes a été choisi en fonction de trois critères: la magnitude de la maladie ou du traumatisme en tant que cause de décès ou d'invalidité selon l'évaluation décrite au début de l'étude; les conditions de santé pour lesquelles un nombre considérable de services de santé est offert, telle l'appendicite aiguë; et les conditions qui sont au centre du débat actuel des politiques de santé.

La catégorie des signes, symptômes et conditions mal définies—Chapitre XVI de la Neuvième Révision de la Classification Internationale des Maladies, Traumatismes et Causes de Décès (CIM-9) (Chapitre XVIII dans la Dixième Révision de la CIM)—n'ayant aucune pertinence à l'intervention en santé publique, elle n'a pas été introduite comme cause majeure dans notre système de classification. Les décès attribués à cette catégorie, ainsi qu'à certains autres codes utilisés pour les diagnostics mal définis, ont été réassignés à des causes spécifiques de décès. L'attribution de décès à des catégories mal définies est peu salutaire, et potentiellement fallacieuse, lorsqu'il s'agit de générer des données ayant pour but d'informer les choix entre des stratégies et politiques de santé alternatives. Chaque décès survient à la suite d'une cause spécifique et, de ce fait, la meilleure estimation possible de la magnitude de chacune de ces causes est requise pour la formulation de politiques de santé. [2]

Le Tableau I catalogue les codes de la CIM-9 à quatre chiffres correspondant à chacune des causes de décès de notre classification ramifiée. La Neuvième Révision de la CIM a été utilisée comme base de référence pour le développement de la liste de causes, étant donné qu'elle était en usage en 1990, l'année de base pour l'Etude de la Charge Globale des Maladies. Du fait que les pays introduisent progressivement l'usage de la CIM-10 au cours des années 1990, les codes correspondants à la CIM-10 sont également indiqués. Une ou plusieures séquelles ont aussi été évaluées pour chacune des maladies ou traumatismes. Par exemple, pour le diabète sucré, nous avons inclus les ulcères du pied diabétique, les amputations, les neuropathies, et la cécité secondaire à la rétinopathie, en plus du seul diabète même. Par commodité, nous avons également attribué un code à chacune des séquelles, soit le code de la maladie suivi d'un tiret et d'un chiffre correspondant à chaque séquelle. Par exemple le pied diabétique est codé comme IIC-2. La place disponible dans ce volume ne nous a pas permis d'inclure l'évaluation de toutes les séquelles. Ceci s'applique tout particulièrement au grand nombre de séquelles survenant à la suite de chacune des causes cataloguées dans le Groupe III (Traumatismes). Les décès pour 1990 et les projections à l'an 2000 sont donnés pour chaque maladie et traumatisme, mais ne sont pas ventilés par séquelle. Afin de faciliter la présentation des tableaux, les décès ont été rapportés soit avec la présentation primaire de la maladie ou traumatisme, soit avec celle de l'issue la plus importante. Ce choix est arbitraire, mais néanmoins nécessaire, afin d'éviter d'avoir de nombreux tableaux différentes pour chacune des maladies et leurs séquelles.

Régions

L'analyse de la CGM a été effectuée pour huit régions spécialement définies par la Banque Mondiale dans son *Rapport sur le Développement dans le Monde 1993*. Ces régions et leurs abréviations sont les suivantes: les économies de marché bien établies (EMBE), les anciennes économies socialistes d'Europe (AESE), l'Amérique latine et les Caraïbes (ALC), la Chine (CHN), l'Inde (IND), les autres pays d'Asie et îles (APAI), le croissant moyen-oriental (qui inclut l'Afrique du Nord, le Moyen-orient, le Pakistan et les Républiques d'Asie centrale de l'ancienne Union Soviétique) (CMO) et l'Afrique sub-saharienne (ASS). L'allocation des pays aux différentes régions par la Banque Mondiale est donnée dans le Tableau II. Le niveau de développement socio-économique, l'homogénéité épidémiologique, et la contiguïté géographique furent les critères utilisés pour définir ces régions. La carte en couleur incluse dans ce volume illustre la localisation et composition de chaque région.

ESTIMATIONS DÉMOGRAPHIQUES RÉGIONALES

Une évaluation fiable de la taille et de la distribution de la population, et de la répartition des décès selon l'âge et le sexe, constitue le point de départ de toute estimation globale, nationale, ou régionale, de la charge des maladies. Grâce aux efforts conjoints de nombreux individus, organisations, et gouvernements, une bonne partie de la démographie de base est actuellement connue pour chacune des régions du monde. Indiscutablement, dans toutes les régions, les données disponibles pour évaluer le niveau de mortalité infanto-juvénile sont plus amples que pour la mortalité adulte (Nations Unies 1992, Hill et Yazbeck 1994). Le niveau de mortalité adulte reste en effet très controversé entre démographes pour certaines régions en voie de développement dépourvues de bons enregistrements de l'état civil, où la mortalité est mesurée indirectement à partir de données de recensements et d'enquêtes (Timaeus 1991). Par exemple, les estimations de la mortalité adulte selon l'âge et le sexe établies par la Banque Mondiale peuvent différer de celles de la Division de Population des Nations Unies jusqu'à 50%, bien que les incertitudes soient le plus souvent moins extrêmes que cela. Les estimations démographiques de la population et des décès en 1990 selon l'âge et le sexe, furent développees spécifiquement pour le *Rapport sur le Développement dans le Monde 1993*. Nous avons continué à utiliser ces estimations dans notre Etude de la Charge Globale des Maladies, ceci afin d'assurer la comparaison avec d'autres publications comprenant des résultats de la charge des maladies. Les Tableaux 1–9 donnent les estimations de la population et des décès, selon les groupes d'âges quinquennaux et le sexe, pour chacune des huit régions et pour le monde entier en 1990. Nous présentons également les données de population et les décès non ventilés selon les cinq grands groupes d'âge pour lesquels les évaluations épidémiologiques ont été faites.[3]

ESTIMATION DES CAUSES DE DÉCÈS

Cette section survole brièvement les sources de données disponibles pour estimer les différents types de répartition des décès selon les grands groupes de cause, et les méthodes appliquées pour dériver les décès selon la cause spécifique à partir de cette information. Le premier volume de la *Série sur la Charge Globale des Maladies et Traumatismes*, intitulé *La Charge Globale des Maladies* fournit une description beaucoup plus détaillée des méthodes et des approches suivies pour estimer les différents paramètres épidémiologiques rapportés dans ce volume, y compris celles appliquées aux projections de la mortalité.

Sources de Données

L'état civil, les systèmes d'enregistrement des décès à partir de zones d'échantillonnage, les évaluations épidémiologiques, et les modèles de

Tableau II   Etats et territoires inclus dans l'Etude de la Charge Globale des Maladies, selon la région démographique

Régions démographiquement developpées

Économies de marché bien établies (EMBE)	Anciennes économies socialistes d'Europe (AESE)
Allemagne	Albanie
Andorre	Bélarus
Australie	Bosnie-Herzégovine
Autriche	Bulgarie
Belgique	Croatie
Bermudes	Estonie
Canada	Fédération de Russie
Danemark	Hongrie
Espagne	Lettonie
Etats-Unis	Lituanie
Finlande	Macédoine, L'ex République yougoslave de
France	Moldova
Gibraltar	Pologne
Grèce	République tchèque
Groenland	Roumanie
Ile de Man	Slovaquie
Iles Anglo-Normandes	Slovénie
Iles Féroé	Ukraine
Irlande	Yougoslavie
Islande	
Italie	
Japon	
Liechtenstein	
Luxembourg	
Monaco	
Norvège	
Nouvelle-Zélande	
Pays-Bas	
Portugal	
Royaume-Uni	
Saint-Marin	
Saint-Pierre-et-Miquelon	
Saint-Siège	
Suède	
Suisse	

Régions en transition démographique

Inde (IND)

Chine (CHN)

Autres pays d'Asie et îles (APAI)

Bangladesh
Bhoutan
Brunéi Darussalam
Cambodge
Corée, République de
Corée, République populaire démocratique de
Etats fédérés de Micronésie
Fidji
Guam
Hong Kong
Ile de Wake
Ile Johnston
Ile Pitcairn
Ile Tokelau
Iles Cook
Iles Mariannes septentrionales
Iles Marshall
Iles Midway
Iles Salomon
Iles Wallis et Futuna
Indonésie
Kiribati
Macao
Malaisie
Maldives
Maurice
Mongolie
Myanmar
Nauru
Népal
Nioué
Nouvelle-Calédonie
Palaos
Papouasie-Nouvelle-Guinée
Philippines
Polynésie française
République démocratique populaire Lao
Réunion
Samoa américaines
Samoa-Occidental
Seychelles
Singapour
Sri Lanka
Taiwan
Thaïlande
Tonga
Tuvalu
Vanuatu
Viet Nam

Tableau II (suite)

Régions en transition démographique, suite

Afrique subsaharienne (ASS)	Amérique latine et Caraïbes (ALC)	Croissant moyen-oriental (CMO)
Afrique du Sud	Anguilla	Afghanistan
Angola	Antigua-et-Barbuda	Algérie
Ascension	Antilles néerlandaises	Arabie saoudite
Bénin	Argentine	Arménie
Botswana	Aruba	Azerbaïdjan
Burkina Faso	Bahamas	Bahreïn
Burundi	Barbade	Chypre
Cameroun	Belize	Cisjordanie et Bande de Gaza
Cap-Vert	Bolivie	Egypte
Comores	Brésil	Emirats arabes unis
Congo	Chili	Géorgie
Côte d'Ivoire	Colombie	Iran, République islamique d'
Djibouti	Costa Rica	Iraq
Erythrée	Cuba	Israël
Ethiopie	Dominique	Jamahiriya arabe lybienne
Gabon	El Salvador	Jordanie
Gambie	Equateur	Kazakhstan
Ghana	Grenade	Kirghizistan
Guinée	Guadeloupe	Koweït
Guinée équatoriale	Guatemala	Liban
Guinée-Bissau	Guyana	Malte
Kenya	Guyane française	Maroc
Lesotho	Haïti	Oman
Libéria	Honduras	Ouzbékistan
Madagascar	Iles Caïmans	Pakistan
Malawi	Iles Turques et Caïques	Qatar
Mali	Iles Vierges britanniques	République arabe syrienne
Mauritanie	Iles Vierges (EU)	Sahara Occidental
Mayotte	Jamaïque	Tadjikistan
Mozambique	Martinique	Tunisie
Namibie	Mexique	Turkménistan
Niger	Montserrat	Turquie
Nigéria	Nicaragua	Yémen
Ouganda	Panama	
République centrafricaine	Paraguay	
Rwanda	Pérou	
Sainte-Hélène	Porto Rico	
São Tomé-et-Principe	République dominicaine	
Sénégal	Sainte-Lucie	
Sierra Leone	Saint-Kitts-et-Nevis	
Somalie	Saint-Vincent-et-les-Grenadines	
Soudan	Suriname	
Swaziland	Trinité-et-Tobago	
Tanzanie	Uruguay	
Tchad	Venezuela	
Togo		
Tristan da Cunha		
Zaïre		
Zambie		
Zimbabwe		

causes de décès sont les quatre grandes sources d'information à partir desquelles il est possible d'estimer la distribution des causes de décès. Le Tableau III résume les données fiables d'état civil selon l'âge et la région qui étaient disponibles en 1990. Seules les EMBE et les AESE ont des systèmes d'état civil complets; pour les régions en voie de développement, d'autres sources ont été utilisées pour complémenter l'information de l'état civil, à savoir, les systèmes d'enregistrement à partir de zones d'échantillonnage, les laboratoires de population, les estimations épidémiologiques, et les modèles.

Bien que l'enregistrement de routine des décès soit peu répandu en Inde et en Chine, les systèmes d'enregistrement à partir de zones d'échantillonnage qui sont en place peuvent être utilisés comme base pour l'estimation des causes de décès. Ainsi en Chine, l'Académie Chinoise de Médecine Préventive opère un système connu sous le nom de Points de Surveillance des Maladies (PSM). Etabli au début des années 1980, le système de surveillance couvre un échantillon représentatif de 10 millions d'habitants dans des régions urbaines et rurales de Chine. Chaque point de surveillance maintient une équipe comprenant un médecin qui investigue chaque décès rapporté et lui assigne une cause à partir de dossiers médicaux et entretiens avec la famille de la personne décédée.

En Inde, comme en Chine, il n'y a pas d'enregistrement complet de l'état civil, ni d'attribution fiable des causes de décès. Deux systèmes donnent néanmoins des informations qui peuvent être utilisées pour estimer la distribution des causes de décès. Dans les zones urbaines, les décès certifiés médicalement (DCM), survenus en milieu hospitalier, sont tabulés et publiés chaque année par le *Registrar-General*. Bien que dans la plupart des états la qualité des données obtenues ainsi soit mauvaise, la couverture des décès certifiés médicalement dans l'état de Maharashtra dépasse 80% (Office du *Registrar-General*, 1992a). Cette information a été utilisée comme base pour établir la distribution des causes de décès urbains en Inde. Dans les zones rurales de l'Inde, un système d'enregistre-

Tableau III   Sources et méthodes utilisées pour estimer la mortalité selon la cause pour chaque région en 1990

	Etat civil (% de couverture)			Enregistrement par zone d'échantillonnage	
	Moins de 5 ans	**5+ ans**	**TOTAL**	**Urbain**	**Rural**
EMBE	99	99	99		
AESE	99	99	99		
IND				DMC	ECD(R)
CHN				PSM	PSM
APAI	2	14	10		
ASS	<1	2	1		
ALC	28	47	43		
CMO	12	27	22		

ment à partir de zones d'échantillonnage des causes de décès, à partir d'autopsies verbales, établi dans les Centres de Soins de Santé Primaires (CSSP) des villages, fonctionne depuis 1965. Connu sous le nom d'Enquête des Causes de Décès (Rurale), ECD(R), le système comprend actuellement plus de 1300 CSSP (Office du *Registrar-General* 1992b) et donne des informations utiles quant aux grandes causes de mortalité dans les zones rurales. Du fait que les causes de décès sont établies par des personnes non-médicales, les données récoltées par ce système permettent l'estimation des grands groupes de causes mais ne sont pas adéquates pour définir les catégories spécifiques des maladies ou traumatismes.

Bien qu'aucun système d'enregistrement n'existe pour une grande partie de la population de l'Afrique sub-saharienne, plusieurs laboratoires de population de petite envergure tels que ceux de Niakhar (Sénégal), de Keneba (Gambie), de Machakos (Kenya), et de Morogoro Hai et Dar es-Salaam (Tanzanie) fournissent une information limitée relative aux causes de décès, à partir d'autopsies verbales. Bien que ces systèmes d'enregistrement contribuent à décrire la distribution locale des causes de décès, ils sont d'utilité limitée pour l'estimation de la distribution régionale des décès.

Pour un certain nombre de conditions spécifiques, les épidémiologues ont développé des estimations de mortalité selon la cause, à partir de l'histoire naturelle de maladies données. Des taux de mortalité approximatifs ont été obtenus en combinant les taux d'incidence et/ou de prévalence, estimés à partir d'enquêtes spécifiques, à l'information relative aux taux de létalité chez les sujets traités et non-traités. Pour d'autres causes de décès, telles les infections respiratoires aiguës, les maladies diarrhéiques, et le paludisme, des enquêtes ont été menées pour mesurer plus directement la mortalité selon la cause, souvent avec un succès limité (pour plus de détails, référez-vous aux chapitres pertinents dans d'autres volumes de la *Série sur la Charge Globale des Maladies et Traumatismes*). La limitation principale des estimations épidémiologiques est leur tendance à surestimer la charge de mortalité attribuée à une maladie particulière. En effet, lorsque l'on additionne le nombre de décès obtenu à partir d'estimations épidémiologiques pour les causes majeures, le total estimé ainsi excède (parfois considérablement) le nombre de décès dus à toutes les causes estimé à partir d'analyses démographiques. La tendance des estimations épidémiologiques à surestimer le niveau des maladies provient de plusieures sources de biais. Tout d'abord, de nombreux décès dus à des causes multiples, sont attribués entièrement à chacune des causes. Deuxièmement, lorsqu'il existe une incertitude quant à l'incidence, à la prévalence, ou au taux de létalité, les analystes tendent à élever les taux, ceci en dépit de fréquentes affirmations du contraire. Troisièmement, du fait que les évaluations épidémiologiques sont, en général, entreprises sans tenir compte d'autres causes de décès, les auteurs d'évaluations épidémiologiques ignorent souvent la magnitude comparative de leurs revendications de mortalité. Bien que les évaluations épidémiologiques relatives à la magnitude des problèmes de santé puissent être très informatives, elles peuvent néanmoins induire en erreur lorsqu'elles sont considérées indépendamment d'autres causes de décès et d'incapacité.

Là où il n'existe ni enregistrement d'état civil, ni enregistrement à partir de zones d'échantillonnage, ni estimation épidémiologique, les modèles des causes de décès peuvent être utiles pour estimer le type de répartition des causes de décès. Preston (1976) fut le premier à développer des techniques d'estimations indirectes de la structure des causes de décès. Il modela la relation existant entre la mortalité totale et la mortalité spécifique pour 12 grands groupes de causes, à partir d'une analyse des données historiques d'état civil pour les pays développés et pour un petit nombre de pays en voie de développement. En particulier, il postula que la mortalité cause-spécifique était une fonction linéaire de la mortalité totale. Les travaux de Preston ont établi les fondements de presque toutes les approches ultérieures pour estimer la répartition des causes de décès dans des régions dépourvues de statistiques vitales. Typiquement ces raffinements ont inclus des équations d'estimation pour des groupes d'âges spécifiques, incorporant des données plus récentes ou examinant une liste plus détaillée (Haukulinen et al. 1986, Hull et al. 1981, Lopez et Hull 1983, Murray et al. 1993).

Les tentatives préalables d'application ces modèles pour estimer la structure des causes de décès dans des régions ou pays dépourvus de données fiables sur la répartition de la mortalité ont été entravées par plusieures préoccupations, y compris la diversité de la répartition des causes de décès selon l'âge et le sexe, le nombre limité d'observations fiables sur la structure des causes de décès dans un contexte de mortalité élevée, les complications analytiques provenant de l'usage du chapitre XVI (Signes, Symptomes, et Conditions Mal Définies), et la forme fonctionnelle réelle de la relation entre la mortalité cause-spécifique et la mortalité générale. Nous avons essayé d'adresser chacune de ces limitations dans les modèles développés pour cette étude—pour plus de détails quant aux méthodes et bases de données utilisées, veuillez vous référer à Murray et Lopez (1996b). Etant donné que l'Etude de la Charge Globale des Maladies exigeait une analyse de la répartitions des causes de décès selon l'âge et le sexe pour plusieurs grands groupes d'âge, des modèles d'estimation des causes de décès furent développés séparément pour le sexe masculin et féminin, pour chacun des sept groupes d'âges: 0–4, 5–14, 15–29, 30–44, 45–59, 60–69, 70+.[4]

Méthodes

Les procédures successives utilisées pour l'estimation des taux de mortalité selon l'âge, le sexe, et les causes spécifiques, pour chacune des régions peuvent être décrites de la manière suivante: (1) les estimations initiales furent développées largement à partir des données d'état civil et d'enregistrements à partir de zones d'échantillonnage; (2) les estimations pour des groupes de causes particulières, tels les tumeurs malignes et l'asthme, furent alors corrigées en appliquant des méthodes spécifiques; (3) les taux de mortalité pour certaines causes spécifiques furent ajustés à partir d'analyses épidémiologiques; et (4) des ajustements finaux furent apportés afin d'assurer que la somme des taux de mortalité par cause soit identique à la mortalité totale spécifique estimée pour chacun des groupes d'âge à partir de méthodes démographiques. L'application de chacune de ces étapes a varié en fonction de la région; la description qui suit souligne certaines de ces différences—pour une description plus complète, référez-vous à Murray et Lopez (1996b).

Pour les EMBE et les AESE, les estimations initiales furent dérivées uniquement à partir de données d'état civil (qui couvrent virtuellement l'ensemble des décès dans les deux régions). Pour la Chine, les estimations initiales furent calculées à partir des Points de Surveillance des Maladies en 1991 couvrant 52,734 décès survenus dans une population de 10 millions, ajustés pour égaler le nombre total de décès dans chacun des groupes d'âge et sexe en Chine. Pour l'Inde, les estimations initiales furent dérivées à partir des données des causes de décès médicalement certifiées selon la classification CIM-9, augmentées pour égaler le nombre de décès urbains survenus dans chaque groupe d'âge et sexe (à partir des résultats du Système Indien d'Enregistrement des Décès à partir de Zones d'Echantillonnage). Les estimations de la mortalité dans les zones rurales furent basées sur les résultats pour les années 1991–1993 de l'Enquête des Causes de Décès (Rurale), augmentées pour égaler le nombre de décès ruraux estimés pour le pays entier.

Pour les quatre régions restantes, l'ALC, les APAI, le CMO et l'ASS, bien qu'il existe quelques données d'état civil, la majorité des décès n'est pas captée par les systèmes existants (voir Tableau III). De plus, les décès qui sont rapportés ne peuvent être considérés comme étant représentatifs de la mortalité de la région dans son ensemble. Chacune de ces régions peut être divisée en une zone ayant des données d'état civil et une zone résiduelle. Pour développer des estimations plausibles de mortalité selon la cause dans les zones résiduelles, une approche en deux étapes successives fut adoptée. Tout d'abord, une nouvelle méthode de courbe de Lorenz fut développée à partir de l'inégalité géographique de la distribution des décès; cette approche fournit des estimations des taux de mortalité selon l'âge et le sexe pour toutes les causes combinées dans les zones résiduelles—pour plus de détails voir Murray et Lopez (1996b). Deuxièmement, pour les zones ayant des données, la distribution proportionnelle des décès enregistrés pour chaque groupe d'âge attribués aux Groupes I, II, et III, fut comparée au pourcentage prédit par les modèles des causes de décès. Le nombre d'écarts-types au-dessus ou au-dessous de la valeur prédite pour chaque Groupe mesure l'écart existant entre la structure de la mortalité des zones de la région ayant des données et celle fournie par les modèles. Pour distribuer l'ensemble de la mortalité de la zone résiduelle aux Groupes I, II, et III, nous avons supposé que la déviation de la structure des causes de décès d'avec le modèle des causes de décès était similaire à celle observée dans les zones avec enregistrement. En d'autres termes, si la zone avec enregistrement en ALC donnait un pourcentage de la mortalité pour l'ensemble des causes du Groupe I supérieure aux résultats attendus de 2.3 écarts-types, nous avons supposé que le pourcentage de l'ensemble des causes de décès du Groupe I dans les zones résiduelles était également supérieur aux valeurs prédites de 2.3 écarts-types.

Pour l'ASS, nous avons utilisé une méthode un peu différente de par le fait que les données d'état civil n'étaient disponibles que pour l'Afrique du Sud.[5] La région fut divisée en deux composantes. La partie Sud qui comprend l'Afrique du Sud, le Botswana, la Namibie, le Mozambique, le Zimbabwe, le Swaziland, la Zambie, le Malawi et la partie Nord qui comprend tous les autres pays de l'Afrique sub-saharienne. La méthode de la courbe de Lorenz fut alors appliquée pour estimer la distribution pour l'Afrique du Sud à partir des données d'état civil en Afrique du Sud. Pour le reste de l'ASS, la distribution de la mortalité fut basée sur la différence observée entre les estimations régionales et celles de la sub-région sud de l'ASS. La distribution des décès entre les Groupes I, II, et III pour les décès enregistrés en Afrique du Sud était égale ou inférieure à 1 écart-type de celui prédite par les modèles. Pour le reste de la région sub-saharienne, nous avons appliqué la distribution des écarts-types observée dans les zones avec enregistrement en Afrique du Sud.

Afin d'estimer la mortalité pour les causes plus détaillées à l'intérieur de chaque Groupe dans les zones résiduelles, nous avons supposé que pour l'ALC, le CMO, l'ASS et les APAI, la distribution proportionnelle pour un groupe âge-sexe donné était la même que dans les régions avec enregistrements. L'alternative aurait été d'appliquer les modèles de régression pour les petites causes discutées auparavant. Nous pensons néanmoins qu'il est préférable d'estimer la distribution plus détaillée des causes de décès à partir des données locales, plutôt qu'à partir des données d'état civil des pays industrialisés.

Pour un certain nombre de catégories de maladies, telles les tumeurs malignes, les maladies cardiovasculaires, les affections neuro-psychiatriques, et les affections respiratoires chroniques, nous avons également appliqué une série de corrections standards. Celles-ci sont décrites en détail dans Murray et Lopez (1996b).

Des experts ont également généré des estimations épidémiologiques pour toutes les régions en voie de développement à partir de revues épidémiologiques détaillées entreprises pour de nombreuses maladies. Ces estimations épidémiologiques furent utilisées pour ajuster les estimations de mortalité préalables pour un certain nombre de causes sélectionnées. Du fait que l'épidémiologie était concentrée avant tout sur les maladies transmissibles dans la plupart des pays en voie de développement, il y a beaucoup plus d'estimations de mortalité basées sur des données épidémiologiques pour les maladies du Groupe I que pour celles du Groupe II. Cette approche a tendance à biaiser les résultats finaux en faveur des maladies du Groupe I et à minimiser l'importance des maladies du Groupe II, du fait que les estimations épidémiologiques tendent à donner des taux plus élevés que ceux basés sur l'état civil. Pour obtenir les bases détaillées de chaque évaluation épidémiologique, le lecteur est prié de se référer aux chapitres pertinents dans le(s) volume(s) de la *Série sur la Charge Globale des Maladies et Traumatismes.*

A cause de la nature sporadique mais intense des traumatismes dûs aux guerres, les estimations épidémiologiques des décès liés aux guerres ont été incluses de manière un peu différente. En bref, nous avons choisi de considérer comme décès de guerre, les décès additionnels qui dépassaient les estimations de décès selon l'âge et le sexe, établies à partir des analyses démographiques de base utilisées pour déterminer le nombre de décès pour chaque groupe âge-sexe dans chacune des régions. De ce fait les estimations des décès de guerre n'ont pas été soumises à l'algorithme d'ajustement final décrit ci-dessous.

Selon la pratique de la CIM, chaque décès a été attribué à une seule cause sous-jacente dans les tabulations primaires (Murray et Lopez 1996b) préparées pour l'Etude de la Charge Globale des Maladies. Par exemple, les décès survenus à la suite d'une tumeur maligne du foie causé par une hépatite infectieuse chronique B sont attribués aux cancers du foie dans les tabulations primaires. De même, les décès dûs à la tuberculose survenant chez des sujets séropositifs pour le VIH sont attribués au VIH dans les tabulations primaires selon les conventions de la CIM. Dans ce volume, la plupart des tableaux indiquent le nombre de décès assignés à une cause dans les tabulations primaires; toutefois, certaines tableaux, telles celles pour la tuberculose/VIH, indiquent le nombres de décès associés à la condition commune. Les notes techniques qui accompagnent les tableaux indiquent clairement le type de mortalité inclus.

Même après correction de nombreuses causes basées sur des données épidémiologiques, la somme de la mortalité par cause excédait souvent la mortalité totale pour certains groupes âge-sexe dans plusieures régions. Dans certains cas, la somme des causes spécifiques à l'intérieur d'un Groupe excédait la mortalité totale pour ce Groupe dans un groupe d'âge donné—un problème commun pour le Groupe I dans les groupes d'âges adultes par exemple. Pour forcer l'addition des décès cause-spécifiques à égaler le nombre total des décès dans tout les groupes âge-sexe donné, deux algorithmes additionnels furent appliqués, l'un pour les causes néonatales, et l'autre pour tous les autres groupes d'âges.

Dans la plupart des régions, 80–90% des décès néonataux sont dûs à un nombre limité de causes: la syphilis congénitale, le tétanos néonatal, les conditions survenant pendant la période néonatale, et les anomalies congénitales. Nous avons d'abord estimé le nombre de décès néonataux dans chaque région, à partir des résultats de projets démographiques majeurs tels le Projet d'Enquêtes Démographiques et de Santé. Nous avons ensuite exigé que la somme des décès attribués à la syphilis congénitale, le tétanos néonatal, les conditions survenant pendant la période néonatale, et les anomalies congénitales soit égale à 85% du nombre estimé de décès pour la période néonatale. Lorsque les estimations basées sur des données épidémiologiques dépassaient 85% du nombre total de décès néonataux estimés, chacune de ces causes fut proportionnellement réduite.

Le degré de surestimation de la mortalité à l'intérieur de chacun des 14 groupes âge-sexe, et pour chacune des régions, fut évalué en comparant le nombre d'écarts-types au-dessus ou au-dessous de la mortalité proportionnelle pour un Groupe, selon les prédictions à partir des modèles de causes de décès, au nombre d'écarts-types au-dessus ou au-dessous obtenues dans les estimations initiales. Pour ajuster la surestimation à partir de l'approche épidémiologique, nous avons arbitrairement choisi l'algorithme suivant. Si les premières estimations pour les Groupes I et II faites à partir des données de l'état civil, ou des enquêtes à partir de zones d'échantillonnage, étaient déjà inférieures ou plus de 2.5 écarts-types par rapport aux estimations attendues, nous ne permettions pas aux estimations épidémiologiques d'augmenter le degré de déviation. Lorsque l'estimation initiale pour le Groupe I était plus de 2.5 écarts-types au-dessus de la valeur attendue ou, pour le Groupe II, plus de 2.5 écarts-types au dessous de la valeur attendue, les résultats des évaluations épidémiologiques pouvaient modifier la proportion dans chacun des deux Groupes de 2 écarts-types. Si un changement de 2 écarts-types augmentait le pourcentage des décès du Groupe I de plus de 2.5 écarts-types au dessus de la moyenne, ou diminuait le pourcentage de décès du Groupe II de plus de 2.5 écarts-types au-dessous de la moyenne, le pourcentage des décès du Groupe I était fixé comme étant égal à 2.5 écarts-types au dessus de la moyenne, et le pourcentage des décès du Groupe II était fixé comme étant égal à 2.5 écarts-types au-dessous de la moyenne.

Incidence, Prévalence, Taux de Létalité et Durée

Des estimations de l'incidence, de la prévalence, de la durée, du taux de létalité et de la mortalité pour chacune des maladies ou traumatismes, et leurs séquelles, étaient requises pour l'Etude de la Charge Globale des Maladies. Toutefois, dans certaines régions, il n'existait aucune étude épidémiologique fiable au niveau de la communauté à partir de laquelle ces paramètres épidémiologiques puissent être estimés. Afin d'identifier toutes les sources de données et d'information utiles, et afin de suppléer les données empiriques d'un jugement bien informé, les estimations présentées dans ce volume furent obtenues en collaboration étroite avec un grand nombre d'experts familiers avec des maladies ou traumatismes spécifiques, et représentent l'aboutissement d'un processus itératif qui s'est déroulé au cours de plus de 4 ans (1992–1996). Les étapes suivantes résument le mécanisme véritable utilisé pour générer les estimations pour chacune des maladies et traumatismes.

1. Des experts en maladies particulières ou, dans certains cas, des groupes d'experts furent identifiés pour chacun des plus de 100 conditions incluses dans l'Etude de la Charge Globale des Maladies. Les participants à cette étude furent choisis à l'Organisation Mondiale de la

Santé, à l'Agence Internationale de Recherche sur le Cancer, à la Banque Mondiale, aux *Centers for Disease Control* (Etats-Unis), et à des institutions académiques dans plusieurs pays, y compris les Etats-Unis d'Amérique, la Grande-Bretagne, la France, le Mexique, la Nouvelle-Zélande, l'Inde, le Sri Lanka et la Chine.

2. Les estimations initiales furent faites par les experts à partir d'études publiées et non-publiées de l'incidence, de la rémission, du taux de létalité, de la prévalence, de la durée, et des décès. Lorsqu'aucune donnée n'était disponible, les experts furent encouragés à faire des estimations selon leur meilleur jugement. Ainsi, la distribution de l'incidence ou de la rémission selon l'âge fut souvent basée sur la supposition que les profils épidémiologiques étaient vraisemblablement similaires dans les différentes régions. Dans le pire des cas, lorsqu'aucune information n'était disponible, toutes les estimations préliminaires furent basées sur des données et informations d'autres régions.

3. Ces estimations furent revues de manière critique et la cohérence interne entre incidence, rémission, taux de létalité, durée et prévalence fut établie à l'aide de DISMOD.[6] Ces vérifications ont permis d'identifier les incohérences majeures de nombreuses estimations. Les experts en maladies particulières furent alors invités à réviser leurs estimations, en consultation avec les auteurs, afin d'obtenir une cohérence interne.

4. Les estimations révisées furent utilisées pour générer les résultats préliminaires. Ces estimations furent soigneusement examinées par un grand groupe d'experts en santé internationaux lors d'une réunion, organisée à l'Organisation Mondiale de la Santé à Genève du 8 au 11 Décembre 1992. Les révisions ultérieures furent à nouveau soumises à une validation de leur cohérence interne, et constituent la base des résultats publiés dans le *Rapport sur le Développement dans le Monde 1993: Investir dans la Santé*.

5. Les experts en maladies particulières furent invités à écrire des chapitres détaillés au sujet des données et des méthodes utilisées pour produire leurs estimations comme une activité faisant partie du suivi du *Rapport sur le Développement dans le Monde 1993*. Ces auteurs eurent ainsi l'occasion de passer par trois itérations supplémentaires de leurs estimations de l'incidence, de la prévalence, de la durée, du taux de létalité, de la rémission, et des décès. Ces révisions ont bénéficié de discussions approfondies, et les révisions des résultats furent publiées en 1993 et 1994. Chacune de ces révisions a été examinée à des fins de cohérence interne. Pour certaines constellations de conditions, telles les maladies neuro-psychiatriques, des séminaires internationaux spécifiques furent organisés afin de réviser les estimations épidémiologiques.

PROJECTIONS DES CAUSES DE DÉCÈS 1990-2020

Les stratégies et politiques visant à promouvoir la santé et la prévention des maladies doivent adopter une perspective d'avenir. Pour répondre à ce besoin, nous avons également inclus dans ce volume les projections de la mortalité d'ici à l'an 2000 pour chacune des causes. La méthode de projection développée pour l'Etude de la Charge Globale des Maladies est entièrement décrite dans un autre volume (Murray et Lopez 1996a). Brièvement, l'approche utilisée était de développer un modèle statistique ou économétrique afin de prédire différents scénarios de mortalité selon la cause, à partir d'un nombre très restreint de variables indépendantes. Cette approche pourrait bien être trop simpliste, mais génère des prédictions plausibles, largement basées sur des observations empiriques dans un large spectre de pays, au cours de nombreuses décennies. Plutôt que de projeter la mortalité totale, et de décomposer ensuite la mortalité totale selon les causes à partir d'un ensemble de relations entre la mortalité totale et la mortalité par cause, nous avons choisi de modeler les différents groupes de causes indépendamment. Nos projections de la mortalité totale pour chaque groupe d'âge et sexe représentent ainsi la somme des projections de chacune des causes. Les causes de décès ont été réparties en 9 regroupements de causes: toutes les maladies du Groupe I, les cancers, les maladies cardiovasculaires, les affections digestives, les affections respiratoires chroniques, les autres maladies du Groupe II, les accidents de la voie publique, les autres traumatismes non-intentionnels, et intentionnels. Ces neuf causes s'additionnent pour donner la mortalité totale à l'intérieur de chaque groupe d'âge et sexe. Nous avons choisi ces regroupements particuliers de causes parce que les tendances de mortalité, dans des pays qui ont de bonnes données d'état civil, au cours des quarante dernières années, suggèrent que les causes plus spécifiques à l'intérieur de chaque regroupement ont suivi des tendances similaires. Il y a toutefois des exceptions évidentes, telle l'augmentation des cas de tuberculose dans les EMBE au cours des 5-10 dernières années, et l'épidémie de VIH, pour lesquelles des méthodes séparées ont été utilisées. En général, toutefois, ces neuf constellations de causes semblent capter raisonnablement la gamme des différentes tendances selon les causes spécifiques.

Quatre variables indépendantes furent incluses dans le modèle prédictif: le revenu par habitant, le capital humain, l'intensité du tabagisme, et le temps. Le revenu par habitant, mesuré en dollars internationaux, ajusté pour les différences de pouvoir d'achat non représentées par les taux de change officiels, fut utilisé comme mesure d'évaluation pour de nombreux aspects du développement économique. Le nombre moyen d'années de scolarité de la population, une mesure du niveau d'éducation et de formation du capital humain, a été utilisé pour capter les déterminantes clé de l'état de santé, et la capacité de la population à faire usage des connaissances disponibles en matière de santé et d'interventions. Un facteur déterminant dominant de l'état de santé adulte, qui n'est pas bien capté par le gain ou le niveau d'éducation, est l'exposition cumulative au tabac, puisque le fait de fumer est l'une des causes principales de plusieures maladies majeures.

Le taux de prévalence du tabagisme, relevé par des enquêtes, n'est pas une mesure fiable de l'impact du fait de fumer. D'autres facteurs, y compris la durée, le type, la quantité, et le mode de fumer, sont des déterminantes critiques de l'exposition cumulative dans le passé. Suivant l'exemple de Peto et Lopez, nous avons pris les taux estimés de cancers du poumon pour chaque groupe âge-sexe comme paramètre de l'intensité du tabagisme (voir Peto et al. 1994 pour plus de détails sur cette méthode).[7] L'intensité du tabagisme est alors utilisée comme une variable indépendante dans les équation prédictives pour les cancers, les maladies cardio-vasculaires, et les affections respiratoires chroniques. La quatrième variable indépendante utilisée dans les projections est le temps lui-même. Ainsi les tendances séculaires de mortalité qui ne sont pas expliquées par le gain, le niveau d'éducation, ou le tabagisme, peuvent être attribuées aux changements de technologies ou de connaissances, que nous captons grossièrement en utilisant le temps comme une variable. En plus, comme nous le discutons plus loin, les projections indépendantes de l'épidémie VIH furent ajoutées aux projections de base générées par le modèle prédictif.

Pour chacune des neuf constellations de causes de décès, et pour chacun des 7 groupes d'âge et chaque sexe, différentes équations de régression furent évaluées. L'équation finale utilisée fut basée sur le plus petit ensemble de variables indépendantes qui avaient une capacité prédictive raisonnable, mesurée par la proportion de variance expliquée. En plus, si un paramètre d'estimation pour une variable avait le signe opposé à celui attendu, et que le coefficient n'était pas significatif au niveau de 1%, cette variable fut éliminée de l'équation. Les projections pour les causes plus détaillées furent basées sur des équations de régression pour chacune des causes détaillées, comme une fonction du taux de mortalité pour l'agglomérat de causes.

Les équations établissant la relation entre le taux de mortalité par âge et sexe et le Produit National Brut (PNB) par habitant, le capital humain, l'intensité du tabagisme, et le temps, étant donnés, des projections de chacune des variables indépendantes furent requises. Pour chaque variable indépendante, différents scénarios—pessimiste, de base, et optimiste—furent développés. Toutefois, en raison du manque de place, seuls les résultats des scénarios de base sont présentés dans ce volume. Les projections du PNB par habitant pour chaque région furent basées sur les prévisions économiques de la Banque Mondiale et les hypothèses plausibles relatives à la croissance du PNB par habitant à long terme. Le capital humain fut projeté selon le taux d'accroissement moyen du capital humain enregistré durant la période de 1950–1990, pour chaque région. Nous avons également supposé que les taux diminuent avec l'accroissement du niveau du capital humain. Pour projeter l'intensité du tabagisme de 1990 à l'an 2000, nous avons examiné la relation entre la consommation de cigarettes par adulte en Grande-Bretagne de 1900 à 1990, et les estimations de l'intensité du tabagisme au cours de la même période. Pour projeter l'intensité du tabagisme, nous avons assumé que le déroulement temporel de l'épidémie de tabagisme en Grande-Bretagne serait répété dans chaque région. Utilisant des estimations de la consommation de cigarettes par habitant pour le sexe masculin et le sexe féminin, nous avons appliqué la relation observée en Grande-Bretagne pour estimer l'intensité du tabagisme trente ans après qu'un seuil donné ait été atteint. Ce nombre fut alors utilisé comme étant la valeur projetée de l'intensité du tabagisme en l'an 2020. Pour les années intermédiaires, nous supposons que les valeurs actuelles de la variable intensité du tabagisme augmentera ou diminuera de façon linéaire en direction de la valeur projetée à l'an 2020.

Comme nous l'avions mentionné auparavant, l'expérience dans le passé des pays ayant de bonnes données d'état civil, incorporées dans les équations prédictives décrites ci-dessus, ne capte pas le cours de l'épidémie de VIH de manière adéquate. Pour estimer l'impact possible de l'épidémie de VIH dans chacune des régions entre 1990 et 2020, nous avons préparé des projections indépendantes de l'incidence du VIH, et de la mortalité due au VIH chaque année, pour chaque âge, sexe, et région. Ces projections concordent étroitement avec celles de l'ancien Programme Global sur le SIDA de l'OMS (GPA) pour la phase de l'épidémie au cours de laquelle l'incidence augmente. Pour la phase au cours de laquelle l'incidence diminue, le modèle de projection du GPA suppose que l'incidence tombe rapidement à zéro dans toutes les régions, si bien que, l'an 2020, il n'y aurait essentiellement que très peu ou pas du tout d'incidence VIH. Ceci nous paraît être un scénario trop optimiste. Nos projections sont basées sur la supposition que l'incidence diminuera en direction d'une valeur d'équilibre égale à la moitié de l'incidence de pointe. Du fait qu'aucune région autre que les EMBE n'est proche du point où l'incidence est égale à la moitié de l'incidence de pointe, nous ne savons pas à quel niveau l'épidémie de VIH se stabilisera dans chaque région. Pour estimer la mortalité due au VIH, nous avons utilisé les mêmes suppositions que celles incluses dans le modèle de projection du GPA en ce qui concerne le temps nécessaire pour progresser du VIH au SIDA, et la distribution des décès dûs au SIDA au cours du temps. Ces projections sont probablement très pessimistes, particulièrement pour des régions telles que l'Inde, les APAI et la Chine.

ORGANISATION DES TABLEAUX

Le Tableau IV donne la liste complète de toutes les séquelles pour chaque maladie et traumatisme inclus dans l'Etude de la Charge Globale des Maladies, pour lesquelles une évaluation épidémiologique détaillée a été entreprise. Du fait du manque de place, l'ensemble des séquelles n'a pas pu être présenté dans ce volume. Le Tableau IV indique les séquelles incluses. Pour chacune des séquelles incluses dans ce volume, il y a trois pages de tableaux contenant des groupes d'estimations identiques pour

Tableau IV Groupes de causes, maladies et traumatismes, et séquelles inclus dans l'Etude de la Charge Globale des Maladies (Version 5) et séquelles pour lesquelles des données sont presentées dans ce volume

CGM Code de Classification	Groupes de causes, maladie, traumatisme, ou séquelle	Données presentées dans ce volume (numéro du tableau)
I	Affections transmissibles, périnatales, maternelles, et nutritionnelles	
IA	Maladies infectieuses et parasitaires	
IA1	Tuberculose	
IA1-1	Cas séro-négatifs pour VIH	10
IA1-2	Cas séro-positifs pour VIH	11
IA2	Maladies sexuellement transmissibles hormis VIH	
IA2a	Syphilis	
IA2a-1	Syphilis congénitale	12
IA2a-2	Poids insuffisant à la naissance	13
IA2a-3	Primaire	14
IA2a-4	Secondaire	15
IA2a-5	Tertiaire – cardio-vasculaire	16
IA2a-6	Tertiaire – gommes	17
IA2a-7	Tertiaire – nerveuse	18
IA2b	Chlamydiose	
IA2b-1	Ophtalmie néonatale	19
IA2b-2	Poids insuffisant à la naissance	20
IA2b-3	Cicatrice de la cornée – cécité	21
IA2b-4	Cicatrice de la cornée – baisse de la vision	22
IA2b-5	Cervicite	23
IA2b-6	Pneumonie néonatale	24
IA2b-7	Inflammation des organes pelviens	25
IA2b-8	Grossesse ectopique	26
IA2b-9	Abcès tubo-ovarien	27
IA2b-10	Douleur pelvienne chronique	28
IA2b-11	Stérilité	29
IA2b-12	Urétrite symptomatique	30
IA2b-13	Epididymite	31
IA2b-14	Rétrécissement urétral	32
IA2c	Gonorrhée	
IA2c-1	Ophtalmie néonatale	33
IA2c-2	Poids insuffisant à la naissance	34
IA2c-3	Cicatrice de la cornée – cécité	35
IA2c-4	Cicatrice de la cornée – baisse de la vision	36
IA2c-5	Cervicite	37
IA2c-6	Inflammation des organes pelviens	38
IA2c-7	Grossesse ectopique	39
IA2c-8	Abcès tubo-ovarien	40
IA2c-9	Douleur pelvienne chronique	41
IA2c-10	Stérilité	42
IA2c-11	Urétrite symptomatique	43
IA2c-12	Epididymite	44
IA2c-13	Rétrécissement urétral	45
IA3	VIH	
IA3-1	Cas	46
IA3-2	SIDA	47
IA4	Maladies diarrhéiques	
IA4-1	Episodes	48

Tableau IV   (suite)

CGM Code de Classification	Groupes de causes, maladie, traumatisme, ou séquelle	Données presentées dans ce volume (numéro du tableau)
IA5	Maladies infantiles	
IA5a	Coqueluche	
IA5a-1	Episodes	49
IA5a-2	Retard mental	50
IA5b	Poliomyélite	
IA5b-1	Paralytique	51
IA5c	Diphtérie	
IA5c-1	Episodes	52
IA5c-2	Complications neurologiques	53
IA5c-3	Myocardite	54
IA5d	Rougeole	
IA5d-1	Episodes	55
IA5e	Tétanos	
IA5e-1	Episodes	56
IA6	Méningite bactérienne et méningococcémie	
IA6-1	Toutes les formes – épisodes	57
IA6-2	Streptococcus pneumoniae – épisodes	58
IA6-3	Haemophilus influenzae – épisodes	59
IA6-4	Neisseria meningitidis – épisodes	60
IA6-5	Méningococcémie sans méningite – épisodes	61
IA6-6	Surdité	62
IA6-7	Atteintes convulsives	63
IA6-8	Déficit moteur	64
IA6-9	Retard mental	65
IA7	Hépatite B et hépatite C	
IA7-1	Episodes	66
IA7-2	Cirrhose du foie – cas symptomatiques	67
IA7-3	Hépatome	68
IA8	Paludisme	
IA8-1	Episodes	69
IA8-2	Anémie	70
IA8-3	Séquelles neurologiques	71
IA9	Maladies tropicales	
IA9a	Trypanosomiase	
IA9a-1	Episodes	72
IA9b	Maladie de Chagas	
IA9b-1	Infection	73
IA9b-2	Cardiomyopathie sans insuffisance cardiaque congestive	74
IA9b-3	Cardiomyopathie avec insuffisance cardiaque congestive	75
IA9b-4	Mégaviscerose	76
IA9c	Schistosomiase	
IA9c-1	Infection	77
IA9d	Leishmaniose	
IA9d-1	Viscerale	78
IA9d-2	Cutanée	79
IA9e	Filariose lymphatique	
IA9e-1	Hydrocèle > 15 cm	80
IA9e-2	Lymphoedème bancroftien	81
IA9e-3	Lymphoedème brugien	82
IA9f	Onchocercose	
IA9f-1	Cécité	83

Tableau IV (suite)

CGM Code de Classification	Groupes de causes, maladie, traumatisme, ou séquelle	Données presentées dans ce volume (numéro du tableau)
IA9f-2	Prurit	84
IA9f-3	Baisse de la vision	85
IA10	Lèpre	
IA10-1	Cas	86
IA10-2	Lèpre avec incapacité	87
IA11	Dengue	
IA11-1	Fièvre hémorragique de la dengue	88
IA12	Encéphalite japonaise	
IA12-1	Episodes	89
IA12-2	Déficience cognitive	90
IA12-3	Séquelles neurologiques	91
IA13	Trachome	
IA13-1	Cécité	92
IA13-2	Baisse de la vision	93
IA14	Infections à nématodes intestinaux	
IA14a	Ascaridose	
IA14a-1	Infection de forte intensité	94
IA14a-2	Déficit cognitif simultané	95
IA14a-3	Déficience cognitive	96
IA14a-4	Obstruction intestinale	97
IA14b	Tricocéphalose	
IA14b-1	Infection de forte intensité	98
IA14b-2	Deficit cognitif simultané	99
IA14b-3	Syndrome dysentérique massif	100
IA14b-4	Déficience cognitive	101
IA14c	Ankylostomiase et nécatoriase	
IA14c-1	Infection de forte intensité	102
IA14c-2	Anémie	103
IA14c-3	Déficience cognitive	104
IB	Infections des voies respiratoires	
IB1	Infections des voies respiratoires inférieures	
IB1-1	Episodes	105
IB1-2	Séquelles chroniques	106
IB2	Infections des voies respiratoires supérieures	
IB2-1	Episodes	107
IB2-2	Pharyngite	108
IB3	Otite moyenne	
IB3-1	Episodes	109
IB3-2	Surdité	110
IC	Affections maternelles	
IC1	Hémorragie maternelle	
IC1-1	Episodes	111
IC1-2	Syndrome de Sheehan	112
IC1-3	Anémie grave	113
IC2	Septicémie maternelle	
IC2-1	Episodes	114
IC2-2	Stérilité	115
IC3	Troubles hypertensifs de la grossesse	
IC3-1	Episodes	116
IC3-2	Séquelles neurologiques	117
IC4	Dystocie d'obstacle	
IC4-1	Episodes	118

Tableau IV   (suite)

CGM Code de Classification	Groupes de causes, maladie, traumatisme, ou séquelle	Données presentées dans ce volume (numéro du tableau)
IC4-2	Incontinence urinaire de stress	119
IC4-3	Fistule recto-vaginale	120
IC5	Avortement	
IC5-1	Episodes	121
IC5-2	Stérilité	122
ID	Affections de la période périnatale	
ID1	Poids insuffisant à la naissance	
ID1-1	Toutes les séquelles	123
ID2	Asphyxie néonatale et traumatismes de l'accouchement	
ID2-1	Toutes les séquelles	124
IE	Carences nutritionnelles	
IE1	Malnutrition protéino-calorique	
IE1-1	Insuffisance pondérale	125
IE1-2	Insuffisance staturale	126
IE1-3	Déficit du développement	127
IE2	Déficience en iode	
IE2-1	Goitre – grade 0	128
IE2-2	Goitre – grade 1	129
IE2-3	Goitre – grade 2	130
IE2-4	Déficit léger du développement	131
IE2-5	Crétinoidisme	132
IE2-6	Crétinisme	133
IE3	Avitaminose A	
IE3-1	Xérophtalmie	134
IE3-2	Cicatrice de la cornée	135
IE4	Anémie ferriprive	
IE4-1	Toutes les formes	136
IE4-2	Légère	137
IE4-3	Modérée	138
IE4-4	Grave	139
IE4-5	Très grave	140
IE4-6	Déficience cognitive	141
II	Maladies non-transmissibles	
IIA	Tumeurs malignes	
IIA1	Cancers de la bouche et de l'oropharynx	
IIA1-1	Cas	142
IIA2	Cancer de l'oesophage	
IIA2-1	Cas	143
IIA3	Cancer de l'estomac	
IIA3-1	Cas	144
IIA4	Cancers du côlon et du rectum	
IIA4-1	Cas	145
IIA5	Cancer du foie	
IIA5-1	Cas	146
IIA6	Cancer du pancréas	
IIA6-1	Cas	147
IIA7	Cancers de la trachée, des bronches et du poumon	
IIA7-1	Cas	148
IIA8	Mélanome et autres tumeurs cutanées	
IIA8-1	Cas	149
IIA9	Cancer du sein	
IIA9-1	Cas	150

Tableau IV   (suite)

CGM Code de Classification	Groupes de causes, maladie, traumatisme, ou séquelle	Données presentées dans ce volume (numéro du tableau)
IIA10	Cancer du col de l'utérus	
IIA10-1	Cas	151
IIA11	Cancer du corps de l'utérus	
IIA11-1	Cas	152
IIA12	Cancer de l'ovaire	
IIA12-1	Cas	153
IIA13	Cancer de la prostate	
IIA13-1	Cas	154
IIA14	Cancer de la vessie	
IIA14-1	Cas	155
IIA15	Lymphomes et myélome multiple	
IIA15-1	Cas	156
IIA16	Leucémie	
IIA16-1	Cas	157
IIB	Autres néoplasmes	
IIC	Diabète sucré	
IIC-1	Cas	158
IIC-2	Pied diabétique	159
IIC-3	Neuropathie	160
IIC-4	Rétinopathie – cécité	161
IIC-5	Amputation	162
IID	Troubles endocriniens	
IIE	Affections neuro-psychiatriques	
IIE1	Dépression unipolaire majeure	
IIE1-1	Episodes dépressifs	163
IIE2	Trouble bipolaire	
IIE2-1	Cas	164
IIE3	Schizophrénie	
IIE3-1	Cas	165
IIE4	Epilepsie	
IIE4-1	Cas	166
IIE5	Usage d'alcool	
IIE5-1	Syndrome de dépendance alcoolique	167
IIE6	Démence et autres troubles dégénératifs et héréditaires du SNC	
IIE6-1	Cas	168
IIE7	Maladie de Parkinson	
IIE7-1	Cas	169
IIE8	Sclérose en plaques	
IIE8-1	Cas	170
IIE9	Usage de drogues	
IIE9-1	Usage disfonctionnel et nocif de drogues	171
IIE10	Troubles anxieux post-traumatiques	
IIE10-1	Cas	172
IIE11	Troubles obsessionnels et compulsifs	
IIE11-1	Cas	173
IIE12	Trouble d'angoisse	
IIE12-1	Cas	174
IIF	Maladies des organes des sens	
IIF1	Glaucome	
IIF1-1	Cécité	175

Tableau IV   (suite)

CGM Code de Classification	Groupes de causes, maladie, traumatisme, ou séquelle	Données presentées dans ce volume (numéro du tableau)
IIF2	Cataractes	
IIF2-1	Cécité	176
IIG	Maladies cardio-vasculaires	
IIG1	Cardiopathie rhumatismale	
IIG1-1	Insuffisance cardiaque congestive	177
IIG2	Cardiopathie ischémique	
IIG2-1	Infarctus aigu du myocarde	178
IIG2-2	Angine de poitrine	179
IIG2-3	Insuffisance cardiaque congestive	180
IIG3	Maladie cérébrovasculaire	
IIG3-1	Premier accident vasculaire cérébral	181
IIG4	Maladies cardiaques inflammatoires	
IIG4-1	Myocardite	182
IIG4-2	Péricardite	183
IIG4-3	Endocardite	184
IIG4-4	Cardiomyopathie	185
IIH	Affections de voies respiratoires	
IIH1	Maladie pulmonaire obstructive chronique	
IIH1-1	Cas symptomatiques	186
IIH2	Asthme	
IIH2-1	Cas	187
III	Maladies de l'appareil digestif	
III1	Ulcère peptique	
III1-1	Cas	188
III2	Cirrhose du foie	
III2-1	Cas symptomatiques	189
III3	Appendicite	
III3-1	Episodes	190
IIJ	Maladies de l'appareil génito-urinaire	
IIJ1	Néphrite et néphrose	
IIJ1-1	Glomerulonéphrite aiguë	191
IIJ1-2	Maladie rénale terminale	192
IIJ2	Hypertrophie bénigne de la prostate	
IIJ2-1	Cas symptomatiques	193
IIK	Maladies de la peau	
IIL	Maladies ostéo-musculaires	
IIL1	Arthrite rhumatoïde	
IIL1-1	Cas	194
IIL2	Ostéoarthrite	
IIL2-1	Hanche	195
IIL2-2	Genou	196
IIM	Anomalies congénitales	
IIM1	Anomalie de la paroi abdominale	
IIM1-1	Cas	197
IIM2	Anencéphalie	
IIM2-1	Cas	198
IIM3	Atrésie anorectale	
IIM3-1	Cas	199
IIM4	Bec de lièvre	
IIM4-1	Cas	200
IIM5	Fissure du palais	
IIM5-1	Cas	201

Tableau IV (suite)

CGM Code de Classification	Groupes de causes, maladie, traumatisme, ou séquelle	Données presentées dans ce volume (numéro du tableau)
IIM6	Atrésie de l'oesophage	
IIM6-1	Cas	202
IIM7	Agénésie rénale	
IIM7-1	Cas	203
IIM8	Syndrome de Down	
IIM8-1	Cas	204
IIM9	Anomalies congénitales du coeur	
IIM9-1	Cas	205
IIM10	Spina bifida	
IIM10-1	Cas	206
IIN	Affections de la cavité buccale	
IIN1	Caries dentaires	
IIN1-1	Episodes	207
IIN2	Maladie périodontale	
IIN2-1	Episodes	208
IIN3	Edentation	
IIN3-1	Cas	209
III	Traumatismes	
IIIA	Traumatismes non-intentionnels	
IIIA1	Accidents de la voie publique	
IIIA1-1	Episodes	210
IIIA1-2	Fracture du crâne – court terme	
IIIA1-3	Fracture du crâne – long terme	211
IIIA1-4	Fracture des os de la face	
IIIA1-5	Fracture de la colonne vertébrale	
IIIA1-6	Lésion de la moelle épinière	212
IIIA1-7	Fracture des côtes ou du sternum	
IIIA1-8	Fracture du bassin	
IIIA1-9	Fracture de la clavicule, de l'omoplate, ou de l'humérus	
IIIA1-10	Fracture du radius ou du cubitus	
IIIA1-11	Fracture des os de la main	
IIIA1-12	Fracture du fémur – court terme	
IIIA1-13	Fracture du fémur – long terme	213
IIIA1-14	Fracture de la rotule, du tibia, ou du péroné	
IIIA1-15	Fracture de la cheville	
IIIA1-16	Fracture des os du pied	
IIIA1-17	Autres dislocations	
IIIA1-18	Dislocation de l'épaule, du coude, ou de la hanche	
IIIA1-19	Fissures	
IIIA1-20	Lésions intra-crâniennes – court terme	214
IIIA1-21	Lésions intra-crâniennes – long terme	215
IIIA1-22	Lésions internes	
IIIA1-23	Plaie ouverte	
IIIA1-24	Lésion du globe oculaire	
IIIA1-25	Amputation du pouce	
IIIA1-26	Amputation d'un doigt	
IIIA1-27	Amputation d'un bras	
IIIA1-28	Amputation d'un orteil	
IIIA1-29	Amputation d'un pied	
IIIA1-30	Amputation d'une jambe	
IIIA1-31	Contusion	
IIIA1-32	Brûlures < 20 % – court terme	

Tableau IV   (suite)

CGM Code de Classification	Groupes de causes, maladie, traumatisme, ou séquelle	Données presentées dans ce volume (numéro du tableau)
IIIA1-33	Brûlures < 20 % – long terme	
IIIA1-34	Brûlures > 20 % et <60% – court terme	
IIIA1-35	Brûlures > 20 % et <60% – long terme	
IIIA1-36	Brûlures > 60 % – court terme	
IIIA1-37	Brûlures > 60 % – long terme	
IIIA1-38	Lésions des nerfs	
IIIA1-39	Empoisonnement	
IIIA1-40	Résiduel	
IIIA2	Empoisonnements	
IIIA2-1	Episodes	216
IIIA3	Chutes	
IIIA3-1	Episodes	217
IIIA3-2	Fracture du crâne – court terme	
IIIA3-3	Fracture du crâne – long terme	218
IIIA3-4	Fracture des os de la face	
IIIA3-5	Fracture de la colonne vertébrale	
IIIA3-6	Lésion de la moelle épinière	219
IIIA3-7	Fracture des côtes ou du sternum	
IIIA3-8	Fracture du bassin	
IIIA3-9	Fracture de la clavicule, de l'omoplate, ou de l'humérus	
IIIA3-10	Fracture du radius ou du cubitus	
IIIA3-11	Fracture des os de la main	
IIIA3-12	Fracture du fémur – court terme	220
IIIA3-13	Fracture du fémur – long terme	221
IIIA3-14	Fracture de la rotule, du tibia, ou du péroné	
IIIA3-15	Fracture de la cheville	
IIIA3-16	Fracture des os du pied	
IIIA3-17	Autres dislocations	
IIIA3-18	Dislocation de l'épaule, du coude, ou de la hanche	
IIIA3-19	Fissures	
IIIA3-20	Lésions intra-crâniennes – court terme	
IIIA3-21	Lésions intra-crâniennes – long terme	222
IIIA3-22	Lésions internes	
IIIA3-23	Plaie ouverte	
IIIA3-24	Lésion du globe oculaire	
IIIA3-25	Amputation du pouce	
IIIA3-26	Amputation d'un doigt	
IIIA3-27	Amputation d'un bras	
IIIA3-28	Amputation d'un orteil	
IIIA3-29	Amputation d'un pied	
IIIA3-30	Amputation d'une jambe	
IIIA3-31	Contusion	
IIIA3-32	Brûlures < 20 % – court terme	
IIIA3-33	Brûlures < 20 % – long terme	
IIIA3-34	Brûlures > 20 % et < 60% – court terme	
IIIA3-35	Brûlures > 20 % et < 60% – long terme	
IIIA3-36	Brûlures > 60 % – court terme	
IIIA3-37	Brûlures > 60 % – long terme	
IIIA3-38	Lésions des nerfs	
IIIA3-39	Empoisonnement	
IIIA4-40	Résiduel	

Tableau IV (suite)

CGM Code de Classification	Groupes de causes, maladie, traumatisme, ou séquelle	Données presentées dans ce volume (numéro du tableau)
IIIA4	Incendies	
IIIA4-1	Episodes	223
IIIA4-2	Fracture du crâne – court terme	
IIIA4-3	Fracture du crâne – long terme	
IIIA4-4	Fracture des os de la face	
IIIA4-5	Fracture de la colonne vertébrale	
IIIA4-6	Lésion de la moelle épinière	224
IIIA4-7	Fracture des côtes ou du sternum	
IIIA4-8	Fracture du bassin	
IIIA4-9	Fracture de la clavicule, de l'omoplate, ou de l'humérus	
IIIA4-10	Fracture du radius ou du cubitus	
IIIA4-11	Fracture des os de la main	
IIIA4-12	Fracture du fémur – court terme	
IIIA4-13	Fracture du fémur – long terme	
IIIA4-14	Fracture de la rotule, du tibia, ou du péroné	
IIIA4-15	Fracture de la cheville	
IIIA4-16	Fracture des os du pied	
IIIA4-17	Autres dislocations	
IIIA4-18	Dislocation de l'épaule, du coude, ou de la hanche	
IIIA4-19	Fissures	
IIIA4-20	Lésions intra-crâniennes – court terme	
IIIA4-21	Lésions intra-crâniennes – long terme	
IIIA4-22	Lésions internes	
IIIA4-23	Plaie ouverte	
IIIA4-24	Lésion du globe oculaire	
IIIA4-25	Amputation du pouce	
IIIA4-26	Amputation d'un doigt	
IIIA4-27	Amputation d'un bras	
IIIA4-28	Amputation d'un orteil	
IIIA4-29	Amputation d'un pied	
IIIA4-30	Amputation d'une jambe	
IIIA4-31	Contusion	
IIIA4-32	Brûlures < 20 % – court terme	225
IIIA4-33	Brûlures < 20 % – long terme	226
IIIA4-34	Brûlures > 20 % et < 60% – court terme	227
IIIA4-35	Brûlures > 20 % et < 60% – long terme	228
IIIA4-36	Brûlures > 60 % – court terme	
IIIA4-37	Brûlures > 60 % – long terme	
IIIA4-38	Lésions des nerfs	
IIIA4-39	Empoisonnement	
IIIA4-40	Résiduel	
IIIA5	Noyades	
IIIA5-1	Episodes	229
IIIA5-2	Quadriplégie	230
IIIA6	Autres traumatismes non-intentionnels	
IIIA6-1	Episodes	231
IIIA6-2	Fracture du crâne – court terme	
IIIA6-3	Fracture du crâne – long terme	
IIIA6-4	Fracture des os de la face	
IIIA6-5	Fracture de la colonne vertébrale	
IIIA6-6	Lésion de la moelle épinière	232
IIIA6-7	Fracture des côtes ou du sternum	

Tableau IV (suite)

CGM Code de Classification	Groupes de causes, maladie, traumatisme, ou séquelle	Données presentées dans ce volume (numéro du tableau)
IIIA6-8	Fracture du bassin	
IIIA6-9	Fracture de la clavicule, de l'omoplate, ou de l'humérus	
IIIA6-10	Fracture du radius ou du cubitus	
IIIA6-11	Fracture des os de la main	
IIIA6-12	Fracture du fémur – court terme	
IIIA6-13	Fracture du fémur – long terme	
IIIA6-14	Fracture de la rotule, du tibia, ou du péroné	
IIIA6-15	Fracture de la cheville	
IIIA6-16	Fracture des os du pied	
IIIA6-17	Autres dislocations	
IIIA6-18	Dislocation de l'épaule, du coude, ou de la hanche	
IIIA6-19	Fissures	
IIIA6-20	Lésions intra-crâniennes – court terme	
IIIA6-21	Lésions intra-crâniennes – long terme	233
IIIA6-22	Lésions internes	
IIIA6-23	Plaie ouverte	
IIIA6-24	Lésion du globe oculaire	
IIIA6-25	Amputation du pouce	
IIIA6-26	Amputation d'un doigt	234
IIIA6-27	Amputation d'un bras	
IIIA6-28	Amputation d'un orteil	
IIIA6-29	Amputation d'un pied	
IIIA6-30	Amputation d'une jambe	
IIIA6-31	Contusion	
IIIA6-32	Brûlures < 20 % – court terme	
IIIA6-33	Brûlures < 20 % – long terme	235
IIIA6-34	Brûlures > 20 % et <60% – court terme	
IIIA6-35	Brûlures > 20 % et <60% – long terme	
IIIA6-36	Brûlures > 60 % – court terme	
IIIA6-37	Brûlures > 60 % – long terme	
IIIA6-38	Lésions des nerfs	236
IIIA6-39	Empoisonnement	
IIIA6-40	Résiduel	
IIIB	Traumatismes intentionnels	
IIIB1	Traumatismes auto-infligés	
IIIB1-1	Episodes	237
IIIB1-2	Fracture du crâne – court terme	
IIIB1-3	Fracture du crâne – long terme	
IIIB1-4	Fracture des os de la face	
IIIB1-5	Fracture de la colonne vertébrale	
IIIB1-6	Lésion de la moelle épinière	
IIIB1-7	Fracture des côtes ou du sternum	
IIIB1-8	Fracture du bassin	
IIIB1-9	Fracture de la clavicule, de l'omoplate, ou de l'humérus	
IIIB1-10	Fracture du radius ou du cubitus	
IIIB1-11	Fracture des os de la main	
IIIB1-12	Fracture du fémur – court terme	
IIIB1-13	Fracture du fémur – long terme	
IIIB1-14	Fracture de la rotule, du tibia, ou du péroné	
IIIB1-15	Fracture de la cheville	
IIIB1-16	Fracture des os du pied	
IIIB1-17	Autres dislocations	

Tableau IV (suite)

CGM Code de Classification	Groupes de causes, maladie, traumatisme, ou séquelle	Données presentées dans ce volume (numéro du tableau)
IIIB1-18	Dislocation de l'épaule, du coude, ou de la hanche	
IIIB1-19	Fissures	
IIIB1-20	Lésions intra-crâniennes – court terme	
IIIB1-21	Lésions intra-crâniennes – long terme	
IIIB1-22	Lésions internes	
IIIB1-23	Plaie ouverte	
IIIB1-24	Lésion du globe oculaire	
IIIB1-25	Amputation du pouce	
IIIB1-26	Amputation d'un doigt	
IIIB1-27	Amputation d'un bras	
IIIB1-28	Amputation d'un orteil	
IIIB1-29	Amputation d'un pied	
IIIB1-30	Amputation d'une jambe	
IIIB1-31	Contusion	
IIIB1-32	Brûlures < 20 % – court terme	
IIIB1-33	Brûlures < 20 % – long terme	
IIIB1-34	Brûlures > 20 % et <60% – court terme	
IIIB1-35	Brûlures > 20 % et <60% – long terme	
IIIB1-36	Brûlures > 60 % – court terme	
IIIB1-37	Brûlures > 60 % – long terme	
IIIB1-38	Lésions des nerfs	
IIIB1-39	Empoisonnement	
IIIB1-40	Résiduel	
IIIB2	Violence	
IIIB2-1	Episodes	238
IIIB2-2	Fracture du crâne – court terme	
IIIB2-3	Fracture du crâne – long terme	239
IIIB2-4	Fracture des os de la face	
IIIB2-5	Fracture de la colonne vertébrale	
IIIB2-6	Lésion de la moelle épinière	240
IIIB2-7	Fracture des côtes ou du sternum	
IIIB2-8	Fracture du bassin	
IIIB2-9	Fracture de la clavicule, de l'omoplate, ou de l'humérus	
IIIB2-10	Fracture du radius ou du cubitus	
IIIB2-11	Fracture des os de la main	
IIIB2-12	Fracture du fémur – court terme	
IIIB2-13	Fracture du fémur – long terme	
IIIB2-14	Fracture de la rotule, du tibia, ou du péroné	
IIIB2-15	Fracture de la cheville	
IIIB2-16	Fracture des os du pied	
IIIB2-17	Autres dislocations	
IIIB2-18	Dislocation de l'épaule, du coude, ou de la hanche	
IIIB2-19	Fissures	
IIIB2-20	Lésions intra-crâniennes – court terme	241
IIIB2-21	Lésions intra-crâniennes – long terme	242
IIIB2-22	Lésions internes	
IIIB2-23	Plaie ouverte	
IIIB2-24	Lésion du globe oculaire	
IIIB2-25	Amputation du pouce	
IIIB2-26	Amputation d'un doigt	
IIIB2-27	Amputation d'un bras	
IIIB2-28	Amputation d'un orteil	

Tableau IV   (suite)

CGM Code de Classification		Groupes de causes, maladie, traumatisme, ou séquelle	Données presentées dans ce volume (numéro du tableau)
IIIB2-29		Amputation d'un pied	
IIIB2-30		Amputation d'une jambe	
IIIB2-31		Contusion	
IIIB2-32		Brûlures < 20 % – court terme	
IIIB2-33		Brûlures < 20 % – long terme	
IIIB2-34		Brûlures > 20 % et <60% – court terme	
IIIB2-35		Brûlures > 20 % et <60% – long terme	
IIIB2-36		Brûlures > 60 % – court terme	
IIIB2-37		Brûlures > 60 % – long terme	
IIIB2-38		Lésions des nerfs	243
IIIB2-39		Empoisonnement	
IIIB2-40		Résiduel	
IIIB3	Guerre		
IIIB3-1		Episodes	244
IIIB3-2		Fracture du crâne – court terme	
IIIB3-3		Fracture du crâne – long terme	
IIIB3-4		Fracture des os de la face	
IIIB3-5		Fracture de la colonne vertébrale	
IIIB3-6		Lésion de la moelle épinière	
IIIB3-7		Fracture des côtes ou du sternum	
IIIB3-8		Fracture du bassin	
IIIB3-9		Fracture de la clavicule, de l'omoplate, ou de l'humérus	
IIIB3-10		Fracture du radius ou du cubitus	
IIIB3-11		Fracture des os de la main	
IIIB3-12		Fracture du fémur – court terme	
IIIB3-13		Fracture du fémur – long terme	
IIIB3-14		Fracture de la rotule, du tibia, ou du péroné	
IIIB3-15		Fracture de la cheville	
IIIB3-16		Fracture des os du pied	
IIIB3-17		Autres dislocations	
IIIB3-18		Dislocation de l'épaule, du coude, ou de la hanche	
IIIB3-19		Fissures	
IIIB3-20		Lésions intra-crâniennes – court terme	
IIIB3-21		Lésions intra-crâniennes – long terme	245
IIIB3-22		Lésions internes	
IIIB3-23		Plaie ouverte	
IIIB3-24		Lésion du globe oculaire	
IIIB3-25		Amputation du pouce	
IIIB3-26		Amputation d'un doigt	
IIIB3-27		Amputation d'un bras	246
IIIB3-28		Amputation d'un orteil	
IIIB3-29		Amputation d'un pied	247
IIIB3-30		Amputation d'une jambe	
IIIB3-31		Contusion	
IIIB3-32		Brûlures < 20 % – court terme	
IIIB3-33		Brûlures < 20 % – long terme	248
IIIB3-34		Brûlures > 20 % et <60% – court terme	
IIIB3-35		Brûlures > 20 % et <60% – long terme	
IIIB3-36		Brûlures > 60 % – court terme	
IIIB3-37		Brûlures > 60 % – long terme	
IIIB3-38		Lésions des nerfs	249
IIIB3-39		Empoisonnement	
IIIB3-40		Résiduel	

chacune des huit régions géographiques utilisées pour le *Rapport sur le Développement dans le Monde 1993*, ainsi qu'un tableau résumant les estimations agrégées pour le monde entier. Les données relatives aux différents indicateurs épidémiologiques inclus dans les tableaux représentent les données de base nécessaires au calcul des AVCI pour chaque maladie ou traumatisme. Les véritables estimations AVCI ne sont pas incluses dans les tableaux mais sont présentées sous forme de résumé dans le volume I de cette série, et sont rapportées de manière plus détaillée dans les chapitres spécifiques à chaque maladie et traumatisme dans les volumes suivants de cette série.

Les indicateurs épidémiologiques inclus dans les tableaux ont pour but de fournir l'information essentielle que les décideurs en santé, et d'autres professionnels de santé publique, requièrent pour formuler, exécuter et évaluer des stratégies adéquates pour la prévention et le traitement des maladies et traumatismes. De ce fait les tableaux présentent des données sur la charge actuelle des maladies et traumatismes (en 1990) dans la région, la manière dont la charge des maladies est répartie entre les différents groupes d'âge et entre les sexes masculin et féminin, combien rapidement l'affection augmente (ou diminue), si l'affection se présente tôt ou plus tardivement au cours de la vie, combien de temps en moyenne l'affection persiste, et le nombre de personnes qui décèdent de cette affection dans les différents sous-groupes de la population.

La description qui suit fournit une explication détaillée du format des tableaux. Le nom court de la maladie ou traumatisme est indiqué au haut de chaque page. Le nom de la séquelle est indiqué immédiatement en-dessous du nom de la maladie ou du traumatisme. Trois termes différents sont utilisés de manière répétitive pour décrire certaines séquelles: épisode, cas, et cas symptomatique. Pour les affections diarrhéiques, une seule séquelle est incluse, soit l'épisode de diarrhée lui même. Pour être cohérent, toute atteinte résultant d'une maladie, y compris la manifestation initiale de la maladie ou du traumatisme, est appelée séquelle. Lorsque le terme épisode est utilisé, il indique que nous donnons des estimations d'incidence et de prévalence d'épisodes de la maladie ou du traumatisme. Pour des conditions plus chroniques, nous donnons parfois des estimations de l'incidence et de la prévalence d'individus avec une maladie chronique telle le diabète—ceci est indiqué par le terme cas. Finalement, pour les autres affections tels les BPOC ou les cirrhoses, nous avons donné des estimations d'incidence ou de prévalence d'individus ayant des symptômes de la maladie, appelés cas symptomatiques.

Spécifiquement, le format des tableaux est le suivant:

Année de référence: toutes les estimations se réfèrent à l'année 1990, l'année de base pour l'Etude de la Charge Globale des Maladies. La seule exception est la projection de la mortalité qui est donnée pour l'an 2000.

Variables démographiques: les estimations sont présentées séparément pour le sexe féminin et le sexe masculin au vu de leurs risques très différents de contracter une maladie ou de subir un traumatisme. Les estimations sont d'abord indiquées pour le sexe masculin dans la moitié supérieure de chaque tableau, et ensuite pour le sexe féminin dans la moitié inférieure de chaque tableau. L'âge est peut-être la variable la plus importante dans la description de la distribution des maladies et des traumatismes, du fait que virtuellement toutes les affections rapportées dans ce livre sont très dépendantes de l'âge. Les estimations sont présentées pour cinq grands groupes d'âge qui décrivent approximativement les phases du cycle de vie au cours des desquelles la distribution des maladies et des traumatismes sera probablement similaire. Les estimations sont aussi présentées pour tous les âges combinés, sans aucune tentative de standardisation selon l'âge. Au bas de chaque tableau, les estimations se rapportent à la population totale de la région, comprenant tous les groupes d'âge et combinant les deux sexes.

Incidence: cet indicateur mesure l'apparition de nouveaux cas de maladies ou de traumatismes en 1990. Le *nombre* estimé de nouveaux cas (en milliers) est présenté avec les estimations des taux d'incidence de la région, soit le nombre de nouveaux cas pour une population de 100 000 par an, dans le groupe âge-sexe respectif.

Prévalence: en plus de l'estimation du nombre de nouveaux cas, il est important de pouvoir estimer la charge des maladies ou des traumatismes qui était réellement présente dans chaque région en 1990, soit à la suite de nouveaux cas (incidence) en 1990, ou de cas des années précédentes. L'estimation du *nombre* (en millier) de cas prévalents de la maladie ou du traumatisme en 1990 est indiqué dans le tableau, ainsi que le *taux* de prévalence, exprimé comme le nombre de cas prévalents pour une population de 100 000.

Âge de début moyen: ce paramètre mesure l'âge moyen (en années) auquel de nouveaux cas de maladies ou de traumatismes se produirent en 1990, à l'intérieur de chaque groupe âge-sexe spécifique, et pour tous les âges combinés.

Durée moyenne: une donnée importante pour le calcul des AVCI est la durée moyenne du temps (en années) que les nouveaux cas peuvent s'attendre à passer dans un état de mauvaise santé à la suite d'une maladie ou d'un traumatisme. Ces durées moyennes de maladie ont été calculées pour chaque groupe d'âge spécifique, et pour tous les âges combinés (sans pondération). La durée est mesurée comme le temps entre le début d'une maladie ou d'un traumatisme et l'absence de cette affection, soit après rémission, soit à la suite de décès.

Décès: la mortalité estimée à la suite de chaque cause est présentée en quatre colonnes, et pour deux périodes temporelles. Tout d'abord le nombre estimé de décès en 1990 (en milliers), à l'intérieur de chacun des groupes âge-sexe, est indiqué ainsi que le taux de mortalité âge-sexe-spécifique pour la région (exprimé pour une population 100 000). Finalement le nombre de décès *projetés* à l'an 2000, et les taux de mortalité pour 100 000 *projetés* à la même année, ont été inclus dans le cadre à l'extrême droite de chaque tableau. Ces projections sont basées sur les méthodes et suppositions décrites plus haut, et sont incluses pour donner une perspective d'avenir du profil épidémiologique probable d'ici à la fin du siècle.

DISCUSSION

Il est nécessaire de décrire en détail, et avec un certain degré de confiance, l'état de santé des populations, que ce soit pour mieux suivre la progression du développement de la santé, pour informer le débat au sujet des politiques de santé, pour la recherche, ou à vrai dire, pour de nombreux autres buts de santé publique. Ce livre essaie de répondre à ce besoin. Les estimations et projections présentées ici sont délibérément ambitieuses et étendues: plus de 200 conditions ont été révisées, des estimations ont été préparées pour chaque sexe séparément, pour cinq grands groupes d'âge, et pour les différents indicateurs épidémiologiques majeurs couramment utilisés pour décrire l'état de santé. A ce régard, le livre apporte un compendium de données, pour les régions géographiques majeures du monde, qui devrait aider à informer le travail de ceux qui s'intéressent à améliorer la santé publique.

Grâce à l'application d'un modèle sophistiqué de l'occurence des maladies, de leur prévalence, de leur létalité, et de leur rémission, les estimations présentées ici pour chaque maladie et traumatisme sont à la fois compatibles entre elles, et compatibles avec ce qui est connu de leur histoire naturelle. D'autre part la *fiabilité* des estimations est très variable et nécessite un usage prudent. En appliquant plusieures méthodes et approches différentes nous avons essayé de confirmer la plausibilité des estimations. Toutefois, aucun degré de rigueur méthodologique ne peut compenser l'extrêmement mauvaise qualité de certaines données et le manque d'informations épidémiologiques auquel nous avons souvent été confrontés lors de la préparation de ces chiffres. Pour de grandes *populations,* y compris une grande partie de l'Afrique sub-saharienne, de l'Inde, des APAI et pour certaines parties d'ALC, il n'y a que très peu de connaissances fiables au sujet des causes de décès, ou à vrai dire, au sujet de l'incidence, de la prévalence et de la durée des maladies. Pour ces régions aucun degré de manipulation épidémiologique, extrapolation ou supposition, ne peut changer le fait que les estimations épidémiologiques rapportées ici sont imprécises. Pour d'autres régions, davantage de données sont disponibles et le degré de confiance dans les estimations est proportionnellement plus grand, bien que, même pour les régions industrialisées, les différences existant au niveau du diagnostic et de la codification entre les différents pays jettent un doute sur la fiabilité des estimations pour certaines conditions spécifiques.

Plutôt que de limiter cette évaluation aux régions et conditions pour lesquelles nous avions d'assez bonnes données pour nos estimations, nous avons opté pour la préparation d'estimations réellement globales et, à notre avis exhaustives, de l'état de santé en 1990 et au delà. Nous avons fait ce choix tout en connaissant le degré substantiel d'incertitude sous-jacent à de nombreuses estimations. Nous sommes aussi conscient qu'une évaluation globale de cette nature sera utilisée avec un degré de confiance beaucoup plus élevé que les données sous-jacentes ne le justifient, ceci en dépit de tous les avertissements exprimés (et non exprimés). Ceci est inévitable étant donné le besoin d'une telle évaluation. La disponibilité des estimations ne devrait toutefois pas détracter du besoin urgent d'améliorer les systèmes d'information épidémiologique dans la plupart des pays, afin de permettre que l'évaluation et le suivi de l'état de santé soient faits avec une plus grande fiabilité, et que les politiques de développement dans le domaine de la santé deviennent plus effectives.

L'une des conséquences d'un renfort des systèmes nationaux de statistiques en santé serait d'augmenter la fiabilité des évaluations globales de ce type dans le futur et, de ce fait, leur utilité. Dans l'intervalle, nous espérons que les estimations et projections présentées ici seront utilisées, revues de façon critique, et en son temps, révisées à partir de ces revues et critiques. Ayant le choix entre des estimations épidémiologiques partielles mais plus sûres et l'incertitude des estimations globales présentées ici, nous avons opté pour cette dernière, trouvant quelque consolation dans la remarque de Greenwood disant que: «Faisant du mieux l'ennemi du bien est un sûr moyen d'empêcher tout progrès statistique. Le puriste scientifique qui attendra jusqu'à ce qu'il obtienne des statistiques médicales nosologiquement exactes, n'est pas plus sage que l'attente d'Horace que la rivière s'en aille».

NOTES

1. Dans les versions antérieures de l'Etude de la Charge Globale des Maladies, les carences nutritionnelles, à savoir la malnutrition protéino-calorique, la déficience en vitamine A, les troubles liés à la déficience en iode et les anémies étaient incluses dans le Groupe II. Ces conditions remplissent les critères définissant le groupe pré-transitionnel dans le Groupe I. Elles n'avaient toutefois pas été incluses dans le Groupe I dans les versions antérieures du fait de la difficulté inhérente à distinguer certains de ces décès des décès dûs à d'autres causes nutritionnelles et endocrines à partir des bases de données alors disponibles. Des efforts beaucoup plus importants ont été fournis pour l'analyse de ces conditions dans cette cinquième et dernière version de l'étude, permettant le transfert de ces causes dans le Groupe I.

2. Les décès inclus dans le chapitre XVI ont été redistribués proportionnellement à toutes les causes du Groupe I en-dessous de l'âge de 5 ans et, au-dessus de 5 ans, à toutes les causes du Groupe II. Des algorithmes spécifiques ont été développés pour traiter la codification imprécise des décès de causes cardiovasculaires, tels que ceux attribués à l'insuffisance cardiaque ainsi que les décès mal définis attribués aux traumatismes intentionnels et non-intentionnels.

3. Le nombre de décès a été légèrement modifié pour certaines régions par rapport à celui rapporté dans le *Rapport sur le Développement dans le Monde 1993*, ceci afin de prendre en compte le haut niveau de mortalité survenu à la suite de guerres autour de 1990 dans certaines régions. A notre avis, les méthodes

d'estimation à partir desquelles les évaluations démographiques ont été faites ne tenaient pas compte de la mortalité due aux guerres de manière adéquate.

4. Les modèles des causes de décès utilisés dans des versions antérieures de l'Etude de la Charge Globale des Maladies et ne sont pas exactement les mêmes que ceux présentés ici pour la Version 5. Bien que la forme fonctionnelle des deux ensembles de modèles soient similaires, les résultats spécifiques diffèrent en raison de l'addition de données plus récentes et du raffinement des procédures d'estimation décrites dans Murray et Lopez (1996b).

5. L'analyse de l'Afrique du Sud a été basée en grande partie sur le travail de Stephen Hendrix, que nous remercions de nous avoir donné accès à son travail avant qu'il ne soit publié.

6. Afin d'assurer la cohérence interne entre les différentes estimations épidémiologiques présentées dans ce volume, nous avons développé un programme de computer, DISMOD, qui formalise la relation entre l'incidence, la rémission, le taux de létalité et la prévalence. On assume que les personnes susceptibles dans la population contractent une maladie ou une invalidité à un taux i et meurent à un taux de mortalité générale m. Les cas de maladie peuvent, soit entrer en rémission au taux r, soit décéder de causes générales au même taux m que les susceptibles, soit décéder de mortalité cause-spécifique au taux f. DISMOD utilise la méthode des différences limitées pour résoudre l'ensemble des équations différentielles linéaires définies par ces relations.

7. Les taux de cancers du poumon chez des non-fumeurs pour toutes les régions sauf la Chine et les APAI sont supposés être les mêmes que les taux de cancers du poumon relevés dans l'enquête CPS-II aux Etats Unis. Pour la Chine et les APAI, le taux de cancers du poumon chez les femmes non-fumeuses est supposé être considérablement plus élevé, comme l'indique les résultats de plusieures études épidémiologiques (Murray et Lopez 1996a).

DEMOGRAPHIC TABLES

Table 1
Distribution of population
and deaths by age and sex
1990

Cuadro 1
Distribución de la población
y de las muertes por edad y sexo
1990

Tableau 1
Distribution de la population et
des décès selon l'âge et le sexe
1990

EME

PEMC

EMBE

Age group	Males			Females			Both Sexes		
	Population	Deaths	Death rates	Population	Deaths	Death rates	Population	Deaths	Death rates
(years)	('000s)	('000s)	(per 100 000)	('000s)	('000s)	(per 100 000)	('000s)	('000s)	(per 100 000)
Five-year age groups									
0-4	26 384	60	228	25 065	45	181	51 449	105	205
5-9	26 490	7	26	25 167	5	19	51 657	12	23
10-14	26 858	7	26	25 513	4	15	52 371	11	21
15-19	29 308	28	95	27 883	10	36	57 191	38	67
20-24	31 495	41	130	30 160	13	43	61 655	54	88
25-29	32 904	45	137	31 980	16	50	64 884	61	94
30-34	31 371	50	160	30 754	21	68	62 125	71	114
35-39	29 951	60	201	29 585	28	94	59 536	88	148
40-44	29 034	76	263	28 837	39	134	57 871	115	199
45-49	24 136	100	415	24 252	53	218	48 388	153	316
50-54	21 908	145	663	22 397	77	343	44 305	222	501
55-59	20 095	222	1 106	21 150	114	538	41 245	336	815
60-64	18 613	325	1 746	20 807	179	860	39 420	504	1 278
65-69	15 555	417	2 680	19 721	269	1 363	35 276	686	1 944
70-74	10 655	449	4 213	14 831	337	2 271	25 486	786	3 083
75+	15 725	1 627	10 344	29 206	2 253	7 714	44 931	3 880	8 634
Total	390 482	3 659	937	407 308	3 462	850	797 790	7 121	893
GBD standard age groups									
0-4	26 384	60	228	25 065	45	181	51 449	105	205
5-14	53 348	14	26	50 680	9	17	104 028	23	22
15-44	184 063	300	163	179 199	127	71	363 262	427	118
45-59	66 139	468	707	67 799	244	359	133 938	711	531
60+	60 548	2 817	4 653	84 565	3 037	3 592	145 113	5 855	4 035
Total	390 482	3 659	937	407 308	3 462	850	797 790	7 121	893

Table 2
Distribution of population
and deaths by age and sex
1990

Cuadro 2
Distribución de la población
y de las muertes por edad y sexo
1990

Tableau 2
Distribution de la population et
des décès selon l'âge et le sexe
1990

FSE

PEAS

AESE

Age group	Males			Females			Both Sexes		
	Population	Deaths	Death rates	Population	Deaths	Death rates	Population	Deaths	Death rates
(years)	('000s)	('000s)	(per 100 000)	('000s)	('000s)	(per 100 000)	('000s)	('000s)	(per 100 000)
Five-year age groups									
0-4	13 759	66	479	13 135	48	366	26 894	114	424
5-9	13 744	9	65	13 343	5	39	27 087	14	52
10-14	13 605	8	57	13 078	4	32	26 683	12	45
15-19	12 702	17	137	12 251	8	68	24 953	26	103
20-24	12 055	27	226	11 528	8	72	23 583	35	150
25-29	11 512	39	340	11 203	11	95	22 715	50	219
30-34	13 826	49	352	13 575	15	107	27 401	63	231
35-39	13 895	61	438	13 869	20	142	27 764	81	290
40-44	12 288	65	528	12 533	24	190	24 821	89	357
45-49	8 591	88	1 020	9 033	33	365	17 624	121	684
50-54	8 848	148	1 677	9 877	61	617	18 725	209	1 118
55-59	9 534	184	1 932	11 096	86	774	20 630	270	1 309
60-64	7 850	244	3 109	10 041	145	1 444	17 891	389	2 175
65-69	6 356	196	3 088	10 089	175	1 733	16 445	371	2 256
70-74	2 833	167	5 912	5 920	198	3 336	8 753	365	4 170
75+	3 924	539	13 744	10 344	1 043	10 084	14 268	1 582	11 090
Total	165 322	1 908	1 154	180 915	1 883	1 041	346 237	3 791	1 095
GBD standard age groups									
0-4	13 759	66	479	13 135	48	366	26 894	114	424
5-14	27 349	17	61	26 421	9	36	53 770	26	49
15-44	76 278	258	338	74 959	85	114	151 237	343	227
45-59	26 973	420	1 558	30 006	180	599	56 979	600	1 053
60+	20 963	1 147	5 472	36 394	1 560	4 287	57 357	2 708	4 720
Total	165 322	1 908	1 154	242 739	1 883	776	408 061	3 791	929

Table 3
Distribution of population
and deaths by age and sex
1990

IND

Cuadro 3
Distribución de la población
y de las muertes por edad y sexo
1990

IND

Tableau 3
Distribution de la population et
des décès selon l'âge et le sexe
1990

IND

| Age group | Males | | | Females | | | Both Sexes | | |
(years)	Population ('000s)	Deaths ('000s)	Death rates (per 100 000)	Population ('000s)	Deaths ('000s)	Death rates (per 100 000)	Population ('000s)	Deaths ('000s)	Death rates (per 100 000)
Five-year age groups									
0-4	59 789	1 600	2 676	56 679	1 650	2 911	116 468	3 250	2 790
5-9	54 590	171	313	51 318	194	378	105 908	365	345
10-14	47 162	85	180	43 945	100	228	91 107	185	203
15-19	45 014	78	173	41 427	102	246	86 441	180	208
20-24	40 573	86	212	37 156	108	291	77 729	194	250
25-29	35 892	87	242	32 705	96	294	68 597	183	267
30-34	31 387	94	299	28 350	87	307	59 737	181	303
35-39	26 281	114	434	23 678	84	355	49 959	198	396
40-44	21 378	135	631	19 926	90	452	41 304	225	545
45-49	18 075	167	924	17 359	114	657	35 434	281	793
50-54	15 837	217	1 370	15 419	156	1 012	31 256	373	1 193
55-59	13 655	281	2 058	13 227	209	1 580	26 882	490	1 823
60-64	10 974	348	3 171	10 577	263	2 487	21 551	611	2 835
65-69	8 172	390	4 772	7 928	306	3 860	16 100	696	4 323
70-74	5 536	386	6 973	5 437	326	5 996	10 973	712	6 489
75+	5 086	636	12 505	4 982	611	12 264	10 068	1 247	12 386
Total	439 401	4 875	1 109	410 113	4 496	1 096	849 514	9 371	1 103
GBD standard age groups									
0-4	59 789	1 600	2 676	56 679	1 650	2 911	116 468	3 250	2 790
5-14	101 752	256	252	95 263	294	309	197 015	550	279
15-44	200 525	594	296	183 242	567	309	383 767	1 161	303
45-59	47 567	665	1 398	46 005	479	1 041	93 572	1 144	1 223
60+	29 768	1 760	5 912	28 924	1 506	5 207	58 692	3 266	5 565
Total	439 401	4 875	1 109	410 113	4 496	1 096	849 514	9 371	1 103

Table 4
Distribution of population
and deaths by age and sex
1990

CHN

Cuadro 4
Distribución de la población
y de las muertes por edad y sexo
1990

CHN

Tableau 4
Distribution de la population et
des décès selon l'âge et le sexe
1990

CHN

	Males			Females			Both Sexes		
Age group	Population	Deaths	Death rates	Population	Deaths	Death rates	Population	Deaths	Death rates
(years)	('000s)	('000s)	(per 100 000)	('000s)	('000s)	(per 100 000)	('000s)	('000s)	(per 100 000)
Five-year age groups									
0-4	60 243	505	838	57 946	565	975	118 189	1 070	905
5-9	47 467	47	99	44 152	34	77	91 619	81	88
10-14	49 530	39	79	46 249	29	63	95 779	68	71
15-19	63 349	81	128	59 405	67	113	122 754	148	121
20 24	65 728	109	166	61 412	93	151	127 140	202	159
25-29	55 048	89	162	50 757	71	140	105 805	160	151
30-34	43 876	97	221	40 380	68	168	84 256	165	196
35-39	44 901	122	273	41 906	81	193	86 807	203	234
40-44	33 403	127	382	30 218	84	278	63 621	211	332
45-49	26 191	157	599	23 083	100	433	49 274	257	522
50-54	24 345	238	978	21 391	148	692	45 736	386	844
55-59	22 138	351	1 586	19 929	214	1 074	42 067	565	1 343
60-64	17 908	479	2 675	16 619	300	1 805	34 527	779	2 256
65-69	13 518	582	4 305	13 521	395	2 921	27 039	977	3 613
70-74	9 089	640	7 041	9 973	501	5 024	19 062	1 141	5 986
75+	8 465	1 165	13 763	11 553	1 306	11 304	20 018	2 471	12 344
Total	585 199	4 829	825	548 494	4 056	739	1 133 693	8 885	784
GBD standard age groups									
0-4	60 243	505	838	57 946	565	975	118 189	1 070	905
5-14	96 997	86	89	90 401	63	70	187 398	149	80
15-44	306 305	626	204	284 078	464	163	590 383	1 090	185
45-59	72 674	746	1 027	64 403	462	717	137 077	1 208	881
60+	48 980	2 866	5 851	51 666	2 502	4 843	100 646	5 368	5 334
Total	585 199	4 829	825	548 494	4 056	739	1 133 693	8 885	784

Table 5
Distribution of population
and deaths by age and sex
1990

OAI

Cuadro 5
Distribución de la población
y de las muertes por edad y sexo
1990

OPAI

Tableau 5
Distribution de la population et
des décès selon l'âge et le sexe
1990

APIA

Age group	Males			Females			Both Sexes		
	Population	Deaths	Death rates	Population	Deaths	Death rates	Population	Deaths	Death rates
(years)	('000s)	('000s)	(per 100 000)	('000s)	('000s)	(per 100 000)	('000s)	('000s)	(per 100 000)
Five-year age groups									
0-4	43 763	901	2 058	41 988	716	1 704	85 751	1 616	1 885
5-9	43 939	173	393	42 061	123	293	86 000	296	344
10-14	40 093	57	143	38 156	48	126	78 249	105	135
15-19	37 037	60	162	35 601	46	128	72 638	106	146
20-24	33 033	71	216	32 762	51	155	65 795	122	185
25-29	29 141	77	265	29 675	62	209	58 816	139	237
30-34	25 268	78	307	25 630	60	236	50 898	138	271
35-39	20 686	83	399	20 361	59	292	41 047	142	346
40-44	15 660	88	560	15 582	64	413	31 242	152	487
45-49	13 168	105	798	13 358	73	547	26 526	178	672
50-54	11 647	131	1 126	11 913	92	773	23 560	223	948
55-59	9 323	162	1 740	9 819	113	1 152	19 142	275	1 438
60-64	7 768	203	2 615	8 091	143	1 769	15 859	346	2 183
65-69	5 338	218	4 086	5 920	171	2 891	11 258	389	3 457
70-74	3 603	210	5 829	4 112	178	4 329	7 715	388	5 030
75+	3 499	427	12 205	4 539	490	10 797	8 038	917	11 410
Total	342 966	3 044	887	339 568	2 490	733	682 534	5 534	811
GBD standard age groups									
0-4	43 763	901	2 058	41 988	716	1 704	85 751	1 616	1 885
5-14	84 032	230	274	80 217	172	214	164 249	402	244
15-44	160 825	456	284	159 611	343	215	320 436	799	249
45-59	34 138	398	1 167	35 090	278	793	69 228	677	978
60+	20 208	1 058	5 237	22 662	982	4 335	42 870	2 041	4 760
Total	342 966	3 044	887	339 568	2 490	733	682 534	5 534	811

Table 6
Distribution of population and deaths by age and sex 1990

Cuadro 6
Distribución de la población y de las muertes por edad y sexo 1990

Tableau 6
Distribution de la population et des décès selon l'âge et le sexe 1990

SSA   ASS   ASS

Age group	Males			Females			Both Sexes		
	Population	Deaths	Death rates	Population	Deaths	Death rates	Population	Deaths	Death rates
(years)	('000s)	('000s)	(per 100 000)	('000s)	('000s)	(per 100 000)	('000s)	('000s)	(per 100 000)
Five-year age groups									
0-4	47 484	2 169	4 568	47 030	1 861	3 957	94 514	4 030	4 264
5-9	38 434	252	655	38 146	231	606	76 580	483	630
10-14	31 824	134	420	31 672	124	391	63 496	257	405
15-19	26 555	145	546	26 619	122	460	53 174	267	503
20-24	22 212	159	716	22 465	124	550	44 677	283	632
25-29	18 045	150	830	18 342	121	661	36 387	271	745
30-34	14 858	124	836	15 383	110	712	30 241	234	773
35-39	12 075	115	956	12 721	105	827	24 796	221	890
40-44	10 019	113	1 131	10 727	100	931	20 746	213	1 027
45-49	8 210	108	1 310	8 825	91	1 028	17 035	198	1 164
50-54	6 771	113	1 664	7 377	94	1 271	14 148	206	1 459
55-59	5 327	120	2 250	5 915	104	1 757	11 242	224	1 991
60-64	4 111	128	3 113	4 655	120	2 576	8 766	248	2 828
65-69	2 910	134	4 607	3 468	135	3 897	6 378	269	4 221
70-74	1 880	128	6 834	2 346	141	6 029	4 226	270	6 387
75+	1 607	232	14 429	2 261	296	13 088	3 868	528	13 645
Total	252 322	4 324	1 714	257 952	3 878	1 504	510 274	8 202	1 607
GBD standard age groups									
0-4	47 484	2 169	4 568	47 030	1 861	3 957	94 514	4 030	4 264
5-14	70 258	385	548	69 818	355	508	140 076	740	528
15-44	103 764	807	778	106 257	682	642	210 021	1 489	709
45-59	20 308	340	1 675	22 117	288	1 304	42 425	629	1 481
60+	10 508	622	5 923	12 730	692	5 439	23 238	1 315	5 658
Total	252 322	4 324	1 714	257 952	3 878	1 504	510 274	8 202	1 607

Table 7
Distribution of population
and deaths by age and sex
1990

Cuadro 7
Distribución de la población
y de las muertes por edad y sexo
1990

Tableau 7
Distribution de la population et
des décès selon l'âge et le sexe
1990

LAC   ALC   ALC

	Males			Females			Both Sexes		
Age group	Population	Deaths	Death rates	Population	Deaths	Death rates	Population	Deaths	Death rates
(years)	('000s)	('000s)	(per 100 000)	('000s)	('000s)	(per 100 000)	('000s)	('000s)	(per 100 000)
Five-year age groups									
0-4	28 721	403	1 402	27 676	306	1 105	56 397	708	1 256
5-9	27 072	40	146	26 295	30	116	53 367	70	131
10-14	25 052	33	134	24 449	24	99	49 501	58	117
15-19	23 583	44	187	23 100	29	125	46 683	73	156
20-24	21 382	54	255	21 040	34	161	42 422	88	208
25-29	19 126	55	290	19 078	36	189	38 204	92	240
30-34	15 956	54	336	16 105	35	220	32 061	89	278
35-39	13 432	55	407	13 687	36	266	27 119	91	336
40-44	10 807	59	543	11 075	41	366	21 882	99	454
45-49	8 801	64	729	9 091	47	518	17 892	111	622
50-54	7 360	75	1 021	7 723	56	727	15 083	131	870
55-59	6 088	88	1 449	6 541	67	1 026	12 629	155	1 230
60-64	5 016	103	2 056	5 526	81	1 468	10 542	184	1 748
65-69	3 773	115	3 052	4 327	95	2 199	8 100	210	2 596
70-74	2 580	121	4 691	3 109	109	3 507	5 689	230	4 044
75+	2 862	290	10 135	3 862	328	8 495	6 724	618	9 193
Total	221 611	1 654	746	222 684	1 355	609	444 295	3 009	677
GBD standard age groups									
0-4	28 721	403	1 402	27 676	306	1 105	56 397	708	1 256
5-14	52 124	73	140	50 744	55	108	102 868	128	124
15-44	104 286	321	308	104 085	211	203	208 371	532	256
45-59	22 249	228	1 023	23 355	170	729	45 604	398	872
60+	14 231	629	4 422	16 824	613	3 646	31 055	1 243	4 002
Total	221 611	1 654	746	222 684	1 355	609	444 295	3 009	677

Table 8
**Distribution of population
and deaths by age and sex
1990**

Cuadro 8
**Distribución de la población
y de las muertes por edad y sexo
1990**

Tableau 8
**Distribution de la population et
des décès selon l'âge et le sexe
1990**

MEC   **AOM**   **CMO**

	Males			Females			Both Sexes		
Age group	Population	Deaths	Death rates	Population	Deaths	Death rates	Population	Deaths	Death rates
(years)	('000s)	('000s)	(per 100 000)	('000s)	('000s)	(per 100 000)	('000s)	('000s)	(per 100 000)
Five-year age groups									
0-4	41 161	955	2 320	39 734	908	2 285	80 895	1 863	2 303
5-9	35 057	115	329	33 510	103	307	68 567	218	319
10-14	30 288	43	141	28 489	38	133	58 777	81	137
15-19	26 617	51	190	25 044	44	175	51 661	94	183
20-24	23 464	56	238	21 986	46	211	45 450	102	225
25-29	20 120	59	291	19 091	45	236	39 211	104	264
30-34	17 880	49	275	16 688	41	243	34 568	90	260
35-39	14 789	54	364	13 887	39	284	28 676	93	325
40-44	11 025	60	540	10 515	41	386	21 540	100	465
45-49	8 339	62	747	8 191	42	511	16 530	104	630
50-54	7 437	82	1 098	7 477	56	750	14 914	138	924
55-59	6 561	108	1 649	6 624	74	1 124	13 185	183	1 386
60-64	5 205	128	2 463	5 502	94	1 711	10 707	222	2 077
65-69	3 749	141	3 770	4 083	114	2 802	7 832	256	3 265
70-74	2 278	140	6 158	2 681	130	4 858	4 959	271	5 455
75+	2 419	297	12 260	3 184	338	10 604	5 603	634	11 319
Total	256 389	2 399	936	246 686	2 154	873	503 075	4 553	905
GBD standard age groups									
0-4	41 161	955	2 320	39 734	908	2 285	80 895	1 863	2 303
5-14	65 345	158	242	61 999	141	227	127 344	299	235
15-44	113 895	328	288	107 211	256	239	221 106	584	264
45-59	22 337	252	1 129	22 292	172	773	44 629	425	951
60+	13 651	706	5 175	15 450	676	4 378	29 101	1 383	4 752
Total	256 389	2 399	936	246 686	2 154	873	503 075	4 553	905

Table 9
Distribution of population
and deaths by age and sex
1990

Cuadro 9
Distribución de la población
y de las muertes por edad y sexo
1990

Tableau 9
Distribution de la population et
des décès selon l'âge et le sexe
1990

World   Mundo   Monde

| Age group | Males | | | Females | | | Both Sexes | | |
| | Population | Deaths | Death rates | Population | Deaths | Death rates | Population | Deaths | Death rates |
(years)	('000s)	('000s)	(per 100 000)	('000s)	('000s)	(per 100 000)	('000s)	('000s)	(per 100 000)
Five-year age groups									
0-4	321 304	6 658	2 072	309 253	6 099	1 972	630 557	12 757	2 023
5-9	286 793	813	284	273 992	726	265	560 785	1 539	274
10-14	264 412	406	153	251 551	371	148	515 963	777	151
15-19	264 165	504	191	251 330	428	170	515 495	932	181
20-24	249 942	604	242	238 509	477	200	488 451	1 081	221
25-29	221 788	601	271	212 831	458	215	434 619	1 059	244
30-34	194 422	595	306	186 865	436	233	381 287	1 031	270
35-39	176 010	664	377	169 694	453	267	345 704	1 117	323
40-44	143 614	723	503	139 413	482	346	283 027	1 205	426
45-49	115 511	851	737	113 192	553	488	228 703	1 403	614
50-54	104 153	1 149	1 103	103 574	740	714	207 727	1 889	909
55-59	92 721	1 517	1 636	94 301	981	1 041	187 022	2 498	1 336
60-64	77 445	1 958	2 529	81 818	1 325	1 620	159 263	3 284	2 062
65-69	59 371	2 194	3 695	69 057	1 660	2 404	128 428	3 854	3 001
70-74	38 454	2 242	5 831	48 409	1 920	3 966	86 863	4 162	4 792
75+	43 587	5 212	11 959	69 931	6 665	9 530	113 518	11 877	10 463
Total	2 653 692	26 692	1 006	2 613 720	23 775	910	5 267 412	50 467	958
GBD standard age groups									
0-4	321 304	6 658	2 072	309 253	6 099	1 972	630 557	12 757	2 023
5-14	551 205	1 219	221	525 543	1 097	209	1 076 748	2 316	215
15-44	1 249 941	3 691	295	1 198 642	2 734	228	2 448 583	6 425	262
45-59	312 385	3 517	1 126	311 067	2 274	731	623 452	5 791	929
60+	218 857	11 607	5 303	269 215	11 570	4 298	488 072	23 177	4 749
Total	2 653 692	26 692	1 006	2 613 720	23 775	910	5 267 412	50 467	958

Epidemiological Tables

Table 10
Tuberculosis

Cuadro 10
Tuberculosis

Tableau 10
Tuberculose

HIV sero-negative cases   Casos sero-negativos para VIH   Cas séro-négatifs pour VIH

Table 10a   EME - PEMC - EMBE   Tuberculosis - HIV sero-negative cases

Age group (years)	Incidence 1990 Number ('000s)	Rate (per 100 000)	Prevalence 1990 Number ('000s)	Rate (per 100 000)	Avg. age at onset (years)	Average duration (years)	Deaths 1990 Number ('000s)	Rate (per 100 000)	Deaths 2000 (Projected) Number ('000s)	Rate (per 100 000)
Males										
0-4	1	3.4	0	0.8	2.5	0.25	0	0.0	0	0.0
5-14	1	2.4	0	0.6	10.0	0.25	0	0.0	0	0.0
15-44	40	21.6	10	5.4	29.9	0.25	1	0.4	0	0.2
45-59	28	41.8	7	10.4	52.4	0.25	2	2.4	1	1.5
60+	35	57.5	9	14.4	71.1	0.25	8	12.6	8	11.2
All ages	104	26.7	26	6.7	49.1	0.25	10	2.6	10	2.4
Females										
0-4	1	3.1	0	0.8	2.5	0.25	0	0.0	0	0.0
5-14	2	3.3	0	0.8	10.0	0.25	0	0.0	0	0.0
15-44	18	10.0	4	2.5	30.0	0.25	0	0.1	0	0.1
45-59	9	12.8	2	3.2	52.4	0.25	0	0.7	0	0.4
60+	18	21.5	5	5.3	72.4	0.25	4	4.6	4	4.1
All ages	47	11.6	12	2.9	49.3	0.25	5	1.1	4	1.0
Total	152	19.0	38	4.7	49.2	0.25	15	1.8	14	1.7

Table 10b   FSE - PEAS - AESE   Tuberculosis - HIV sero-negative cases

Age group (years)	Incidence 1990 Number ('000s)	Rate (per 100 000)	Prevalence 1990 Number ('000s)	Rate (per 100 000)	Avg. age at onset (years)	Average duration (years)	Deaths 1990 Number ('000s)	Rate (per 100 000)	Deaths 2000 (Projected) Number ('000s)	Rate (per 100 000)
Males										
0-4	1	6.0	0	2.8	2.5	0.50	0	0.5	0	0.4
5-14	1	4.7	1	2.4	10.0	0.50	0	0.0	0	0.0
15-44	64	84.4	32	41.7	29.8	0.50	6	7.5	3	4.3
45-59	32	119.0	16	59.4	52.2	0.50	7	27.4	6	18.0
60+	18	84.7	9	43.9	70.0	0.50	6	28.2	6	22.7
All ages	116	70.4	58	35.1	41.7	0.50	19	11.6	15	8.6
Females										
0-4	1	5.5	0	2.6	2.5	0.50	0	0.3	0	0.2
5-14	3	12.0	2	5.9	10.0	0.50	0	0.1	0	0.1
15-44	26	34.4	13	17.1	29.9	0.50	1	1.0	0	0.5
45-59	6	19.9	3	10.2	52.4	0.50	1	2.8	1	1.8
60+	11	29.4	5	14.9	71.5	0.50	2	6.3	2	5.4
All ages	46	25.6	23	12.8	40.6	0.50	4	2.2	3	1.7
Total	163	47.0	81	23.5	41.4	0.50	23	6.7	18	5.0

Table 10c   India - India - Inde   Tuberculosis - HIV sero-negative cases

Age group (years)	Incidence 1990 Number ('000s)	Rate (per 100 000)	Prevalence 1990 Number ('000s)	Rate (per 100 000)	Avg. age at onset (years)	Average duration (years)	Deaths 1990 Number ('000s)	Rate (per 100 000)	Deaths 2000 (Projected) Number ('000s)	Rate (per 100 000)
Males										
0-4	47	79	49	83	3.0	2.0	15	24.5	14	24.5
5-14	56	55	155	152	10.0	2.7	9	9.1	10	9.1
15-44	435	217	1 029	513	29.7	2.5	138	69.1	176	70.8
45-59	214	449	468	983	52.2	2.4	152	319.3	190	319.3
60+	278	934	669	2 247	70.0	2.2	188	630.8	240	649.6
All ages	1 030	234	2 370	539	43.0	2.4	502	114.3	630	123.0
Females										
0-4	30	52	38	66	3.0	2.4	11	19.5	10	19.5
5-14	47	49	117	123	10.0	2.4	7	7.5	8	7.5
15-44	360	197	846	462	29.8	2.5	73	39.7	92	40.1
45-59	92	199	208	452	52.3	2.2	84	181.7	104	181.7
60+	97	337	194	672	72.6	1.8	75	260.2	105	269.1
All ages	625	152	1 403	342	37.0	2.3	250	60.9	319	65.9
Total	1 656	195	3 772	444	40.7	2.4	752	88.5	948	95.3

For epidemiological sources see Kumaresan et al. 1996. For the methods used to estimate and project incidence, prevalence, and deaths see Murray and Lopez 1996a. See explanatory notes for definitions and caveats.

Table 10 Tuberculosis	Cuadro 10 Tuberculosis	Tableau 10 Tuberculose
HIV sero-negative cases	Casos sero-negativos para VIH	Cas séro-négatifs pour VIH

Table 10d — China - China - Chine — Tuberculosis - HIV sero-negative cases

Age group (years)	Incidence 1990 Number ('000s)	Rate (per 100 000)	Prevalence 1990 Number ('000s)	Rate (per 100 000)	Avg. age at onset (years)	Average duration (years)	Deaths 1990 Number ('000s)	Rate (per 100 000)	Deaths 2000 (Projected) Number ('000s)	Rate (per 100 000)
Males										
0-4	9	15.5	13	22	2.5	2.5	3	4.5	1	2.3
5-14	8	8.0	23	24	10.2	2.5	1	0.6	0	0.2
15-44	244	79.6	543	177	33.0	2.5	25	8.2	10	3.0
45-59	161	221.4	370	509	53.3	2.5	47	64.2	24	24.7
60+	179	364.9	469	958	69.7	2.3	98	200.9	83	137.8
All ages	601	102.6	1 418	242	48.6	2.4	173	29.6	119	18.1
Females										
0-4	21	37.0	31	53	2.5	2.5	3	5.1	1	2.5
5-14	21	23.1	57	63	9.8	2.5	2	2.0	1	0.7
15-44	159	56.0	372	131	31.9	2.5	22	7.7	7	2.3
45-59	66	102.5	157	244	53.3	2.5	24	36.6	13	14.5
60+	75	144.4	163	316	71.3	1.9	54	104.9	46	71.5
All ages	342	62.4	781	142	41.4	2.4	104	19.0	68	10.9
Total	943	83.1	2 199	194	46.0	2.4	278	24.5	187	14.6

Table 10e — OAI - OPAI - APAI — Tuberculosis - HIV sero-negative cases

Age group (years)	Incidence 1990 Number ('000s)	Rate (per 100 000)	Prevalence 1990 Number ('000s)	Rate (per 100 000)	Avg. age at onset (years)	Average duration (years)	Deaths 1990 Number ('000s)	Rate (per 100 000)	Deaths 2000 (Projected) Number ('000s)	Rate (per 100 000)
Males										
0-4	4	8.7	5	12	2.5	2.5	1	2.5	1	1.6
5-14	37	44.6	76	90	10.0	2.5	2	2.3	1	1.1
15-44	390	242.5	919	572	29.7	2.5	34	21.1	20	9.7
45-59	174	509.8	404	1 184	52.2	2.5	46	135.8	31	68.0
60+	142	701.3	377	1 866	69.4	2.5	80	394.3	80	288.8
All ages	747	217.8	1 781	519	41.3	2.5	163	47.5	133	32.8
Females										
0-4	3	7.0	4	10	2.5	2.5	0	0.9	0	0.6
5-14	29	36.1	59	74	10.0	2.5	2	2.6	1	1.2
15-44	302	189.2	696	436	29.8	2.5	34	21.3	17	8.3
45-59	134	382.9	306	872	52.3	2.5	45	128.2	30	64.4
60+	111	488.5	262	1 157	70.2	2.5	75	332.6	79	244.2
All ages	579	170.5	1 327	391	41.6	2.5	157	46.2	128	31.6
Total	1 326	194.3	3 109	455	41.5	2.5	320	46.9	260	32.2

Table 10f — SSA - ASS - ASS — Tuberculosis - HIV sero-negative cases

Age group (years)	Incidence 1990 Number ('000s)	Rate (per 100 000)	Prevalence 1990 Number ('000s)	Rate (per 100 000)	Avg. age at onset (years)	Average duration (years)	Deaths 1990 Number ('000s)	Rate (per 100 000)	Deaths 2000 (Projected) Number ('000s)	Rate (per 100 000)
Males										
0-4	39	82	50	105	2.4	2.0	18	38	25	38
5-14	78	111	150	214	10.0	2.0	11	15	14	15
15-44	345	333	691	666	29.5	2.0	84	81	115	81
45-59	82	405	166	815	52.1	2.0	44	216	57	216
60+	41	393	97	923	69.1	2.0	29	273	39	274
All ages	586	232	1 154	457	31.1	2.0	186	74	251	73
Females										
0-4	40	85	51	108	2.4	2.0	20	42	27	42
5-14	94	135	175	251	10.0	2.0	16	22	21	22
15-44	302	284	587	552	29.9	2.0	97	92	133	92
45-59	75	339	148	670	52.2	2.0	40	182	53	182
60+	38	295	89	699	69.6	2.0	27	212	37	212
All ages	549	213	1 050	407	30.3	2.0	200	78	271	78
Total	1 134	222	2 205	432	30.7	2.0	386	76	522	75

For epidemiological sources see Kumaresan et al. 1996. For the methods used to estimate and project incidence, prevalence, and deaths see Murray and Lopez 1996a. See explanatory notes for definitions and caveats.

Table 10
Tuberculosis

Cuadro 10
Tuberculosis

Tableau 10
Tuberculose

HIV sero-negative cases | Casos sero-negativos para VIH | Cas séro-négatifs pour VIH

Table 10g   LAC - ALC - ALC   Tuberculosis - HIV sero-negative cases

Age group (years)	Incidence 1990 Number ('000s)	Rate (per 100 000)	Prevalence 1990 Number ('000s)	Rate (per 100 000)	Avg. age at onset (years)	Average duration (years)	Deaths 1990 Number ('000s)	Rate (per 100 000)	Deaths 2000 (Projected) Number ('000s)	Rate (per 100 000)
Males										
0-4	9	31	10	33	2.5	1.5	1	5.1	1	3.6
5-14	21	41	30	57	10.0	1.5	1	2.8	1	1.6
15-44	106	102	160	153	29.8	1.5	17	16.2	11	8.3
45-59	35	155	50	226	52.3	1.5	10	44.4	8	24.9
60+	34	237	53	374	70.3	1.5	14	101.5	14	72.8
All ages	204	92	303	137	37.1	1.5	44	19.9	35	13.1
Females										
0-4	8	27	8	30	2.5	1.5	1	4.2	1	2.9
5-14	28	55	39	77	10.0	1.5	2	4.4	1	2.4
15-44	89	85	133	128	29.8	1.5	16	15.1	8	6.6
45-59	21	90	32	138	52.4	1.5	6	25.7	5	14.4
60+	20	121	32	192	71.1	1.5	9	51.6	9	36.9
All ages	166	74	245	110	33.1	1.5	34	15.2	24	9.0
Total	370	83	548	123	35.3	1.5	78	17.5	59	11.0

Table 10h   MEC - AOM - CMO   Tuberculosis - HIV sero-negative cases

Age group (years)	Incidence 1990 Number ('000s)	Rate (per 100 000)	Prevalence 1990 Number ('000s)	Rate (per 100 000)	Avg. age at onset (years)	Average duration (years)	Deaths 1990 Number ('000s)	Rate (per 100 000)	Deaths 2000 (Projected) Number ('000s)	Rate (per 100 000)
Males										
0-4	19	47	20	50	2.5	1.5	5	12.4	5	9.1
5-14	23	36	37	57	10.0	1.5	3	4.1	2	2.3
15-44	187	164	234	206	30.1	1.5	28	24.3	19	12.6
45-59	54	243	78	347	52.3	1.5	17	76.3	14	42.6
60+	32	236	54	395	39.7	1.5	16	117.9	15	80.1
All ages	316	123	423	165	31.7	1.5	69	26.7	54	16.1
Females										
0-4	16	41	18	45	2.5	1.5	3	7.9	3	5.7
5-14	15	24	24	39	10.0	1.5	2	2.7	1	1.5
15-44	99	93	142	132	30.1	1.5	15	14.4	9	6.2
45-59	30	133	43	194	52.3	1.5	9	41.9	7	22.8
60+	24	153	37	236	70.6	1.5	11	69.7	10	48.2
All ages	184	74	264	107	34.9	1.5	40	16.4	30	9.3
Total	500	99	687	137	32.9	1.5	109	21.7	84	12.8

Table 10i   World - Mundo - Monde   Tuberculosis - HIV sero-negative cases

Age group (years)	Incidence 1990 Number ('000s)	Rate (per 100 000)	Prevalence 1990 Number ('000s)	Rate (per 100 000)	Avg. age at onset (years)	Average duration (years)	Deaths 1990 Number ('000s)	Rate (per 100 000)	Deaths 2000 (Projected) Number ('000s)	Rate (per 100 000)
Males										
0-4	129	40	149	46	2.7	1.9	43	13.5	47	13.5
5-14	226	41	472	86	10.0	2.1	26	4.8	28	4.5
15-44	1 812	145	3 618	289	30.2	2.1	333	26.6	354	24.5
45-59	780	250	1 558	499	52.4	2.1	325	103.9	331	82.2
60+	758	346	1 737	794	68.5	2.1	439	200.4	485	176.3
All ages	3 705	140	7 534	284	40.5	2.1	1 166	43.9	1 245	40.2
Females										
0-4	119	39	151	49	2.6	2.1	39	12.5	42	12.8
5-14	238	45	474	90	10.0	2.1	31	5.8	33	5.5
15-44	1 355	113	2 793	233	30.1	2.2	258	21.5	266	19.2
45-59	432	139	900	289	52.4	2.2	209	67.2	213	52.9
60+	393	146	788	293	71.2	1.9	257	95.6	293	86.8
All ages	2 538	97	5 105	195	37.1	2.1	794	30.4	847	27.6
Total	6 243	119	12 639	240	39.1	2.1	1 960	37.2	2 092	34.0

For epidemiological sources see Kumaresan et al. 1996. For the methods used to estimate and project incidence, prevalence, and deaths see Murray and Lopez 1996a. See explanatory notes for definitions and caveats.

Table 11	Cuadro 11	Tableau 11
Tuberculosis	Tuberculosis	Tuberculose
HIV sero-positive cases	Casos sero-positivos para VIH	Cas séro-positifs pour VIH

Table 11a EME - PEMC - EMBE — Tuberculosis - HIV sero-positive cases

Age group (years)	Incidence 1990 Number ('000s)	Rate (per 100 000)	Prevalence 1990 Number ('000s)	Rate (per 100 000)	Avg. age at onset (years)	Average duration (years)	Deaths 1990 Number ('000s)	Rate (per 100 000)	Deaths 2000 (Projected) Number ('000s)	Rate (per 100 000)
Males										
0-4	0	0.0	0	0.0	2.5	0.25	0	0.0	0	0.0
5-14	0	0.0	0	0.0	10.0	0.25	0	0.0	0	0.0
15-44	1	0.8	0	0.2	29.9	0.25	1	0.3	0	0.2
45-59	1	1.7	0	0.4	52.4	0.25	1	0.9	0	0.4
60+	0	0.5	0	0.1	71.1	0.25	0	0.3	0	0.2
All ages	3	0.7	1	0.2	43.1	0.25	1	0.4	1	0.2
Females										
0-4	0	0.0	0	0.0	2.5	0.25	0	0.0	0	0.0
5-14	0	0.0	0	0.0	10.0	0.25	0	0.0	0	0.0
15-44	0	0.2	0	0.0	30.0	0.25	0	0.1	0	0.0
45-59	0	0.2	0	0.1	52.4	0.25	0	0.1	0	0.0
60+	0	0.0	0	0.0	72.4	0.25	0	0.0	0	0.0
All ages	0	0.1	0	0.0	38.5	0.25	0	0.1	0	0.0
Total	3	0.4	1	0.1	42.4	0.25	2	0.2	1	0.1

Table 11b FSE - PEAS - AESE — Tuberculosis - HIV sero-positive cases

Age group (years)	Incidence 1990 Number ('000s)	Rate (per 100 000)	Prevalence 1990 Number ('000s)	Rate (per 100 000)	Avg. age at onset (years)	Average duration (years)	Deaths 1990 Number ('000s)	Rate (per 100 000)	Deaths 2000 (Projected) Number ('000s)	Rate (per 100 000)
Males										
0-4	0	0	0	0	-	-	0	0	0	0
5-14	0	0	0	0	-	-	0	0	0	0
15-44	0	0	0	0	-	-	0	0	0	0
45-59	0	0	0	0	-	-	0	0	0	0
60+	0	0	0	0	-	-	0	0	0	0
All ages	0	0	0	0	-	-	0	0	0	0
Females										
0-4	0	0	0	0	-	-	0	0	0	0
5-14	0	0	0	0	-	-	0	0	0	0
15-44	0	0	0	0	-	-	0	0	0	0
45-59	0	0	0	0	-	-	0	0	0	0
60+	0	0	0	0	-	-	0	0	0	0
All ages	0	0	0	0	-	-	0	0	0	0
Total	0	0	0	0	-	-	0	0	0	0

Table 11c India - India - Inde — Tuberculosis - HIV sero-positive cases

Age group (years)	Incidence 1990 Number ('000s)	Rate (per 100 000)	Prevalence 1990 Number ('000s)	Rate (per 100 000)	Avg. age at onset (years)	Average duration (years)	Deaths 1990 Number ('000s)	Rate (per 100 000)	Deaths 2000 (Projected) Number ('000s)	Rate (per 100 000)
Males										
0-4	0	0	0	0	-	-	0	0	0	0.2
5-14	0	0	0	0	-	-	0	0	0	0.0
15-44	0	0	0	0	-	-	0	0	38	15.2
45-59	0	0	0	0	-	-	0	0	3	5.3
60+	0	0	0	0	-	-	0	0	1	3.1
All ages	0	0	0	0	-	-	0	0	42	8.2
Females										
0-4	0	0	0	0	-	-	0	0	0	0.2
5-14	0	0	0	0	-	-	0	0	0	0.1
15-44	0	0	0	0	-	-	0	0	27	11.9
45-59	0	0	0	0	-	-	0	0	1	1.8
60+	0	0	0	0	-	-	0	0	0	0.7
All ages	0	0	0	0	-	-	0	0	29	6.0
Total	0	0	0	0	-	-	0	0	71	7.1

For epidemiological sources see Kumaresan et al. 1996. For the methods used to estimate and project incidence, prevalence, and deaths see Murray and Lopez 1996a. See explanatory notes for definitions and caveats.

Table 11   **Cuadro 11**   **Tableau 11**
Tuberculosis   **Tuberculosis**   **Tuberculose**

HIV sero-positive cases   Casos sero-positivos para VIH   Cas séro-positifs pour VIH

Table 11d   China - China - Chine   Tuberculosis - HIV sero-positive cases

Age group (years)	Incidence 1990 Number ('000s)	Rate (per 100 000)	Prevalence 1990 Number ('000s)	Rate (per 100 000)	Avg. age at onset (years)	Average duration (years)	Deaths 1990 Number ('000s)	Rate (per 100 000)	Deaths 2000 (Projected) Number ('000s)	Rate (per 100 000)
Males										
0-4	0	0	0	0	-	-	0	0	0	0.0
5-14	0	0	0	0	-	-	0	0	0	0.0
15-44	0	0	0	0	-	-	0	0	0	0.1
45-59	0	0	0	0	-	-	0	0	0	0.1
60+	0	0	0	0	-	-	0	0	0	0.0
All ages	0	0	0	0	-	-	0	0	1	0.1
Females										
0-4	0	0	0	0	-	-	0	0	0	0.0
5-14	0	0	0	0	-	-	0	0	0	0.0
15-44	0	0	0	0	-	-	0	0	0	0.1
45-59	0	0	0	0	-	-	0	0	0	0.0
60+	0	0	0	0	-	-	0	0	0	0.0
All ages	0	0	0	0	-	-	0	0	0	0.1
Total	0	0	0	0	-	-	0	0	1	0.1

Table 11e   OAI - OPAI - APAI   Tuberculosis - HIV sero-positive cases

Age group (years)	Incidence 1990 Number ('000s)	Rate (per 100 000)	Prevalence 1990 Number ('000s)	Rate (per 100 000)	Avg. age at onset (years)	Average duration (years)	Deaths 1990 Number ('000s)	Rate (per 100 000)	Deaths 2000 (Projected) Number ('000s)	Rate (per 100 000)
Males										
0-4	0	0	0	0	-	-	0	0	0	0.1
5-14	0	0	0	0	-	-	0	0	0	0.0
15-44	0	0	0	0	-	-	0	0	21	10.5
45-59	0	0	0	0	-	-	0	0	2	4.4
60+	0	0	0	0	-	-	0	0	1	2.5
All ages	0	0	0	0	-	-	0	0	24	6.0
Females										
0-4	0	0	0	0	-	-	0	0	0	0.1
5-14	0	0	0	0	-	-	0	0	0	0.0
15-44	0	0	0	0	-	-	0	0	16	7.7
45-59	0	0	0	0	-	-	0	0	1	1.4
60+	0	0	0	0	-	-	0	0	0	0.5
All ages	0	0	0	0	-	-	0	0	16	4.1
Total	0	0	0	0	-	-	0	0	41	5.0

Table 11f   SSA - ASS - ASS   Tuberculosis - HIV sero-positive cases

Age group (years)	Incidence 1990 Number ('000s)	Rate (per 100 000)	Prevalence 1990 Number ('000s)	Rate (per 100 000)	Avg. age at onset (years)	Average duration (years)	Deaths 1990 Number ('000s)	Rate (per 100 000)	Deaths 2000 (Projected) Number ('000s)	Rate (per 100 000)
Males										
0-4	1	1.1	0	0.9	2.4	1.0	0	0.9	1	1.9
5-14	0	0.0	0	0.3	10.0	1.6	0	0.0	0	0.1
15-44	42	40.2	40	38.3	29.4	1.0	34	32.6	96	67.3
45-59	2	10.0	3	15.3	52.2	1.3	2	8.4	5	18.9
60+	0	3.5	1	6.7	69.2	1.5	0	3.0	1	7.3
All ages	45	17.7	44	17.5	30.4	1.0	36	14.4	103	30.0
Females										
0-4	1	1.2	0	0.9	2.4	1.0	0	0.9	1	2.2
5-14	0	0.3	0	0.4	10.0	1.3	0	0.2	0	0.5
15-44	42	39.2	40	32.6	29.5	1.0	34	31.8	106	73.2
45-59	2	7.9	3	12.5	52.2	1.4	1	6.6	5	16.0
60+	0	1.1	0	3.2	69.7	1.7	0	1.0	0	2.3
All ages	44	17.1	44	14.9	30.1	1.0	36	13.9	113	32.4
Total	89	17.4	88	16.2	30.3	1.0	72	14.2	216	31.2

For epidemiological sources see Kumaresan et al. 1996. For the methods used to estimate and project incidence, prevalence, and deaths see Murray and Lopez 1996a. See explanatory notes for definitions and caveats.

Table 11	Cuadro 11	Tableau 11
Tuberculosis	Tuberculosis	Tuberculose

HIV sero-positive cases	Casos sero-positivos para VIH	Cas séro-positifs pour VIH

Table 11g   LAC - ALC - ALC — Tuberculosis - HIV sero-positive cases

Age group (years)	Incidence 1990 Number ('000s)	Rate (per 100 000)	Prevalence 1990 Number ('000s)	Rate (per 100 000)	Avg. age at onset (years)	Average duration (years)	Deaths 1990 Number ('000s)	Rate (per 100 000)	Deaths 2000 (Projected) Number ('000s)	Rate (per 100 000)
Males										
0-4	0	0.1	0	0.0	2.5	1.0	0	0.0	0	0.1
5-14	0	0.0	0	0.0	10.0	1.0	0	0.0	0	0.0
15-44	7	7.1	7	7.1	29.8	1.0	4	4.1	15	11.4
45-59	1	3.5	1	3.6	52.3	1.0	1	2.3	2	6.3
60+	0	0.7	0	1.0	70.3	1.0	0	0.5	0	1.6
All ages	8	3.7	8	3.8	32.4	1.0	5	2.2	17	6.4
Females										
0-4	0	0.0	0	0.0	2.5	1.0	0	0.0	0	0.0
5-14	0	0.0	0	0.0	10.0	1.0	0	0.0	0	0.0
15-44	2	2.1	2	1.9	29.8	1.0	1	1.2	4	2.7
45-59	0	1.0	0	1.1	52.4	1.0	0	0.7	0	1.5
60+	0	0.3	0	0.3	71.1	1.0	0	0.2	0	0.5
All ages	2	1.1	2	1.0	32.7	1.0	1	0.7	4	1.5
Total	11	2.4	11	2.4	32.4	1.0	6	1.4	21	3.9

Table 11h   MEC - AOM - CMO — Tuberculosis - HIV sero-positive cases

Age group (years)	Incidence 1990 Number ('000s)	Rate (per 100 000)	Prevalence 1990 Number ('000s)	Rate (per 100 000)	Avg. age at onset (years)	Average duration (years)	Deaths 1990 Number ('000s)	Rate (per 100 000)	Deaths 2000 (Projected) Number ('000s)	Rate (per 100 000)
Males										
0-4	0	0.0	0	0.0	2.5	1.0	0	0.0	0	0.0
5-14	0	0.0	0	0.0	10.0	1.0	0	0.0	0	0.0
15-44	0	0.1	0	0.1	29.8	1.0	0	0.1	1	0.9
45-59	0	0.1	0	0.1	52.3	1.0	0	0.1	0	0.7
60+	0	0.0	0	0.0	69.7	1.0	0	0.0	0	0.2
All ages	0	0.1	0	0.1	32.8	1.0	0	0.0	2	0.5
Females										
0-4	0	0.0	0	0.0	2.5	1.0	0	0.0	0	0.0
5-14	0	0.0	0	0.0	10.0	1.0	0	0.0	0	0.0
15-44	0	0.0	0	0.0	29.8	1.0	0	0.0	0	0.2
45-59	0	0.0	0	0.0	52.3	1.0	0	0.0	0	0.1
60+	0	0.0	0	0.0	70.4	1.0	0	0.0	0	0.0
All ages	0	0.0	0	0.0	31.9	1.0	0	0.0	0	0.1
Total	0	0.0	0	0.0	32.7	1.0	0	0.0	2	0.3

Table 11i   World - Mundo - Monde — Tuberculosis - HIV sero-positive cases

Age group (years)	Incidence 1990 Number ('000s)	Rate (per 100 000)	Prevalence 1990 Number ('000s)	Rate (per 100 000)	Avg. age at onset (years)	Average duration (years)	Deaths 1990 Number ('000s)	Rate (per 100 000)	Deaths 2000 (Projected) Number ('000s)	Rate (per 100 000)
Males										
0-4	1	0.2	0	0.1	2.4	1.00	0	0.1	1	0.4
5-14	0	0.0	0	0.0	10.0	1.57	0	0.0	0	0.0
15-44	51	4.1	48	3.8	29.5	0.98	39	3.1	171	11.9
45-59	4	1.3	4	1.3	52.3	0.94	3	0.9	13	3.2
60+	1	0.4	1	0.4	70.1	0.94	1	0.3	3	1.3
All ages	56	2.1	53	2.0	31.4	0.98	43	1.6	189	6.1
Females										
0-4	1	0.2	0	0.1	2.4	1.00	0	0.1	2	0.5
5-14	0	0.0	0	0.1	10.0	1.29	0	0.0	1	0.1
15-44	44	3.7	42	3.1	29.5	0.99	35	2.9	153	11.0
45-59	2	0.7	3	1.0	52.2	1.27	2	0.5	7	1.7
60+	0	0.1	0	0.2	70.2	1.43	0	0.1	1	0.3
All ages	47	1.8	47	1.6	30.3	1.01	38	1.4	163	5.3
Total	103	2.0	100	1.8	30.9	0.99	80	1.5	352	5.7

For epidemiological sources see Kumaresan et al. 1996. For the methods used to estimate and project incidence, prevalence, and deaths see Murray and Lopez 1996a. See explanatory notes for definitions and caveats.

Table 12
Syphilis

Cuadro 12
Sífilis

Tableau 12
Syphilis

Congenital syphilis   Sífilis congénita   Syphilis congénitale

Table 12a EME - PEMC - EMBE   Syphilis - Congenital syphilis

Age group (years)	Incidence 1990 Number ('000s)	Rate (per 100 000)	Prevalence 1990 Number ('000s)	Rate (per 100 000)	Avg. age at onset (years)	Average duration (years)	Deaths 1990 Number ('000s)	Rate (per 100 000)	Deaths 2000 (Projected) Number ('000s)	Rate (per 100 000)
Males										
0-4	0	1.7	1	3.9	0.0	3.0	0	0.1	0	0
5-14	0	0.0	0	0.6	-	-	0	0.0	0	0
15-44	0	0.0	0	0.0	-	-	0	0.0	0	0
45-59	0	0.0	0	0.0	-	-	0	0.0	0	0
60+	0	0.0	0	0.0	-	-	0	0.0	0	0
All ages	0	0.1	1	0.3	0.0	3.0	0	0.0	0	0
Females										
0-4	0	1.7	1	3.9	0.0	3.0	0	0.0	0	0
5-14	0	0.0	0	0.6	-	-	0	0.0	0	0
15-44	0	0.0	0	0.0	-	-	0	0.0	0	0
45-59	0	0.0	0	0.0	-	-	0	0.0	0	0
60+	0	0.0	0	0.0	-	-	0	0.0	0	0
All ages	0	0.1	1	0.3	0.0	3.0	0	0.0	0	0
Total	1	0.1	3	0.3	0.0	3.0	0	0.0	0	0

Table 12b FSE - PEAS - AESE   Syphilis - Congenital syphilis

Age group (years)	Incidence 1990 Number ('000s)	Rate (per 100 000)	Prevalence 1990 Number ('000s)	Rate (per 100 000)	Avg. age at onset (years)	Average duration (years)	Deaths 1990 Number ('000s)	Rate (per 100 000)	Deaths 2000 (Projected) Number ('000s)	Rate (per 100 000)
Males										
0-4	0	1.9	1	4.4	0.0	3.0	0	0	0	0
5-14	0	0.0	0	0.6	-	-	0	0	0	0
15-44	0	0.0	0	0.0	-	-	0	0	0	0
45-59	0	0.0	0	0.0	-	-	0	0	0	0
60+	0	0.0	0	0.0	-	-	0	0	0	0
All ages	0	0.2	1	0.5	0.0	3.0	0	0	0	0
Females										
0-4	0	1.9	1	4.4	0.0	3.0	0	0	0	0
5-14	0	0.0	0	0.6	-	-	0	0	0	0
15-44	0	0.0	0	0.1	-	-	0	0	0	0
45-59	0	0.0	0	0.0	-	-	0	0	0	0
60+	0	0.0	0	0.0	-	-	0	0	0	0
All ages	0	0.1	1	0.4	0.0	3.0	0	0	0	0
Total	1	0.1	2	0.5	0.0	3.0	0	0	0	0

Table 12c India - India - Inde   Syphilis - Congenital syphilis

Age group (years)	Incidence 1990 Number ('000s)	Rate (per 100 000)	Prevalence 1990 Number ('000s)	Rate (per 100 000)	Avg. age at onset (years)	Average duration (years)	Deaths 1990 Number ('000s)	Rate (per 100 000)	Deaths 2000 (Projected) Number ('000s)	Rate (per 100 000)
Males										
0-4	34	56.8	78	130.4	0.0	3.0	22	36.6	11	19.9
5-14	0	0.0	21	21.0	-	-	0	0.0	0	0.0
15-44	0	0.0	1	0.4	-	-	0	0.0	0	0.0
45-59	0	0.0	0	0.0	-	-	0	0.0	0	0.0
60+	0	0.0	0	0.0	-	-	0	0.0	0	0.0
All ages	34	7.7	100	22.8	0.0	3.0	22	5.0	11	2.2
Females										
0-4	32	57.1	74	130.7	0.0	3.0	23	41.2	12	21.8
5-14	0	0.0	20	21.2	-	-	0	0.0	0	0.0
15-44	0	0.0	1	0.4	-	-	0	0.0	0	0.0
45-59	0	0.0	0	0.0	-	-	0	0.0	0	0.0
60+	0	0.0	0	0.0	-	-	0	0.0	0	0.0
All ages	32	7.9	95	23.2	0.0	3.0	23	5.7	12	2.4
Total	66	7.8	195	23.0	0.0	3.0	45	5.3	23	2.3

For epidemiological sources see Berkley et al. 1996. For the methods used to estimate and project incidence, prevalence, and deaths see Murray and Lopez 1996a. See explanatory notes for definitions and caveats.

Table 12	Cuadro 12	Tableau 12
Syphilis	Sífilis	Syphilis

Congenital syphilis	Sífilis congénita	Syphilis congénitale

Table 12d China - China - Chine Syphilis - Congenital syphilis

Age group (years)	Incidence 1990 Number ('000s)	Rate (per 100 000)	Prevalence 1990 Number ('000s)	Rate (per 100 000)	Avg. age at onset (years)	Average duration (years)	Deaths 1990 Number ('000s)	Rate (per 100 000)	Deaths 2000 (Projected) Number ('000s)	Rate (per 100 000)
Males										
0-4	0	0.1	0	0.2	0.0	3.0	0	0	0	0
5-14	0	0.0	0	0.0	-	-	0	0	0	0
15-44	0	0.0	0	0.0	-	-	0	0	0	0
45-59	0	0.0	0	0.0	-	-	0	0	0	0
60+	0	0.0	0	0.0	-	-	0	0	0	0
All ages	0	0.0	0	0.0	0.0	3.0	0	0	0	0
Females										
0-4	0	0.1	0	0.2	0.0	3.0	0	0	0	0
5-14	0	0.0	0	0.0	-	-	0	0	0	0
15-44	0	0.0	0	0.0	-	-	0	0	0	0
45-59	0	0.0	0	0.0	-	-	0	0	0	0
60+	0	0.0	0	0.0	-	-	0	0	0	0
All ages	0	0.0	0	0.0	0.0	3.0	0	0	0	0
Total	0	0.0	0	0.0	0.0	3.0	0	0	0	0

Table 12e OAI - OPAI - APAI Syphilis - Congenital syphilis

Age group (years)	Incidence 1990 Number ('000s)	Rate (per 100 000)	Prevalence 1990 Number ('000s)	Rate (per 100 000)	Avg. age at onset (years)	Average duration (years)	Deaths 1990 Number ('000s)	Rate (per 100 000)	Deaths 2000 (Projected) Number ('000s)	Rate (per 100 000)
Males										
0-4	21	46.9	47	107.6	0.0	3.0	17	39.1	10	22.7
5-14	0	0.0	14	16.8	-	-	0	0.0	0	0.0
15-44	0	0.0	0	0.3	-	-	0	0.0	0	0.0
45-59	0	0.0	0	0.0	-	-	0	0.0	0	0.0
60+	0	0.0	0	0.0	-	-	0	0.0	0	0.0
All ages	21	6.0	62	18.0	0.0	3.0	17	5.0	10	2.5
Females										
0-4	20	46.6	45	107.1	0.0	3.0	12	28.6	7	15.5
5-14	0	0.0	13	16.5	-	-	0	0.0	0	0.0
15-44	0	0.0	0	0.3	-	-	0	0.0	0	0.0
45-59	0	0.0	0	0.0	-	-	0	0.0	0	0.0
60+	0	0.0	0	0.0	-	-	0	0.0	0	0.0
All ages	20	5.8	59	17.3	0.0	3.0	12	3.5	7	1.6
Total	40	5.9	120	17.6	0.0	3.0	29	4.3	17	2.0

Table 12f SSA - ASS - ASS Syphilis - Congenital syphilis

Age group (years)	Incidence 1990 Number ('000s)	Rate (per 100 000)	Prevalence 1990 Number ('000s)	Rate (per 100 000)	Avg. age at onset (years)	Average duration (years)	Deaths 1990 Number ('000s)	Rate (per 100 000)	Deaths 2000 (Projected) Number ('000s)	Rate (per 100 000)
Males										
0-4	63	133	143	302.2	0.0	3.0	33	70	28	41.9
5-14	0	0	38	53.5	-	-	0	0	0	0.0
15-44	0	0	1	1.1	-	-	0	0	0	0.0
45-59	0	0	0	0.0	-	-	0	0	0	0.0
60+	0	0	0	0.0	-	-	0	0	0	0.0
All ages	63	25	182	72.2	0.0	3.0	33	13	28	8.0
Females										
0-4	62	131	141	299.1	0.0	3.0	31	66	25	38.5
5-14	0	0	36	51.5	-	-	0	0	0	0.0
15-44	0	0	1	1.0	-	-	0	0	0	0.0
45-59	0	0	0	0.0	-	-	0	0	0	0.0
60+	0	0	0	0.0	-	-	0	0	0	0.0
All ages	62	24	178	68.9	0.0	3.0	31	12	25	7.0
Total	125	24	360	70.5	0.0	3.0	64	13	52	7.5

For epidemiological sources see Berkley et al. 1996. For the methods used to estimate and project incidence, prevalence, and deaths see Murray and Lopez 1996a. See explanatory notes for definitions and caveats.

Table 12 / **Cuadro 12** / **Tableau 12**
Syphilis / **Sífilis** / **Syphilis**

Congenital syphilis / Sífilis congénita / Syphilis congénitale

Table 12g   LAC - ALC - ALC   Syphilis - Congenital syphilis

Age group (years)	Incidence 1990 Number ('000s)	Rate (per 100 000)	Prevalence 1990 Number ('000s)	Rate (per 100 000)	Avg. age at onset (years)	Average duration (years)	Deaths 1990 Number ('000s)	Rate (per 100 000)	Deaths 2000 (Projected) Number ('000s)	Rate (per 100 000)
Males										
0-4	7	23.2	15	53.4	0.0	3.0	5	18.0	3	11.8
5-14	0	0.0	4	8.1	-	-	0	0.0	0	0.0
15-44	0	0.0	0	0.1	-	-	0	0.0	0	0.0
45-59	0	0.0	0	0.0	-	-	0	0.0	0	0.0
60+	0	0.0	0	0.0	-	-	0	0.0	0	0.0
All ages	7	3.0	20	8.9	0.0	3.0	5	2.3	3	1.3
Females										
0-4	6	23.1	15	53.2	0.0	3.0	4	15.5	3	9.8
5-14	0	0.0	4	8.0	-	-	0	0.0	0	0.0
15-44	0	0.0	0	0.1	-	-	0	0.0	0	0.0
45-59	0	0.0	0	0.0	-	-	0	0.0	0	0.0
60+	0	0.0	0	0.0	-	-	0	0.0	0	0.0
All ages	6	2.9	19	8.5	0.0	3.0	4	1.9	3	1.0
Total	13	2.9	39	8.7	0.0	3.0	9	2.1	6	1.2

Table 12h   MEC - AOM - CMO   Syphilis - Congenital syphilis

Age group (years)	Incidence 1990 Number ('000s)	Rate (per 100 000)	Prevalence 1990 Number ('000s)	Rate (per 100 000)	Avg. age at onset (years)	Average duration (years)	Deaths 1990 Number ('000s)	Rate (per 100 000)	Deaths 2000 (Projected) Number ('000s)	Rate (per 100 000)
Males										
0-4	8	18.4	17	42.2	0.0	3.0	6	15.3	5	10.7
5-14	0	0.0	4	6.7	-	-	0	0.0	0	0.0
15-44	0	0.0	0	0.1	-	-	0	0.0	0	0.0
45-59	0	0.0	0	0.0	-	-	0	0.0	0	0.0
60+	0	0.0	0	0.0	-	-	0	0.0	0	0.0
All ages	8	3.0	22	8.5	0.0	3.0	6	2.5	5	1.6
Females										
0-4	7	18.4	17	42.2	0.0	3.0	6	15.2	5	10.2
5-14	0	0.0	4	6.7	-	-	0	0.0	0	0.0
15-44	0	0.0	0	0.1	-	-	0	0.0	0	0.0
45-59	0	0.0	0	0.0	-	-	0	0.0	0	0.0
60+	0	0.0	0	0.0	-	-	0	0.0	0	0.0
All ages	7	3.0	21	8.5	0.0	3.0	6	2.4	5	1.5
Total	15	3.0	43	8.5	0.0	3.0	12	2.5	10	1.6

Table 12i   World - Mundo - Monde   Syphilis - Congenital syphilis

Age group (years)	Incidence 1990 Number ('000s)	Rate (per 100 000)	Prevalence 1990 Number ('000s)	Rate (per 100 000)	Avg. age at onset (years)	Average duration (years)	Deaths 1990 Number ('000s)	Rate (per 100 000)	Deaths 2000 (Projected) Number ('000s)	Rate (per 100 000)
Males										
0-4	133	41.3	303	94.3	0.0	3.0	84	26.0	58	16.7
5-14	0	0.0	82	14.9	-	-	0	0.0	0	0.0
15-44	0	0.0	3	0.2	-	-	0	0.0	0	0.0
45-59	0	0.0	0	0.0	-	-	0	0.0	0	0.0
60+	0	0.0	0	0.0	-	-	0	0.0	0	0.0
All ages	133	5.0	388	14.6	0.0	3.0	84	3.1	58	1.9
Females										
0-4	128	41.4	293	94.7	0.0	3.0	77	24.9	51	15.3
5-14	0	0.0	78	14.9	-	-	0	0.0	0	0.0
15-44	0	0.0	3	0.2	-	-	0	0.0	0	0.0
45-59	0	0.0	0	0.0	-	-	0	0.0	0	0.0
60+	0	0.0	0	0.0	-	-	0	0.0	0	0.0
All ages	128	4.9	373	14.3	0.0	3.0	77	2.9	51	1.7
Total	261	4.9	761	14.5	0.0	3.0	160	3.0	108	1.8

For epidemiological sources see Berkley et al. 1996. For the methods used to estimate and project incidence, prevalence, and deaths see Murray and Lopez 1996a. See explanatory notes for definitions and caveats.

Table 13	Cuadro 13	Tableau 13
Syphilis	Sífilis	Syphilis
Low birth weight	Bajo peso al nacer	Poids insuffisant à la naissance

Table 13a — EME - PEMC - EMBE — Syphilis - Low birth weight

Age group (years)	Incidence 1990 Number ('000s)	Rate (per 100 000)	Prevalence 1990 Number ('000s)	Rate (per 100 000)	Avg. age at onset (years)	Average duration (years)	Deaths 1990 Number ('000s)	Rate (per 100 000)	Deaths 2000 (Projected) Number ('000s)	Rate (per 100 000)
Males										
0-4	0	1.7	0	0.9	0.0	0.50	0	0	0	0
5-14	0	0.0	0	0.0	-	-	0	0	0	0
15-44	0	0.0	0	0.0	-	-	0	0	0	0
45-59	0	0.0	0	0.0	-	-	0	0	0	0
60+	0	0.0	0	0.0	-	-	0	0	0	0
All ages	0	0.1	0	0.1	0.0	0.50	0	0	0	0
Females										
0-4	0	1.7	0	0.9	0.0	0.50	0	0	0	0
5-14	0	0.0	0	0.0	-	-	0	0	0	0
15-44	0	0.0	0	0.0	-	-	0	0	0	0
45-59	0	0.0	0	0.0	-	-	0	0	0	0
60+	0	0.0	0	0.0	-	-	0	0	0	0
All ages	0	0.1	0	0.1	0.0	0.50	0	0	0	0
Total	1	0.1	0	0.1	0.0	0.50	0	0	0	0

Table 13b — FSE - PEAS - AESE — Syphilis - Low birth weight

Age group (years)	Incidence 1990 Number ('000s)	Rate (per 100 000)	Prevalence 1990 Number ('000s)	Rate (per 100 000)	Avg. age at onset (years)	Average duration (years)	Deaths 1990 Number ('000s)	Rate (per 100 000)	Deaths 2000 (Projected) Number ('000s)	Rate (per 100 000)
Males										
0-4	0	1.9	0	1.0	0.0	0.50	0	0.1	0	0
5-14	0	0.0	0	0.0	-	-	0	0.0	0	0
15-44	0	0.0	0	0.0	-	-	0	0.0	0	0
45-59	0	0.0	0	0.0	-	-	0	0.0	0	0
60+	0	0.0	0	0.0	-	-	0	0.0	0	0
All ages	0	0.2	0	0.1	0.0	0.50	0	0.0	0	0
Females										
0-4	0	1.9	0	1.0	0.0	0.50	0	0.1	0	0
5-14	0	0.0	0	0.0	-	-	0	0.0	0	0
15-44	0	0.0	0	0.0	-	-	0	0.0	0	0
45-59	0	0.0	0	0.0	-	-	0	0.0	0	0
60+	0	0.0	0	0.0	-	-	0	0.0	0	0
All ages	0	0.1	0	0.1	0.0	0.50	0	0.0	0	0
Total	1	0.1	0	0.1	0.0	0.50	0	0.0	0	0

Table 13c — India - India - Inde — Syphilis - Low birth weight

Age group (years)	Incidence 1990 Number ('000s)	Rate (per 100 000)	Prevalence 1990 Number ('000s)	Rate (per 100 000)	Avg. age at onset (years)	Average duration (years)	Deaths 1990 Number ('000s)	Rate (per 100 000)	Deaths 2000 (Projected) Number ('000s)	Rate (per 100 000)
Males										
0-4	34	56.9	17	28.3	0.0	0.50	3	5.4	2	3.0
5-14	0	0.0	0	0.0	-	-	0	0.0	0	0.0
15-44	0	0.0	0	0.0	-	-	0	0.0	0	0.0
45-59	0	0.0	0	0.0	-	-	0	0.0	0	0.0
60+	0	0.0	0	0.0	-	-	0	0.0	0	0.0
All ages	34	7.7	17	3.9	0.0	0.50	3	0.7	2	0.3
Females										
0-4	32	57.1	16	28.4	0.0	0.50	3	5.4	2	2.9
5-14	0	0.0	0	0.0	-	-	0	0.0	0	0.0
15-44	0	0.0	0	0.0	-	-	0	0.0	0	0.0
45-59	0	0.0	0	0.0	-	-	0	0.0	0	0.0
60+	0	0.0	0	0.0	-	-	0	0.0	0	0.0
All ages	32	7.9	16	3.9	0.0	0.50	3	0.8	2	0.3
Total	66	7.8	33	3.9	0.0	0.50	6	0.7	3	0.3

For epidemiological sources see Berkley et al. 1996. For the methods used to estimate and project incidence, prevalence, and deaths see Murray and Lopez 1996a. See explanatory notes for definitions and caveats.

Table 13   Cuadro 13   Tableau 13
Syphilis   Sífilis   Syphilis

Low birth weight   Bajo peso al nacer   Poids insuffisant à la naissance

Table 13d   China - China - Chine   Syphilis - Low birth weight

Age group (years)	Incidence 1990 Number ('000s)	Rate (per 100 000)	Prevalence 1990 Number ('000s)	Rate (per 100 000)	Avg. age at onset (years)	Average duration (years)	Deaths 1990 Number ('000s)	Rate (per 100 000)	Deaths 2000 (Projected) Number ('000s)	Rate (per 100 000)
Males										
0-4	0	0.1	0	0	0.0	0.50	0	0	0	0
5-14	0	0.0	0	0	-	-	0	0	0	0
15-44	0	0.0	0	0	-	-	0	0	0	0
45-59	0	0.0	0	0	-	-	0	0	0	0
60+	0	0.0	0	0	-	-	0	0	0	0
All ages	0	0.0	0	0	0.0	0.50	0	0	0	0
Females										
0-4	0	0.1	0	0	0.0	0.50	0	0	0	0
5-14	0	0.0	0	0	-	-	0	0	0	0
15-44	0	0.0	0	0	-	-	0	0	0	0
45-59	0	0.0	0	0	-	-	0	0	0	0
60+	0	0.0	0	0	-	-	0	0	0	0
All ages	0	0.0	0	0	0.0	0.50	0	0	0	0
Total	0	0.0	0	0	0.0	0.50	0	0	0	0

Table 13e   OAI - OPAI - APAI   Syphilis - Low birth weight

Age group (years)	Incidence 1990 Number ('000s)	Rate (per 100 000)	Prevalence 1990 Number ('000s)	Rate (per 100 000)	Avg. age at onset (years)	Average duration (years)	Deaths 1990 Number ('000s)	Rate (per 100 000)	Deaths 2000 (Projected) Number ('000s)	Rate (per 100 000)
Males										
0-4	21	46.9	10	23.4	0.0	0.50	2	4.3	1	2.5
5-14	0	0.0	0	0.0	-	-	0	0.0	0	0.0
15-44	0	0.0	0	0.0	-	-	0	0.0	0	0.0
45-59	0	0.0	0	0.0	-	-	0	0.0	0	0.0
60+	0	0.0	0	0.0	-	-	0	0.0	0	0.0
All ages	21	6.0	10	3.0	0.0	0.50	2	0.6	1	0.3
Females										
0-4	20	46.6	10	23.3	0.0	0.50	2	4.3	1	2.3
5-14	0	0.0	0	0.0	-	-	0	0.0	0	0.0
15-44	0	0.0	0	0.0	-	-	0	0.0	0	0.0
45-59	0	0.0	0	0.0	-	-	0	0.0	0	0.0
60+	0	0.0	0	0.0	-	-	0	0.0	0	0.0
All ages	20	5.8	10	2.9	0.0	0.50	2	0.5	1	0.2
Total	40	5.9	20	2.9	0.0	0.50	4	0.5	2	0.3

Table 13f   SSA - ASS - ASS   Syphilis - Low birth weight

Age group (years)	Incidence 1990 Number ('000s)	Rate (per 100 000)	Prevalence 1990 Number ('000s)	Rate (per 100 000)	Avg. age at onset (years)	Average duration (years)	Deaths 1990 Number ('000s)	Rate (per 100 000)	Deaths 2000 (Projected) Number ('000s)	Rate (per 100 000)
Males										
0-4	63	133	32	67	0.0	0.50	6	13.5	5	8.1
5-14	0	0	0	0	-	-	0	0.0	0	0.0
15-44	0	0	0	0	-	-	0	0.0	0	0.0
45-59	0	0	0	0	-	-	0	0.0	0	0.0
60+	0	0	0	0	-	-	0	0.0	0	0.0
All ages	63	25	32	13	0.0	0.50	6	2.5	5	1.6
Females										
0-4	62	131	31	66	0.0	0.50	6	13.0	5	7.5
5-14	0	0	0	0	-	-	0	0.0	0	0.0
15-44	0	0	0	0	-	-	0	0.0	0	0.0
45-59	0	0	0	0	-	-	0	0.0	0	0.0
60+	0	0	0	0	-	-	0	0.0	0	0.0
All ages	62	24	31	12	0.0	0.50	6	2.4	5	1.4
Total	125	24	63	12	0.0	0.50	13	2.5	10	1.5

For epidemiological sources see Berkley et al. 1996. For the methods used to estimate and project incidence, prevalence, and deaths see Murray and Lopez 1996a. See explanatory notes for definitions and caveats.

Table 13
Syphilis

Cuadro 13
Sífilis

Tableau 13
Syphilis

Low birth weight

Bajo peso al nacer

Poids insuffisant à la naissance

Table 13g LAC - ALC - ALC Syphilis - Low birth weight

Age group (years)	Incidence 1990 Number ('000s)	Rate (per 100 000)	Prevalence 1990 Number ('000s)	Rate (per 100 000)	Avg. age at onset (years)	Average duration (years)	Deaths 1990 Number ('000s)	Rate (per 100 000)	Deaths 2000 (Projected) Number ('000s)	Rate (per 100 000)
Males										
0-4	7	23.2	3	11.6	0.0	0.50	0	1.2	0	0.8
5-14	0	0.0	0	0.0	-	-	0	0.0	0	0.0
15-44	0	0.0	0	0.0	-	-	0	0.0	0	0.0
45-59	0	0.0	0	0.0	-	-	0	0.0	0	0.0
60+	0	0.0	0	0.0	-	-	0	0.0	0	0.0
All ages	7	3.0	3	1.5	0.0	0.50	0	0.1	0	0.1
Females										
0-4	6	23.1	3	11.6	0.0	0.50	0	1.1	0	0.7
5-14	0	0.0	0	0.0	-	-	0	0.0	0	0.0
15-44	0	0.0	0	0.0	-	-	0	0.0	0	0.0
45-59	0	0.0	0	0.0	-	-	0	0.0	0	0.0
60+	0	0.0	0	0.0	-	-	0	0.0	0	0.0
All ages	6	2.9	3	1.4	0.0	0.50	0	0.1	0	0.1
Total	13	2.9	7	1.5	0.0	0.50	1	0.1	0	0.1

Table 13h MEC - AOM - CMO Syphilis - Low birth weight

Age group (years)	Incidence 1990 Number ('000s)	Rate (per 100 000)	Prevalence 1990 Number ('000s)	Rate (per 100 000)	Avg. age at onset (years)	Average duration (years)	Deaths 1990 Number ('000s)	Rate (per 100 000)	Deaths 2000 (Projected) Number ('000s)	Rate (per 100 000)
Males										
0-4	8	18.4	4	9.2	0.0	0.50	0	0.9	0	0.7
5-14	0	0.0	0	0.0	-	-	0	0.0	0	0.0
15-44	0	0.0	0	0.0	-	-	0	0.0	0	0.0
45-59	0	0.0	0	0.0	-	-	0	0.0	0	0.0
60+	0	0.0	0	0.0	-	-	0	0.0	0	0.0
All ages	8	3.0	4	1.5	0.0	0.50	0	0.2	0	0.1
Females										
0-4	7	18.4	4	9.2	0.0	0.50	0	0.9	0	0.6
5-14	0	0.0	0	0.0	-	-	0	0.0	0	0.0
15-44	0	0.0	0	0.0	-	-	0	0.0	0	0.0
45-59	0	0.0	0	0.0	-	-	0	0.0	0	0.0
60+	0	0.0	0	0.0	-	-	0	0.0	0	0.0
All ages	7	3.0	4	1.5	0.0	0.50	0	0.2	0	0.1
Total	15	3.0	7	1.5	0.0	0.50	1	0.2	1	0.1

Table 13i World - Mundo - Monde Syphilis - Low birth weight

Age group (years)	Incidence 1990 Number ('000s)	Rate (per 100 000)	Prevalence 1990 Number ('000s)	Rate (per 100 000)	Avg. age at onset (years)	Average duration (years)	Deaths 1990 Number ('000s)	Rate (per 100 000)	Deaths 2000 (Projected) Number ('000s)	Rate (per 100 000)
Males										
0-4	133	41.3	66	20.7	0.0	0.50	12	3.8	9	2.5
5-14	0	0.0	0	0.0	-	-	0	0.0	0	0.0
15-44	0	0.0	0	0.0	-	-	0	0.0	0	0.0
45-59	0	0.0	0	0.0	-	-	0	0.0	0	0.0
60+	0	0.0	0	0.0	-	-	0	0.0	0	0.0
All ages	133	5.0	66	2.5	0.0	0.50	12	0.5	9	0.3
Females										
0-4	128	41.4	64	20.8	0.0	0.50	12	3.8	8	2.3
5-14	0	0.0	0	0.0	-	-	0	0.0	0	0.0
15-44	0	0.0	0	0.0	-	-	0	0.0	0	0.0
45-59	0	0.0	0	0.0	-	-	0	0.0	0	0.0
60+	0	0.0	0	0.0	-	-	0	0.0	0	0.0
All ages	128	4.9	64	2.5	0.0	0.50	12	0.4	8	0.3
Total	261	5.0	131	2.5	0.0	0.50	24	0.5	16	0.3

For epidemiological sources see Berkley et al. 1996. For the methods used to estimate and project incidence, prevalence, and deaths see Murray and Lopez 1996a. See explanatory notes for definitions and caveats.

Table 14	Cuadro 14	Tableau 14
Syphilis	Sífilis	Syphilis
Primary	Primaria	Primaire

Table 14a   EME - PEMC - EMBE   Syphilis - Primary

Age group (years)	Incidence 1990 Number ('000s)	Rate (per 100 000)	Prevalence 1990 Number ('000s)	Rate (per 100 000)	Avg. age at onset (years)	Average duration (years)	Deaths 1990 Number ('000s)	Rate (per 100 000)	Deaths 2000 (Projected) Number ('000s)	Rate (per 100 000)
Males										
0-4	0	0.0	0	0.0	-	-	0	0	0	0
5-14	1	2.6	0	0.1	13.0	0.04	0	0	0	0
15-44	192	104.2	8	4.3	25.0	0.04	0	0	0	0
45-59	3	5.2	0	0.2	52.4	0.04	0	0	0	0
60+	2	2.6	0	0.1	71.1	0.04	0	0	0	0
All ages	198	50.8	8	2.1	25.8	0.04	0	0	0	0
Females										
0-4	0	0.0	0	0.0	-	-	0	0	0	0
5-14	1	2.6	0	0.1	13.0	0.04	0	0	0	0
15-44	187	104.1	8	4.2	25.0	0.04	0	0	0	0
45-59	4	5.2	0	0.2	52.4	0.04	0	0	0	0
60+	2	2.6	0	0.1	72.4	0.04	0	0	0	0
All ages	194	47.5	8	1.9	26.0	0.04	0	0	0	0
Total	392	49.1	16	2.0	25.9	0.04	0	0	0	0

Table 14b   FSE - PEAS - AESE   Syphilis - Primary

Age group (years)	Incidence 1990 Number ('000s)	Rate (per 100 000)	Prevalence 1990 Number ('000s)	Rate (per 100 000)	Avg. age at onset (years)	Average duration (years)	Deaths 1990 Number ('000s)	Rate (per 100 000)	Deaths 2000 (Projected) Number ('000s)	Rate (per 100 000)
Males										
0-4	0	0.0	0	0.0	-	-	0	0	0	0
5-14	0	1.3	0	0.1	13.0	0.05	0	0	0	0
15-44	40	52.2	2	2.4	25.0	0.05	0	0	0	0
45-59	1	2.6	0	0.1	52.2	0.05	0	0	0	0
60+	0	1.3	0	0.1	70.0	0.05	0	0	0	0
All ages	41	24.9	2	1.1	25.7	0.05	0	0	0	0
Females										
0-4	0	0.0	0	0.0	-	-	0	0	0	0
5-14	0	1.3	0	0.1	13.0	0.05	0	0	0	0
15-44	39	52.2	2	2.4	25.0	0.05	0	0	0	0
45-59	1	2.6	0	0.1	52.4	0.05	0	0	0	0
60+	0	1.3	0	0.1	71.5	0.05	0	0	0	0
All ages	41	22.5	2	1.0	26.0	0.05	0	0	0	0
Total	82	23.7	4	1.1	25.8	0.05	0	0	0	0

Table 14c   India - India - Inde   Syphilis - Primary

Age group (years)	Incidence 1990 Number ('000s)	Rate (per 100 000)	Prevalence 1990 Number ('000s)	Rate (per 100 000)	Avg. age at onset (years)	Average duration (years)	Deaths 1990 Number ('000s)	Rate (per 100 000)	Deaths 2000 (Projected) Number ('000s)	Rate (per 100 000)
Males										
0-4	0	0	0	0.0	-	-	0	0	0	0
5-14	15	15	1	0.8	13.0	0.05	0	0	0	0
15-44	1 219	608	62	31.0	25.0	0.05	0	0	0	0
45-59	14	30	1	1.6	52.3	0.05	0	0	0	0
60+	5	15	0	0.8	69.7	0.05	0	0	0	0
All ages	1 254	285	64	14.5	25.3	0.05	0	0	0	0
Females										
0-4	0	0	0	0.0	-	-	0	0	0	0
5-14	18	19	1	1.0	13.0	0.05	0	0	0	0
15-44	1 393	760	71	38.7	25.0	0.05	0	0	0	0
45-59	17	38	1	1.9	52.4	0.05	0	0	0	0
60+	5	19	0	1.0	70.1	0.05	0	0	0	0
All ages	1 434	350	73	17.8	25.4	0.05	0	0	0	0
Total	2 688	316	137	16.1	25.3	0.05	0	0	0	0

For epidemiological sources see Berkley et al. 1996. For the methods used to estimate and project incidence, prevalence, and deaths see Murray and Lopez 1996a. See explanatory notes for definitions and caveats.

Table 14	Cuadro 14	Tableau 14
Syphilis	Sífilis	Syphilis
Primary	Primaria	Primaire

Table 14d — China - China - Chine — Syphilis - Primary

Age group (years)	Incidence 1990 Number ('000s)	Rate (per 100 000)	Prevalence 1990 Number ('000s)	Rate (per 100 000)	Avg. age at onset (years)	Average duration (years)	Deaths 1990 Number ('000s)	Rate (per 100 000)	Deaths 2000 (Projected) Number ('000s)	Rate (per 100 000)
Males										
0-4	0	0.0	0	0.0	-	-	0	0	0	0
5-14	0	0.0	0	0.0	13.0	0.05	0	0	0	0
15-44	4	1.3	0	0.1	25.0	0.05	0	0	0	0
45-59	0	0.1	0	0.0	52.3	0.05	0	0	0	0
60+	0	0.0	0	0.0	69.8	0.05	0	0	0	0
All ages	4	0.7	0	0.0	25.4	0.05	0	0	0	0
Females										
0-4	0	0.0	0	0.0	-	-	0	0	0	0
5-14	0	0.1	0	0.0	13.0	0.05	0	0	0	0
15-44	6	2.0	0	0.1	25.0	0.05	0	0	0	0
45-59	0	0.1	0	0.0	52.4	0.05	0	0	0	0
60+	0	0.1	0	0.0	70.6	0.05	0	0	0	0
All ages	6	1.1	0	0.0	25.4	0.05	0	0	0	0
Total	10	0.9	0	0.0	25.4	0.05	0	0	0	0

Table 14e — OAI - OPAI - APAI — Syphilis - Primary

Age group (years)	Incidence 1990 Number ('000s)	Rate (per 100 000)	Prevalence 1990 Number ('000s)	Rate (per 100 000)	Avg. age at onset (years)	Average duration (years)	Deaths 1990 Number ('000s)	Rate (per 100 000)	Deaths 2000 (Projected) Number ('000s)	Rate (per 100 000)
Males										
0-4	0	0	0	0.0	-	-	0	0	0	0
5-14	10	12	1	0.6	13.0	0.05	0	0	0	0
15-44	782	486	40	24.8	25.0	0.05	0	0	0	0
45-59	8	24	0	1.2	52.3	0.05	0	0	0	0
60+	2	12	0	0.6	69.6	0.05	0	0	0	0
All ages	803	234	41	11.9	25.2	0.05	0	0	0	0
Females										
0-4	0	0	0	0.0	-	-	0	0	0	0
5-14	12	15	1	0.8	13.0	0.05	0	0	0	0
15-44	971	608	49	31.0	25.0	0.05	0	0	0	0
45-59	11	30	1	1.6	52.3	0.05	0	0	0	0
60+	3	15	0	0.8	70.3	0.05	0	0	0	0
All ages	997	294	51	14.9	25.3	0.05	0	0	0	0
Total	1 800	264	92	13.4	25.3	0.05	0	0	0	0

Table 14f — SSA - ASS - ASS — Syphilis - Primary

Age group (years)	Incidence 1990 Number ('000s)	Rate (per 100 000)	Prevalence 1990 Number ('000s)	Rate (per 100 000)	Avg. age at onset (years)	Average duration (years)	Deaths 1990 Number ('000s)	Rate (per 100 000)	Deaths 2000 (Projected) Number ('000s)	Rate (per 100 000)
Males										
0-4	0	0	0	0.0	-	-	0	0	0	0
5-14	22	31	1	1.6	13.0	0.05	0	0	0	0
15-44	1 279	1 232	65	62.8	25.0	0.05	0	0	0	0
45-59	13	62	1	3.1	52.2	0.05	0	0	0	0
60+	3	31	0	1.6	69.2	0.05	0	0	0	0
All ages	1 316	522	67	26.6	25.1	0.05	0	0	0	0
Females										
0-4	0	0	0	0.0	-	-	0	0	0	0
5-14	27	39	1	2.0	13.0	0.05	0	0	0	0
15-44	1 637	1 541	83	78.4	25.0	0.05	0	0	0	0
45-59	17	77	1	3.9	52.2	0.05	0	0	0	0
60+	2	39	0	2.0	69.7	0.05	0	0	0	0
All ages	1 683	652	86	33.2	25.1	0.05	0	0	0	0
Total	2 999	588	153	29.9	25.1	0.05	0	0	0	0

For epidemiological sources see Berkley et al. 1996. For the methods used to estimate and project incidence, prevalence, and deaths see Murray and Lopez 1996a. See explanatory notes for definitions and caveats.

Table 14
Syphilis

Cuadro 14
Sífilis

Tableau 14
Syphilis

Primary

Primaria

Primaire

Table 14g   LAC - ALC - ALC   Syphilis - Primary

Age group (years)	Incidence 1990 Number ('000s)	Rate (per 100 000)	Prevalence 1990 Number ('000s)	Rate (per 100 000)	Avg. age at onset (years)	Average duration (years)	Deaths 1990 Number ('000s)	Rate (per 100 000)	Deaths 2000 (Projected) Number ('000s)	Rate (per 100 000)
Males										
0-4	0	0	0	0.0	-	-	0	0	0	0
5-14	6	12	0	0.5	13.0	0.05	0	0	0	0
15-44	483	463	22	20.8	25.0	0.05	0	0	0	0
45-59	5	23	0	1.1	52.3	0.05	0	0	0	0
60+	2	12	0	0.5	70.3	0.05	0	0	0	0
All ages	496	224	22	10.1	25.3	0.05	0	0	0	0
Females										
0-4	0	0	0	0.0	-	-	0	0	0	0
5-14	7	14	0	0.6	13.0	0.05	0	0	0	0
15-44	586	563	27	25.8	25.0	0.05	0	0	0	0
45-59	7	28	0	1.3	52.4	0.05	0	0	0	0
60+	2	14	0	0.6	71.1	0.05	0	0	0	0
All ages	602	270	28	12.4	25.3	0.05	0	0	0	0
Total	1 097	247	50	11.2	25.3	0.05	0	0	0	0

Table 14h   MEC - AOM - CMO   Syphilis - Primary

Age group (years)	Incidence 1990 Number ('000s)	Rate (per 100 000)	Prevalence 1990 Number ('000s)	Rate (per 100 000)	Avg. age at onset (years)	Average duration (years)	Deaths 1990 Number ('000s)	Rate (per 100 000)	Deaths 2000 (Projected) Number ('000s)	Rate (per 100 000)
Males										
0-4	0	0.0	0	0.0	-	-	0	0	0	0
5-14	5	8.4	0	0.4	13.0	0.05	0	0	0	0
15-44	383	336.2	18	15.4	25.0	0.05	0	0	0	0
45-59	4	16.8	0	0.8	52.3	0.05	0	0	0	0
60+	1	8.4	0	0.4	69.7	0.05	0	0	0	0
All ages	393	153.4	18	7.0	25.2	0.05	0	0	0	0
Females										
0-4	0	0.0	0	0.0	-	-	0	0	0	0
5-14	7	10.5	0	0.5	13.0	0.05	0	0	0	0
15-44	452	421.9	21	19.3	25.0	0.05	0	0	0	0
45-59	5	21.1	0	1.0	52.3	0.05	0	0	0	0
60+	2	10.5	0	0.5	70.4	0.05	0	0	0	0
All ages	465	188.6	21	8.6	25.3	0.05	0	0	0	0
Total	858	170.6	39	7.8	25.2	0.05	0	0	0	0

Table 14i   World - Mundo - Monde   Syphilis - Primary

Age group (years)	Incidence 1990 Number ('000s)	Rate (per 100 000)	Prevalence 1990 Number ('000s)	Rate (per 100 000)	Avg. age at onset (years)	Average duration (years)	Deaths 1990 Number ('000s)	Rate (per 100 000)	Deaths 2000 (Projected) Number ('000s)	Rate (per 100 000)
Males										
0-4	0	0.0	0	0.0	-	-	0	0	0	0
5-14	61	11.0	3	0.5	13.0	0.05	0	0	0	0
15-44	4 381	350.5	216	17.3	25.0	0.05	0	0	0	0
45-59	48	15.5	2	0.8	52.3	0.05	0	0	0	0
60+	15	6.8	1	0.3	69.8	0.05	0	0	0	0
All ages	4 505	169.8	222	8.4	25.2	0.05	0	0	0	0
Females										
0-4	0	0.0	0	0.0	-	-	0	0	0	0
5-14	73	13.8	4	0.7	13.0	0.05	0	0	0	0
15-44	5 270	439.7	261	21.8	25.0	0.05	0	0	0	0
45-59	61	19.6	3	1.0	52.3	0.05	0	0	0	0
60+	17	6.4	1	0.3	70.6	0.05	0	0	0	0
All ages	5 421	207.4	268	10.3	25.3	0.05	0	0	0	0
Total	9 926	188.5	491	9.3	25.3	0.05	0	0	0	0

For epidemiological sources see Berkley et al. 1996. For the methods used to estimate and project incidence, prevalence, and deaths see Murray and Lopez 1996a. See explanatory notes for definitions and caveats.

Table 15 Syphilis	Cuadro 15 Sífilis	Tableau 15 Syphilis
Secondary	Secundaria	Secondaire

Table 15a   EME - PEMC - EMBE   Syphilis - Secondary

Age group (years)	Incidence 1990 Number ('000s)	Rate (per 100 000)	Prevalence 1990 Number ('000s)	Rate (per 100 000)	Avg. age at onset (years)	Average duration (years)	Deaths 1990 Number ('000s)	Rate (per 100 000)	Deaths 2000 (Projected) Number ('000s)	Rate (per 100 000)
Males										
0-4	0	0.0	0	0.0	-	-	0	0	0	0
5-14	0	0.4	0	0.0	13.0	0.07	0	0	0	0
15-44	30	16.4	2	1.1	25.2	0.07	0	0	0	0
45-59	1	0.8	0	0.1	52.4	0.07	0	0	0	0
60+	0	0.4	0	0.0	71.1	0.07	0	0	0	0
All ages	31	8.0	2	0.5	26.0	0.07	0	0	0	0
Females										
0-4	0	0.0	0	0.0	-	-	0	0	0	0
5-14	0	0.4	0	0.0	13.0	0.07	0	0	0	0
15-44	29	16.3	2	1.1	25.2	0.07	0	0	0	0
45-59	1	0.8	0	0.1	52.4	0.07	0	0	0	0
60+	0	0.4	0	0.0	72.4	0.07	0	0	0	0
All ages	30	7.4	2	0.5	26.1	0.07	0	0	0	0
Total	62	7.7	4	0.5	26.0	0.07	0	0	0	0

Table 15b   FSE - PEAS - AESE   Syphilis - Secondary

Age group (years)	Incidence 1990 Number ('000s)	Rate (per 100 000)	Prevalence 1990 Number ('000s)	Rate (per 100 000)	Avg. age at onset (years)	Average duration (years)	Deaths 1990 Number ('000s)	Rate (per 100 000)	Deaths 2000 (Projected) Number ('000s)	Rate (per 100 000)
Males										
0-4	0	0.0	0	0.0	-	-	0	0	0	0
5-14	0	0.4	0	0.0	13.0	0.08	0	0	0	0
15-44	12	16.0	1	1.3	25.2	0.08	0	0	0	0
45-59	0	0.8	0	0.1	52.2	0.08	0	0	0	0
60+	0	0.4	0	0.0	70.0	0.08	0	0	0	0
All ages	13	7.6	1	0.6	25.9	0.08	0	0	0	0
Females										
0-4	0	0.0	0	0.0	-	-	0	0	0	0
5-14	0	0.4	0	0.0	13.0	0.08	0	0	0	0
15-44	12	16.0	1	1.3	25.2	0.08	0	0	0	0
45-59	0	0.8	0	0.1	52.4	0.08	0	0	0	0
60+	0	0.4	0	0.0	71.5	0.08	0	0	0	0
All ages	12	6.9	1	0.6	26.2	0.08	0	0	0	0
Total	25	7.2	2	0.6	26.0	0.08	0	0	0	0

Table 15c   India - India - Inde   Syphilis - Secondary

Age group (years)	Incidence 1990 Number ('000s)	Rate (per 100 000)	Prevalence 1990 Number ('000s)	Rate (per 100 000)	Avg. age at onset (years)	Average duration (years)	Deaths 1990 Number ('000s)	Rate (per 100 000)	Deaths 2000 (Projected) Number ('000s)	Rate (per 100 000)
Males										
0-4	0	0.0	0	0.0	-	-	0	0	0	0
5-14	7	7.0	1	0.7	13.0	0.10	0	0	0	0
15-44	557	278.0	53	26.4	25.2	0.10	0	0	0	0
45-59	7	13.9	1	1.3	52.3	0.10	0	0	0	0
60+	2	7.0	0	0.7	69.7	0.10	0	0	0	0
All ages	573	130.5	54	12.4	25.5	0.10	0	0	0	0
Females										
0-4	0	0.0	0	0.0	-	-	0	0	0	0
5-14	8	8.7	1	0.8	13.0	0.10	0	0	0	0
15-44	636	347.2	60	33.0	25.2	0.10	0	0	0	0
45-59	8	17.4	1	1.7	52.4	0.10	0	0	0	0
60+	3	8.7	0	0.8	70.1	0.10	0	0	0	0
All ages	655	159.7	62	15.2	25.5	0.10	0	0	0	0
Total	1 228	144.6	117	13.7	25.5	0.10	0	0	0	0

For epidemiological sources see Berkley et al. 1996. For the methods used to estimate and project incidence, prevalence, and deaths see Murray and Lopez 1996a. See explanatory notes for definitions and caveats.

Table 15 — **Cuadro 15** — **Tableau 15**
Syphilis — **Sífilis** — **Syphilis**

Secondary — Secundaria — Secondaire

Table 15d China - China - Chine — Syphilis - Secondary

Age group (years)	Incidence 1990 Number ('000s)	Rate (per 100 000)	Prevalence 1990 Number ('000s)	Rate (per 100 000)	Avg. age at onset (years)	Average duration (years)	Deaths 1990 Number ('000s)	Rate (per 100 000)	Deaths 2000 (Projected) Number ('000s)	Rate (per 100 000)
Males										
0-4	0	0.0	0	0	-	-	0	0	0	0
5-14	0	0.0	0	0	13.0	0.09	0	0	0	0
15-44	1	0.4	0	0	25.2	0.09	0	0	0	0
45-59	0	0.0	0	0	52.3	0.09	0	0	0	0
60+	0	0.0	0	0	69.8	0.09	0	0	0	0
All ages	1	0.2	0	0	25.6	0.09	0	0	0	0
Females										
0-4	0	0.0	0	0	-	-	0	0	0	0
5-14	0	0.0	0	0	13.0	0.08	0	0	0	0
15-44	2	0.6	0	0	25.2	0.08	0	0	0	0
45-59	0	0.0	0	0	52.4	0.08	0	0	0	0
60+	0	0.0	0	0	70.6	0.08	0	0	0	0
All ages	2	0.3	0	0	25.6	0.08	0	0	0	0
Total	3	0.3	0	0	25.6	0.08	0	0	0	0

Table 15e OAI - OPAI - APAI — Syphilis - Secondary

Age group (years)	Incidence 1990 Number ('000s)	Rate (per 100 000)	Prevalence 1990 Number ('000s)	Rate (per 100 000)	Avg. age at onset (years)	Average duration (years)	Deaths 1990 Number ('000s)	Rate (per 100 000)	Deaths 2000 (Projected) Number ('000s)	Rate (per 100 000)
Males										
0-4	0	0.0	0	0.0	-	-	0	0	0	0
5-14	5	5.6	0	0.5	13.0	0.09	0	0	0	0
15-44	357	222.1	34	21.1	25.2	0.09	0	0	0	0
45-59	4	11.1	0	1.1	52.3	0.09	0	0	0	0
60+	1	5.6	0	0.5	69.6	0.09	0	0	0	0
All ages	367	106.9	35	10.2	25.5	0.09	0	0	0	0
Females										
0-4	0	0.0	0	0.0	-	-	0	0	0	0
5-14	6	6.9	1	0.7	13.0	0.10	0	0	0	0
15-44	443	277.8	42	26.4	25.2	0.10	0	0	0	0
45-59	5	13.9	0	1.3	52.3	0.10	0	0	0	0
60+	2	6.9	0	0.7	70.3	0.10	0	0	0	0
All ages	455	134.1	43	12.7	25.5	0.10	0	0	0	0
Total	822	120.5	78	11.4	25.5	0.10	0	0	0	0

Table 15f SSA - ASS - ASS — Syphilis - Secondary

Age group (years)	Incidence 1990 Number ('000s)	Rate (per 100 000)	Prevalence 1990 Number ('000s)	Rate (per 100 000)	Avg. age at onset (years)	Average duration (years)	Deaths 1990 Number ('000s)	Rate (per 100 000)	Deaths 2000 (Projected) Number ('000s)	Rate (per 100 000)
Males										
0-4	0	0	0	0.0	-	-	0	0	0	0
5-14	10	14	1	1.3	13.0	0.10	0	0	0	0
15-44	584	563	56	53.5	25.2	0.10	0	0	0	0
45-59	6	28	1	2.7	52.2	0.10	0	0	0	0
60+	1	14	0	1.3	69.2	0.10	0	0	0	0
All ages	602	238	57	22.6	25.4	0.10	0	0	0	0
Females										
0-4	0	0	0	0.0	-	-	0	0	0	0
5-14	12	18	1	1.7	13.0	0.10	0	0	0	0
15-44	748	703	71	66.8	25.2	0.10	0	0	0	0
45-59	8	35	1	3.3	52.2	0.10	0	0	0	0
60+	0	18	0	1.7	69.7	0.10	0	0	0	0
All ages	768	298	73	28.3	25.3	0.10	0	0	0	0
Total	1 369	268	130	25.5	25.3	0.10	0	0	0	0

For epidemiological sources see Berkley et al. 1996. For the methods used to estimate and project incidence, prevalence, and deaths see Murray and Lopez 1996a. See explanatory notes for definitions and caveats.

Table 15	Cuadro 15	Tableau 15
Syphilis	Sífilis	Syphilis
Secondary	Secundaria	Secondaire

Table 15g — LAC - ALC - ALC — Syphilis - Secondary

Age group (years)	Incidence 1990 Number ('000s)	Rate (per 100 000)	Prevalence 1990 Number ('000s)	Rate (per 100 000)	Avg. age at onset (years)	Average duration (years)	Deaths 1990 Number ('000s)	Rate (per 100 000)	Deaths 2000 (Projected) Number ('000s)	Rate (per 100 000)
Males										
0-4	0	0.0	0	0.0	-	-	0	0	0	0
5-14	2	3.5	0	0.3	13.0	0.08	0	0	0	0
15-44	145	139.0	12	11.2	25.2	0.08	0	0	0	0
45-59	2	6.9	0	0.6	52.3	0.08	0	0	0	0
60+	0	3.5	0	0.3	70.3	0.08	0	0	0	0
All ages	149	67.1	12	5.4	25.5	0.08	0	0	0	0
Females										
0-4	0	0.0	0	0.0	-	-	0	0	0	0
5-14	2	4.3	0	0.3	13.0	0.08	0	0	0	0
15-44	180	172.5	14	13.9	25.2	0.08	0	0	0	0
45-59	2	8.6	0	0.7	52.4	0.08	0	0	0	0
60+	1	4.3	0	0.3	71.1	0.08	0	0	0	0
All ages	184	82.8	15	6.7	25.5	0.08	0	0	0	0
Total	333	75.0	27	6.1	25.5	0.08	0	0	0	0

Table 15h — MEC - AOM - CMO — Syphilis - Secondary

Age group (years)	Incidence 1990 Number ('000s)	Rate (per 100 000)	Prevalence 1990 Number ('000s)	Rate (per 100 000)	Avg. age at onset (years)	Average duration (years)	Deaths 1990 Number ('000s)	Rate (per 100 000)	Deaths 2000 (Projected) Number ('000s)	Rate (per 100 000)
Males										
0-4	0	0.0	0	0.0	-	-	0	0	0	0
5-14	2	2.6	0	0.2	13.0	0.08	0	0	0	0
15-44	117	103.0	9	8.3	25.2	0.08	0	0	0	0
45-59	1	5.2	0	0.4	52.3	0.08	0	0	0	0
60+	0	2.6	0	0.2	69.7	0.08	0	0	0	0
All ages	121	47.0	10	3.8	25.4	0.08	0	0	0	0
Females										
0-4	0	0.0	0	0.0	-	-	0	0	0	0
5-14	2	3.2	0	0.3	13.0	0.08	0	0	0	0
15-44	139	129.3	11	10.4	25.2	0.08	0	0	0	0
45-59	1	6.5	0	0.5	52.3	0.08	0	0	0	0
60+	0	3.2	0	0.3	70.4	0.08	0	0	0	0
All ages	143	57.8	12	4.7	25.5	0.08	0	0	0	0
Total	263	52.3	21	4.2	25.4	0.08	0	0	0	0

Table 15i — World - Mundo - Monde — Syphilis - Secondary

Age group (years)	Incidence 1990 Number ('000s)	Rate (per 100 000)	Prevalence 1990 Number ('000s)	Rate (per 100 000)	Avg. age at onset (years)	Average duration (years)	Deaths 1990 Number ('000s)	Rate (per 100 000)	Deaths 2000 (Projected) Number ('000s)	Rate (per 100 000)
Males										
0-4	0	0.0	0	0.0	-	-	0	0	0	0
5-14	25	4.6	2	0.4	13.0	0.09	0	0	0	0
15-44	1 805	144.4	167	13.3	25.2	0.09	0	0	0	0
45-59	20	6.3	2	0.6	52.3	0.09	0	0	0	0
60+	6	2.7	1	0.2	69.7	0.09	0	0	0	0
All ages	1 856	69.9	171	6.5	25.5	0.09	0	0	0	0
Females										
0-4	0	0.0	0	0.0	-	-	0	0	0	0
5-14	31	5.8	3	0.5	13.0	0.09	0	0	0	0
15-44	2 188	182.6	202	16.9	25.2	0.09	0	0	0	0
45-59	25	8.0	2	0.7	52.3	0.09	0	0	0	0
60+	6	2.2	1	0.2	70.5	0.09	0	0	0	0
All ages	2 250	86.1	208	8.0	25.5	0.09	0	0	0	0
Total	4 105	77.9	379	7.2	25.5	0.09	0	0	0	0

For epidemiological sources see Berkley et al. 1996. For the methods used to estimate and project incidence, prevalence, and deaths see Murray and Lopez 1996a. See explanatory notes for definitions and caveats.

Table 16
Syphilis

Cuadro 16
Sífilis

Tableau 16
Syphilis

Tertiary - cardiovascular

Terciaria - cardiovascular

Tertiaire - cardio-vasculaire

Table 16a   EME - PEMC - EMBE   Syphilis - Tertiary - cardiovascular

Age group (years)	Incidence 1990 Number ('000s)	Rate (per 100 000)	Prevalence 1990 Number ('000s)	Rate (per 100 000)	Avg. age at onset (years)	Average duration (years)	Deaths 1990 Number ('000s)	Rate (per 100 000)	Deaths 2000 (Projected) Number ('000s)	Rate (per 100 000)
Males										
0-4	0	0.0	0	0.0	-	-	0	0.0	0	0.0
5-14	0	0.0	0	0.0	13.0	10.0	0	0.0	0	0.0
15-44	0	0.1	1	0.3	35.0	10.0	0	0.0	0	0.0
45-59	0	0.0	0	0.5	52.4	10.0	0	0.0	0	0.0
60+	0	0.0	0	0.1	71.1	10.0	0	0.1	0	0.1
All ages	0	0.0	1	0.3	35.4	10.0	0	0.0	0	0.0
Females										
0-4	0	0.0	0	0.0	-	-	0	0.0	0	0.0
5-14	0	0.0	0	0.0	13.0	10.0	0	0.0	0	0.0
15-44	0	0.1	1	0.3	35.0	10.0	0	0.0	0	0.0
45-59	0	0.0	0	0.4	52.4	10.0	0	0.0	0	0.0
60+	0	0.0	0	0.1	72.4	10.0	0	0.1	0	0.1
All ages	0	0.0	1	0.2	35.6	10.0	0	0.0	0	0.0
Total	0	0.0	2	0.2	35.5	10.0	0	0.0	0	0.0

Table 16b   FSE - PEAS - AESE   Syphilis - Tertiary - cardiovascular

Age group (years)	Incidence 1990 Number ('000s)	Rate (per 100 000)	Prevalence 1990 Number ('000s)	Rate (per 100 000)	Avg. age at onset (years)	Average duration (years)	Deaths 1990 Number ('000s)	Rate (per 100 000)	Deaths 2000 (Projected) Number ('000s)	Rate (per 100 000)
Males										
0-4	0	0.0	0	0.0	-	-	0	0	0	0
5-14	0	0.0	0	0.1	13.0	10.0	0	0	0	0
15-44	0	0.2	1	1.3	35.0	10.0	0	0	0	0
45-59	0	0.0	1	1.9	52.2	10.0	0	0	0	0
60+	0	0.0	0	0.4	70.0	10.0	0	0	0	0
All ages	0	0.1	2	1.0	35.3	10.0	0	0	0	0
Females										
0-4	0	0.0	0	0.0	-	-	0	0	0	0
5-14	0	0.0	0	0.1	13.0	10.0	0	0	0	0
15-44	0	0.2	1	1.3	35.0	10.0	0	0	0	0
45-59	0	0.0	1	1.7	52.4	10.0	0	0	0	0
60+	0	0.0	0	0.3	71.5	10.0	0	0	0	0
All ages	0	0.1	2	0.9	35.5	10.0	0	0	0	0
Total	0	0.1	3	0.9	35.4	10.0	0	0	0	0

Table 16c   India - India - Inde   Syphilis - Tertiary - cardiovascular

Age group (years)	Incidence 1990 Number ('000s)	Rate (per 100 000)	Prevalence 1990 Number ('000s)	Rate (per 100 000)	Avg. age at onset (years)	Average duration (years)	Deaths 1990 Number ('000s)	Rate (per 100 000)	Deaths 2000 (Projected) Number ('000s)	Rate (per 100 000)
Males										
0-4	0	0.0	0	0.0	-	-	0	0.0	0	0.0
5-14	0	0.2	2	2.1	13.0	10.0	0	0.0	0	0.0
15-44	16	8.2	93	46.6	35.0	10.0	1	0.3	0	0.1
45-59	0	0.4	32	67.2	52.3	10.0	1	1.3	0	0.6
60+	0	0.2	5	15.2	69.7	10.0	3	10.2	3	7.8
All ages	17	3.8	132	30.0	35.0	10.0	4	1.0	4	0.7
Females										
0-4	0	0.0	0	0.0	-	-	0	0.0	0	0.0
5-14	0	0.3	2	2.6	13.0	10.0	0	0.0	0	0.0
15-44	19	10.3	106	57.9	35.0	10.0	1	0.3	0	0.1
45-59	0	0.5	38	82.8	52.4	10.0	1	1.6	0	0.7
60+	0	0.3	5	17.9	70.1	10.0	3	12.0	4	9.2
All ages	19	4.7	152	37.0	35.0	10.0	5	1.2	4	0.9
Total	36	4.3	284	33.4	35.0	10.0	9	1.1	8	0.8

For epidemiological sources see Berkley et al. 1996. For the methods used to estimate and project incidence, prevalence, and deaths see Murray and Lopez 1996a. See explanatory notes for definitions and caveats.

Table 16	Cuadro 16	Tableau 16
Syphilis	Sífilis	Syphilis

Tertiary - cardiovascular	Terciaria - cardiovascular	Tertiaire - cardio-vasculaire

Table 16d — China - China - Chine — Syphilis - Tertiary - cardiovascular

Age group (years)	Incidence 1990 Number ('000s)	Rate (per 100 000)	Prevalence 1990 Number ('000s)	Rate (per 100 000)	Avg. age at onset (years)	Average duration (years)	Deaths 1990 Number ('000s)	Rate (per 100 000)	Deaths 2000 (Projected) Number ('000s)	Rate (per 100 000)
Males										
0-4	0	0	0	0.0	-	-	0	0.0	0	0.0
5-14	0	0	0	0.0	13.0	10.0	0	0.0	0	0.0
15-44	0	0	0	0.1	35.0	10.0	0	0.0	0	0.0
45-59	0	0	0	0.1	52.3	10.0	0	0.0	0	0.0
60+	0	0	0	0.0	69.8	10.0	0	0.3	0	0.2
All ages	0	0	0	0.0	35.1	10.0	0	0.0	0	0.0
Females										
0-4	0	0	0	0.0	-	-	0	0.0	0	0.0
5-14	0	0	0	0.0	13.0	10.0	0	0.0	0	0.0
15-44	0	0	0	0.1	35.0	10.0	0	0.0	0	0.0
45-59	0	0	0	0.1	52.4	10.0	0	0.0	0	0.0
60+	0	0	0	0.0	70.6	10.0	0	0.2	0	0.1
All ages	0	0	0	0.0	35.2	10.0	0	0.0	0	0.0
Total	0	0	0	0.0	35.1	10.0	0	0.0	0	0.0

Table 16e — OAI - OPAI - APAI — Syphilis - Tertiary - cardiovascular

Age group (years)	Incidence 1990 Number ('000s)	Rate (per 100 000)	Prevalence 1990 Number ('000s)	Rate (per 100 000)	Avg. age at onset (years)	Average duration (years)	Deaths 1990 Number ('000s)	Rate (per 100 000)	Deaths 2000 (Projected) Number ('000s)	Rate (per 100 000)
Males										
0-4	0	0.0	0	0.0	-	-	0	0.0	0	0.0
5-14	0	0.2	1	1.7	13.0	10.0	0	0.0	0	0.0
15-44	11	6.6	61	37.7	35.0	10.0	0	0.2	0	0.1
45-59	0	0.3	19	55.2	52.3	10.0	0	1.2	0	0.6
60+	0	0.2	3	12.8	69.6	10.0	2	10.0	2	8.1
All ages	11	3.2	83	24.3	35.0	10.0	3	0.8	3	0.7
Females										
0-4	0	0.0	0	0.0	-	-	0	0.0	0	0.0
5-14	0	0.2	2	2.1	13.0	10.0	0	0.0	0	0.0
15-44	13	8.2	74	46.6	35.0	10.0	0	0.2	0	0.1
45-59	0	0.4	23	66.5	52.3	10.0	1	1.5	0	0.7
60+	0	0.2	3	14.3	70.3	10.0	2	10.2	3	8.3
All ages	14	4.0	103	30.2	35.0	10.0	3	0.9	3	0.8
Total	24	3.6	186	27.2	35.0	10.0	6	0.9	6	0.7

Table 16f — SSA - ASS - ASS — Syphilis - Tertiary - cardiovascular

Age group (years)	Incidence 1990 Number ('000s)	Rate (per 100 000)	Prevalence 1990 Number ('000s)	Rate (per 100 000)	Avg. age at onset (years)	Average duration (years)	Deaths 1990 Number ('000s)	Rate (per 100 000)	Deaths 2000 (Projected) Number ('000s)	Rate (per 100 000)
Males										
0-4	0	0.0	0	0.0	-	-	0	0.0	0	0.0
5-14	0	0.4	3	4.2	13.0	10.0	0	0.0	0	0.0
15-44	17	16.7	99	95.5	35.0	10.0	0	0.4	0	0.2
45-59	0	0.8	32	155.3	52.2	10.0	1	3.3	0	1.8
60+	0	0.4	4	39.4	69.2	10.0	3	31.1	3	23.6
All ages	18	7.1	138	54.6	34.8	10.0	4	1.7	4	1.2
Females										
0-4	0	0.0	0	0.0	-	-	0	0.0	0	0.0
5-14	0	0.5	4	5.2	13.0	10.0	0	0.0	0	0.0
15-44	22	20.8	126	118.3	35.0	10.0	1	0.6	0	0.3
45-59	0	1.0	41	184.2	52.2	10.0	1	4.0	1	2.0
60+	0	0.5	6	43.9	69.7	10.0	4	33.2	4	24.7
All ages	23	8.8	176	68.1	34.8	10.0	6	2.2	5	1.5
Total	41	8.0	313	61.4	34.8	10.0	10	2.0	9	1.4

For epidemiological sources see Berkley et al. 1996. For the methods used to estimate and project incidence, prevalence, and deaths see Murray and Lopez 1996a. See explanatory notes for definitions and caveats.

Table 16
Syphilis

Cuadro 16
Sífilis

Tableau 16
Syphilis

Tertiary - cardiovascular

Terciaria - cardiovascular

Tertiaire - cardio-vasculaire

Table 16g   **LAC - ALC - ALC**   Syphilis - Tertiary - cardiovascular

Age group (years)	Incidence 1990 Number ('000s)	Incidence 1990 Rate (per 100 000)	Prevalence 1990 Number ('000s)	Prevalence 1990 Rate (per 100 000)	Avg. age at onset (years)	Average duration (years)	Deaths 1990 Number ('000s)	Deaths 1990 Rate (per 100 000)	Deaths 2000 (Projected) Number ('000s)	Deaths 2000 (Projected) Rate (per 100 000)
Males										
0-4	0	0.0	0	0.0	-	-	0	0.0	0	0.0
5-14	0	0.0	0	0.5	13.0	10.0	0	0.0	0	0.0
15-44	2	2.0	12	11.3	35.0	10.0	0	0.1	0	0.0
45-59	0	0.1	4	16.1	52.3	10.0	0	0.4	0	0.2
60+	0	0.0	0	3.5	70.3	10.0	0	2.6	0	2.2
All ages	2	1.0	16	7.3	35.0	10.0	1	0.2	1	0.2
Females										
0-4	0	0.0	0	0.0	-	-	0	0.0	0	0.0
5-14	0	0.1	0	0.6	13.0	10.0	0	0.0	0	0.0
15-44	3	2.5	15	14.0	35.0	10.0	0	0.1	0	0.0
45-59	0	0.1	5	19.4	52.4	10.0	0	0.4	0	0.2
60+	0	0.1	1	3.8	71.1	10.0	0	2.8	1	2.3
All ages	3	1.2	20	9.0	35.0	10.0	1	0.3	1	0.2
Total	5	1.1	36	8.1	35.0	10.0	1	0.3	1	0.2

Table 16h   **MEC - AOM - CMO**   Syphilis - Tertiary - cardiovascular

Age group (years)	Incidence 1990 Number ('000s)	Incidence 1990 Rate (per 100 000)	Prevalence 1990 Number ('000s)	Prevalence 1990 Rate (per 100 000)	Avg. age at onset (years)	Average duration (years)	Deaths 1990 Number ('000s)	Deaths 1990 Rate (per 100 000)	Deaths 2000 (Projected) Number ('000s)	Deaths 2000 (Projected) Rate (per 100 000)
Males										
0-4	0	0.0	0	0.0	-	-	0	0.0	0	0.0
5-14	0	0.0	0	0.4	13.0	10.0	0	0.0	0	0.0
15-44	2	1.5	10	8.5	35.0	10.0	0	0.0	0	0.0
45-59	0	0.1	3	12.2	52.3	10.0	0	0.3	0	0.2
60+	0	0.0	0	2.8	69.7	10.0	0	2.2	0	1.8
All ages	2	0.7	13	5.1	34.9	10.0	0	0.2	0	0.1
Females										
0-4	0	0.0	0	0.0	-	-	0	0.0	0	0.0
5-14	0	0.0	0	0.5	13.0	10.0	0	0.0	0	0.0
15-44	2	1.9	11	10.7	35.0	10.0	0	0.0	0	0.0
45-59	0	0.1	3	15.0	52.3	10.0	0	0.3	0	0.2
60+	0	0.0	0	3.1	70.4	10.0	0	2.2	0	1.8
All ages	2	0.8	16	6.3	34.9	10.0	0	0.2	0	0.1
Total	4	0.8	29	5.7	34.9	10.0	1	0.2	1	0.1

Table 16i   **World - Mundo - Monde**   Syphilis - Tertiary - cardiovascular

Age group (years)	Incidence 1990 Number ('000s)	Incidence 1990 Rate (per 100 000)	Prevalence 1990 Number ('000s)	Prevalence 1990 Rate (per 100 000)	Avg. age at onset (years)	Average duration (years)	Deaths 1990 Number ('000s)	Deaths 1990 Rate (per 100 000)	Deaths 2000 (Projected) Number ('000s)	Deaths 2000 (Projected) Rate (per 100 000)
Males										
0-4	0	0.0	0	0.0	-	-	0	0.0	0	0.0
5-14	1	0.1	7	1.3	13.0	10.0	0	0.0	0	0.0
15-44	49	3.9	276	22.1	35.0	10.0	1	0.1	1	0.1
45-59	1	0.2	90	28.7	52.3	10.0	2	0.6	1	0.3
60+	0	0.1	12	5.6	70.1	10.0	9	4.2	10	3.5
All ages	50	1.9	385	14.5	35.1	10.0	13	0.5	12	0.4
Females										
0-4	0	0.0	0	0.0	-	-	0	0.0	0	0.0
5-14	1	0.2	8	1.6	13.0	10.0	0	0.0	0	0.0
15-44	59	4.9	334	27.9	35.0	10.0	2	0.1	1	0.1
45-59	1	0.2	111	35.7	52.4	10.0	2	0.7	1	0.4
60+	0	0.1	15	5.7	71.3	10.0	11	4.1	12	3.5
All ages	61	2.3	469	17.9	35.2	10.0	15	0.6	14	0.5
Total	111	2.1	854	16.2	35.1	10.0	28	0.5	26	0.4

For epidemiological sources see Berkley et al. 1996. For the methods used to estimate and project incidence, prevalence, and deaths see Murray and Lopez 1996a. See explanatory notes for definitions and caveats.

Table 17	Cuadro 17	Tableau 17
Syphilis	Sífilis	Syphilis
Tertiary - gummas	Terciaria - gomas	Tertiaire - gommes

Table 17a   EME - PEMC - EMBE   Syphilis - Tertiary - gummas

Age group (years)	Incidence 1990 Number ('000s)	Rate (per 100 000)	Prevalence 1990 Number ('000s)	Rate (per 100 000)	Avg. age at onset (years)	Average duration (years)	Deaths 1990 Number ('000s)	Rate (per 100 000)	Deaths 2000 (Projected) Number ('000s)	Rate (per 100 000)
Males										
0-4	0	0.0	0	0.0	-	-	0	0	0	0
5-14	0	0.0	0	0.0	13.0	2.0	0	0	0	0
15-44	0	0.1	0	0.1	35.0	2.0	0	0	0	0
45-59	0	0.0	0	0.0	52.4	2.0	0	0	0	0
60+	0	0.0	0	0.0	71.1	2.0	0	0	0	0
All ages	0	0.0	0	0.1	35.4	2.0	0	0	0	0
Females										
0-4	0	0.0	0	0.0	-	-	0	0	0	0
5-14	0	0.0	0	0.0	13.0	2.0	0	0	0	0
15-44	0	0.1	0	0.2	35.0	2.0	0	0	0	0
45-59	0	0.0	0	0.0	52.4	2.0	0	0	0	0
60+	0	0.0	0	0.0	72.4	2.0	0	0	0	0
All ages	0	0.0	0	0.1	35.7	2.0	0	0	0	0
Total	0	0.0	1	0.1	35.6	2.0	0	0	0	0

Table 17b   FSE - PEAS - AESE   Syphilis - Tertiary - gummas

Age group (years)	Incidence 1990 Number ('000s)	Rate (per 100 000)	Prevalence 1990 Number ('000s)	Rate (per 100 000)	Avg. age at onset (years)	Average duration (years)	Deaths 1990 Number ('000s)	Rate (per 100 000)	Deaths 2000 (Projected) Number ('000s)	Rate (per 100 000)
Males										
0-4	0	0.0	0	0.0	-	-	0	0	0	0
5-14	0	0.0	0	0.0	13.0	2.0	0	0	0	0
15-44	0	0.3	0	0.5	35.0	2.0	0	0	0	0
45-59	0	0.0	0	0.0	52.2	2.0	0	0	0	0
60+	0	0.0	0	0.0	70.0	2.0	0	0	0	0
All ages	0	0.1	0	0.3	35.3	2.0	0	0	0	0
Females										
0-4	0	0.0	0	0.0	-	-	0	0	0	0
5-14	0	0.0	0	0.0	13.0	2.0	0	0	0	0
15-44	0	0.3	0	0.5	35.0	2.0	0	0	0	0
45-59	0	0.0	0	0.0	52.4	2.0	0	0	0	0
60+	0	0.0	0	0.0	71.5	2.0	0	0	0	0
All ages	0	0.1	0	0.2	35.6	2.0	0	0	0	0
Total	0	0.1	1	0.2	35.5	2.0	0	0	0	0

Table 17c   India - India - Inde   Syphilis - Tertiary - gummas

Age group (years)	Incidence 1990 Number ('000s)	Rate (per 100 000)	Prevalence 1990 Number ('000s)	Rate (per 100 000)	Avg. age at onset (years)	Average duration (years)	Deaths 1990 Number ('000s)	Rate (per 100 000)	Deaths 2000 (Projected) Number ('000s)	Rate (per 100 000)
Males										
0-4	0	0.0	0	0.0	-	-	0	0	0	0
5-14	0	0.3	1	0.5	13.0	2.0	0	0	0	0
15-44	22	11.0	39	19.6	35.0	2.0	0	0	0	0
45-59	0	0.5	1	1.1	52.3	2.0	0	0	0	0
60+	0	0.3	0	0.5	69.7	2.0	0	0	0	0
All ages	23	5.1	41	9.2	35.0	2.0	0	0	0	0
Females										
0-4	0	0.0	0	0.0	-	-	0	0	0	0
5-14	0	0.3	1	0.7	13.0	2.0	0	0	0	0
15-44	25	13.7	45	24.5	35.0	2.0	0	0	0	0
45-59	0	0.7	1	1.4	52.4	2.0	0	0	0	0
60+	0	0.3	0	0.7	70.1	2.0	0	0	0	0
All ages	26	6.3	46	11.3	35.0	2.0	0	0	0	0
Total	48	5.7	87	10.2	35.0	2.0	0	0	0	0

For epidemiological sources see Berkley et al. 1996. For the methods used to estimate and project incidence, prevalence, and deaths see Murray and Lopez 1996a. See explanatory notes for definitions and caveats.

Table 17	Cuadro 17	Tableau 17
Syphilis	**Sífilis**	**Syphilis**
Tertiary - gummas	Terciaria - gomas	Tertiaire - gommes

Table 17d   China - China - Chine   Syphilis - Tertiary - gummas

Age group (years)	Incidence 1990 Number ('000s)	Rate (per 100 000)	Prevalence 1990 Number ('000s)	Rate (per 100 000)	Avg. age at onset (years)	Average duration (years)	Deaths 1990 Number ('000s)	Rate (per 100 000)	Deaths 2000 (Projected) Number ('000s)	Rate (per 100 000)
Males										
0-4	0	0	0	0	-	-	0	0	0	0
5-14	0	0	0	0	13.0	2.0	0	0	0	0
15-44	0	0	0	0	35.0	2.0	0	0	0	0
45-59	0	0	0	0	52.3	2.0	0	0	0	0
60+	0	0	0	0	69.8	2.0	0	0	0	0
All ages	0	0	0	0	35.1	2.0	0	0	0	0
Females										
0-4	0	0	0	0	-	-	0	0	0	0
5-14	0	0	0	0	13.0	2.0	0	0	0	0
15-44	0	0	0	0	35.0	2.0	0	0	0	0
45-59	0	0	0	0	52.4	2.0	0	0	0	0
60+	0	0	0	0	70.6	2.0	0	0	0	0
All ages	0	0	0	0	35.3	2.0	0	0	0	0
Total	0	0	0	0	35.2	2.0	0	0	0	0

Table 17e   OAI - OPAI - APAI   Syphilis - Tertiary - gummas

Age group (years)	Incidence 1990 Number ('000s)	Rate (per 100 000)	Prevalence 1990 Number ('000s)	Rate (per 100 000)	Avg. age at onset (years)	Average duration (years)	Deaths 1990 Number ('000s)	Rate (per 100 000)	Deaths 2000 (Projected) Number ('000s)	Rate (per 100 000)
Males										
0-4	0	0.0	0	0.0	-	-	0	0	0	0
5-14	0	0.2	0	0.4	13.0	2.0	0	0	0	0
15-44	14	8.8	25	15.8	35.0	2.0	0	0	0	0
45-59	0	0.4	0	0.9	52.3	2.0	0	0	0	0
60+	0	0.2	0	0.4	69.6	2.0	0	0	0	0
All ages	15	4.3	26	7.6	35.0	2.0	0	0	0	0
Females										
0-4	0	0.0	0	0.0	-	-	0	0	0	0
5-14	0	0.3	0	0.5	13.0	2.0	0	0	0	0
15-44	17	10.8	31	19.3	35.0	2.0	0	0	0	0
45-59	0	0.5	0	1.1	52.3	2.0	0	0	0	0
60+	0	0.3	0	0.5	70.3	2.0	0	0	0	0
All ages	18	5.2	32	9.3	35.0	2.0	0	0	0	0
Total	32	4.7	58	8.5	35.0	2.0	0	0	0	0

Table 17f   SSA - ASS - ASS   Syphilis - Tertiary - gummas

Age group (years)	Incidence 1990 Number ('000s)	Rate (per 100 000)	Prevalence 1990 Number ('000s)	Rate (per 100 000)	Avg. age at onset (years)	Average duration (years)	Deaths 1990 Number ('000s)	Rate (per 100 000)	Deaths 2000 (Projected) Number ('000s)	Rate (per 100 000)
Males										
0-4	0	0.0	0	0.0	-	-	0	0	0	0
5-14	0	0.6	1	1.1	13.0	2.0	0	0	0	0
15-44	23	22.1	41	39.6	35.0	2.0	0	0	0	0
45-59	0	1.1	0	2.2	52.2	2.0	0	0	0	0
60+	0	0.6	0	1.1	69.2	2.0	0	0	0	0
All ages	24	9.3	42	16.8	34.8	2.0	0	0	0	0
Females										
0-4	0	0.0	0	0.0	-	-	0	0	0	0
5-14	0	0.7	1	1.4	13.0	2.0	0	0	0	0
15-44	29	27.8	53	50.0	35.0	2.0	0	0	0	0
45-59	0	1.4	1	2.8	52.2	2.0	0	0	0	0
60+	0	0.7	0	1.4	-	2.0	0	0	0	0
All ages	30	27.1	55	48.8	34.7	2.0	0	0	0	0
Total	54	21.3	97	38.5	34.7	2.0	0	0	0	0

For epidemiological sources see Berkley et al. 1996. For the methods used to estimate and project incidence, prevalence, and deaths see Murray and Lopez 1996a. See explanatory notes for definitions and caveats.

Table 17   **Cuadro 17**   **Tableau 17**
Syphilis   **Sífilis**   **Syphilis**

Tertiary - gummas   Terciaria - gomas   Tertiaire - gommes

Table 17g   LAC - ALC - ALC   Syphilis - Tertiary - gummas

Age group (years)	Incidence 1990 Number ('000s)	Rate (per 100 000)	Prevalence 1990 Number ('000s)	Rate (per 100 000)	Avg. age at onset (years)	Average duration (years)	Deaths 1990 Number ('000s)	Rate (per 100 000)	Deaths 2000 (Projected) Number ('000s)	Rate (per 100 000)
Males										
0-4	0	0.0	0	0.0	-	-	0	0	0	0
5-14	0	0.1	0	0.1	13.0	2.0	0	0	0	0
15-44	3	2.7	5	4.8	35.0	2.0	0	0	0	0
45-59	0	0.1	0	0.3	52.3	2.0	0	0	0	0
60+	0	0.1	0	0.1	70.3	2.0	0	0	0	0
All ages	3	1.3	5	2.3	35.0	2.0	0	0	0	0
Females										
0-4	0	0.0	0	0.0	-	-	0	0	0	0
5-14	0	0.1	0	0.2	13.0	2.0	0	0	0	0
15-44	3	3.3	6	5.9	35.0	2.0	0	0	0	0
45-59	0	0.2	0	0.3	52.4	2.0	0	0	0	0
60+	0	0.1	0	0.2	71.1	2.0	0	0	0	0
All ages	4	1.6	6	2.9	35.0	2.0	0	0	0	0
Total	6	1.4	12	2.6	35.0	2.0	0	0	0	0

Table 17h   MEC - AOM - CMO   Syphilis - Tertiary - gummas

Age group (years)	Incidence 1990 Number ('000s)	Rate (per 100 000)	Prevalence 1990 Number ('000s)	Rate (per 100 000)	Avg. age at onset (years)	Average duration (years)	Deaths 1990 Number ('000s)	Rate (per 100 000)	Deaths 2000 (Projected) Number ('000s)	Rate (per 100 000)
Males										
0-4	0	0.0	0	0.0	-	-	0	0	0	0
5-14	0	0.0	0	0.1	13.0	2.0	0	0	0	0
15-44	2	2.0	4	3.6	35.0	2.0	0	0	0	0
45-59	0	0.1	0	0.2	52.3	2.0	0	0	0	0
60+	0	0.0	0	0.1	69.7	2.0	0	0	0	0
All ages	2	0.9	4	1.6	34.9	2.0	0	0	0	0
Females										
0-4	0	0.0	0	0.0	-	-	0	0	0	0
5-14	0	0.1	0	0.1	13.0	2.0	0	0	0	0
15-44	3	2.5	5	4.4	35.0	2.0	0	0	0	0
45-59	0	0.1	0	0.2	52.3	2.0	0	0	0	0
60+	0	0.1	0	0.1	70.4	2.0	0	0	0	0
All ages	3	1.1	5	2.0	34.9	2.0	0	0	0	0
Total	5	1.0	9	1.8	34.9	2.0	0	0	0	0

Table 17i   World - Mundo - Monde   Syphilis - Tertiary - gummas

Age group (years)	Incidence 1990 Number ('000s)	Rate (per 100 000)	Prevalence 1990 Number ('000s)	Rate (per 100 000)	Avg. age at onset (years)	Average duration (years)	Deaths 1990 Number ('000s)	Rate (per 100 000)	Deaths 2000 (Projected) Number ('000s)	Rate (per 100 000)
Males										
0-4	0	0.0	0	0.0	-	-	0	0	0	0
5-14	1	0.2	2	0.3	13.0	2.0	0	0	0	0
15-44	65	5.2	116	9.2	35.0	2.0	0	0	0	0
45-59	1	0.2	1	0.4	52.3	2.0	0	0	0	0
60+	0	0.1	0	0.2	69.6	2.0	0	0	0	0
All ages	66	2.5	119	4.5	34.9	2.0	0	0	0	0
Females										
0-4	0	0.0	0	0.0	-	-	0	0	0	0
5-14	1	0.2	2	0.4	13.0	2.0	0	0	0	0
15-44	78	6.5	141	11.7	35.0	2.0	0	0	0	0
45-59	1	0.3	2	0.6	52.3	2.0	0	0	0	0
60+	0	0.1	0	0.1	70.3	2.0	0	0	0	0
All ages	81	3.1	145	5.5	34.9	2.0	0	0	0	0
Total	147	2.8	264	5.0	34.9	2.0	0	0	0	0

For epidemiological sources see Berkley et al. 1996. For the methods used to estimate and project incidence, prevalence, and deaths see Murray and Lopez 1996a. See explanatory notes for definitions and caveats.

Table 18   **Cuadro 18**   **Tableau 18**
Syphilis   **Sífilis**   **Syphilis**

Tertiary - neurologic   Terciaria - neurosífilis   Tertiaire - nerveuse

Table 18a   EME - PEMC - EMBE   Syphilis - Tertiary - neurologic

Age group (years)	Incidence 1990 Number ('000s)	Rate (per 100 000)	Prevalence 1990 Number ('000s)	Rate (per 100 000)	Avg. age at onset (years)	Average duration (years)	Deaths 1990 Number ('000s)	Rate (per 100 000)	Deaths 2000 (Projected) Number ('000s)	Rate (per 100 000)
Males										
0-4	0	0.0	0	0.0	-	-	0	0.0	0	0.0
5-14	0	0.0	0	0.0	13.0	10.0	0	0.0	0	0.0
15-44	0	0.1	1	0.3	35.0	10.0	0	0.0	0	0.0
45-59	0	0.0	0	0.5	52.4	10.0	0	0.0	0	0.0
60+	0	0.0	0	0.1	71.1	10.0	0	0.1	0	0.1
All ages	0	0.0	1	0.3	35.4	10.0	0	0.0	0	0.0
Females										
0-4	0	0.0	0	0.0	-	-	0	0.0	0	0.0
5-14	0	0.0	0	0.0	13.0	10.0	0	0.0	0	0.0
15-44	0	0.1	1	0.3	35.0	10.0	0	0.0	0	0.0
45-59	0	0.0	0	0.4	52.4	10.0	0	0.0	0	0.0
60+	0	0.0	0	0.1	72.4	10.0	0	0.0	0	0.0
All ages	0	0.0	1	0.2	35.6	10.0	0	0.0	0	0.0
Total	0	0.0	2	0.2	35.5	10.0	0	0.0	0	0.0

Table 18b   FSE - PEAS - AESE   Syphilis - Tertiary - neurologic

Age group (years)	Incidence 1990 Number ('000s)	Rate (per 100 000)	Prevalence 1990 Number ('000s)	Rate (per 100 000)	Avg. age at onset (years)	Average duration (years)	Deaths 1990 Number ('000s)	Rate (per 100 000)	Deaths 2000 (Projected) Number ('000s)	Rate (per 100 000)
Males										
0-4	0	0.0	0	0.0	-	-	0	0	0	0
5-14	0	0.0	0	0.0	13.0	10.0	0	0	0	0
15-44	0	0.2	1	1.3	35.0	10.0	0	0	0	0
45-59	0	0.0	1	1.9	52.2	10.0	0	0	0	0
60+	0	0.0	0	0.4	70.0	10.0	0	0	0	0
All ages	0	0.1	2	1.0	35.3	10.0	0	0	0	0
Females										
0-4	0	0.0	0	0.0	-	-	0	0	0	0
5-14	0	0.0	0	0.0	13.0	10.0	0	0	0	0
15-44	0	0.2	1	1.3	35.0	10.0	0	0	0	0
45-59	0	0.0	1	1.7	52.4	10.0	0	0	0	0
60+	0	0.0	0	0.3	71.5	10.0	0	0	0	0
All ages	0	0.1	2	0.9	35.6	10.0	0	0	0	0
Total	0	0.1	3	0.9	35.5	10.0	0	0	0	0

Table 18c   India - India - Inde   Syphilis - Tertiary - neurologic

Age group (years)	Incidence 1990 Number ('000s)	Rate (per 100 000)	Prevalence 1990 Number ('000s)	Rate (per 100 000)	Avg. age at onset (years)	Average duration (years)	Deaths 1990 Number ('000s)	Rate (per 100 000)	Deaths 2000 (Projected) Number ('000s)	Rate (per 100 000)
Males										
0-4	0	0.0	0	0.0	-	-	0	0.0	0	0.0
5-14	0	0.2	0	0.4	13.0	10.0	0	0.0	0	0.0
15-44	16	8.2	93	46.6	35.0	10.0	0	0.2	0	0.1
45-59	0	0.4	32	67.2	52.3	10.0	0	0.8	0	0.4
60+	0	0.2	5	15.2	69.7	10.0	2	6.1	2	4.7
All ages	17	3.8	130	29.7	35.1	10.0	3	0.6	2	0.4
Females										
0-4	0	0.0	0	0.0	-	-	0	0.0	0	0.0
5-14	0	0.3	0	0.5	13.0	10.0	0	0.0	0	0.0
15-44	19	10.3	106	57.9	35.0	10.0	0	0.2	0	0.1
45-59	0	0.5	38	82.8	52.4	10.0	0	0.9	0	0.4
60+	0	0.3	5	17.9	70.1	10.0	2	7.2	2	5.5
All ages	19	4.7	150	36.6	35.1	10.0	3	0.7	3	0.5
Total	36	4.3	280	33.0	35.1	10.0	5	0.6	5	0.5

For epidemiological sources see Berkley et al. 1996. For the methods used to estimate and project incidence, prevalence, and deaths see Murray and Lopez 1996a. See explanatory notes for definitions and caveats.

Table 18	Cuadro 18	Tableau 18
Syphilis	Sífilis	Syphilis

Tertiary - neurologic   Terciaria - neurosífilis   Tertiaire - nerveuse

Table 18d   China - China - Chine   Syphilis - Tertiary - neurologic

Age group (years)	Incidence 1990 Number ('000s)	Rate (per 100 000)	Prevalence 1990 Number ('000s)	Rate (per 100 000)	Avg. age at onset (years)	Average duration (years)	Deaths 1990 Number ('000s)	Rate (per 100 000)	Deaths 2000 (Projected) Number ('000s)	Rate (per 100 000)
Males										
0-4	0	0	0	0.0	-	-	0	0.0	0	0.0
5-14	0	0	0	0.0	13.0	10.0	0	0.0	0	0.0
15-44	0	0	0	0.1	35.0	10.0	0	0.0	0	0.0
45-59	0	0	0	0.1	52.3	10.0	0	0.0	0	0.0
60+	0	0	0	0.0	69.8	10.0	0	0.0	0	0.0
All ages	0	0	0	0.0	35.2	10.0	0	0.0	0	0.0
Females										
0-4	0	0	0	0.0	-	-	0	0.0	0	0.0
5-14	0	0	0	0.0	13.0	10.0	0	0.0	0	0.0
15-44	0	0	0	0.1	35.0	10.0	0	0.0	0	0.0
45-59	0	0	0	0.1	52.4	10.0	0	0.0	0	0.0
60+	0	0	0	0.0	70.6	10.0	0	0.0	0	0.0
All ages	0	0	0	0.0	35.2	10.0	0	0.0	0	0.0
Total	0	0	0	0.0	35.2	10.0	0	0.0	0	0.0

Table 18e   OAI - OPAI - APAI   Syphilis - Tertiary - neurologic

Age group (years)	Incidence 1990 Number ('000s)	Rate (per 100 000)	Prevalence 1990 Number ('000s)	Rate (per 100 000)	Avg. age at onset (years)	Average duration (years)	Deaths 1990 Number ('000s)	Rate (per 100 000)	Deaths 2000 (Projected) Number ('000s)	Rate (per 100 000)
Males										
0-4	0	0.0	0	0.0	-	-	0	0.0	0	0.0
5-14	0	0.2	0	0.3	13.0	10.0	0	0.0	0	0.0
15-44	11	6.6	61	37.7	35.0	10.0	0	0.1	0	0.0
45-59	0	0.3	19	55.2	52.3	10.0	0	0.7	0	0.4
60+	0	0.2	3	12.8	69.6	10.0	1	6.0	1	4.8
All ages	11	3.2	82	24.0	35.0	10.0	2	0.5	2	0.4
Females										
0-4	0	0.0	0	0.0	-	-	0	0.0	0	0.0
5-14	0	0.2	0	0.4	13.0	10.0	0	0.0	0	0.0
15-44	13	8.2	74	46.6	35.0	10.0	0	0.1	0	0.0
45-59	0	0.4	23	66.5	52.3	10.0	0	0.9	0	0.4
60+	0	0.2	3	14.3	70.3	10.0	1	6.1	2	5.0
All ages	14	4.0	101	29.8	35.0	10.0	2	0.6	2	0.5
Total	24	3.6	183	26.9	35.0	10.0	4	0.5	4	0.4

Table 18f   SSA - ASS - ASS   Syphilis - Tertiary - neurologic

Age group (years)	Incidence 1990 Number ('000s)	Rate (per 100 000)	Prevalence 1990 Number ('000s)	Rate (per 100 000)	Avg. age at onset (years)	Average duration (years)	Deaths 1990 Number ('000s)	Rate (per 100 000)	Deaths 2000 (Projected) Number ('000s)	Rate (per 100 000)
Males										
0-4	0	0.0	0	0.0	-	-	0	0.0	0	0.0
5-14	0	0.4	1	0.8	13.0	10.0	0	0.0	0	0.0
15-44	17	16.7	99	95.5	35.0	10.0	0	0.2	0	0.1
45-59	0	0.8	32	155.3	52.2	10.0	0	2.0	0	1.1
60+	0	0.4	4	39.4	69.2	10.0	2	18.6	2	14.2
All ages	18	7.1	135	53.6	34.9	10.0	3	1.0	2	0.7
Females										
0-4	0	0.0	0	0.0	-	-	0	0.0	0	0.0
5-14	0	0.5	1	1.0	13.0	10.0	0	0.0	0	0.0
15-44	22	20.8	126	118.3	35.0	10.0	0	0.4	0	0.2
45-59	0	1.0	41	184.2	52.2	10.0	1	2.4	0	1.2
60+	0	0.5	0	43.9	69.7	10.0	3	19.9	3	14.8
All ages	23	8.8	167	64.8	34.8	10.0	3	1.3	3	0.9
Total	41	7.9	303	59.3	34.9	10.0	6	1.2	6	0.8

For epidemiological sources see Berkley et al. 1996. For the methods used to estimate and project incidence, prevalence, and deaths see Murray and Lopez 1996a. See explanatory notes for definitions and caveats.

Table 18　　　　　　　　**Cuadro 18**　　　　　　　　**Tableau 18**
Syphilis　　　　　　　　**Sífilis**　　　　　　　　　**Syphilis**

Tertiary - neurologic　　　　Terciaria - neurosífilis　　　Tertiaire - nerveuse

Table 18g　　　LAC - ALC - ALC　　　　　　　　　Syphilis - Tertiary - neurologic

Age group (years)	Incidence 1990 Number ('000s)	Rate (per 100 000)	Prevalence 1990 Number ('000s)	Rate (per 100 000)	Avg. age at onset (years)	Average duration (years)	Deaths 1990 Number ('000s)	Rate (per 100 000)	Deaths 2000 (Projected) Number ('000s)	Rate (per 100 000)
Males										
0-4	0	0.0	0	0.0	-	-	0	0.0	0	0.0
5-14	0	0.0	0	0.1	13.0	10.0	0	0.0	0	0.0
15-44	2	2.0	12	11.3	35.0	10.0	0	0.0	0	0.0
45-59	0	0.1	4	16.1	52.3	10.0	0	0.2	0	0.1
60+	0	0.0	0	3.5	70.3	10.0	0	1.6	0	1.3
All ages	2	1.0	16	7.2	35.0	10.0	0	0.1	0	0.1
Females										
0-4	0	0.0	0	0.0	-	-	0	0.0	0	0.0
5-14	0	0.1	0	0.1	13.0	10.0	0	0.0	0	0.0
15-44	3	2.5	15	14.0	35.0	10.0	0	0.0	0	0.0
45-59	0	0.1	5	19.4	52.4	10.0	0	0.3	0	0.1
60+	0	0.1	1	3.8	71.1	10.0	0	1.7	0	1.4
All ages	3	1.2	20	8.9	35.1	10.0	0	0.2	0	0.1
Total	5	1.1	36	8.0	35.1	10.0	1	0.2	1	0.1

Table 18h　　　MEC - AOM - CMO　　　　　　　　　Syphilis - Tertiary - neurologic

Age group (years)	Incidence 1990 Number ('000s)	Rate (per 100 000)	Prevalence 1990 Number ('000s)	Rate (per 100 000)	Avg. age at onset (years)	Average duration (years)	Deaths 1990 Number ('000s)	Rate (per 100 000)	Deaths 2000 (Projected) Number ('000s)	Rate (per 100 000)
Males										
0-4	0	0.0	0	0.0	-	-	0	0.0	0	0.0
5-14	0	0.0	0	0.1	13.0	10.0	0	0.0	0	0.0
15-44	2	1.5	10	8.5	35.0	10.0	0	0.0	0	0.0
45-59	0	0.1	3	12.2	52.3	10.0	0	0.2	0	0.1
60+	0	0.0	0	2.8	69.7	10.0	0	1.3	0	1.1
All ages	2	0.7	13	5.0	35.0	10.0	0	0.1	0	0.1
Females										
0-4	0	0.0	0	0.0	-	-	0	0.0	0	0.0
5-14	0	0.0	0	0.5	13.0	10.0	0	0.0	0	0.0
15-44	2	1.9	11	10.7	35.0	10.0	0	0.0	0	0.0
45-59	0	0.1	3	15.0	52.3	10.0	0	0.2	0	0.1
60+	0	0.0	0	3.1	70.4	10.0	0	1.3	0	1.1
All ages	2	0.8	16	6.3	35.0	10.0	0	0.1	0	0.1
Total	4	0.8	28	5.7	35.0	10.0	1	0.1	1	0.1

Table 18i　　　World - Mundo - Monde　　　　　　　Syphilis - Tertiary - neurologic

Age group (years)	Incidence 1990 Number ('000s)	Rate (per 100 000)	Prevalence 1990 Number ('000s)	Rate (per 100 000)	Avg. age at onset (years)	Average duration (years)	Deaths 1990 Number ('000s)	Rate (per 100 000)	Deaths 2000 (Projected) Number ('000s)	Rate (per 100 000)
Males										
0-4	0	0.0	0	0.0	-	-	0	0.0	0	0.0
5-14	1	0.1	1	0.3	13.0	10.0	0	0.0	0	0.0
15-44	49	3.9	276	22.1	35.0	10.0	1	0.1	0	0.0
45-59	1	0.2	90	28.7	52.3	10.0	1	0.4	1	0.2
60+	0	0.1	12	5.6	70.1	10.0	6	2.5	6	2.1
All ages	50	1.9	380	14.3	35.1	10.0	8	0.3	7	0.2
Females										
0-4	0	0.0	0	0.0	-	-	0	0.0	0	0.0
5-14	1	0.2	2	0.4	13.0	10.0	0	0.0	0	0.0
15-44	59	4.9	334	27.9	35.0	10.0	1	0.1	0	0.0
45-59	1	0.2	111	35.7	52.4	10.0	1	0.4	1	0.2
60+	0	0.1	10	3.6	71.3	10.0	7	2.4	7	2.1
All ages	61	2.3	456	17.5	35.2	10.0	9	0.3	8	0.3
Total	111	2.1	836	15.9	35.2	10.0	17	0.3	15	0.2

For epidemiological sources see Berkley et al. 1996. For the methods used to estimate and project incidence, prevalence, and deaths see Murray and Lopez 1996a. See explanatory notes for definitions and caveats.

Table 19
Chlamydia

Cuadro 19
Clamidia

Tableau 19
Chlamydiose

Ophthalmia neonatorum

Oftalmía neonatal

Ophtalmie néonatale

Table 19a   EME - PEMC - EMBE   Chlamydia - Ophthalmia neonatorum

Age group (years)	Incidence 1990 Number ('000s)	Rate (per 100 000)	Prevalence 1990 Number ('000s)	Rate (per 100 000)	Avg. age at onset (years)	Average duration (years)	Deaths 1990 Number ('000s)	Rate (per 100 000)	Deaths 2000 (Projected) Number ('000s)	Rate (per 100 000)
Males										
0-4	8	28.9	0	1.1	0.0	0.04	0	0	0	0
5-14	0	0.0	0	0.0	-	-	0	0	0	0
15-44	0	0.0	0	0.0	-	-	0	0	0	0
45-59	0	0.0	0	0.0	-	-	0	0	0	0
60+	0	0.0	0	0.0	-	-	0	0	0	0
All ages	8	1.9	0	0.1	0.0	0.04	0	0	0	0
Females										
0-4	7	28.8	0	1.1	0.0	0.04	0	0	0	0
5-14	0	0.0	0	0.0	-	-	0	0	0	0
15-44	0	0.0	0	0.0	-	-	0	0	0	0
45-59	0	0.0	0	0.0	-	-	0	0	0	0
60+	0	0.0	0	0.0	-	-	0	0	0	0
All ages	7	1.8	0	0.1	0.0	0.04	0	0	0	0
Total	15	1.9	1	0.1	0.0	0.04	0	0	0	0

Table 19b   FSE - PEAS - AESE   Chlamydia - Ophthalmia neonatorum

Age group (years)	Incidence 1990 Number ('000s)	Rate (per 100 000)	Prevalence 1990 Number ('000s)	Rate (per 100 000)	Avg. age at onset (years)	Average duration (years)	Deaths 1990 Number ('000s)	Rate (per 100 000)	Deaths 2000 (Projected) Number ('000s)	Rate (per 100 000)
Males										
0-4	22	163	1	6.3	0.0	0.04	0	0	0	0
5-14	0	0	0	0.0	-	-	0	0	0	0
15-44	0	0	0	0.0	-	-	0	0	0	0
45-59	0	0	0	0.0	-	-	0	0	0	0
60+	0	0	0	0.0	-	-	0	0	0	0
All ages	22	14	1	0.5	0.0	0.04	0	0	0	0
Females										
0-4	21	163	1	6.3	0.0	0.04	0	0	0	0
5-14	0	0	0	0.0	-	-	0	0	0	0
15-44	0	0	0	0.0	-	-	0	0	0	0
45-59	0	0	0	0.0	-	-	0	0	0	0
60+	0	0	0	0.0	-	-	0	0	0	0
All ages	21	12	1	0.5	0.0	0.04	0	0	0	0
Total	44	13	2	0.5	0.0	0.04	0	0	0	0

Table 19c   India - India - Inde   Chlamydia - Ophthalmia neonatorum

Age group (years)	Incidence 1990 Number ('000s)	Rate (per 100 000)	Prevalence 1990 Number ('000s)	Rate (per 100 000)	Avg. age at onset (years)	Average duration (years)	Deaths 1990 Number ('000s)	Rate (per 100 000)	Deaths 2000 (Projected) Number ('000s)	Rate (per 100 000)
Males										
0-4	354	593	14	22.9	0.0	0.04	0	0	0	0
5-14	0	0	0	0.0	-	-	0	0	0	0
15-44	0	0	0	0.0	-	-	0	0	0	0
45-59	0	0	0	0.0	-	-	0	0	0	0
60+	0	0	0	0.0	-	-	0	0	0	0
All ages	354	81	14	3.1	0.0	0.04	0	0	0	0
Females										
0-4	338	596	13	23.0	0.0	0.04	0	0	0	0
5-14	0	0	0	0.0	-	-	0	0	0	0
15-44	0	0	0	0.0	-	-	0	0	0	0
45-59	0	0	0	0.0	-	-	0	0	0	0
60+	0	0	0	0.0	-	-	0	0	0	0
All ages	338	82	13	3.2	0.0	0.04	0	0	0	0
Total	692	81	27	3.1	0.0	0.04	0	0	0	0

For epidemiological sources see Berkley et al. 1996. For the methods used to estimate and project incidence, prevalence, and deaths see Murray and Lopez 1996a. See explanatory notes for definitions and caveats.

Table 19   **Cuadro 19**   **Tableau 19**
Chlamydia   **Clamidia**   **Chlamydiose**

Ophthalmia neonatorum   Oftalmía neonatal   Ophtalmie néonatale

Table 19d   China - China - Chine   Chlamydia - Ophthalmia neonatorum

Age group (years)	Incidence 1990 Number ('000s)	Rate (per 100 000)	Prevalence 1990 Number ('000s)	Rate (per 100 000)	Avg. age at onset (years)	Average duration (years)	Deaths 1990 Number ('000s)	Rate (per 100 000)	Deaths 2000 (Projected) Number ('000s)	Rate (per 100 000)
Males										
0-4	5	8.8	0	0.3	0.0	0.04	0	0	0	0
5-14	0	0.0	0	0.0	-	-	0	0	0	0
15-44	0	0.0	0	0.0	-	-	0	0	0	0
45-59	0	0.0	0	0.0	-	-	0	0	0	0
60+	0	0.0	0	0.0	-	-	0	0	0	0
All ages	5	0.9	0	0.0	0.0	0.04	0	0	0	0
Females										
0-4	5	8.8	0	0.3	0.0	0.04	0	0	0	0
5-14	0	0.0	0	0.0	-	-	0	0	0	0
15-44	0	0.0	0	0.0	-	-	0	0	0	0
45-59	0	0.0	0	0.0	-	-	0	0	0	0
60+	0	0.0	0	0.0	-	-	0	0	0	0
All ages	5	0.9	0	0.0	0.0	0.04	0	0	0	0
Total	10	0.9	0	0.0	0.0	0.04	0	0	0	0

Table 19e   OAI - OPAI - APAI   Chlamydia - Ophthalmia neonatorum

Age group (years)	Incidence 1990 Number ('000s)	Rate (per 100 000)	Prevalence 1990 Number ('000s)	Rate (per 100 000)	Avg. age at onset (years)	Average duration (years)	Deaths 1990 Number ('000s)	Rate (per 100 000)	Deaths 2000 (Projected) Number ('000s)	Rate (per 100 000)
Males										
0-4	238	543	9	21.0	0.0	0.04	0	0	0	0
5-14	0	0	0	0.0	-	-	0	0	0	0
15-44	0	0	0	0.0	-	-	0	0	0	0
45-59	0	0	0	0.0	-	-	0	0	0	0
60+	0	0	0	0.0	-	-	0	0	0	0
All ages	238	69	9	2.7	0.0	0.04	0	0	0	0
Females										
0-4	227	540	9	20.8	0.0	0.04	0	0	0	0
5-14	0	0	0	0.0	-	-	0	0	0	0
15-44	0	0	0	0.0	-	-	0	0	0	0
45-59	0	0	0	0.0	-	-	0	0	0	0
60+	0	0	0	0.0	-	-	0	0	0	0
All ages	227	67	9	2.6	0.0	0.04	0	0	0	0
Total	464	68	18	2.6	0.0	0.04	0	0	0	0

Table 19f   SSA - ASS - ASS   Chlamydia - Ophthalmia neonatorum

Age group (years)	Incidence 1990 Number ('000s)	Rate (per 100 000)	Prevalence 1990 Number ('000s)	Rate (per 100 000)	Avg. age at onset (years)	Average duration (years)	Deaths 1990 Number ('000s)	Rate (per 100 000)	Deaths 2000 (Projected) Number ('000s)	Rate (per 100 000)
Males										
0-4	457	963	18	37.1	0.0	0.04	0	0	0	0
5-14	0	0	0	0.0	-	-	0	0	0	0
15-44	0	0	0	0.0	-	-	0	0	0	0
45-59	0	0	0	0.0	-	-	0	0	0	0
60+	0	0	0	0.0	-	-	0	0	0	0
All ages	457	181	18	7.0	0.0	0.04	0	0	0	0
Females										
0-4	447	951	17	36.7	0.0	0.04	0	0	0	0
5-14	0	0	0	0.0	-	-	0	0	0	0
15-44	0	0	0	0.0	-	-	0	0	0	0
45-59	0	0	0	0.0	-	-	0	0	0	0
60+	0	0	0	0.0	-	-	0	0	0	0
All ages	447	173	17	6.7	0.0	0.04	0	0	0	0
Total	904	177	35	6.8	0.0	0.04	0	0	0	0

For epidemiological sources see Berkley et al. 1996. For the methods used to estimate and project incidence, prevalence, and deaths see Murray and Lopez 1996a. See explanatory notes for definitions and caveats.

Table 19
Chlamydia

Cuadro 19
Clamidia

Tableau 19
Chlamydiose

Ophthalmia neonatorum

Oftalmía neonatal

Ophtalmie néonatale

Table 19g LAC - ALC - ALC Chlamydia - Ophthalmia neonatorum

Age group (years)	Incidence 1990 Number ('000s)	Rate (per 100 000)	Prevalence 1990 Number ('000s)	Rate (per 100 000)	Avg. age at onset (years)	Average duration (years)	Deaths 1990 Number ('000s)	Rate (per 100 000)	Deaths 2000 (Projected) Number ('000s)	Rate (per 100 000)
Males										
0-4	70	243	3	9.4	0.0	0.04	0	0	0	0
5-14	0	0	0	0.0	-	-	0	0	0	0
15-44	0	0	0	0.0	-	-	0	0	0	0
45-59	0	0	0	0.0	-	-	0	0	0	0
60+	0	0	0	0.0	-	-	0	0	0	0
All ages	70	31	3	1.2	0.0	0.04	0	0	0	0
Females										
0-4	67	242	3	9.3	0.0	0.04	0	0	0	0
5-14	0	0	0	0.0	-	-	0	0	0	0
15-44	0	0	0	0.0	-	-	0	0	0	0
45-59	0	0	0	0.0	-	-	0	0	0	0
60+	0	0	0	0.0	-	-	0	0	0	0
All ages	67	30	3	1.2	0.0	0.04	0	0	0	0
Total	137	31	5	1.2	0.0	0.04	0	0	0	0

Table 19h MEC - AOM - CMO Chlamydia - Ophthalmia neonatorum

Age group (years)	Incidence 1990 Number ('000s)	Rate (per 100 000)	Prevalence 1990 Number ('000s)	Rate (per 100 000)	Avg. age at onset (years)	Average duration (years)	Deaths 1990 Number ('000s)	Rate (per 100 000)	Deaths 2000 (Projected) Number ('000s)	Rate (per 100 000)
Males										
0-4	42	103	2	4.0	0.0	0.04	0	0	0	0
5-14	0	0	0	0.0	-	-	0	0	0	0
15-44	0	0	0	0.0	-	-	0	0	0	0
45-59	0	0	0	0.0	-	-	0	0	0	0
60+	0	0	0	0.0	-	-	0	0	0	0
All ages	42	17	2	0.6	0.0	0.04	0	0	0	0
Females										
0-4	41	103	2	4.0	0.0	0.04	0	0	0	0
5-14	0	0	0	0.0	-	-	0	0	0	0
15-44	0	0	0	0.0	-	-	0	0	0	0
45-59	0	0	0	0.0	-	-	0	0	0	0
60+	0	0	0	0.0	-	-	0	0	0	0
All ages	41	17	2	0.6	0.0	0.04	0	0	0	0
Total	83	17	3	0.6	0.0	0.04	0	0	0	0

Table 19i World - Mundo - Monde Chlamydia - Ophthalmia neonatorum

Age group (years)	Incidence 1990 Number ('000s)	Rate (per 100 000)	Prevalence 1990 Number ('000s)	Rate (per 100 000)	Avg. age at onset (years)	Average duration (years)	Deaths 1990 Number ('000s)	Rate (per 100 000)	Deaths 2000 (Projected) Number ('000s)	Rate (per 100 000)
Males										
0-4	1 197	373	46	14.4	0.0	0.04	0	0	0	0
5-14	0	0	0	0.0	-	-	0	0	0	0
15-44	0	0	0	0.0	-	-	0	0	0	0
45-59	0	0	0	0.0	-	-	0	0	0	0
60+	0	0	0	0.0	-	-	0	0	0	0
All ages	1 197	45	46	1.7	0.0	0.04	0	0	0	0
Females										
0-4	1 153	373	44	14.4	0.0	0.04	0	0	0	0
5-14	0	0	0	0.0	-	-	0	0	0	0
15-44	0	0	0	0.0	-	-	0	0	0	0
45-59	0	0	0	0.0	-	-	0	0	0	0
60+	0	0	0	0.0	-	-	0	0	0	0
All ages	1 153	44	44	1.7	0.0	0.04	0	0	0	0
Total	2 350	45	91	1.7	0.0	0.04	0	0	0	0

For epidemiological sources see Berkley et al. 1996. For the methods used to estimate and project incidence, prevalence, and deaths see Murray and Lopez 1996a. See explanatory notes for definitions and caveats.

Table 20
Chlamydia

Cuadro 20
Clamidia

Tableau 20
Chlamydiose

Low birth weight

Bajo peso al nacer

Poids insuffisant à la naissance

Table 20a EME - PEMC - EMBE

Chlamydia - Low birth weight

Age group (years)	Incidence 1990 Number ('000s)	Rate (per 100 000)	Prevalence 1990 Number ('000s)	Rate (per 100 000)	Avg. age at onset (years)	Average duration (years)	Deaths 1990 Number ('000s)	Rate (per 100 000)	Deaths 2000 (Projected) Number ('000s)	Rate (per 100 000)
Males										
0-4	13	48.1	6	24.1	0.0	0.50	0	0.5	0	0.4
5-14	0	0.0	0	0.0	-	-	0	0.0	0	0.0
15-44	0	0.0	0	0.0	-	-	0	0.0	0	0.0
45-59	0	0.0	0	0.0	-	-	0	0.0	0	0.0
60+	0	0.0	0	0.0	-	-	0	0.0	0	0.0
All ages	13	3.2	6	1.6	0.0	0.50	0	0.0	0	0.0
Females										
0-4	12	48.0	6	24.1	0.0	0.50	0	0.5	0	0.4
5-14	0	0.0	0	0.0	-	-	0	0.0	0	0.0
15-44	0	0.0	0	0.0	-	-	0	0.0	0	0.0
45-59	0	0.0	0	0.0	-	-	0	0.0	0	0.0
60+	0	0.0	0	0.0	-	-	0	0.0	0	0.0
All ages	12	3.0	6	1.5	0.0	0.50	0	0.0	0	0.0
Total	25	3.1	12	1.6	0.0	0.50	0	0.0	0	0.0

Table 20b FSE - PEAS - AESE

Chlamydia - Low birth weight

Age group (years)	Incidence 1990 Number ('000s)	Rate (per 100 000)	Prevalence 1990 Number ('000s)	Rate (per 100 000)	Avg. age at onset (years)	Average duration (years)	Deaths 1990 Number ('000s)	Rate (per 100 000)	Deaths 2000 (Projected) Number ('000s)	Rate (per 100 000)
Males										
0-4	7	54.4	4	27.3	0.0	0.50	0	2.7	0	1.9
5-14	0	0.0	0	0.0	-	-	0	0.0	0	0.0
15-44	0	0.0	0	0.0	-	-	0	0.0	0	0.0
45-59	0	0.0	0	0.0	-	-	0	0.0	0	0.0
60+	0	0.0	0	0.0	-	-	0	0.0	0	0.0
All ages	7	4.5	4	2.3	0.0	0.50	0	0.2	0	0.2
Females										
0-4	7	54.3	4	27.3	0.0	0.50	0	2.7	0	1.9
5-14	0	0.0	0	0.0	-	-	0	0.0	0	0.0
15-44	0	0.0	0	0.0	-	-	0	0.0	0	0.0
45-59	0	0.0	0	0.0	-	-	0	0.0	0	0.0
60+	0	0.0	0	0.0	-	-	0	0.0	0	0.0
All ages	7	3.9	4	2.0	0.0	0.50	0	0.2	0	0.1
Total	15	4.2	7	2.1	0.0	0.50	1	0.2	1	0.1

Table 20c India - India - Inde

Chlamydia - Low birth weight

Age group (years)	Incidence 1990 Number ('000s)	Rate (per 100 000)	Prevalence 1990 Number ('000s)	Rate (per 100 000)	Avg. age at onset (years)	Average duration (years)	Deaths 1990 Number ('000s)	Rate (per 100 000)	Deaths 2000 (Projected) Number ('000s)	Rate (per 100 000)
Males										
0-4	66	110	33	55.2	0.0	0.50	6	10.5	4	6.3
5-14	0	0	0	0.0	-	-	0	0.0	0	0.0
15-44	0	0	0	0.0	-	-	0	0.0	0	0.0
45-59	0	0	0	0.0	-	-	0	0.0	0	0.0
60+	0	0	0	0.0	-	-	0	0.0	0	0.0
All ages	66	15	33	7.5	0.0	0.50	6	1.4	4	0.9
Females										
0-4	62	110	31	55.4	0.0	0.50	6	10.5	3	6.2
5-14	0	0	0	0.0	-	-	0	0.0	0	0.0
15-44	0	0	0	0.0	-	-	0	0.0	0	0.0
45-59	0	0	0	0.0	-	-	0	0.0	0	0.0
60+	0	0	0	0.0	-	-	0	0.0	0	0.0
All ages	62	15	31	7.7	0.0	0.50	6	1.5	3	0.9
Total	128	15	64	7.6	0.0	0.50	12	1.4	7	0.9

For epidemiological sources see Berkley et al. 1996. For the methods used to estimate and project incidence, prevalence, and deaths see Murray and Lopez 1996a. See explanatory notes for definitions and caveats.

Table 20	Cuadro 20	Tableau 20
Chlamydia	Clamidia	Chlamydiose
Low birth weight	Bajo peso al nacer	Poids insuffisant à la naissance

Table 20d China - China - Chine Chlamydia - Low birth weight

Age group (years)	Incidence 1990 Number ('000s)	Rate (per 100 000)	Prevalence 1990 Number ('000s)	Rate (per 100 000)	Avg. age at onset (years)	Average duration (years)	Deaths 1990 Number ('000s)	Rate (per 100 000)	Deaths 2000 (Projected) Number ('000s)	Rate (per 100 000)
Males										
0-4	2	2.9	1	1.5	0.0	0.50	0	0.2	0	0.1
5-14	0	0.0	0	0.0	-	-	0	0.0	0	0.0
15-44	0	0.0	0	0.0	-	-	0	0.0	0	0.0
45-59	0	0.0	0	0.0	-	-	0	0.0	0	0.0
60+	0	0.0	0	0.0	-	-	0	0.0	0	0.0
All ages	2	0.3	1	0.2	0.0	0.50	0	0.0	0	0.0
Females										
0-4	2	2.9	1	1.5	0.0	0.50	0	0.2	0	0.1
5-14	0	0.0	0	0.0	-	-	0	0.0	0	0.0
15-44	0	0.0	0	0.0	-	-	0	0.0	0	0.0
45-59	0	0.0	0	0.0	-	-	0	0.0	0	0.0
60+	0	0.0	0	0.0	-	-	0	0.0	0	0.0
All ages	2	0.3	1	0.2	0.0	0.50	0	0.0	0	0.0
Total	3	0.3	2	0.2	0.0	0.50	0	0.0	0	0.0

Table 20e OAI - OPAI - APAI Chlamydia - Low birth weight

Age group (years)	Incidence 1990 Number ('000s)	Rate (per 100 000)	Prevalence 1990 Number ('000s)	Rate (per 100 000)	Avg. age at onset (years)	Average duration (years)	Deaths 1990 Number ('000s)	Rate (per 100 000)	Deaths 2000 (Projected) Number ('000s)	Rate (per 100 000)
Males										
0-4	44	101	22	50.5	0.0	0.50	4	9.3	3	6.1
5-14	0	0	0	0.0	-	-	0	0.0	0	0.0
15-44	0	0	0	0.0	-	-	0	0.0	0	0.0
45-59	0	0	0	0.0	-	-	0	0.0	0	0.0
60+	0	0	0	0.0	-	-	0	0.0	0	0.0
All ages	44	13	22	6.4	0.0	0.50	4	1.2	3	0.8
Females										
0-4	42	100	21	50.3	0.0	0.50	4	9.2	3	6.0
5-14	0	0	0	0.0	-	-	0	0.0	0	0.0
15-44	0	0	0	0.0	-	-	0	0.0	0	0.0
45-59	0	0	0	0.0	-	-	0	0.0	0	0.0
60+	0	0	0	0.0	-	-	0	0.0	0	0.0
All ages	42	12	21	6.2	0.0	0.50	4	1.1	3	0.7
Total	86	13	43	6.3	0.0	0.50	8	1.2	5	0.8

Table 20f SSA - ASS - ASS Chlamydia - Low birth weight

Age group (years)	Incidence 1990 Number ('000s)	Rate (per 100 000)	Prevalence 1990 Number ('000s)	Rate (per 100 000)	Avg. age at onset (years)	Average duration (years)	Deaths 1990 Number ('000s)	Rate (per 100 000)	Deaths 2000 (Projected) Number ('000s)	Rate (per 100 000)
Males										
0-4	85	178	42	89	0.0	0.50	8	17.7	9	18.0
5-14	0	0	0	0	-	-	0	0.0	0	0.0
15-44	0	0	0	0	-	-	0	0.0	0	0.0
45-59	0	0	0	0	-	-	0	0.0	0	0.0
60+	0	0	0	0	-	-	0	0.0	0	0.0
All ages	85	34	42	17	0.0	0.50	8	3.3	9	3.4
Females										
0-4	83	176	42	88	0.0	0.50	8	17.7	8	17.0
5-14	0	0	0	0	-	-	0	0.0	0	0.0
15-44	0	0	0	0	-	-	0	0.0	0	0.0
45-59	0	0	0	0	-	-	0	0.0	0	0.0
60+	0	0	0	0	-	-	0	0.0	0	0.0
All ages	83	32	42	16	0.0	0.50	8	3.2	8	3.1
Total	167	33	84	16	0.0	0.50	17	3.3	17	3.2

For epidemiological sources see Berkley et al. 1996. For the methods used to estimate and project incidence, prevalence, and deaths see Murray and Lopez 1996a. See explanatory notes for definitions and caveats.

Table 20
Chlamydia

Cuadro 20
Clamidia

Tableau 20
Chlamydiose

Low birth weight

Bajo peso al nacer

Poids insuffisant à la naissance

Table 20g   LAC - ALC - ALC   Chlamydia - Low birth weight

Age group (years)	Incidence 1990 Number ('000s)	Rate (per 100 000)	Prevalence 1990 Number ('000s)	Rate (per 100 000)	Avg. age at onset (years)	Average duration (years)	Deaths 1990 Number ('000s)	Rate (per 100 000)	Deaths 2000 (Projected) Number ('000s)	Rate (per 100 000)
Males										
0-4	23	81	12	40.7	0.0	0.50	1	4.0	1	2.9
5-14	0	0	0	0.0	-	-	0	0.0	0	0.0
15-44	0	0	0	0.0	-	-	0	0.0	0	0.0
45-59	0	0	0	0.0	-	-	0	0.0	0	0.0
60+	0	0	0	0.0	-	-	0	0.0	0	0.0
All ages	23	10	12	5.3	0.0	0.50	1	0.5	1	0.4
Females										
0-4	22	80	11	40.5	0.0	0.50	1	4.0	1	2.8
5-14	0	0	0	0.0	-	-	0	0.0	0	0.0
15-44	0	0	0	0.0	-	-	0	0.0	0	0.0
45-59	0	0	0	0.0	-	-	0	0.0	0	0.0
60+	0	0	0	0.0	-	-	0	0.0	0	0.0
All ages	22	10	11	5.0	0.0	0.50	1	0.5	1	0.3
Total	46	10	23	5.2	0.0	0.50	2	0.5	2	0.4

Table 20h   MEC - AOM - CMO   Chlamydia - Low birth weight

Age group (years)	Incidence 1990 Number ('000s)	Rate (per 100 000)	Prevalence 1990 Number ('000s)	Rate (per 100 000)	Avg. age at onset (years)	Average duration (years)	Deaths 1990 Number ('000s)	Rate (per 100 000)	Deaths 2000 (Projected) Number ('000s)	Rate (per 100 000)
Males										
0-4	14	34.3	7	17.2	0.0	0.50	1	1.7	1	1.6
5-14	0	0.0	0	0.0	-	-	0	0.0	0	0.0
15-44	0	0.0	0	0.0	-	-	0	0.0	0	0.0
45-59	0	0.0	0	0.0	-	-	0	0.0	0	0.0
60+	0	0.0	0	0.0	-	-	0	0.0	0	0.0
All ages	14	5.5	7	2.8	0.0	0.50	1	0.3	1	0.3
Females										
0-4	14	34.3	7	17.2	0.0	0.50	1	1.7	1	1.5
5-14	0	0.0	0	0.0	-	-	0	0.0	0	0.0
15-44	0	0.0	0	0.0	-	-	0	0.0	0	0.0
45-59	0	0.0	0	0.0	-	-	0	0.0	0	0.0
60+	0	0.0	0	0.0	-	-	0	0.0	0	0.0
All ages	14	5.5	7	2.8	0.0	0.50	1	0.3	1	0.2
Total	28	5.5	14	2.8	0.0	0.50	1	0.3	1	0.2

Table 20i   World - Mundo - Monde   Chlamydia - Low birth weight

Age group (years)	Incidence 1990 Number ('000s)	Rate (per 100 000)	Prevalence 1990 Number ('000s)	Rate (per 100 000)	Avg. age at onset (years)	Average duration (years)	Deaths 1990 Number ('000s)	Rate (per 100 000)	Deaths 2000 (Projected) Number ('000s)	Rate (per 100 000)
Males										
0-4	254	78.9	127	39.6	0.0	0.50	21	6.6	16	5.1
5-14	0	0.0	0	0.0	-	-	0	0.0	0	0.0
15-44	0	0.0	0	0.0	-	-	0	0.0	0	0.0
45-59	0	0.0	0	0.0	-	-	0	0.0	0	0.0
60+	0	0.0	0	0.0	-	-	0	0.0	0	0.0
All ages	254	9.6	127	4.8	0.0	0.50	21	0.8	16	0.6
Females										
0-4	244	78.9	123	39.7	0.0	0.50	21	6.6	15	4.9
5-14	0	0.0	0	0.0	-	-	0	0.0	0	0.0
15-44	0	0.0	0	0.0	-	-	0	0.0	0	0.0
45-59	0	0.0	0	0.0	-	-	0	0.0	0	0.0
60+	0	0.0	0	0.0	-	-	0	0.0	0	0.0
All ages	244	9.3	123	4.7	0.0	0.50	21	0.8	15	0.6
Total	498	9.4	250	4.7	0.0	0.50	42	0.8	32	0.6

For epidemiological sources see Berkley et al. 1996. For the methods used to estimate and project incidence, prevalence, and deaths see Murray and Lopez 1996a. See explanatory notes for definitions and caveats.

Table 21	Cuadro 21	Tableau 21
Chlamydia	**Clamidia**	**Chlamydiose**
Corneal scar - blindness	Cicatriz de la córnea - ceguera	Cicatrice de la cornée - cécité

Table 21a   EME - PEMC - EMBE   Chlamydia - Corneal scar - blindness

Age group (years)	Incidence 1990 Number ('000s)	Rate (per 100 000)	Prevalence 1990 Number ('000s)	Rate (per 100 000)	Avg. age at onset (years)	Average duration (years)	Deaths 1990 Number ('000s)	Rate (per 100 000)	Deaths 2000 (Projected) Number ('000s)	Rate (per 100 000)
Males										
0-4	0	0	0	0	-	-	0	0	0	0
5-14	0	0	0	0	-	-	0	0	0	0
15-44	0	0	0	0	-	-	0	0	0	0
45-59	0	0	0	0	-	-	0	0	0	0
60+	0	0	0	0	-	-	0	0	0	0
All ages	0	0	0	0	-	-	0	0	0	0
Females										
0-4	0	0	0	0	-	-	0	0	0	0
5-14	0	0	0	0	-	-	0	0	0	0
15-44	0	0	0	0	-	-	0	0	0	0
45-59	0	0	0	0	-	-	0	0	0	0
60+	0	0	0	0	-	-	0	0	0	0
All ages	0	0	0	0	-	-	0	0	0	0
Total	0	0	0	0	-	-	0	0	0	0

Table 21b   FSE - PEAS - AESE   Chlamydia - Corneal scar - blindness

Age group (years)	Incidence 1990 Number ('000s)	Rate (per 100 000)	Prevalence 1990 Number ('000s)	Rate (per 100 000)	Avg. age at onset (years)	Average duration (years)	Deaths 1990 Number ('000s)	Rate (per 100 000)	Deaths 2000 (Projected) Number ('000s)	Rate (per 100 000)
Males										
0-4	0	0	0	0	-	-	0	0	0	0
5-14	0	0	0	0	-	-	0	0	0	0
15-44	0	0	0	0	-	-	0	0	0	0
45-59	0	0	0	0	-	-	0	0	0	0
60+	0	0	0	0	-	-	0	0	0	0
All ages	0	0	0	0	-	-	0	0	0	0
Females										
0-4	0	0	0	0	-	-	0	0	0	0
5-14	0	0	0	0	-	-	0	0	0	0
15-44	0	0	0	0	-	-	0	0	0	0
45-59	0	0	0	0	-	-	0	0	0	0
60+	0	0	0	0	-	-	0	0	0	0
All ages	0	0	0	0	-	-	0	0	0	0
Total	0	0	0	0	-	-	0	0	0	0

Table 21c   India - India - Inde   Chlamydia - Corneal scar - blindness

Age group (years)	Incidence 1990 Number ('000s)	Rate (per 100 000)	Prevalence 1990 Number ('000s)	Rate (per 100 000)	Avg. age at onset (years)	Average duration (years)	Deaths 1990 Number ('000s)	Rate (per 100 000)	Deaths 2000 (Projected) Number ('000s)	Rate (per 100 000)
Males										
0-4	1	2.2	5	8.3	0.0	36.8	0	0	0	0
5-14	0	0.0	8	8.1	-	-	0	0	0	0
15-44	0	0.0	15	7.4	-	-	0	0	0	0
45-59	0	0.0	3	5.9	-	-	0	0	0	0
60+	0	0.0	1	2.8	-	-	0	0	0	0
All ages	1	0.3	32	7.2	0.0	36.8	0	0	0	0
Females										
0-4	1	2.2	5	8.2	0.0	36.5	0	0	0	0
5-14	0	0.0	8	7.9	-	-	0	0	0	0
15-44	0	0.0	13	7.2	-	-	0	0	0	0
45-59	0	0.0	3	5.9	-	-	0	0	0	0
60+	0	0.0	1	3.1	-	-	0	0	0	0
All ages	1	0.3	29	7.1	0.0	36.5	0	0	0	0
Total	3	0.3	61	7.2	0.0	36.7	0	0	0	0

For epidemiological sources see Berkley et al. 1996. For the methods used to estimate and project incidence, prevalence, and deaths see Murray and Lopez 1996a. See explanatory notes for definitions and caveats.

Table 21
Chlamydia

Corneal scar - blindness

Cuadro 21
Clamidia

Cicatriz de la córnea - ceguera

Tableau 21
Chlamydiose

Cicatrice de la cornée - cécité

Table 21d — China - China - Chine — Chlamydia - Corneal scar - blindness

Age group (years)	Incidence 1990 Number ('000s)	Rate (per 100 000)	Prevalence 1990 Number ('000s)	Rate (per 100 000)	Avg. age at onset (years)	Average duration (years)	Deaths 1990 Number ('000s)	Rate (per 100 000)	Deaths 2000 (Projected) Number ('000s)	Rate (per 100 000)
Males										
0-4	0	0.0	0	0.1	0.0	50.7	0	0	0	0
5-14	0	0.0	0	0.1	-	-	0	0	0	0
15-44	0	0.0	0	0.1	-	-	0	0	0	0
45-59	0	0.0	0	0.0	-	-	0	0	0	0
60+	0	0.0	0	0.0	-	-	0	0	0	0
All ages	0	0.0	0	0.1	0.0	50.7	0	0	0	0
Females										
0-4	0	0.0	0	0.1	0.0	53.2	0	0	0	0
5-14	0	0.0	0	0.1	-	-	0	0	0	0
15-44	0	0.0	0	0.1	-	-	0	0	0	0
45-59	0	0.0	0	0.0	-	-	0	0	0	0
60+	0	0.0	0	0.0	-	-	0	0	0	0
All ages	0	0.0	0	0.1	0.0	53.2	0	0	0	0
Total	0	0.0	1	0.1	0.0	51.9	0	0	0	0

Table 21e — OAI - OPAI - APAI — Chlamydia - Corneal scar - blindness

Age group (years)	Incidence 1990 Number ('000s)	Rate (per 100 000)	Prevalence 1990 Number ('000s)	Rate (per 100 000)	Avg. age at onset (years)	Average duration (years)	Deaths 1990 Number ('000s)	Rate (per 100 000)	Deaths 2000 (Projected) Number ('000s)	Rate (per 100 000)
Males										
0-4	1	2.0	4	8.6	0.0	39.0	0	0	0	0
5-14	0	0.0	7	8.0	-	-	0	0	0	0
15-44	0	0.0	12	7.3	-	-	0	0	0	0
45-59	0	0.0	2	5.5	-	-	0	0	0	0
60+	0	0.0	0	2.4	-	-	0	0	0	0
All ages	1	0.3	24	7.1	0.0	39.0	0	0	0	0
Females										
0-4	1	2.0	4	8.8	0.0	43.1	0	0	0	0
5-14	0	0.0	7	8.2	-	-	0	0	0	0
15-44	0	0.0	12	7.6	-	-	0	0	0	0
45-59	0	0.0	2	6.1	-	-	0	0	0	0
60+	0	0.0	1	3.0	-	-	0	0	0	0
All ages	1	0.3	25	7.3	0.0	43.1	0	0	0	0
Total	2	0.3	49	7.2	0.0	41.0	0	0	0	0

Table 21f — SSA - ASS - ASS — Chlamydia - Corneal scar - blindness

Age group (years)	Incidence 1990 Number ('000s)	Rate (per 100 000)	Prevalence 1990 Number ('000s)	Rate (per 100 000)	Avg. age at onset (years)	Average duration (years)	Deaths 1990 Number ('000s)	Rate (per 100 000)	Deaths 2000 (Projected) Number ('000s)	Rate (per 100 000)
Males										
0-4	2	3.6	6	11.9	0.0	21.5	0	0	0	0
5-14	0	0.0	7	10.3	-	-	0	0	0	0
15-44	0	0.0	8	8.2	-	-	0	0	0	0
45-59	0	0.0	1	5.1	-	-	0	0	0	0
60+	0	0.0	0	2.1	-	-	0	0	0	0
All ages	2	0.7	23	9.0	0.0	21.5	0	0	0	0
Females										
0-4	2	3.6	6	12.2	0.0	24.8	0	0	0	0
5-14	0	0.0	8	10.9	-	-	0	0	0	0
15-44	0	0.0	9	8.9	-	-	0	0	0	0
45-59	0	0.0	1	6.0	-	-	0	0	0	0
60+	0	0.0	0	2.6	-	-	0	0	0	0
All ages	2	0.7	24	9.5	0.0	24.8	0	0	0	0
Total	3	0.7	47	9.2	0.0	23.1	0	0	0	0

For epidemiological sources see Berkley et al. 1996. For the methods used to estimate and project incidence, prevalence, and deaths see Murray and Lopez 1996a. See explanatory notes for definitions and caveats.

Table 21
Chlamydia

Cuadro 21
Clamidia

Tableau 21
Chlamydiose

Corneal scar - blindness

Cicatriz de la córnea - ceguera

Cicatrice de la cornée - cécité

Table 21g   LAC - ALC - ALC   Chlamydia - Corneal scar - blindness

Age group (years)	Incidence 1990 Number ('000s)	Rate (per 100 000)	Prevalence 1990 Number ('000s)	Rate (per 100 000)	Avg. age at onset (years)	Average duration (years)	Deaths 1990 Number ('000s)	Rate (per 100 000)	Deaths 2000 (Projected) Number ('000s)	Rate (per 100 000)
Males										
0-4	0	0.4	0	1.6	0.0	45.0	0	0	0	0
5-14	0	0.0	1	1.5	-	-	0	0	0	0
15-44	0	0.0	1	1.4	-	-	0	0	0	0
45-59	0	0.0	0	1.1	-	-	0	0	0	0
60+	0	0.0	0	0.6	-	-	0	0	0	0
All ages	0	0.0	3	1.4	0.0	45.0	0	0	0	0
Females										
0-4	0	0.4	0	1.7	0.0	50.5	0	0	0	0
5-14	0	0.0	1	1.6	-	-	0	0	0	0
15-44	0	0.0	2	1.5	-	-	0	0	0	0
45-59	0	0.0	0	1.3	-	-	0	0	0	0
60+	0	0.0	0	0.7	-	-	0	0	0	0
All ages	0	0.0	3	1.4	0.0	50.5	0	0	0	0
Total	0	0.0	6	1.4	0.0	47.7	0	0	0	0

Table 21h   MEC - AOM - CMO   Chlamydia - Corneal scar - blindness

Age group (years)	Incidence 1990 Number ('000s)	Rate (per 100 000)	Prevalence 1990 Number ('000s)	Rate (per 100 000)	Avg. age at onset (years)	Average duration (years)	Deaths 1990 Number ('000s)	Rate (per 100 000)	Deaths 2000 (Projected) Number ('000s)	Rate (per 100 000)
Males										
0-4	0	0.2	0	0.6	0.0	39.3	0	0	0	0
5-14	0	0.0	0	0.6	-	-	0	0	0	0
15-44	0	0.0	1	0.5	-	-	0	0	0	0
45-59	0	0.0	0	0.4	-	-	0	0	0	0
60+	0	0.0	0	0.2	-	-	0	0	0	0
All ages	0	0.0	1	0.5	0.0	39.3	0	0	0	0
Females										
0-4	0	0.2	0	0.6	0.0	41.5	0	0	0	0
5-14	0	0.0	0	0.6	-	-	0	0	0	0
15-44	0	0.0	1	0.6	-	-	0	0	0	0
45-59	0	0.0	0	0.5	-	-	0	0	0	0
60+	0	0.0	0	0.2	-	-	0	0	0	0
All ages	0	0.0	1	0.5	0.0	41.5	0	0	0	0
Total	0	0.0	3	0.5	0.0	40.4	0	0	0	0

Table 21i   World - Mundo - Monde   Chlamydia - Corneal scar - blindness

Age group (years)	Incidence 1990 Number ('000s)	Rate (per 100 000)	Prevalence 1990 Number ('000s)	Rate (per 100 000)	Avg. age at onset (years)	Average duration (years)	Deaths 1990 Number ('000s)	Rate (per 100 000)	Deaths 2000 (Projected) Number ('000s)	Rate (per 100 000)
Males										
0-4	4	1.3	15	4.7	0.0	31.2	0	0	0	0
5-14	0	0.0	23	4.2	-	-	0	0	0	0
15-44	0	0.0	37	3.0	-	-	0	0	0	0
45-59	0	0.0	6	2.0	-	-	0	0	0	0
60+	0	0.0	2	0.8	-	-	0	0	0	0
All ages	4	0.2	83	3.1	0.0	31.2	0	0	0	0
Females										
0-4	4	1.3	15	4.8	0.0	33.4	0	0	0	0
5-14	0	0.0	23	4.4	-	-	0	0	0	0
15-44	0	0.0	37	3.1	-	-	0	0	0	0
45-59	0	0.0	7	2.1	-	-	0	0	0	0
60+	0	0.0	2	0.8	-	-	0	0	0	0
All ages	4	0.2	83	3.2	0.0	33.4	0	0	0	0
Total	8	0.2	167	3.2	0.0	32.3	0	0	0	0

For epidemiological sources see Berkley et al. 1996. For the methods used to estimate and project incidence, prevalence, and deaths see Murray and Lopez 1996a. See explanatory notes for definitions and caveats.

Table 22	Cuadro 22	Tableau 22
Chlamydia	Clamidia	Chlamydiose
	Cicatriz de la córnea - disminución	Cicatrice de la cornée - baisse
Corneal scar - low vision	de la agudeza visual	de la vision

Table 22a   EME - PEMC - EMBE   Chlamydia - Corneal scar - low vision

Age group (years)	Incidence 1990 Number ('000s)	Rate (per 100 000)	Prevalence 1990 Number ('000s)	Rate (per 100 000)	Avg. age at onset (years)	Average duration (years)	Deaths 1990 Number ('000s)	Rate (per 100 000)	Deaths 2000 (Projected) Number ('000s)	Rate (per 100 000)
Males										
0-4	0	0	0	0	-	-	0	0	0	0
5-14	0	0	0	0	-	-	0	0	0	0
15-44	0	0	0	0	-	-	0	0	0	0
45-59	0	0	0	0	-	-	0	0	0	0
60+	0	0	0	0	-	-	0	0	0	0
All ages	0	0	0	0	-	-	0	0	0	0
Females										
0-4	0	0	0	0	-	-	0	0	0	0
5-14	0	0	0	0	-	-	0	0	0	0
15-44	0	0	0	0	-	-	0	0	0	0
45-59	0	0	0	0	-	-	0	0	0	0
60+	0	0	0	0	-	-	0	0	0	0
All ages	0	0	0	0	-	-	0	0	0	0
Total	0	0	0	0	-	-	0	0	0	0

Table 22b   FSE - PEAS - AESE   Chlamydia - Corneal scar - low vision

Age group (years)	Incidence 1990 Number ('000s)	Rate (per 100 000)	Prevalence 1990 Number ('000s)	Rate (per 100 000)	Avg. age at onset (years)	Average duration (years)	Deaths 1990 Number ('000s)	Rate (per 100 000)	Deaths 2000 (Projected) Number ('000s)	Rate (per 100 000)
Males										
0-4	0	2.4	1	3.9	0.0	21.2	0	0	0	0
5-14	0	0.0	1	3.9	-	-	0	0	0	0
15-44	0	0.0	3	3.9	-	-	0	0	0	0
45-59	0	0.0	1	3.9	-	-	0	0	0	0
60+	0	0.0	1	3.9	-	-	0	0	0	0
All ages	0	0.2	6	3.9	0.0	21.2	0	0	0	0
Females										
0-4	0	2.4	1	3.9	0.0	24.1	0	0	0	0
5-14	0	0.0	1	3.9	-	-	0	0	0	0
15-44	0	0.0	3	3.9	-	-	0	0	0	0
45-59	0	0.0	1	3.9	-	-	0	0	0	0
60+	0	0.0	1	3.9	-	-	0	0	0	0
All ages	0	0.2	7	3.9	0.0	24.1	0	0	0	0
Total	1	0.2	14	3.9	0.0	22.6	0	0	0	0

Table 22c   India - India - Inde   Chlamydia - Corneal scar - low vision

Age group (years)	Incidence 1990 Number ('000s)	Rate (per 100 000)	Prevalence 1990 Number ('000s)	Rate (per 100 000)	Avg. age at onset (years)	Average duration (years)	Deaths 1990 Number ('000s)	Rate (per 100 000)	Deaths 2000 (Projected) Number ('000s)	Rate (per 100 000)
Males										
0-4	12	20.0	14	24	0.0	14.9	0	0	0	0
5-14	0	0.0	24	24	-	-	0	0	0	0
15-44	0	0.0	48	24	-	-	0	0	0	0
45-59	0	0.0	11	24	-	-	0	0	0	0
60+	0	0.0	7	24	-	-	0	0	0	0
All ages	12	2.7	105	24	0.0	14.9	0	0	0	0
Females										
0-4	11	20.1	14	24	0.0	15.1	0	0	0	0
5-14	0	0.0	23	24	-	-	0	0	0	0
15-44	0	0.0	44	24	-	-	0	0	0	0
45-59	0	0.0	11	24	-	-	0	0	0	0
60+	0	0.0	7	24	-	-	0	0	0	0
All ages	11	2.8	98	24	0.0	15.1	0	0	0	0
Total	23	2.8	203	24	0.0	15.0	0	0	0	0

For epidemiological sources see Berkley et al. 1996. For the methods used to estimate and project incidence, prevalence, and deaths see Murray and Lopez 1996a. See explanatory notes for definitions and caveats.

Table 22
Chlamydia

Corneal scar - low vision

Cuadro 22
Clamidia
Cicatriz de la córnea - disminución
de la agudeza visual

Tableau 22
Chlamydiose
Cicatrice de la cornée - baisse
de la vision

Table 22d — China - China - Chine — Chlamydia - Corneal scar - low vision

Age group (years)	Incidence 1990 Number ('000s)	Rate (per 100 000)	Prevalence 1990 Number ('000s)	Rate (per 100 000)	Avg. age at onset (years)	Average duration (years)	Deaths 1990 Number ('000s)	Rate (per 100 000)	Deaths 2000 (Projected) Number ('000s)	Rate (per 100 000)
Males										
0-4	0	0.1	0	0.1	0.0	17.1	0	0	0	0
5-14	0	0.0	0	0.1	-	-	0	0	0	0
15-44	0	0.0	0	0.1	-	-	0	0	0	0
45-59	0	0.0	0	0.1	-	-	0	0	0	0
60+	0	0.0	0	0.1	-	-	0	0	0	0
All ages	0	0.0	1	0.1	0.0	17.1	0	0	0	0
Females										
0-4	0	0.1	0	0.1	0.0	17.7	0	0	0	0
5-14	0	0.0	0	0.1	-	-	0	0	0	0
15-44	0	0.0	0	0.1	-	-	0	0	0	0
45-59	0	0.0	0	0.1	-	-	0	0	0	0
60+	0	0.0	0	0.1	-	-	0	0	0	0
All ages	0	0.0	1	0.1	0.0	17.7	0	0	0	0
Total	0	0.0	2	0.1	0.0	17.4	0	0	0	0

Table 22e — OAI - OPAI - APAI — Chlamydia - Corneal scar - low vision

Age group (years)	Incidence 1990 Number ('000s)	Rate (per 100 000)	Prevalence 1990 Number ('000s)	Rate (per 100 000)	Avg. age at onset (years)	Average duration (years)	Deaths 1990 Number ('000s)	Rate (per 100 000)	Deaths 2000 (Projected) Number ('000s)	Rate (per 100 000)
Males										
0-4	8	18.3	10	22	0.0	15.1	0	0	0	0
5-14	0	0.0	19	22	-	-	0	0	0	0
15-44	0	0.0	36	22	-	-	0	0	0	0
45-59	0	0.0	8	22	-	-	0	0	0	0
60+	0	0.0	4	22	-	-	0	0	0	0
All ages	8	2.3	76	22	0.0	15.1	0	0	0	0
Females										
0-4	8	18.2	9	22	0.0	16.0	0	0	0	0
5-14	0	0.0	18	22	-	-	0	0	0	0
15-44	0	0.0	36	22	-	-	0	0	0	0
45-59	0	0.0	8	22	-	-	0	0	0	0
60+	0	0.0	5	22	-	-	0	0	0	0
All ages	8	2.3	76	22	0.0	16.0	0	0	0	0
Total	16	2.3	152	22	0.0	15.6	0	0	0	0

Table 22f — SSA - ASS - ASS — Chlamydia - Corneal scar - low vision

Age group (years)	Incidence 1990 Number ('000s)	Rate (per 100 000)	Prevalence 1990 Number ('000s)	Rate (per 100 000)	Avg. age at onset (years)	Average duration (years)	Deaths 1990 Number ('000s)	Rate (per 100 000)	Deaths 2000 (Projected) Number ('000s)	Rate (per 100 000)
Males										
0-4	15	32.5	18	37	0.0	11.7	0	0	0	0
5-14	0	0.0	26	37	-	-	0	0	0	0
15-44	0	0.0	39	37	-	-	0	0	0	0
45-59	0	0.0	8	37	-	-	0	0	0	0
60+	0	0.0	4	37	-	-	0	0	0	0
All ages	15	6.1	94	37	0.0	11.7	0	0	0	0
Females										
0-4	15	32.1	18	37	0.0	12.6	0	0	0	0
5-14	0	0.0	26	37	-	-	0	0	0	0
15-44	0	0.0	40	37	-	-	0	0	0	0
45-59	0	0.0	8	37	-	-	0	0	0	0
60+	0	0.0	5	37	-	-	0	0	0	0
All ages	15	5.9	96	37	0.0	12.6	0	0	0	0
Total	31	6.0	191	37	0.0	12.2	0	0	0	0

For epidemiological sources see Berkley et al. 1996. For the methods used to estimate and project incidence, prevalence, and deaths see Murray and Lopez 1996a. See explanatory notes for definitions and caveats.

Table 22
Chlamydia

Corneal scar - low vision

Cuadro 22
Clamidia
Cicatriz de la córnea - disminución
de la agudeza visual

Tableau 22
Chlamydiose
Cicatrice de la cornée - baisse
de la vision

Table 22g LAC - ALC - ALC — Chlamydia - Corneal scar - low vision

Age group (years)	Incidence 1990 Number ('000s)	Rate (per 100 000)	Prevalence 1990 Number ('000s)	Rate (per 100 000)	Avg. age at onset (years)	Average duration (years)	Deaths 1990 Number ('000s)	Rate (per 100 000)	Deaths 2000 (Projected) Number ('000s)	Rate (per 100 000)
Males										
0-4	1	3.3	1	4.0	0.0	16.3	0	0	0	0
5-14	0	0.0	2	4.0	-	-	0	0	0	0
15-44	0	0.0	4	4.0	-	-	0	0	0	0
45-59	0	0.0	1	4.0	-	-	0	0	0	0
60+	0	0.0	1	4.0	-	-	0	0	0	0
All ages	1	0.4	9	4.0	0.0	16.3	0	0	0	0
Females										
0-4	1	3.3	1	4.0	0.0	17.4	0	0	0	0
5-14	0	0.0	2	4.0	-	-	0	0	0	0
15-44	0	0.0	4	4.0	-	-	0	0	0	0
45-59	0	0.0	1	4.0	-	-	0	0	0	0
60+	0	0.0	1	4.0	-	-	0	0	0	0
All ages	1	0.4	9	4.0	0.0	17.4	0	0	0	0
Total	2	0.4	18	4.0	0.0	16.8	0	0	0	0

Table 22h MEC - AOM - CMO — Chlamydia - Corneal scar - low vision

Age group (years)	Incidence 1990 Number ('000s)	Rate (per 100 000)	Prevalence 1990 Number ('000s)	Rate (per 100 000)	Avg. age at onset (years)	Average duration (years)	Deaths 1990 Number ('000s)	Rate (per 100 000)	Deaths 2000 (Projected) Number ('000s)	Rate (per 100 000)
Males										
0-4	1	1.4	1	1.7	0.0	15.3	0	0	0	0
5-14	0	0.0	1	1.7	-	-	0	0	0	0
15-44	0	0.0	2	1.7	-	-	0	0	0	0
45-59	0	0.0	0	1.7	-	-	0	0	0	0
60+	0	0.0	0	1.7	-	-	0	0	0	0
All ages	1	0.2	4	1.7	0.0	15.3	0	0	0	0
Females										
0-4	1	1.4	1	1.7	0.0	15.9	0	0	0	0
5-14	0	0.0	1	1.7	-	-	0	0	0	0
15-44	0	0.0	2	1.7	-	-	0	0	0	0
45-59	0	0.0	0	1.7	-	-	0	0	0	0
60+	0	0.0	0	1.7	-	-	0	0	0	0
All ages	1	0.2	4	1.7	0.0	15.9	0	0	0	0
Total	1	0.2	8	1.7	0.0	15.6	0	0	0	0

Table 22i World - Mundo - Monde — Chlamydia - Corneal scar - low vision

Age group (years)	Incidence 1990 Number ('000s)	Rate (per 100 000)	Prevalence 1990 Number ('000s)	Rate (per 100 000)	Avg. age at onset (years)	Average duration (years)	Deaths 1990 Number ('000s)	Rate (per 100 000)	Deaths 2000 (Projected) Number ('000s)	Rate (per 100 000)
Males										
0-4	37	11.6	44	13.8	0.0	13.7	0	0	0	0
5-14	0	0.0	74	13.4	-	-	0	0	0	0
15-44	0	0.0	132	10.6	-	-	0	0	0	0
45-59	0	0.0	29	9.3	-	-	0	0	0	0
60+	0	0.0	17	7.9	-	-	0	0	0	0
All ages	37	1.4	296	11.2	0.0	13.7	0	0	0	0
Females										
0-4	36	11.6	43	13.9	0.0	14.4	0	0	0	0
5-14	0	0.0	71	15.3	-	-	0	0	0	0
15-44	0	0.0	128	12.9	-	-	0	0	0	0
45-59	0	0.0	30	13.0	-	-	0	0	0	0
60+	0	0.0	19	11.9	-	-	0	0	0	0
All ages	36	1.4	291	11.1	0.0	14.4	0	0	0	0
Total	73	1.4	587	11.2	0.0	14.1	0	0	0	0

For epidemiological sources see Berkley et al. 1996. For the methods used to estimate and project incidence, prevalence, and deaths see Murray and Lopez 1996a. See explanatory notes for definitions and caveats.

Table 23	Cuadro 23	Tableau 23
Chlamydia	Clamidia	Chlamydiose
Cervicitis	Cervicitis	Cervicite

Table 23a   EME - PEMC - EMBE   Chlamydia - Cervicitis

Age group (years)	Incidence 1990 Number ('000s)	Rate (per 100 000)	Prevalence 1990 Number ('000s)	Rate (per 100 000)	Avg. age at onset (years)	Average duration (years)	Deaths 1990 Number ('000s)	Rate (per 100 000)	Deaths 2000 (Projected) Number ('000s)	Rate (per 100 000)
Males										
0-4	0	0	0	0	-	-	0	0	0	0
5-14	0	0	0	0	-	-	0	0	0	0
15-44	0	0	0	0	-	-	0	0	0	0
45-59	0	0	0	0	-	-	0	0	0	0
60+	0	0	0	0	-	-	0	0	0	0
All ages	0	0	0	0	-	-	0	0	0	0
Females										
0-4	0	0	0	0.0	-	-	0	0	0	0
5-14	13	26	0	0.9	13.0	0.03	0	0	0	0
15-44	1 838	1 026	61	33.8	22.0	0.03	0	0	0	0
45-59	35	51	1	1.7	52.4	0.03	0	0	0	0
60+	22	26	1	0.9	72.4	0.03	0	0	0	0
All ages	1 908	468	63	15.5	23.1	0.03	0	0	0	0
Total	1 908	239	63	7.9	23.1	0.03	0	0	0	0

Table 23b   FSE - PEAS - AESE   Chlamydia - Cervicitis

Age group (years)	Incidence 1990 Number ('000s)	Rate (per 100 000)	Prevalence 1990 Number ('000s)	Rate (per 100 000)	Avg. age at onset (years)	Average duration (years)	Deaths 1990 Number ('000s)	Rate (per 100 000)	Deaths 2000 (Projected) Number ('000s)	Rate (per 100 000)
Males										
0-4	0	0	0	0	-	-	0	0	0	0
5-14	0	0	0	0	-	-	0	0	0	0
15-44	0	0	0	0	-	-	0	0	0	0
45-59	0	0	0	0	-	-	0	0	0	0
60+	0	0	0	0	-	-	0	0	0	0
All ages	0	0	0	0	-	-	0	0	0	0
Females										
0-4	0	0	0	0.0	-	-	0	0	0	0
5-14	7	26	0	1.1	13.0	0.04	0	0	0	0
15-44	771	1 029	32	43.0	22.0	0.04	0	0	0	0
45-59	15	51	1	2.2	52.4	0.04	0	0	0	0
60+	9	26	0	1.1	71.5	0.04	0	0	0	0
All ages	803	444	34	18.6	23.1	0.04	0	0	0	0
Total	803	232	34	9.7	23.1	0.04	0	0	0	0

Table 23c   India - India - Inde   Chlamydia - Cervicitis

Age group (years)	Incidence 1990 Number ('000s)	Rate (per 100 000)	Prevalence 1990 Number ('000s)	Rate (per 100 000)	Avg. age at onset (years)	Average duration (years)	Deaths 1990 Number ('000s)	Rate (per 100 000)	Deaths 2000 (Projected) Number ('000s)	Rate (per 100 000)
Males										
0-4	0	0	0	0	-	-	0	0	0	0
5-14	0	0	0	0	-	-	0	0	0	0
15-44	0	0	0	0	-	-	0	0	0	0
45-59	0	0	0	0	-	-	0	0	0	0
60+	0	0	0	0	-	-	0	0	0	0
All ages	0	0	0	0	-	-	0	0	0	0
Females										
0-4	0	0	0	0.0	-	-	0	0	0	0
5-14	37	39	2	2.0	13.0	0.05	0	0	0	0
15-44	2 866	1 564	145	79.2	22.0	0.05	0	0	0	0
45-59	36	78	2	4.0	52.4	0.05	0	0	0	0
60+	11	39	1	2.0	70.1	0.05	0	0	0	0
All ages	2 951	720	149	36.4	22.4	0.05	0	0	0	0
Total	2 951	347	149	17.6	22.4	0.05	0	0	0	0

For epidemiological sources see Berkley et al. 1996. For the methods used to estimate and project incidence, prevalence, and deaths see Murray and Lopez 1996a. See explanatory notes for definitions and caveats.

Table 23 — **Cuadro 23** — **Tableau 23**
Chlamydia — **Clamidia** — **Chlamydiose**

Cervicitis — Cervicitis — Cervicite

Table 23d China - China - Chine — Chlamydia - Cervicitis

Age group (years)	Incidence 1990 Number ('000s)	Rate (per 100 000)	Prevalence 1990 Number ('000s)	Rate (per 100 000)	Avg. age at onset (years)	Average duration (years)	Deaths 1990 Number ('000s)	Rate (per 100 000)	Deaths 2000 (Projected) Number ('000s)	Rate (per 100 000)
Males										
0-4	0	0	0	0	-	-	0	0	0	0
5-14	0	0	0	0	-	-	0	0	0	0
15-44	0	0	0	0	-	-	0	0	0	0
45-59	0	0	0	0	-	-	0	0	0	0
60+	0	0	0	0	-	-	0	0	0	0
All ages	0	0	0	0	-	-	0	0	0	0
Females										
0-4	0	0.0	0	0.0	-	-	0	0	0	0
5-14	1	1.5	0	0.1	13.0	0.04	0	0	0	0
15-44	170	60.0	7	2.5	22.0	0.04	0	0	0	0
45-59	2	3.0	0	0.1	52.4	0.04	0	0	0	0
60+	1	1.5	0	0.1	70.6	0.04	0	0	0	0
All ages	175	31.8	7	1.3	22.5	0.04	0	0	0	0
Total	175	15.4	7	0.6	22.5	0.04	0	0	0	0

Table 23e OAI - OPAI - APAI — Chlamydia - Cervicitis

Age group (years)	Incidence 1990 Number ('000s)	Rate (per 100 000)	Prevalence 1990 Number ('000s)	Rate (per 100 000)	Avg. age at onset (years)	Average duration (years)	Deaths 1990 Number ('000s)	Rate (per 100 000)	Deaths 2000 (Projected) Number ('000s)	Rate (per 100 000)
Males										
0-4	0	0	0	0	-	-	0	0	0	0
5-14	0	0	0	0	-	-	0	0	0	0
15-44	0	0	0	0	-	-	0	0	0	0
45-59	0	0	0	0	-	-	0	0	0	0
60+	0	0	0	0	-	-	0	0	0	0
All ages	0	0	0	0	-	-	0	0	0	0
Females										
0-4	0	0	0	0.0	-	-	0	0	0	0
5-14	28	35	1	1.8	13.0	0.05	0	0	0	0
15-44	2 219	1 390	112	70.4	22.0	0.05	0	0	0	0
45-59	24	70	1	3.5	52.3	0.05	0	0	0	0
60+	8	35	0	1.8	70.3	0.05	0	0	0	0
All ages	2 279	671	115	34.0	22.4	0.05	0	0	0	0
Total	2 279	334	115	16.9	22.4	0.05	0	0	0	0

Table 23f SSA - ASS - ASS — Chlamydia - Cervicitis

Age group (years)	Incidence 1990 Number ('000s)	Rate (per 100 000)	Prevalence 1990 Number ('000s)	Rate (per 100 000)	Avg. age at onset (years)	Average duration (years)	Deaths 1990 Number ('000s)	Rate (per 100 000)	Deaths 2000 (Projected) Number ('000s)	Rate (per 100 000)
Males										
0-4	0	0	0	0	-	-	0	0	0	0
5-14	0	0	0	0	-	-	0	0	0	0
15-44	0	0	0	0	-	-	0	0	0	0
45-59	0	0	0	0	-	-	0	0	0	0
60+	0	0	0	0	-	-	0	0	0	0
All ages	0	0	0	0	-	-	0	0	0	0
Females										
0-4	0	0	0	0.0	-	-	0	0	0	0
5-14	38	55	2	2.8	13.0	0.05	0	0	0	0
15-44	2 337	2 200	118	111.3	22.0	0.05	0	0	0	0
45-59	24	110	1	5.6	52.2	0.05	0	0	0	0
60+	7	55	0	2.8	69.7	0.05	0	0	0	0
All ages	2 407	933	122	47.2	22.3	0.05	0	0	0	0
Total	2 407	472	122	23.9	22.3	0.05	0	0	0	0

For epidemiological sources see Berkley et al. 1996. For the methods used to estimate and project incidence, prevalence, and deaths see Murray and Lopez 1996a. See explanatory notes for definitions and caveats.

Table 23 Chlamydia	Cuadro 23 Clamidia	Tableau 23 Chlamydiose
Cervicitis	Cervicitis	Cervicite

Table 23g   LAC - ALC - ALC   Chlamydia - Cervicitis

Age group (years)	Incidence 1990 Number ('000s)	Rate (per 100 000)	Prevalence 1990 Number ('000s)	Rate (per 100 000)	Avg. age at onset (years)	Average duration (years)	Deaths 1990 Number ('000s)	Rate (per 100 000)	Deaths 2000 (Projected) Number ('000s)	Rate (per 100 000)
Males										
0-4	0	0	0	0	-	-	0	0	0	0
5-14	0	0	0	0	-	-	0	0	0	0
15-44	0	0	0	0	-	-	0	0	0	0
45-59	0	0	0	0	-	-	0	0	0	0
60+	0	0	0	0	-	-	0	0	0	0
All ages	0	0	0	0	-	-	0	0	0	0
Females										
0-4	0	0	0	0.0	-	-	0	0	0	0
5-14	17	34	1	1.4	13.0	0.04	0	0	0	0
15-44	1 415	1 360	59	56.8	22.0	0.04	0	0	0	0
45-59	16	68	1	2.9	52.4	0.04	0	0	0	0
60+	6	34	0	1.4	71.1	0.04	0	0	0	0
All ages	1 454	653	61	27.3	22.4	0.04	0	0	0	0
Total	1 454	327	61	13.7	22.4	0.04	0	0	0	0

Table 23h   MEC - AOM - CMO   Chlamydia - Cervicitis

Age group (years)	Incidence 1990 Number ('000s)	Rate (per 100 000)	Prevalence 1990 Number ('000s)	Rate (per 100 000)	Avg. age at onset (years)	Average duration (years)	Deaths 1990 Number ('000s)	Rate (per 100 000)	Deaths 2000 (Projected) Number ('000s)	Rate (per 100 000)
Males										
0-4	0	0	0	0	-	-	0	0	0	0
5-14	0	0	0	0	-	-	0	0	0	0
15-44	0	0	0	0	-	-	0	0	0	0
45-59	0	0	0	0	-	-	0	0	0	0
60+	0	0	0	0	-	-	0	0	0	0
All ages	0	0	0	0	-	-	0	0	0	0
Females										
0-4	0	0	0	0.0	-	-	0	0	0	0
5-14	8	14	0	0.6	13.0	0.04	0	0	0	0
15-44	583	544	24	22.7	22.0	0.04	0	0	0	0
45-59	6	27	0	1.1	52.3	0.04	0	0	0	0
60+	2	14	0	0.6	70.4	0.04	0	0	0	0
All ages	600	243	25	10.2	22.3	0.04	0	0	0	0
Total	600	119	25	5.0	22.3	0.04	0	0	0	0

Table 23i   World - Mundo - Monde   Chlamydia - Cervicitis

Age group (years)	Incidence 1990 Number ('000s)	Rate (per 100 000)	Prevalence 1990 Number ('000s)	Rate (per 100 000)	Avg. age at onset (years)	Average duration (years)	Deaths 1990 Number ('000s)	Rate (per 100 000)	Deaths 2000 (Projected) Number ('000s)	Rate (per 100 000)
Males										
0-4	0	0	0	0	-	-	0	0	0	0
5-14	0	0	0	0	-	-	0	0	0	0
15-44	0	0	0	0	-	-	0	0	0	0
45-59	0	0	0	0	-	-	0	0	0	0
60+	0	0	0	0	-	-	0	0	0	0
All ages	0	0	0	0	-	-	0	0	0	0
Females										
0-4	0	0	0	0.0	-	-	0	0	0	0
5-14	150	29	7	1.4	13.0	0.05	0	0	0	0
15-44	12 201	1 018	559	46.7	22.0	0.05	0	0	0	0
45-59	159	51	7	2.3	52.4	0.04	0	0	0	0
60+	66	24	3	1.0	71.1	0.04	0	0	0	0
All ages	12 576	481	576	22.0	22.5	0.05	0	0	0	0
Total	12 576	239	576	10.9	22.5	0.05	0	0	0	0

For epidemiological sources see Berkley et al. 1996. For the methods used to estimate and project incidence, prevalence, and deaths see Murray and Lopez 1996a. See explanatory notes for definitions and caveats.

Table 24	Cuadro 24	Tableau 24
Chlamydia	Clamidia	Chlamydiose

Neonatal pneumonia   Neumonía neonatal   Pneumonie néonatale

Table 24a   EME - PEMC - EMBE   Chlamydia - Neonatal pneumonia

Age group (years)	Incidence 1990 Number ('000s)	Rate (per 100 000)	Prevalence 1990 Number ('000s)	Rate (per 100 000)	Avg. age at onset (years)	Average duration (years)	Deaths 1990 Number ('000s)	Rate (per 100 000)	Deaths 2000 (Projected) Number ('000s)	Rate (per 100 000)
Males										
0-4	13	48.1	6	24.1	0.0	0.50	0	0.5	0	0.3
5-14	0	0.0	0	0.0	-	-	0	0.0	0	0.0
15-44	0	0.0	0	0.0	-	-	0	0.0	0	0.0
45-59	0	0.0	0	0.0	-	-	0	0.0	0	0.0
60+	0	0.0	0	0.0	-	-	0	0.0	0	0.0
All ages	13	3.2	6	1.6	0.0	0.50	0	0.0	0	0.0
Females										
0-4	12	48.0	6	24.1	0.0	0.50	0	0.5	0	0.3
5-14	0	0.0	0	0.0	-	-	0	0.0	0	0.0
15-44	0	0.0	0	0.0	-	-	0	0.0	0	0.0
45-59	0	0.0	0	0.0	-	-	0	0.0	0	0.0
60+	0	0.0	0	0.0	-	-	0	0.0	0	0.0
All ages	12	3.0	6	1.5	0.0	0.50	0	0.0	0	0.0
Total	25	3.1	12	1.6	0.0	0.50	0	0.0	0	0.0

Table 24b   FSE - PEAS - AESE   Chlamydia - Neonatal pneumonia

Age group (years)	Incidence 1990 Number ('000s)	Rate (per 100 000)	Prevalence 1990 Number ('000s)	Rate (per 100 000)	Avg. age at onset (years)	Average duration (years)	Deaths 1990 Number ('000s)	Rate (per 100 000)	Deaths 2000 (Projected) Number ('000s)	Rate (per 100 000)
Males										
0-4	7	54.4	4	27.3	0.0	0.50	0	2.7	0	2.0
5-14	0	0.0	0	0.0	-	-	0	0.0	0	0.0
15-44	0	0.0	0	0.0	-	-	0	0.0	0	0.0
45-59	0	0.0	0	0.0	-	-	0	0.0	0	0.0
60+	0	0.0	0	0.0	-	-	0	0.0	0	0.0
All ages	7	4.5	4	2.3	0.0	0.50	0	0.2	0	0.2
Females										
0-4	7	54.3	4	27.3	0.0	0.50	0	2.7	0	2.0
5-14	0	0.0	0	0.0	-	-	0	0.0	0	0.0
15-44	0	0.0	0	0.0	-	-	0	0.0	0	0.0
45-59	0	0.0	0	0.0	-	-	0	0.0	0	0.0
60+	0	0.0	0	0.0	-	-	0	0.0	0	0.0
All ages	7	3.9	4	2.0	0.0	0.50	0	0.2	0	0.2
Total	15	4.2	7	2.1	0.0	0.50	1	0.2	1	0.2

Table 24c   India - India - Inde   Chlamydia - Neonatal pneumonia

Age group (years)	Incidence 1990 Number ('000s)	Rate (per 100 000)	Prevalence 1990 Number ('000s)	Rate (per 100 000)	Avg. age at onset (years)	Average duration (years)	Deaths 1990 Number ('000s)	Rate (per 100 000)	Deaths 2000 (Projected) Number ('000s)	Rate (per 100 000)
Males										
0-4	66	110	33	55.2	0.0	0.50	6	10.5	4	6.5
5-14	0	0	0	0.0	-	-	0	0.0	0	0.0
15-44	0	0	0	0.0	-	-	0	0.0	0	0.0
45-59	0	0	0	0.0	-	-	0	0.0	0	0.0
60+	0	0	0	0.0	-	-	0	0.0	0	0.0
All ages	66	15	33	7.5	0.0	0.50	6	1.4	4	0.8
Females										
0-4	62	110	31	55.4	0.0	0.50	6	10.5	3	6.3
5-14	0	0	0	0.0	-	-	0	0.0	0	0.0
15-44	0	0	0	0.0	-	-	0	0.0	0	0.0
45-59	0	0	0	0.0	-	-	0	0.0	0	0.0
60+	0	0	0	0.0	-	-	0	0.0	0	0.0
All ages	62	15	31	7.7	0.0	0.50	6	1.5	4	0.8
Total	128	15	64	7.6	0.0	0.50	12	1.4	8	0.8

For epidemiological sources see Berkley et al. 1996. For the methods used to estimate and project incidence, prevalence, and deaths see Murray and Lopez 1996a. See explanatory notes for definitions and caveats.

Table 24
Chlamydia

Cuadro 24
Clamidia

Tableau 24
Chlamydiose

Neonatal pneumonia

Neumonía neonatal

Pneumonie néonatale

Table 24d China - China - Chine — Chlamydia - Neonatal pneumonia

Age group (years)	Incidence 1990 Number ('000s)	Rate (per 100 000)	Prevalence 1990 Number ('000s)	Rate (per 100 000)	Avg. age at onset (years)	Average duration (years)	Deaths 1990 Number ('000s)	Rate (per 100 000)	Deaths 2000 (Projected) Number ('000s)	Rate (per 100 000)
Males										
0-4	2	2.9	1	1.5	0.0	0.50	0	0.2	0	0.1
5-14	0	0.0	0	0.0	-	-	0	0.0	0	0.0
15-44	0	0.0	0	0.0	-	-	0	0.0	0	0.0
45-59	0	0.0	0	0.0	-	-	0	0.0	0	0.0
60+	0	0.0	0	0.0	-	-	0	0.0	0	0.0
All ages	2	0.3	1	0.2	0.0	0.50	0	0.0	0	0.0
Females										
0-4	2	2.9	1	1.5	0.0	0.50	0	0.2	0	0.1
5-14	0	0.0	0	0.0	-	-	0	0.0	0	0.0
15-44	0	0.0	0	0.0	-	-	0	0.0	0	0.0
45-59	0	0.0	0	0.0	-	-	0	0.0	0	0.0
60+	0	0.0	0	0.0	-	-	0	0.0	0	0.0
All ages	2	0.3	1	0.2	0.0	0.50	0	0.0	0	0.0
Total	3	0.3	2	0.2	0.0	0.50	0	0.0	0	0.0

Table 24e OAI - OPAI - APAI — Chlamydia - Neonatal pneumonia

Age group (years)	Incidence 1990 Number ('000s)	Rate (per 100 000)	Prevalence 1990 Number ('000s)	Rate (per 100 000)	Avg. age at onset (years)	Average duration (years)	Deaths 1990 Number ('000s)	Rate (per 100 000)	Deaths 2000 (Projected) Number ('000s)	Rate (per 100 000)
Males										
0-4	44	101	22	50.5	0.0	0.50	4	9.3	3	7.0
5-14	0	0	0	0.0	-	-	0	0.0	0	0.0
15-44	0	0	0	0.0	-	-	0	0.0	0	0.0
45-59	0	0	0	0.0	-	-	0	0.0	0	0.0
60+	0	0	0	0.0	-	-	0	0.0	0	0.0
All ages	44	13	22	6.4	0.0	0.50	4	1.2	4	1.1
Females										
0-4	42	100	21	50.3	0.0	0.50	4	9.2	3	6.8
5-14	0	0	0	0.0	-	-	0	0.0	0	0.0
15-44	0	0	0	0.0	-	-	0	0.0	0	0.0
45-59	0	0	0	0.0	-	-	0	0.0	0	0.0
60+	0	0	0	0.0	-	-	0	0.0	0	0.0
All ages	42	12	21	6.2	0.0	0.50	4	1.1	4	1.1
Total	86	13	43	6.3	0.0	0.50	8	1.2	8	1.1

Table 24f SSA - ASS - ASS — Chlamydia - Neonatal pneumonia

Age group (years)	Incidence 1990 Number ('000s)	Rate (per 100 000)	Prevalence 1990 Number ('000s)	Rate (per 100 000)	Avg. age at onset (years)	Average duration (years)	Deaths 1990 Number ('000s)	Rate (per 100 000)	Deaths 2000 (Projected) Number ('000s)	Rate (per 100 000)
Males										
0-4	85	178	42	89	0.0	0.50	9	18.1	5	11.3
5-14	0	0	0	0	-	-	0	0.0	0	0.0
15-44	0	0	0	0	-	-	0	0.0	0	0.0
45-59	0	0	0	0	-	-	0	0.0	0	0.0
60+	0	0	0	0	-	-	0	0.0	0	0.0
All ages	85	34	42	17	0.0	0.50	9	3.4	6	2.0
Females										
0-4	83	176	42	88	0.0	0.50	8	17.4	5	10.4
5-14	0	0	0	0	-	-	0	0.0	0	0.0
15-44	0	0	0	0	-	-	0	0.0	0	0.0
45-59	0	0	0	0	-	-	0	0.0	0	0.0
60+	0	0	0	0	-	-	0	0.0	0	0.0
All ages	83	32	42	16	0.0	0.50	8	3.2	5	1.8
Total	167	33	84	16	0.0	0.50	17	3.3	11	1.9

For epidemiological sources see Berkley et al. 1996. For the methods used to estimate and project incidence, prevalence, and deaths see Murray and Lopez 1996a. See explanatory notes for definitions and caveats.

Table 24	Cuadro 24	Tableau 24
Chlamydia	Clamidia	Chlamydiose

Neonatal pneumonia	Neumonía neonatal	Pneumonie néonatale

Table 24g LAC - ALC - ALC Chlamydia - Neonatal pneumonia

Age group (years)	Incidence 1990 Number ('000s)	Rate (per 100 000)	Prevalence 1990 Number ('000s)	Rate (per 100 000)	Avg. age at onset (years)	Average duration (years)	Deaths 1990 Number ('000s)	Rate (per 100 000)	Deaths 2000 (Projected) Number ('000s)	Rate (per 100 000)
Males										
0-4	23	81	12	40.7	0.0	0.50	1	4.0	1	2.8
5-14	0	0	0	0.0	-	-	0	0.0	0	0.0
15-44	0	0	0	0.0	-	-	0	0.0	0	0.0
45-59	0	0	0	0.0	-	-	0	0.0	0	0.0
60+	0	0	0	0.0	-	-	0	0.0	0	0.0
All ages	23	10	12	5.3	0.0	0.50	1	0.5	1	0.4
Females										
0-4	22	80	11	40.5	0.0	0.50	1	4.0	1	2.7
5-14	0	0	0	0.0	-	-	0	0.0	0	0.0
15-44	0	0	0	0.0	-	-	0	0.0	0	0.0
45-59	0	0	0	0.0	-	-	0	0.0	0	0.0
60+	0	0	0	0.0	-	-	0	0.0	0	0.0
All ages	22	10	11	5.0	0.0	0.50	1	0.5	1	0.3
Total	46	10	23	5.2	0.0	0.50	2	0.5	2	0.4

Table 24h MEC - AOM - CMO Chlamydia - Neonatal pneumonia

Age group (years)	Incidence 1990 Number ('000s)	Rate (per 100 000)	Prevalence 1990 Number ('000s)	Rate (per 100 000)	Avg. age at onset (years)	Average duration (years)	Deaths 1990 Number ('000s)	Rate (per 100 000)	Deaths 2000 (Projected) Number ('000s)	Rate (per 100 000)
Males										
0-4	14	34.3	7	17.2	0.0	0.50	1	1.8	1	1.3
5-14	0	0.0	0	0.0	-	-	0	0.0	0	0.0
15-44	0	0.0	0	0.0	-	-	0	0.0	0	0.0
45-59	0	0.0	0	0.0	-	-	0	0.0	0	0.0
60+	0	0.0	0	0.0	-	-	0	0.0	0	0.0
All ages	14	5.5	7	2.8	0.0	0.50	1	0.3	1	0.2
Females										
0-4	14	34.3	7	17.2	0.0	0.50	1	1.7	1	1.2
5-14	0	0.0	0	0.0	-	-	0	0.0	0	0.0
15-44	0	0.0	0	0.0	-	-	0	0.0	0	0.0
45-59	0	0.0	0	0.0	-	-	0	0.0	0	0.0
60+	0	0.0	0	0.0	-	-	0	0.0	0	0.0
All ages	14	5.5	7	2.8	0.0	0.50	1	0.3	1	0.2
Total	28	5.5	14	2.8	0.0	0.50	1	0.3	1	0.2

Table 24i World - Mundo - Monde Chlamydia - Neonatal pneumonia

Age group (years)	Incidence 1990 Number ('000s)	Rate (per 100 000)	Prevalence 1990 Number ('000s)	Rate (per 100 000)	Avg. age at onset (years)	Average duration (years)	Deaths 1990 Number ('000s)	Rate (per 100 000)	Deaths 2000 (Projected) Number ('000s)	Rate (per 100 000)
Males										
0-4	254	78.9	127	39.6	0.0	0.50	21	6.6	16	4.7
5-14	0	0.0	0	0.0	-	-	0	0.0	0	0.0
15-44	0	0.0	0	0.0	-	-	0	0.0	0	0.0
45-59	0	0.0	0	0.0	-	-	0	0.0	0	0.0
60+	0	0.0	0	0.0	-	-	0	0.0	0	0.0
All ages	254	9.6	127	4.8	0.0	0.50	21	0.8	17	0.6
Females										
0-4	244	78.9	123	39.7	0.0	0.50	21	6.6	15	4.4
5-14	0	0.0	0	0.0	-	-	0	0.0	0	0.0
15-44	0	0.0	0	0.0	-	-	0	0.0	0	0.0
45-59	0	0.0	0	0.0	-	-	0	0.0	0	0.0
60+	0	0.0	0	0.0	-	-	0	0.0	0	0.0
All ages	244	9.3	123	4.7	0.0	0.50	21	0.8	45	1.5
Total	498	9.4	250	4.7	0.0	0.50	42	0.8	63	1.0

For epidemiological sources see Berkley et al. 1996. For the methods used to estimate and project incidence, prevalence, and deaths see Murray and Lopez 1996a. See explanatory notes for definitions and caveats.

Table 25	Cuadro 25	Tableau 25
Chlamydia	Clamidia	Chlamydiose
Pelvic inflammatory disease	Enfermedad inflamatoria pélvica	Inflammation des organes pelviens

Table 25a   EME - PEMC - EMBE   Chlamydia - Pelvic inflammatory disease

Age group (years)	Incidence 1990 Number ('000s)	Rate (per 100 000)	Prevalence 1990 Number ('000s)	Rate (per 100 000)	Avg. age at onset (years)	Average duration (years)	Deaths 1990 Number ('000s)	Rate (per 100 000)	Deaths 2000 (Projected) Number ('000s)	Rate (per 100 000)
Males										
0-4	0	0	0	0	-	-	-	-	-	-
5-14	0	0	0	0	-	-	-	-	-	-
15-44	0	0	0	0	-	-	-	-	-	-
45-59	0	0	0	0	-	-	-	-	-	-
60+	0	0	0	0	-	-	-	-	-	-
All ages	0	0	0	0	-	-	-	-	-	-
Females										
0-4	0	0	0	0.0	-	-	-	-	-	-
5-14	10	20	0	0.4	13.0	0.02	-	-	-	-
15-44	1 421	793	31	17.4	22.2	0.02	-	-	-	-
45-59	27	40	1	0.9	52.4	0.02	-	-	-	-
60+	17	20	0	0.4	72.4	0.02	-	-	-	-
All ages	1 475	362	32	8.0	23.3	0.02	-	-	-	-
Total	1 475	185	32	4.1	23.3	0.02	-	-	-	-

Table 25b   FSE - PEAS - AESE   Chlamydia - Pelvic inflammatory disease

Age group (years)	Incidence 1990 Number ('000s)	Rate (per 100 000)	Prevalence 1990 Number ('000s)	Rate (per 100 000)	Avg. age at onset (years)	Average duration (years)	Deaths 1990 Number ('000s)	Rate (per 100 000)	Deaths 2000 (Projected) Number ('000s)	Rate (per 100 000)
Males										
0-4	0	0	0	0	-	-	-	-	-	-
5-14	0	0	0	0	-	-	-	-	-	-
15-44	0	0	0	0	-	-	-	-	-	-
45-59	0	0	0	0	-	-	-	-	-	-
60+	0	0	0	0	-	-	-	-	-	-
All ages	0	0	0	0	-	-	-	-	-	-
Females										
0-4	0	0	0	0.0	-	-	-	-	-	-
5-14	7	25	0	0.7	13.0	0.03	-	-	-	-
15-44	747	996	21	27.9	22.2	0.03	-	-	-	-
45-59	15	50	0	1.4	52.4	0.03	-	-	-	-
60+	9	25	0	0.7	71.5	0.03	-	-	-	-
All ages	777	430	22	12.0	23.3	0.03	-	-	-	-
Total	777	224	22	6.3	23.3	0.03	-	-	-	-

Table 25c   India - India - Inde   Chlamydia - Pelvic inflammatory disease

Age group (years)	Incidence 1990 Number ('000s)	Rate (per 100 000)	Prevalence 1990 Number ('000s)	Rate (per 100 000)	Avg. age at onset (years)	Average duration (years)	Deaths 1990 Number ('000s)	Rate (per 100 000)	Deaths 2000 (Projected) Number ('000s)	Rate (per 100 000)
Males										
0-4	0	0	0	0	-	-	-	-	-	-
5-14	0	0	0	0	-	-	-	-	-	-
15-44	0	0	0	0	-	-	-	-	-	-
45-59	0	0	0	0	-	-	-	-	-	-
60+	0	0	0	0	-	-	-	-	-	-
All ages	0	0	0	0	-	-	-	-	-	-
Females										
0-4	0	0	0	0.0	-	-	-	-	-	-
5-14	44	46	1	1.5	13.0	0.03	-	-	-	-
15-44	3 382	1 846	112	61.2	22.2	0.03	-	-	-	-
45-59	42	92	1	3.1	52.4	0.03	-	-	-	-
60+	13	46	0	1.5	70.1	0.03	-	-	-	-
All ages	3 482	849	116	28.2	22.6	0.03	-	-	-	-
Total	3 482	410	116	13.6	22.6	0.03	-	-	-	-

For epidemiological sources see Berkley et al. 1996. For the methods used to estimate and project incidence, prevalence, and deaths see Murray and Lopez 1996a. See explanatory notes for definitions and caveats.

Table 25	Cuadro 25	Tableau 25
Chlamydia	Clamidia	Chlamydiose

Pelvic inflammatory disease	Enfermedad inflamatoria pélvica	Inflammation des organes pelviens

Table 25d China - China - Chine — Chlamydia - Pelvic inflammatory disease

Age group (years)	Incidence 1990 Number ('000s)	Rate (per 100 000)	Prevalence 1990 Number ('000s)	Rate (per 100 000)	Avg. age at onset (years)	Average duration (years)	Deaths 1990 Number ('000s)	Rate (per 100 000)	Deaths 2000 (Projected) Number ('000s)	Rate (per 100 000)
Males										
0-4	0	0	0	0	-	-	-	-	-	-
5-14	0	0	0	0	-	-	-	-	-	-
15-44	0	0	0	0	-	-	-	-	-	-
45-59	0	0	0	0	-	-	-	-	-	-
60+	0	0	0	0	-	-	-	-	-	-
All ages	0	0	0	0	-	-	-	-	-	-
Females										
0-4	0	0.0	0	0.0	-	-	-	-	-	-
5-14	1	1.4	0	0.0	13.0	0.03	-	-	-	-
15-44	162	57.0	5	1.6	22.2	0.03	-	-	-	-
45-59	2	2.9	0	0.1	52.4	0.03	-	-	-	-
60+	1	1.4	0	0.0	70.6	0.03	-	-	-	-
All ages	166	30.2	5	0.8	22.7	0.03	-	-	-	-
Total	166	14.6	5	0.4	22.7	0.03	-	-	-	-

Table 25e OAI - OPAI - APAI — Chlamydia - Pelvic inflammatory disease

Age group (years)	Incidence 1990 Number ('000s)	Rate (per 100 000)	Prevalence 1990 Number ('000s)	Rate (per 100 000)	Avg. age at onset (years)	Average duration (years)	Deaths 1990 Number ('000s)	Rate (per 100 000)	Deaths 2000 (Projected) Number ('000s)	Rate (per 100 000)
Males										
0-4	0	0	0	0	-	-	-	-	-	-
5-14	0	0	0	0	-	-	-	-	-	-
15-44	0	0	0	0	-	-	-	-	-	-
45-59	0	0	0	0	-	-	-	-	-	-
60+	0	0	0	0	-	-	-	-	-	-
All ages	0	0	0	0	-	-	-	-	-	-
Females										
0-4	0	0	0	0.0	-	-	-	-	-	-
5-14	33	41	1	1.4	13.0	0.03	-	-	-	-
15-44	2 620	1 642	87	54.5	22.2	0.03	-	-	-	-
45-59	29	82	1	2.7	52.3	0.03	-	-	-	-
60+	9	41	0	1.4	70.3	0.03	-	-	-	-
All ages	2 691	793	89	26.3	22.6	0.03	-	-	-	-
Total	2 691	394	89	13.1	22.6	0.03	-	-	-	-

Table 25f SSA - ASS - ASS — Chlamydia - Pelvic inflammatory disease

Age group (years)	Incidence 1990 Number ('000s)	Rate (per 100 000)	Prevalence 1990 Number ('000s)	Rate (per 100 000)	Avg. age at onset (years)	Average duration (years)	Deaths 1990 Number ('000s)	Rate (per 100 000)	Deaths 2000 (Projected) Number ('000s)	Rate (per 100 000)
Males										
0-4	0	0	0	0	-	-	-	-	-	-
5-14	0	0	0	0	-	-	-	-	-	-
15-44	0	0	0	0	-	-	-	-	-	-
45-59	0	0	0	0	-	-	-	-	-	-
60+	0	0	0	0	-	-	-	-	-	-
All ages	0	0	0	0	-	-	-	-	-	-
Females										
0-4	0	0	0	0.0	-	-	-	-	-	-
5-14	45	65	2	2.2	13.0	0.03	-	-	-	-
15-44	2 759	2 596	92	86.1	22.2	0.03	-	-	-	-
45-59	29	130	1	4.3	52.2	0.03	-	-	-	-
60+	8	65	0	2.2	69.7	0.03	-	-	-	-
All ages	2 841	1 101	94	36.5	22.5	0.03	-	-	-	-
Total	2 841	557	94	18.5	22.5	0.03	-	-	-	-

For epidemiological sources see Berkley et al. 1996. For the methods used to estimate and project incidence, prevalence, and deaths see Murray and Lopez 1996a. See explanatory notes for definitions and caveats.

Table 25
Chlamydia

Cuadro 25
Clamidia

Tableau 25
Chlamydiose

Pelvic inflammatory disease

Enfermedad inflamatoria pélvica

Inflammation des organes pelviens

Table 25g LAC - ALC - ALC Chlamydia - Pelvic inflammatory disease

Age group (years)	Incidence 1990 Number ('000s)	Rate (per 100 000)	Prevalence 1990 Number ('000s)	Rate (per 100 000)	Avg. age at onset (years)	Average duration (years)	Deaths 1990 Number ('000s)	Rate (per 100 000)	Deaths 2000 (Projected) Number ('000s)	Rate (per 100 000)
Males										
0-4	0	0	0	0	-	-	-	-	-	-
5-14	0	0	0	0	-	-	-	-	-	-
15-44	0	0	0	0	-	-	-	-	-	-
45-59	0	0	0	0	-	-	-	-	-	-
60+	0	0	0	0	-	-	-	-	-	-
All ages	0	0	0	0	-	-	-	-	-	-
Females										
0-4	0	0	0	0.0	-	-	-	-	-	-
5-14	17	33	0	0.9	13.0	0.03	-	-	-	-
15-44	1 368	1 314	38	36.8	22.2	0.03	-	-	-	-
45-59	15	66	0	1.8	52.4	0.03	-	-	-	-
60+	6	33	0	0.9	71.1	0.03	-	-	-	-
All ages	1 405	631	39	17.7	22.6	0.03	-	-	-	-
Total	1 405	316	39	8.8	22.6	0.03	-	-	-	-

Table 25h MEC - AOM - CMO Chlamydia - Pelvic inflammatory disease

Age group (years)	Incidence 1990 Number ('000s)	Rate (per 100 000)	Prevalence 1990 Number ('000s)	Rate (per 100 000)	Avg. age at onset (years)	Average duration (years)	Deaths 1990 Number ('000s)	Rate (per 100 000)	Deaths 2000 (Projected) Number ('000s)	Rate (per 100 000)
Males										
0-4	0	0	0	0	-	-	-	-	-	-
5-14	0	0	0	0	-	-	-	-	-	-
15-44	0	0	0	0	-	-	-	-	-	-
45-59	0	0	0	0	-	-	-	-	-	-
60+	0	0	0	0	-	-	-	-	-	-
All ages	0	0	0	0	-	-	-	-	-	-
Females										
0-4	0	0	0	0.0	-	-	-	-	-	-
5-14	8	13	0	0.4	13.0	0.03	-	-	-	-
15-44	564	526	16	14.7	22.2	0.03	-	-	-	-
45-59	6	26	0	0.7	52.3	0.03	-	-	-	-
60+	2	13	0	0.4	70.4	0.03	-	-	-	-
All ages	580	235	16	6.6	22.5	0.03	-	-	-	-
Total	580	115	16	3.2	22.5	0.03	-	-	-	-

Table 25i World - Mundo - Monde Chlamydia - Pelvic inflammatory disease

Age group (years)	Incidence 1990 Number ('000s)	Rate (per 100 000)	Prevalence 1990 Number ('000s)	Rate (per 100 000)	Avg. age at onset (years)	Average duration (years)	Deaths 1990 Number ('000s)	Rate (per 100 000)	Deaths 2000 (Projected) Number ('000s)	Rate (per 100 000)
Males										
0-4	0	0	0	0	-	-	-	-	-	-
5-14	0	0	0	0	-	-	-	-	-	-
15-44	0	0	0	0	-	-	-	-	-	-
45-59	0	0	0	0	-	-	-	-	-	-
60+	0	0	0	0	-	-	-	-	-	-
All ages	0	0	0	0	-	-	-	-	-	-
Females										
0-4	0	0	0	0.0	-	-	-	-	-	-
5-14	165	31	5	1.0	13.0	0.03	-	-	-	-
15-44	13 022	1 086	401	33.5	22.2	0.03	-	-	-	-
45-59	165	53	5	1.6	52.4	0.03	-	-	-	-
60+	65	24	2	0.7	71.2	0.03	-	-	-	-
All ages	13 416	513	413	15.8	22.8	0.03	-	-	-	-
Total	13 416	255	413	7.8	22.8	0.03	-	-	-	-

For epidemiological sources see Berkley et al. 1996. For the methods used to estimate and project incidence, prevalence, and deaths see Murray and Lopez 1996a. See explanatory notes for definitions and caveats.

Table 26
Chlamydia

Cuadro 26
Clamidia

Tableau 26
Chlamydiose

Ectopic pregnancy

Embarazo ectópico

Grossesse ectopique

Table 26a EME - PEMC - EMBE Chlamydia - Ectopic pregnancy

Age group (years)	Incidence 1990 Number ('000s)	Incidence 1990 Rate (per 100 000)	Prevalence 1990 Number ('000s)	Prevalence 1990 Rate (per 100 000)	Avg. age at onset (years)	Average duration (years)	Deaths 1990 Number ('000s)	Deaths 1990 Rate (per 100 000)	Deaths 2000 (Projected) Number ('000s)	Deaths 2000 (Projected) Rate (per 100 000)
Males										
0-4	0	0	0	0	-	-	0	0	0	0
5-14	0	0	0	0	-	-	0	0	0	0
15-44	0	0	0	0	-	-	0	0	0	0
45-59	0	0	0	0	-	-	0	0	0	0
60+	0	0	0	0	-	-	0	0	0	0
All ages	0	0	0	0	-	-	0	0	0	0
Females										
0-4	0	0.0	0	0.0	-	-	0	0	0	0
5-14	0	0.0	0	0.0	13.0	0.08	0	0	0	0
15-44	3	1.5	0	0.1	25.0	0.08	0	0	0	0
45-59	0	0.1	0	0.0	52.4	0.08	0	0	0	0
60+	0	0.0	0	0.0	72.4	0.08	0	0	0	0
All ages	3	0.7	0	0.1	26.0	0.08	0	0	0	0
Total	3	0.3	0	0.0	26.0	0.08	0	0	0	0

Table 26b FSE - PEAS - AESE Chlamydia - Ectopic pregnancy

Age group (years)	Incidence 1990 Number ('000s)	Incidence 1990 Rate (per 100 000)	Prevalence 1990 Number ('000s)	Prevalence 1990 Rate (per 100 000)	Avg. age at onset (years)	Average duration (years)	Deaths 1990 Number ('000s)	Deaths 1990 Rate (per 100 000)	Deaths 2000 (Projected) Number ('000s)	Deaths 2000 (Projected) Rate (per 100 000)
Males										
0-4	0	0	0	0	-	-	0	0	0	0
5-14	0	0	0	0	-	-	0	0	0	0
15-44	0	0	0	0	-	-	0	0	0	0
45-59	0	0	0	0	-	-	0	0	0	0
60+	0	0	0	0	-	-	0	0	0	0
All ages	0	0	0	0	-	-	0	0	0	0
Females										
0-4	0	0.0	0	0.0	-	-	0	0.0	0	0.0
5-14	0	0.1	0	0.0	13.0	0.08	0	0.0	0	0.0
15-44	3	3.4	0	0.3	25.0	0.08	0	0.3	0	0.2
45-59	0	0.2	0	0.0	52.4	0.08	0	0.0	0	0.0
60+	0	0.1	0	0.0	71.5	0.08	0	0.0	0	0.0
All ages	3	1.5	0	0.1	26.0	0.08	0	0.1	0	0.1
Total	3	0.8	0	0.1	26.0	0.08	0	0.1	0	0.0

Table 26c India - India - Inde Chlamydia - Ectopic pregnancy

Age group (years)	Incidence 1990 Number ('000s)	Incidence 1990 Rate (per 100 000)	Prevalence 1990 Number ('000s)	Prevalence 1990 Rate (per 100 000)	Avg. age at onset (years)	Average duration (years)	Deaths 1990 Number ('000s)	Deaths 1990 Rate (per 100 000)	Deaths 2000 (Projected) Number ('000s)	Deaths 2000 (Projected) Rate (per 100 000)
Males										
0-4	0	0	0	0	-	-	0	0	0	0
5-14	0	0	0	0	-	-	0	0	0	0
15-44	0	0	0	0	-	-	0	0	0	0
45-59	0	0	0	0	-	-	0	0	0	0
60+	0	0	0	0	-	-	0	0	0	0
All ages	0	0	0	0	-	-	0	0	0	0
Females										
0-4	0	0.0	0	0.0	-	-	0	0.0	0	0.0
5-14	0	0.4	0	0.0	13.0	0.08	0	0.0	0	0.0
15-44	30	16.6	2	1.3	25.0	0.08	6	3.3	3	1.3
45-59	0	0.8	0	0.1	52.4	0.08	0	0.0	0	0.0
60+	0	0.4	0	0.0	70.1	0.08	0	0.0	0	0.0
All ages	31	7.6	2	0.6	25.4	0.08	6	1.5	3	0.6
Total	31	3.7	2	0.3	25.4	0.08	6	0.7	3	0.3

For epidemiological sources see Berkley et al. 1996. For the methods used to estimate and project incidence, prevalence, and deaths see Murray and Lopez 1996a. See explanatory notes for definitions and caveats.

Table 26	Cuadro 26	Tableau 26
Chlamydia	Clamidia	Chlamydiose
Ectopic pregnancy	Embarazo ectópico	Grossesse ectopique

Table 26d China - China - Chine — Chlamydia - Ectopic pregnancy

Age group (years)	Incidence 1990 Number ('000s)	Rate (per 100 000)	Prevalence 1990 Number ('000s)	Rate (per 100 000)	Avg. age at onset (years)	Average duration (years)	Deaths 1990 Number ('000s)	Rate (per 100 000)	Deaths 2000 (Projected) Number ('000s)	Rate (per 100 000)
Males										
0-4	0	0	0	0	-	-	0	0	0	0
5-14	0	0	0	0	-	-	0	0	0	0
15-44	0	0	0	0	-	-	0	0	0	0
45-59	0	0	0	0	-	-	0	0	0	0
60+	0	0	0	0	-	-	0	0	0	0
All ages	0	0	0	0	-	-	0	0	0	0
Females										
0-4	0	0.0	0	0	-	-	0	0	0	0
5-14	0	0.0	0	0	13.0	0.08	0	0	0	0
15-44	1	0.2	0	0	25.0	0.08	0	0	0	0
45-59	0	0.0	0	0	52.4	0.08	0	0	0	0
60+	0	0.0	0	0	70.6	0.08	0	0	0	0
All ages	1	0.1	0	0	25.4	0.08	0	0	0	0
Total	1	0.1	0	0	25.4	0.08	0	0	0	0

Table 26e OAI - OPAI - APAI — Chlamydia - Ectopic pregnancy

Age group (years)	Incidence 1990 Number ('000s)	Rate (per 100 000)	Prevalence 1990 Number ('000s)	Rate (per 100 000)	Avg. age at onset (years)	Average duration (years)	Deaths 1990 Number ('000s)	Rate (per 100 000)	Deaths 2000 (Projected) Number ('000s)	Rate (per 100 000)
Males										
0-4	0	0	0	0	-	-	0	0	0	0
5-14	0	0	0	0	-	-	0	0	0	0
15-44	0	0	0	0	-	-	0	0	0	0
45-59	0	0	0	0	-	-	0	0	0	0
60+	0	0	0	0	-	-	0	0	0	0
All ages	0	0	0	0	-	-	0	0	0	0
Females										
0-4	0	0.0	0	0.0	-	-	0	0.0	0	0.0
5-14	0	0.3	0	0.0	13.0	0.08	0	0.0	0	0.0
15-44	20	12.4	2	1.0	25.0	0.08	4	2.5	2	1.1
45-59	0	0.6	0	0.0	52.3	0.08	0	0.0	0	0.0
60+	0	0.3	0	0.0	70.3	0.08	0	0.0	0	0.0
All ages	20	6.0	2	0.5	25.3	0.08	4	1.2	2	0.5
Total	20	3.0	2	0.2	25.3	0.08	4	0.6	2	0.3

Table 26f SSA - ASS - ASS — Chlamydia - Ectopic pregnancy

Age group (years)	Incidence 1990 Number ('000s)	Rate (per 100 000)	Prevalence 1990 Number ('000s)	Rate (per 100 000)	Avg. age at onset (years)	Average duration (years)	Deaths 1990 Number ('000s)	Rate (per 100 000)	Deaths 2000 (Projected) Number ('000s)	Rate (per 100 000)
Males										
0-4	0	0	0	0	-	-	0	0	0	0
5-14	0	0	0	0	-	-	0	0	0	0
15-44	0	0	0	0	-	-	0	0	0	0
45-59	0	0	0	0	-	-	0	0	0	0
60+	0	0	0	0	-	-	0	0	0	0
All ages	0	0	0	0	-	-	0	0	0	0
Females										
0-4	0	0.0	0	0.0	-	-	0	0.0	0	0.0
5-14	1	1.0	0	0.1	13.0	0.08	0	0.0	0	0.0
15-44	42	39.3	3	3.0	25.0	0.08	8	7.9	5	3.6
45-59	0	2.0	0	0.2	52.2	0.08	0	0.0	0	0.0
60+	0	1.0	0	0.1	69.7	0.08	0	0.0	0	0.0
All ages	43	16.7	3	1.3	25.2	0.08	8	3.2	5	1.5
Total	43	8.4	3	0.6	25.2	0.08	8	1.6	5	0.8

For epidemiological sources see Berkley et al. 1996. For the methods used to estimate and project incidence, prevalence, and deaths see Murray and Lopez 1996a. See explanatory notes for definitions and caveats.

Table 26	Cuadro 26	Tableau 26
Chlamydia	Clamidia	Chlamydiose

Ectopic pregnancy	Embarazo ectópico	Grossesse ectopique

Table 26g   LAC - ALC - ALC   Chlamydia - Ectopic pregnancy

Age group (years)	Incidence 1990 Number ('000s)	Rate (per 100 000)	Prevalence 1990 Number ('000s)	Rate (per 100 000)	Avg. age at onset (years)	Average duration (years)	Deaths 1990 Number ('000s)	Rate (per 100 000)	Deaths 2000 (Projected) Number ('000s)	Rate (per 100 000)
Males										
0-4	0	0	0	0	-	-	0	0	0	0
5-14	0	0	0	0	-	-	0	0	0	0
15-44	0	0	0	0	-	-	0	0	0	0
45-59	0	0	0	0	-	-	0	0	0	0
60+	0	0	0	0	-	-	0	0	0	0
All ages	0	0	0	0	-	-	0	0	0	0
Females										
0-4	0	0.0	0	0.0	-	-	0	0.0	0	0.0
5-14	0	0.2	0	0.0	13.0	0.08	0	0.0	0	0.0
15-44	8	7.7	1	0.6	25.0	0.08	1	0.8	0	0.4
45-59	0	0.4	0	0.0	52.4	0.08	0	0.0	0	0.0
60+	0	0.2	0	0.0	71.1	0.08	0	0.0	0	0.0
All ages	8	3.7	1	0.3	25.3	0.08	1	0.4	0	0.2
Total	8	1.9	1	0.1	25.3	0.08	1	0.2	0	0.1

Table 26h   MEC - AOM - CMO   Chlamydia - Ectopic pregnancy

Age group (years)	Incidence 1990 Number ('000s)	Rate (per 100 000)	Prevalence 1990 Number ('000s)	Rate (per 100 000)	Avg. age at onset (years)	Average duration (years)	Deaths 1990 Number ('000s)	Rate (per 100 000)	Deaths 2000 (Projected) Number ('000s)	Rate (per 100 000)
Males										
0-4	0	0	0	0	-	-	0	0	0	0
5-14	0	0	0	0	-	-	0	0	0	0
15-44	0	0	0	0	-	-	0	0	0	0
45-59	0	0	0	0	-	-	0	0	0	0
60+	0	0	0	0	-	-	0	0	0	0
All ages	0	0	0	0	-	-	0	0	0	0
Females										
0-4	0	0.0	0	0.0	-	-	0	0.0	0	0.0
5-14	0	0.1	0	0.0	13.0	0.08	0	0.0	0	0.0
15-44	5	4.7	0	0.4	25.0	0.08	1	0.5	0	0.2
45-59	0	0.2	0	0.0	52.3	0.08	0	0.0	0	0.0
60+	0	0.1	0	0.0	70.4	0.08	0	0.0	0	0.0
All ages	5	2.1	0	0.2	25.3	0.08	1	0.2	0	0.1
Total	5	1.0	0	0.1	25.3	0.08	1	0.1	0	0.1

Table 26i   World - Mundo - Monde   Chlamydia - Ectopic pregnancy

Age group (years)	Incidence 1990 Number ('000s)	Rate (per 100 000)	Prevalence 1990 Number ('000s)	Rate (per 100 000)	Avg. age at onset (years)	Average duration (years)	Deaths 1990 Number ('000s)	Rate (per 100 000)	Deaths 2000 (Projected) Number ('000s)	Rate (per 100 000)
Males										
0-4	0	0	0	0	-	-	0	0	0	0
5-14	0	0	0	0	-	-	0	0	0	0
15-44	0	0	0	0	-	-	0	0	0	0
45-59	0	0	0	0	-	-	0	0	0	0
60+	0	0	0	0	-	-	0	0	0	0
All ages	0	0	0	0	-	-	0	0	0	0
Females										
0-4	0	0.0	0	0.0	-	-	0	0.0	0	0.0
5-14	2	0.3	0	0.0	13.0	0.08	0	0.0	0	0.0
15-44	111	9.2	9	0.7	25.0	0.08	20	1.7	11	0.8
45-59	1	0.4	0	0.0	52.3	0.08	0	0.0	0	0.0
60+	0	0.2	0	0.0	70.4	0.08	0	0.0	0	0.0
All ages	114	4.4	9	0.3	25.3	0.08	20	0.8	11	0.4
Total	114	2.2	9	0.2	25.3	0.08	20	0.4	11	0.2

For epidemiological sources see Berkley et al. 1996. For the methods used to estimate and project incidence, prevalence, and deaths see Murray and Lopez 1996a. See explanatory notes for definitions and caveats.

Table 27	Cuadro 27	Tableau 27
Chlamydia	Clamidia	Chlamydiose
Tubo-ovarian abscess	Absceso tuboovárico	Abcès tubo-ovarien

Table 27a　　EME - PEMC - EMBE　　　　　　Chlamydia - Tubo-ovarian abscess

Age group (years)	Incidence 1990 Number ('000s)	Rate (per 100 000)	Prevalence 1990 Number ('000s)	Rate (per 100 000)	Avg. age at onset (years)	Average duration (years)	Deaths 1990 Number ('000s)	Rate (per 100 000)	Deaths 2000 (Projected) Number ('000s)	Rate (per 100 000)
Males										
0-4	0	0	0	0	-	-	0	0	0	0
5-14	0	0	0	0	-	-	0	0	0	0
15-44	0	0	0	0	-	-	0	0	0	0
45-59	0	0	0	0	-	-	0	0	0	0
60+	0	0	0	0	-	-	0	0	0	0
All ages	0	0	0	0	-	-	0	0	0	0
Females										
0-4	0	0.0	0	0.0	-	-	0	0	0	0
5-14	0	0.3	0	0.0	13.0	0.08	0	0	0	0
15-44	23	13.0	2	1.0	25.0	0.08	0	0	0	0
45-59	0	0.7	0	0.1	52.4	0.08	0	0	0	0
60+	0	0.3	0	0.0	72.4	0.08	0	0	0	0
All ages	24	5.9	2	0.5	26.0	0.08	0	0	0	0
Total	24	3.0	2	0.2	26.0	0.08	0	0	0	0

Table 27b　　FSE - PEAS - AESE　　　　　　Chlamydia - Tubo-ovarian abscess

Age group (years)	Incidence 1990 Number ('000s)	Rate (per 100 000)	Prevalence 1990 Number ('000s)	Rate (per 100 000)	Avg. age at onset (years)	Average duration (years)	Deaths 1990 Number ('000s)	Rate (per 100 000)	Deaths 2000 (Projected) Number ('000s)	Rate (per 100 000)
Males										
0-4	0	0	0	0	-	-	0	0	0	0
5-14	0	0	0	0	-	-	0	0	0	0
15-44	0	0	0	0	-	-	0	0	0	0
45-59	0	0	0	0	-	-	0	0	0	0
60+	0	0	0	0	-	-	0	0	0	0
All ages	0	0	0	0	-	-	0	0	0	0
Females										
0-4	0	0.0	0	0.0	-	-	0	0.0	0	0.0
5-14	0	0.6	0	0.0	13.0	0.08	0	0.0	0	0.0
15-44	18	24.0	1	1.8	25.0	0.08	0	0.0	0	0.0
45-59	0	1.2	0	0.1	52.4	0.08	0	0.1	0	0.1
60+	0	0.6	0	0.0	71.5	0.08	0	0.0	0	0.0
All ages	19	10.4	1	0.8	26.0	0.08	0	0.0	0	0.0
Total	19	5.4	1	0.4	26.0	0.08	0	0.0	0	0.0

Table 27c　　India - India - Inde　　　　　　Chlamydia - Tubo-ovarian abscess

Age group (years)	Incidence 1990 Number ('000s)	Rate (per 100 000)	Prevalence 1990 Number ('000s)	Rate (per 100 000)	Avg. age at onset (years)	Average duration (years)	Deaths 1990 Number ('000s)	Rate (per 100 000)	Deaths 2000 (Projected) Number ('000s)	Rate (per 100 000)
Males										
0-4	0	0	0	0	-	-	0	0	0	0
5-14	0	0	0	0	-	-	0	0	0	0
15-44	0	0	0	0	-	-	0	0	0	0
45-59	0	0	0	0	-	-	0	0	0	0
60+	0	0	0	0	-	-	0	0	0	0
All ages	0	0	0	0	-	-	0	0	0	0
Females										
0-4	0	0.0	0	0.0	-	-	0	0.0	0	0.0
5-14	1	1.5	0	0.1	13.0	0.08	0	0.1	0	0.1
15-44	108	59.0	8	4.5	25.0	0.08	6	3.1	2	1.0
45-59	1	3.0	0	0.2	52.4	0.08	0	0.3	0	0.1
60+	0	1.5	0	0.1	70.1	0.08	0	0.0	0	0.0
All ages	111	27.1	9	2.1	25.4	0.08	6	1.4	3	0.5
Total	111	13.1	9	1.0	25.4	0.08	6	0.7	3	0.3

For epidemiological sources see Berkley et al. 1996. For the methods used to estimate and project incidence, prevalence, and deaths see Murray and Lopez 1996a. See explanatory notes for definitions and caveats.

Table 27	Cuadro 27	Tableau 27
Chlamydia	Clamidia	Chlamydiose
Tubo-ovarian abscess	Absceso tuboovárico	Abcès tubo-ovarien

Table 27d   China - China - Chine   Chlamydia - Tubo-ovarian abscess

Age group (years)	Incidence 1990 Number ('000s)	Rate (per 100 000)	Prevalence 1990 Number ('000s)	Rate (per 100 000)	Avg. age at onset (years)	Average duration (years)	Deaths 1990 Number ('000s)	Rate (per 100 000)	Deaths 2000 (Projected) Number ('000s)	Rate (per 100 000)
Males										
0-4	0	0	0	0	-	-	0	0	0	0
5-14	0	0	0	0	-	-	0	0	0	0
15-44	0	0	0	0	-	-	0	0	0	0
45-59	0	0	0	0	-	-	0	0	0	0
60+	0	0	0	0	-	-	0	0	0	0
All ages	0	0	0	0	-	-	0	0	0	0
Females										
0-4	0	0.0	0	0.0	-	-	0	0	0	0
5-14	0	0.0	0	0.0	13.0	0.08	0	0	0	0
15-44	4	1.4	0	0.1	25.0	0.08	0	0	0	0
45-59	0	0.1	0	0.0	52.4	0.08	0	0	0	0
60+	0	0.0	0	0.0	70.6	0.08	0	0	0	0
All ages	4	0.7	0	0.1	25.4	0.08	0	0	0	0
Total	4	0.4	0	0.0	25.4	0.08	0	0	0	0

Table 27e   OAI - OPAI - APAI   Chlamydia - Tubo-ovarian abscess

Age group (years)	Incidence 1990 Number ('000s)	Rate (per 100 000)	Prevalence 1990 Number ('000s)	Rate (per 100 000)	Avg. age at onset (years)	Average duration (years)	Deaths 1990 Number ('000s)	Rate (per 100 000)	Deaths 2000 (Projected) Number ('000s)	Rate (per 100 000)
Males										
0-4	0	0	0	0	-	-	0	0	0	0
5-14	0	0	0	0	-	-	0	0	0	0
15-44	0	0	0	0	-	-	0	0	0	0
45-59	0	0	0	0	-	-	0	0	0	0
60+	0	0	0	0	-	-	0	0	0	0
All ages	0	0	0	0	-	-	0	0	0	0
Females										
0-4	0	0.0	0	0.0	-	-	0	0.0	0	0.0
5-14	1	1.3	0	0.1	13.0	0.08	0	0.1	0	0.1
15-44	83	52.0	6	4.0	25.0	0.08	4	2.3	2	0.9
45-59	1	2.6	0	0.2	52.3	0.08	0	0.3	0	0.2
60+	0	1.3	0	0.1	70.3	0.08	0	0.0	0	0.0
All ages	85	25.1	7	1.9	25.3	0.08	4	1.2	2	0.5
Total	85	12.5	7	1.0	25.3	0.08	4	0.6	2	0.2

Table 27f   SSA - ASS - ASS   Chlamydia - Tubo-ovarian abscess

Age group (years)	Incidence 1990 Number ('000s)	Rate (per 100 000)	Prevalence 1990 Number ('000s)	Rate (per 100 000)	Avg. age at onset (years)	Average duration (years)	Deaths 1990 Number ('000s)	Rate (per 100 000)	Deaths 2000 (Projected) Number ('000s)	Rate (per 100 000)
Males										
0-4	0	0	0	0	-	-	0	0	0	0
5-14	0	0	0	0	-	-	0	0	0	0
15-44	0	0	0	0	-	-	0	0	0	0
45-59	0	0	0	0	-	-	0	0	0	0
60+	0	0	0	0	-	-	0	0	0	0
All ages	0	0	0	0	-	-	0	0	0	0
Females										
0-4	0	0.0	0	0.0	-	-	0	0.0	0	0.0
5-14	1	2.1	0	0.2	13.0	0.08	0	0.2	0	0.1
15-44	88	83.0	7	6.4	25.0	0.08	5	4.4	3	1.8
45-59	1	4.2	0	0.3	52.2	0.08	0	0.7	0	0.4
60+	0	2.1	0	0.2	69.7	0.08	0	0.0	0	0.0
All ages	91	35.2	7	2.7	25.2	0.08	5	1.9	3	0.8
Total	91	17.8	7	1.4	25.2	0.08	5	1.0	3	0.4

For epidemiological sources see Berkley et al. 1996. For the methods used to estimate and project incidence, prevalence, and deaths see Murray and Lopez 1996a. See explanatory notes for definitions and caveats.

Table 27
Chlamydia

Cuadro 27
Clamidia

Tableau 27
Chlamydiose

Tubo-ovarian abscess　　　Absceso tuboovárico　　　Abcès tubo-ovarien

Table 27g　　LAC - ALC - ALC　　　Chlamydia - Tubo-ovarian abscess

Age group (years)	Incidence 1990 Number ('000s)	Rate (per 100 000)	Prevalence 1990 Number ('000s)	Rate (per 100 000)	Avg. age at onset (years)	Average duration (years)	Deaths 1990 Number ('000s)	Rate (per 100 000)	Deaths 2000 (Projected) Number ('000s)	Rate (per 100 000)
Males										
0-4	0	0	0	0	-	-	0	0	0	0
5-14	0	0	0	0	-	-	0	0	0	0
15-44	0	0	0	0	-	-	0	0	0	0
45-59	0	0	0	0	-	-	0	0	0	0
60+	0	0	0	0	-	-	0	0	0	0
All ages	0	0	0	0	-	-	0	0	0	0
Females										
0-4	0	0.0	0	0.0	-	-	0	0.0	0	0.0
5-14	0	0.8	0	0.1	13.0	0.08	0	0.0	0	0.0
15-44	33	32.0	3	2.5	25.0	0.08	1	0.6	0	0.3
45-59	0	1.6	0	0.1	52.4	0.08	0	0.1	0	0.0
60+	0	0.8	0	0.1	71.1	0.08	0	0.0	0	0.0
All ages	34	15.4	3	1.2	25.3	0.08	1	0.3	0	0.1
Total	34	7.7	3	0.6	25.3	0.08	1	0.1	0	0.1

Table 27h　　MEC - AOM - CMO　　　Chlamydia - Tubo-ovarian abscess

Age group (years)	Incidence 1990 Number ('000s)	Rate (per 100 000)	Prevalence 1990 Number ('000s)	Rate (per 100 000)	Avg. age at onset (years)	Average duration (years)	Deaths 1990 Number ('000s)	Rate (per 100 000)	Deaths 2000 (Projected) Number ('000s)	Rate (per 100 000)
Males										
0-4	0	0	0	0	-	-	0	0	0	0
5-14	0	0	0	0	-	-	0	0	0	0
15-44	0	0	0	0	-	-	0	0	0	0
45-59	0	0	0	0	-	-	0	0	0	0
60+	0	0	0	0	-	-	0	0	0	0
All ages	0	0	0	0	-	-	0	0	0	0
Females										
0-4	0	0.0	0	0.0	-	-	0	0.0	0	0.0
5-14	0	0.3	0	0.0	13.0	0.08	0	0.0	0	0.0
15-44	14	13.0	1	1.0	25.0	0.08	0	0.2	0	0.1
45-59	0	0.7	0	0.1	52.3	0.08	0	0.0	0	0.0
60+	0	0.3	0	0.0	70.4	0.08	0	0.0	0	0.0
All ages	14	5.8	1	0.4	25.3	0.08	0	0.1	0	0.0
Total	14	2.8	1	0.2	25.3	0.08	0	0.0	0	0.0

Table 27i　　World - Mundo - Monde　　　Chlamydia - Tubo-ovarian abscess

Age group (years)	Incidence 1990 Number ('000s)	Rate (per 100 000)	Prevalence 1990 Number ('000s)	Rate (per 100 000)	Avg. age at onset (years)	Average duration (years)	Deaths 1990 Number ('000s)	Rate (per 100 000)	Deaths 2000 (Projected) Number ('000s)	Rate (per 100 000)
Males										
0-4	0	0	0	0	-	-	0	0	0	0
5-14	0	0	0	0	-	-	0	0	0	0
15-44	0	0	0	0	-	-	0	0	0	0
45-59	0	0	0	0	-	-	0	0	0	0
60+	0	0	0	0	-	-	0	0	0	0
All ages	0	0	0	0	-	-	0	0	0	0
Females										
0-4	0	0.0	0	0.0	-	-	0	0.0	0	0.0
5-14	5	0.9	0	0.1	13.0	0.08	0	0.1	0	0.0
15-44	372	31.0	29	2.4	25.0	0.08	15	1.3	4	0.3
45-59	5	1.5	0	0.1	52.3	0.08	0	0.1	0	0.0
60+	2	0.6	0	0.0	70.7	0.08	0	0.0	0	0.0
All ages	383	14.7	29	1.1	25.4	0.08	16	0.6	4	0.1
Total	383	7.3	29	0.6	25.4	0.08	16	0.3	4	0.1

For epidemiological sources see Berkley et al. 1996. For the methods used to estimate and project incidence, prevalence, and deaths see Murray and Lopez 1996a. See explanatory notes for definitions and caveats.

Table 28	Cuadro 28	Tableau 28
Chlamydia	Clamidia	Chlamydiose
Chronic pelvic pain	Dolor pélvico crónico	Douleur pelvienne chronique

Table 28a   EME - PEMC - EMBE   Chlamydia - Chronic pelvic pain

Age group (years)	Incidence 1990 Number ('000s)	Rate (per 100 000)	Prevalence 1990 Number ('000s)	Rate (per 100 000)	Avg. age at onset (years)	Average duration (years)	Deaths 1990 Number ('000s)	Rate (per 100 000)	Deaths 2000 (Projected) Number ('000s)	Rate (per 100 000)
Males										
0-4	0	0	0	0	-	-	0	0	0	0
5-14	0	0	0	0	-	-	0	0	0	0
15-44	0	0	0	0	-	-	0	0	0	0
45-59	0	0	0	0	-	-	0	0	0	0
60+	0	0	0	0	-	-	0	0	0	0
All ages	0	0	0	0	-	-	0	0	0	0
Females										
0-4	0	0.0	0	0.0	-	-	0	0	0	0
5-14	1	1.6	2	4.7	13.0	3.0	0	0	0	0
15-44	113	62.9	305	170.5	23.0	3.0	0	0	0	0
45-59	2	3.1	6	9.4	52.4	3.0	0	0	0	0
60+	1	1.6	4	4.7	72.4	3.0	0	0	0	0
All ages	117	28.7	318	78.1	24.0	3.0	0	0	0	0
Total	117	14.7	318	39.9	24.0	3.0	0	0	0	0

Table 28b   FSE - PEAS - AESE   Chlamydia - Chronic pelvic pain

Age group (years)	Incidence 1990 Number ('000s)	Rate (per 100 000)	Prevalence 1990 Number ('000s)	Rate (per 100 000)	Avg. age at onset (years)	Average duration (years)	Deaths 1990 Number ('000s)	Rate (per 100 000)	Deaths 2000 (Projected) Number ('000s)	Rate (per 100 000)
Males										
0-4	0	0	0	0	-	-	0	0	0	0
5-14	0	0	0	0	-	-	0	0	0	0
15-44	0	0	0	0	-	-	0	0	0	0
45-59	0	0	0	0	-	-	0	0	0	0
60+	0	0	0	0	-	-	0	0	0	0
All ages	0	0	0	0	-	-	0	0	0	0
Females										
0-4	0	0.0	0	0.0	-	-	0	0	0	0
5-14	1	3.0	2	9.1	13.0	3.0	0	0	0	0
15-44	91	121.6	247	329.8	23.0	3.0	0	0	0	0
45-59	2	6.1	5	18.2	52.4	3.0	0	0	0	0
60+	1	3.0	3	9.1	71.5	3.0	0	0	0	0
All ages	95	52.4	258	142.8	24.0	3.0	0	0	0	0
Total	95	27.4	258	74.6	24.0	3.0	0	0	0	0

Table 28c   India - India - Inde   Chlamydia - Chronic pelvic pain

Age group (years)	Incidence 1990 Number ('000s)	Rate (per 100 000)	Prevalence 1990 Number ('000s)	Rate (per 100 000)	Avg. age at onset (years)	Average duration (years)	Deaths 1990 Number ('000s)	Rate (per 100 000)	Deaths 2000 (Projected) Number ('000s)	Rate (per 100 000)
Males										
0-4	0	0	0	0	-	-	0	0	0	0
5-14	0	0	0	0	-	-	0	0	0	0
15-44	0	0	0	0	-	-	0	0	0	0
45-59	0	0	0	0	-	-	0	0	0	0
60+	0	0	0	0	-	-	0	0	0	0
All ages	0	0	0	0	-	-	0	0	0	0
Females										
0-4	0	0.0	0	0	-	-	0	0	0	0
5-14	7	7.4	21	22	13.0	3.0	0	0	0	0
15-44	540	294.9	1 470	802	23.0	3.0	0	0	0	0
45-59	7	14.7	20	44	52.4	3.0	0	0	0	0
60+	2	7.4	6	22	70.1	3.0	0	0	0	0
All ages	556	135.7	1 518	370	23.4	3.0	0	0	0	0
Total	556	65.5	1 518	179	23.4	3.0	0	0	0	0

For epidemiological sources see Berkley et al. 1996. For the methods used to estimate and project incidence, prevalence, and deaths see Murray and Lopez 1996a. See explanatory notes for definitions and caveats.

Table 28   **Cuadro 28**   **Tableau 28**
Chlamydia   **Clamidia**   **Chlamydiose**

Chronic pelvic pain   Dolor pélvico crónico   Douleur pelvienne chronique

Table 28d   China - China - Chine   Chlamydia - Chronic pelvic pain

Age group (years)	Incidence 1990 Number ('000s)	Rate (per 100 000)	Prevalence 1990 Number ('000s)	Rate (per 100 000)	Avg. age at onset (years)	Average duration (years)	Deaths 1990 Number ('000s)	Rate (per 100 000)	Deaths 2000 (Projected) Number ('000s)	Rate (per 100 000)
Males										
0-4	0	0	0	0	-	-	0	0	0	0
5-14	0	0	0	0	-	-	0	0	0	0
15-44	0	0	0	0	-	-	0	0	0	0
45-59	0	0	0	0	-	-	0	0	0	0
60+	0	0	0	0	-	-	0	0	0	0
All ages	0	0	0	0	-	-	0	0	0	0
Females										
0-4	0	0.0	0	0.0	-	-	0	0	0	0
5-14	0	0.2	0	0.5	13.0	3.0	0	0	0	0
15-44	20	7.0	54	19.0	23.0	3.0	0	0	0	0
45-59	0	0.4	1	1.1	52.4	3.0	0	0	0	0
60+	0	0.2	0	0.5	70.6	3.0	0	0	0	0
All ages	20	3.7	55	10.1	23.5	3.0	0	0	0	0
Total	20	1.8	55	4.9	23.5	3.0	0	0	0	0

Table 28e   OAI - OPAI - APAI   Chlamydia - Chronic pelvic pain

Age group (years)	Incidence 1990 Number ('000s)	Rate (per 100 000)	Prevalence 1990 Number ('000s)	Rate (per 100 000)	Avg. age at onset (years)	Average duration (years)	Deaths 1990 Number ('000s)	Rate (per 100 000)	Deaths 2000 (Projected) Number ('000s)	Rate (per 100 000)
Males										
0-4	0	0	0	0	-	-	0	0	0	0
5-14	0	0	0	0	-	-	0	0	0	0
15-44	0	0	0	0	-	-	0	0	0	0
45-59	0	0	0	0	-	-	0	0	0	0
60+	0	0	0	0	-	-	0	0	0	0
All ages	0	0	0	0	-	-	0	0	0	0
Females										
0-4	0	0.0	0	0	-	-	0	0	0	0
5-14	5	6.6	16	20	13.0	3.0	0	0	0	0
15-44	418	262.1	1 138	713	23.0	3.0	0	0	0	0
45-59	5	13.1	14	39	52.3	3.0	0	0	0	0
60+	1	6.6	4	20	70.3	3.0	0	0	0	0
All ages	430	126.6	1 172	345	23.4	3.0	0	0	0	0
Total	430	63.0	1 172	172	23.4	3.0	0	0	0	0

Table 28f   SSA - ASS - ASS   Chlamydia - Chronic pelvic pain

Age group (years)	Incidence 1990 Number ('000s)	Rate (per 100 000)	Prevalence 1990 Number ('000s)	Rate (per 100 000)	Avg. age at onset (years)	Average duration (years)	Deaths 1990 Number ('000s)	Rate (per 100 000)	Deaths 2000 (Projected) Number ('000s)	Rate (per 100 000)
Males										
0-4	0	0	0	0	-	-	0	0	0	0
5-14	0	0	0	0	-	-	0	0	0	0
15-44	0	0	0	0	-	-	0	0	0	0
45-59	0	0	0	0	-	-	0	0	0	0
60+	0	0	0	0	-	-	0	0	0	0
All ages	0	0	0	0	-	-	0	0	0	0
Females										
0-4	0	0	0	0	-	-	0	0	0	0
5-14	7	10	22	31	13.0	3.0	0	0	0	0
15-44	441	415	1 209	1 138	23.0	3.0	0	0	0	0
45-59	5	21	14	62	52.2	3.0	0	0	0	0
60+	1	10	4	31	69.7	3.0	0	0	0	0
All ages	454	176	1 248	484	23.3	3.0	0	0	0	0
Total	454	89	1 248	245	23.3	3.0	0	0	0	0

For epidemiological sources see Berkley et al. 1996. For the methods used to estimate and project incidence, prevalence, and deaths see Murray and Lopez 1996a. See explanatory notes for definitions and caveats.

Table 28	Cuadro 28	Tableau 28
Chlamydia	Clamidia	Chlamydiose
Chronic pelvic pain	Dolor pélvico crónico	Douleur pelvienne chronique

Table 28g   LAC - ALC - ALC   Chlamydia - Chronic pelvic pain

Age group (years)	Incidence 1990 Number ('000s)	Rate (per 100 000)	Prevalence 1990 Number ('000s)	Rate (per 100 000)	Avg. age at onset (years)	Average duration (years)	Deaths 1990 Number ('000s)	Rate (per 100 000)	Deaths 2000 (Projected) Number ('000s)	Rate (per 100 000)
Males										
0-4	0	0	0	0	-	-	0	0	0	0
5-14	0	0	0	0	-	-	0	0	0	0
15-44	0	0	0	0	-	-	0	0	0	0
45-59	0	0	0	0	-	-	0	0	0	0
60+	0	0	0	0	-	-	0	0	0	0
All ages	0	0	0	0	-	-	0	0	0	0
Females										
0-4	0	0.0	0	0	-	-	0	0	0	0
5-14	2	4.0	6	12	13.0	3.0	0	0	0	0
15-44	168	161.3	456	438	23.0	3.0	0	0	0	0
45-59	2	8.1	6	24	52.4	3.0	0	0	0	0
60+	1	4.0	2	12	71.1	3.0	0	0	0	0
All ages	172	77.5	470	211	23.4	3.0	0	0	0	0
Total	172	38.8	470	106	23.4	3.0	0	0	0	0

Table 28h   MEC - AOM - CMO   Chlamydia - Chronic pelvic pain

Age group (years)	Incidence 1990 Number ('000s)	Rate (per 100 000)	Prevalence 1990 Number ('000s)	Rate (per 100 000)	Avg. age at onset (years)	Average duration (years)	Deaths 1990 Number ('000s)	Rate (per 100 000)	Deaths 2000 (Projected) Number ('000s)	Rate (per 100 000)
Males										
0-4	0	0	0	0	-	-	0	0	0	0
5-14	0	0	0	0	-	-	0	0	0	0
15-44	0	0	0	0	-	-	0	0	0	0
45-59	0	0	0	0	-	-	0	0	0	0
60+	0	0	0	0	-	-	0	0	0	0
All ages	0	0	0	0	-	-	0	0	0	0
Females										
0-4	0	0.0	0	0.0	-	-	0	0	0	0
5-14	1	1.6	3	4.8	13.0	3.0	0	0	0	0
15-44	68	63.9	186	173.7	23.0	3.0	0	0	0	0
45-59	1	3.2	2	9.6	52.3	3.0	0	0	0	0
60+	0	1.6	1	4.8	70.4	3.0	0	0	0	0
All ages	70	28.6	192	77.9	23.3	3.0	0	0	0	0
Total	70	14.0	192	38.2	23.3	3.0	0	0	0	0

Table 28i   World - Mundo - Monde   Chlamydia - Chronic pelvic pain

Age group (years)	Incidence 1990 Number ('000s)	Rate (per 100 000)	Prevalence 1990 Number ('000s)	Rate (per 100 000)	Avg. age at onset (years)	Average duration (years)	Deaths 1990 Number ('000s)	Rate (per 100 000)	Deaths 2000 (Projected) Number ('000s)	Rate (per 100 000)
Males										
0-4	0	0	0	0	-	-	0	0	0	0
5-14	0	0	0	0	-	-	0	0	0	0
15-44	0	0	0	0	-	-	0	0	0	0
45-59	0	0	0	0	-	-	0	0	0	0
60+	0	0	0	0	-	-	0	0	0	0
All ages	0	0	0	0	-	-	0	0	0	0
Females										
0-4	0	0.0	0	0.0	-	-	0	0	0	0
5-14	24	4.6	73	13.9	13.0	3.0	0	0	0	0
15-44	1 860	155.2	5 066	422.7	23.0	3.0	0	0	0	0
45-59	23	7.3	68	21.9	52.3	3.0	0	0	0	0
60+	8	3.1	25	9.3	70.7	3.0	0	0	0	0
All ages	1 916	73.3	5 232	200.2	23.4	3.0	0	0	0	0
Total	1 916	36.4	5 232	99.3	23.4	3.0	0	0	0	0

For epidemiological sources see Berkley et al. 1996. For the methods used to estimate and project incidence, prevalence, and deaths see Murray and Lopez 1996a. See explanatory notes for definitions and caveats.

Table 29 Chlamydia	Cuadro 29 Clamidia	Tableau 29 Chlamydiose
Infertility	Infertilidad	Stérilité

Table 29a — EME - PEMC - EMBE — Chlamydia - Infertility

Age group (years)	Incidence 1990 Number ('000s)	Rate (per 100 000)	Prevalence 1990 Number ('000s)	Rate (per 100 000)	Avg. age at onset (years)	Average duration (years)	Deaths 1990 Number ('000s)	Rate (per 100 000)	Deaths 2000 (Projected) Number ('000s)	Rate (per 100 000)
Males										
0-4	0	0.0	0	0.0	-	-	0	0	0	0
5-14	0	0.0	0	0.0	13.0	27.0	0	0	0	0
15-44	0	0.0	1	0.3	27.0	13.0	0	0	0	0
45-59	0	0.0	0	0.0	-	-	0	0	0	0
60+	0	0.0	0	0.0	-	-	0	0	0	0
All ages	0	0.0	1	0.2	26.9	13.1	0	0	0	0
Females										
0-4	0	0.0	0	0.0	-	-	0	0	0	0
5-14	0	0.8	12	23.6	13.0	27.0	0	0	0	0
15-44	57	31.8	817	456.2	23.0	17.0	0	0	0	0
45-59	0	0.0	0	0.0	-	-	0	0	0	0
60+	0	0.0	0	0.0	-	-	0	0	0	0
All ages	57	14.1	829	203.6	22.9	17.1	0	0	0	0
Total	57	7.2	830	104.0	22.9	17.1	0	0	0	0

Table 29b — FSE - PEAS - AESE — Chlamydia - Infertility

Age group (years)	Incidence 1990 Number ('000s)	Rate (per 100 000)	Prevalence 1990 Number ('000s)	Rate (per 100 000)	Avg. age at onset (years)	Average duration (years)	Deaths 1990 Number ('000s)	Rate (per 100 000)	Deaths 2000 (Projected) Number ('000s)	Rate (per 100 000)
Males										
0-4	0	0.0	0	0.0	-	-	0	0	0	0
5-14	0	0.1	0	1.6	13.0	27.0	0	0	0	0
15-44	2	2.1	18	24.0	27.0	13.0	0	0	0	0
45-59	0	0.0	0	0.0	-	-	0	0	0	0
60+	0	0.0	0	0.0	-	-	0	0	0	0
All ages	2	1.0	19	11.3	26.8	13.2	0	0	0	0
Females										
0-4	0	0.0	0	0.0	-	-	0	0	0	0
5-14	0	1.5	12	45.7	13.0	27.0	0	0	0	0
15-44	46	61.6	668	891.6	23.0	17.0	0	0	0	0
45-59	0	0.0	0	0.0	-	-	0	0	0	0
60+	0	0.0	0	0.0	-	-	0	0	0	0
All ages	47	25.7	680	376.1	22.9	17.1	0	0	0	0
Total	48	13.9	699	201.9	23.0	17.0	0	0	0	0

Table 29c — India - India - Inde — Chlamydia - Infertility

Age group (years)	Incidence 1990 Number ('000s)	Rate (per 100 000)	Prevalence 1990 Number ('000s)	Rate (per 100 000)	Avg. age at onset (years)	Average duration (years)	Deaths 1990 Number ('000s)	Rate (per 100 000)	Deaths 2000 (Projected) Number ('000s)	Rate (per 100 000)
Males										
0-4	0	0.0	0	0	-	-	0	0	0	0
5-14	0	0.4	13	13	13.0	27.0	0	0	0	0
15-44	35	17.6	401	200	27.0	13.0	0	0	0	0
45-59	0	0.0	0	0	-	-	0	0	0	0
60+	0	0.0	0	0	-	-	0	0	0	0
All ages	36	8.1	415	94	26.8	13.2	0	0	0	0
Females										
0-4	0	0.0	0	0	-	-	0	0	0	0
5-14	4	3.8	105	111	13.0	27.0	0	0	0	0
15-44	276	150.7	4 024	2 196	23.0	17.0	0	0	0	0
45-59	0	0.0	0	0	-	-	0	0	0	0
60+	0	0.0	0	0	-	-	0	0	0	0
All ages	280	68.2	4 129	1 007	22.8	17.2	0	0	0	0
Total	315	37.1	4 544	535	23.3	16.7	0	0	0	0

For epidemiological sources see Berkley et al. 1996. For the methods used to estimate and project incidence, prevalence, and deaths see Murray and Lopez 1996a. See explanatory notes for definitions and caveats.

Table 29	Cuadro 29	Tableau 29
Chlamydia	Clamidia	Chlamydiose
Infertility	Infertilidad	Stérilité

Table 29d   China - China - Chine   Chlamydia - Infertility

Age group (years)	Incidence 1990 Number ('000s)	Rate (per 100 000)	Prevalence 1990 Number ('000s)	Rate (per 100 000)	Avg. age at onset (years)	Average duration (years)	Deaths 1990 Number ('000s)	Rate (per 100 000)	Deaths 2000 (Projected) Number ('000s)	Rate (per 100 000)
Males										
0-4	0	0.0	0	0.0	-	-	0	0	0	0
5-14	0	0.0	0	0.1	13.0	27.0	0	0	0	0
15-44	1	0.2	7	2.2	27.0	13.0	0	0	0	0
45-59	0	0.0	0	0.0	-	-	0	0	0	0
60+	0	0.0	0	0.0	-	-	0	0	0	0
All ages	1	0.1	7	1.2	26.9	13.1	0	0	0	0
Females										
0-4	0	0.0	0	0.0	-	-	0	0	0	0
5-14	0	0.1	2	2.6	13.0	27.0	0	0	0	0
15-44	10	3.6	147	51.9	23.0	17.0	0	0	0	0
45-59	0	0.0	0	0.0	-	-	0	0	0	0
60+	0	0.0	0	0.0	-	-	0	0	0	0
All ages	10	1.9	150	27.3	22.9	17.1	0	0	0	0
Total	11	1.0	157	13.8	23.1	16.9	0	0	0	0

Table 29e   OAI - OPAI - APAI   Chlamydia - Infertility

Age group (years)	Incidence 1990 Number ('000s)	Rate (per 100 000)	Prevalence 1990 Number ('000s)	Rate (per 100 000)	Avg. age at onset (years)	Average duration (years)	Deaths 1990 Number ('000s)	Rate (per 100 000)	Deaths 2000 (Projected) Number ('000s)	Rate (per 100 000)
Males										
0-4	0	0.0	0	0	-	-	0	0	0	0
5-14	0	0.4	10	12	13.0	27.0	0	0	0	0
15-44	25	15.7	289	180	27.0	13.0	0	0	0	0
45-59	0	0.0	0	0	-	-	0	0	0	0
60+	0	0.0	0	0	-	-	0	0	0	0
All ages	26	7.5	299	87	26.8	13.2	0	0	0	0
Females										
0-4	0	0.0	0	0	-	-	0	0	0	0
5-14	3	3.3	79	98	13.0	27.0	0	0	0	0
15-44	213	133.5	3 118	1 954	23.0	17.0	0	0	0	0
45-59	0	0.0	0	0	-	-	0	0	0	0
60+	0	0.0	0	0	-	-	0	0	0	0
All ages	216	63.5	3 197	942	22.8	17.2	0	0	0	0
Total	241	35.4	3 496	512	23.3	16.7	0	0	0	0

Table 29f   SSA - ASS - ASS   Chlamydia - Infertility

Age group (years)	Incidence 1990 Number ('000s)	Rate (per 100 000)	Prevalence 1990 Number ('000s)	Rate (per 100 000)	Avg. age at onset (years)	Average duration (years)	Deaths 1990 Number ('000s)	Rate (per 100 000)	Deaths 2000 (Projected) Number ('000s)	Rate (per 100 000)
Males										
0-4	0	0.0	0	0	-	-	0	0	0	0
5-14	0	0.5	12	16	13.0	27.0	0	0	0	0
15-44	23	22.0	261	252	27.0	13.0	0	0	0	0
45-59	0	0.0	0	0	-	-	0	0	0	0
60+	0	0.0	0	0	-	-	0	0	0	0
All ages	23	9.2	273	108	26.7	13.3	0	0	0	0
Females										
0-4	0	0.0	0	0	-	-	0	0	0	0
5-14	4	5.4	108	155	13.0	27.0	0	0	0	0
15-44	228	214.9	3 348	3 151	23.0	17.0	0	0	0	0
45-59	0	0.0	0	0	-	-	0	0	0	0
60+	0	0.0	0	0	-	-	0	0	0	0
All ages	232	90.0	3 456	1 340	22.8	17.2	0	0	0	0
Total	255	50.0	3 729	731	23.1	16.9	0	0	0	0

For epidemiological sources see Berkley et al. 1996. For the methods used to estimate and project incidence, prevalence, and deaths see Murray and Lopez 1996a. See explanatory notes for definitions and caveats.

Table 29	Cuadro 29	Tableau 29
Chlamydia	Clamidia	Chlamydiose
Infertility	Infertilidad	Stérilité

Table 29g — LAC - ALC - ALC — Chlamydia - Infertility

Age group (years)	Incidence 1990 Number ('000s)	Rate (per 100 000)	Prevalence 1990 Number ('000s)	Rate (per 100 000)	Avg. age at onset (years)	Average duration (years)	Deaths 1990 Number ('000s)	Rate (per 100 000)	Deaths 2000 (Projected) Number ('000s)	Rate (per 100 000)
Males										
0-4	0	0.0	0	0.0	-	-	0	0	0	0
5-14	0	0.1	1	2.8	13.0	27.0	0	0	0	0
15-44	4	3.7	44	41.8	27.0	13.0	0	0	0	0
45-59	0	0.0	0	0.0	-	-	0	0	0	0
60+	0	0.0	0	0.0	-	-	0	0	0	0
All ages	4	1.8	45	20.3	26.8	13.2	0	0	0	0
Females										
0-4	0	0.0	0	0.0	-	-	0	0	0	0
5-14	1	2.0	31	60.3	13.0	27.0	0	0	0	0
15-44	85	81.9	1 238	1 189.6	23.0	17.0	0	0	0	0
45-59	0	0.0	0	0.0	-	-	0	0	0	0
60+	0	0.0	0	0.0	-	-	0	0	0	0
All ages	86	38.8	1 269	569.8	22.8	17.2	0	0	0	0
Total	90	20.3	1 314	295.7	23.0	17.0	0	0	0	0

Table 29h — MEC - AOM - CMO — Chlamydia - Infertility

Age group (years)	Incidence 1990 Number ('000s)	Rate (per 100 000)	Prevalence 1990 Number ('000s)	Rate (per 100 000)	Avg. age at onset (years)	Average duration (years)	Deaths 1990 Number ('000s)	Rate (per 100 000)	Deaths 2000 (Projected) Number ('000s)	Rate (per 100 000)
Males										
0-4	0	0.0	0	0.0	-	-	0	0	0	0
5-14	0	0.0	1	1.4	13.0	27.0	0	0	0	0
15-44	2	1.9	25	21.7	27.0	13.0	0	0	0	0
45-59	0	0.0	0	0.0	-	-	0	0	0	0
60+	0	0.0	0	0.0	-	-	0	0	0	0
All ages	2	0.9	26	10.0	26.8	13.2	0	0	0	0
Females										
0-4	0	0.0	0	0.0	-	-	0	0	0	0
5-14	1	0.8	15	24.0	13.0	27.0	0	0	0	0
15-44	35	33.0	516	481.7	23.0	17.0	0	0	0	0
45-59	0	0.0	0	0.0	-	-	0	0	0	0
60+	0	0.0	0	0.0	-	-	0	0	0	0
All ages	36	14.5	531	215.4	22.8	17.2	0	0	0	0
Total	38	7.6	557	110.7	23.0	17.0	0	0	0	0

Table 29i — World - Mundo - Monde — Chlamydia - Infertility

Age group (years)	Incidence 1990 Number ('000s)	Rate (per 100 000)	Prevalence 1990 Number ('000s)	Rate (per 100 000)	Avg. age at onset (years)	Average duration (years)	Deaths 1990 Number ('000s)	Rate (per 100 000)	Deaths 2000 (Projected) Number ('000s)	Rate (per 100 000)
Males										
0-4	0	0.0	0	0.0	-	-	0	0	0	0
5-14	1	0.0	38	0.0	13.0	27.0	0	0	0	0
15-44	92	0.0	1 046	0.1	27.0	13.0	0	0	0	0
45-59	0	0.0	0	0.0	-	-	0	0	0	0
60+	0	0.0	0	0.0	-	-	0	0	0	0
All ages	93	0.0	1 084	0.0	26.8	13.2	0	0	0	0
Females										
0-4	0	0.0	0	0.0	-	-	0	0	0	0
5-14	12	0.0	364	0.1	13.0	27.0	0	0	0	0
15-44	951	0.1	13 878	1.2	23.0	17.0	0	0	0	0
45-59	0	0.0	0	0.0	-	-	0	0	0	0
60+	0	0.0	0	0.0	-	-	0	0	0	0
All ages	964	0.0	14 243	0.5	22.9	17.2	0	0	0	0
Total	1 057	0.1	15 326	1.2	23.2	16.8	0	0	0	0

For epidemiological sources see Berkley et al. 1996. For the methods used to estimate and project incidence, prevalence, and deaths see Murray and Lopez 1996a. See explanatory notes for definitions and caveats.

Table 30　　　　　　　　**Cuadro 30**　　　　　　　　　**Tableau 30**
Chlamydia　　　　　　　　**Clamidia**　　　　　　　　　**Chlamydiose**

Symptomatic urethritis　　　　Uretritis sintomática　　　　　Urétrite symptomatique

Table 30a　　　EME - PEMC - EMBE　　　　　　　Chlamydia - Symptomatic urethritis

Age group (years)	Incidence 1990 Number ('000s)	Rate (per 100 000)	Prevalence 1990 Number ('000s)	Rate (per 100 000)	Avg. age at onset (years)	Average duration (years)	Deaths 1990 Number ('000s)	Rate (per 100 000)	Deaths 2000 (Projected) Number ('000s)	Rate (per 100 000)
Males										
0-4	0	0	0	0.0	-	-	0	0	0	0
5-14	26	48	1	1.5	13.0	0.03	0	0	0	0
15-44	3 523	1 914	111	60.3	25.0	0.03	0	0	0	0
45-59	63	96	2	3.1	52.4	0.03	0	0	0	0
60+	29	48	1	1.5	71.1	0.03	0	0	0	0
All ages	3 641	932	115	29.4	25.8	0.03	0	0	0	0
Females										
0-4	0	0	0	0	-	-	0	0	0	0
5-14	0	0	0	0	-	-	0	0	0	0
15-44	0	0	0	0	-	-	0	0	0	0
45-59	0	0	0	0	-	-	0	0	0	0
60+	0	0	0	0	-	-	0	0	0	0
All ages	0	0	0	0	-	-	0	0	0	0
Total	3 641	456	115	14.4	25.8	0.03	0	0	0	0

Table 30b　　　FSE - PEAS - AESE　　　　　　　　Chlamydia - Symptomatic urethritis

Age group (years)	Incidence 1990 Number ('000s)	Rate (per 100 000)	Prevalence 1990 Number ('000s)	Rate (per 100 000)	Avg. age at onset (years)	Average duration (years)	Deaths 1990 Number ('000s)	Rate (per 100 000)	Deaths 2000 (Projected) Number ('000s)	Rate (per 100 000)
Males										
0-4	0	0	0	0.0	-	-	0	0	0	0
5-14	14	50	1	2.0	13.0	0.04	0	0	0	0
15-44	1 539	2 018	60	78.4	25.0	0.04	0	0	0	0
45-59	27	101	1	3.9	52.2	0.04	0	0	0	0
60+	11	50	0	2.0	70.0	0.04	0	0	0	0
All ages	1 591	962	62	37.4	25.7	0.04	0	0	0	0
Females										
0-4	0	0	0	0	-	-	0	0	0	0
5-14	0	0	0	0	-	-	0	0	0	0
15-44	0	0	0	0	-	-	0	0	0	0
45-59	0	0	0	0	-	-	0	0	0	0
60+	0	0	0	0	-	-	0	0	0	0
All ages	0	0	0	0	-	-	0	0	0	0
Total	1 591	459	62	17.9	25.7	0.04	0	0	0	0

Table 30c　　　India - India - Inde　　　　　　　　Chlamydia - Symptomatic urethritis

Age group (years)	Incidence 1990 Number ('000s)	Rate (per 100 000)	Prevalence 1990 Number ('000s)	Rate (per 100 000)	Avg. age at onset (years)	Average duration (years)	Deaths 1990 Number ('000s)	Rate (per 100 000)	Deaths 2000 (Projected) Number ('000s)	Rate (per 100 000)
Males										
0-4	0	0	0	0.0	-	-	0	0	0	0
5-14	100	98	5	4.5	13.0	0.05	0	0	0	0
15-44	7 847	3 913	363	180.8	25.0	0.05	0	0	0	0
45-59	93	196	4	9.1	52.3	0.05	0	0	0	0
60+	29	98	1	4.5	69.7	0.05	0	0	0	0
All ages	8 068	1 836	373	84.9	25.3	0.05	0	0	0	0
Females										
0-4	0	0	0	0	-	-	0	0	0	0
5-14	0	0	0	0	-	-	0	0	0	0
15-44	0	0	0	0	-	-	0	0	0	0
45-59	0	0	0	0	-	-	0	0	0	0
60+	0	0	0	0	-	-	0	0	0	0
All ages	0	0	0	0	-	-	0	0	0	0
Total	8 068	950	373	43.9	25.3	0.05	0	0	0	0

For epidemiological sources see Berkley et al. 1996. For the methods used to estimate and project incidence, prevalence, and deaths see Murray and Lopez 1996a. See explanatory notes for definitions and caveats.

Table 30
Chlamydia

Cuadro 30
Clamidia

Tableau 30
Chlamydiose

Symptomatic urethritis

Uretritis sintomática

Urétrite symptomatique

Table 30d   China - China - Chine   Chlamydia - Symptomatic urethritis

Age group (years)	Incidence 1990 Number ('000s)	Rate (per 100 000)	Prevalence 1990 Number ('000s)	Rate (per 100 000)	Avg. age at onset (years)	Average duration (years)	Deaths 1990 Number ('000s)	Rate (per 100 000)	Deaths 2000 (Projected) Number ('000s)	Rate (per 100 000)
Males										
0-4	0	0.0	0	0.0	-	-	0	0	0	0
5-14	5	4.7	0	0.2	13.0	0.04	0	0	0	0
15-44	576	188.0	22	7.3	25.0	0.04	0	0	0	0
45-59	7	9.4	0	0.4	52.3	0.04	0	0	0	0
60+	2	4.7	0	0.2	69.8	0.04	0	0	0	0
All ages	590	100.7	23	3.9	25.4	0.04	0	0	0	0
Females										
0-4	0	0	0	0	-	-	0	0	0	0
5-14	0	0	0	0	-	-	0	0	0	0
15-44	0	0	0	0	-	-	0	0	0	0
45-59	0	0	0	0	-	-	0	0	0	0
60+	0	0	0	0	-	-	0	0	0	0
All ages	0	0	0	0	-	-	0	0	0	0
Total	590	52.0	23	2.0	25.4	0.04	0	0	0	0

Table 30e   OAI - OPAI - APAI   Chlamydia - Symptomatic urethritis

Age group (years)	Incidence 1990 Number ('000s)	Rate (per 100 000)	Prevalence 1990 Number ('000s)	Rate (per 100 000)	Avg. age at onset (years)	Average duration (years)	Deaths 1990 Number ('000s)	Rate (per 100 000)	Deaths 2000 (Projected) Number ('000s)	Rate (per 100 000)
Males										
0-4	0	0	0	0.0	-	-	0	0	0	0
5-14	73	87	3	4.0	13.0	0.05	0	0	0	0
15-44	5 594	3 478	258	160.7	25.0	0.05	0	0	0	0
45-59	59	174	3	8.1	52.3	0.05	0	0	0	0
60+	18	87	1	4.0	69.6	0.05	0	0	0	0
All ages	5 744	1 675	265	77.4	25.3	0.05	0	0	0	0
Females										
0-4	0	0	0	0	-	-	0	0	0	0
5-14	0	0	0	0	-	-	0	0	0	0
15-44	0	0	0	0	-	-	0	0	0	0
45-59	0	0	0	0	-	-	0	0	0	0
60+	0	0	0	0	-	-	0	0	0	0
All ages	0	0	0	0	-	-	0	0	0	0
Total	5 744	842	265	38.9	25.3	0.05	0	0	0	0

Table 30f   SSA - ASS - ASS   Chlamydia - Symptomatic urethritis

Age group (years)	Incidence 1990 Number ('000s)	Rate (per 100 000)	Prevalence 1990 Number ('000s)	Rate (per 100 000)	Avg. age at onset (years)	Average duration (years)	Deaths 1990 Number ('000s)	Rate (per 100 000)	Deaths 2000 (Projected) Number ('000s)	Rate (per 100 000)
Males										
0-4	0	0	0	0.0	-	-	0	0	0	0
5-14	86	122	4	5.7	13.0	0.05	0	0	0	0
15-44	5 074	4 890	234	226.0	25.0	0.05	0	0	0	0
45-59	50	245	2	11.3	52.2	0.05	0	0	0	0
60+	13	122	1	5.7	69.2	0.05	0	0	0	0
All ages	5 223	2 070	241	95.6	25.2	0.05	0	0	0	0
Females										
0-4	0	0	0	0	-	-	0	0	0	0
5-14	0	0	0	0	-	-	0	0	0	0
15-44	0	0	0	0	-	-	0	0	0	0
45-59	0	0	0	0	-	-	0	0	0	0
60+	0	0	0	0	-	-	0	0	0	0
All ages	0	0	0	0	-	-	0	0	0	0
Total	5 223	1 023	241	47.3	25.2	0.05	0	0	0	0

For epidemiological sources see Berkley et al. 1996. For the methods used to estimate and project incidence, prevalence, and deaths see Murray and Lopez 1996a. See explanatory notes for definitions and caveats.

Table 30   **Cuadro 30**   **Tableau 30**
Chlamydia   **Clamidia**   **Chlamydiose**

Symptomatic urethritis   Uretritis sintomática   Urétrite symptomatique

Table 30g   LAC - ALC - ALC   Chlamydia - Symptomatic urethritis

Age group (years)	Incidence 1990 Number ('000s)	Rate (per 100 000)	Prevalence 1990 Number ('000s)	Rate (per 100 000)	Avg. age at onset (years)	Average duration (years)	Deaths 1990 Number ('000s)	Rate (per 100 000)	Deaths 2000 (Projected) Number ('000s)	Rate (per 100 000)
Males										
0-4	0	0	0	0.0	-	-	0	0	0	0
5-14	46	89	2	3.5	13.0	0.04	0	0	0	0
15-44	3 709	3 556	144	138.2	25.0	0.04	0	0	0	0
45-59	40	178	2	7.0	52.3	0.04	0	0	0	0
60+	13	89	0	3.5	70.3	0.04	0	0	0	0
All ages	3 807	1 718	148	66.8	25.3	0.04	0	0	0	0
Females										
0-4	0	0	0	0	-	-	0	0	0	0
5-14	0	0	0	0	-	-	0	0	0	0
15-44	0	0	0	0	-	-	0	0	0	0
45-59	0	0	0	0	-	-	0	0	0	0
60+	0	0	0	0	-	-	0	0	0	0
All ages	0	0	0	0	-	-	0	0	0	0
Total	3 807	857	148	33.3	25.3	0.04	0	0	0	0

Table 30h   MEC - AOM - CMO   Chlamydia - Symptomatic urethritis

Age group (years)	Incidence 1990 Number ('000s)	Rate (per 100 000)	Prevalence 1990 Number ('000s)	Rate (per 100 000)	Avg. age at onset (years)	Average duration (years)	Deaths 1990 Number ('000s)	Rate (per 100 000)	Deaths 2000 (Projected) Number ('000s)	Rate (per 100 000)
Males										
0-4	0	0	0	0.0	-	-	0	0	0	0
5-14	29	44	1	1.7	13.0	0.04	0	0	0	0
15-44	2 025	1 778	79	69.1	25.0	0.04	0	0	0	0
45-59	20	89	1	3.5	52.3	0.04	0	0	0	0
60+	6	44	0	1.7	69.7	0.04	0	0	0	0
All ages	2 080	811	81	31.5	25.2	0.04	0	0	0	0
Females										
0-4	0	0	0	0	-	-	0	0	0	0
5-14	0	0	0	0	-	-	0	0	0	0
15-44	0	0	0	0	-	-	0	0	0	0
45-59	0	0	0	0	-	-	0	0	0	0
60+	0	0	0	0	-	-	0	0	0	0
All ages	0	0	0	0	-	-	0	0	0	0
Total	2 080	413	81	16.1	25.2	0.04	0	0	0	0

Table 30i   World - Mundo - Monde   Chlamydia - Symptomatic urethritis

Age group (years)	Incidence 1990 Number ('000s)	Rate (per 100 000)	Prevalence 1990 Number ('000s)	Rate (per 100 000)	Avg. age at onset (years)	Average duration (years)	Deaths 1990 Number ('000s)	Rate (per 100 000)	Deaths 2000 (Projected) Number ('000s)	Rate (per 100 000)
Males										
0-4	0	0	0	0.0	-	-	0	0	0	0
5-14	378	69	16	3.0	13.0	0.04	0	0	0	0
15-44	29 886	2 391	1 272	101.7	25.0	0.04	0	0	0	0
45-59	359	115	15	4.8	52.3	0.04	0	0	0	0
60+	120	55	5	2.2	70.1	0.04	0	0	0	0
All ages	30 742	1 158	1 308	49.3	25.3	0.04	0	0	0	0
Females										
0-4	0	0	0	0	-	-	0	0	0	0
5-14	0	0	0	0	-	-	0	0	0	0
15-44	0	0	0	0	-	-	0	0	0	0
45-59	0	0	0	0	-	-	0	0	0	0
60+	0	0	0	0	-	-	0	0	0	0
All ages	0	0	0	0	-	-	0	0	0	0
Total	30 742	584	1 308	24.8	25.3	0.04	0	0	0	0

For epidemiological sources see Berkley et al. 1996. For the methods used to estimate and project incidence, prevalence, and deaths see Murray and Lopez 1996a. See explanatory notes for definitions and caveats.

Table 31	Cuadro 31	Tableau 31
Chlamydia	Clamidia	Chlamydiose
Epididymitis	Epidedimitis	Epididymite

Table 31a EME - PEMC - EMBE Chlamydia - Epididymitis

Age group (years)	Incidence 1990 Number ('000s)	Rate (per 100 000)	Prevalence 1990 Number ('000s)	Rate (per 100 000)	Avg. age at onset (years)	Average duration (years)	Deaths 1990 Number ('000s)	Rate (per 100 000)	Deaths 2000 (Projected) Number ('000s)	Rate (per 100 000)
Males										
0-4	0	0.0	0	0.0	-	-	0	0	0	0
5-14	0	0.5	0	0.0	13.0	0.04	0	0	0	0
15-44	35	19.2	1	0.7	25.2	0.04	0	0	0	0
45-59	1	1.0	0	0.0	52.4	0.04	0	0	0	0
60+	0	0.5	0	0.0	71.1	0.04	0	0	0	0
All ages	37	9.3	1	0.4	25.9	0.04	0	0	0	0
Females										
0-4	0	0	0	0	-	-	0	0	0	0
5-14	0	0	0	0	-	-	0	0	0	0
15-44	0	0	0	0	-	-	0	0	0	0
45-59	0	0	0	0	-	-	0	0	0	0
60+	0	0	0	0	-	-	0	0	0	0
All ages	0	0	0	0	-	-	0	0	0	0
Total	37	4.6	1	0.2	25.9	0.04	0	0	0	0

Table 31b FSE - PEAS - AESE Chlamydia - Epididymitis

Age group (years)	Incidence 1990 Number ('000s)	Rate (per 100 000)	Prevalence 1990 Number ('000s)	Rate (per 100 000)	Avg. age at onset (years)	Average duration (years)	Deaths 1990 Number ('000s)	Rate (per 100 000)	Deaths 2000 (Projected) Number ('000s)	Rate (per 100 000)
Males										
0-4	0	0.0	0	0.0	-	-	0	0	0	0
5-14	0	1.8	0	0.1	13.0	0.05	0	0	0	0
15-44	54	70.6	3	3.5	25.2	0.05	0	0	0	0
45-59	1	3.5	0	0.2	52.2	0.05	0	0	0	0
60+	0	1.8	0	0.1	70.0	0.05	0	0	0	0
All ages	56	33.7	3	1.7	25.8	0.05	0	0	0	0
Females										
0-4	0	0	0	0	-	-	0	0	0	0
5-14	0	0	0	0	-	-	0	0	0	0
15-44	0	0	0	0	-	-	0	0	0	0
45-59	0	0	0	0	-	-	0	0	0	0
60+	0	0	0	0	-	-	0	0	0	0
All ages	0	0	0	0	-	-	0	0	0	0
Total	56	16.1	3	0.8	25.8	0.05	0	0	0	0

Table 31c India - India - Inde Chlamydia - Epididymitis

Age group (years)	Incidence 1990 Number ('000s)	Rate (per 100 000)	Prevalence 1990 Number ('000s)	Rate (per 100 000)	Avg. age at onset (years)	Average duration (years)	Deaths 1990 Number ('000s)	Rate (per 100 000)	Deaths 2000 (Projected) Number ('000s)	Rate (per 100 000)
Males										
0-4	0	0.0	0	0.0	-	-	0	0	0	0
5-14	6	5.9	0	0.4	13.0	0.07	0	0	0	0
15-44	471	234.7	42	21.2	25.2	0.07	0	0	0	0
45-59	6	11.7	0	0.8	52.3	0.07	0	0	0	0
60+	2	5.9	0	0.4	69.7	0.07	0	0	0	0
All ages	484	110.2	43	9.9	25.5	0.07	0	0	0	0
Females										
0-4	0	0	0	0	-	-	0	0	0	0
5-14	0	0	0	0	-	-	0	0	0	0
15-44	0	0	0	0	-	-	0	0	0	0
45-59	0	0	0	0	-	-	0	0	0	0
60+	0	0	0	0	-	-	0	0	0	0
All ages	0	0	0	0	-	-	0	0	0	0
Total	484	57.0	43	5.1	25.5	0.07	0	0	0	0

For epidemiological sources see Berkley et al. 1996. For the methods used to estimate and project incidence, prevalence, and deaths see Murray and Lopez 1996a. See explanatory notes for definitions and caveats.

Table 31   **Cuadro 31**   **Tableau 31**
Chlamydia   **Clamidia**   **Chlamydiose**

Epididymitis   Epidedimitis   Epididymite

Table 31d	**China - China - Chine**								Chlamydia - Epididymitis	
Age group (years)	Incidence 1990		Prevalence 1990		Avg. age at onset (years)	Average duration (years)	Deaths 1990		Deaths 2000 (Projected)	
	Number ('000s)	Rate (per 100 000)	Number ('000s)	Rate (per 100 000)			Number ('000s)	Rate (per 100 000)	Number ('000s)	Rate (per 100 000)
Males										
0-4	0	0.0	0	0.0	-	-	0	0	0	0
5-14	0	0.2	0	0.0	13.0	0.05	0	0	0	0
15-44	20	6.6	1	0.3	25.2	0.05	0	0	0	0
45-59	0	0.3	0	0.0	52.3	0.05	0	0	0	0
60+	0	0.2	0	0.0	69.8	0.05	0	0	0	0
All ages	21	3.5	1	0.2	25.6	0.05	0	0	0	0
Females										
0-4	0	0	0	0	-	-	0	0	0	0
5-14	0	0	0	0	-	-	0	0	0	0
15-44	0	0	0	0	-	-	0	0	0	0
45-59	0	0	0	0	-	-	0	0	0	0
60+	0	0	0	0	-	-	0	0	0	0
All ages	0	0	0	0	-	-	0	0	0	0
Total	21	1.8	1	0.1	25.6	0.05	0	0	0	0

Table 31e	**OAI - OPAI - APAI**								Chlamydia - Epididymitis	
Age group (years)	Incidence 1990		Prevalence 1990		Avg. age at onset (years)	Average duration (years)	Deaths 1990		Deaths 2000 (Projected)	
	Number ('000s)	Rate (per 100 000)	Number ('000s)	Rate (per 100 000)			Number ('000s)	Rate (per 100 000)	Number ('000s)	Rate (per 100 000)
Males										
0-4	0	0.0	0	0.0	-	-	0	0	0	0
5-14	4	5.2	0	0.3	13.0	0.07	0	0	0	0
15-44	336	208.6	22	14.0	25.2	0.07	0	0	0	0
45-59	4	10.4	0	0.7	52.3	0.07	0	0	0	0
60+	1	5.2	0	0.3	69.6	0.07	0	0	0	0
All ages	345	100.5	23	6.7	25.4	0.07	0	0	0	0
Females										
0-4	0	0	0	0	-	-	0	0	0	0
5-14	0	0	0	0	-	-	0	0	0	0
15-44	0	0	0	0	-	-	0	0	0	0
45-59	0	0	0	0	-	-	0	0	0	0
60+	0	0	0	0	-	-	0	0	0	0
All ages	0	0	0	0	-	-	0	0	0	0
Total	345	50.5	23	3.4	25.4	0.07	0	0	0	0

Table 31f	**SSA - ASS - ASS**								Chlamydia - Epididymitis	
Age group (years)	Incidence 1990		Prevalence 1990		Avg. age at onset (years)	Average duration (years)	Deaths 1990		Deaths 2000 (Projected)	
	Number ('000s)	Rate (per 100 000)	Number ('000s)	Rate (per 100 000)			Number ('000s)	Rate (per 100 000)	Number ('000s)	Rate (per 100 000)
Males										
0-4	0	0.0	0	0.0	-	-	0	0	0	0
5-14	5	7.3	0	0.5	13.0	0.07	0	0	0	0
15-44	304	293.4	20	19.7	25.2	0.07	0	0	0	0
45-59	3	14.7	0	1.0	52.2	0.07	0	0	0	0
60+	1	7.3	0	0.5	69.2	0.07	0	0	0	0
All ages	313	124.2	21	8.3	25.3	0.07	0	0	0	0
Females										
0-4	0	0	0	0	-	-	0	0	0	0
5-14	0	0	0	0	-	-	0	0	0	0
15-44	0	0	0	0	-	-	0	0	0	0
45-59	0	0	0	0	-	-	0	0	0	0
60+	0	0	0	0	-	-	0	0	0	0
All ages	0	0	0	0	-	-	0	0	0	0
Total	313	61.4	21	4.1	25.3	0.07	0	0	0	0

For epidemiological sources see Berkley et al. 1996. For the methods used to estimate and project incidence, prevalence, and deaths see Murray and Lopez 1996a. See explanatory notes for definitions and caveats.

Table 31 Chlamydia	Cuadro 31 Clamidia	Tableau 31 Chlamydiose
Epididymitis	Epidedimitis	Epididymite

Table 31g LAC - ALC - ALC Chlamydia - Epididymitis

Age group (years)	Incidence 1990 Number ('000s)	Rate (per 100 000)	Prevalence 1990 Number ('000s)	Rate (per 100 000)	Avg. age at onset (years)	Average duration (years)	Deaths 1990 Number ('000s)	Rate (per 100 000)	Deaths 2000 (Projected) Number ('000s)	Rate (per 100 000)
Males										
0-4	0	0.0	0	0.0	-	-	0	0	0	0
5-14	2	3.1	0	0.2	13.0	0.05	0	0	0	0
15-44	130	124.5	6	6.2	25.2	0.05	0	0	0	0
45-59	1	6.2	0	0.3	52.3	0.05	0	0	0	0
60+	0	3.1	0	0.2	70.3	0.05	0	0	0	0
All ages	133	60.1	7	3.0	25.4	0.05	0	0	0	0
Females										
0-4	0	0	0	0	-	-	0	0	0	0
5-14	0	0	0	0	-	-	0	0	0	0
15-44	0	0	0	0	-	-	0	0	0	0
45-59	0	0	0	0	-	-	0	0	0	0
60+	0	0	0	0	-	-	0	0	0	0
All ages	0	0	0	0	-	-	0	0	0	0
Total	133	30.0	7	1.5	25.4	0.05	0	0	0	0

Table 31h MEC - AOM - CMO Chlamydia - Epididymitis

Age group (years)	Incidence 1990 Number ('000s)	Rate (per 100 000)	Prevalence 1990 Number ('000s)	Rate (per 100 000)	Avg. age at onset (years)	Average duration (years)	Deaths 1990 Number ('000s)	Rate (per 100 000)	Deaths 2000 (Projected) Number ('000s)	Rate (per 100 000)
Males										
0-4	0	0.0	0	0.0	-	-	0	0	0	0
5-14	1	1.6	0	0.1	13.0	0.05	0	0	0	0
15-44	71	62.2	4	3.1	25.2	0.05	0	0	0	0
45-59	1	3.1	0	0.2	52.3	0.05	0	0	0	0
60+	0	1.6	0	0.1	69.7	0.05	0	0	0	0
All ages	73	28.4	4	1.4	25.4	0.05	0	0	0	0
Females										
0-4	0	0	0	0	-	-	0	0	0	0
5-14	0	0	0	0	-	-	0	0	0	0
15-44	0	0	0	0	-	-	0	0	0	0
45-59	0	0	0	0	-	-	0	0	0	0
60+	0	0	0	0	-	-	0	0	0	0
All ages	0	0	0	0	-	-	0	0	0	0
Total	73	14.5	4	0.7	25.4	0.05	0	0	0	0

Table 31i World - Mundo - Monde Chlamydia - Epididymitis

Age group (years)	Incidence 1990 Number ('000s)	Rate (per 100 000)	Prevalence 1990 Number ('000s)	Rate (per 100 000)	Avg. age at onset (years)	Average duration (years)	Deaths 1990 Number ('000s)	Rate (per 100 000)	Deaths 2000 (Projected) Number ('000s)	Rate (per 100 000)
Males										
0-4	0	0.0	0	0.0	-	-	0	0	0	0
5-14	19	3.5	1	0.2	13.0	0.06	0	0	0	0
15-44	1 421	113.7	100	8.0	25.2	0.06	0	0	0	0
45-59	16	5.1	1	0.3	52.3	0.06	0	0	0	0
60+	5	2.3	0	0.1	69.8	0.06	0	0	0	0
All ages	1 461	55.1	103	3.9	25.5	0.06	0	0	0	0
Females										
0-4	0	0	0	0	-	-	0	0	0	0
5-14	0	0	0	0	-	-	0	0	0	0
15-44	0	0	0	0	-	-	0	0	0	0
45-59	0	0	0	0	-	-	0	0	0	0
60+	0	0	0	0	-	-	0	0	0	0
All ages	0	0	0	0	-	-	0	0	0	0
Total	1 461	27.7	103	2.0	25.5	0.06	0	0	0	0

For epidemiological sources see Berkley et al. 1996. For the methods used to estimate and project incidence, prevalence, and deaths see Murray and Lopez 1996a. See explanatory notes for definitions and caveats.

Table 32   **Cuadro 32**   **Tableau 32**
Chlamydia   **Clamidia**   **Chlamydiose**

Stricture   Obstrucción ureteral   Rétrécissement urétral

Table 32a   EME - PEMC - EMBE   Chlamydia - Stricture

Age group (years)	Incidence 1990 Number ('000s)	Rate (per 100 000)	Prevalence 1990 Number ('000s)	Rate (per 100 000)	Avg. age at onset (years)	Average duration (years)	Deaths 1990 Number ('000s)	Rate (per 100 000)	Deaths 2000 (Projected) Number ('000s)	Rate (per 100 000)
Males										
0-4	0	0.0	0	0.0	-	-	0	0	0	0
5-14	0	0.1	0	0.1	13.0	0.55	0	0	0	0
15-44	11	5.8	6	3.1	25.2	0.55	0	0	0	0
45-59	0	0.3	0	0.2	52.4	0.55	0	0	0	0
60+	0	0.1	0	0.1	71.1	0.55	0	0	0	0
All ages	11	2.8	6	1.5	25.9	0.55	0	0	0	0
Females										
0-4	0	0	0	0	-	-	0	0	0	0
5-14	0	0	0	0	-	-	0	0	0	0
15-44	0	0	0	0	-	-	0	0	0	0
45-59	0	0	0	0	-	-	0	0	0	0
60+	0	0	0	0	-	-	0	0	0	0
All ages	0	0	0	0	-	-	0	0	0	0
Total	11	1.4	6	0.8	25.9	0.55	0	0	0	0

Table 32b   FSE - PEAS - AESE   Chlamydia - Stricture

Age group (years)	Incidence 1990 Number ('000s)	Rate (per 100 000)	Prevalence 1990 Number ('000s)	Rate (per 100 000)	Avg. age at onset (years)	Average duration (years)	Deaths 1990 Number ('000s)	Rate (per 100 000)	Deaths 2000 (Projected) Number ('000s)	Rate (per 100 000)
Males										
0-4	0	0.0	0	0.0	-	-	0	0	0	0
5-14	0	0.5	0	0.7	13.0	1.4	0	0	0	0
15-44	16	21.3	22	28.4	25.2	1.4	0	0	0	0
45-59	0	1.1	0	1.5	52.2	1.4	0	0	0	0
60+	0	0.5	0	0.7	70.0	1.4	0	0	0	0
All ages	17	10.1	22	13.6	25.8	1.4	0	0	0	0
Females										
0-4	0	0	0	0	-	-	0	0	0	0
5-14	0	0	0	0	-	-	0	0	0	0
15-44	0	0	0	0	-	-	0	0	0	0
45-59	0	0	0	0	-	-	0	0	0	0
60+	0	0	0	0	-	-	0	0	0	0
All ages	0	0	0	0	-	-	0	0	0	0
Total	17	4.8	22	6.5	25.8	1.4	0	0	0	0

Table 32c   India - India - Inde   Chlamydia - Stricture

Age group (years)	Incidence 1990 Number ('000s)	Rate (per 100 000)	Prevalence 1990 Number ('000s)	Rate (per 100 000)	Avg. age at onset (years)	Average duration (years)	Deaths 1990 Number ('000s)	Rate (per 100 000)	Deaths 2000 (Projected) Number ('000s)	Rate (per 100 000)
Males										
0-4	0	0.0	0	0.0	-	-	0	0	0	0
5-14	2	1.8	4	4.1	13.0	2.3	0	0	0	0
15-44	141	70.5	306	152.7	25.2	2.3	0	0	0	0
45-59	2	3.5	4	8.1	52.3	2.3	0	0	0	0
60+	1	1.8	1	4.1	69.7	2.3	0	0	0	0
All ages	145	33.1	315	71.8	25.5	2.3	0	0	0	0
Females										
0-4	0	0	0	0	-	-	0	0	0	0
5-14	0	0	0	0	-	-	0	0	0	0
15-44	0	0	0	0	-	-	0	0	0	0
45-59	0	0	0	0	-	-	0	0	0	0
60+	0	0	0	0	-	-	0	0	0	0
All ages	0	0	0	0	-	-	0	0	0	0
Total	145	17.1	315	37.1	25.5	2.3	0	0	0	0

For epidemiological sources see Berkley et al. 1996. For the methods used to estimate and project incidence, prevalence, and deaths see Murray and Lopez 1996a. See explanatory notes for definitions and caveats.

Table 32 / **Cuadro 32** / **Tableau 32**
Chlamydia / **Clamidia** / **Chlamydiose**

Stricture / Obstrucción ureteral / Rétrécissement urétral

Table 32d China - China - Chine — Chlamydia - Stricture

Age group (years)	Incidence 1990 Number ('000s)	Rate (per 100 000)	Prevalence 1990 Number ('000s)	Rate (per 100 000)	Avg. age at onset (years)	Average duration (years)	Deaths 1990 Number ('000s)	Rate (per 100 000)	Deaths 2000 (Projected) Number ('000s)	Rate (per 100 000)
Males										
0-4	0	0.0	0	0.0	-	-	0	0	0	0
5-14	0	0.1	0	0.1	13.0	1.4	0	0	0	0
15-44	6	2.0	8	2.6	25.2	1.4	0	0	0	0
45-59	0	0.1	0	0.1	52.3	1.4	0	0	0	0
60+	0	0.1	0	0.1	69.8	1.4	0	0	0	0
All ages	6	1.1	8	1.4	25.6	1.4	0	0	0	0
Females										
0-4	0	0	0	0	-	-	0	0	0	0
5-14	0	0	0	0	-	-	0	0	0	0
15-44	0	0	0	0	-	-	0	0	0	0
45-59	0	0	0	0	-	-	0	0	0	0
60+	0	0	0	0	-	-	0	0	0	0
All ages	0	0	0	0	-	-	0	0	0	0
Total	6	0.6	8	0.7	25.6	1.4	0	0	0	0

Table 32e OAI - OPAI - APAI — Chlamydia - Stricture

Age group (years)	Incidence 1990 Number ('000s)	Rate (per 100 000)	Prevalence 1990 Number ('000s)	Rate (per 100 000)	Avg. age at onset (years)	Average duration (years)	Deaths 1990 Number ('000s)	Rate (per 100 000)	Deaths 2000 (Projected) Number ('000s)	Rate (per 100 000)
Males										
0-4	0	0.0	0	0.0	-	-	0	0	0	0
5-14	1	1.6	3	3.6	13.0	2.3	0	0	0	0
15-44	101	62.7	219	136.0	25.2	2.3	0	0	0	0
45-59	1	3.1	2	7.2	52.3	2.3	0	0	0	0
60+	0	1.6	1	3.6	69.6	2.3	0	0	0	0
All ages	103	30.2	225	65.6	25.4	2.3	0	0	0	0
Females										
0-4	0	0	0	0	-	-	0	0	0	0
5-14	0	0	0	0	-	-	0	0	0	0
15-44	0	0	0	0	-	-	0	0	0	0
45-59	0	0	0	0	-	-	0	0	0	0
60+	0	0	0	0	-	-	0	0	0	0
All ages	0	0	0	0	-	-	0	0	0	0
Total	103	15.2	225	33.0	25.4	2.3	0	0	0	0

Table 32f SSA - ASS - ASS — Chlamydia - Stricture

Age group (years)	Incidence 1990 Number ('000s)	Rate (per 100 000)	Prevalence 1990 Number ('000s)	Rate (per 100 000)	Avg. age at onset (years)	Average duration (years)	Deaths 1990 Number ('000s)	Rate (per 100 000)	Deaths 2000 (Projected) Number ('000s)	Rate (per 100 000)
Males										
0-4	0	0.0	0	0.0	-	-	0	0	0	0
5-14	2	2.2	4	5.1	13.0	2.3	0	0	0	0
15-44	91	88.0	199	191.4	25.2	2.3	0	0	0	0
45-59	1	4.4	2	10.2	52.2	2.3	0	0	0	0
60+	0	2.2	1	5.1	69.2	2.3	0	0	0	0
All ages	94	37.3	205	81.2	25.3	2.3	0	0	0	0
Females										
0-4	0	0	0	0	-	-	0	0	0	0
5-14	0	0	0	0	-	-	0	0	0	0
15-44	0	0	0	0	-	-	0	0	0	0
45-59	0	0	0	0	-	-	0	0	0	0
60+	0	0	0	0	-	-	0	0	0	0
All ages	0	0	0	0	-	-	0	0	0	0
Total	94	18.4	205	40.1	25.3	2.3	0	0	0	0

For epidemiological sources see Berkley et al. 1996. For the methods used to estimate and project incidence, prevalence, and deaths see Murray and Lopez 1996a. See explanatory notes for definitions and caveats.

Table 32
Chlamydia

Cuadro 32
Clamidia

Tableau 32
Chlamydiose

Stricture

Obstrucción ureteral

Rétrécissement urétral

Table 32g LAC - ALC - ALC

Chlamydia - Stricture

Age group (years)	Incidence 1990 Number ('000s)	Rate (per 100 000)	Prevalence 1990 Number ('000s)	Rate (per 100 000)	Avg. age at onset (years)	Average duration (years)	Deaths 1990 Number ('000s)	Rate (per 100 000)	Deaths 2000 (Projected) Number ('000s)	Rate (per 100 000)
Males										
0-4	0	0.0	0	0.0	-	-	0	0	0	0
5-14	0	0.9	1	1.3	13.0	1.4	0	0	0	0
15-44	39	37.4	52	50.0	25.2	1.4	0	0	0	0
45-59	0	1.9	1	2.6	52.3	1.4	0	0	0	0
60+	0	0.9	0	1.3	70.3	1.4	0	0	0	0
All ages	40	18.1	54	24.2	25.4	1.4	0	0	0	0
Females										
0-4	0	0	0	0	-	-	0	0	0	0
5-14	0	0	0	0	-	-	0	0	0	0
15-44	0	0	0	0	-	-	0	0	0	0
45-59	0	0	0	0	-	-	0	0	0	0
60+	0	0	0	0	-	-	0	0	0	0
All ages	0	0	0	0	-	-	0	0	0	0
Total	40	9.0	54	12.1	25.4	1.4	0	0	0	0

Table 32h MEC - AOM - CMO

Chlamydia - Stricture

Age group (years)	Incidence 1990 Number ('000s)	Rate (per 100 000)	Prevalence 1990 Number ('000s)	Rate (per 100 000)	Avg. age at onset (years)	Average duration (years)	Deaths 1990 Number ('000s)	Rate (per 100 000)	Deaths 2000 (Projected) Number ('000s)	Rate (per 100 000)
Males										
0-4	0	0.0	0	0.0	-	-	0	0	0	0
5-14	0	0.5	0	0.7	13.0	1.4	0	0	0	0
15-44	21	18.7	28	25.0	25.2	1.4	0	0	0	0
45-59	0	0.9	0	1.3	52.3	1.4	0	0	0	0
60+	0	0.5	0	0.7	69.7	1.4	0	0	0	0
All ages	22	8.5	29	11.4	25.4	1.4	0	0	0	0
Females										
0-4	0	0	0	0	-	-	0	0	0	0
5-14	0	0	0	0	-	-	0	0	0	0
15-44	0	0	0	0	-	-	0	0	0	0
45-59	0	0	0	0	-	-	0	0	0	0
60+	0	0	0	0	-	-	0	0	0	0
All ages	0	0	0	0	-	-	0	0	0	0
Total	22	4.3	29	5.8	25.4	1.4	0	0	0	0

Table 32i World - Mundo - Monde

Chlamydia - Stricture

Age group (years)	Incidence 1990 Number ('000s)	Rate (per 100 000)	Prevalence 1990 Number ('000s)	Rate (per 100 000)	Avg. age at onset (years)	Average duration (years)	Deaths 1990 Number ('000s)	Rate (per 100 000)	Deaths 2000 (Projected) Number ('000s)	Rate (per 100 000)
Males										
0-4	0	0.0	0	0.0	-	-	0	0	0	0
5-14	6	1.0	12	2.2	13.0	2.1	0	0	0	0
15-44	427	34.1	840	67.2	25.2	2.1	0	0	0	0
45-59	5	1.5	10	3.2	52.3	2.1	0	0	0	0
60+	1	0.7	3	1.4	69.8	2.0	0	0	0	0
All ages	439	16.5	865	32.6	25.5	2.1	0	0	0	0
Females										
0-4	0	0	0	0	-	-	0	0	0	0
5-14	0	0	0	0	-	-	0	0	0	0
15-44	0	0	0	0	-	-	0	0	0	0
45-59	0	0	0	0	-	-	0	0	0	0
60+	0	0	0	0	-	-	0	0	0	0
All ages	0	0	0	0	-	-	0	0	0	0
Total	439	8.3	865	16.4	25.5	2.1	0	0	0	0

For epidemiological sources see Berkley et al. 1996. For the methods used to estimate and project incidence, prevalence, and deaths see Murray and Lopez 1996a. See explanatory notes for definitions and caveats.

Table 33	Cuadro 33	Tableau 33
Gonorrhoea	Gonorrea	Gonorrhée

Ophthalmia neonatorum	Oftalmía neonatal	Ophtalmie néonatale

Table 33a EME - PEMC - EMBE   Gonorrhoea - Ophthalmia neonatorum

Age group (years)	Incidence 1990 Number ('000s)	Rate (per 100 000)	Prevalence 1990 Number ('000s)	Rate (per 100 000)	Avg. age at onset (years)	Average duration (years)	Deaths 1990 Number ('000s)	Rate (per 100 000)	Deaths 2000 (Projected) Number ('000s)	Rate (per 100 000)
Males										
0-4	1	3.5	0	0.1	0.0	0.04	0	0	0	0
5-14	0	0.0	0	0.0	-	-	0	0	0	0
15-44	0	0.0	0	0.0	-	-	0	0	0	0
45-59	0	0.0	0	0.0	-	-	0	0	0	0
60+	0	0.0	0	0.0	-	-	0	0	0	0
All ages	1	0.2	0	0.0	0.0	0.04	0	0	0	0
Females										
0-4	1	3.5	0	0.1	0.0	0.04	0	0	0	0
5-14	0	0.0	0	0.0	-	-	0	0	0	0
15-44	0	0.0	0	0.0	-	-	0	0	0	0
45-59	0	0.0	0	0.0	-	-	0	0	0	0
60+	0	0.0	0	0.0	-	-	0	0	0	0
All ages	1	0.2	0	0.0	0.0	0.04	0	0	0	0
Total	2	0.2	0	0.0	0.0	0.04	0	0	0	0

Table 33b FSE - PEAS - AESE   Gonorrhoea - Ophthalmia neonatorum

Age group (years)	Incidence 1990 Number ('000s)	Rate (per 100 000)	Prevalence 1990 Number ('000s)	Rate (per 100 000)	Avg. age at onset (years)	Average duration (years)	Deaths 1990 Number ('000s)	Rate (per 100 000)	Deaths 2000 (Projected) Number ('000s)	Rate (per 100 000)
Males										
0-4	5	32.8	0	1.3	0.0	0.04	0	0	0	0
5-14	0	0.0	0	0.0	-	-	0	0	0	0
15-44	0	0.0	0	0.0	-	-	0	0	0	0
45-59	0	0.0	0	0.0	-	-	0	0	0	0
60+	0	0.0	0	0.0	-	-	0	0	0	0
All ages	5	2.7	0	0.1	0.0	0.04	0	0	0	0
Females										
0-4	4	32.8	0	1.3	0.0	0.04	0	0	0	0
5-14	0	0.0	0	0.0	-	-	0	0	0	0
15-44	0	0.0	0	0.0	-	-	0	0	0	0
45-59	0	0.0	0	0.0	-	-	0	0	0	0
60+	0	0.0	0	0.0	-	-	0	0	0	0
All ages	4	2.4	0	0.1	0.0	0.04	0	0	0	0
Total	9	2.5	0	0.1	0.0	0.04	0	0	0	0

Table 33c India - India - Inde   Gonorrhoea - Ophthalmia neonatorum

Age group (years)	Incidence 1990 Number ('000s)	Rate (per 100 000)	Prevalence 1990 Number ('000s)	Rate (per 100 000)	Avg. age at onset (years)	Average duration (years)	Deaths 1990 Number ('000s)	Rate (per 100 000)	Deaths 2000 (Projected) Number ('000s)	Rate (per 100 000)
Males										
0-4	137	229	5	8.8	0.0	0.04	0	0	0	0
5-14	0	0	0	0.0	-	-	0	0	0	0
15-44	0	0	0	0.0	-	-	0	0	0	0
45-59	0	0	0	0.0	-	-	0	0	0	0
60+	0	0	0	0.0	-	-	0	0	0	0
All ages	137	31	5	1.2	0.0	0.04	0	0	0	0
Females										
0-4	130	230	5	8.9	0.0	0.04	0	0	0	0
5-14	0	0	0	0.0	-	-	0	0	0	0
15-44	0	0	0	0.0	-	-	0	0	0	0
45-59	0	0	0	0.0	-	-	0	0	0	0
60+	0	0	0	0.0	-	-	0	0	0	0
All ages	130	32	5	1.2	0.0	0.04	0	0	0	0
Total	267	31	10	1.2	0.0	0.04	0	0	0	0

For epidemiological sources see Berkley et al. 1996. For the methods used to estimate and project incidence, prevalence, and deaths see Murray and Lopez 1996a. See explanatory notes for definitions and caveats.

Table 33
Gonorrhoea

Cuadro 33
Gonorrea

Tableau 33
Gonorrhée

Ophthalmia neonatorum   Oftalmía neonatal   Ophtalmie néonatale

Table 33d	China - China - Chine										Gonorrhoea - Ophthalmia neonatorum
Age group (years)	Incidence 1990		Prevalence 1990		Avg. age at onset (years)	Average duration (years)	Deaths 1990		Deaths 2000 (Projected)	
	Number ('000s)	Rate (per 100 000)	Number ('000s)	Rate (per 100 000)			Number ('000s)	Rate (per 100 000)	Number ('000s)	Rate (per 100 000)
Males										
0-4	2	2.9	0	0.1	0.0	0.04	0	0	0	0
5-14	0	0.0	0	0.0	-	-	0	0	0	0
15-44	0	0.0	0	0.0	-	-	0	0	0	0
45-59	0	0.0	0	0.0	-	-	0	0	0	0
60+	0	0.0	0	0.0	-	-	0	0	0	0
All ages	2	0.3	0	0.0	0.0	0.04	0	0	0	0
Females										
0-4	2	2.9	0	0.1	0.0	0.04	0	0	0	0
5-14	0	0.0	0	0.0	-	-	0	0	0	0
15-44	0	0.0	0	0.0	-	-	0	0	0	0
45-59	0	0.0	0	0.0	-	-	0	0	0	0
60+	0	0.0	0	0.0	-	-	0	0	0	0
All ages	2	0.3	0	0.0	0.0	0.04	0	0	0	0
Total	3	0.3	0	0.0	0.0	0.04	0	0	0	0

Table 33e	OAI - OPAI - APAI										Gonorrhoea - Ophthalmia neonatorum
Age group (years)	Incidence 1990		Prevalence 1990		Avg. age at onset (years)	Average duration (years)	Deaths 1990		Deaths 2000 (Projected)	
	Number ('000s)	Rate (per 100 000)	Number ('000s)	Rate (per 100 000)			Number ('000s)	Rate (per 100 000)	Number ('000s)	Rate (per 100 000)
Males										
0-4	97	221	4	8.5	0.0	0.04	0	0	0	0
5-14	0	0	0	0.0	-	-	0	0	0	0
15-44	0	0	0	0.0	-	-	0	0	0	0
45-59	0	0	0	0.0	-	-	0	0	0	0
60+	0	0	0	0.0	-	-	0	0	0	0
All ages	97	28	4	1.1	0.0	0.04	0	0	0	0
Females										
0-4	92	220	4	8.5	0.0	0.04	0	0	0	0
5-14	0	0	0	0.0	-	-	0	0	0	0
15-44	0	0	0	0.0	-	-	0	0	0	0
45-59	0	0	0	0.0	-	-	0	0	0	0
60+	0	0	0	0.0	-	-	0	0	0	0
All ages	92	27	4	1.1	0.0	0.04	0	0	0	0
Total	189	28	7	1.1	0.0	0.04	0	0	0	0

Table 33f	SSA - ASS - ASS										Gonorrhoea - Ophthalmia neonatorum
Age group (years)	Incidence 1990		Prevalence 1990		Avg. age at onset (years)	Average duration (years)	Deaths 1990		Deaths 2000 (Projected)	
	Number ('000s)	Rate (per 100 000)	Number ('000s)	Rate (per 100 000)			Number ('000s)	Rate (per 100 000)	Number ('000s)	Rate (per 100 000)
Males										
0-4	251	529	10	20.4	0.0	0.04	0	0	0	0
5-14	0	0	0	0.0	-	-	0	0	0	0
15-44	0	0	0	0.0	-	-	0	0	0	0
45-59	0	0	0	0.0	-	-	0	0	0	0
60+	0	0	0	0.0	-	-	0	0	0	0
All ages	251	100	10	3.8	0.0	0.04	0	0	0	0
Females										
0-4	246	523	9	20.2	0.0	0.04	0	0	0	0
5-14	0	0	0	0.0	-	-	0	0	0	0
15-44	0	0	0	0.0	-	-	0	0	0	0
45-59	0	0	0	0.0	-	-	0	0	0	0
60+	0	0	0	0.0	-	-	0	0	0	0
All ages	246	95	9	3.7	0.0	0.04	0	0	0	0
Total	497	97	19	3.8	0.0	0.04	0	0	0	0

For epidemiological sources see Berkley et al. 1996. For the methods used to estimate and project incidence, prevalence, and deaths see Murray and Lopez 1996a. See explanatory notes for definitions and caveats.

Table 33	Cuadro 33	Tableau 33
Gonorrhoea	Gonorrea	Gonorrhée
Ophthalmia neonatorum	Oftalmía neonatal	Ophtalmie néonatale

Table 33g   LAC - ALC - ALC   Gonorrhoea - Ophthalmia neonatorum

Age group (years)	Incidence 1990 Number ('000s)	Rate (per 100 000)	Prevalence 1990 Number ('000s)	Rate (per 100 000)	Avg. age at onset (years)	Average duration (years)	Deaths 1990 Number ('000s)	Rate (per 100 000)	Deaths 2000 (Projected) Number ('000s)	Rate (per 100 000)
Males										
0-4	26	89	1	3.4	0.0	0.04	0	0	0	0
5-14	0	0	0	0.0	-	-	0	0	0	0
15-44	0	0	0	0.0	-	-	0	0	0	0
45-59	0	0	0	0.0	-	-	0	0	0	0
60+	0	0	0	0.0	-	-	0	0	0	0
All ages	26	12	1	0.4	0.0	0.04	0	0	0	0
Females										
0-4	24	88	1	3.4	0.0	0.04	0	0	0	0
5-14	0	0	0	0.0	-	-	0	0	0	0
15-44	0	0	0	0.0	-	-	0	0	0	0
45-59	0	0	0	0.0	-	-	0	0	0	0
60+	0	0	0	0.0	-	-	0	0	0	0
All ages	24	11	1	0.4	0.0	0.04	0	0	0	0
Total	50	11	2	0.4	0.0	0.04	0	0	0	0

Table 33h   MEC - AOM - CMO   Gonorrhoea - Ophthalmia neonatorum

Age group (years)	Incidence 1990 Number ('000s)	Rate (per 100 000)	Prevalence 1990 Number ('000s)	Rate (per 100 000)	Avg. age at onset (years)	Average duration (years)	Deaths 1990 Number ('000s)	Rate (per 100 000)	Deaths 2000 (Projected) Number ('000s)	Rate (per 100 000)
Males										
0-4	13	31.4	0	1.2	0.0	0.04	0	0	0	0
5-14	0	0.0	0	0.0	-	-	0	0	0	0
15-44	0	0.0	0	0.0	-	-	0	0	0	0
45-59	0	0.0	0	0.0	-	-	0	0	0	0
60+	0	0.0	0	0.0	-	-	0	0	0	0
All ages	13	5.0	0	0.2	0.0	0.04	0	0	0	0
Females										
0-4	12	31.3	0	1.2	0.0	0.04	0	0	0	0
5-14	0	0.0	0	0.0	-	-	0	0	0	0
15-44	0	0.0	0	0.0	-	-	0	0	0	0
45-59	0	0.0	0	0.0	-	-	0	0	0	0
60+	0	0.0	0	0.0	-	-	0	0	0	0
All ages	12	5.0	0	0.2	0.0	0.04	0	0	0	0
Total	25	5.0	1	0.2	0.0	0.04	0	0	0	0

Table 33i   World - Mundo - Monde   Gonorrhoea - Ophthalmia neonatorum

Age group (years)	Incidence 1990 Number ('000s)	Rate (per 100 000)	Prevalence 1990 Number ('000s)	Rate (per 100 000)	Avg. age at onset (years)	Average duration (years)	Deaths 1990 Number ('000s)	Rate (per 100 000)	Deaths 2000 (Projected) Number ('000s)	Rate (per 100 000)
Males										
0-4	531	165	20	6.4	0.0	0.04	0	0	0	0
5-14	0	0	0	0.0	-	-	0	0	0	0
15-44	0	0	0	0.0	-	-	0	0	0	0
45-59	0	0	0	0.0	-	-	0	0	0	0
60+	0	0	0	0.0	-	-	0	0	0	0
All ages	531	20	20	0.8	0.0	0.04	0	0	0	0
Females										
0-4	512	166	20	6.4	0.0	0.04	0	0	0	0
5-14	0	0	0	0.0	-	-	0	0	0	0
15-44	0	0	0	0.0	-	-	0	0	0	0
45-59	0	0	0	0.0	-	-	0	0	0	0
60+	0	0	0	0.0	-	-	0	0	0	0
All ages	512	20	20	0.8	0.0	0.04	0	0	0	0
Total	1 043	20	40	0.8	0.0	0.04	0	0	0	0

For epidemiological sources see Berkley et al. 1996. For the methods used to estimate and project incidence, prevalence, and deaths see Murray and Lopez 1996a. See explanatory notes for definitions and caveats.

Table 34
Gonorrhoea

Cuadro 34
Gonorrea

Tableau 34
Gonorrhée

Low birth weight   Bajo peso al nacer   Poids insuffisant à la naissance

Table 34a   EME - PEMC - EMBE   Gonorrhoea - Low birth weight

Age group (years)	Incidence 1990 Number ('000s)	Rate (per 100 000)	Prevalence 1990 Number ('000s)	Rate (per 100 000)	Avg. age at onset (years)	Average duration (years)	Deaths 1990 Number ('000s)	Rate (per 100 000)	Deaths 2000 (Projected) Number ('000s)	Rate (per 100 000)
Males										
0-4	4	15.2	2	7.6	0.0	0.50	0	0.1	0	0.1
5-14	0	0.0	0	0.0	-	-	0	0.0	0	0.0
15-44	0	0.0	0	0.0	-	-	0	0.0	0	0.0
45-59	0	0.0	0	0.0	-	-	0	0.0	0	0.0
60+	0	0.0	0	0.0	-	-	0	0.0	0	0.0
All ages	4	1.0	2	0.5	0.0	0.50	0	0.0	0	0.0
Females										
0-4	4	15.2	2	7.6	0.0	0.50	0	0.1	0	0.1
5-14	0	0.0	0	0.0	-	-	0	0.0	0	0.0
15-44	0	0.0	0	0.0	-	-	0	0.0	0	0.0
45-59	0	0.0	0	0.0	-	-	0	0.0	0	0.0
60+	0	0.0	0	0.0	-	-	0	0.0	0	0.0
All ages	4	0.9	2	0.5	0.0	0.50	0	0.0	0	0.0
Total	8	1.0	4	0.5	0.0	0.50	0	0.0	0	0.0

Table 34b   FSE - PEAS - AESE   Gonorrhoea - Low birth weight

Age group (years)	Incidence 1990 Number ('000s)	Rate (per 100 000)	Prevalence 1990 Number ('000s)	Rate (per 100 000)	Avg. age at onset (years)	Average duration (years)	Deaths 1990 Number ('000s)	Rate (per 100 000)	Deaths 2000 (Projected) Number ('000s)	Rate (per 100 000)
Males										
0-4	4	28.1	2	14.1	0.0	0.50	0	1.4	0	1.0
5-14	0	0.0	0	0.0	-	-	0	0.0	0	0.0
15-44	0	0.0	0	0.0	-	-	0	0.0	0	0.0
45-59	0	0.0	0	0.0	-	-	0	0.0	0	0.0
60+	0	0.0	0	0.0	-	-	0	0.0	0	0.0
All ages	4	2.3	2	1.2	0.0	0.50	0	0.1	0	0.1
Females										
0-4	4	28.1	2	14.0	0.0	0.50	0	1.4	0	1.0
5-14	0	0.0	0	0.0	-	-	0	0.0	0	0.0
15-44	0	0.0	0	0.0	-	-	0	0.0	0	0.0
45-59	0	0.0	0	0.0	-	-	0	0.0	0	0.0
60+	0	0.0	0	0.0	-	-	0	0.0	0	0.0
All ages	4	2.0	2	1.0	0.0	0.50	0	0.1	0	0.1
Total	8	2.2	4	1.1	0.0	0.50	0	0.1	0	0.1

Table 34c   India - India - Inde   Gonorrhoea - Low birth weight

Age group (years)	Incidence 1990 Number ('000s)	Rate (per 100 000)	Prevalence 1990 Number ('000s)	Rate (per 100 000)	Avg. age at onset (years)	Average duration (years)	Deaths 1990 Number ('000s)	Rate (per 100 000)	Deaths 2000 (Projected) Number ('000s)	Rate (per 100 000)
Males										
0-4	65	109	32	54.0	0.0	0.50	6	10.4	4	6.3
5-14	0	0	0	0.0	-	-	0	0.0	0	0.0
15-44	0	0	0	0.0	-	-	0	0.0	0	0.0
45-59	0	0	0	0.0	-	-	0	0.0	0	0.0
60+	0	0	0	0.0	-	-	0	0.0	0	0.0
All ages	65	15	32	7.3	0.0	0.50	6	1.4	4	0.9
Females										
0-4	62	110	31	54.2	0.0	0.50	6	10.4	3	6.1
5-14	0	0	0	0.0	-	-	0	0.0	0	0.0
15-44	0	0	0	0.0	-	-	0	0.0	0	0.0
45-59	0	0	0	0.0	-	-	0	0.0	0	0.0
60+	0	0	0	0.0	-	-	0	0.0	0	0.0
All ages	62	15	31	7.5	0.0	0.50	6	1.4	3	0.8
Total	127	15	63	7.4	0.0	0.50	12	1.4	7	0.9

For epidemiological sources see Berkley et al. 1996. For the methods used to estimate and project incidence, prevalence, and deaths see Murray and Lopez 1996a. See explanatory notes for definitions and caveats.

Table 34	Cuadro 34	Tableau 34
Gonorrhoea	Gonorrea	Gonorrhée
Low birth weight	Bajo peso al nacer	Poids insuffisant à la naissance

Table 34d   China - China - Chine   Gonorrhoea - Low birth weight

Age group (years)	Incidence 1990 Number ('000s)	Rate (per 100 000)	Prevalence 1990 Number ('000s)	Rate (per 100 000)	Avg. age at onset (years)	Average duration (years)	Deaths 1990 Number ('000s)	Rate (per 100 000)	Deaths 2000 (Projected) Number ('000s)	Rate (per 100 000)
Males										
0-4	1	2.5	1	1.2	0.0	0.50	0	0.1	0	0.1
5-14	0	0.0	0	0.0	-	-	0	0.0	0	0.0
15-44	0	0.0	0	0.0	-	-	0	0.0	0	0.0
45-59	0	0.0	0	0.0	-	-	0	0.0	0	0.0
60+	0	0.0	0	0.0	-	-	0	0.0	0	0.0
All ages	1	0.3	1	0.1	0.0	0.50	0	0.0	0	0.0
Females										
0-4	1	2.5	1	1.2	0.0	0.50	0	0.1	0	0.1
5-14	0	0.0	0	0.0	-	-	0	0.0	0	0.0
15-44	0	0.0	0	0.0	-	-	0	0.0	0	0.0
45-59	0	0.0	0	0.0	-	-	0	0.0	0	0.0
60+	0	0.0	0	0.0	-	-	0	0.0	0	0.0
All ages	1	0.3	1	0.1	0.0	0.50	0	0.0	0	0.0
Total	3	0.3	1	0.1	0.0	0.50	0	0.0	0	0.0

Table 34e   OAI - OPAI - APAI   Gonorrhoea - Low birth weight

Age group (years)	Incidence 1990 Number ('000s)	Rate (per 100 000)	Prevalence 1990 Number ('000s)	Rate (per 100 000)	Avg. age at onset (years)	Average duration (years)	Deaths 1990 Number ('000s)	Rate (per 100 000)	Deaths 2000 (Projected) Number ('000s)	Rate (per 100 000)
Males										
0-4	46	105	23	52.4	0.0	0.50	4	9.7	3	6.4
5-14	0	0	0	0.0	-	-	0	0.0	0	0.0
15-44	0	0	0	0.0	-	-	0	0.0	0	0.0
45-59	0	0	0	0.0	-	-	0	0.0	0	0.0
60+	0	0	0	0.0	-	-	0	0.0	0	0.0
All ages	46	13	23	6.7	0.0	0.50	4	1.2	3	0.8
Females										
0-4	44	105	22	52.1	0.0	0.50	4	9.7	3	6.2
5-14	0	0	0	0.0	-	-	0	0.0	0	0.0
15-44	0	0	0	0.0	-	-	0	0.0	0	0.0
45-59	0	0	0	0.0	-	-	0	0.0	0	0.0
60+	0	0	0	0.0	-	-	0	0.0	0	0.0
All ages	44	13	22	6.4	0.0	0.50	4	1.2	3	0.8
Total	90	13	45	6.6	0.0	0.50	8	1.2	5	0.8

Table 34f   SSA - ASS - ASS   Gonorrhoea - Low birth weight

Age group (years)	Incidence 1990 Number ('000s)	Rate (per 100 000)	Prevalence 1990 Number ('000s)	Rate (per 100 000)	Avg. age at onset (years)	Average duration (years)	Deaths 1990 Number ('000s)	Rate (per 100 000)	Deaths 2000 (Projected) Number ('000s)	Rate (per 100 000)
Males										
0-4	119	251	59	124	0.0	0.50	12	25.1	12	25.4
5-14	0	0	0	0	-	-	0	0.0	0	0.0
15-44	0	0	0	0	-	-	0	0.0	0	0.0
45-59	0	0	0	0	-	-	0	0.0	0	0.0
60+	0	0	0	0	-	-	0	0.0	0	0.0
All ages	119	47	59	23	0.0	0.50	12	4.7	12	4.8
Females										
0-4	117	248	58	122	0.0	0.50	12	25.1	11	24.0
5-14	0	0	0	0	-	-	0	0.0	0	0.0
15-44	0	0	0	0	-	-	0	0.0	0	0.0
45-59	0	0	0	0	-	-	0	0.0	0	0.0
60+	0	0	0	0	-	-	0	0.0	0	0.0
All ages	117	45	58	22	0.0	0.50	12	4.6	11	4.4
Total	236	46	116	23	0.0	0.50	24	4.6	23	4.6

For epidemiological sources see Berkley et al. 1996. For the methods used to estimate and project incidence, prevalence, and deaths see Murray and Lopez 1996a. See explanatory notes for definitions and caveats.

Table 34	Cuadro 34	Tableau 34
Gonorrhoea	Gonorrea	Gonorrhée
Low birth weight	Bajo peso al nacer	Poids insuffisant à la naissance

Table 34g   LAC - ALC - ALC   Gonorrhoea - Low birth weight

Age group (years)	Incidence 1990 Number ('000s)	Rate (per 100 000)	Prevalence 1990 Number ('000s)	Rate (per 100 000)	Avg. age at onset (years)	Average duration (years)	Deaths 1990 Number ('000s)	Rate (per 100 000)	Deaths 2000 (Projected) Number ('000s)	Rate (per 100 000)
Males										
0-4	22	76.1	11	37.9	0.0	0.50	1	3.8	1	2.7
5-14	0	0.0	0	0.0	-	-	0	0.0	0	0.0
15-44	0	0.0	0	0.0	-	-	0	0.0	0	0.0
45-59	0	0.0	0	0.0	-	-	0	0.0	0	0.0
60+	0	0.0	0	0.0	-	-	0	0.0	0	0.0
All ages	22	9.9	11	4.9	0.0	0.50	1	0.5	1	0.4
Females										
0-4	21	75.6	10	37.7	0.0	0.50	1	3.7	1	2.6
5-14	0	0.0	0	0.0	-	-	0	0.0	0	0.0
15-44	0	0.0	0	0.0	-	-	0	0.0	0	0.0
45-59	0	0.0	0	0.0	-	-	0	0.0	0	0.0
60+	0	0.0	0	0.0	-	-	0	0.0	0	0.0
All ages	21	9.4	10	4.7	0.0	0.50	1	0.5	1	0.3
Total	43	9.6	21	4.8	0.0	0.50	2	0.5	2	0.3

Table 34h   MEC - AOM - CMO   Gonorrhoea - Low birth weight

Age group (years)	Incidence 1990 Number ('000s)	Rate (per 100 000)	Prevalence 1990 Number ('000s)	Rate (per 100 000)	Avg. age at onset (years)	Average duration (years)	Deaths 1990 Number ('000s)	Rate (per 100 000)	Deaths 2000 (Projected) Number ('000s)	Rate (per 100 000)
Males										
0-4	11	26.9	5	13.3	0.0	0.50	1	1.4	1	1.2
5-14	0	0.0	0	0.0	-	-	0	0.0	0	0.0
15-44	0	0.0	0	0.0	-	-	0	0.0	0	0.0
45-59	0	0.0	0	0.0	-	-	0	0.0	0	0.0
60+	0	0.0	0	0.0	-	-	0	0.0	0	0.0
All ages	11	4.3	5	2.1	0.0	0.50	1	0.2	1	0.2
Females										
0-4	11	26.9	5	13.3	0.0	0.50	1	1.4	0	1.2
5-14	0	0.0	0	0.0	-	-	0	0.0	0	0.0
15-44	0	0.0	0	0.0	-	-	0	0.0	0	0.0
45-59	0	0.0	0	0.0	-	-	0	0.0	0	0.0
60+	0	0.0	0	0.0	-	-	0	0.0	0	0.0
All ages	11	4.3	5	2.1	0.0	0.50	1	0.2	0	0.2
Total	22	4.3	11	2.1	0.0	0.50	1	0.2	1	0.2

Table 34i   World - Mundo - Monde   Gonorrhoea - Low birth weight

Age group (years)	Incidence 1990 Number ('000s)	Rate (per 100 000)	Prevalence 1990 Number ('000s)	Rate (per 100 000)	Avg. age at onset (years)	Average duration (years)	Deaths 1990 Number ('000s)	Rate (per 100 000)	Deaths 2000 (Projected) Number ('000s)	Rate (per 100 000)
Males										
0-4	273	85	135	42.0	0.0	0.50	24	7.6	19	5.8
5-14	0	0	0	0.0	-	-	0	0.0	0	0.0
15-44	0	0	0	0.0	-	-	0	0.0	0	0.0
45-59	0	0	0	0.0	-	-	0	0.0	0	0.0
60+	0	0	0	0.0	-	-	0	0.0	0	0.0
All ages	273	10	135	5.1	0.0	0.50	24	0.9	19	0.7
Females										
0-4	263	85	130	42.1	0.0	0.50	24	7.6	18	5.7
5-14	0	0	0	0.0	-	-	0	0.0	0	0.0
15-44	0	0	0	0.0	-	-	0	0.0	0	0.0
45-59	0	0	0	0.0	-	-	0	0.0	0	0.0
60+	0	0	0	0.0	-	-	0	0.0	0	0.0
All ages	263	10	130	5.0	0.0	0.50	24	0.9	18	0.7
Total	536	10	265	5.0	0.0	0.50	48	0.9	36	0.7

For epidemiological sources see Berkley et al. 1996. For the methods used to estimate and project incidence, prevalence, and deaths see Murray and Lopez 1996a. See explanatory notes for definitions and caveats.

Table 35	Cuadro 35	Tableau 35
Gonorrhoea	Gonorrea	Gonorrhée
Corneal scar - blindness	Cicatriz de la córnea - ceguera	Cicatrice de la cornée - cécité

Table 35a EME - PEMC - EMBE Gonorrhoea - Corneal scar - blindness

Age group (years)	Incidence 1990 Number ('000s)	Rate (per 100 000)	Prevalence 1990 Number ('000s)	Rate (per 100 000)	Avg. age at onset (years)	Average duration (years)	Deaths 1990 Number ('000s)	Rate (per 100 000)	Deaths 2000 (Projected) Number ('000s)	Rate (per 100 000)
Males										
0-4	0	0	0	0	-	-	0	0	0	0
5-14	0	0	0	0	-	-	0	0	0	0
15-44	0	0	0	0	-	-	0	0	0	0
45-59	0	0	0	0	-	-	0	0	0	0
60+	0	0	0	0	-	-	0	0	0	0
All ages	0	0	0	0	-	-	0	0	0	0
Females										
0-4	0	0	0	0	-	-	0	0	0	0
5-14	0	0	0	0	-	-	0	0	0	0
15-44	0	0	0	0	-	-	0	0	0	0
45-59	0	0	0	0	-	-	0	0	0	0
60+	0	0	0	0	-	-	0	0	0	0
All ages	0	0	0	0	-	-	0	0	0	0
Total	0	0	0	0	-	-	0	0	0	0

Table 35b FSE - PEAS - AESE Gonorrhoea - Corneal scar - blindness

Age group (years)	Incidence 1990 Number ('000s)	Rate (per 100 000)	Prevalence 1990 Number ('000s)	Rate (per 100 000)	Avg. age at onset (years)	Average duration (years)	Deaths 1990 Number ('000s)	Rate (per 100 000)	Deaths 2000 (Projected) Number ('000s)	Rate (per 100 000)
Males										
0-4	0	0	0	0	-	-	0	0	0	0
5-14	0	0	0	0	-	-	0	0	0	0
15-44	0	0	0	0	-	-	0	0	0	0
45-59	0	0	0	0	-	-	0	0	0	0
60+	0	0	0	0	-	-	0	0	0	0
All ages	0	0	0	0	-	-	0	0	0	0
Females										
0-4	0	0	0	0	-	-	0	0	0	0
5-14	0	0	0	0	-	-	0	0	0	0
15-44	0	0	0	0	-	-	0	0	0	0
45-59	0	0	0	0	-	-	0	0	0	0
60+	0	0	0	0	-	-	0	0	0	0
All ages	0	0	0	0	-	-	0	0	0	0
Total	0	0	0	0	-	-	0	0	0	0

Table 35c India - India - Inde Gonorrhoea - Corneal scar - blindness

Age group (years)	Incidence 1990 Number ('000s)	Rate (per 100 000)	Prevalence 1990 Number ('000s)	Rate (per 100 000)	Avg. age at onset (years)	Average duration (years)	Deaths 1990 Number ('000s)	Rate (per 100 000)	Deaths 2000 (Projected) Number ('000s)	Rate (per 100 000)
Males										
0-4	4	6.9	15	25.7	0.0	36.8	0	0	0	0
5-14	0	0.0	26	25.1	-	-	0	0	0	0
15-44	0	0.0	46	23.0	-	-	0	0	0	0
45-59	0	0.0	9	18.1	-	-	0	0	0	0
60+	0	0.0	3	8.6	-	-	0	0	0	0
All ages	4	0.9	98	22.3	0.0	36.8	0	0	0	0
Females										
0-4	4	6.9	14	25.4	0.0	36.5	0	0	0	0
5-14	0	0.0	23	24.5	-	-	0	0	0	0
15-44	0	0.0	41	22.3	-	-	0	0	0	0
45-59	0	0.0	8	18.3	-	-	0	0	0	0
60+	0	0.0	3	9.5	-	-	0	0	0	0
All ages	4	1.0	90	21.9	0.0	36.5	0	0	0	0
Total	8	0.9	188	22.1	0.0	36.7	0	0	0	0

For epidemiological sources see Berkley et al. 1996. For the methods used to estimate and project incidence, prevalence, and deaths see Murray and Lopez 1996a. See explanatory notes for definitions and caveats.

Table 35
Gonorrhoea

Cuadro 35
Gonorrea

Tableau 35
Gonorrhée

Corneal scar - blindness   Cicatriz de la córnea - ceguera   Cicatrice de la cornée - cécité

Table 35d   China - China - Chine   Gonorrhoea - Corneal scar - blindness

Age group (years)	Incidence 1990 Number ('000s)	Rate (per 100 000)	Prevalence 1990 Number ('000s)	Rate (per 100 000)	Avg. age at onset (years)	Average duration (years)	Deaths 1990 Number ('000s)	Rate (per 100 000)	Deaths 2000 (Projected) Number ('000s)	Rate (per 100 000)
Males										
0-4	0	0.0	0	0.2	0.0	50.7	0	0	0	0
5-14	0	0.0	0	0.2	-	-	0	0	0	0
15-44	0	0.0	0	0.1	-	-	0	0	0	0
45-59	0	0.0	0	0.1	-	-	0	0	0	0
60+	0	0.0	0	0.1	-	-	0	0	0	0
All ages	0	0.0	1	0.1	0.0	50.7	0	0	0	0
Females										
0-4	0	0.0	0	0.2	0.0	53.2	0	0	0	0
5-14	0	0.0	0	0.2	-	-	0	0	0	0
15-44	0	0.0	0	0.1	-	-	0	0	0	0
45-59	0	0.0	0	0.1	-	-	0	0	0	0
60+	0	0.0	0	0.1	-	-	0	0	0	0
All ages	0	0.0	1	0.1	0.0	53.2	0	0	0	0
Total	0	0.0	2	0.1	0.0	51.9	0	0	0	0

Table 35e   OAI - OPAI - APAI   Gonorrhoea - Corneal scar - blindness

Age group (years)	Incidence 1990 Number ('000s)	Rate (per 100 000)	Prevalence 1990 Number ('000s)	Rate (per 100 000)	Avg. age at onset (years)	Average duration (years)	Deaths 1990 Number ('000s)	Rate (per 100 000)	Deaths 2000 (Projected) Number ('000s)	Rate (per 100 000)
Males										
0-4	3	6.6	12	26.3	0.0	39.0	0	0	0	0
5-14	0	0.0	22	26.1	-	-	0	0	0	0
15-44	0	0.0	38	23.7	-	-	0	0	0	0
45-59	0	0.0	6	18.1	-	-	0	0	0	0
60+	0	0.0	2	7.9	-	-	0	0	0	0
All ages	3	0.8	79	23.1	0.0	39.0	0	0	0	0
Females										
0-4	3	6.6	11	27.0	0.0	43.1	0	0	0	0
5-14	0	0.0	22	26.8	-	-	0	0	0	0
15-44	0	0.0	40	24.8	-	-	0	0	0	0
45-59	0	0.0	7	20.0	-	-	0	0	0	0
60+	0	0.0	2	9.9	-	-	0	0	0	0
All ages	3	0.8	81	24.0	0.0	43.1	0	0	0	0
Total	6	0.8	160	23.5	0.0	41.0	0	0	0	0

Table 35f   SSA - ASS - ASS   Gonorrhoea - Corneal scar - blindness

Age group (years)	Incidence 1990 Number ('000s)	Rate (per 100 000)	Prevalence 1990 Number ('000s)	Rate (per 100 000)	Avg. age at onset (years)	Average duration (years)	Deaths 1990 Number ('000s)	Rate (per 100 000)	Deaths 2000 (Projected) Number ('000s)	Rate (per 100 000)
Males										
0-4	8	15.9	25	52.5	0.0	21.5	0	0	0	0
5-14	0	0.0	32	45.1	-	-	0	0	0	0
15-44	0	0.0	37	35.9	-	-	0	0	0	0
45-59	0	0.0	5	22.3	-	-	0	0	0	0
60+	0	0.0	1	8.9	-	-	0	0	0	0
All ages	8	3.0	99	39.4	0.0	21.5	0	0	0	0
Females										
0-4	7	15.7	25	53.8	0.0	24.8	0	0	0	0
5-14	0	0.0	33	47.7	-	-	0	0	0	0
15-44	0	0.0	42	39.1	-	-	0	0	0	0
45-59	0	0.0	6	26.4	-	-	0	0	0	0
60+	0	0.0	1	11.6	-	-	0	0	0	0
All ages	7	2.9	107	41.7	0.0	24.8	0	0	0	0
Total	15	2.9	207	40.5	0.0	23.1	0	0	0	0

For epidemiological sources see Berkley et al. 1996. For the methods used to estimate and project incidence, prevalence, and deaths see Murray and Lopez 1996a. See explanatory notes for definitions and caveats.

Table 35	Cuadro 35	Tableau 35
Gonorrhoea	Gonorrea	Gonorrhée

Corneal scar - blindness	Cicatriz de la córnea - ceguera	Cicatrice de la cornée - cécité

Table 35g — LAC - ALC - ALC — Gonorrhoea - Corneal scar - blindness

Age group (years)	Incidence 1990 Number ('000s)	Rate (per 100 000)	Prevalence 1990 Number ('000s)	Rate (per 100 000)	Avg. age at onset (years)	Average duration (years)	Deaths 1990 Number ('000s)	Rate (per 100 000)	Deaths 2000 (Projected) Number ('000s)	Rate (per 100 000)
Males										
0-4	0	1.1	1	4.7	0.0	45.0	0	0	0	0
5-14	0	0.0	2	4.5	-	-	0	0	0	0
15-44	0	0.0	4	4.1	-	-	0	0	0	0
45-59	0	0.0	1	3.4	-	-	0	0	0	0
60+	0	0.0	0	1.6	-	-	0	0	0	0
All ages	0	0.1	9	4.0	0.0	45.0	0	0	0	0
Females										
0-4	0	1.1	1	4.8	0.0	50.5	0	0	0	0
5-14	0	0.0	2	4.6	-	-	0	0	0	0
15-44	0	0.0	5	4.3	-	-	0	0	0	0
45-59	0	0.0	1	3.7	-	-	0	0	0	0
60+	0	0.0	0	2.1	-	-	0	0	0	0
All ages	0	0.1	9	4.2	0.0	50.5	0	0	0	0
Total	1	0.1	18	4.1	0.0	47.7	0	0	0	0

Table 35h — MEC - AOM - CMO — Gonorrhoea - Corneal scar - blindness

Age group (years)	Incidence 1990 Number ('000s)	Rate (per 100 000)	Prevalence 1990 Number ('000s)	Rate (per 100 000)	Avg. age at onset (years)	Average duration (years)	Deaths 1990 Number ('000s)	Rate (per 100 000)	Deaths 2000 (Projected) Number ('000s)	Rate (per 100 000)
Males										
0-4	0	0.4	1	1.4	0.0	39.3	0	0	0	0
5-14	0	0.0	1	1.4	-	-	0	0	0	0
15-44	0	0.0	2	1.3	-	-	0	0	0	0
45-59	0	0.0	0	1.1	-	-	0	0	0	0
60+	0	0.0	0	0.5	-	-	0	0	0	0
All ages	0	0.1	3	1.3	0.0	39.3	0	0	0	0
Females										
0-4	0	0.4	1	1.4	0.0	41.5	0	0	0	0
5-14	0	0.0	1	1.4	-	-	0	0	0	0
15-44	0	0.0	1	1.3	-	-	0	0	0	0
45-59	0	0.0	0	1.1	-	-	0	0	0	0
60+	0	0.0	0	0.6	-	-	0	0	0	0
All ages	0	0.1	3	1.3	0.0	41.5	0	0	0	0
Total	0	0.1	7	1.3	0.0	40.4	0	0	0	0

Table 35i — World - Mundo - Monde — Gonorrhoea - Corneal scar - blindness

Age group (years)	Incidence 1990 Number ('000s)	Rate (per 100 000)	Prevalence 1990 Number ('000s)	Rate (per 100 000)	Avg. age at onset (years)	Average duration (years)	Deaths 1990 Number ('000s)	Rate (per 100 000)	Deaths 2000 (Projected) Number ('000s)	Rate (per 100 000)
Males										
0-4	15	4.7	54	16.7	0.0	29.8	0	0	0	0
5-14	0	0.0	83	15.0	-	-	0	0	0	0
15-44	0	0.0	128	10.2	-	-	0	0	0	0
45-59	0	0.0	20	6.5	-	-	0	0	0	0
60+	0	0.0	5	2.5	-	-	0	0	0	0
All ages	15	0.6	290	10.9	0.0	29.8	0	0	0	0
Females										
0-4	15	4.7	53	17.0	0.0	32.2	0	0	0	0
5-14	0	0.0	82	15.5	-	-	0	0	0	0
15-44	0	0.0	128	10.7	-	-	0	0	0	0
45-59	0	0.0	22	7.2	-	-	0	0	0	0
60+	0	0.0	7	2.6	-	-	0	0	0	0
All ages	15	0.6	292	11.2	0.0	32.2	0	0	0	0
Total	30	0.6	582	11.0	0.0	31.0	0	0	0	0

For epidemiological sources see Berkley et al. 1996. For the methods used to estimate and project incidence, prevalence, and deaths see Murray and Lopez 1996a. See explanatory notes for definitions and caveats.

Table 36
Gonorrhoea

Corneal scar - low vision

Cuadro 36
Gonorrea
Cicatriz de la córnea - disminución
de la agudeza visual

Tableau 36
Gonorrhée
Cicatrice de la cornée - baisse
de la vision

Table 36a   EME - PEMC - EMBE

Gonorrhoea - Corneal scar - low vision

Age group (years)	Incidence 1990 Number ('000s)	Rate (per 100 000)	Prevalence 1990 Number ('000s)	Rate (per 100 000)	Avg. age at onset (years)	Average duration (years)	Deaths 1990 Number ('000s)	Rate (per 100 000)	Deaths 2000 (Projected) Number ('000s)	Rate (per 100 000)
Males										
0-4	0	0	0	0	-	-	0	0	0	0
5-14	0	0	0	0	-	-	0	0	0	0
15-44	0	0	0	0	-	-	0	0	0	0
45-59	0	0	0	0	-	-	0	0	0	0
60+	0	0	0	0	-	-	0	0	0	0
All ages	0	0	0	0	-	-	0	0	0	0
Females										
0-4	0	0	0	0	-	-	0	0	0	0
5-14	0	0	0	0	-	-	0	0	0	0
15-44	0	0	0	0	-	-	0	0	0	0
45-59	0	0	0	0	-	-	0	0	0	0
60+	0	0	0	0	-	-	0	0	0	0
All ages	0	0	0	0	-	-	0	0	0	0
Total	0	0	0	0	-	-	0	0	0	0

Table 36b   FSE - PEAS - AESE

Gonorrhoea - Corneal scar - low vision

Age group (years)	Incidence 1990 Number ('000s)	Rate (per 100 000)	Prevalence 1990 Number ('000s)	Rate (per 100 000)	Avg. age at onset (years)	Average duration (years)	Deaths 1990 Number ('000s)	Rate (per 100 000)	Deaths 2000 (Projected) Number ('000s)	Rate (per 100 000)
Males										
0-4	0	2.6	1	6.3	0.0	31.8	0	0	0	0
5-14	0	0.0	2	6.3	-	-	0	0	0	0
15-44	0	0.0	5	6.3	-	-	0	0	0	0
45-59	0	0.0	2	6.3	-	-	0	0	0	0
60+	0	0.0	1	6.3	-	-	0	0	0	0
All ages	0	0.2	10	6.3	0.0	31.8	0	0	0	0
Females										
0-4	0	2.6	1	6.3	0.0	36.1	0	0	0	0
5-14	0	0.0	2	6.3	-	-	0	0	0	0
15-44	0	0.0	5	6.3	-	-	0	0	0	0
45-59	0	0.0	2	6.3	-	-	0	0	0	0
60+	0	0.0	2	6.3	-	-	0	0	0	0
All ages	0	0.2	11	6.3	0.0	36.1	0	0	0	0
Total	1	0.2	22	6.3	0.0	33.9	0	0	0	0

Table 36c   India - India - Inde

Gonorrhoea - Corneal scar - low vision

Age group (years)	Incidence 1990 Number ('000s)	Rate (per 100 000)	Prevalence 1990 Number ('000s)	Rate (per 100 000)	Avg. age at onset (years)	Average duration (years)	Deaths 1990 Number ('000s)	Rate (per 100 000)	Deaths 2000 (Projected) Number ('000s)	Rate (per 100 000)
Males										
0-4	23	39.0	44	74	0.0	23.7	0	0	0	0
5-14	0	0.0	75	74	-	-	0	0	0	0
15-44	0	0.0	148	74	-	-	0	0	0	0
45-59	0	0.0	35	74	-	-	0	0	0	0
60+	0	0.0	22	74	-	-	0	0	0	0
All ages	23	5.3	325	74	0.0	23.7	0	0	0	0
Females										
0-4	22	39.1	42	74	0.0	23.9	0	0	0	0
5-14	0	0.0	71	74	-	-	0	0	0	0
15-44	0	0.0	136	74	-	-	0	0	0	0
45-59	0	0.0	34	74	-	-	0	0	0	0
60+	0	0.0	21	74	-	-	0	0	0	0
All ages	22	5.4	304	74	0.0	23.9	0	0	0	0
Total	45	5.4	629	74	0.0	23.8	0	0	0	0

For epidemiological sources see Berkley et al. 1996. For the methods used to estimate and project incidence, prevalence, and deaths see Murray and Lopez 1996a. See explanatory notes for definitions and caveats.

Table 36 Gonorrhoea	Cuadro 36 Gonorrea	Tableau 36 Gonorrhée
Corneal scar - low vision	Cicatriz de la córnea - disminución de la agudeza visual	Cicatrice de la cornée - baisse de la vision

Table 36d China - China - Chine — Gonorrhoea - Corneal scar - low vision

Age group (years)	Incidence 1990 Number ('000s)	Rate (per 100 000)	Prevalence 1990 Number ('000s)	Rate (per 100 000)	Avg. age at onset (years)	Average duration (years)	Deaths 1990 Number ('000s)	Rate (per 100 000)	Deaths 2000 (Projected) Number ('000s)	Rate (per 100 000)
Males										
0-4	0	0.2	0	0.4	0.0	26.8	0	0	0	0
5-14	0	0.0	0	0.4	-	-	0	0	0	0
15-44	0	0.0	1	0.4	-	-	0	0	0	0
45-59	0	0.0	0	0.4	-	-	0	0	0	0
60+	0	0.0	0	0.4	-	-	0	0	0	0
All ages	0	0.0	2	0.4	0.0	26.8	0	0	0	0
Females										
0-4	0	0.2	0	0.4	0.0	27.9	0	0	0	0
5-14	0	0.0	0	0.4	-	-	0	0	0	0
15-44	0	0.0	1	0.4	-	-	0	0	0	0
45-59	0	0.0	0	0.4	-	-	0	0	0	0
60+	0	0.0	0	0.4	-	-	0	0	0	0
All ages	0	0.0	2	0.4	0.0	27.9	0	0	0	0
Total	0	0.0	4	0.4	0.0	27.4	0	0	0	0

Table 36e OAI - OPAI - APAI — Gonorrhoea - Corneal scar - low vision

Age group (years)	Incidence 1990 Number ('000s)	Rate (per 100 000)	Prevalence 1990 Number ('000s)	Rate (per 100 000)	Avg. age at onset (years)	Average duration (years)	Deaths 1990 Number ('000s)	Rate (per 100 000)	Deaths 2000 (Projected) Number ('000s)	Rate (per 100 000)
Males										
0-4	16	37.7	32	73	0.0	24.0	0	0	0	0
5-14	0	0.0	61	73	-	-	0	0	0	0
15-44	0	0.0	117	73	-	-	0	0	0	0
45-59	0	0.0	25	73	-	-	0	0	0	0
60+	0	0.0	15	73	-	-	0	0	0	0
All ages	16	4.8	249	73	0.0	24.0	0	0	0	0
Females										
0-4	16	37.4	30	73	0.0	25.4	0	0	0	0
5-14	0	0.0	58	73	-	-	0	0	0	0
15-44	0	0.0	116	73	-	-	0	0	0	0
45-59	0	0.0	25	73	-	-	0	0	0	0
60+	0	0.0	16	73	-	-	0	0	0	0
All ages	16	4.6	246	73	0.0	25.4	0	0	0	0
Total	32	4.7	495	73	0.0	24.7	0	0	0	0

Table 36f SSA - ASS - ASS — Gonorrhoea - Corneal scar - low vision

Age group (years)	Incidence 1990 Number ('000s)	Rate (per 100 000)	Prevalence 1990 Number ('000s)	Rate (per 100 000)	Avg. age at onset (years)	Average duration (years)	Deaths 1990 Number ('000s)	Rate (per 100 000)	Deaths 2000 (Projected) Number ('000s)	Rate (per 100 000)
Males										
0-4	43	90	78	164	0.0	18.6	0	0	0	0
5-14	0	0	115	164	-	-	0	0	0	0
15-44	0	0	170	164	-	-	0	0	0	0
45-59	0	0	33	164	-	-	0	0	0	0
60+	0	0	17	164	-	-	0	0	0	0
All ages	43	17	414	164	0.0	18.6	0	0	0	0
Females										
0-4	42	89	77	164	0.0	20.0	0	0	0	0
5-14	0	0	115	164	-	-	0	0	0	0
15-44	0	0	174	164	-	-	0	0	0	0
45-59	0	0	36	164	-	-	0	0	0	0
60+	0	0	21	164	-	-	0	0	0	0
All ages	42	16	423	164	0.0	20.0	0	0	0	0
Total	85	17	837	164	0.0	19.3	0	0	0	0

For epidemiological sources see Berkley et al. 1996. For the methods used to estimate and project incidence, prevalence, and deaths see Murray and Lopez 1996a. See explanatory notes for definitions and caveats.

Table 36	Cuadro 36	Tableau 36
Gonorrhoea	Gonorrea	Gonorrhée
	Cicatriz de la córnea - disminución	Cicatrice de la cornée - baisse
Corneal scar - low vision	de la agudeza visual	de la vision

Table 36g LAC - ALC - ALC — Gonorrhoea - Corneal scar - low vision

Age group (years)	Incidence 1990 Number ('000s)	Rate (per 100 000)	Prevalence 1990 Number ('000s)	Rate (per 100 000)	Avg. age at onset (years)	Average duration (years)	Deaths 1990 Number ('000s)	Rate (per 100 000)	Deaths 2000 (Projected) Number ('000s)	Rate (per 100 000)
Males										
0-4	2	6.0	3	12	0.0	25.8	0	0	0	0
5-14	0	0.0	6	12	-	-	0	0	0	0
15-44	0	0.0	12	12	-	-	0	0	0	0
45-59	0	0.0	3	12	-	-	0	0	0	0
60+	0	0.0	2	12	-	-	0	0	0	0
All ages	2	0.8	26	12	0.0	25.8	0	0	0	0
Females										
0-4	2	6.0	3	12	0.0	27.6	0	0	0	0
5-14	0	0.0	6	12	-	-	0	0	0	0
15-44	0	0.0	12	12	-	-	0	0	0	0
45-59	0	0.0	3	12	-	-	0	0	0	0
60+	0	0.0	2	12	-	-	0	0	0	0
All ages	2	0.7	26	12	0.0	27.6	0	0	0	0
Total	3	0.8	52	12	0.0	26.7	0	0	0	0

Table 36h MEC - AOM - CMO — Gonorrhoea - Corneal scar - low vision

Age group (years)	Incidence 1990 Number ('000s)	Rate (per 100 000)	Prevalence 1990 Number ('000s)	Rate (per 100 000)	Avg. age at onset (years)	Average duration (years)	Deaths 1990 Number ('000s)	Rate (per 100 000)	Deaths 2000 (Projected) Number ('000s)	Rate (per 100 000)
Males										
0-4	1	2.1	2	4.1	0.0	24.3	0	0	0	0
5-14	0	0.0	3	4.1	-	-	0	0	0	0
15-44	0	0.0	5	4.1	-	-	0	0	0	0
45-59	0	0.0	1	4.1	-	-	0	0	0	0
60+	0	0.0	1	4.1	-	-	0	0	0	0
All ages	1	0.3	10	4.1	0.0	24.3	0	0	0	0
Females										
0-4	1	2.1	2	4.1	0.0	25.3	0	0	0	0
5-14	0	0.0	3	4.1	-	-	0	0	0	0
15-44	0	0.0	4	4.1	-	-	0	0	0	0
45-59	0	0.0	1	4.1	-	-	0	0	0	0
60+	0	0.0	1	4.1	-	-	0	0	0	0
All ages	1	0.3	10	4.1	0.0	25.3	0	0	0	0
Total	2	0.3	20	4.1	0.0	24.7	0	0	0	0

Table 36i World - Mundo - Monde — Gonorrhoea - Corneal scar - low vision

Age group (years)	Incidence 1990 Number ('000s)	Rate (per 100 000)	Prevalence 1990 Number ('000s)	Rate (per 100 000)	Avg. age at onset (years)	Average duration (years)	Deaths 1990 Number ('000s)	Rate (per 100 000)	Deaths 2000 (Projected) Number ('000s)	Rate (per 100 000)
Males										
0-4	86	26.6	160	50	0.0	21.3	0	0	0	0
5-14	0	0.0	262	48	-	-	0	0	0	0
15-44	0	0.0	458	37	-	-	0	0	0	0
45-59	0	0.0	99	32	-	-	0	0	0	0
60+	0	0.0	58	26	-	-	0	0	0	0
All ages	86	3.2	1 037	39	0.0	21.3	0	0	0	0
Females										
0-4	83	26.7	155	50	0.0	22.4	0	0	0	0
5-14	0	0.0	254	48	-	-	0	0	0	0
15-44	0	0.0	448	37	-	-	0	0	0	0
45-59	0	0.0	102	33	-	-	0	0	0	0
60+	0	0.0	64	24	-	-	0	0	0	0
All ages	83	3.2	1 023	39	0.0	22.4	0	0	0	0
Total	168	3.2	2 060	39	0.0	21.8	0	0	0	0

For epidemiological sources see Berkley et al. 1996. For the methods used to estimate and project incidence, prevalence, and deaths see Murray and Lopez 1996a. See explanatory notes for definitions and caveats.

Table 37	Cuadro 37	Tableau 37
Gonorrhoea	Gonorrea	Gonorrhée
Cervicitis	Cervicitis	Cervicite

Table 37a — EME - PEMC - EMBE — Gonorrhoea - Cervicitis

Age group (years)	Incidence 1990 Number ('000s)	Rate (per 100 000)	Prevalence 1990 Number ('000s)	Rate (per 100 000)	Avg. age at onset (years)	Average duration (years)	Deaths 1990 Number ('000s)	Rate (per 100 000)	Deaths 2000 (Projected) Number ('000s)	Rate (per 100 000)
Males										
0-4	0	0	0	0	-	-	0	0	0	0
5-14	0	0	0	0	-	-	0	0	0	0
15-44	0	0	0	0	-	-	0	0	0	0
45-59	0	0	0	0	-	-	0	0	0	0
60+	0	0	0	0	-	-	0	0	0	0
All ages	0	0	0	0	-	-	0	0	0	0
Females										
0-4	0	0	0	0.0	-	-	0	0	0	0
5-14	6	12	0	0.4	13.0	0.03	0	0	0	0
15-44	829	463	27	15.3	22.0	0.03	0	0	0	0
45-59	16	23	1	0.8	52.4	0.03	0	0	0	0
60+	10	12	0	0.4	72.4	0.03	0	0	0	0
All ages	861	211	28	7.0	23.1	0.03	0	0	0	0
Total	861	108	28	3.6	23.1	0.03	0	0	0	0

Table 37b — FSE - PEAS - AESE — Gonorrhoea - Cervicitis

Age group (years)	Incidence 1990 Number ('000s)	Rate (per 100 000)	Prevalence 1990 Number ('000s)	Rate (per 100 000)	Avg. age at onset (years)	Average duration (years)	Deaths 1990 Number ('000s)	Rate (per 100 000)	Deaths 2000 (Projected) Number ('000s)	Rate (per 100 000)
Males										
0-4	0	0	0	0	-	-	0	0	0	0
5-14	0	0	0	0	-	-	0	0	0	0
15-44	0	0	0	0	-	-	0	0	0	0
45-59	0	0	0	0	-	-	0	0	0	0
60+	0	0	0	0	-	-	0	0	0	0
All ages	0	0	0	0	-	-	0	0	0	0
Females										
0-4	0	0	0	0.0	-	-	0	0	0	0
5-14	4	17	0	0.7	13.0	0.04	0	0	0	0
15-44	507	676	21	28.3	22.0	0.04	0	0	0	0
45-59	10	34	0	1.4	52.4	0.04	0	0	0	0
60+	6	17	0	0.7	71.5	0.04	0	0	0	0
All ages	527	292	22	12.2	23.1	0.04	0	0	0	0
Total	527	152	22	6.4	23.1	0.04	0	0	0	0

Table 37c — India - India - Inde — Gonorrhoea - Cervicitis

Age group (years)	Incidence 1990 Number ('000s)	Rate (per 100 000)	Prevalence 1990 Number ('000s)	Rate (per 100 000)	Avg. age at onset (years)	Average duration (years)	Deaths 1990 Number ('000s)	Rate (per 100 000)	Deaths 2000 (Projected) Number ('000s)	Rate (per 100 000)
Males										
0-4	0	0	0	0	-	-	0	0	0	0
5-14	0	0	0	0	-	-	0	0	0	0
15-44	0	0	0	0	-	-	0	0	0	0
45-59	0	0	0	0	-	-	0	0	0	0
60+	0	0	0	0	-	-	0	0	0	0
All ages	0	0	0	0	-	-	0	0	0	0
Females										
0-4	0	0	0	0.0	-	-	0	0	0	0
5-14	43	45	2	2.3	13.0	0.05	0	0	0	0
15-44	3 331	1 818	169	92.0	22.0	0.05	0	0	0	0
45-59	42	91	2	4.6	52.4	0.05	0	0	0	0
60+	13	45	1	2.3	70.1	0.05	0	0	0	0
All ages	3 429	836	174	42.3	22.4	0.05	0	0	0	0
Total	3 429	404	174	20.4	22.4	0.05	0	0	0	0

For epidemiological sources see Berkley et al. 1996. For the methods used to estimate and project incidence, prevalence, and deaths see Murray and Lopez 1996a. See explanatory notes for definitions and caveats.

Table 37
Gonorrhoea

Cuadro 37
Gonorrea

Tableau 37
Gonorrhée

Cervicitis

Cervicitis

Cervicite

Table 37d — China - China - Chine — Gonorrhoea - Cervicitis

Age group (years)	Incidence 1990 Number ('000s)	Rate (per 100 000)	Prevalence 1990 Number ('000s)	Rate (per 100 000)	Avg. age at onset (years)	Average duration (years)	Deaths 1990 Number ('000s)	Rate (per 100 000)	Deaths 2000 (Projected) Number ('000s)	Rate (per 100 000)
Males										
0-4	0	0	0	0	-	-	0	0	0	0
5-14	0	0	0	0	-	-	0	0	0	0
15-44	0	0	0	0	-	-	0	0	0	0
45-59	0	0	0	0	-	-	0	0	0	0
60+	0	0	0	0	-	-	0	0	0	0
All ages	0	0	0	0	-	-	0	0	0	0
Females										
0-4	0	0.0	0	0.0	-	-	0	0	0	0
5-14	1	1.6	0	0.1	13.0	0.04	0	0	0	0
15-44	179	63.1	7	2.6	22.0	0.04	0	0	0	0
45-59	2	3.2	0	0.1	52.4	0.04	0	0	0	0
60+	1	1.6	0	0.1	70.6	0.04	0	0	0	0
All ages	184	33.5	8	1.4	22.5	0.04	0	0	0	0
Total	184	16.2	8	0.7	22.5	0.04	0	0	0	0

Table 37e — OAI - OPAI - APAI — Gonorrhoea - Cervicitis

Age group (years)	Incidence 1990 Number ('000s)	Rate (per 100 000)	Prevalence 1990 Number ('000s)	Rate (per 100 000)	Avg. age at onset (years)	Average duration (years)	Deaths 1990 Number ('000s)	Rate (per 100 000)	Deaths 2000 (Projected) Number ('000s)	Rate (per 100 000)
Males										
0-4	0	0	0	0	-	-	0	0	0	0
5-14	0	0	0	0	-	-	0	0	0	0
15-44	0	0	0	0	-	-	0	0	0	0
45-59	0	0	0	0	-	-	0	0	0	0
60+	0	0	0	0	-	-	0	0	0	0
All ages	0	0	0	0	-	-	0	0	0	0
Females										
0-4	0	0	0	0.0	-	-	0	0	0	0
5-14	34	43	2	2.2	13.0	0.05	0	0	0	0
15-44	2 720	1 704	138	86.3	22.0	0.05	0	0	0	0
45-59	30	85	2	4.3	52.3	0.05	0	0	0	0
60+	10	43	0	2.2	70.3	0.05	0	0	0	0
All ages	2 794	823	141	41.7	22.4	0.05	0	0	0	0
Total	2 794	409	141	20.7	22.4	0.05	0	0	0	0

Table 37f — SSA - ASS - ASS — Gonorrhoea - Cervicitis

Age group (years)	Incidence 1990 Number ('000s)	Rate (per 100 000)	Prevalence 1990 Number ('000s)	Rate (per 100 000)	Avg. age at onset (years)	Average duration (years)	Deaths 1990 Number ('000s)	Rate (per 100 000)	Deaths 2000 (Projected) Number ('000s)	Rate (per 100 000)
Males										
0-4	0	0	0	0	-	-	0	0	0	0
5-14	0	0	0	0	-	-	0	0	0	0
15-44	0	0	0	0	-	-	0	0	0	0
45-59	0	0	0	0	-	-	0	0	0	0
60+	0	0	0	0	-	-	0	0	0	0
All ages	0	0	0	0	-	-	0	0	0	0
Females										
0-4	0	0	0	0.0	-	-	0	0	0	0
5-14	63	91	3	4.6	13.0	0.05	0	0	0	0
15-44	3 866	3 638	196	184.1	22.0	0.05	0	0	0	0
45-59	40	182	2	9.2	52.2	0.05	0	0	0	0
60+	12	91	1	4.6	69.7	0.05	0	0	0	0
All ages	3 981	1 543	202	78.1	22.3	0.05	0	0	0	0
Total	3 981	780	202	39.5	22.3	0.05	0	0	0	0

For epidemiological sources see Berkley et al. 1996. For the methods used to estimate and project incidence, prevalence, and deaths see Murray and Lopez 1996a. See explanatory notes for definitions and caveats.

Table 37	Cuadro 37	Tableau 37
Gonorrhoea	Gonorrea	Gonorrhée
Cervicitis	Cervicitis	Cervicite

Table 37g LAC - ALC - ALC   Gonorrhoea - Cervicitis

Age group (years)	Incidence 1990		Prevalence 1990		Avg. age at onset (years)	Average duration (years)	Deaths 1990		Deaths 2000 (Projected)	
	Number ('000s)	Rate (per 100 000)	Number ('000s)	Rate (per 100 000)			Number ('000s)	Rate (per 100 000)	Number ('000s)	Rate (per 100 000)
Males										
0-4	0	0	0	0	-	-	0	0	0	0
5-14	0	0	0	0	-	-	0	0	0	0
15-44	0	0	0	0	-	-	0	0	0	0
45-59	0	0	0	0	-	-	0	0	0	0
60+	0	0	0	0	-	-	0	0	0	0
All ages	0	0	0	0	-	-	0	0	0	0
Females										
0-4	0	0	0	0.0	-	-	0	0	0	0
5-14	21	41	1	1.7	13.0	0.04	0	0	0	0
15-44	1 688	1 622	71	67.8	22.0	0.04	0	0	0	0
45-59	19	81	1	3.4	52.4	0.04	0	0	0	0
60+	7	41	0	1.7	71.1	0.04	0	0	0	0
All ages	1 734	779	72	32.6	22.4	0.04	0	0	0	0
Total	1 734	390	72	16.3	22.4	0.04	0	0	0	0

Table 37h MEC - AOM - CMO   Gonorrhoea - Cervicitis

Age group (years)	Incidence 1990		Prevalence 1990		Avg. age at onset (years)	Average duration (years)	Deaths 1990		Deaths 2000 (Projected)	
	Number ('000s)	Rate (per 100 000)	Number ('000s)	Rate (per 100 000)			Number ('000s)	Rate (per 100 000)	Number ('000s)	Rate (per 100 000)
Males										
0-4	0	0	0	0	-	-	0	0	0	0
5-14	0	0	0	0	-	-	0	0	0	0
15-44	0	0	0	0	-	-	0	0	0	0
45-59	0	0	0	0	-	-	0	0	0	0
60+	0	0	0	0	-	-	0	0	0	0
All ages	0	0	0	0	-	-	0	0	0	0
Females										
0-4	0	0	0	0.0	-	-	0	0	0	0
5-14	8	14	0	0.6	13.0	0.04	0	0	0	0
15-44	580	541	24	22.6	22.0	0.04	0	0	0	0
45-59	6	27	0	1.1	52.3	0.04	0	0	0	0
60+	2	14	0	0.6	70.4	0.04	0	0	0	0
All ages	596	242	25	10.1	22.3	0.04	0	0	0	0
Total	596	118	25	5.0	22.3	0.04	0	0	0	0

Table 37i World - Mundo - Monde   Gonorrhoea - Cervicitis

Age group (years)	Incidence 1990		Prevalence 1990		Avg. age at onset (years)	Average duration (years)	Deaths 1990		Deaths 2000 (Projected)	
	Number ('000s)	Rate (per 100 000)	Number ('000s)	Rate (per 100 000)			Number ('000s)	Rate (per 100 000)	Number ('000s)	Rate (per 100 000)
Males										
0-4	0	0	0	0	-	-	0	0	0	0
5-14	0	0	0	0	-	-	0	0	0	0
15-44	0	0	0	0	-	-	0	0	0	0
45-59	0	0	0	0	-	-	0	0	0	0
60+	0	0	0	0	-	-	0	0	0	0
All ages	0	0	0	0	-	-	0	0	0	0
Females										
0-4	0	0	0	0.0	-	-	0	0	0	0
5-14	182	35	9	1.7	13.0	0.05	0	0	0	0
15-44	13 700	1 143	653	54.5	22.0	0.05	0	0	0	0
45-59	165	53	8	2.5	52.3	0.05	0	0	0	0
60+	60	22	3	1.0	70.7	0.05	0	0	0	0
All ages	14 106	540	672	25.7	22.4	0.05	0	0	0	0
Total	14 106	268	672	12.8	22.4	0.05	0	0	0	0

For epidemiological sources see Berkley et al. 1996. For the methods used to estimate and project incidence, prevalence, and deaths see Murray and Lopez 1996a. See explanatory notes for definitions and caveats.

Table 38
Gonorrhoea

Pelvic inflammatory disease

Cuadro 38
Gonorrea

Enfermedad inflamatoria pélvica

Tableau 38
Gonorrhée

Inflammation des organes pelviens

Table 38a   EME - PEMC - EMBE   Gonorrhoea - Pelvic inflammatory disease

Age group (years)	Incidence 1990 Number ('000s)	Rate (per 100 000)	Prevalence 1990 Number ('000s)	Rate (per 100 000)	Avg. age at onset (years)	Average duration (years)	Deaths 1990 Number ('000s)	Rate (per 100 000)	Deaths 2000 (Projected) Number ('000s)	Rate (per 100 000)
Males										
0-4	0	0	0	0	-	-	-	-	-	-
5-14	0	0	0	0	-	-	-	-	-	-
15-44	0	0	0	0	-	-	-	-	-	-
45-59	0	0	0	0	-	-	-	-	-	-
60+	0	0	0	0	-	-	-	-	-	-
All ages	0	0	0	0	-	-	-	-	-	-
Females										
0-4	0	0.0	0	0.0	-	-	-	-	-	-
5-14	1	2.1	0	0.0	13.0	0.02	-	-	-	-
15-44	149	83.4	3	1.8	22.2	0.02	-	-	-	-
45-59	3	4.2	0	0.1	52.4	0.02	-	-	-	-
60+	2	2.1	0	0.0	72.4	0.02	-	-	-	-
All ages	155	38.1	3	0.8	23.3	0.02	-	-	-	-
Total	155	19.4	3	0.4	23.3	0.02	-	-	-	-

Table 38b   FSE - PEAS - AESE   Gonorrhoea - Pelvic inflammatory disease

Age group (years)	Incidence 1990 Number ('000s)	Rate (per 100 000)	Prevalence 1990 Number ('000s)	Rate (per 100 000)	Avg. age at onset (years)	Average duration (years)	Deaths 1990 Number ('000s)	Rate (per 100 000)	Deaths 2000 (Projected) Number ('000s)	Rate (per 100 000)
Males										
0-4	0	0	0	0	-	-	-	-	-	-
5-14	0	0	0	0	-	-	-	-	-	-
15-44	0	0	0	0	-	-	-	-	-	-
45-59	0	0	0	0	-	-	-	-	-	-
60+	0	0	0	0	-	-	-	-	-	-
All ages	0	0	0	0	-	-	-	-	-	-
Females										
0-4	0	0.0	0	0.0	-	-	-	-	-	-
5-14	1	4.3	0	0.1	13.0	0.03	-	-	-	-
15-44	129	171.7	4	4.8	22.2	0.03	-	-	-	-
45-59	3	8.6	0	0.2	52.4	0.03	-	-	-	-
60+	2	4.3	0	0.1	71.5	0.03	-	-	-	-
All ages	134	74.1	4	2.1	23.3	0.03	-	-	-	-
Total	134	38.7	4	1.1	23.3	0.03	-	-	-	-

Table 38c   India - India - Inde   Gonorrhoea - Pelvic inflammatory disease

Age group (years)	Incidence 1990 Number ('000s)	Rate (per 100 000)	Prevalence 1990 Number ('000s)	Rate (per 100 000)	Avg. age at onset (years)	Average duration (years)	Deaths 1990 Number ('000s)	Rate (per 100 000)	Deaths 2000 (Projected) Number ('000s)	Rate (per 100 000)
Males										
0-4	0	0	0	0	-	-	-	-	-	-
5-14	0	0	0	0	-	-	-	-	-	-
15-44	0	0	0	0	-	-	-	-	-	-
45-59	0	0	0	0	-	-	-	-	-	-
60+	0	0	0	0	-	-	-	-	-	-
All ages	0	0	0	0	-	-	-	-	-	-
Females										
0-4	0	0	0	0.0	-	-	-	-	-	-
5-14	15	15	0	0.5	13.0	0.03	-	-	-	-
15-44	1 121	612	37	20.3	22.2	0.03	-	-	-	-
45-59	14	31	0	1.0	52.4	0.03	-	-	-	-
60+	4	15	0	0.5	70.1	0.03	-	-	-	-
All ages	1 154	281	38	9.3	22.6	0.03	-	-	-	-
Total	1 154	136	38	4.5	22.6	0.03	-	-	-	-

For epidemiological sources see Berkley et al. 1996. For the methods used to estimate and project incidence, prevalence, and deaths see Murray and Lopez 1996a. See explanatory notes for definitions and caveats.

Table 38
Gonorrhoea

Cuadro 38
Gonorrea

Tableau 38
Gonorrhée

Pelvic inflammatory disease

Enfermedad inflamatoria pélvica

Inflammation des organes pelviens

Table 38d   China - China - Chine   Gonorrhoea - Pelvic inflammatory disease

Age group (years)	Incidence 1990 Number ('000s)	Rate (per 100 000)	Prevalence 1990 Number ('000s)	Rate (per 100 000)	Avg. age at onset (years)	Average duration (years)	Deaths 1990 Number ('000s)	Rate (per 100 000)	Deaths 2000 (Projected) Number ('000s)	Rate (per 100 000)
Males										
0-4	0	0	0	0	-	-	-	-	-	-
5-14	0	0	0	0	-	-	-	-	-	-
15-44	0	0	0	0	-	-	-	-	-	-
45-59	0	0	0	0	-	-	-	-	-	-
60+	0	0	0	0	-	-	-	-	-	-
All ages	0	0	0	0	-	-	-	-	-	-
Females										
0-4	0	0.0	0	0.0	-	-	-	-	-	-
5-14	0	0.4	0	0.0	13.0	0.03	-	-	-	-
15-44	45	15.9	1	0.4	22.2	0.03	-	-	-	-
45-59	1	0.8	0	0.0	52.4	0.03	-	-	-	-
60+	0	0.4	0	0.0	70.6	0.03	-	-	-	-
All ages	46	8.4	1	0.2	22.7	0.03	-	-	-	-
Total	46	4.1	1	0.1	22.7	0.03	-	-	-	-

Table 38e   OAI - OPAI - APAI   Gonorrhoea - Pelvic inflammatory disease

Age group (years)	Incidence 1990 Number ('000s)	Rate (per 100 000)	Prevalence 1990 Number ('000s)	Rate (per 100 000)	Avg. age at onset (years)	Average duration (years)	Deaths 1990 Number ('000s)	Rate (per 100 000)	Deaths 2000 (Projected) Number ('000s)	Rate (per 100 000)
Males										
0-4	0	0	0	0	-	-	-	-	-	-
5-14	0	0	0	0	-	-	-	-	-	-
15-44	0	0	0	0	-	-	-	-	-	-
45-59	0	0	0	0	-	-	-	-	-	-
60+	0	0	0	0	-	-	-	-	-	-
All ages	0	0	0	0	-	-	-	-	-	-
Females										
0-4	0	0	0	0.0	-	-	-	-	-	-
5-14	11	14	0	0.5	13.0	0.03	-	-	-	-
15-44	915	573	30	19.0	22.2	0.03	-	-	-	-
45-59	10	29	0	1.0	52.3	0.03	-	-	-	-
60+	3	14	0	0.5	70.3	0.03	-	-	-	-
All ages	940	277	31	9.2	22.6	0.03	-	-	-	-
Total	940	138	31	4.6	22.6	0.03	-	-	-	-

Table 38f   SSA - ASS - ASS   Gonorrhoea - Pelvic inflammatory disease

Age group (years)	Incidence 1990 Number ('000s)	Rate (per 100 000)	Prevalence 1990 Number ('000s)	Rate (per 100 000)	Avg. age at onset (years)	Average duration (years)	Deaths 1990 Number ('000s)	Rate (per 100 000)	Deaths 2000 (Projected) Number ('000s)	Rate (per 100 000)
Males										
0-4	0	0	0	0	-	-	-	-	-	-
5-14	0	0	0	0	-	-	-	-	-	-
15-44	0	0	0	0	-	-	-	-	-	-
45-59	0	0	0	0	-	-	-	-	-	-
60+	0	0	0	0	-	-	-	-	-	-
All ages	0	0	0	0	-	-	-	-	-	-
Females										
0-4	0	0	0	0.0	-	-	-	-	-	-
5-14	21	31	1	1.0	13.0	0.03	-	-	-	-
15-44	1 300	1 224	43	40.6	22.2	0.03	-	-	-	-
45-59	14	61	0	2.0	52.2	0.03	-	-	-	-
60+	4	31	0	1.0	69.7	0.03	-	-	-	-
All ages	1 339	519	44	17.2	22.5	0.03	-	-	-	-
Total	1 339	262	44	8.7	22.5	0.03	-	-	-	-

For epidemiological sources see Berkley et al. 1996. For the methods used to estimate and project incidence, prevalence, and deaths see Murray and Lopez 1996a. See explanatory notes for definitions and caveats.

Table 38 / **Cuadro 38** / **Tableau 38**
Gonorrhoea / Gonorrea / Gonorrhée

Pelvic inflammatory disease / Enfermedad inflamatoria pélvica / Inflammation des organes pelviens

Table 38g LAC - ALC - ALC Gonorrhoea - Pelvic inflammatory disease

Age group (years)	Incidence 1990 Number ('000s)	Rate (per 100 000)	Prevalence 1990 Number ('000s)	Rate (per 100 000)	Avg. age at onset (years)	Average duration (years)	Deaths 1990 Number ('000s)	Rate (per 100 000)	Deaths 2000 (Projected) Number ('000s)	Rate (per 100 000)
Males										
0-4	0	0	0	0	-	-	-	-	-	-
5-14	0	0	0	0	-	-	-	-	-	-
15-44	0	0	0	0	-	-	-	-	-	-
45-59	0	0	0	0	-	-	-	-	-	-
60+	0	0	0	0	-	-	-	-	-	-
All ages	0	0	0	0	-	-	-	-	-	-
Females										
0-4	0	0.0	0	0.0	-	-	-	-	-	-
5-14	5	10.3	0	0.3	13.0	0.03	-	-	-	-
15-44	429	412.0	12	11.5	22.2	0.03	-	-	-	-
45-59	5	20.6	0	0.6	52.4	0.03	-	-	-	-
60+	2	10.3	0	0.3	71.1	0.03	-	-	-	-
All ages	441	197.9	12	5.5	22.6	0.03	-	-	-	-
Total	441	99.2	12	2.8	22.6	0.03	-	-	-	-

Table 38h MEC - AOM - CMO Gonorrhoea - Pelvic inflammatory disease

Age group (years)	Incidence 1990 Number ('000s)	Rate (per 100 000)	Prevalence 1990 Number ('000s)	Rate (per 100 000)	Avg. age at onset (years)	Average duration (years)	Deaths 1990 Number ('000s)	Rate (per 100 000)	Deaths 2000 (Projected) Number ('000s)	Rate (per 100 000)
Males										
0-4	0	0	0	0	-	-	-	-	-	-
5-14	0	0	0	0	-	-	-	-	-	-
15-44	0	0	0	0	-	-	-	-	-	-
45-59	0	0	0	0	-	-	-	-	-	-
60+	0	0	0	0	-	-	-	-	-	-
All ages	0	0	0	0	-	-	-	-	-	-
Females										
0-4	0	0.0	0	0.0	-	-	-	-	-	-
5-14	2	3.4	0	0.1	13.0	0.03	-	-	-	-
15-44	147	137.3	4	3.8	22.2	0.03	-	-	-	-
45-59	2	6.9	0	0.2	52.3	0.03	-	-	-	-
60+	1	3.4	0	0.1	70.4	0.03	-	-	-	-
All ages	151	61.4	4	1.7	22.5	0.03	-	-	-	-
Total	151	30.1	4	0.8	22.5	0.03	-	-	-	-

Table 38i World - Mundo - Monde Gonorrhoea - Pelvic inflammatory disease

Age group (years)	Incidence 1990 Number ('000s)	Rate (per 100 000)	Prevalence 1990 Number ('000s)	Rate (per 100 000)	Avg. age at onset (years)	Average duration (years)	Deaths 1990 Number ('000s)	Rate (per 100 000)	Deaths 2000 (Projected) Number ('000s)	Rate (per 100 000)
Males										
0-4	0	0	0	0	-	-	-	-	-	-
5-14	0	0	0	0	-	-	-	-	-	-
15-44	0	0	0	0	-	-	-	-	-	-
45-59	0	0	0	0	-	-	-	-	-	-
60+	0	0	0	0	-	-	-	-	-	-
All ages	0	0	0	0	-	-	-	-	-	-
Females										
0-4	0	0.0	0	0.0	-	-	-	-	-	-
5-14	57	10.9	2	0.4	13.0	0.03	-	-	-	-
15-44	4 236	353.4	135	11.3	22.2	0.03	-	-	-	-
45-59	50	16.0	2	0.5	52.4	0.03	-	-	-	-
60+	17	6.4	1	0.2	71.2	0.03	-	-	-	-
All ages	4 360	166.8	139	5.3	22.6	0.03	-	-	-	-
Total	4 360	82.8	139	2.6	22.6	0.03	-	-	-	-

For epidemiological sources see Berkley et al. 1996. For the methods used to estimate and project incidence, prevalence, and deaths see Murray and Lopez 1996a. See explanatory notes for definitions and caveats.

Table 39
Gonorrhoea

Cuadro 39
Gonorrea

Tableau 39
Gonorrhée

Ectopic pregnancy

Embarazo ectópico

Grossesse ectopique

Table 39a **EME - PEMC - EMBE** Gonorrhoea - Ectopic pregnancy

Age group (years)	Incidence 1990 Number ('000s)	Rate (per 100 000)	Prevalence 1990 Number ('000s)	Rate (per 100 000)	Avg. age at onset (years)	Average duration (years)	Deaths 1990 Number ('000s)	Rate (per 100 000)	Deaths 2000 (Projected) Number ('000s)	Rate (per 100 000)
Males										
0-4	0	0	0	0	-	-	0	0	0	0
5-14	0	0	0	0	-	-	0	0	0	0
15-44	0	0	0	0	-	-	0	0	0	0
45-59	0	0	0	0	-	-	0	0	0	0
60+	0	0	0	0	-	-	0	0	0	0
All ages	0	0	0	0	-	-	0	0	0	0
Females										
0-4	0	0.0	0	0.0	-	-	0	0	0	0
5-14	0	0.0	0	0.0	13.0	0.08	0	0	0	0
15-44	0	0.2	0	0.0	25.0	0.08	0	0	0	0
45-59	0	0.0	0	0.0	52.4	0.08	0	0	0	0
60+	0	0.0	0	0.0	72.4	0.08	0	0	0	0
All ages	0	0.1	0	0.0	25.9	0.08	0	0	0	0
Total	0	0.0	0	0.0	25.9	0.08	0	0	0	0

Table 39b **FSE - PEAS - AESE** Gonorrhoea - Ectopic pregnancy

Age group (years)	Incidence 1990 Number ('000s)	Rate (per 100 000)	Prevalence 1990 Number ('000s)	Rate (per 100 000)	Avg. age at onset (years)	Average duration (years)	Deaths 1990 Number ('000s)	Rate (per 100 000)	Deaths 2000 (Projected) Number ('000s)	Rate (per 100 000)
Males										
0-4	0	0	0	0	-	-	0	0	0	0
5-14	0	0	0	0	-	-	0	0	0	0
15-44	0	0	0	0	-	-	0	0	0	0
45-59	0	0	0	0	-	-	0	0	0	0
60+	0	0	0	0	-	-	0	0	0	0
All ages	0	0	0	0	-	-	0	0	0	0
Females										
0-4	0	0.0	0	0.0	-	-	0	0.0	0	0
5-14	0	0.0	0	0.0	13.0	0.08	0	0.0	0	0
15-44	0	0.6	0	0.0	25.0	0.08	0	0.1	0	0
45-59	0	0.0	0	0.0	52.4	0.08	0	0.0	0	0
60+	0	0.0	0	0.0	71.5	0.08	0	0.0	0	0
All ages	0	0.3	0	0.0	25.9	0.08	0	0.0	0	0
Total	0	0.1	0	0.0	25.9	0.08	0	0.0	0	0

Table 39c **India - India - Inde** Gonorrhoea - Ectopic pregnancy

Age group (years)	Incidence 1990 Number ('000s)	Rate (per 100 000)	Prevalence 1990 Number ('000s)	Rate (per 100 000)	Avg. age at onset (years)	Average duration (years)	Deaths 1990 Number ('000s)	Rate (per 100 000)	Deaths 2000 (Projected) Number ('000s)	Rate (per 100 000)
Males										
0-4	0	0	0	0	-	-	0	0	0	0
5-14	0	0	0	0	-	-	0	0	0	0
15-44	0	0	0	0	-	-	0	0	0	0
45-59	0	0	0	0	-	-	0	0	0	0
60+	0	0	0	0	-	-	0	0	0	0
All ages	0	0	0	0	-	-	0	0	0	0
Females										
0-4	0	0.0	0	0.0	-	-	0	0.0	0	0.0
5-14	0	0.1	0	0.0	13.0	0.08	0	0.0	0	0.0
15-44	10	5.5	1	0.4	25.0	0.08	2	1.1	1	0.4
45-59	0	0.3	0	0.0	52.4	0.08	0	0.0	0	0.0
60+	0	0.1	0	0.0	70.1	0.08	0	0.0	0	0.0
All ages	10	2.5	1	0.2	25.3	0.08	2	0.5	1	0.2
Total	10	1.2	1	0.1	25.3	0.08	2	0.2	1	0.1

For epidemiological sources see Berkley et al. 1996. For the methods used to estimate and project incidence, prevalence, and deaths see Murray and Lopez 1996a. See explanatory notes for definitions and caveats.

Table 39   **Cuadro 39**   **Tableau 39**
Gonorrhoea   **Gonorrea**   **Gonorrhée**

Ectopic pregnancy   Embarazo ectópico   Grossesse ectopique

Table 39d   China - China - Chine   Gonorrhoea - Ectopic pregnancy

Age group (years)	Incidence 1990 Number ('000s)	Rate (per 100 000)	Prevalence 1990 Number ('000s)	Rate (per 100 000)	Avg. age at onset (years)	Average duration (years)	Deaths 1990 Number ('000s)	Rate (per 100 000)	Deaths 2000 (Projected) Number ('000s)	Rate (per 100 000)
Males										
0-4	0	0	0	0	-	-	0	0	0	0
5-14	0	0	0	0	-	-	0	0	0	0
15-44	0	0	0	0	-	-	0	0	0	0
45-59	0	0	0	0	-	-	0	0	0	0
60+	0	0	0	0	-	-	0	0	0	0
All ages	0	0	0	0	-	-	0	0	0	0
Females										
0-4	0	0.0	0	0.0	-	-	0	0	0	0
5-14	0	0.0	0	0.0	13.0	0.08	0	0	0	0
15-44	0	0.1	0	0.0	25.0	0.08	0	0	0	0
45-59	0	0.0	0	0.0	52.4	0.08	0	0	0	0
60+	0	0.0	0	0.0	70.6	0.08	0	0	0	0
All ages	0	0.0	0	0.0	25.4	0.08	0	0	0	0
Total	0	0.0	0	0.0	25.4	0.08	0	0	0	0

Table 39e   OAI - OPAI - APAI   Gonorrhoea - Ectopic pregnancy

Age group (years)	Incidence 1990 Number ('000s)	Rate (per 100 000)	Prevalence 1990 Number ('000s)	Rate (per 100 000)	Avg. age at onset (years)	Average duration (years)	Deaths 1990 Number ('000s)	Rate (per 100 000)	Deaths 2000 (Projected) Number ('000s)	Rate (per 100 000)
Males										
0-4	0	0	0	0	-	-	0	0	0	0
5-14	0	0	0	0	-	-	0	0	0	0
15-44	0	0	0	0	-	-	0	0	0	0
45-59	0	0	0	0	-	-	0	0	0	0
60+	0	0	0	0	-	-	0	0	0	0
All ages	0	0	0	0	-	-	0	0	0	0
Females										
0-4	0	0.0	0	0.0	-	-	0	0.0	0	0.0
5-14	0	0.1	0	0.0	13.0	0.08	0	0.0	0	0.0
15-44	7	4.3	1	0.3	25.0	0.08	1	0.9	1	0.4
45-59	0	0.2	0	0.0	52.3	0.08	0	0.0	0	0.0
60+	0	0.1	0	0.0	70.3	0.08	0	0.0	0	0.0
All ages	7	2.1	1	0.2	25.3	0.08	1	0.4	1	0.2
Total	7	1.0	1	0.1	25.3	0.08	1	0.2	1	0.1

Table 39f   SSA - ASS - ASS   Gonorrhoea - Ectopic pregnancy

Age group (years)	Incidence 1990 Number ('000s)	Rate (per 100 000)	Prevalence 1990 Number ('000s)	Rate (per 100 000)	Avg. age at onset (years)	Average duration (years)	Deaths 1990 Number ('000s)	Rate (per 100 000)	Deaths 2000 (Projected) Number ('000s)	Rate (per 100 000)
Males										
0-4	0	0	0	0	-	-	0	0	0	0
5-14	0	0	0	0	-	-	0	0	0	0
15-44	0	0	0	0	-	-	0	0	0	0
45-59	0	0	0	0	-	-	0	0	0	0
60+	0	0	0	0	-	-	0	0	0	0
All ages	0	0	0	0	-	-	0	0	0	0
Females										
0-4	0	0.0	0	0.0	-	-	0	0.0	0	0.0
5-14	0	0.5	0	0.0	13.0	0.08	0	0.0	0	0.0
15-44	20	18.5	2	1.4	25.0	0.08	4	3.7	2	1.7
45-59	0	0.9	0	0.1	52.2	0.08	0	0.0	0	0.0
60+	0	0.5	0	0.0	69.7	0.08	0	0.0	0	0.0
All ages	20	7.9	2	0.6	25.2	0.08	4	1.5	2	0.7
Total	20	4.0	2	0.3	25.2	0.08	4	0.8	2	0.4

For epidemiological sources see Berkley et al. 1996. For the methods used to estimate and project incidence, prevalence, and deaths see Murray and Lopez 1996a. See explanatory notes for definitions and caveats.

Table 39	Cuadro 39	Tableau 39
Gonorrhoea	Gonorrea	Gonorrhée
Ectopic pregnancy	Embarazo ectópico	Grossesse ectopique

Table 39g — LAC - ALC - ALC — Gonorrhoea - Ectopic pregnancy

Age group (years)	Incidence 1990 Number ('000s)	Rate (per 100 000)	Prevalence 1990 Number ('000s)	Rate (per 100 000)	Avg. age at onset (years)	Average duration (years)	Deaths 1990 Number ('000s)	Rate (per 100 000)	Deaths 2000 (Projected) Number ('000s)	Rate (per 100 000)
Males										
0-4	0	0	0	0	-	-	0	0	0	0
5-14	0	0	0	0	-	-	0	0	0	0
15-44	0	0	0	0	-	-	0	0	0	0
45-59	0	0	0	0	-	-	0	0	0	0
60+	0	0	0	0	-	-	0	0	0	0
All ages	0	0	0	0	-	-	0	0	0	0
Females										
0-4	0	0.0	0	0.0	-	-	0	0.0	0	0.0
5-14	0	0.1	0	0.0	13.0	0.08	0	0.0	0	0.0
15-44	3	2.4	0	0.2	25.0	0.08	0	0.2	0	0.1
45-59	0	0.1	0	0.0	52.4	0.08	0	0.0	0	0.0
60+	0	0.1	0	0.0	71.1	0.08	0	0.0	0	0.0
All ages	3	1.2	0	0.1	25.3	0.08	0	0.1	0	0.1
Total	3	0.6	0	0.0	25.3	0.08	0	0.1	0	0.0

Table 39h — MEC - AOM - CMO — Gonorrhoea - Ectopic pregnancy

Age group (years)	Incidence 1990 Number ('000s)	Rate (per 100 000)	Prevalence 1990 Number ('000s)	Rate (per 100 000)	Avg. age at onset (years)	Average duration (years)	Deaths 1990 Number ('000s)	Rate (per 100 000)	Deaths 2000 (Projected) Number ('000s)	Rate (per 100 000)
Males										
0-4	0	0	0	0	-	-	0	0	0	0
5-14	0	0	0	0	-	-	0	0	0	0
15-44	0	0	0	0	-	-	0	0	0	0
45-59	0	0	0	0	-	-	0	0	0	0
60+	0	0	0	0	-	-	0	0	0	0
All ages	0	0	0	0	-	-	0	0	0	0
Females										
0-4	0	0.0	0	0.0	-	-	0	0.0	0	0.0
5-14	0	0.0	0	0.0	13.0	0.08	0	0.0	0	0.0
15-44	1	1.2	0	0.1	25.0	0.08	0	0.1	0	0.1
45-59	0	0.1	0	0.0	52.3	0.08	0	0.0	0	0.0
60+	0	0.0	0	0.0	70.4	0.08	0	0.0	0	0.0
All ages	1	0.5	0	0.0	25.2	0.08	0	0.1	0	0.0
Total	1	0.3	0	0.0	25.2	0.08	0	0.0	0	0.0

Table 39i — World - Mundo - Monde — Gonorrhoea - Ectopic pregnancy

Age group (years)	Incidence 1990 Number ('000s)	Rate (per 100 000)	Prevalence 1990 Number ('000s)	Rate (per 100 000)	Avg. age at onset (years)	Average duration (years)	Deaths 1990 Number ('000s)	Rate (per 100 000)	Deaths 2000 (Projected) Number ('000s)	Rate (per 100 000)
Males										
0-4	0	0	0	0	-	-	0	0	0	0
5-14	0	0	0	0	-	-	0	0	0	0
15-44	0	0	0	0	-	-	0	0	0	0
45-59	0	0	0	0	-	-	0	0	0	0
60+	0	0	0	0	-	-	0	0	0	0
All ages	0	0	0	0	-	-	0	0	0	0
Females										
0-4	0	0.0	0	0.0	-	-	0	0.0	0	0.0
5-14	1	0.1	0	0.0	13.0	0.08	0	0.0	0	0.0
15-44	41	3.5	3	0.3	25.0	0.08	8	0.6	4	0.3
45-59	0	0.1	0	0.0	52.3	0.08	0	0.0	0	0.0
60+	0	0.1	0	0.0	70.2	0.08	0	0.0	0	0.0
All ages	43	1.6	3	0.1	25.2	0.08	8	0.3	4	0.1
Total	43	0.8	3	0.1	25.2	0.08	8	0.1	4	0.1

For epidemiological sources see Berkley et al. 1996. For the methods used to estimate and project incidence, prevalence, and deaths see Murray and Lopez 1996a. See explanatory notes for definitions and caveats.

Table 40
Gonorrhoea

Cuadro 40
Gonorrea

Tableau 40
Gonorrhée

Tubo-ovarian abscess | Absceso tuboovárico | Abcès tubo-ovarien

---

Table 40a EME - PEMC - EMBE   Gonorrhoea - Tubo-ovarian abscess

Age group (years)	Incidence 1990 Number ('000s)	Rate (per 100 000)	Prevalence 1990 Number ('000s)	Rate (per 100 000)	Avg. age at onset (years)	Average duration (years)	Deaths 1990 Number ('000s)	Rate (per 100 000)	Deaths 2000 (Projected) Number ('000s)	Rate (per 100 000)
Males										
0-4	0	0	0	0	-	-	0	0	0	0
5-14	0	0	0	0	-	-	0	0	0	0
15-44	0	0	0	0	-	-	0	0	0	0
45-59	0	0	0	0	-	-	0	0	0	0
60+	0	0	0	0	-	-	0	0	0	0
All ages	0	0	0	0	-	-	0	0	0	0
Females										
0-4	0	0.0	0	0.0	-	-	0	0	0	0
5-14	0	0.1	0	0.0	13.0	0.08	0	0	0	0
15-44	4	2.0	0	0.2	25.0	0.08	0	0	0	0
45-59	0	0.1	0	0.0	52.4	0.08	0	0	0	0
60+	0	0.1	0	0.0	72.4	0.08	0	0	0	0
All ages	4	0.9	0	0.1	26.0	0.08	0	0	0	0
Total	4	0.5	0	0.0	26.0	0.08	0	0	0	0

Table 40b FSE - PEAS - AESE   Gonorrhoea - Tubo-ovarian abscess

Age group (years)	Incidence 1990 Number ('000s)	Rate (per 100 000)	Prevalence 1990 Number ('000s)	Rate (per 100 000)	Avg. age at onset (years)	Average duration (years)	Deaths 1990 Number ('000s)	Rate (per 100 000)	Deaths 2000 (Projected) Number ('000s)	Rate (per 100 000)
Males										
0-4	0	0	0	0	-	-	0	0	0	0
5-14	0	0	0	0	-	-	0	0	0	0
15-44	0	0	0	0	-	-	0	0	0	0
45-59	0	0	0	0	-	-	0	0	0	0
60+	0	0	0	0	-	-	0	0	0	0
All ages	0	0	0	0	-	-	0	0	0	0
Females										
0-4	0	0.0	0	0.0	-	-	0	0	0	0
5-14	0	0.2	0	0.0	13.0	0.08	0	0	0	0
15-44	5	6.3	0	0.5	25.0	0.08	0	0	0	0
45-59	0	0.3	0	0.0	52.4	0.08	0	0	0	0
60+	0	0.2	0	0.0	71.5	0.08	0	0	0	0
All ages	5	2.7	0	0.2	26.0	0.08	0	0	0	0
Total	5	1.4	0	0.1	26.0	0.08	0	0	0	0

Table 40c India - India - Inde   Gonorrhoea - Tubo-ovarian abscess

Age group (years)	Incidence 1990 Number ('000s)	Rate (per 100 000)	Prevalence 1990 Number ('000s)	Rate (per 100 000)	Avg. age at onset (years)	Average duration (years)	Deaths 1990 Number ('000s)	Rate (per 100 000)	Deaths 2000 (Projected) Number ('000s)	Rate (per 100 000)
Males										
0-4	0	0	0	0	-	-	0	0	0	0
5-14	0	0	0	0	-	-	0	0	0	0
15-44	0	0	0	0	-	-	0	0	0	0
45-59	0	0	0	0	-	-	0	0	0	0
60+	0	0	0	0	-	-	0	0	0	0
All ages	0	0	0	0	-	-	0	0	0	0
Females										
0-4	0	0.0	0	0.0	-	-	0	0.0	0	0.0
5-14	1	0.7	0	0.1	13.0	0.08	0	0.1	0	0.0
15-44	54	29.3	4	2.3	25.0	0.08	3	1.5	1	0.5
45-59	1	1.5	0	0.1	52.4	0.08	0	0.2	0	0.1
60+	0	0.7	0	0.1	70.1	0.08	0	0.0	0	0.0
All ages	55	13.5	4	1.0	25.4	0.08	3	0.7	1	0.3
Total	55	6.5	4	0.5	25.4	0.08	3	0.3	1	0.1

For epidemiological sources see Berkley et al. 1996. For the methods used to estimate and project incidence, prevalence, and deaths see Murray and Lopez 1996a. See explanatory notes for definitions and caveats.

Table 40
Gonorrhoea

Cuadro 40
Gonorrea

Tableau 40
Gonorrhée

Tubo-ovarian abscess

Absceso tuboovárico

Abcès tubo-ovarien

Table 40d — China - China - Chine — Gonorrhoea - Tubo-ovarian abscess

Age group (years)	Incidence 1990 Number ('000s)	Rate (per 100 000)	Prevalence 1990 Number ('000s)	Rate (per 100 000)	Avg. age at onset (years)	Average duration (years)	Deaths 1990 Number ('000s)	Rate (per 100 000)	Deaths 2000 (Projected) Number ('000s)	Rate (per 100 000)
Males										
0-4	0	0	0	0	-	-	0	0	0	0
5-14	0	0	0	0	-	-	0	0	0	0
15-44	0	0	0	0	-	-	0	0	0	0
45-59	0	0	0	0	-	-	0	0	0	0
60+	0	0	0	0	-	-	0	0	0	0
All ages	0	0	0	0	-	-	0	0	0	0
Females										
0-4	0	0.0	0	0.0	-	-	0	0	0	0
5-14	0	0.0	0	0.0	13.0	0.08	0	0	0	0
15-44	2	0.6	0	0.0	25.0	0.08	0	0	0	0
45-59	0	0.0	0	0.0	52.4	0.08	0	0	0	0
60+	0	0.0	0	0.0	70.6	0.08	0	0	0	0
All ages	2	0.3	0	0.0	25.4	0.08	0	0	0	0
Total	2	0.2	0	0.0	25.4	0.08	0	0	0	0

Table 40e — OAI - OPAI - APAI — Gonorrhoea - Tubo-ovarian abscess

Age group (years)	Incidence 1990 Number ('000s)	Rate (per 100 000)	Prevalence 1990 Number ('000s)	Rate (per 100 000)	Avg. age at onset (years)	Average duration (years)	Deaths 1990 Number ('000s)	Rate (per 100 000)	Deaths 2000 (Projected) Number ('000s)	Rate (per 100 000)
Males										
0-4	0	0	0	0	-	-	0	0	0	0
5-14	0	0	0	0	-	-	0	0	0	0
15-44	0	0	0	0	-	-	0	0	0	0
45-59	0	0	0	0	-	-	0	0	0	0
60+	0	0	0	0	-	-	0	0	0	0
All ages	0	0	0	0	-	-	0	0	0	0
Females										
0-4	0	0.0	0	0.0	-	-	0	0.0	0	0.0
5-14	1	0.7	0	0.1	13.0	0.08	0	0.1	0	0.0
15-44	44	27.5	3	2.1	25.0	0.08	2	1.2	1	0.5
45-59	0	1.4	0	0.1	52.3	0.08	0	0.2	0	0.1
60+	0	0.7	0	0.1	70.3	0.08	0	0.0	0	0.0
All ages	45	13.3	3	1.0	25.3	0.08	2	0.6	1	0.3
Total	45	6.6	3	0.5	25.3	0.08	2	0.3	1	0.1

Table 40f — SSA - ASS - ASS — Gonorrhoea - Tubo-ovarian abscess

Age group (years)	Incidence 1990 Number ('000s)	Rate (per 100 000)	Prevalence 1990 Number ('000s)	Rate (per 100 000)	Avg. age at onset (years)	Average duration (years)	Deaths 1990 Number ('000s)	Rate (per 100 000)	Deaths 2000 (Projected) Number ('000s)	Rate (per 100 000)
Males										
0-4	0	0	0	0	-	-	0	0	0	0
5-14	0	0	0	0	-	-	0	0	0	0
15-44	0	0	0	0	-	-	0	0	0	0
45-59	0	0	0	0	-	-	0	0	0	0
60+	0	0	0	0	-	-	0	0	0	0
All ages	0	0	0	0	-	-	0	0	0	0
Females										
0-4	0	0.0	0	0.0	-	-	0	0.0	0	0.0
5-14	1	1.5	0	0.1	13.0	0.08	0	0.1	0	0.1
15-44	62	58.6	5	4.5	25.0	0.08	3	3.1	2	1.3
45-59	1	2.9	0	0.2	52.2	0.08	0	0.5	0	0.3
60+	0	1.5	0	0.1	69.7	0.08	0	0.0	0	0.0
All ages	64	24.9	5	1.9	25.2	0.08	4	1.4	2	0.6
Total	64	12.6	5	1.0	25.2	0.08	4	0.7	2	0.3

For epidemiological sources see Berkley et al. 1996. For the methods used to estimate and project incidence, prevalence, and deaths see Murray and Lopez 1996a. See explanatory notes for definitions and caveats.

Table 40　　　　　　　　**Cuadro 40**　　　　　　　　**Tableau 40**
Gonorrhoea　　　　　　　**Gonorrea**　　　　　　　　**Gonorrhée**

Tubo-ovarian abscess　　　　　Absceso tuboovárico　　　　　Abcès tubo-ovarien

Table 40g　　LAC - ALC - ALC　　　　　　　Gonorrhoea - Tubo-ovarian abscess

Age group (years)	Incidence 1990 Number ('000s)	Rate (per 100 000)	Prevalence 1990 Number ('000s)	Rate (per 100 000)	Avg. age at onset (years)	Average duration (years)	Deaths 1990 Number ('000s)	Rate (per 100 000)	Deaths 2000 (Projected) Number ('000s)	Rate (per 100 000)
Males										
0-4	0	0	0	0	-	-	0	0	0	0
5-14	0	0	0	0	-	-	0	0	0	0
15-44	0	0	0	0	-	-	0	0	0	0
45-59	0	0	0	0	-	-	0	0	0	0
60+	0	0	0	0	-	-	0	0	0	0
All ages	0	0	0	0	-	-	0	0	0	0
Females										
0-4	0	0.0	0	0.0	-	-	0	0.0	0	0.0
5-14	0	0.4	0	0.0	13.0	0.08	0	0.0	0	0.0
15-44	16	15.1	1	1.2	25.0	0.08	0	0.3	0	0.1
45-59	0	0.8	0	0.1	52.4	0.08	0	0.0	0	0.0
60+	0	0.4	0	0.0	71.1	0.08	0	0.0	0	0.0
All ages	16	7.3	1	0.6	25.3	0.08	0	0.1	0	0.1
Total	16	3.6	1	0.3	25.3	0.08	0	0.1	0	0.0

Table 40h　　MEC - AOM - CMO　　　　　　　Gonorrhoea - Tubo-ovarian abscess

Age group (years)	Incidence 1990 Number ('000s)	Rate (per 100 000)	Prevalence 1990 Number ('000s)	Rate (per 100 000)	Avg. age at onset (years)	Average duration (years)	Deaths 1990 Number ('000s)	Rate (per 100 000)	Deaths 2000 (Projected) Number ('000s)	Rate (per 100 000)
Males										
0-4	0	0	0	0	-	-	0	0	0	0
5-14	0	0	0	0	-	-	0	0	0	0
15-44	0	0	0	0	-	-	0	0	0	0
45-59	0	0	0	0	-	-	0	0	0	0
60+	0	0	0	0	-	-	0	0	0	0
All ages	0	0	0	0	-	-	0	0	0	0
Females										
0-4	0	0.0	0	0.0	-	-	0	0.0	0	0
5-14	0	0.1	0	0.0	13.0	0.08	0	0.0	0	0
15-44	5	5.0	0	0.4	25.0	0.08	0	0.1	0	0
45-59	0	0.3	0	0.0	52.3	0.08	0	0.0	0	0
60+	0	0.1	0	0.0	70.4	0.08	0	0.0	0	0
All ages	6	2.2	0	0.2	25.3	0.08	0	0.0	0	0
Total	6	1.1	0	0.1	25.3	0.08	0	0.0	0	0

Table 40i　　World - Mundo - Monde　　　　　　　Gonorrhoea - Tubo-ovarian abscess

Age group (years)	Incidence 1990 Number ('000s)	Rate (per 100 000)	Prevalence 1990 Number ('000s)	Rate (per 100 000)	Avg. age at onset (years)	Average duration (years)	Deaths 1990 Number ('000s)	Rate (per 100 000)	Deaths 2000 (Projected) Number ('000s)	Rate (per 100 000)
Males										
0-4	0	0	0	0	-	-	0	0	0	0
5-14	0	0	0	0	-	-	0	0	0	0
15-44	0	0	0	0	-	-	0	0	0	0
45-59	0	0	0	0	-	-	0	0	0	0
60+	0	0	0	0	-	-	0	0	0	0
All ages	0	0	0	0	-	-	0	0	0	0
Females										
0-4	0	0.0	0	0.0	-	-	0	0.0	0	0.0
5-14	3	0.5	0	0.0	13.0	0.08	0	0.0	0	0.0
15-44	191	15.9	15	1.2	25.0	0.08	9	0.7	4	0.3
45-59	2	0.7	0	0.1	52.3	0.08	0	0.1	0	0.0
60+	1	0.3	0	0.0	70.4	0.08	0	0.0	0	0.0
All ages	197	7.5	15	0.6	25.3	0.08	9	0.3	4	0.1
Total	197	3.7	15	0.3	25.3	0.08	9	0.2	4	0.1

For epidemiological sources see Berkley et al. 1996. For the methods used to estimate and project incidence, prevalence, and deaths see Murray and Lopez 1996a. See explanatory notes for definitions and caveats.

Table 41
Gonorrhoea

Cuadro 41
Gonorrea

Tableau 41
Infections gonococciques

Chronic pelvic pain

Dolor pélvico crónico

Douleur pelvienne chronique

Table 41a EME - PEMC - EMBE Gonorrhoea - Chronic pelvic pain

Age group (years)	Incidence 1990 Number ('000s)	Rate (per 100 000)	Prevalence 1990 Number ('000s)	Rate (per 100 000)	Avg. age at onset (years)	Average duration (years)	Deaths 1990 Number ('000s)	Rate (per 100 000)	Deaths 2000 (Projected) Number ('000s)	Rate (per 100 000)
Males										
0-4	0	0	0	0	-	-	0	0	0	0
5-14	0	0	0	0	-	-	0	0	0	0
15-44	0	0	0	0	-	-	0	0	0	0
45-59	0	0	0	0	-	-	0	0	0	0
60+	0	0	0	0	-	-	0	0	0	0
All ages	0	0	0	0	-	-	0	0	0	0
Females										
0-4	0	0.0	0	0.0	-	-	0	0	0	0
5-14	0	0.2	0	0.5	13.0	3.0	0	0	0	0
15-44	12	6.6	32	17.9	23.0	3.0	0	0	0	0
45-59	0	0.3	1	1.0	52.4	3.0	0	0	0	0
60+	0	0.2	0	0.5	72.4	3.0	0	0	0	0
All ages	12	3.0	33	8.2	24.0	3.0	0	0	0	0
Total	12	1.5	33	4.2	24.0	3.0	0	0	0	0

Table 41b FSE - PEAS - AESE Gonorrhoea - Chronic pelvic pain

Age group (years)	Incidence 1990 Number ('000s)	Rate (per 100 000)	Prevalence 1990 Number ('000s)	Rate (per 100 000)	Avg. age at onset (years)	Average duration (years)	Deaths 1990 Number ('000s)	Rate (per 100 000)	Deaths 2000 (Projected) Number ('000s)	Rate (per 100 000)
Males										
0-4	0	0	0	0	-	-	0	0	0	0
5-14	0	0	0	0	-	-	0	0	0	0
15-44	0	0	0	0	-	-	0	0	0	0
45-59	0	0	0	0	-	-	0	0	0	0
60+	0	0	0	0	-	-	0	0	0	0
All ages	0	0	0	0	-	-	0	0	0	0
Females										
0-4	0	0.0	0	0.0	-	-	0	0	0	0
5-14	0	0.5	0	1.6	13.0	3.0	0	0	0	0
15-44	16	21.0	43	57.1	23.0	3.0	0	0	0	0
45-59	0	1.1	1	3.2	52.4	3.0	0	0	0	0
60+	0	0.5	1	1.6	71.5	3.0	0	0	0	0
All ages	16	9.1	45	24.7	24.0	3.0	0	0	0	0
Total	16	4.7	45	12.9	24.0	3.0	0	0	0	0

Table 41c India - India - Inde Gonorrhoea - Chronic pelvic pain

Age group (years)	Incidence 1990 Number ('000s)	Rate (per 100 000)	Prevalence 1990 Number ('000s)	Rate (per 100 000)	Avg. age at onset (years)	Average duration (years)	Deaths 1990 Number ('000s)	Rate (per 100 000)	Deaths 2000 (Projected) Number ('000s)	Rate (per 100 000)
Males										
0-4	0	0	0	0	-	-	0	0	0	0
5-14	0	0	0	0	-	-	0	0	0	0
15-44	0	0	0	0	-	-	0	0	0	0
45-59	0	0	0	0	-	-	0	0	0	0
60+	0	0	0	0	-	-	0	0	0	0
All ages	0	0	0	0	-	-	0	0	0	0
Females										
0-4	0	0.0	0	0.0	-	-	0	0	0	0
5-14	2	2.4	7	7.3	13.0	3.0	0	0	0	0
15-44	179	97.7	487	265.6	23.0	3.0	0	0	0	0
45-59	2	4.9	7	14.6	52.4	3.0	0	0	0	0
60+	1	2.4	2	7.3	70.1	3.0	0	0	0	0
All ages	184	44.9	503	122.5	23.4	3.0	0	0	0	0
Total	184	21.7	503	59.2	23.4	3.0	0	0	0	0

For epidemiological sources see Berkley et al. 1996. For the methods used to estimate and project incidence, prevalence, and deaths see Murray and Lopez 1996a. See explanatory notes for definitions and caveats.

Table 41   **Cuadro 41**   **Tableau 41**
Gonorrhoea   **Gonorrea**   **Infections gonococciques**

Chronic pelvic pain   Dolor pélvico crónico   Douleur pelvienne chronique

Table 41d   China - China - Chine   Gonorrhoea - Chronic pelvic pain

Age group (years)	Incidence 1990 Number ('000s)	Rate (per 100 000)	Prevalence 1990 Number ('000s)	Rate (per 100 000)	Avg. age at onset (years)	Average duration (years)	Deaths 1990 Number ('000s)	Rate (per 100 000)	Deaths 2000 (Projected) Number ('000s)	Rate (per 100 000)
Males										
0-4	0	0	0	0	-	-	0	0	0	0
5-14	0	0	0	0	-	-	0	0	0	0
15-44	0	0	0	0	-	-	0	0	0	0
45-59	0	0	0	0	-	-	0	0	0	0
60+	0	0	0	0	-	-	0	0	0	0
All ages	0	0	0	0	-	-	0	0	0	0
Females										
0-4	0	0.0	0	0.0	-	-	0	0	0	0
5-14	0	0.1	0	0.2	13.0	3.0	0	0	0	0
15-44	6	2.0	15	5.4	23.0	3.0	0	0	0	0
45-59	0	0.1	0	0.3	52.4	3.0	0	0	0	0
60+	0	0.1	0	0.2	70.6	3.0	0	0	0	0
All ages	6	1.1	16	2.9	23.5	3.0	0	0	0	0
Total	6	0.5	16	1.4	23.5	3.0	0	0	0	0

Table 41e   OAI - OPAI - APAI   Gonorrhoea - Chronic pelvic pain

Age group (years)	Incidence 1990 Number ('000s)	Rate (per 100 000)	Prevalence 1990 Number ('000s)	Rate (per 100 000)	Avg. age at onset (years)	Average duration (years)	Deaths 1990 Number ('000s)	Rate (per 100 000)	Deaths 2000 (Projected) Number ('000s)	Rate (per 100 000)
Males										
0-4	0	0	0	0	-	-	0	0	0	0
5-14	0	0	0	0	-	-	0	0	0	0
15-44	0	0	0	0	-	-	0	0	0	0
45-59	0	0	0	0	-	-	0	0	0	0
60+	0	0	0	0	-	-	0	0	0	0
All ages	0	0	0	0	-	-	0	0	0	0
Females										
0-4	0	0.0	0	0.0	-	-	0	0	0	0
5-14	2	2.3	6	6.9	13.0	3.0	0	0	0	0
15-44	146	91.6	398	249.2	23.0	3.0	0	0	0	0
45-59	2	4.6	5	13.7	52.3	3.0	0	0	0	0
60+	1	2.3	2	6.9	70.3	3.0	0	0	0	0
All ages	150	44.2	410	120.6	23.4	3.0	0	0	0	0
Total	150	22.0	410	60.0	23.4	3.0	0	0	0	0

Table 41f   SSA - ASS - ASS   Gonorrhoea - Chronic pelvic pain

Age group (years)	Incidence 1990 Number ('000s)	Rate (per 100 000)	Prevalence 1990 Number ('000s)	Rate (per 100 000)	Avg. age at onset (years)	Average duration (years)	Deaths 1990 Number ('000s)	Rate (per 100 000)	Deaths 2000 (Projected) Number ('000s)	Rate (per 100 000)
Males										
0-4	0	0	0	0	-	-	0	0	0	0
5-14	0	0	0	0	-	-	0	0	0	0
15-44	0	0	0	0	-	-	0	0	0	0
45-59	0	0	0	0	-	-	0	0	0	0
60+	0	0	0	0	-	-	0	0	0	0
All ages	0	0	0	0	-	-	0	0	0	0
Females										
0-4	0	0.0	0	0	-	-	0	0	0	0
5-14	3	4.9	10	15	13.0	3.0	0	0	0	0
15-44	208	195.4	568	534	23.0	3.0	0	0	0	0
45-59	2	9.8	6	29	52.2	3.0	0	0	0	0
60+	1	4.9	2	15	69.7	3.0	0	0	0	0
All ages	214	82.9	586	227	23.3	3.0	0	0	0	0
Total	214	41.9	586	115	23.3	3.0	0	0	0	0

For epidemiological sources see Berkley et al. 1996. For the methods used to estimate and project incidence, prevalence, and deaths see Murray and Lopez 1996a. See explanatory notes for definitions and caveats.

Table 41	Cuadro 41	Tableau 41
Gonorrhoea	Gonorrea	Infections gonococciques
Chronic pelvic pain	Dolor pélvico crónico	Douleur pelvienne chronique

Table 41g LAC - ALC - ALC Gonorrhoea - Chronic pelvic pain

Age group (years)	Incidence 1990 Number ('000s)	Rate (per 100 000)	Prevalence 1990 Number ('000s)	Rate (per 100 000)	Avg. age at onset (years)	Average duration (years)	Deaths 1990 Number ('000s)	Rate (per 100 000)	Deaths 2000 (Projected) Number ('000s)	Rate (per 100 000)
Males										
0-4	0	0	0	0	-	-	0	0	0	0
5-14	0	0	0	0	-	-	0	0	0	0
15-44	0	0	0	0	-	-	0	0	0	0
45-59	0	0	0	0	-	-	0	0	0	0
60+	0	0	0	0	-	-	0	0	0	0
All ages	0	0	0	0	-	-	0	0	0	0
Females										
0-4	0	0.0	0	0.0	-	-	0	0	0	0
5-14	1	1.3	2	3.8	13.0	3.0	0	0	0	0
15-44	52	50.4	143	137.2	23.0	3.0	0	0	0	0
45-59	1	2.5	2	7.6	52.4	3.0	0	0	0	0
60+	0	1.3	1	3.8	71.1	3.0	0	0	0	0
All ages	54	24.2	147	66.1	23.4	3.0	0	0	0	0
Total	54	12.1	147	33.1	23.4	3.0	0	0	0	0

Table 41h MEC - AOM - CMO Gonorrhoea - Chronic pelvic pain

Age group (years)	Incidence 1990 Number ('000s)	Rate (per 100 000)	Prevalence 1990 Number ('000s)	Rate (per 100 000)	Avg. age at onset (years)	Average duration (years)	Deaths 1990 Number ('000s)	Rate (per 100 000)	Deaths 2000 (Projected) Number ('000s)	Rate (per 100 000)
Males										
0-4	0	0	0	0	-	-	0	0	0	0
5-14	0	0	0	0	-	-	0	0	0	0
15-44	0	0	0	0	-	-	0	0	0	0
45-59	0	0	0	0	-	-	0	0	0	0
60+	0	0	0	0	-	-	0	0	0	0
All ages	0	0	0	0	-	-	0	0	0	0
Females										
0-4	0	0.0	0	0.0	-	-	0	0	0	0
5-14	0	0.4	1	1.3	13.0	3.0	0	0	0	0
15-44	18	16.8	49	45.7	23.0	3.0	0	0	0	0
45-59	0	0.8	1	2.5	52.3	3.0	0	0	0	0
60+	0	0.4	0	1.3	70.4	3.0	0	0	0	0
All ages	19	7.5	51	20.5	23.3	3.0	0	0	0	0
Total	19	3.7	51	10.1	23.3	3.0	0	0	0	0

Table 41i World - Mundo - Monde Gonorrhoea - Chronic pelvic pain

Age group (years)	Incidence 1990 Number ('000s)	Rate (per 100 000)	Prevalence 1990 Number ('000s)	Rate (per 100 000)	Avg. age at onset (years)	Average duration (years)	Deaths 1990 Number ('000s)	Rate (per 100 000)	Deaths 2000 (Projected) Number ('000s)	Rate (per 100 000)
Males										
0-4	0	0	0	0	-	-	0	0	0	0
5-14	0	0	0	0	-	-	0	0	0	0
15-44	0	0	0	0	-	-	0	0	0	0
45-59	0	0	0	0	-	-	0	0	0	0
60+	0	0	0	0	-	-	0	0	0	0
All ages	0	0	0	0	-	-	0	0	0	0
Females										
0-4	0	0.0	0	0.0	-	-	0	0	0	0
5-14	9	1.7	26	5.0	13.0	3.0	0	0	0	0
15-44	637	53.1	1 734	144.7	23.0	3.0	0	0	0	0
45-59	7	2.4	22	7.1	52.3	3.0	0	0	0	0
60+	2	0.9	7	2.8	70.4	3.0	0	0	0	0
All ages	655	25.1	1 790	68.5	23.4	3.0	0	0	0	0
Total	655	12.4	1 790	34.0	23.4	3.0	0	0	0	0

For epidemiological sources see Berkley et al. 1996. For the methods used to estimate and project incidence, prevalence, and deaths see Murray and Lopez 1996a. See explanatory notes for definitions and caveats.

Table 42	Cuadro 42	Tableau 42
Gonorrhoea	Gonorrea	Gonorrhée
Infertility	Infertilidad	Stérilité

Table 42a   EME - PEMC - EMBE   Gonorrhoea - Infertility

Age group (years)	Incidence 1990 Number ('000s)	Rate (per 100 000)	Prevalence 1990 Number ('000s)	Rate (per 100 000)	Avg. age at onset (years)	Average duration (years)	Deaths 1990 Number ('000s)	Rate (per 100 000)	Deaths 2000 (Projected) Number ('000s)	Rate (per 100 000)
Males										
0-4	0	0.0	0	0.0	-	-	0	0	0	0
5-14	0	0.0	0	0.0	13.0	27.0	0	0	0	0
15-44	0	0.0	0	0.2	27.0	13.0	0	0	0	0
45-59	0	0.0	0	0.0	-	-	0	0	0	0
60+	0	0.0	0	0.0	-	-	0	0	0	0
All ages	0	0.0	0	0.1	26.9	13.1	0	0	0	0
Females										
0-4	0	0.0	0	0.0	-	-	0	0	0	0
5-14	0	0.1	1	2.5	13.0	27.0	0	0	0	0
15-44	6	3.3	86	47.8	23.0	17.0	0	0	0	0
45-59	0	0.0	0	0.0	-	-	0	0	0	0
60+	0	0.0	0	0.0	-	-	0	0	0	0
All ages	6	1.5	87	21.4	22.9	17.1	0	0	0	0
Total	6	0.8	87	11.0	22.9	17.1	0	0	0	0

Table 42b   FSE - PEAS - AESE   Gonorrhoea - Infertility

Age group (years)	Incidence 1990 Number ('000s)	Rate (per 100 000)	Prevalence 1990 Number ('000s)	Rate (per 100 000)	Avg. age at onset (years)	Average duration (years)	Deaths 1990 Number ('000s)	Rate (per 100 000)	Deaths 2000 (Projected) Number ('000s)	Rate (per 100 000)
Males										
0-4	0	0.0	0	0.0	-	-	0	0	0	0
5-14	0	0.1	0	1.5	13.0	27.0	0	0	0	0
15-44	2	2.1	18	23.5	27.0	13.0	0	0	0	0
45-59	0	0.0	0	0.0	-	-	0	0	0	0
60+	0	0.0	0	0.0	-	-	0	0	0	0
All ages	2	1.0	18	11.1	26.8	13.2	0	0	0	0
Females										
0-4	0	0.0	0	0.0	-	-	0	0	0	0
5-14	0	0.3	2	8.0	13.0	27.0	0	0	0	0
15-44	8	10.6	115	154.0	23.0	17.0	0	0	0	0
45-59	0	0.0	0	0.0	-	-	0	0	0	0
60+	0	0.0	0	0.0	-	-	0	0	0	0
All ages	8	4.4	118	65.0	22.9	17.1	0	0	0	0
Total	10	2.8	136	39.2	23.5	16.5	0	0	0	0

Table 42c   India - India - Inde   Gonorrhoea - Infertility

Age group (years)	Incidence 1990 Number ('000s)	Rate (per 100 000)	Prevalence 1990 Number ('000s)	Rate (per 100 000)	Avg. age at onset (years)	Average duration (years)	Deaths 1990 Number ('000s)	Rate (per 100 000)	Deaths 2000 (Projected) Number ('000s)	Rate (per 100 000)
Males										
0-4	0	0.0	0	0	-	-	0	0	0	0
5-14	1	0.6	17	17	13.0	27.0	0	0	0	0
15-44	44	22.0	502	250	27.0	13.0	0	0	0	0
45-59	0	0.0	0	0	-	-	0	0	0	0
60+	0	0.0	0	0	-	-	0	0	0	0
All ages	45	10.2	518	118	26.8	13.2	0	0	0	0
Females										
0-4	0	0.0	0	0	-	-	0	0	0	0
5-14	1	1.2	36	37	13.0	27.0	0	0	0	0
15-44	91	49.9	1 335	729	23.0	17.0	0	0	0	0
45-59	0	0.0	0	0	-	-	0	0	0	0
60+	0	0.0	0	0	-	-	0	0	0	0
All ages	93	22.6	1 371	334	22.8	17.2	0	0	0	0
Total	137	16.2	1 889	222	24.1	15.9	0	0	0	0

For epidemiological sources see Berkley et al. 1996. For the methods used to estimate and project incidence, prevalence, and deaths see Murray and Lopez 1996a. See explanatory notes for definitions and caveats.

Table 42   **Cuadro 42**   **Tableau 42**
Gonorrhoea   **Gonorrea**   **Gonorrhée**

Infertility   Infertilidad   Stérilité

Table 42d   China - China - Chine   Gonorrhoea - Infertility

Age group (years)	Incidence 1990 Number ('000s)	Rate (per 100 000)	Prevalence 1990 Number ('000s)	Rate (per 100 000)	Avg. age at onset (years)	Average duration (years)	Deaths 1990 Number ('000s)	Rate (per 100 000)	Deaths 2000 (Projected) Number ('000s)	Rate (per 100 000)
Males										
0-4	0	0.0	0	0.0	-	-	0	0	0	0
5-14	0	0.0	0	0.2	13.0	27.0	0	0	0	0
15-44	1	0.2	8	2.6	27.0	13.0	0	0	0	0
45-59	0	0.0	0	0.0	-	-	0	0	0	0
60+	0	0.0	0	0.0	-	-	0	0	0	0
All ages	1	0.1	8	1.4	26.9	13.1	0	0	0	0
Females										
0-4	0	0.0	0	0.0	-	-	0	0	0	0
5-14	0	0.0	1	0.8	13.0	27.0	0	0	0	0
15-44	3	1.0	42	14.9	23.0	17.0	0	0	0	0
45-59	0	0.0	0	0.0	-	-	0	0	0	0
60+	0	0.0	0	0.0	-	-	0	0	0	0
All ages	3	0.5	43	7.8	22.9	17.1	0	0	0	0
Total	4	0.3	51	4.5	23.7	16.3	0	0	0	0

Table 42e   OAI - OPAI - APAI   Gonorrhoea - Infertility

Age group (years)	Incidence 1990 Number ('000s)	Rate (per 100 000)	Prevalence 1990 Number ('000s)	Rate (per 100 000)	Avg. age at onset (years)	Average duration (years)	Deaths 1990 Number ('000s)	Rate (per 100 000)	Deaths 2000 (Projected) Number ('000s)	Rate (per 100 000)
Males										
0-4	0	0.0	0	0	-	-	0	0	0	0
5-14	0	0.5	13	16	13.0	27.0	0	0	0	0
15-44	33	20.7	380	237	27.0	13.0	0	0	0	0
45-59	0	0.0	0	0	-	-	0	0	0	0
60+	0	0.0	0	0	-	-	0	0	0	0
All ages	34	9.8	393	115	26.8	13.2	0	0	0	0
Females										
0-4	0	0.0	0	0	-	-	0	0	0	0
5-14	1	1.2	28	35	13.0	27.0	0	0	0	0
15-44	74	46.7	1 093	685	23.0	17.0	0	0	0	0
45-59	0	0.0	0	0	-	-	0	0	0	0
60+	0	0.0	0	0	-	-	0	0	0	0
All ages	75	22.2	1 121	330	22.8	17.2	0	0	0	0
Total	109	16.0	1 514	222	24.1	15.9	0	0	0	0

Table 42f   SSA - ASS - ASS   Gonorrhoea - Infertility

Age group (years)	Incidence 1990 Number ('000s)	Rate (per 100 000)	Prevalence 1990 Number ('000s)	Rate (per 100 000)	Avg. age at onset (years)	Average duration (years)	Deaths 1990 Number ('000s)	Rate (per 100 000)	Deaths 2000 (Projected) Number ('000s)	Rate (per 100 000)
Males										
0-4	0	0.0	0	0	-	-	0	0	0	0
5-14	1	1.0	22	31	13.0	27.0	0	0	0	0
15-44	43	41.1	488	470	27.0	13.0	0	0	0	0
45-59	0	0.0	0	0	-	-	0	0	0	0
60+	0	0.0	0	0	-	-	0	0	0	0
All ages	43	17.2	510	202	26.7	13.3	0	0	0	0
Females										
0-4	0	0.0	0	0	-	-	0	0	0	0
5-14	2	2.5	53	76	13.0	27.0	0	0	0	0
15-44	108	101.4	1 587	1 494	23.0	17.0	0	0	0	0
45-59	0	0.0	0	0	-	-	0	0	0	0
60+	0	0.0	0	0	-	-	0	0	0	0
All ages	110	42.5	1 640	636	22.8	17.2	0	0	0	0
Total	153	30.0	2 150	421	23.9	16.1	0	0	0	0

For epidemiological sources see Berkley et al. 1996. For the methods used to estimate and project incidence, prevalence, and deaths see Murray and Lopez 1996a. See explanatory notes for definitions and caveats.

Table 42
Gonorrhoea

Cuadro 42
Gonorrea

Tableau 42
Gonorrhée

Infertility | Infertilidad | Stérilité

Table 42g — LAC - ALC - ALC — Gonorrhoea - Infertility

Age group (years)	Incidence 1990 Number ('000s)	Rate (per 100 000)	Prevalence 1990 Number ('000s)	Rate (per 100 000)	Avg. age at onset (years)	Average duration (years)	Deaths 1990 Number ('000s)	Rate (per 100 000)	Deaths 2000 (Projected) Number ('000s)	Rate (per 100 000)
Males										
0-4	0	0.0	0	0.0	-	-	0	0	0	0
5-14	0	0.1	2	3.4	13.0	27.0	0	0	0	0
15-44	5	4.6	54	51.5	27.0	13.0	0	0	0	0
45-59	0	0.0	0	0.0	-	-	0	0	0	0
60+	0	0.0	0	0.0	-	-	0	0	0	0
All ages	5	2.2	56	25.0	26.8	13.2	0	0	0	0
Females										
0-4	0	0.0	0	0.0	-	-	0	0	0	0
5-14	0	0.6	10	19.3	13.0	27.0	0	0	0	0
15-44	27	25.7	388	373.0	23.0	17.0	0	0	0	0
45-59	0	0.0	0	0.0	-	-	0	0	0	0
60+	0	0.0	0	0.0	-	-	0	0	0	0
All ages	27	12.1	398	178.7	22.8	17.2	0	0	0	0
Total	32	7.2	454	102.1	23.4	16.6	0	0	0	0

Table 42h — MEC - AOM - CMO — Gonorrhoea - Infertility

Age group (years)	Incidence 1990 Number ('000s)	Rate (per 100 000)	Prevalence 1990 Number ('000s)	Rate (per 100 000)	Avg. age at onset (years)	Average duration (years)	Deaths 1990 Number ('000s)	Rate (per 100 000)	Deaths 2000 (Projected) Number ('000s)	Rate (per 100 000)
Males										
0-4	0	0.0	0	0.0	-	-	0	0	0	0
5-14	0	0.0	1	1.1	13.0	27.0	0	0	0	0
15-44	2	1.5	19	17.1	27.0	13.0	0	0	0	0
45-59	0	0.0	0	0.0	-	-	0	0	0	0
60+	0	0.0	0	0.0	-	-	0	0	0	0
All ages	2	0.7	20	7.9	26.8	13.2	0	0	0	0
Females										
0-4	0	0.0	0	0.0	-	-	0	0	0	0
5-14	0	0.2	4	6.5	13.0	27.0	0	0	0	0
15-44	9	8.7	136	126.6	23.0	17.0	0	0	0	0
45-59	0	0.0	0	0.0	-	-	0	0	0	0
60+	0	0.0	0	0.0	-	-	0	0	0	0
All ages	9	3.8	140	56.7	22.8	17.2	0	0	0	0
Total	11	2.2	160	31.8	23.4	16.6	0	0	0	0

Table 42i — World - Mundo - Monde — Gonorrhoea - Infertility

Age group (years)	Incidence 1990 Number ('000s)	Rate (per 100 000)	Prevalence 1990 Number ('000s)	Rate (per 100 000)	Avg. age at onset (years)	Average duration (years)	Deaths 1990 Number ('000s)	Rate (per 100 000)	Deaths 2000 (Projected) Number ('000s)	Rate (per 100 000)
Males										
0-4	0	0.0	0	0	-	-	0	0	0	0
5-14	2	0.3	55	10	13.0	27.0	0	0	0	0
15-44	129	10.3	1 469	118	27.0	13.0	0	0	0	0
45-59	0	0.0	0	0	-	-	0	0	0	0
60+	0	0.0	0	0	-	-	0	0	0	0
All ages	131	4.9	1 524	57	26.8	13.2	0	0	0	0
Females										
0-4	0	0.0	0	0	-	-	0	0	0	0
5-14	4	0.9	135	26	13.0	27.0	0	0	0	0
15-44	327	27.2	4 783	399	23.0	17.0	0	0	0	0
45-59	0	0.0	0	0	-	-	0	0	0	0
60+	0	0.0	0	0	-	-	0	0	0	0
All ages	331	12.7	4 917	188	22.8	17.2	0	0	0	0
Total	462	8.8	6 441	122	23.9	16.1	0	0	0	0

For epidemiological sources see Berkley et al. 1996. For the methods used to estimate and project incidence, prevalence, and deaths see Murray and Lopez 1996a. See explanatory notes for definitions and caveats.

Table 43 / **Cuadro 43** / **Tableau 43**
Gonorrhoea / Gonorrea / Gonorrhée

Symptomatic urethritis / Uretritis sintomática / Urétrite symptomatique

Table 43a — EME - PEMC - EMBE — Gonorrhoea - Symptomatic urethritis

Age group (years)	Incidence 1990 Number ('000s)	Rate (per 100 000)	Prevalence 1990 Number ('000s)	Rate (per 100 000)	Avg. age at onset (years)	Average duration (years)	Deaths 1990 Number ('000s)	Rate (per 100 000)	Deaths 2000 (Projected) Number ('000s)	Rate (per 100 000)
Males										
0-4	0	0	0	0.0	-	-	0	0	0	0
5-14	11	22	0	0.7	13.0	0.03	0	0	0	0
15-44	1 587	862	50	27.2	25.0	0.03	0	0	0	0
45-59	29	43	1	1.4	52.4	0.03	0	0	0	0
60+	13	22	0	0.7	71.1	0.03	0	0	0	0
All ages	1 640	420	52	13.2	25.7	0.03	0	0	0	0
Females										
0-4	0	0	0	0	-	-	0	0	0	0
5-14	0	0	0	0	-	-	0	0	0	0
15-44	0	0	0	0	-	-	0	0	0	0
45-59	0	0	0	0	-	-	0	0	0	0
60+	0	0	0	0	-	-	0	0	0	0
All ages	0	0	0	0	-	-	0	0	0	0
Total	1 640	206	52	6.5	25.7	0.03	0	0	0	0

Table 43b — FSE - PEAS - AESE — Gonorrhoea - Symptomatic urethritis

Age group (years)	Incidence 1990 Number ('000s)	Rate (per 100 000)	Prevalence 1990 Number ('000s)	Rate (per 100 000)	Avg. age at onset (years)	Average duration (years)	Deaths 1990 Number ('000s)	Rate (per 100 000)	Deaths 2000 (Projected) Number ('000s)	Rate (per 100 000)
Males										
0-4	0	0	0	0.0	-	-	0	0	0	0
5-14	9	32	0	1.3	13.0	0.04	0	0	0	0
15-44	991	1 299	39	50.5	25.0	0.04	0	0	0	0
45-59	18	65	1	2.5	52.2	0.04	0	0	0	0
60+	7	32	0	1.3	70.0	0.04	0	0	0	0
All ages	1 024	619	40	24.1	25.6	0.04	0	0	0	0
Females										
0-4	0	0	0	0	-	-	0	0	0	0
5-14	0	0	0	0	-	-	0	0	0	0
15-44	0	0	0	0	-	-	0	0	0	0
45-59	0	0	0	0	-	-	0	0	0	0
60+	0	0	0	0	-	-	0	0	0	0
All ages	0	0	0	0	-	-	0	0	0	0
Total	1 024	296	40	11.5	25.6	0.04	0	0	0	0

Table 43c — India - India - Inde — Gonorrhoea - Symptomatic urethritis

Age group (years)	Incidence 1990 Number ('000s)	Rate (per 100 000)	Prevalence 1990 Number ('000s)	Rate (per 100 000)	Avg. age at onset (years)	Average duration (years)	Deaths 1990 Number ('000s)	Rate (per 100 000)	Deaths 2000 (Projected) Number ('000s)	Rate (per 100 000)
Males										
0-4	0	0	0	0.0	-	-	0	0	0	0
5-14	83	81	4	3.8	13.0	0.05	0	0	0	0
15-44	6 531	3 257	302	150.5	25.0	0.05	0	0	0	0
45-59	77	163	4	7.6	52.3	0.05	0	0	0	0
60+	24	81	1	3.8	69.7	0.05	0	0	0	0
All ages	6 716	1 528	310	70.6	25.3	0.05	0	0	0	0
Females										
0-4	0	0	0	0	-	-	0	0	0	0
5-14	0	0	0	0	-	-	0	0	0	0
15-44	0	0	0	0	-	-	0	0	0	0
45-59	0	0	0	0	-	-	0	0	0	0
60+	0	0	0	0	-	-	0	0	0	0
All ages	0	0	0	0	-	-	0	0	0	0
Total	6 716	791	310	36.5	25.3	0.05	0	0	0	0

For epidemiological sources see Berkley et al. 1996. For the methods used to estimate and project incidence, prevalence, and deaths see Murray and Lopez 1996a. See explanatory notes for definitions and caveats.

Table 43
Gonorrhoea

Cuadro 43
Gonorrea

Tableau 43
Gonorrhée

Symptomatic urethritis

Uretritis sintomática

Urétrite symptomatique

Table 43d — China - China - Chine — Gonorrhoea - Symptomatic urethritis

Age group (years)	Incidence 1990 Number ('000s)	Rate (per 100 000)	Prevalence 1990 Number ('000s)	Rate (per 100 000)	Avg. age at onset (years)	Average duration (years)	Deaths 1990 Number ('000s)	Rate (per 100 000)	Deaths 2000 (Projected) Number ('000s)	Rate (per 100 000)
Males										
0-4	0	0.0	0	0.0	-	-	0	0	0	0
5-14	4	3.8	0	0.1	13.0	0.04	0	0	0	0
15-44	463	151.0	18	5.9	25.0	0.04	0	0	0	0
45-59	5	7.6	0	0.3	52.3	0.04	0	0	0	0
60+	2	3.8	0	0.1	69.8	0.04	0	0	0	0
All ages	474	80.9	18	3.1	25.4	0.04	0	0	0	0
Females										
0-4	0	0	0	0	-	-	0	0	0	0
5-14	0	0	0	0	-	-	0	0	0	0
15-44	0	0	0	0	-	-	0	0	0	0
45-59	0	0	0	0	-	-	0	0	0	0
60+	0	0	0	0	-	-	0	0	0	0
All ages	0	0	0	0	-	-	0	0	0	0
Total	474	41.8	18	1.6	25.4	0.04	0	0	0	0

Table 43e — OAI - OPAI - APAI — Gonorrhoea - Symptomatic urethritis

Age group (years)	Incidence 1990 Number ('000s)	Rate (per 100 000)	Prevalence 1990 Number ('000s)	Rate (per 100 000)	Avg. age at onset (years)	Average duration (years)	Deaths 1990 Number ('000s)	Rate (per 100 000)	Deaths 2000 (Projected) Number ('000s)	Rate (per 100 000)
Males										
0-4	0	0	0	0.0	-	-	0	0	0	0
5-14	65	77	3	3.6	13.0	0.05	0	0	0	0
15-44	4 946	3 075	229	142.1	25.0	0.05	0	0	0	0
45-59	52	154	2	7.1	52.3	0.05	0	0	0	0
60+	16	77	1	3.6	69.6	0.05	0	0	0	0
All ages	5 078	1 481	235	68.4	25.2	0.05	0	0	0	0
Females										
0-4	0	0	0	0	-	-	0	0	0	0
5-14	0	0	0	0	-	-	0	0	0	0
15-44	0	0	0	0	-	-	0	0	0	0
45-59	0	0	0	0	-	-	0	0	0	0
60+	0	0	0	0	-	-	0	0	0	0
All ages	0	0	0	0	-	-	0	0	0	0
Total	5 078	744	235	34.4	25.2	0.05	0	0	0	0

Table 43f — SSA - ASS - ASS — Gonorrhoea - Symptomatic urethritis

Age group (years)	Incidence 1990 Number ('000s)	Rate (per 100 000)	Prevalence 1990 Number ('000s)	Rate (per 100 000)	Avg. age at onset (years)	Average duration (years)	Deaths 1990 Number ('000s)	Rate (per 100 000)	Deaths 2000 (Projected) Number ('000s)	Rate (per 100 000)
Males										
0-4	0	0	0	0.0	-	-	0	0	0	0
5-14	107	152	5	7.1	13.0	0.05	0	0	0	0
15-44	6 324	6 095	292	281.6	25.0	0.05	0	0	0	0
45-59	62	305	3	14.1	52.2	0.05	0	0	0	0
60+	16	152	1	7.1	69.2	0.05	0	0	0	0
All ages	6 509	2 580	301	119.2	25.1	0.05	0	0	0	0
Females										
0-4	0	0	0	0	-	-	0	0	0	0
5-14	0	0	0	0	-	-	0	0	0	0
15-44	0	0	0	0	-	-	0	0	0	0
45-59	0	0	0	0	-	-	0	0	0	0
60+	0	0	0	0	-	-	0	0	0	0
All ages	0	0	0	0	-	-	0	0	0	0
Total	6 509	1 276	301	59.0	25.1	0.05	0	0	0	0

For epidemiological sources see Berkley et al. 1996. For the methods used to estimate and project incidence, prevalence, and deaths see Murray and Lopez 1996a. See explanatory notes for definitions and caveats.

Table 43 **Cuadro 43** **Tableau 43**
Gonorrhoea **Gonorrea** **Gonorrhée**

Symptomatic urethritis Uretritis sintomática Urétrite symptomatique

Table 43g LAC - ALC - ALC — Gonorrhoea - Symptomatic urethritis

Age group (years)	Incidence 1990 Number ('000s)	Rate (per 100 000)	Prevalence 1990 Number ('000s)	Rate (per 100 000)	Avg. age at onset (years)	Average duration (years)	Deaths 1990 Number ('000s)	Rate (per 100 000)	Deaths 2000 (Projected) Number ('000s)	Rate (per 100 000)
Males										
0-4	0	0	0	0.0	-	-	0	0	0	0
5-14	38	72	1	2.8	13.0	0.04	0	0	0	0
15-44	3 016	2 892	117	112.4	25.0	0.04	0	0	0	0
45-59	32	145	1	5.7	52.3	0.04	0	0	0	0
60+	10	72	0	2.8	70.3	0.04	0	0	0	0
All ages	3 096	1 397	120	54.3	25.3	0.04	0	0	0	0
Females										
0-4	0	0	0	0	-	-	0	0	0	0
5-14	0	0	0	0	-	-	0	0	0	0
15-44	0	0	0	0	-	-	0	0	0	0
45-59	0	0	0	0	-	-	0	0	0	0
60+	0	0	0	0	-	-	0	0	0	0
All ages	0	0	0	0	-	-	0	0	0	0
Total	3 096	697	120	27.1	25.3	0.04	0	0	0	0

Table 43h MEC - AOM - CMO — Gonorrhoea - Symptomatic urethritis

Age group (years)	Incidence 1990 Number ('000s)	Rate (per 100 000)	Prevalence 1990 Number ('000s)	Rate (per 100 000)	Avg. age at onset (years)	Average duration (years)	Deaths 1990 Number ('000s)	Rate (per 100 000)	Deaths 2000 (Projected) Number ('000s)	Rate (per 100 000)
Males										
0-4	0	0	0	0.0	-	-	0	0	0	0
5-14	16	24	1	0.9	13.0	0.04	0	0	0	0
15-44	1 097	963	43	37.4	25.0	0.04	0	0	0	0
45-59	11	48	0	1.9	52.3	0.04	0	0	0	0
60+	3	24	0	0.9	69.7	0.04	0	0	0	0
All ages	1 127	439	44	17.1	25.2	0.04	0	0	0	0
Females										
0-4	0	0	0	0	-	-	0	0	0	0
5-14	0	0	0	0	-	-	0	0	0	0
15-44	0	0	0	0	-	-	0	0	0	0
45-59	0	0	0	0	-	-	0	0	0	0
60+	0	0	0	0	-	-	0	0	0	0
All ages	0	0	0	0	-	-	0	0	0	0
Total	1 127	224	44	8.7	25.2	0.04	0	0	0	0

Table 43i World - Mundo - Monde — Gonorrhoea - Symptomatic urethritis

Age group (years)	Incidence 1990 Number ('000s)	Rate (per 100 000)	Prevalence 1990 Number ('000s)	Rate (per 100 000)	Avg. age at onset (years)	Average duration (years)	Deaths 1990 Number ('000s)	Rate (per 100 000)	Deaths 2000 (Projected) Number ('000s)	Rate (per 100 000)
Males										
0-4	0	0	0	0.0	-	-	0	0	0	0
5-14	332	60	15	2.7	13.0	0.04	0	0	0	0
15-44	24 954	1 996	1 089	87.1	25.0	0.04	0	0	0	0
45-59	286	92	12	4.0	52.3	0.04	0	0	0	0
60+	91	42	4	1.8	69.9	0.04	0	0	0	0
All ages	25 664	967	1 120	42.2	25.3	0.04	0	0	0	0
Females										
0-4	0	0	0	0	-	-	0	0	0	0
5-14	0	0	0	0	-	-	0	0	0	0
15-44	0	0	0	0	-	-	0	0	0	0
45-59	0	0	0	0	-	-	0	0	0	0
60+	0	0	0	0	-	-	0	0	0	0
All ages	0	0	0	0	-	-	0	0	0	0
Total	25 664	487	1 120	21.3	25.3	0.04	0	0	0	0

For epidemiological sources see Berkley et al. 1996. For the methods used to estimate and project incidence, prevalence, and deaths see Murray and Lopez 1996a. See explanatory notes for definitions and caveats.

Table 44   **Cuadro 44**   **Tableau 44**
Gonorrhoea   **Gonorrea**   **Gonorrhée**

Epididymitis   Epidedimitis   Epididymite

Table 44a   EME - PEMC - EMBE   Gonorrhoea - Epididymitis

Age group (years)	Incidence 1990 Number ('000s)	Rate (per 100 000)	Prevalence 1990 Number ('000s)	Rate (per 100 000)	Avg. age at onset (years)	Average duration (years)	Deaths 1990 Number ('000s)	Rate (per 100 000)	Deaths 2000 (Projected) Number ('000s)	Rate (per 100 000)
Males										
0-4	0	0.0	0	0.0	-	-	0	0	0	0
5-14	0	0.3	0	0.0	13.0	0.04	0	0	0	0
15-44	24	13.1	1	0.5	25.2	0.04	0	0	0	0
45-59	0	0.7	0	0.0	52.4	0.04	0	0	0	0
60+	0	0.3	0	0.0	71.1	0.04	0	0	0	0
All ages	25	6.4	1	0.2	25.9	0.04	0	0	0	0
Females										
0-4	0	0	0	0	-	-	0	0	0	0
5-14	0	0	0	0	-	-	0	0	0	0
15-44	0	0	0	0	-	-	0	0	0	0
45-59	0	0	0	0	-	-	0	0	0	0
60+	0	0	0	0	-	-	0	0	0	0
All ages	0	0	0	0	-	-	0	0	0	0
Total	25	3.1	1	0.1	25.9	0.04	0	0	0	0

Table 44b   FSE - PEAS - AESE   Gonorrhoea - Epididymitis

Age group (years)	Incidence 1990 Number ('000s)	Rate (per 100 000)	Prevalence 1990 Number ('000s)	Rate (per 100 000)	Avg. age at onset (years)	Average duration (years)	Deaths 1990 Number ('000s)	Rate (per 100 000)	Deaths 2000 (Projected) Number ('000s)	Rate (per 100 000)
Males										
0-4	0	0.0	0	0.0	-	-	0	0	0	0
5-14	0	1.7	0	0.1	13.0	0.05	0	0	0	0
15-44	52	68.7	3	3.4	25.2	0.05	0	0	0	0
45-59	1	3.4	0	0.2	52.2	0.05	0	0	0	0
60+	0	1.7	0	0.1	70.0	0.05	0	0	0	0
All ages	54	32.7	3	1.6	25.8	0.05	0	0	0	0
Females										
0-4	0	0	0	0	-	-	0	0	0	0
5-14	0	0	0	0	-	-	0	0	0	0
15-44	0	0	0	0	-	-	0	0	0	0
45-59	0	0	0	0	-	-	0	0	0	0
60+	0	0	0	0	-	-	0	0	0	0
All ages	0	0	0	0	-	-	0	0	0	0
Total	54	15.6	3	0.8	25.8	0.05	0	0	0	0

Table 44c   India - India - Inde   Gonorrhoea - Epididymitis

Age group (years)	Incidence 1990 Number ('000s)	Rate (per 100 000)	Prevalence 1990 Number ('000s)	Rate (per 100 000)	Avg. age at onset (years)	Average duration (years)	Deaths 1990 Number ('000s)	Rate (per 100 000)	Deaths 2000 (Projected) Number ('000s)	Rate (per 100 000)
Males										
0-4	0	0.0	0	0.0	-	-	0	0	0	0
5-14	7	7.4	1	0.5	13.0	0.07	0	0	0	0
15-44	590	294.1	40	19.7	25.2	0.07	0	0	0	0
45-59	7	14.7	0	1.0	52.3	0.07	0	0	0	0
60+	2	7.4	0	0.5	69.7	0.07	0	0	0	0
All ages	606	138.0	41	9.2	25.5	0.07	0	0	0	0
Females										
0-4	0	0	0	0	-	-	0	0	0	0
5-14	0	0	0	0	-	-	0	0	0	0
15-44	0	0	0	0	-	-	0	0	0	0
45-59	0	0	0	0	-	-	0	0	0	0
60+	0	0	0	0	-	-	0	0	0	0
All ages	0	0	0	0	-	-	0	0	0	0
Total	606	71.4	41	4.8	25.5	0.07	0	0	0	0

For epidemiological sources see Berkley et al. 1996. For the methods used to estimate and project incidence, prevalence, and deaths see Murray and Lopez 1996a. See explanatory notes for definitions and caveats.

Table 44	Cuadro 44	Tableau 44
Gonorrhoea	Gonorrea	Gonorrhée
Epididymitis	Epidedimitis	Epididymite

Table 44d   China - China - Chine   Gonorrhoea - Epididymitis

Age group (years)	Incidence 1990 Number ('000s)	Rate (per 100 000)	Prevalence 1990 Number ('000s)	Rate (per 100 000)	Avg. age at onset (years)	Average duration (years)	Deaths 1990 Number ('000s)	Rate (per 100 000)	Deaths 2000 (Projected) Number ('000s)	Rate (per 100 000)
Males										
0-4	0	0.0	0	0.0	-	-	0	0	0	0
5-14	0	0.2	0	0.0	13.0	0.05	0	0	0	0
15-44	24	8.0	1	0.4	25.2	0.05	0	0	0	0
45-59	0	0.4	0	0.0	52.3	0.05	0	0	0	0
60+	0	0.2	0	0.0	69.8	0.05	0	0	0	0
All ages	25	4.3	1	0.2	25.6	0.05	0	0	0	0
Females										
0-4	0	0	0	0	-	-	0	0	0	0
5-14	0	0	0	0	-	-	0	0	0	0
15-44	0	0	0	0	-	-	0	0	0	0
45-59	0	0	0	0	-	-	0	0	0	0
60+	0	0	0	0	-	-	0	0	0	0
All ages	0	0	0	0	-	-	0	0	0	0
Total	25	2.2	1	0.1	25.6	0.05	0	0	0	0

Table 44e   OAI - OPAI - APAI   Gonorrhoea - Epididymitis

Age group (years)	Incidence 1990 Number ('000s)	Rate (per 100 000)	Prevalence 1990 Number ('000s)	Rate (per 100 000)	Avg. age at onset (years)	Average duration (years)	Deaths 1990 Number ('000s)	Rate (per 100 000)	Deaths 2000 (Projected) Number ('000s)	Rate (per 100 000)
Males										
0-4	0	0.0	0	0.0	-	-	0	0	0	0
5-14	6	6.9	0	0.5	13.0	0.07	0	0	0	0
15-44	445	276.6	43	26.6	25.2	0.07	0	0	0	0
45-59	5	13.8	0	0.9	52.3	0.07	0	0	0	0
60+	1	6.9	0	0.5	69.6	0.07	0	0	0	0
All ages	457	133.2	44	12.7	25.4	0.07	0	0	0	0
Females										
0-4	0	0	0	0	-	-	0	0	0	0
5-14	0	0	0	0	-	-	0	0	0	0
15-44	0	0	0	0	-	-	0	0	0	0
45-59	0	0	0	0	-	-	0	0	0	0
60+	0	0	0	0	-	-	0	0	0	0
All ages	0	0	0	0	-	-	0	0	0	0
Total	457	66.9	44	6.4	25.4	0.07	0	0	0	0

Table 44f   SSA - ASS - ASS   Gonorrhoea - Epididymitis

Age group (years)	Incidence 1990 Number ('000s)	Rate (per 100 000)	Prevalence 1990 Number ('000s)	Rate (per 100 000)	Avg. age at onset (years)	Average duration (years)	Deaths 1990 Number ('000s)	Rate (per 100 000)	Deaths 2000 (Projected) Number ('000s)	Rate (per 100 000)
Males										
0-4	0	0	0	0.0	-	-	0	0	0	0
5-14	10	14	1	0.9	13.0	0.07	0	0	0	0
15-44	569	548	38	36.7	25.2	0.07	0	0	0	0
45-59	6	27	0	1.8	52.2	0.07	0	0	0	0
60+	1	14	0	0.9	69.2	0.07	0	0	0	0
All ages	586	232	39	15.5	25.3	0.07	0	0	0	0
Females										
0-4	0	0	0	0	-	-	0	0	0	0
5-14	0	0	0	0	-	-	0	0	0	0
15-44	0	0	0	0	-	-	0	0	0	0
45-59	0	0	0	0	-	-	0	0	0	0
60+	0	0	0	0	-	-	0	0	0	0
All ages	0	0	0	0	-	-	0	0	0	0
Total	586	115	39	7.7	25.3	0.07	0	0	0	0

For epidemiological sources see Berkley et al. 1996. For the methods used to estimate and project incidence, prevalence, and deaths see Murray and Lopez 1996a. See explanatory notes for definitions and caveats.

Table 44
Gonorrhoea

Cuadro 44
Gonorrea

Tableau 44
Gonorrhée

Epididymitis

Epidedimitis

Epididymite

Table 44g LAC - ALC - ALC   Gonorrhoea - Epididymitis

Age group (years)	Incidence 1990 Number ('000s)	Rate (per 100 000)	Prevalence 1990 Number ('000s)	Rate (per 100 000)	Avg. age at onset (years)	Average duration (years)	Deaths 1990 Number ('000s)	Rate (per 100 000)	Deaths 2000 (Projected) Number ('000s)	Rate (per 100 000)
Males										
0-4	0	0.0	0	0.0	-	-	0	0	0	0
5-14	2	3.8	0	0.2	13.0	0.05	0	0	0	0
15-44	158	151.4	8	7.5	25.2	0.05	0	0	0	0
45-59	2	7.6	0	0.4	52.3	0.05	0	0	0	0
60+	1	3.8	0	0.2	70.3	0.05	0	0	0	0
All ages	162	73.1	8	3.6	25.4	0.05	0	0	0	0
Females										
0-4	0	0	0	0	-	-	0	0	0	0
5-14	0	0	0	0	-	-	0	0	0	0
15-44	0	0	0	0	-	-	0	0	0	0
45-59	0	0	0	0	-	-	0	0	0	0
60+	0	0	0	0	-	-	0	0	0	0
All ages	0	0	0	0	-	-	0	0	0	0
Total	162	36.5	8	1.8	25.4	0.05	0	0	0	0

Table 44h MEC - AOM - CMO   Gonorrhoea - Epididymitis

Age group (years)	Incidence 1990 Number ('000s)	Rate (per 100 000)	Prevalence 1990 Number ('000s)	Rate (per 100 000)	Avg. age at onset (years)	Average duration (years)	Deaths 1990 Number ('000s)	Rate (per 100 000)	Deaths 2000 (Projected) Number ('000s)	Rate (per 100 000)
Males										
0-4	0	0.0	0	0.0	-	-	0	0	0	0
5-14	1	1.3	0	0.1	13.0	0.05	0	0	0	0
15-44	58	50.6	3	2.5	25.2	0.05	0	0	0	0
45-59	1	2.5	0	0.1	52.3	0.05	0	0	0	0
60+	0	1.3	0	0.1	69.7	0.05	0	0	0	0
All ages	59	23.1	3	1.1	25.4	0.05	0	0	0	0
Females										
0-4	0	0	0	0	-	-	0	0	0	0
5-14	0	0	0	0	-	-	0	0	0	0
15-44	0	0	0	0	-	-	0	0	0	0
45-59	0	0	0	0	-	-	0	0	0	0
60+	0	0	0	0	-	-	0	0	0	0
All ages	0	0	0	0	-	-	0	0	0	0
Total	59	11.8	3	0.6	25.4	0.05	0	0	0	0

Table 44i World - Mundo - Monde   Gonorrhoea - Epididymitis

Age group (years)	Incidence 1990 Number ('000s)	Rate (per 100 000)	Prevalence 1990 Number ('000s)	Rate (per 100 000)	Avg. age at onset (years)	Average duration (years)	Deaths 1990 Number ('000s)	Rate (per 100 000)	Deaths 2000 (Projected) Number ('000s)	Rate (per 100 000)
Males										
0-4	0	0.0	0	0.0	-	-	0	0	0	0
5-14	27	4.8	2	0.3	13.0	0.06	0	0	0	0
15-44	1 920	153.6	136	10.9	25.2	0.06	0	0	0	0
45-59	21	6.8	1	0.4	52.3	0.06	0	0	0	0
60+	6	2.9	0	0.2	69.7	0.06	0	0	0	0
All ages	1 974	74.4	139	5.2	25.4	0.06	0	0	0	0
Females										
0-4	0	0	0	0	-	-	0	0	0	0
5-14	0	0	0	0	-	-	0	0	0	0
15-44	0	0	0	0	-	-	0	0	0	0
45-59	0	0	0	0	-	-	0	0	0	0
60+	0	0	0	0	-	-	0	0	0	0
All ages	0	0	0	0	-	-	0	0	0	0
Total	1 974	37.5	139	2.6	25.4	0.06	0	0	0	0

For epidemiological sources see Berkley et al. 1996. For the methods used to estimate and project incidence, prevalence, and deaths see Murray and Lopez 1996a. See explanatory notes for definitions and caveats.

Table 45	Cuadro 45	Tableau 45
Gonorrhoea	Gonorrea	Gonorrhée
Stricture	Obstrucción ureteral	Rétrécissement urétral

Table 45a EME - PEMC - EMBE — Gonorrhoea - Stricture

Age group (years)	Incidence 1990 Number ('000s)	Rate (per 100 000)	Prevalence 1990 Number ('000s)	Rate (per 100 000)	Avg. age at onset (years)	Average duration (years)	Deaths 1990 Number ('000s)	Rate (per 100 000)	Deaths 2000 (Projected) Number ('000s)	Rate (per 100 000)
Males										
0-4	0	0.0	0	0.0	-	-	0	0	0	0
5-14	0	0.2	0	0.1	13.0	0.55	0	0	0	0
15-44	16	8.6	9	4.7	25.2	0.55	0	0	0	0
45-59	0	0.4	0	0.2	52.4	0.55	0	0	0	0
60+	0	0.2	0	0.1	71.1	0.55	0	0	0	0
All ages	16	4.2	9	2.3	25.9	0.55	0	0	0	0
Females										
0-4	0	0	0	0	-	-	0	0	0	0
5-14	0	0	0	0	-	-	0	0	0	0
15-44	0	0	0	0	-	-	0	0	0	0
45-59	0	0	0	0	-	-	0	0	0	0
60+	0	0	0	0	-	-	0	0	0	0
All ages	0	0	0	0	-	-	0	0	0	0
Total	16	2.1	9	1.1	25.9	0.55	0	0	0	0

Table 45b FSE - PEAS - AESE — Gonorrhoea - Stricture

Age group (years)	Incidence 1990 Number ('000s)	Rate (per 100 000)	Prevalence 1990 Number ('000s)	Rate (per 100 000)	Avg. age at onset (years)	Average duration (years)	Deaths 1990 Number ('000s)	Rate (per 100 000)	Deaths 2000 (Projected) Number ('000s)	Rate (per 100 000)
Males										
0-4	0	0.0	0	0.0	-	-	0	0	0	0
5-14	0	1.1	0	1.6	13.0	1.4	0	0	0	0
15-44	35	45.5	46	60.8	25.2	1.4	0	0	0	0
45-59	1	2.3	1	3.2	52.2	1.4	0	0	0	0
60+	0	1.1	0	1.6	70.0	1.4	0	0	0	0
All ages	36	21.7	48	29.1	25.8	1.4	0	0	0	0
Females										
0-4	0	0	0	0	-	-	0	0	0	0
5-14	0	0	0	0	-	-	0	0	0	0
15-44	0	0	0	0	-	-	0	0	0	0
45-59	0	0	0	0	-	-	0	0	0	0
60+	0	0	0	0	-	-	0	0	0	0
All ages	0	0	0	0	-	-	0	0	0	0
Total	36	10.4	48	13.9	25.8	1.4	0	0	0	0

Table 45c India - India - Inde — Gonorrhoea - Stricture

Age group (years)	Incidence 1990 Number ('000s)	Rate (per 100 000)	Prevalence 1990 Number ('000s)	Rate (per 100 000)	Avg. age at onset (years)	Average duration (years)	Deaths 1990 Number ('000s)	Rate (per 100 000)	Deaths 2000 (Projected) Number ('000s)	Rate (per 100 000)
Males										
0-4	0	0.0	0	0	-	-	0	0	0	0
5-14	5	4.9	11	11	13.0	2.3	0	0	0	0
15-44	392	195.3	852	425	25.2	2.3	0	0	0	0
45-59	5	9.8	11	23	52.3	2.3	0	0	0	0
60+	1	4.9	3	11	69.7	2.3	0	0	0	0
All ages	403	91.6	878	200	25.5	2.3	0	0	0	0
Females										
0-4	0	0	0	0	-	-	0	0	0	0
5-14	0	0	0	0	-	-	0	0	0	0
15-44	0	0	0	0	-	-	0	0	0	0
45-59	0	0	0	0	-	-	0	0	0	0
60+	0	0	0	0	-	-	0	0	0	0
All ages	0	0	0	0	-	-	0	0	0	0
Total	403	47.4	878	103	25.5	2.3	0	0	0	0

For epidemiological sources see Berkley et al. 1996. For the methods used to estimate and project incidence, prevalence, and deaths see Murray and Lopez 1996a. See explanatory notes for definitions and caveats.

Table 45   Cuadro 45   Tableau 45
Gonorrhoea   Gonorrea   Gonorrhée

Stricture   Obstrucción ureteral   Rétrécissement urétral

Table 45d   China - China - Chine   Gonorrhoea - Stricture

Age group (years)	Incidence 1990 Number ('000s)	Rate (per 100 000)	Prevalence 1990 Number ('000s)	Rate (per 100 000)	Avg. age at onset (years)	Average duration (years)	Deaths 1990 Number ('000s)	Rate (per 100 000)	Deaths 2000 (Projected) Number ('000s)	Rate (per 100 000)
Males										
0-4	0	0.0	0	0.0	-	-	0	0	0	0
5-14	0	0.1	0	0.2	13.0	1.4	0	0	0	0
15-44	16	5.3	22	7.2	25.2	1.4	0	0	0	0
45-59	0	0.3	0	0.4	52.3	1.4	0	0	0	0
60+	0	0.1	0	0.2	69.8	1.4	0	0	0	0
All ages	17	2.8	23	3.9	25.6	1.4	0	0	0	0
Females										
0-4	0	0	0	0	-	-	0	0	0	0
5-14	0	0	0	0	-	-	0	0	0	0
15-44	0	0	0	0	-	-	0	0	0	0
45-59	0	0	0	0	-	-	0	0	0	0
60+	0	0	0	0	-	-	0	0	0	0
All ages	0	0	0	0	-	-	0	0	0	0
Total	17	1.5	23	2.0	25.6	1.4	0	0	0	0

Table 45e   OAI - OPAI - APAI   Gonorrhoea - Stricture

Age group (years)	Incidence 1990 Number ('000s)	Rate (per 100 000)	Prevalence 1990 Number ('000s)	Rate (per 100 000)	Avg. age at onset (years)	Average duration (years)	Deaths 1990 Number ('000s)	Rate (per 100 000)	Deaths 2000 (Projected) Number ('000s)	Rate (per 100 000)
Males										
0-4	0	0.0	0	0	-	-	0	0	0	0
5-14	4	4.6	9	11	13.0	2.3	0	0	0	0
15-44	297	184.6	644	400	25.2	2.3	0	0	0	0
45-59	3	9.2	7	21	52.3	2.3	0	0	0	0
60+	1	4.6	2	11	69.6	2.3	0	0	0	0
All ages	305	88.9	662	193	25.4	2.3	0	0	0	0
Females										
0-4	0	0	0	0	-	-	0	0	0	0
5-14	0	0	0	0	-	-	0	0	0	0
15-44	0	0	0	0	-	-	0	0	0	0
45-59	0	0	0	0	-	-	0	0	0	0
60+	0	0	0	0	-	-	0	0	0	0
All ages	0	0	0	0	-	-	0	0	0	0
Total	305	44.7	662	97	25.4	2.3	0	0	0	0

Table 45f   SSA - ASS - ASS   Gonorrhoea - Stricture

Age group (years)	Incidence 1990 Number ('000s)	Rate (per 100 000)	Prevalence 1990 Number ('000s)	Rate (per 100 000)	Avg. age at onset (years)	Average duration (years)	Deaths 1990 Number ('000s)	Rate (per 100 000)	Deaths 2000 (Projected) Number ('000s)	Rate (per 100 000)
Males										
0-4	0	0.0	0	0	-	-	0	0	0	0
5-14	6	9.1	15	21	13.0	2.3	0	0	0	0
15-44	379	365.1	823	793	25.2	2.3	0	0	0	0
45-59	4	18.3	9	42	52.2	2.3	0	0	0	0
60+	1	9.1	2	21	69.2	2.3	0	0	0	0
All ages	390	154.5	848	336	25.3	2.3	0	0	0	0
Females										
0-4	0	0	0	0	-	-	0	0	0	0
5-14	0	0	0	0	-	-	0	0	0	0
15-44	0	0	0	0	-	-	0	0	0	0
45-59	0	0	0	0	-	-	0	0	0	0
60+	0	0	0	0	-	-	0	0	0	0
All ages	0	0	0	0	-	-	0	0	0	0
Total	390	76.4	848	166	25.3	2.3	0	0	0	0

For epidemiological sources see Berkley et al. 1996. For the methods used to estimate and project incidence, prevalence, and deaths see Murray and Lopez 1996a. See explanatory notes for definitions and caveats.

Table 45   **Cuadro 45**   **Tableau 45**
Gonorrhoea   **Gonorrea**   **Gonorrhée**

Stricture   Obstrucción ureteral   Rétrécissement urétral

Table 45g   LAC - ALC - ALC   Gonorrhoea - Stricture

Age group (years)	Incidence 1990 Number ('000s)	Rate (per 100 000)	Prevalence 1990 Number ('000s)	Rate (per 100 000)	Avg. age at onset (years)	Average duration (years)	Deaths 1990 Number ('000s)	Rate (per 100 000)	Deaths 2000 (Projected) Number ('000s)	Rate (per 100 000)
Males										
0-4	0	0.0	0	0.0	-	-	0	0	0	0
5-14	1	2.5	2	3.5	13.0	1.4	0	0	0	0
15-44	106	101.2	141	135.0	25.2	1.4	0	0	0	0
45-59	1	5.1	2	7.1	52.3	1.4	0	0	0	0
60+	0	2.5	1	3.5	70.3	1.4	0	0	0	0
All ages	108	48.9	145	65.3	25.4	1.4	0	0	0	0
Females										
0-4	0	0	0	0	-	-	0	0	0	0
5-14	0	0	0	0	-	-	0	0	0	0
15-44	0	0	0	0	-	-	0	0	0	0
45-59	0	0	0	0	-	-	0	0	0	0
60+	0	0	0	0	-	-	0	0	0	0
All ages	0	0	0	0	-	-	0	0	0	0
Total	108	24.4	145	32.6	25.4	1.4	0	0	0	0

Table 45h   MEC - AOM - CMO   Gonorrhoea - Stricture

Age group (years)	Incidence 1990 Number ('000s)	Rate (per 100 000)	Prevalence 1990 Number ('000s)	Rate (per 100 000)	Avg. age at onset (years)	Average duration (years)	Deaths 1990 Number ('000s)	Rate (per 100 000)	Deaths 2000 (Projected) Number ('000s)	Rate (per 100 000)
Males										
0-4	0	0.0	0	0.0	-	-	0	0	0	0
5-14	1	0.8	1	1.2	13.0	1.4	0	0	0	0
15-44	38	33.7	51	45.0	25.2	1.4	0	0	0	0
45-59	0	1.7	1	2.4	52.3	1.4	0	0	0	0
60+	0	0.8	0	1.2	69.7	1.4	0	0	0	0
All ages	39	15.4	53	20.6	25.4	1.4	0	0	0	0
Females										
0-4	0	0	0	0	-	-	0	0	0	0
5-14	0	0	0	0	-	-	0	0	0	0
15-44	0	0	0	0	-	-	0	0	0	0
45-59	0	0	0	0	-	-	0	0	0	0
60+	0	0	0	0	-	-	0	0	0	0
All ages	0	0	0	0	-	-	0	0	0	0
Total	39	7.8	53	10.5	25.4	1.4	0	0	0	0

Table 45i   World - Mundo - Monde   Gonorrhoea - Stricture

Age group (years)	Incidence 1990 Number ('000s)	Rate (per 100 000)	Prevalence 1990 Number ('000s)	Rate (per 100 000)	Avg. age at onset (years)	Average duration (years)	Deaths 1990 Number ('000s)	Rate (per 100 000)	Deaths 2000 (Projected) Number ('000s)	Rate (per 100 000)
Males										
0-4	0	0.0	0	0.0	-	-	0	0	0	0
5-14	18	3.2	39	7.0	13.0	2.2	0	0	0	0
15-44	1 278	102.2	2 588	207.1	25.2	2.1	0	0	0	0
45-59	14	4.5	30	9.6	52.3	2.1	0	0	0	0
60+	4	1.9	9	4.1	69.7	2.1	0	0	0	0
All ages	1 314	49.5	2 666	100.5	25.4	2.1	0	0	0	0
Females										
0-4	0	0	0	0	-	-	0	0	0	0
5-14	0	0	0	0	-	-	0	0	0	0
15-44	0	0	0	0	-	-	0	0	0	0
45-59	0	0	0	0	-	-	0	0	0	0
60+	0	0	0	0	-	-	0	0	0	0
All ages	0	0	0	0	-	-	0	0	0	0
Total	1 314	24.9	2 666	50.6	25.4	2.1	0	0	0	0

For epidemiological sources see Berkley et al. 1996. For the methods used to estimate and project incidence, prevalence, and deaths see Murray and Lopez 1996a. See explanatory notes for definitions and caveats.

Table 46	Cuadro 46	Tableau 46
HIV	VIH	VIH
Cases	Casos	Cas

Table 46a   EME - PEMC - EMBE   HIV - Cases

Age group (years)	Incidence 1990 Number ('000s)	Rate (per 100 000)	Prevalence 1990 Number ('000s)	Rate (per 100 000)	Avg. age at onset (years)	Average duration (years)	Deaths 1990 Number ('000s)	Rate (per 100 000)	Deaths 2000 (Projected) Number ('000s)	Rate (per 100 000)
Males										
0-4	1	4.6	3	10.1	0.0	4.0	0	0	0	0
5-14	0	0.2	0	0.5	13.0	10.0	0	0	0	0
15-44	102	55.7	1 012	550.1	30.0	10.0	0	0	0	0
45-59	9	13.6	89	134.1	52.0	10.0	0	0	0	0
60+	1	1.3	8	12.8	68.0	10.0	0	0	0	0
All ages	114	29.1	1 112	284.7	31.7	9.9	0	0	0	0
Females										
0-4	1	4.8	3	10.7	0.0	4.0	0	0	0	0
5-14	0	0.2	0	0.8	13.0	10.0	0	0	0	0
15-44	22	12.5	178	99.1	30.0	10.0	0	0	0	0
45-59	1	1.7	10	15.3	52.0	10.0	0	0	0	0
60+	0	0.1	0	0.4	68.0	10.0	0	0	0	0
All ages	25	6.1	191	47.0	29.6	9.7	0	0	0	0
Total	138	17.3	1 303	163.3	31.3	9.9	0	0	0	0

Table 46b   FSE - PEAS - AESE   HIV - Cases

Age group (years)	Incidence 1990 Number ('000s)	Rate (per 100 000)	Prevalence 1990 Number ('000s)	Rate (per 100 000)	Avg. age at onset (years)	Average duration (years)	Deaths 1990 Number ('000s)	Rate (per 100 000)	Deaths 2000 (Projected) Number ('000s)	Rate (per 100 000)
Males										
0-4	0	0.2	1	3.6	0.0	2.0	0	0	0	0
5-14	0	0.0	0	0.4	13.0	7.0	0	0	0	0
15-44	6	8.2	9	11.2	30.0	7.0	0	0	0	0
45-59	1	2.0	1	2.8	52.0	7.0	0	0	0	0
60+	0	0.2	0	0.3	68.0	7.0	0	0	0	0
All ages	7	4.2	10	6.0	31.9	7.0	0	0	0	0
Females										
0-4	0	0.2	1	3.8	0.0	2.0	0	0	0	0
5-14	0	0.0	0	0.4	13.0	7.0	0	0	0	0
15-44	1	1.3	1	1.7	30.0	7.0	0	0	0	0
45-59	0	0.2	0	0.2	52.0	7.0	0	0	0	0
60+	0	0.0	0	0.0	68.0	7.0	0	0	0	0
All ages	1	0.6	2	1.1	30.3	6.9	0	0	0	0
Total	8	2.3	12	3.4	31.7	7.0	0	0	0	0

Table 46c   India - India - Inde   HIV - Cases

Age group (years)	Incidence 1990 Number ('000s)	Rate (per 100 000)	Prevalence 1990 Number ('000s)	Rate (per 100 000)	Avg. age at onset (years)	Average duration (years)	Deaths 1990 Number ('000s)	Rate (per 100 000)	Deaths 2000 (Projected) Number ('000s)	Rate (per 100 000)
Males										
0-4	0	0.8	1	0.8	0.0	2.0	0	0	0	0
5-14	0	0.2	0	0.3	13.0	7.0	0	0	0	0
15-44	108	53.8	183	91.4	30.0	7.0	0	0	0	0
45-59	6	12.2	10	20.6	52.0	7.0	0	0	0	0
60+	2	5.8	3	9.9	68.0	7.0	0	0	0	0
All ages	116	26.4	197	44.8	31.5	7.0	0	0	0	0
Females										
0-4	0	0.8	1	0.9	0.0	2.0	0	0	0	0
5-14	0	0.3	0	0.4	13.0	7.0	0	0	0	0
15-44	61	33.3	64	34.7	30.0	7.0	0	0	0	0
45-59	1	1.4	1	2.1	52.0	7.0	0	0	0	0
60+	0	1.1	0	1.1	68.0	7.0	0	0	0	0
All ages	63	15.3	66	16.0	30.1	7.0	0	0	0	0
Total	179	21.0	262	30.9	31.0	7.0	0	0	0	0

For epidemiological sources see Low-Beer et al. 1996. For the methods used to estimate and project incidence, prevalence, and deaths see Murray and Lopez 1996a. See explanatory notes for definitions and caveats.

Table 46	Cuadro 46	Tableau 46
HIV	VIH	VIH
Cases	Casos	Cas

Table 46d — China - China - Chine — HIV - Cases

Age group (years)	Incidence 1990 Number ('000s)	Rate (per 100 000)	Prevalence 1990 Number ('000s)	Rate (per 100 000)	Avg. age at onset (years)	Average duration (years)	Deaths 1990 Number ('000s)	Rate (per 100 000)	Deaths 2000 (Projected) Number ('000s)	Rate (per 100 000)
Males										
0-4	0	0.0	0	0.0	0.0	2.0	0	0	0	0
5-14	0	0.0	0	0.0	13.0	7.0	0	0	0	0
15-44	2	0.7	2	0.7	30.0	7.0	0	0	0	0
45-59	0	0.2	0	0.2	52.0	7.0	0	0	0	0
60+	0	0.1	0	0.1	68.0	7.0	0	0	0	0
All ages	2	0.4	2	0.4	31.6	7.0	0	0	0	0
Females										
0-4	0	0.0	0	0.0	0.0	2.0	0	0	0	0
5-14	0	0.0	0	0.0	13.0	7.0	0	0	0	0
15-44	0	0.1	0	0.1	30.0	7.0	0	0	0	0
45-59	0	0.0	0	0.0	52.0	7.0	0	0	0	0
60+	0	0.0	0	0.0	68.0	7.0	0	0	0	0
All ages	0	0.1	0	0.1	30.0	7.0	0	0	0	0
Total	3	0.2	3	0.2	31.4	7.0	0	0	0	0

Table 46e — OAI - OPAI - APAI — HIV - Cases

Age group (years)	Incidence 1990 Number ('000s)	Rate (per 100 000)	Prevalence 1990 Number ('000s)	Rate (per 100 000)	Avg. age at onset (years)	Average duration (years)	Deaths 1990 Number ('000s)	Rate (per 100 000)	Deaths 2000 (Projected) Number ('000s)	Rate (per 100 000)
Males										
0-4	0	0.6	0	0.6	0.0	2.0	0	0	0	0
5-14	0	0.1	0	0.1	13.0	7.0	0	0	0	0
15-44	54	33.6	78	48.5	30.0	7.0	0	0	0	0
45-59	3	8.5	4	12.2	52.0	7.0	0	0	0	0
60+	1	4.3	1	6.2	68.0	7.0	0	0	0	0
All ages	58	16.9	84	24.4	31.5	7.0	0	0	0	0
Females										
0-4	0	0.6	0	0.7	0.0	2.0	0	0	0	0
5-14	0	0.2	0	0.2	13.0	7.0	0	0	0	0
15-44	31	19.1	41	25.8	30.0	7.0	0	0	0	0
45-59	0	0.9	0	1.2	52.0	7.0	0	0	0	0
60+	0	0.7	0	0.9	68.0	7.0	0	0	0	0
All ages	31	9.2	42	12.4	30.1	7.0	0	0	0	0
Total	89	13.1	126	18.5	31.0	7.0	0	0	0	0

Table 46f — SSA - ASS - ASS — HIV - Cases

Age group (years)	Incidence 1990 Number ('000s)	Rate (per 100 000)	Prevalence 1990 Number ('000s)	Rate (per 100 000)	Avg. age at onset (years)	Average duration (years)	Deaths 1990 Number ('000s)	Rate (per 100 000)	Deaths 2000 (Projected) Number ('000s)	Rate (per 100 000)
Males										
0-4	57	119.7	114	240	0.0	2.0	0	0	0	0
5-14	1	1.4	7	10	13.0	7.0	0	0	0	0
15-44	460	442.9	2 401	2 314	30.0	7.0	0	0	0	0
45-59	16	77.8	157	771	52.0	7.0	0	0	0	0
60+	2	22.8	52	497	68.0	7.0	0	0	0	0
All ages	536	212.3	2 731	1 082	27.7	6.5	0	0	0	0
Females										
0-4	57	120.9	114	243	0.0	2.0	0	0	0	0
5-14	5	6.9	11	15	13.0	7.0	0	0	0	0
15-44	460	432.5	2 432	2 289	30.0	7.0	0	0	0	0
45-59	13	60.6	130	590	52.0	7.0	0	0	0	0
60+	1	7.5	47	369	68.0	7.0	0	0	0	0
All ages	536	207.6	2 735	1 060	27.3	6.5	0	0	0	0
Total	1 071	209.9	5 465	1 071	27.5	6.5	0	0	0	0

For epidemiological sources see Low-Beer et al. 1996. For the methods used to estimate and project incidence, prevalence, and deaths see Murray and Lopez 1996a. See explanatory notes for definitions and caveats.

Table 46	Cuadro 46	Tableau 46
HIV	VIH	VIH
Cases	Casos	Cas

Table 46g — LAC - ALC - ALC — HIV - Cases

Age group (years)	Incidence 1990 Number ('000s)	Incidence 1990 Rate (per 100 000)	Prevalence 1990 Number ('000s)	Prevalence 1990 Rate (per 100 000)	Avg. age at onset (years)	Average duration (years)	Deaths 1990 Number ('000s)	Deaths 1990 Rate (per 100 000)	Deaths 2000 (Projected) Number ('000s)	Deaths 2000 (Projected) Rate (per 100 000)
Males										
0-4	2	7.0	4	12.6	0.0	2.0	0	0	0	0
5-14	0	0.3	0	0.7	13.0	7.0	0	0	0	0
15-44	164	157.6	761	730.2	30.0	7.0	0	0	0	0
45-59	9	39.0	40	180.5	52.0	7.0	0	0	0	0
60+	0	2.4	2	11.3	68.0	7.0	0	0	0	0
All ages	176	79.2	807	364.2	30.8	6.9	0	0	0	0
Females										
0-4	2	7.3	4	13.1	0.0	2.0	0	0	0	0
5-14	0	0.5	0	0.9	13.0	7.0	0	0	0	0
15-44	47	44.8	193	185.4	30.0	7.0	0	0	0	0
45-59	3	12.9	8	34.8	52.0	7.0	0	0	0	0
60+	1	3.0	2	12.1	68.0	7.0	0	0	0	0
All ages	52	23.5	207	93.0	30.4	6.8	0	0	0	0
Total	228	51.3	1 014	228.3	30.7	6.9	0	0	0	0

Table 46h — MEC - AOM - CMO — HIV - Cases

Age group (years)	Incidence 1990 Number ('000s)	Incidence 1990 Rate (per 100 000)	Prevalence 1990 Number ('000s)	Prevalence 1990 Rate (per 100 000)	Avg. age at onset (years)	Average duration (years)	Deaths 1990 Number ('000s)	Deaths 1990 Rate (per 100 000)	Deaths 2000 (Projected) Number ('000s)	Deaths 2000 (Projected) Rate (per 100 000)
Males										
0-4	0	0.3	0	0.4	0.0	2.0	0	0	0	0
5-14	0	0.0	0	0.0	13.0	7.0	0	0	0	0
15-44	19	17.1	59	51.9	30.0	7.0	0	0	0	0
45-59	2	7.6	5	23.2	52.0	7.0	0	0	0	0
60+	0	0.9	0	3.3	68.0	7.0	0	0	0	0
All ages	21	8.4	65	25.3	31.8	7.0	0	0	0	0
Females										
0-4	0	0.3	0	0.4	0.0	2.0	0	0	0	0
5-14	0	0.0	0	0.0	13.0	7.0	0	0	0	0
15-44	3	3.1	9	8.8	30.0	7.0	0	0	0	0
45-59	0	0.9	1	2.5	52.0	7.0	0	0	0	0
60+	0	0.0	0	0.1	68.0	7.0	0	0	0	0
All ages	4	1.5	10	4.1	30.3	6.9	0	0	0	0
Total	25	5.0	75	14.9	31.6	7.0	0	0	0	0

Table 46i — World - Mundo - Monde — HIV - Cases

Age group (years)	Incidence 1990 Number ('000s)	Incidence 1990 Rate (per 100 000)	Prevalence 1990 Number ('000s)	Prevalence 1990 Rate (per 100 000)	Avg. age at onset (years)	Average duration (years)	Deaths 1990 Number ('000s)	Deaths 1990 Rate (per 100 000)	Deaths 2000 (Projected) Number ('000s)	Deaths 2000 (Projected) Rate (per 100 000)
Males										
0-4	61	19.0	122	37.9	0.0	2.0	0	0	0	0
5-14	2	0.3	8	1.5	13.0	7.2	0	0	0	0
15-44	916	73.3	4 506	360.5	30.0	7.3	0	0	0	0
45-59	45	14.2	305	97.8	52.0	7.6	0	0	0	0
60+	6	2.9	66	30.3	68.0	7.4	0	0	0	0
All ages	1 030	38.8	5 008	188.7	29.4	7.0	0	0	0	0
Females										
0-4	61	19.7	122	39.4	0.0	2.0	0	0	0	0
5-14	6	1.1	12	2.3	13.0	7.1	0	0	0	0
15-44	625	52.1	2 918	243.5	30.0	7.1	0	0	0	0
45-59	19	6.0	151	48.5	52.0	7.2	0	0	0	0
60+	2	0.7	50	18.6	68.0	7.1	0	0	0	0
All ages	712	27.2	3 253	124.5	28.0	6.7	0	0	0	0
Total	1 742	33.1	8 261	156.8	28.8	6.9	0	0	0	0

For epidemiological sources see Low-Beer et al. 1996. For the methods used to estimate and project incidence, prevalence, and deaths see Murray and Lopez 1996a. See explanatory notes for definitions and caveats.

Table 47	Cuadro 47	Tableau 47
HIV	VIH	VIH
AIDS	SIDA	SIDA

Table 47a — EME - PEMC - EMBE — HIV - AIDS

Age group (years)	Incidence 1990 Number ('000s)	Rate (per 100 000)	Prevalence 1990 Number ('000s)	Rate (per 100 000)	Avg. age at onset (years)	Average duration (years)	Deaths 1990 Number ('000s)	Rate (per 100 000)	Deaths 2000 (Projected) Number ('000s)	Rate (per 100 000)
Males										
0-4	1	3.0	1	4.6	2.5	2.0	0	1.9	1	4.4
5-14	0	0.2	0	0.3	10.0	2.0	0	0.1	0	0.3
15-44	51	27.5	82	44.3	35.0	2.0	25	13.6	63	36.0
45-59	10	15.1	16	24.4	57.0	2.0	9	12.9	22	27.2
60+	2	3.1	3	5.0	73.0	2.0	2	2.7	4	5.8
All ages	63	16.3	102	26.1	39.2	2.0	36	9.2	91	22.0
Females										
0-4	1	3.2	1	4.8	2.5	2.0	0	1.4	1	3.3
5-14	0	0.2	0	0.3	10.0	2.0	0	0.1	0	0.4
15-44	8	4.6	18	10.0	35.0	2.0	4	2.2	10	5.8
45-59	1	1.6	2	3.4	57.0	2.0	1	1.3	2	2.8
60+	0	0.5	1	1.0	73.0	2.0	0	0.4	1	0.8
All ages	10	2.6	23	5.5	36.0	2.0	6	1.4	14	3.3
Total	74	9.3	125	15.6	38.7	2.0	41	5.2	105	12.5

Table 47b — FSE - PEAS - AESE — HIV - AIDS

Age group (years)	Incidence 1990 Number ('000s)	Rate (per 100 000)	Prevalence 1990 Number ('000s)	Rate (per 100 000)	Avg. age at onset (years)	Average duration (years)	Deaths 1990 Number ('000s)	Rate (per 100 000)	Deaths 2000 (Projected) Number ('000s)	Rate (per 100 000)
Males										
0-4	0	2.5	0	2.8	1.5	0.50	0	2.2	1	9.5
5-14	0	0.2	0	0.2	10.0	1.00	0	0.2	0	0.6
15-44	0	0.3	0	0.3	33.5	1.00	0	0.2	1	0.8
45-59	0	0.1	0	0.1	55.5	1.00	0	0.1	0	0.3
60+	0	0.0	0	0.1	71.5	1.00	0	0.0	0	0.1
All ages	1	0.4	1	0.4	16.1	0.73	1	0.3	2	1.2
Females										
0-4	0	2.7	0	2.9	1.5	0.50	0	2.3	1	9.9
5-14	0	0.2	0	0.2	10.0	1.00	0	0.2	0	0.7
15-44	0	0.1	0	0.2	33.5	1.00	0	0.1	0	0.4
45-59	0	0.1	0	0.1	55.5	1.00	0	0.0	0	0.2
60+	0	0.0	0	0.0	71.5	1.00	0	0.0	0	0.0
All ages	1	0.3	1	0.3	11.8	0.67	0	0.2	2	0.9
Total	1	0.3	1	0.4	14.1	0.70	1	0.3	4	1.1

Table 47c — India - India - Inde — HIV - AIDS

Age group (years)	Incidence 1990 Number ('000s)	Rate (per 100 000)	Prevalence 1990 Number ('000s)	Rate (per 100 000)	Avg. age at onset (years)	Average duration (years)	Deaths 1990 Number ('000s)	Rate (per 100 000)	Deaths 2000 (Projected) Number ('000s)	Rate (per 100 000)
Males										
0-4	0	0.2	0	0.2	1.5	0.50	0	0.2	27	48.2
5-14	0	0.0	0	0.0	10.0	1.00	0	0.0	5	4.1
15-44	0	0.2	0	0.2	33.5	1.00	0	0.1	99	39.7
45-59	0	0.1	0	0.1	55.5	1.00	0	0.0	17	28.2
60+	0	0.0	0	0.0	71.5	1.00	0	0.0	9	23.8
All ages	1	0.1	1	0.1	27.6	0.88	0	0.1	156	30.5
Females										
0-4	0	0.3	0	0.3	1.5	0.50	0	0.3	28	51.1
5-14	0	0.0	0	0.0	10.0	1.00	0	0.0	5	4.5
15-44	0	0.0	0	0.0	33.5	1.00	0	0.0	70	30.5
45-59	0	0.0	0	0.0	55.5	1.00	0	0.0	7	11.5
60+	0	0.0	0	0.0	-	-	0	0.0	3	6.9
All ages	0	0.0	0	0.0	6.5	0.60	0	0.0	111	23.0
Total	1	0.1	1	0.1	22.6	0.81	1	0.1	267	26.9

For epidemiological sources see Low-Beer et al. 1996. For the methods used to estimate and project incidence, prevalence, and deaths see Murray and Lopez 1996a. See explanatory notes for definitions and caveats.

Table 47	Cuadro 47	Tableau 47
HIV	VIH	VIH
AIDS	SIDA	SIDA

Table 47d — China - China - Chine — HIV - AIDS

Age group (years)	Incidence 1990 Number ('000s)	Rate (per 100 000)	Prevalence 1990 Number ('000s)	Rate (per 100 000)	Avg. age at onset (years)	Average duration (years)	Deaths 1990 Number ('000s)	Rate (per 100 000)	Deaths 2000 (Projected) Number ('000s)	Rate (per 100 000)
Males										
0-4	0	0	0	0	-	-	0	0	1	1.3
5-14	0	0	0	0	-	-	0	0	0	0.1
15-44	0	0	0	0	33.5	1.0	0	0	1	0.4
45-59	0	0	0	0	-	-	0	0	0	0.2
60+	0	0	0	0	-	-	0	0	0	0.2
All ages	0	0	0	0	33.5	1.0	0	0	2	0.4
Females										
0-4	0	0	0	0	-	-	0	0	1	1.6
5-14	0	0	0	0	-	-	0	0	0	0.1
15-44	0	0	0	0	33.5	1.0	0	0	1	0.2
45-59	0	0	0	0	-	-	0	0	0	0.1
60+	0	0	0	0	-	-	0	0	0	0.0
All ages	0	0	0	0	33.5	1.0	0	0	2	0.3
Total	0	0	0	0	33.5	1.0	0	0	4	0.3

Table 47e — OAI - OPAI - APAI — HIV - AIDS

Age group (years)	Incidence 1990 Number ('000s)	Rate (per 100 000)	Prevalence 1990 Number ('000s)	Rate (per 100 000)	Avg. age at onset (years)	Average duration (years)	Deaths 1990 Number ('000s)	Rate (per 100 000)	Deaths 2000 (Projected) Number ('000s)	Rate (per 100 000)
Males										
0-4	0	0.2	0	0.2	1.5	0.50	0	0.2	12	27.9
5-14	0	0.0	0	0.0	10.0	1.00	0	0.0	2	2.3
15-44	0	0.0	0	0.0	33.5	1.00	0	0.0	46	22.4
45-59	0	0.0	0	0.0	55.5	1.00	0	0.0	7	15.6
60+	0	0.0	0	0.0	-	-	0	0.0	3	12.5
All ages	0	0.0	0	0.0	14.4	0.72	0	0.0	70	17.4
Females										
0-4	0	0.2	0	0.2	1.5	0.50	0	0.2	7	17.6
5-14	0	0.0	0	0.0	10.0	1.00	0	0.0	1	1.6
15-44	0	0.0	0	0.0	33.5	1.00	0	0.0	37	18.5
45-59	0	0.0	0	0.0	55.5	1.00	0	0.0	3	6.8
60+	0	0.0	0	0.0	-	-	0	0.0	1	3.9
All ages	0	0.0	0	0.0	14.4	0.72	0	0.0	50	12.5
Total	0	0.0	0	0.0	14.4	0.72	0	0.0	121	14.9

Table 47f — SSA - ASS - ASS — HIV - AIDS

Age group (years)	Incidence 1990 Number ('000s)	Rate (per 100 000)	Prevalence 1990 Number ('000s)	Rate (per 100 000)	Avg. age at onset (years)	Average duration (years)	Deaths 1990 Number ('000s)	Rate (per 100 000)	Deaths 2000 (Projected) Number ('000s)	Rate (per 100 000)
Males										
0-4	34	71.6	35	74.4	1.5	0.50	32	67.2	88	134
5-14	4	5.4	4	5.6	10.0	1.00	4	6.2	12	13
15-44	97	93.0	133	128.5	33.5	1.00	64	61.8	177	125
45-59	9	45.9	13	63.4	55.5	1.00	8	41.7	23	88
60+	4	36.5	5	50.5	71.5	1.00	4	33.3	10	67
All ages	147	58.5	191	75.6	28.0	0.88	112	44.5	310	90
Females										
0-4	34	72.3	35	75.1	1.5	0.50	30	64.1	83	131
5-14	4	5.4	4	5.6	10.0	1.00	4	6.4	12	13
15-44	101	95.0	139	131.2	33.5	1.00	84	78.6	230	159
45-59	7	29.8	9	41.1	55.5	1.00	6	27.3	17	57
60+	2	17.2	3	23.8	71.5	1.00	2	16.2	6	33
All ages	147	57.2	191	74.0	27.2	0.88	126	48.9	348	100
Total	295	57.8	382	74.8	27.6	0.88	239	46.8	658	95

For epidemiological sources see Low-Beer et al. 1996. For the methods used to estimate and project incidence, prevalence, and deaths see Murray and Lopez 1996a. See explanatory notes for definitions and caveats.

Table 47
HIV

Cuadro 47
VIH

Tableau 47
VIH

AIDS

SIDA

SIDA

Table 47g LAC - ALC - ALC HIV - AIDS

Age group (years)	Incidence 1990 Number ('000s)	Rate (per 100 000)	Prevalence 1990 Number ('000s)	Rate (per 100 000)	Avg. age at onset (years)	Average duration (years)	Deaths 1990 Number ('000s)	Rate (per 100 000)	Deaths 2000 (Projected) Number ('000s)	Rate (per 100 000)
Males										
0-4	1	3.8	1	3.9	1.5	0.50	1	3.7	5	18.3
5-14	0	0.2	0	0.2	10.0	1.00	0	0.2	0	0.8
15-44	25	24.4	34	33.0	33.5	1.00	19	17.8	93	72.2
45-59	3	13.5	4	18.2	55.5	1.00	3	11.5	13	41.7
60+	1	10.5	2	14.2	71.5	1.00	1	8.9	6	32.4
All ages	31	14.1	42	18.8	36.3	0.98	23	10.6	118	44.4
Females										
0-4	1	3.9	1	4.0	1.5	0.50	1	3.6	5	17.7
5-14	0	0.2	0	0.2	10.0	1.00	0	0.2	1	0.9
15-44	6	5.3	8	7.7	33.5	1.00	4	4.0	21	16.3
45-59	1	2.2	1	3.1	55.5	1.00	0	1.4	2	5.2
60+	0	1.5	0	2.2	71.5	1.00	0	1.1	1	4.1
All ages	8	3.4	10	4.7	31.3	0.93	6	2.6	29	10.9
Total	39	8.7	52	11.7	35.3	0.97	29	6.6	147	27.6

Table 47h MEC - AOM - CMO HIV - AIDS

Age group (years)	Incidence 1990 Number ('000s)	Rate (per 100 000)	Prevalence 1990 Number ('000s)	Rate (per 100 000)	Avg. age at onset (years)	Average duration (years)	Deaths 1990 Number ('000s)	Rate (per 100 000)	Deaths 2000 (Projected) Number ('000s)	Rate (per 100 000)
Males										
0-4	0	0.1	0	0.1	1.5	0.50	0	0.1	1	1.9
5-14	0	0.0	0	0.0	10.0	1.00	0	0.0	0	0.1
15-44	1	0.6	1	0.7	33.5	1.00	0	0.3	7	4.4
45-59	0	0.6	0	0.7	55.5	1.00	0	0.4	2	5.8
60+	0	0.2	0	0.2	71.5	1.00	0	0.1	0	1.8
All ages	1	0.4	1	0.4	36.2	0.98	0	0.2	10	2.9
Females										
0-4	0	0.1	0	0.1	1.5	0.50	0	0.1	1	2.0
5-14	0	0.0	0	0.0	10.0	1.00	0	0.0	0	0.1
15-44	0	0.1	0	0.1	33.5	1.00	0	0.0	1	0.7
45-59	0	0.1	0	0.1	55.5	1.00	0	0.0	0	0.6
60+	0	0.0	0	0.0	71.5	1.00	0	0.0	0	0.3
All ages	0	0.1	0	0.1	27.4	0.87	0	0.0	2	0.7
Total	1	0.2	1	0.3	34.8	0.96	1	0.1	12	1.8

Table 47i World - Mundo - Monde HIV - AIDS

Age group (years)	Incidence 1990 Number ('000s)	Rate (per 100 000)	Prevalence 1990 Number ('000s)	Rate (per 100 000)	Avg. age at onset (years)	Average duration (years)	Deaths 1990 Number ('000s)	Rate (per 100 000)	Deaths 2000 (Projected) Number ('000s)	Rate (per 100 000)
Males										
0-4	37	11.4	38	11.9	1.5	0.53	34	10.6	151	43.6
5-14	4	0.7	4	0.8	10.0	1.02	5	0.8	21	3.4
15-44	174	13.9	251	20.1	33.9	1.29	108	8.7	476	33.0
45-59	23	7.2	33	10.7	56.2	1.44	20	6.3	81	20.1
60+	7	3.3	10	4.8	71.9	1.26	6	2.9	30	11.1
All ages	244	9.2	337	12.7	31.9	1.19	173	6.5	759	24.5
Females										
0-4	37	11.8	38	12.4	1.5	0.53	32	10.4	185	55.8
5-14	4	0.8	4	0.8	10.0	1.02	5	0.9	28	4.6
15-44	115	9.6	166	13.8	33.6	1.07	92	7.7	312	22.5
45-59	8	2.6	12	3.9	55.7	1.13	7	2.3	25	6.2
60+	3	1.1	4	1.6	71.7	1.14	3	1.0	9	2.7
All ages	167	6.4	225	8.6	27.8	0.96	138	5.3	559	18.2
Total	411	7.8	562	10.7	30.3	1.09	312	5.9	1 318	21.4

For epidemiological sources see Low-Beer et al. 1996. For the methods used to estimate and project incidence, prevalence, and deaths see Murray and Lopez 1996a. See explanatory notes for definitions and caveats.

Table 48
Diarrhoeal diseases

Cuadro 48
Enfermedades diarreicas

Tableau 48
Maladies diarrhéiques

Episodes

Episodios

Episodes

Table 48a	EME - PEMC - EMBE								Diarrhoeal diseases - Episodes	
Age group (years)	Incidence 1990		Prevalence 1990		Avg. age at onset (years)	Average duration (years)	Deaths 1990		Deaths 2000 (Projected)	
	Number ('000s)	Rate (per 100 000)	Number ('000s)	Rate (per 100 000)			Number ('000s)	Rate (per 100 000)	Number ('000s)	Rate (per 100 000)
Males										
0-4	47 491	180 000	852	3 230	2.5	0.02	0	0.8	*0*	*0.5*
5-14	5 335	10 000	90	170	10.0	0.02	0	0.0	*0*	*0.0*
15-44	18 406	10 000	310	168	29.9	0.02	0	0.0	*0*	*0.0*
45-59	6 614	10 000	111	168	52.4	0.02	0	0.1	*0*	*0.1*
60+	6 055	10 000	102	168	71.1	0.02	1	1.3	*1*	*1.3*
All ages	83 901	21 487	1 466	376	17.9	0.02	1	0.3	*1*	*0.3*
Females										
0-4	45 117	180 000	810	3 230	2.5	0.02	0	0.5	*0*	*0.4*
5-14	5 068	10 000	86	170	10.0	0.02	0	0.0	*0*	*0.0*
15-44	17 920	10 000	302	168	30.0	0.02	0	0.0	*0*	*0.0*
45-59	6 780	10 000	114	168	52.4	0.02	0	0.1	*0*	*0.0*
60+	8 457	10 000	142	168	72.4	0.02	1	1.6	*1*	*1.5*
All ages	83 341	20 461	1 454	357	20.0	0.02	2	0.4	*2*	*0.4*
Total	167 242	20 963	2 921	366	18.9	0.02	3	0.3	*3*	*0.3*

Table 48b	FSE - PEAS - AESE								Diarrhoeal diseases - Episodes	
Age group (years)	Incidence 1990		Prevalence 1990		Avg. age at onset (years)	Average duration (years)	Deaths 1990		Deaths 2000 (Projected)	
	Number ('000s)	Rate (per 100 000)	Number ('000s)	Rate (per 100 000)			Number ('000s)	Rate (per 100 000)	Number ('000s)	Rate (per 100 000)
Males										
0-4	31 646	230 000	568	4 127	2.5	0.02	2	14.2	*1*	*10.6*
5-14	2 735	10 000	46	170	10.0	0.02	0	0.1	*0*	*0.1*
15-44	7 628	10 000	129	168	29.8	0.02	0	0.1	*0*	*0.0*
45-59	2 697	10 000	45	168	52.2	0.02	0	0.3	*0*	*0.2*
60+	2 096	10 000	35	168	70.0	0.02	0	0.5	*0*	*0.5*
All ages	46 802	28 310	824	498	13.3	0.02	2	1.3	*2*	*0.9*
Females										
0-4	30 211	230 000	542	4 127	2.5	0.02	2	12.7	*1*	*9.4*
5-14	2 642	10 000	45	170	10.0	0.02	0	0.1	*0*	*0.1*
15-44	7 496	10 000	126	168	29.9	0.02	0	0.0	*0*	*0.0*
45-59	3 001	10 000	51	168	52.4	0.02	0	0.1	*0*	*0.1*
60+	3 639	10 000	61	168	71.5	0.02	0	0.5	*0*	*0.4*
All ages	46 989	25 973	825	456	15.8	0.02	2	1.1	*1*	*0.7*
Total	93 791	27 089	1 649	476	14.6	0.02	4	1.2	*3*	*0.8*

Table 48c	India - India - Inde								Diarrhoeal diseases - Episodes	
Age group (years)	Incidence 1990		Prevalence 1990		Avg. age at onset (years)	Average duration (years)	Deaths 1990		Deaths 2000 (Projected)	
	Number ('000s)	Rate (per 100 000)	Number ('000s)	Rate (per 100 000)			Number ('000s)	Rate (per 100 000)	Number ('000s)	Rate (per 100 000)
Males										
0-4	269 051	450 000	4 828	8 075	2.5	0.02	355	594.1	*211*	*371.7*
5-14	61 051	60 000	1 035	1 018	10.0	0.02	23	22.2	*11*	*9.9*
15-44	60 158	30 000	1 014	505	29.8	0.02	19	9.3	*9*	*3.8*
45-59	9 513	20 000	160	337	52.3	0.02	10	20.2	*5*	*9.2*
60+	5 954	20 000	100	337	69.7	0.02	40	134.7	*36*	*96.4*
All ages	405 726	92 336	7 138	1 624	9.8	0.02	446	101.5	*272*	*53.2*
Females										
0-4	255 056	450 000	4 577	8 075	2.5	0.02	378	666.1	*215*	*399.8*
5-14	57 158	60 000	969	1 018	10.0	0.02	32	33.8	*15*	*14.6*
15-44	54 973	30 000	926	505	29.8	0.02	18	9.8	*7*	*3.3*
45-59	9 201	20 000	155	337	52.4	0.02	9	20.1	*5*	*9.1*
60+	5 785	20 000	97	337	70.1	0.02	39	134.2	*38*	*97.3*
All ages	382 172	93 187	6 725	1 640	9.8	0.02	476	116.0	*281*	*58.2*
Total	787 898	92 747	13 863	1 632	9.8	0.02	922	108.5	*553*	*55.6*

For epidemiological sources see Bern et al. 1996. For the methods used to estimate and project incidence, prevalence, and deaths see Murray and Lopez 1996a. See explanatory notes for definitions and caveats.

Table 48
Diarrhoeal diseases

Cuadro 48
Enfermedades diarreicas

Tableau 48
Maladies diarrhéiques

Episodes

Episodios

Episodes

Table 48d   China - China - Chine   Diarrhoeal diseases - Episodes

Age group (years)	Incidence 1990 Number ('000s)	Rate (per 100 000)	Prevalence 1990 Number ('000s)	Rate (per 100 000)	Avg. age at onset (years)	Average duration (years)	Deaths 1990 Number ('000s)	Rate (per 100 000)	Deaths 2000 (Projected) Number ('000s)	Rate (per 100 000)
Males										
0-4	138 559	230 000	2 486	4 127	2.5	0.02	22	36.4	11	18.8
5-14	58 198	60 000	987	1 018	10.0	0.02	1	1.5	1	0.5
15-44	214 414	70 000	3 613	1 179	29.9	0.02	3	0.9	1	0.3
45-59	50 872	70 000	857	1 179	52.3	0.02	2	2.4	1	0.9
60+	34 286	70 000	578	1 179	69.8	0.02	16	33.5	15	25.2
All ages	496 328	84 814	8 521	1 456	25.0	0.02	44	7.6	29	4.4
Females										
0-4	179 633	230 000	2 392	4 127	2.5	0.02	28	48.7	13	24.1
5-14	54 241	60 000	920	1 018	10.0	0.02	1	1.3	1	0.5
15-44	198 855	70 000	3 351	1 179	29.9	0.02	2	0.7	1	0.2
45-59	45 082	70 000	760	1 179	52.4	0.02	1	1.9	1	0.8
60+	36 166	70 000	609	1 179	70.6	0.02	16	30.6	16	24.7
All ages	513 976	93 707	8 031	1 464	23.1	0.02	48	8.8	31	5.0
Total	1 010 305	89 116	16 552	1 460	24.0	0.02	93	8.2	60	4.7

Table 48e   OAI - OPAI - APAI   Diarrhoeal diseases - Episodes

Age group (years)	Incidence 1990 Number ('000s)	Rate (per 100 000)	Prevalence 1990 Number ('000s)	Rate (per 100 000)	Avg. age at onset (years)	Average duration (years)	Deaths 1990 Number ('000s)	Rate (per 100 000)	Deaths 2000 (Projected) Number ('000s)	Rate (per 100 000)
Males										
0-4	175 052	400 000	3 141	7 178	2.5	0.02	202	461.5	131	297.2
5-14	33 613	40 000	570	678	10.0	0.02	13	15.0	6	7.4
15-44	32 165	20 000	542	337	29.7	0.02	2	1.5	1	0.7
45-59	6 828	20 000	115	337	52.3	0.02	2	6.6	2	3.3
60+	4 042	20 000	68	337	69.6	0.02	6	31.4	6	22.6
All ages	251 699	73 389	4 436	1 294	9.4	0.02	226	65.8	146	36.2
Females										
0-4	125 964	400 000	3 014	7 178	2.5	0.02	150	358.3	94	223.3
5-14	32 087	40 000	544	678	10.0	0.02	9	11.6	5	5.6
15-44	63 844	40 000	1 076	674	29.8	0.02	4	2.2	2	0.9
45-59	14 036	40 000	236	674	52.3	0.02	3	7.3	2	3.6
60+	9 065	40 000	153	674	70.3	0.02	5	23.8	6	18.5
All ages	244 996	72 149	5 023	1 479	16.0	0.02	171	50.4	108	26.9
Total	496 695	72 772	9 460	1 386	12.6	0.02	397	58.2	255	31.5

Table 48f   SSA - ASS - ASS   Diarrhoeal diseases - Episodes

Age group (years)	Incidence 1990 Number ('000s)	Rate (per 100 000)	Prevalence 1990 Number ('000s)	Rate (per 100 000)	Avg. age at onset (years)	Average duration (years)	Deaths 1990 Number ('000s)	Rate (per 100 000)	Deaths 2000 (Projected) Number ('000s)	Rate (per 100 000)
Males										
0-4	237 420	500 000	4 261	8 973	2.4	0.02	447	941.9	447	678.0
5-14	63 232	90 000	1 072	1 526	10.0	0.02	34	49.0	25	26.3
15-44	31 129	30 000	525	505	29.4	0.02	9	8.8	6	4.3
45-59	6 092	30 000	103	505	52.2	0.02	4	19.8	3	10.5
60+	3 152	30 000	53	505	69.2	0.02	15	144.7	16	108.1
All ages	341 026	135 155	6 013	2 383	7.8	0.02	510	202.2	496	144.6
Females										
0-4	206 932	500 000	4 220	8 973	2.4	0.02	362	769.1	339	533.5
5-14	62 836	90 000	1 066	1 526	10.0	0.02	37	52.3	25	27.1
15-44	31 877	30 000	537	505	29.5	0.02	19	18.0	11	7.3
45-59	6 635	30 000	112	505	52.2	0.02	5	23.2	4	12.0
60+	3 819	30 000	64	505	69.7	0.02	18	138.3	18	102.0
All ages	312 099	120 991	5 999	2 326	8.6	0.02	440	170.6	397	113.8
Total	653 126	127 995	12 012	2 354	8.2	0.02	950	186.2	892	129.1

For epidemiological sources see Bern et al. 1996. For the methods used to estimate and project incidence, prevalence, and deaths see Murray and Lopez 1996a. See explanatory notes for definitions and caveats.

Table 48
Diarrhoeal diseases

Cuadro 48
Enfermedades diarreicas

Tableau 48
Maladies diarrhéiques

Episodes

Episodios

Episodes

Table 48g   LAC - ALC - ALC

Diarrhoeal diseases - Episodes

Age group (years)	Incidence 1990 Number ('000s)	Rate (per 100 000)	Prevalence 1990 Number ('000s)	Rate (per 100 000)	Avg. age at onset (years)	Average duration (years)	Deaths 1990 Number ('000s)	Rate (per 100 000)	Deaths 2000 (Projected) Number ('000s)	Rate (per 100 000)
Males										
0-4	114 884	400 000	2 062	7 178	2.5	0.02	76	265.3	54	185.4
5-14	62 549	120 000	1 061	2 035	10.0	0.02	2	4.5	1	2.6
15-44	31 286	30 000	527	505	29.8	0.02	2	1.5	1	0.8
45-59	6 675	30 000	112	505	52.3	0.02	1	6.2	1	3.5
60+	4 269	30 000	72	505	70.3	0.02	5	34.3	6	28.4
All ages	219 663	99 121	3 834	1 730	11.4	0.02	86	39.0	64	23.9
Females										
0-4	110 704	400 000	1 987	7 178	2.5	0.02	54	193.5	37	131.7
5-14	60 893	120 000	1 033	2 035	10.0	0.02	3	5.5	2	3.1
15-44	31 226	30 000	526	505	29.9	0.02	3	3.2	2	1.4
45-59	7 007	30 000	118	505	52.4	0.02	2	6.6	1	3.7
60+	5 047	30 000	85	505	71.1	0.02	6	34.2	7	28.2
All ages	214 876	96 494	3 749	1 683	11.8	0.02	67	30.1	48	18.1
Total	434 539	97 804	7 582	1 707	11.6	0.02	153	34.5	112	21.0

Table 48h   MEC - AOM - CMO

Diarrhoeal diseases - Episodes

Age group (years)	Incidence 1990 Number ('000s)	Rate (per 100 000)	Prevalence 1990 Number ('000s)	Rate (per 100 000)	Avg. age at onset (years)	Average duration (years)	Deaths 1990 Number ('000s)	Rate (per 100 000)	Deaths 2000 (Projected) Number ('000s)	Rate (per 100 000)
Males										
0-4	164 644	400 000	2 955	7 178	2.5	0.02	206	501.3	184	369.8
5-14	32 673	50 000	554	848	10.0	0.02	7	11.3	5	6.4
15-44	22 779	20 000	384	337	29.8	0.02	1	0.9	1	0.5
45-59	4 467	20 000	75	337	52.3	0.02	1	2.7	0	1.5
60+	2 730	20 000	46	337	69.7	0.02	1	10.8	1	8.0
All ages	227 293	88 652	4 014	1 565	8.1	0.02	217	84.6	192	57.7
Females										
0-4	143 042	400 000	2 852	7 178	2.5	0.02	196	493.3	167	352.0
5-14	31 000	50 000	526	848	10.0	0.02	8	12.1	5	6.5
15-44	21 442	20 000	361	337	29.8	0.02	2	1.9	1	0.8
45-59	4 458	20 000	75	337	52.3	0.02	1	3.0	1	1.6
60+	3 090	20 000	52	337	70.4	0.02	1	8.7	1	6.7
All ages	203 033	82 304	3 866	1 567	8.7	0.02	208	84.2	176	54.5
Total	430 326	85 539	7 880	1 566	8.4	0.02	424	84.4	368	56.1

Table 48i   World - Mundo - Monde

Diarrhoeal diseases - Episodes

Age group (years)	Incidence 1990 Number ('000s)	Rate (per 100 000)	Prevalence 1990 Number ('000s)	Rate (per 100 000)	Avg. age at onset (years)	Average duration (years)	Deaths 1990 Number ('000s)	Rate (per 100 000)	Deaths 2000 (Projected) Number ('000s)	Rate (per 100 000)
Males										
0-4	1 178 746	366 868	21 153	6 584	2.5	0.02	1 311	408.1	1 040	300.5
5-14	319 385	57 944	5 416	983	10.0	0.02	81	14.7	49	7.8
15-44	417 964	33 439	7 042	563	29.8	0.02	36	2.9	20	1.4
45-59	93 759	30 015	1 580	506	52.3	0.02	20	6.3	12	3.1
60+	62 584	28 596	1 055	482	69.9	0.02	85	39.0	81	29.3
All ages	2 072 439	78 098	36 246	1 366	13.4	0.02	1 533	57.8	1 202	38.8
Females										
0-4	1 096 658	354 620	20 393	6 594	2.5	0.02	1 169	378.1	868	262.5
5-14	305 924	58 212	5 188	987	10.0	0.02	90	17.0	53	8.7
15-44	427 632	35 677	7 205	601	29.8	0.02	48	4.0	23	1.7
45-59	96 200	30 927	1 621	521	52.4	0.02	20	6.6	13	3.2
60+	75 068	27 884	1 265	470	70.8	0.02	86	32.0	87	25.9
All ages	2 001 482	76 578	35 672	1 365	14.4	0.02	1 414	54.1	1 044	34.1
Total	4 073 920	77 344	71 918	1 365	13.9	0.02	2 946	55.9	2 246	36.5

For epidemiological sources see Bern et al. 1996. For the methods used to estimate and project incidence, prevalence, and deaths see Murray and Lopez 1996a. See explanatory notes for definitions and caveats.

Table 49   **Cuadro 49**   **Tableau 49**
Pertussis   **Tosferina**   **Coqueluche**

Episodes   Episodios   Episodes

Table 49a   EME - PEMC - EMBE   Pertussis - Episodes

Age group (years)	Incidence 1990 Number ('000s)	Rate (per 100 000)	Prevalence 1990 Number ('000s)	Rate (per 100 000)	Avg. age at onset (years)	Average duration (years)	Deaths 1990 Number ('000s)	Rate (per 100 000)	Deaths 2000 (Projected) Number ('000s)	Rate (per 100 000)
Males										
0-4	230	873	19	72.8	0.5	0.08	0	0.1	0	0.1
5-14	58	108	5	9.0	10.0	0.08	0	0.0	0	0.0
15-44	0	0	0	0.0	-	-	0	0.0	0	0.0
45-59	0	0	0	0.0	-	-	0	0.0	0	0.0
60+	0	0	0	0.0	-	-	0	0.0	0	0.0
All ages	288	74	24	6.1	2.4	0.08	0	0.0	0	0.0
Females										
0-4	219	876	18	73.0	0.5	0.08	0	0.1	0	0.1
5-14	55	108	5	9.0	10.0	0.08	0	0.0	0	0.0
15-44	0	0	0	0.0	-	-	0	0.0	0	0.0
45-59	0	0	0	0.0	-	-	0	0.0	0	0.0
60+	0	0	0	0.0	-	-	0	0.0	0	0.0
All ages	274	67	23	5.6	2.4	0.08	0	0.0	0	0.0
Total	562	70	47	5.9	2.4	0.08	0	0.0	0	0.0

Table 49b   FSE - PEAS - AESE   Pertussis - Episodes

Age group (years)	Incidence 1990 Number ('000s)	Rate (per 100 000)	Prevalence 1990 Number ('000s)	Rate (per 100 000)	Avg. age at onset (years)	Average duration (years)	Deaths 1990 Number ('000s)	Rate (per 100 000)	Deaths 2000 (Projected) Number ('000s)	Rate (per 100 000)
Males										
0-4	224	1 625	19	135	0.5	0.08	0	0.0	0	0.0
5-14	56	204	5	17	10.0	0.08	0	0.0	0	0.0
15-44	0	0	0	0	-	-	0	0.0	0	0.0
45-59	0	0	0	0	-	-	0	0.0	0	0.0
60+	0	0	0	0	-	-	0	0.0	0	0.0
All ages	279	169	23	14	2.4	0.08	0	0.0	0	0.0
Females										
0-4	213	1 621	18	135	0.5	0.08	0	0.1	0	0.1
5-14	53	201	4	17	10.0	0.08	0	0.0	0	0.0
15-44	0	0	0	0	-	-	0	0.0	0	0.0
45-59	0	0	0	0	-	-	0	0.0	0	0.0
60+	0	0	0	0	-	-	0	0.0	0	0.0
All ages	266	147	22	12	2.4	0.08	0	0.0	0	0.0
Total	546	158	45	13	2.4	0.08	0	0.0	0	0.0

Table 49c   India - India - Inde   Pertussis - Episodes

Age group (years)	Incidence 1990 Number ('000s)	Rate (per 100 000)	Prevalence 1990 Number ('000s)	Rate (per 100 000)	Avg. age at onset (years)	Average duration (years)	Deaths 1990 Number ('000s)	Rate (per 100 000)	Deaths 2000 (Projected) Number ('000s)	Rate (per 100 000)
Males										
0-4	2 437	4 075	203	340	2.0	0.08	37	61.7	22	38.6
5-14	609	599	51	50	8.5	0.08	3	3.1	2	1.4
15-44	0	0	0	0	-	-	0	0.0	0	0.0
45-59	0	0	0	0	-	-	0	0.0	0	0.0
60+	0	0	0	0	-	-	0	0.0	0	0.0
All ages	3 046	693	254	58	3.3	0.08	40	9.1	23	4.6
Females										
0-4	2 321	4 094	193	341	2.0	0.08	36	63.9	21	38.3
5-14	580	609	48	51	8.5	0.08	3	3.4	2	1.5
15-44	0	0	0	0	-	-	0	0.0	0	0.0
45-59	0	0	0	0	-	-	0	0.0	0	0.0
60+	0	0	0	0	-	-	0	0.0	0	0.0
All ages	2 901	707	242	59	3.3	0.08	39	9.6	22	4.6
Total	5 947	700	496	58	3.3	0.08	80	9.4	46	4.6

For epidemiological sources see Galazka 1996b. For the methods used to estimate and project incidence, prevalence, and deaths see Murray and Lopez 1996a. See explanatory notes for definitions and caveats.

Table 49	Cuadro 49	Tableau 49
Pertussis	Tosferina	Coqueluche
Episodes	Episodios	Episodes

Table 49d — China - China - Chine — Pertussis - Episodes

Age group (years)	Incidence 1990 Number ('000s)	Rate (per 100 000)	Prevalence 1990 Number ('000s)	Rate (per 100 000)	Avg. age at onset (years)	Average duration (years)	Deaths 1990 Number ('000s)	Rate (per 100 000)	Deaths 2000 (Projected) Number ('000s)	Rate (per 100 000)
Males										
0-4	1 582	2 625	132	219	2.0	0.08	8	13.4	4	7.0
5-14	395	408	33	34	8.5	0.08	1	0.6	0	0.2
15-44	0	0	0	0	-	-	0	0.0	0	0.0
45-59	0	0	0	0	-	-	0	0.0	0	0.0
60+	0	0	0	0	-	-	0	0.0	0	0.0
All ages	1 977	338	165	28	3.3	0.08	9	1.5	4	0.7
Females										
0-4	1 506	2 600	126	217	2.0	0.08	8	13.1	4	6.5
5-14	377	417	31	35	8.5	0.08	1	0.6	0	0.2
15-44	0	0	0	0	-	-	0	0.0	0	0.0
45-59	0	0	0	0	-	-	0	0.0	0	0.0
60+	0	0	0	0	-	-	0	0.0	0	0.0
All ages	1 883	343	157	29	3.3	0.08	8	1.5	4	0.6
Total	3 860	340	322	28	3.3	0.08	17	1.5	8	0.6

Table 49e — OAI - OPAI - APAI — Pertussis - Episodes

Age group (years)	Incidence 1990 Number ('000s)	Rate (per 100 000)	Prevalence 1990 Number ('000s)	Rate (per 100 000)	Avg. age at onset (years)	Average duration (years)	Deaths 1990 Number ('000s)	Rate (per 100 000)	Deaths 2000 (Projected) Number ('000s)	Rate (per 100 000)
Males										
0-4	1 386	3 166	115	264	2.0	0.08	16	37.1	11	23.9
5-14	346	412	29	34	8.5	0.08	1	1.6	1	0.8
15-44	0	0	0	0	-	-	0	0.0	0	0.0
45-59	0	0	0	0	-	-	0	0.0	0	0.0
60+	0	0	0	0	-	-	0	0.0	0	0.0
All ages	1 732	505	144	42	3.3	0.08	18	5.1	11	2.8
Females										
0-4	1 320	3 143	110	262	2.0	0.08	15	34.5	9	21.5
5-14	330	411	27	34	8.5	0.08	1	1.5	1	0.7
15-44	0	0	0	0	-	-	0	0.0	0	0.0
45-59	0	0	0	0	-	-	0	0.0	0	0.0
60+	0	0	0	0	-	-	0	0.0	0	0.0
All ages	1 650	486	137	40	3.3	0.08	16	4.6	10	2.4
Total	3 382	495	282	41	3.3	0.08	33	4.9	21	2.6

Table 49f — SSA - ASS - ASS — Pertussis - Episodes

Age group (years)	Incidence 1990 Number ('000s)	Rate (per 100 000)	Prevalence 1990 Number ('000s)	Rate (per 100 000)	Avg. age at onset (years)	Average duration (years)	Deaths 1990 Number ('000s)	Rate (per 100 000)	Deaths 2000 (Projected) Number ('000s)	Rate (per 100 000)
Males										
0-4	3 539	7 454	295	621	2.0	0.08	71	150.0	71	108.0
5-14	885	1 259	74	105	8.5	0.08	7	9.4	5	5.0
15-44	0	0	0	0	-	-	0	0.0	0	0.0
45-59	0	0	0	0	-	-	0	0.0	0	0.0
60+	0	0	0	0	-	-	0	0.0	0	0.0
All ages	4 424	1 753	369	146	3.3	0.08	78	30.8	76	22.1
Females										
0-4	3 371	7 167	281	597	2.0	0.08	64	135.8	60	94.2
5-14	843	1 207	70	101	8.5	0.08	6	9.2	4	4.7
15-44	0	0	0	0	-	-	0	0.0	0	0.0
45-59	0	0	0	0	-	-	0	0.0	0	0.0
60+	0	0	0	0	-	-	0	0.0	0	0.0
All ages	4 214	1 633	351	136	3.3	0.08	70	27.2	64	18.5
Total	8 638	1 693	720	141	3.3	0.08	148	29.0	140	20.3

For epidemiological sources see Galazka 1996b. For the methods used to estimate and project incidence, prevalence, and deaths see Murray and Lopez 1996a. See explanatory notes for definitions and caveats.

Table 49	Cuadro 49	Tableau 49
Pertussis	Tosferina	Coqueluche
Episodes	Episodios	Episodes

Table 49g LAC - ALC - ALC   Pertussis - Episodes

Age group (years)	Incidence 1990 Number ('000s)	Rate (per 100 000)	Prevalence 1990 Number ('000s)	Rate (per 100 000)	Avg. age at onset (years)	Average duration (years)	Deaths 1990 Number ('000s)	Rate (per 100 000)	Deaths 2000 (Projected) Number ('000s)	Rate (per 100 000)
Males										
0-4	1 176	4 096	98	341	2.0	0.08	9	29.6	6	20.7
5-14	294	564	25	47	8.5	0.08	0	0.9	0	0.5
15-44	0	0	0	0	-	-	0	0.0	0	0.0
45-59	0	0	0	0	-	-	0	0.0	0	0.0
60+	0	0	0	0	-	-	0	0.0	0	0.0
All ages	1 470	664	123	55	3.3	0.08	9	4.1	6	2.4
Females										
0-4	1 120	4 048	93	337	2.0	0.08	8	27.3	5	18.6
5-14	280	552	23	46	8.5	0.08	1	1.0	0	0.6
15-44	0	0	0	0	-	-	0	0.0	0	0.0
45-59	0	0	0	0	-	-	0	0.0	0	0.0
60+	0	0	0	0	-	-	0	0.0	0	0.0
All ages	1 400	629	117	52	3.3	0.08	8	3.6	6	2.1
Total	2 871	646	239	54	3.3	0.08	17	3.8	12	2.2

Table 49h MEC - AOM - CMO   Pertussis - Episodes

Age group (years)	Incidence 1990 Number ('000s)	Rate (per 100 000)	Prevalence 1990 Number ('000s)	Rate (per 100 000)	Avg. age at onset (years)	Average duration (years)	Deaths 1990 Number ('000s)	Rate (per 100 000)	Deaths 2000 (Projected) Number ('000s)	Rate (per 100 000)
Males										
0-4	1 849	4 491	154	374	2.0	0.08	25	60.3	22	44.5
5-14	462	707	39	59	8.5	0.08	2	3.0	1	1.7
15-44	0	0	0	0	-	-	0	0.0	0	0.0
45-59	0	0	0	0	-	-	0	0.0	0	0.0
60+	0	0	0	0	-	-	0	0.0	0	0.0
All ages	2 311	901	193	75	3.3	0.08	27	10.4	24	7.1
Females										
0-4	1 760	4 431	147	369	2.0	0.08	24	59.5	20	42.4
5-14	440	710	37	59	8.5	0.08	2	3.1	1	1.7
15-44	0	0	0	0	-	-	0	0.0	0	0.0
45-59	0	0	0	0	-	-	0	0.0	0	0.0
60+	0	0	0	0	-	-	0	0.0	0	0.0
All ages	2 201	892	183	74	3.3	0.08	26	10.4	22	6.7
Total	4 511	897	376	75	3.3	0.08	52	10.4	45	6.9

Table 49i World - Mundo - Monde   Pertussis - Episodes

Age group (years)	Incidence 1990 Number ('000s)	Rate (per 100 000)	Prevalence 1990 Number ('000s)	Rate (per 100 000)	Avg. age at onset (years)	Average duration (years)	Deaths 1990 Number ('000s)	Rate (per 100 000)	Deaths 2000 (Projected) Number ('000s)	Rate (per 100 000)
Males										
0-4	12 422	3 866	1 035	322	1.9	0.08	166	51.6	136	39.3
5-14	3 106	563	259	47	8.6	0.08	14	2.6	9	1.4
15-44	0	0	0	0	-	-	0	0.0	0	0.0
45-59	0	0	0	0	-	-	0	0.0	0	0.0
60+	0	0	0	0	-	-	0	0.0	0	0.0
All ages	15 528	585	1 294	49	3.3	0.08	180	6.8	145	4.7
Females										
0-4	11 831	3 826	986	319	1.9	0.08	153	49.6	119	35.9
5-14	2 958	563	246	47	8.6	0.08	14	2.6	8	1.4
15-44	0	0	0	0	-	-	0	0.0	0	0.0
45-59	0	0	0	0	-	-	0	0.0	0	0.0
60+	0	0	0	0	-	-	0	0.0	0	0.0
All ages	14 788	566	1 232	47	3.3	0.08	167	6.4	127	4.2
Total	30 316	576	2 527	48	3.3	0.08	347	6.6	272	4.4

For epidemiological sources see Galazka 1996b. For the methods used to estimate and project incidence, prevalence, and deaths see Murray and Lopez 1996a. See explanatory notes for definitions and caveats.

Table 50
Pertussis

Cuadro 50
Tosferina

Tableau 50
Coqueluche

Mental retardation

Retraso mental

Retard mental

Table 50a		EME - PEMC - EMBE								Pertussis - Mental retardation
Age group (years)	Incidence 1990		Prevalence 1990		Avg. age at onset (years)	Average duration (years)	Deaths 1990		Deaths 2000 (Projected)	
	Number ('000s)	Rate (per 100 000)	Number ('000s)	Rate (per 100 000)			Number ('000s)	Rate (per 100 000)	Number ('000s)	Rate (per 100 000)
Males										
0-4	1	2.6	2	6.5	0.5	70.2	0	0	0	0
5-14	0	0.3	8	14.6	10.0	63.6	0	0	0	0
15-44	0	0.0	30	16.2	-	-	0	0	0	0
45-59	0	0.0	11	16.2	-	-	0	0	0	0
60+	0	0.0	10	16.2	-	-	0	0	0	0
All ages	1	0.2	60	15.4	2.4	68.9	0	0	0	0
Females										
0-4	1	2.6	2	6.6	0.5	76.1	0	0	0	0
5-14	0	0.3	7	14.7	10.0	69.5	0	0	0	0
15-44	0	0.0	29	16.3	-	-	0	0	0	0
45-59	0	0.0	11	16.3	-	-	0	0	0	0
60+	0	0.0	14	16.3	-	-	0	0	0	0
All ages	1	0.2	63	15.5	2.4	74.8	0	0	0	0
Total	2	0.2	123	15.4	2.4	71.8	0	0	0	0

Table 50b		FSE - PEAS - AESE								Pertussis - Mental retardation
Age group (years)	Incidence 1990		Prevalence 1990		Avg. age at onset (years)	Average duration (years)	Deaths 1990		Deaths 2000 (Projected)	
	Number ('000s)	Rate (per 100 000)	Number ('000s)	Rate (per 100 000)			Number ('000s)	Rate (per 100 000)	Number ('000s)	Rate (per 100 000)
Males										
0-4	1	4.9	2	12	0.5	63.5	0	0	0	0
5-14	0	0.6	7	27	10.0	57.3	0	0	0	0
15-44	0	0.0	23	30	-	-	0	0	0	0
45-59	0	0.0	8	30	-	-	0	0	0	0
60+	0	0.0	6	30	-	-	0	0	0	0
All ages	1	0.5	47	28	2.4	62.3	0	0	0	0
Females										
0-4	1	4.9	2	12	0.5	72.4	0	0	0	0
5-14	0	0.6	7	27	10.0	66.0	0	0	0	0
15-44	0	0.0	23	30	-	-	0	0	0	0
45-59	0	0.0	9	30	-	-	0	0	0	0
60+	0	0.0	11	30	-	-	0	0	0	0
All ages	1	0.4	51	28	2.4	71.1	0	0	0	0
Total	2	0.5	98	28	2.4	66.6	0	0	0	0

Table 50c		India - India - Inde								Pertussis - Mental retardation
Age group (years)	Incidence 1990		Prevalence 1990		Avg. age at onset (years)	Average duration (years)	Deaths 1990		Deaths 2000 (Projected)	
	Number ('000s)	Rate (per 100 000)	Number ('000s)	Rate (per 100 000)			Number ('000s)	Rate (per 100 000)	Number ('000s)	Rate (per 100 000)
Males										
0-4	7	12.2	18	30	2.0	59.9	0	0	0	0
5-14	2	1.8	71	70	8.5	57.4	0	0	0	0
15-44	0	0.0	158	79	-	-	0	0	0	0
45-59	0	0.0	37	79	-	-	0	0	0	0
60+	0	0.0	23	79	-	-	0	0	0	0
All ages	9	2.1	308	70	3.3	59.4	0	0	0	0
Females										
0-4	7	12.3	17	30	2.0	60.8	0	0	0	0
5-14	2	1.8	67	70	8.5	59.1	0	0	0	0
15-44	0	0.0	145	79	-	-	0	0	0	0
45-59	0	0.0	37	79	-	-	0	0	0	0
60+	0	0.0	23	79	-	-	0	0	0	0
All ages	9	2.1	289	70	3.3	60.5	0	0	0	0
Total	18	2.1	597	70	3.3	59.9	0	0	0	0

For epidemiological sources see Galazka 1996b. For the methods used to estimate and project incidence, prevalence, and deaths see Murray and Lopez 1996a. See explanatory notes for definitions and caveats.

Table 50	Cuadro 50	Tableau 50
Pertussis	Tosferina	Coqueluche
Mental retardation	Retraso mental	Retard mental

Table 50d — China - China - Chine — Pertussis - Mental retardation

Age group (years)	Incidence 1990 Number ('000s)	Incidence 1990 Rate (per 100 000)	Prevalence 1990 Number ('000s)	Prevalence 1990 Rate (per 100 000)	Avg. age at onset (years)	Average duration (years)	Deaths 1990 Number ('000s)	Deaths 1990 Rate (per 100 000)	Deaths 2000 (Projected) Number ('000s)	Deaths 2000 (Projected) Rate (per 100 000)
Males										
0-4	5	7.9	12	20	2.0	65.5	0	0	0	0
5-14	1	1.2	44	45	8.5	59.9	0	0	0	0
15-44	0	0.0	157	51	-	-	0	0	0	0
45-59	0	0.0	37	51	-	-	0	0	0	0
60+	0	0.0	25	51	-	-	0	0	0	0
All ages	6	1.0	276	47	3.3	64.4	0	0	0	0
Females										
0-4	5	7.8	11	19	2.0	68.5	0	0	0	0
5-14	1	1.2	41	45	8.5	63.2	0	0	0	0
15-44	0	0.0	146	51	-	-	0	0	0	0
45-59	0	0.0	33	51	-	-	0	0	0	0
60+	0	0.0	26	51	-	-	0	0	0	0
All ages	6	1.0	257	47	3.3	67.4	0	0	0	0
Total	12	1.0	533	47	3.3	65.9	0	0	0	0

Table 50e — OAI - OPAI - APAI — Pertussis - Mental retardation

Age group (years)	Incidence 1990 Number ('000s)	Incidence 1990 Rate (per 100 000)	Prevalence 1990 Number ('000s)	Prevalence 1990 Rate (per 100 000)	Avg. age at onset (years)	Average duration (years)	Deaths 1990 Number ('000s)	Deaths 1990 Rate (per 100 000)	Deaths 2000 (Projected) Number ('000s)	Deaths 2000 (Projected) Rate (per 100 000)
Males										
0-4	4	9.5	10	23	2.0	59.8	0	0	0	0
5-14	1	1.2	45	53	8.5	56.2	0	0	0	0
15-44	0	0.0	96	60	-	-	0	0	0	0
45-59	0	0.0	20	60	-	-	0	0	0	0
60+	0	0.0	12	60	-	-	0	0	0	0
All ages	5	1.5	184	54	3.3	59.1	0	0	0	0
Females										
0-4	4	9.4	10	23	2.0	63.2	0	0	0	0
5-14	1	1.2	43	53	8.5	59.2	0	0	0	0
15-44	0	0.0	94	59	-	-	0	0	0	0
45-59	0	0.0	21	59	-	-	0	0	0	0
60+	0	0.0	13	59	-	-	0	0	0	0
All ages	5	1.5	181	53	3.3	62.4	0	0	0	0
Total	10	1.5	365	53	3.3	60.7	0	0	0	0

Table 50f — SSA - ASS - ASS — Pertussis - Mental retardation

Age group (years)	Incidence 1990 Number ('000s)	Incidence 1990 Rate (per 100 000)	Prevalence 1990 Number ('000s)	Prevalence 1990 Rate (per 100 000)	Avg. age at onset (years)	Average duration (years)	Deaths 1990 Number ('000s)	Deaths 1990 Rate (per 100 000)	Deaths 2000 (Projected) Number ('000s)	Deaths 2000 (Projected) Rate (per 100 000)
Males										
0-4	11	22.4	26	54	2.0	48.7	0	0	0	0
5-14	3	3.8	91	130	8.5	49.2	0	0	0	0
15-44	0	0.0	155	149	-	-	0	0	0	0
45-59	0	0.0	30	149	-	-	0	0	0	0
60+	0	0.0	16	149	-	-	0	0	0	0
All ages	13	5.3	317	126	3.3	48.8	0	0	0	0
Females										
0-4	10	21.5	24	52	2.0	51.9	0	0	0	0
5-14	3	3.6	87	125	8.5	51.9	0	0	0	0
15-44	0	0.0	152	143	-	-	0	0	0	0
45-59	0	0.0	32	143	-	-	0	0	0	0
60+	0	0.0	18	143	-	-	0	0	0	0
All ages	13	4.9	314	122	3.3	51.9	0	0	0	0
Total	26	5.1	631	124	3.3	50.3	0	0	0	0

For epidemiological sources see Galazka 1996b. For the methods used to estimate and project incidence, prevalence, and deaths see Murray and Lopez 1996a. See explanatory notes for definitions and caveats.

Table 50	Cuadro 50	Tableau 50
Pertussis	**Tosferina**	**Coqueluche**
Mental retardation	Retraso mental	Retard mental

Table 50g LAC - ALC - ALC — Pertussis - Mental retardation

Age group (years)	Incidence 1990 Number ('000s)	Rate (per 100 000)	Prevalence 1990 Number ('000s)	Rate (per 100 000)	Avg. age at onset (years)	Average duration (years)	Deaths 1990 Number ('000s)	Rate (per 100 000)	Deaths 2000 (Projected) Number ('000s)	Rate (per 100 000)
Males										
0-4	4	12.3	9	30	2.0	63.9	0	0	0	0
5-14	1	1.7	36	70	8.5	59.3	0	0	0	0
15-44	0	0.0	81	78	-	-	0	0	0	0
45-59	0	0.0	17	78	-	-	0	0	0	0
60+	0	0.0	11	78	-	-	0	0	0	0
All ages	4	2.0	155	70	3.3	63.0	0	0	0	0
Females										
0-4	3	12.1	8	30	2.0	67.9	0	0	0	0
5-14	1	1.7	35	69	8.5	63.0	0	0	0	0
15-44	0	0.0	80	77	-	-	0	0	0	0
45-59	0	0.0	18	77	-	-	0	0	0	0
60+	0	0.0	13	77	-	-	0	0	0	0
All ages	4	1.9	154	69	3.3	66.9	0	0	0	0
Total	9	1.9	309	70	3.3	64.9	0	0	0	0

Table 50h MEC - AOM - CMO — Pertussis - Mental retardation

Age group (years)	Incidence 1990 Number ('000s)	Rate (per 100 000)	Prevalence 1990 Number ('000s)	Rate (per 100 000)	Avg. age at onset (years)	Average duration (years)	Deaths 1990 Number ('000s)	Rate (per 100 000)	Deaths 2000 (Projected) Number ('000s)	Rate (per 100 000)
Males										
0-4	6	13.5	14	33	2.0	61.1	0	0	0	0
5-14	1	2.1	51	78	8.5	58.1	0	0	0	0
15-44	0	0.0	100	88	-	-	0	0	0	0
45-59	0	0.0	20	88	-	-	0	0	0	0
60+	0	0.0	12	88	-	-	0	0	0	0
All ages	7	2.7	196	77	3.3	60.5	0	0	0	0
Females										
0-4	5	13.3	13	33	2.0	63.7	0	0	0	0
5-14	1	2.1	48	77	8.5	60.9	0	0	0	0
15-44	0	0.0	94	87	-	-	0	0	0	0
45-59	0	0.0	19	87	-	-	0	0	0	0
60+	0	0.0	14	87	-	-	0	0	0	0
All ages	7	2.7	187	76	3.3	63.1	0	0	0	0
Total	14	2.7	384	76	3.3	61.8	0	0	0	0

Table 50i World - Mundo - Monde — Pertussis - Mental retardation

Age group (years)	Incidence 1990 Number ('000s)	Rate (per 100 000)	Prevalence 1990 Number ('000s)	Rate (per 100 000)	Avg. age at onset (years)	Average duration (years)	Deaths 1990 Number ('000s)	Rate (per 100 000)	Deaths 2000 (Projected) Number ('000s)	Rate (per 100 000)
Males										
0-4	37	11.6	91	28	1.9	58.2	0	0	0	0
5-14	9	1.7	354	64	8.6	55.7	0	0	0	0
15-44	0	0.0	801	64	-	-	0	0	0	0
45-59	0	0.0	181	58	-	-	0	0	0	0
60+	0	0.0	116	53	-	-	0	0	0	0
All ages	47	1.8	1 543	58	3.3	57.7	0	0	0	0
Females										
0-4	35	11.5	87	28	1.9	61.1	0	0	0	0
5-14	9	1.7	335	64	8.6	58.5	0	0	0	0
15-44	0	0.0	763	64	-	-	0	0	0	0
45-59	0	0.0	180	58	-	-	0	0	0	0
60+	0	0.0	132	49	-	-	0	0	0	0
All ages	44	1.7	1 497	57	3.3	60.6	0	0	0	0
Total	91	1.7	3 039	58	3.3	59.1	0	0	0	0

For epidemiological sources see Galazka 1996b. For the methods used to estimate and project incidence, prevalence, and deaths see Murray and Lopez 1996a. See explanatory notes for definitions and caveats.

Table 51	Cuadro 51	Tableau 51
Poliomyelitis	Poliomielitis	Poliomyélite
Lameness	Paralítica	Paralytique

Table 51a EME - PEMC - EMBE — Poliomyelitis - Lameness

Age group (years)	Incidence 1990 Number ('000s)	Rate (per 100 000)	Prevalence 1990 Number ('000s)	Rate (per 100 000)	Avg. age at onset (years)	Average duration (years)	Deaths 1990 Number ('000s)	Rate (per 100 000)	Deaths 2000 (Projected) Number ('000s)	Rate (per 100 000)
Males										
0-4	0	0	-	-	-	-	0	0.0	0	0.0
5-14	0	0	-	-	-	-	0	0.0	0	0.0
15-44	0	0	-	-	-	-	0	0.0	0	0.0
45-59	0	0	-	-	-	-	0	0.0	0	0.0
60+	0	0	-	-	-	-	0	0.2	0	0.2
All ages	0	0	-	-	-	-	0	0.0	0	0.0
Females										
0-4	0	0	-	-	-	-	0	0.0	0	0.0
5-14	0	0	-	-	-	-	0	0.0	0	0.0
15-44	0	0	-	-	-	-	0	0.0	0	0.0
45-59	0	0	-	-	-	-	0	0.0	0	0.0
60+	0	0	-	-	-	-	0	0.1	0	0.1
All ages	0	0	-	-	-	-	0	0.0	0	0.0
Total	0	0	-	-	-	-	0	0.0	0	0.0

Table 51b FSE - PEAS - AESE — Poliomyelitis - Lameness

Age group (years)	Incidence 1990 Number ('000s)	Rate (per 100 000)	Prevalence 1990 Number ('000s)	Rate (per 100 000)	Avg. age at onset (years)	Average duration (years)	Deaths 1990 Number ('000s)	Rate (per 100 000)	Deaths 2000 (Projected) Number ('000s)	Rate (per 100 000)
Males										
0-4	0	0	0	0	-	-	0	0	0	0
5-14	0	0	0	0	-	-	0	0	0	0
15-44	0	0	0	0	-	-	0	0	0	0
45-59	0	0	0	0	-	-	0	0	0	0
60+	0	0	0	0	-	-	0	0	0	0
All ages	0	0	0	0	-	-	0	0	0	0
Females										
0-4	0	0	0	0	-	-	0	0	0	0
5-14	0	0	0	0	-	-	0	0	0	0
15-44	0	0	0	0	-	-	0	0	0	0
45-59	0	0	0	0	-	-	0	0	0	0
60+	0	0	0	0	-	-	0	0	0	0
All ages	0	0	0	0	-	-	0	0	0	0
Total	0	0	0	0	-	-	0	0	0	0

Table 51c India - India - Inde — Poliomyelitis - Lameness

Age group (years)	Incidence 1990 Number ('000s)	Rate (per 100 000)	Prevalence 1990 Number ('000s)	Rate (per 100 000)	Avg. age at onset (years)	Average duration (years)	Deaths 1990 Number ('000s)	Rate (per 100 000)	Deaths 2000 (Projected) Number ('000s)	Rate (per 100 000)
Males										
0-4	46	77.5	141	236	2.5	58.7	6	10.4	4	6.5
5-14	0	0.2	690	678	9.7	56.4	0	0.0	0	0.0
15-44	1	0.7	1 500	748	29.8	38.7	0	0.0	0	0.0
45-59	0	0.3	362	760	52.2	20.0	0	0.0	0	0.0
60+	0	0.0	227	763	69.7	9.8	0	0.0	0	0.0
All ages	48	11.0	2 920	664	3.5	58.0	6	1.4	4	0.7
Females										
0-4	34	59.8	103	181	2.5	59.6	5	8.3	3	5.0
5-14	0	0.2	498	525	9.7	57.8	0	0.0	0	0.0
15-44	1	0.5	1 056	576	29.8	40.7	0	0.0	0	0.0
45-59	0	0.3	270	586	52.3	21.5	0	0.0	0	0.0
60+	0	0.0	170	588	70.1	10.1	0	0.0	0	0.0
All ages	35	8.6	2 096	511	3.5	58.9	5	1.2	3	0.6
Total	83	9.8	5 016	590	3.5	58.4	11	1.3	6	0.6

For epidemiological sources see Shibuya et al. 1996. For the methods used to estimate and project incidence, prevalence, and deaths see Murray and Lopez 1996a. See explanatory notes for definitions and caveats.

Table 51 **Poliomyelitis**

Cuadro 51 **Poliomielitis**

Tableau 51 **Poliomyélite**

Lameness Paralítica Paralytique

Table 51d   China - China - Chine — Poliomyelitis - Lameness

Age group (years)	Incidence 1990 Number ('000s)	Rate (per 100 000)	Prevalence 1990 Number ('000s)	Rate (per 100 000)	Avg. age at onset (years)	Average duration (years)	Deaths 1990 Number ('000s)	Rate (per 100 000)	Deaths 2000 (Projected) Number ('000s)	Rate (per 100 000)
Males										
0-4	13	20.8	32	53	2.5	64.5	1	2.3	1	1.2
5-14	0	0.1	106	109	10.0	59.0	0	0.0	0	0.0
15-44	1	0.3	355	116	29.9	40.5	0	0.0	0	0.0
45-59	0	0.2	89	122	52.3	20.7	0	0.0	0	0.0
60+	0	0.0	60	123	69.6	9.6	0	0.0	0	0.0
All ages	14	2.4	642	110	5.1	62.3	1	0.2	1	0.1
Females										
0-4	9	16.0	24	41	2.5	67.5	1	1.8	0	0.9
5-14	0	0.1	76	84	10.0	62.3	0	0.0	0	0.0
15-44	1	0.3	253	89	29.9	43.6	0	0.0	0	0.0
45-59	0	0.1	61	94	52.4	23.3	0	0.0	0	0.0
60+	0	0.0	49	95	70.6	10.6	0	0.0	0	0.0
All ages	10	1.9	463	84	5.0	65.4	1	0.2	1	0.1
Total	24	2.1	1 104	97	5.0	63.6	3	0.2	1	0.1

Table 51e   OAI - OPAI - APAI — Poliomyelitis - Lameness

Age group (years)	Incidence 1990 Number ('000s)	Rate (per 100 000)	Prevalence 1990 Number ('000s)	Rate (per 100 000)	Avg. age at onset (years)	Average duration (years)	Deaths 1990 Number ('000s)	Rate (per 100 000)	Deaths 2000 (Projected) Number ('000s)	Rate (per 100 000)
Males										
0-4	14	31.2	37	83	2.5	60.8	2	4.2	1	2.7
5-14	0	0.2	180	214	10.0	57.8	0	0.0	0	0.0
15-44	1	0.5	376	234	29.8	40.1	0	0.1	0	0.0
45-59	0	0.3	83	243	52.3	21.2	0	0.0	0	0.0
60+	0	0.0	50	245	70.1	10.1	0	0.0	0	0.0
All ages	15	4.3	725	211	4.4	59.4	2	0.6	1	0.3
Females										
0-4	10	24.0	27	64	2.5	64.9	1	3.0	1	1.9
5-14	0	0.1	132	165	10.0	61.4	0	0.0	0	0.0
15-44	1	0.4	287	180	29.8	43.3	0	0.0	0	0.0
45-59	0	0.2	66	187	52.4	23.6	0	0.0	0	0.0
60+	0	0.0	43	189	70.8	10.8	0	0.0	0	0.0
All ages	11	3.2	555	163	4.5	63.4	1	0.4	1	0.2
Total	26	3.8	1 280	188	4.5	61.1	3	0.5	2	0.3

Table 51f   SSA - ASS - ASS — Poliomyelitis - Lameness

Age group (years)	Incidence 1990 Number ('000s)	Rate (per 100 000)	Prevalence 1990 Number ('000s)	Rate (per 100 000)	Avg. age at onset (years)	Average duration (years)	Deaths 1990 Number ('000s)	Rate (per 100 000)	Deaths 2000 (Projected) Number ('000s)	Rate (per 100 000)
Males										
0-4	21	45.1	58	122	2.4	50.6	3	5.6	3	4.0
5-14	0	0.2	213	303	9.8	50.9	0	0.0	0	0.0
15-44	1	0.5	339	326	29.5	36.1	0	0.1	0	0.0
45-59	0	0.3	68	336	52.2	19.7	0	0.0	0	0.0
60+	0	0.0	36	339	69.5	9.5	0	0.0	0	0.0
All ages	22	8.8	714	283	3.2	50.2	3	1.1	3	0.8
Females										
0-4	16	34.7	44	94	2.4	53.8	2	4.1	2	2.8
5-14	0	0.1	163	234	9.8	53.5	0	0.0	0	0.0
15-44	0	0.4	267	251	29.5	38.2	0	0.1	0	0.0
45-59	0	0.2	57	259	52.3	21.1	0	0.0	0	0.0
60+	0	0.0	33	261	70.0	10.0	0	0.0	0	0.0
All ages	17	6.5	565	219	3.3	53.3	2	0.8	2	0.5
Total	39	7.6	1 279	251	3.2	51.6	5	0.9	5	0.7

For epidemiological sources see Shibuya et al. 1996. For the methods used to estimate and project incidence, prevalence, and deaths see Murray and Lopez 1996a. See explanatory notes for definitions and caveats.

Table 51 **Cuadro 51** **Tableau 51**
Poliomyelitis **Poliomielitis** **Poliomyélite**

Lameness Paralítica Paralytique

Table 51g LAC - ALC - ALC Poliomyelitis - Lameness

Age group (years)	Incidence 1990 Number ('000s)	Rate (per 100 000)	Prevalence 1990 Number ('000s)	Rate (per 100 000)	Avg. age at onset (years)	Average duration (years)	Deaths 1990 Number ('000s)	Rate (per 100 000)	Deaths 2000 (Projected) Number ('000s)	Rate (per 100 000)
Males										
0-4	7	25.8	20	70	2.5	64.0	1	3.1	1	2.1
5-14	0	0.1	87	167	9.8	59.5	0	0.0	0	0.0
15-44	0	0.2	186	178	29.8	41.8	0	0.0	0	0.0
45-59	0	0.1	41	182	52.3	23.0	0	0.0	0	0.0
60+	0	0.0	26	183	70.9	10.9	0	0.0	0	0.0
All ages	8	3.5	360	162	3.5	63.1	1	0.4	1	0.2
Females										
0-4	5	19.9	18	65	2.5	68.2	1	2.2	0	1.5
5-14	0	0.1	119	235	9.8	63.4	0	0.0	0	0.0
15-44	0	0.2	280	269	29.8	45.0	0	0.0	0	0.0
45-59	0	0.1	63	270	52.4	25.3	0	0.0	0	0.0
60+	0	0.0	46	271	71.6	11.6	0	0.0	0	0.0
All ages	6	2.6	526	120	3.6	67.3	1	0.3	0	0.2
Total	13	3.0	886	144	3.6	64.9	2	0.3	1	0.2

Table 51h MEC - AOM - CMO Poliomyelitis - Lameness

Age group (years)	Incidence 1990 Number ('000s)	Rate (per 100 000)	Prevalence 1990 Number ('000s)	Rate (per 100 000)	Avg. age at onset (years)	Average duration (years)	Deaths 1990 Number ('000s)	Rate (per 100 000)	Deaths 2000 (Projected) Number ('000s)	Rate (per 100 000)
Males										
0-4	17	40.3	45	109	2.5	61.6	2	5.2	2	3.8
5-14	0	0.2	172	263	9.8	58.8	0	0.0	0	0.0
15-44	1	0.5	321	282	29.8	40.8	0	0.0	0	0.0
45-59	0	0.2	65	291	52.3	21.5	0	0.0	0	0.0
60+	0	0.0	40	293	70.1	10.1	0	0.0	0	0.0
All ages	17	6.7	643	251	3.5	60.8	2	0.8	2	0.6
Females										
0-4	12	31.0	33	84	2.5	64.4	2	4.0	1	2.8
5-14	0	0.1	125	202	9.8	61.7	0	0.0	0	0.0
15-44	0	0.4	233	217	29.9	43.6	0	0.0	0	0.0
45-59	0	0.2	50	224	52.4	23.7	0	0.0	0	0.0
60+	0	0.0	35	225	70.8	10.8	0	0.0	0	0.0
All ages	13	5.2	476	193	3.5	63.6	2	0.7	1	0.4
Total	30	6.0	1 119	222	3.5	62.0	4	0.7	3	0.5

Table 51i World - Mundo - Monde Poliomyelitis - Lameness

Age group (years)	Incidence 1990 Number ('000s)	Rate (per 100 000)	Prevalence 1990 Number ('000s)	Rate (per 100 000)	Avg. age at onset (years)	Average duration (years)	Deaths 1990 Number ('000s)	Rate (per 100 000)	Deaths 2000 (Projected) Number ('000s)	Rate (per 100 000)
Males										
0-4	118	36.7	332	103	2.5	58.9	15	4.7	11	3.1
5-14	1	0.1	1 448	263	9.8	56.6	0	0.0	0	0.0
15-44	5	0.4	3 076	246	29.8	39.5	0	0.0	0	0.0
45-59	0	0.2	707	226	52.3	20.7	0	0.0	0	0.0
60+	0	0.0	439	201	69.8	9.9	0	0.1	0	0.1
All ages	124	4.7	6 002	226	3.8	58.0	16	0.6	11	0.4
Females										
0-4	87	28.3	249	80	2.5	61.2	11	3.6	8	2.3
5-14	1	0.1	1 114	212	9.8	59.2	0	0.0	0	0.0
15-44	3	0.3	2 377	198	29.8	42.1	0	0.0	0	0.0
45-59	0	0.1	566	182	52.4	22.7	0	0.0	0	0.0
60+	0	0.0	376	140	70.5	10.5	0	0.0	0	0.0
All ages	92	3.5	4 682	179	3.7	60.3	12	0.4	8	0.3
Total	215	4.1	10 684	203	3.8	59.0	27	0.5	19	0.3

For epidemiological sources see Shibuya et al. 1996. For the methods used to estimate and project incidence, prevalence, and deaths see Murray and Lopez 1996a. See explanatory notes for definitions and caveats.

Table 52 | Cuadro 52 | Tableau 52
Diphtheria | Difteria | Diphtérie

Episodes | Episodios | Episodes

Table 52a — EME - PEMC - EMBE — Diphtheria - Episodes

Age group (years)	Incidence 1990 Number ('000s)	Incidence 1990 Rate (per 100 000)	Prevalence 1990 Number ('000s)	Prevalence 1990 Rate (per 100 000)	Avg. age at onset (years)	Average duration (years)	Deaths 1990 Number ('000s)	Deaths 1990 Rate (per 100 000)	Deaths 2000 (Projected) Number ('000s)	Deaths 2000 (Projected) Rate (per 100 000)
Males										
0-4	0	0.0	0	0.0	0.5	0.04	0	0	0	0
5-14	0	0.0	0	0.0	10.0	0.04	0	0	0	0
15-44	0	0.0	0	0.0	35.0	0.04	0	0	0	0
45-59	0	0.0	0	0.0	55.0	0.04	0	0	0	0
60+	0	0.0	0	0.0	-	-	0	0	0	0
All ages	0	0.0	0	0.0	27.7	0.04	0	0	0	0
Females										
0-4	0	0.0	0	0.0	0.5	0.04	0	0	0	0
5-14	0	0.0	0	0.0	10.0	0.04	0	0	0	0
15-44	0	0.0	0	0.0	35.0	0.04	0	0	0	0
45-59	0	0.0	0	0.0	55.0	0.04	0	0	0	0
60+	0	0.0	0	0.0	-	-	0	0	0	0
All ages	0	0.0	0	0.0	27.7	0.04	0	0	0	0
Total	0	0.0	0	0.0	27.7	0.04	0	0	0	0

Table 52b — FSE - PEAS - AESE — Diphtheria - Episodes

Age group (years)	Incidence 1990 Number ('000s)	Incidence 1990 Rate (per 100 000)	Prevalence 1990 Number ('000s)	Prevalence 1990 Rate (per 100 000)	Avg. age at onset (years)	Average duration (years)	Deaths 1990 Number ('000s)	Deaths 1990 Rate (per 100 000)	Deaths 2000 (Projected) Number ('000s)	Deaths 2000 (Projected) Rate (per 100 000)
Males										
0-4	0	0.5	0	0.0	0.5	0.04	0	0.1	0	0.1
5-14	0	0.7	0	0.0	10.0	0.04	0	0.0	0	0.0
15-44	0	0.5	0	0.0	35.0	0.04	0	0.0	0	0.0
45-59	0	0.3	0	0.0	55.0	0.04	0	0.0	0	0.0
60+	0	0.0	0	0.0	-	-	0	0.0	0	0.0
All ages	1	0.4	0	0.0	27.5	0.04	0	0.0	0	0.0
Females										
0-4	0	0.5	0	0.0	0.5	0.04	0	0.1	0	0.1
5-14	0	0.6	0	0.0	10.0	0.04	0	0.0	0	0.0
15-44	0	0.5	0	0.0	35.0	0.04	0	0.0	0	0.0
45-59	0	0.3	0	0.0	55.0	0.04	0	0.0	0	0.0
60+	0	0.0	0	0.0	-	-	0	0.0	0	0.0
All ages	1	0.4	0	0.0	27.6	0.04	0	0.0	0	0.0
Total	1	0.4	0	0.0	27.6	0.04	0	0.0	0	0.0

Table 52c — India - India - Inde — Diphtheria - Episodes

Age group (years)	Incidence 1990 Number ('000s)	Incidence 1990 Rate (per 100 000)	Prevalence 1990 Number ('000s)	Prevalence 1990 Rate (per 100 000)	Avg. age at onset (years)	Average duration (years)	Deaths 1990 Number ('000s)	Deaths 1990 Rate (per 100 000)	Deaths 2000 (Projected) Number ('000s)	Deaths 2000 (Projected) Rate (per 100 000)
Males										
0-4	13	21.7	0	0.8	0.5	0.04	2	3.3	1	2.1
5-14	6	6.4	0	0.2	10.0	0.04	0	0.2	0	0.1
15-44	2	1.0	0	0.0	35.0	0.04	0	0.0	0	0.0
45-59	0	0.4	0	0.0	55.0	0.04	0	0.0	0	0.0
60+	0	0.0	0	0.0	-	-	0	0.0	0	0.0
All ages	22	4.9	1	0.2	7.0	0.04	2	0.5	1	0.3
Females										
0-4	12	21.8	0	0.8	0.5	0.04	2	3.4	1	2.0
5-14	6	6.5	0	0.2	10.0	0.04	0	0.2	0	0.1
15-44	2	1.0	0	0.0	35.0	0.04	0	0.0	0	0.0
45-59	0	0.4	0	0.0	55.0	0.04	0	0.0	0	0.0
60+	0	0.0	0	0.0	-	-	0	0.0	0	0.0
All ages	21	5.0	1	0.2	7.0	0.04	2	0.5	1	0.3
Total	42	5.0	2	0.2	7.0	0.04	4	0.5	3	0.3

For epidemiological sources see Galazka 1996a. For the methods used to estimate and project incidence, prevalence, and deaths see Murray and Lopez 1996a. See explanatory notes for definitions and caveats.

Table 52	Cuadro 52	Tableau 52
Diphtheria	**Difteria**	**Diphtérie**

Episodes	Episodios	Episodes

Table 52d   China - China - Chine   Diphtheria - Episodes

Age group (years)	Incidence 1990 Number ('000s)	Rate (per 100 000)	Prevalence 1990 Number ('000s)	Rate (per 100 000)	Avg. age at onset (years)	Average duration (years)	Deaths 1990 Number ('000s)	Rate (per 100 000)	Deaths 2000 (Projected) Number ('000s)	Rate (per 100 000)
Males										
0-4	1	1.1	0	0.0	0.5	0.04	0	0.2	0	0.1
5-14	0	0.3	0	0.0	10.0	0.04	0	0.0	0	0.0
15-44	0	0.0	0	0.0	35.0	0.04	0	0.0	0	0.0
45-59	0	0.0	0	0.0	55.0	0.04	0	0.0	0	0.0
60+	0	0.0	0	0.0	-	-	0	0.0	0	0.0
All ages	1	0.2	0	0.0	7.0	0.04	0	0.0	0	0.0
Females										
0-4	1	1.1	0	0.0	0.5	0.04	0	0.2	0	0.1
5-14	0	0.3	0	0.0	10.0	0.04	0	0.0	0	0.0
15-44	0	0.0	0	0.0	35.0	0.04	0	0.0	0	0.0
45-59	0	0.0	0	0.0	55.0	0.04	0	0.0	0	0.0
60+	0	0.0	0	0.0	-	-	0	0.0	0	0.0
All ages	1	0.2	0	0.0	7.0	0.04	0	0.0	0	0.0
Total	2	0.2	0	0.0	7.0	0.04	0	0.0	0	0.0

Table 52e   OAI - OPAI - APAI   Diphtheria - Episodes

Age group (years)	Incidence 1990 Number ('000s)	Rate (per 100 000)	Prevalence 1990 Number ('000s)	Rate (per 100 000)	Avg. age at onset (years)	Average duration (years)	Deaths 1990 Number ('000s)	Rate (per 100 000)	Deaths 2000 (Projected) Number ('000s)	Rate (per 100 000)
Males										
0-4	7	16.9	0	0.6	0.5	0.04	1	2.5	1	1.6
5-14	4	4.4	0	0.2	10.0	0.04	0	0.1	0	0.1
15-44	1	0.7	0	0.0	35.0	0.04	0	0.0	0	0.0
45-59	0	0.3	0	0.0	55.0	0.04	0	0.0	0	0.0
60+	0	0.0	0	0.0	-	-	0	0.0	0	0.0
All ages	12	3.6	0	0.1	7.0	0.04	1	0.4	1	0.2
Females										
0-4	7	16.7	0	0.6	0.5	0.04	1	2.4	1	1.5
5-14	4	4.4	0	0.2	10.0	0.04	0	0.1	0	0.1
15-44	1	0.7	0	0.0	35.0	0.04	0	0.0	0	0.0
45-59	0	0.3	0	0.0	55.0	0.04	0	0.0	0	0.0
60+	0	0.0	0	0.0	-	-	0	0.0	0	0.0
All ages	12	3.4	0	0.1	7.0	0.04	1	0.3	1	0.2
Total	24	3.5	1	0.1	7.0	0.04	2	0.3	1	0.2

Table 52f   SSA - ASS - ASS   Diphtheria - Episodes

Age group (years)	Incidence 1990 Number ('000s)	Rate (per 100 000)	Prevalence 1990 Number ('000s)	Rate (per 100 000)	Avg. age at onset (years)	Average duration (years)	Deaths 1990 Number ('000s)	Rate (per 100 000)	Deaths 2000 (Projected) Number ('000s)	Rate (per 100 000)
Males										
0-4	6	12.5	0	0.5	0.5	0.04	1	1.8	1	1.3
5-14	3	4.2	0	0.2	10.0	0.04	0	0.1	0	0.1
15-44	1	0.9	0	0.0	35.0	0.04	0	0.0	0	0.0
45-59	0	0.4	0	0.0	55.0	0.04	0	0.0	0	0.0
60+	0	0.0	0	0.0	-	-	0	0.0	0	0.0
All ages	10	3.9	0	0.2	6.9	0.04	1	0.4	1	0.3
Females										
0-4	6	12.0	0	0.5	0.5	0.04	1	1.6	1	1.1
5-14	3	4.0	0	0.2	10.0	0.04	0	0.1	0	0.1
15-44	1	0.8	0	0.0	35.0	0.04	0	0.0	0	0.0
45-59	0	0.3	0	0.0	55.0	0.04	0	0.0	0	0.0
60+	0	0.0	0	0.0	-	-	0	0.0	0	0.0
All ages	9	3.6	0	0.1	7.0	0.04	1	0.3	1	0.2
Total	19	3.8	1	0.1	6.9	0.04	2	0.4	2	0.2

For epidemiological sources see Galazka 1996a. For the methods used to estimate and project incidence, prevalence, and deaths see Murray and Lopez 1996a. See explanatory notes for definitions and caveats.

Table 52
Diphtheria

Cuadro 52
Difteria

Tableau 52
Diphtérie

Episodes

Episodios

Episodes

Table 52g — LAC - ALC - ALC — Diphtheria - Episodes

Age group (years)	Incidence 1990 Number ('000s)	Rate (per 100 000)	Prevalence 1990 Number ('000s)	Rate (per 100 000)	Avg. age at onset (years)	Average duration (years)	Deaths 1990 Number ('000s)	Rate (per 100 000)	Deaths 2000 (Projected) Number ('000s)	Rate (per 100 000)
Males										
0-4	2	5.4	0	0.2	0.5	0.04	0	0.5	0	0.4
5-14	1	1.5	0	0.1	10.0	0.04	0	0.1	0	0.1
15-44	0	0.2	0	0.0	35.0	0.04	0	0.0	0	0.0
45-59	0	0.1	0	0.0	55.0	0.04	0	0.0	0	0.0
60+	0	0.0	0	0.0	-	-	0	0.0	0	0.0
All ages	3	1.2	0	0.0	7.0	0.04	0	0.1	0	0.1
Females										
0-4	1	5.3	0	0.2	0.5	0.04	0	0.4	0	0.3
5-14	1	1.4	0	0.1	10.0	0.04	0	0.2	0	0.1
15-44	0	0.2	0	0.0	35.0	0.04	0	0.0	0	0.0
45-59	0	0.1	0	0.0	55.0	0.04	0	0.0	0	0.0
60+	0	0.0	0	0.0	-	-	0	0.0	0	0.0
All ages	2	1.1	0	0.0	7.0	0.04	0	0.1	0	0.1
Total	5	1.1	0	0.0	7.0	0.04	0	0.1	0	0.1

Table 52h — MEC - AOM - CMO — Diphtheria - Episodes

Age group (years)	Incidence 1990 Number ('000s)	Rate (per 100 000)	Prevalence 1990 Number ('000s)	Rate (per 100 000)	Avg. age at onset (years)	Average duration (years)	Deaths 1990 Number ('000s)	Rate (per 100 000)	Deaths 2000 (Projected) Number ('000s)	Rate (per 100 000)
Males										
0-4	4	9.0	0	0.3	0.5	0.04	1	1.3	0	1.0
5-14	2	2.8	0	0.1	10.0	0.04	0	0.1	0	0.0
15-44	1	0.5	0	0.0	35.0	0.04	0	0.0	0	0.0
45-59	0	0.2	0	0.0	55.0	0.04	0	0.0	0	0.0
60+	0	0.0	0	0.0	-	-	0	0.0	0	0.0
All ages	6	2.4	0	0.1	6.9	0.04	1	0.2	1	0.2
Females										
0-4	4	8.8	0	0.3	0.5	0.04	1	1.3	0	0.9
5-14	2	2.8	0	0.1	10.0	0.04	0	0.1	0	0.0
15-44	1	0.5	0	0.0	35.0	0.04	0	0.0	0	0.0
45-59	0	0.2	0	0.0	55.0	0.04	0	0.0	0	0.0
60+	0	0.0	0	0.0	-	-	0	0.0	0	0.0
All ages	6	2.4	0	0.1	6.9	0.04	1	0.2	0	0.2
Total	12	2.4	0	0.1	6.9	0.04	1	0.2	1	0.2

Table 52i — World - Mundo - Monde — Diphtheria - Episodes

Age group (years)	Incidence 1990 Number ('000s)	Rate (per 100 000)	Prevalence 1990 Number ('000s)	Rate (per 100 000)	Avg. age at onset (years)	Average duration (years)	Deaths 1990 Number ('000s)	Rate (per 100 000)	Deaths 2000 (Projected) Number ('000s)	Rate (per 100 000)
Males										
0-4	32	10.0	1	0.4	0.5	0.04	5	1.5	3	1.0
5-14	16	2.9	1	0.1	10.0	0.04	1	0.1	0	0.1
15-44	5	0.4	0	0.0	35.0	0.04	0	0.0	0	0.0
45-59	0	0.2	0	0.0	55.0	0.04	0	0.0	0	0.0
60+	0	0.0	0	0.0	-	-	0	0.0	0	0.0
All ages	54	2.0	2	0.1	7.2	0.04	5	0.2	4	0.1
Females										
0-4	31	9.9	1	0.4	0.5	0.04	4	1.4	3	0.9
5-14	15	2.9	1	0.1	10.0	0.04	1	0.1	0	0.1
15-44	5	0.4	0	0.0	35.0	0.04	0	0.0	0	0.0
45-59	0	0.2	0	0.0	55.0	0.04	0	0.0	0	0.0
60+	0	0.0	0	0.0	-	-	0	0.0	0	0.0
All ages	52	2.0	2	0.1	7.2	0.04	5	0.2	3	0.1
Total	106	2.0	4	0.1	7.2	0.04	11	0.2	7	0.1

For epidemiological sources see Galazka 1996a. For the methods used to estimate and project incidence, prevalence, and deaths see Murray and Lopez 1996a. See explanatory notes for definitions and caveats.

Table 53	Cuadro 53	Tableau 53
Diphtheria	Difteria	Diphtérie

Neurological complications   Complicaciones neurológicas   Complications neurologiques

Table 53a   EME - PEMC - EMBE   Diphtheria - Neurological complications

Age group (years)	Incidence 1990 Number ('000s)	Rate (per 100 000)	Prevalence 1990 Number ('000s)	Rate (per 100 000)	Avg. age at onset (years)	Average duration (years)	Deaths 1990 Number ('000s)	Rate (per 100 000)	Deaths 2000 (Projected) Number ('000s)	Rate (per 100 000)
Males										
0-4	0	0.0	0	0.0	0.5	0.17	0	0	0	0
5-14	0	0.0	0	0.0	10.0	0.17	0	0	0	0
15-44	0	0.0	0	0.0	35.0	0.17	0	0	0	0
45-59	0	0.0	0	0.0	55.0	0.17	0	0	0	0
60+	0	0.0	0	0.0	-	-	0	0	0	0
All ages	0	0.0	0	0.0	27.7	0.17	0	0	0	0
Females										
0-4	0	0.0	0	0.0	0.5	0.17	0	0	0	0
5-14	0	0.0	0	0.0	10.0	0.17	0	0	0	0
15-44	0	0.0	0	0.0	35.0	0.17	0	0	0	0
45-59	0	0.0	0	0.0	55.0	0.17	0	0	0	0
60+	0	0.0	0	0.0	-	-	0	0	0	0
All ages	0	0.0	0	0.0	27.7	0.17	0	0	0	0
Total	0	0.0	0	0.0	27.7	0.17	0	0	0	0

Table 53b   FSE - PEAS - AESE   Diphtheria - Neurological complications

Age group (years)	Incidence 1990 Number ('000s)	Rate (per 100 000)	Prevalence 1990 Number ('000s)	Rate (per 100 000)	Avg. age at onset (years)	Average duration (years)	Deaths 1990 Number ('000s)	Rate (per 100 000)	Deaths 2000 (Projected) Number ('000s)	Rate (per 100 000)
Males										
0-4	0	0.1	0	0.0	0.5	0.17	0	0	0	0
5-14	0	0.1	0	0.0	10.0	0.17	0	0	0	0
15-44	0	0.1	0	0.0	35.0	0.17	0	0	0	0
45-59	0	0.1	0	0.0	55.0	0.17	0	0	0	0
60+	0	0.0	0	0.0	-	-	0	0	0	0
All ages	0	0.1	0	0.0	27.5	0.17	0	0	0	0
Females										
0-4	0	0.1	0	0.0	0.5	0.17	0	0	0	0
5-14	0	0.1	0	0.0	10.0	0.17	0	0	0	0
15-44	0	0.1	0	0.0	35.0	0.17	0	0	0	0
45-59	0	0.1	0	0.0	55.0	0.17	0	0	0	0
60+	0	0.0	0	0.0	-	-	0	0	0	0
All ages	0	0.1	0	0.0	27.6	0.17	0	0	0	0
Total	0	0.1	0	0.0	27.6	0.17	0	0	0	0

Table 53c   India - India - Inde   Diphtheria - Neurological complications

Age group (years)	Incidence 1990 Number ('000s)	Rate (per 100 000)	Prevalence 1990 Number ('000s)	Rate (per 100 000)	Avg. age at onset (years)	Average duration (years)	Deaths 1990 Number ('000s)	Rate (per 100 000)	Deaths 2000 (Projected) Number ('000s)	Rate (per 100 000)
Males										
0-4	3	4.3	0	0.7	0.5	0.17	0	0	0	0
5-14	1	1.3	0	0.2	10.0	0.17	0	0	0	0
15-44	0	0.2	0	0.0	35.0	0.17	0	0	0	0
45-59	0	0.1	0	0.0	55.0	0.17	0	0	0	0
60+	0	0.0	0	0.0	-	-	0	0	0	0
All ages	4	1.0	1	0.2	7.0	0.17	0	0	0	0
Females										
0-4	2	4.4	0	0.7	0.5	0.17	0	0	0	0
5-14	1	1.3	0	0.2	10.0	0.17	0	0	0	0
15-44	0	0.2	0	0.0	35.0	0.17	0	0	0	0
45-59	0	0.1	0	0.0	55.0	0.17	0	0	0	0
60+	0	0.0	0	0.0	-	-	0	0	0	0
All ages	4	1.0	1	0.2	7.0	0.17	0	0	0	0
Total	8	1.0	1	0.2	7.0	0.17	0	0	0	0

For epidemiological sources see Galazka 1996a. For the methods used to estimate and project incidence, prevalence, and deaths see Murray and Lopez 1996a. See explanatory notes for definitions and caveats.

Table 53 — Cuadro 53 — Tableau 53
Diphtheria — Difteria — Diphtérie

Neurological complications — Complicaciones neurológicas — Complications neurologiques

Table 53d — China - China - Chine
Diphtheria - Neurological complications

Age group (years)	Incidence 1990 Number ('000s)	Rate (per 100 000)	Prevalence 1990 Number ('000s)	Rate (per 100 000)	Avg. age at onset (years)	Average duration (years)	Deaths 1990 Number ('000s)	Rate (per 100 000)	Deaths 2000 (Projected) Number ('000s)	Rate (per 100 000)
Males										
0-4	0	0.2	0	0.0	0.5	0.17	0	0	0	0
5-14	0	0.1	0	0.0	10.0	0.17	0	0	0	0
15-44	0	0.0	0	0.0	35.0	0.17	0	0	0	0
45-59	0	0.0	0	0.0	55.0	0.17	0	0	0	0
60+	0	0.0	0	0.0	-	-	0	0	0	0
All ages	0	0.0	0	0.0	7.0	0.17	0	0	0	0
Females										
0-4	0	0.2	0	0.0	0.5	0.17	0	0	0	0
5-14	0	0.1	0	0.0	10.0	0.17	0	0	0	0
15-44	0	0.0	0	0.0	35.0	0.17	0	0	0	0
45-59	0	0.0	0	0.0	55.0	0.17	0	0	0	0
60+	0	0.0	0	0.0	-	-	0	0	0	0
All ages	0	0.0	0	0.0	7.0	0.17	0	0	0	0
Total	0	0.0	0	0.0	7.0	0.17	0	0	0	0

Table 53e — OAI - OPAI - APAI
Diphtheria - Neurological complications

Age group (years)	Incidence 1990 Number ('000s)	Rate (per 100 000)	Prevalence 1990 Number ('000s)	Rate (per 100 000)	Avg. age at onset (years)	Average duration (years)	Deaths 1990 Number ('000s)	Rate (per 100 000)	Deaths 2000 (Projected) Number ('000s)	Rate (per 100 000)
Males										
0-4	1	3.4	0	0.6	0.5	0.17	0	0	0	0
5-14	1	0.9	0	0.1	10.0	0.17	0	0	0	0
15-44	0	0.1	0	0.0	35.0	0.17	0	0	0	0
45-59	0	0.1	0	0.0	55.0	0.17	0	0	0	0
60+	0	0.0	0	0.0	-	-	0	0	0	0
All ages	2	0.7	0	0.1	7.0	0.17	0	0	0	0
Females										
0-4	1	3.3	0	0.6	0.5	0.17	0	0	0	0
5-14	1	0.9	0	0.1	10.0	0.17	0	0	0	0
15-44	0	0.1	0	0.0	35.0	0.17	0	0	0	0
45-59	0	0.1	0	0.0	55.0	0.17	0	0	0	0
60+	0	0.0	0	0.0	-	-	0	0	0	0
All ages	2	0.7	0	0.1	7.0	0.17	0	0	0	0
Total	5	0.7	1	0.1	7.0	0.17	0	0	0	0

Table 53f — SSA - ASS - ASS
Diphtheria - Neurological complications

Age group (years)	Incidence 1990 Number ('000s)	Rate (per 100 000)	Prevalence 1990 Number ('000s)	Rate (per 100 000)	Avg. age at onset (years)	Average duration (years)	Deaths 1990 Number ('000s)	Rate (per 100 000)	Deaths 2000 (Projected) Number ('000s)	Rate (per 100 000)
Males										
0-4	1	2.5	0	0.4	0.5	0.17	0	0	0	0
5-14	1	0.8	0	0.1	10.0	0.17	0	0	0	0
15-44	0	0.2	0	0.0	35.0	0.17	0	0	0	0
45-59	0	0.1	0	0.0	55.0	0.17	0	0	0	0
60+	0	0.0	0	0.0	-	-	0	0	0	0
All ages	2	0.8	0	0.1	6.9	0.17	0	0	0	0
Females										
0-4	1	2.4	0	0.4	0.5	0.17	0	0	0	0
5-14	1	0.8	0	0.1	10.0	0.17	0	0	0	0
15-44	0	0.2	0	0.0	35.0	0.17	0	0	0	0
45-59	0	0.1	0	0.0	55.0	0.17	0	0	0	0
60+	0	0.0	0	0.0	-	-	0	0	0	0
All ages	2	0.7	0	0.1	7.0	0.17	0	0	0	0
Total	4	0.8	1	0.1	6.9	0.17	0	0	0	0

For epidemiological sources see Galazka 1996a. For the methods used to estimate and project incidence, prevalence, and deaths see Murray and Lopez 1996a. See explanatory notes for definitions and caveats.

Table 53 / **Cuadro 53** / **Tableau 53**
Diphtheria / **Difteria** / **Diphtérie**

Neurological complications / Complicaciones neurológicas / Complications neurologiques

Table 53g — LAC - ALC - ALC — Diphtheria - Neurological complications

Age group (years)	Incidence 1990 Number ('000s)	Rate (per 100 000)	Prevalence 1990 Number ('000s)	Rate (per 100 000)	Avg. age at onset (years)	Average duration (years)	Deaths 1990 Number ('000s)	Rate (per 100 000)	Deaths 2000 (Projected) Number ('000s)	Rate (per 100 000)
Males										
0-4	0	1.1	0	0.2	0.5	0.17	0	0	0	0
5-14	0	0.3	0	0.0	10.0	0.17	0	0	0	0
15-44	0	0.0	0	0.0	35.0	0.17	0	0	0	0
45-59	0	0.0	0	0.0	55.0	0.17	0	0	0	0
60+	0	0.0	0	0.0	-	-	0	0	0	0
All ages	1	0.2	0	0.0	7.0	0.17	0	0	0	0
Females										
0-4	0	1.1	0	0.2	0.5	0.17	0	0	0	0
5-14	0	0.3	0	0.0	10.0	0.17	0	0	0	0
15-44	0	0.0	0	0.0	35.0	0.17	0	0	0	0
45-59	0	0.0	0	0.0	55.0	0.17	0	0	0	0
60+	0	0.0	0	0.0	-	-	0	0	0	0
All ages	0	0.2	0	0.0	7.0	0.17	0	0	0	0
Total	1	0.2	0	0.0	7.0	0.17	0	0	0	0

Table 53h — MEC - AOM - CMO — Diphtheria - Neurological complications

Age group (years)	Incidence 1990 Number ('000s)	Rate (per 100 000)	Prevalence 1990 Number ('000s)	Rate (per 100 000)	Avg. age at onset (years)	Average duration (years)	Deaths 1990 Number ('000s)	Rate (per 100 000)	Deaths 2000 (Projected) Number ('000s)	Rate (per 100 000)
Males										
0-4	1	1.8	0	0.3	0.5	0.17	0	0	0	0
5-14	0	0.6	0	0.1	10.0	0.17	0	0	0	0
15-44	0	0.1	0	0.0	35.0	0.17	0	0	0	0
45-59	0	0.0	0	0.0	55.0	0.17	0	0	0	0
60+	0	0.0	0	0.0	-	-	0	0	0	0
All ages	1	0.5	0	0.1	6.9	0.17	0	0	0	0
Females										
0-4	1	1.8	0	0.3	0.5	0.17	0	0	0	0
5-14	0	0.6	0	0.1	10.0	0.17	0	0	0	0
15-44	0	0.1	0	0.0	35.0	0.17	0	0	0	0
45-59	0	0.0	0	0.0	55.0	0.17	0	0	0	0
60+	0	0.0	0	0.0	-	-	0	0	0	0
All ages	1	0.5	0	0.1	6.9	0.17	0	0	0	0
Total	2	0.5	0	0.1	6.9	0.17	0	0	0	0

Table 53i — World - Mundo - Monde — Diphtheria - Neurological complications

Age group (years)	Incidence 1990 Number ('000s)	Rate (per 100 000)	Prevalence 1990 Number ('000s)	Rate (per 100 000)	Avg. age at onset (years)	Average duration (years)	Deaths 1990 Number ('000s)	Rate (per 100 000)	Deaths 2000 (Projected) Number ('000s)	Rate (per 100 000)
Males										
0-4	6	2.0	1	0.3	0.5	0.17	0	0	0	0
5-14	3	0.6	1	0.1	10.0	0.17	0	0	0	0
15-44	1	0.1	0	0.0	35.0	0.17	0	0	0	0
45-59	0	0.0	0	0.0	55.0	0.17	0	0	0	0
60+	0	0.0	0	0.0	-	-	0	0	0	0
All ages	11	0.4	2	0.1	7.2	0.17	0	0	0	0
Females										
0-4	6	2.0	1	0.3	0.5	0.17	0	0	0	0
5-14	3	0.6	1	0.1	10.0	0.17	0	0	0	0
15-44	1	0.1	0	0.0	35.0	0.17	0	0	0	0
45-59	0	0.0	0	0.0	55.0	0.17	0	0	0	0
60+	0	0.0	0	0.0	-	-	0	0	0	0
All ages	10	0.4	2	0.1	7.2	0.17	0	0	0	0
Total	21	0.4	4	0.1	7.2	0.17	0	0	0	0

For epidemiological sources see Galazka 1996a. For the methods used to estimate and project incidence, prevalence, and deaths see Murray and Lopez 1996a. See explanatory notes for definitions and caveats.

Table 54	Cuadro 54	Tableau 54
Diphtheria	Difteria	Diphtérie

| Myocarditis | Miocarditis | Myocardite |

Table 54a EME - PEMC - EMBE   Diphtheria - Myocarditis

Age group (years)	Incidence 1990 Number ('000s)	Rate (per 100 000)	Prevalence 1990 Number ('000s)	Rate (per 100 000)	Avg. age at onset (years)	Average duration (years)	Deaths 1990 Number ('000s)	Rate (per 100 000)	Deaths 2000 (Projected) Number ('000s)	Rate (per 100 000)
Males										
0-4	0	0.0	0	0.0	0.5	0.25	-	-	-	-
5-14	0	0.0	0	0.0	10.0	0.25	-	-	-	-
15-44	0	0.0	0	0.0	35.0	0.25	-	-	-	-
45-59	0	0.0	0	0.0	55.0	0.25	-	-	-	-
60+	0	0.0	0	0.0	-	-	-	-	-	-
All ages	0	0.0	0	0.0	29.0	0.25	-	-	-	-
Females										
0-4	0	0.0	0	0.0	0.5	0.25	-	-	-	-
5-14	0	0.0	0	0.0	10.0	0.25	-	-	-	-
15-44	0	0.0	0	0.0	35.0	0.25	-	-	-	-
45-59	0	0.0	0	0.0	55.0	0.25	-	-	-	-
60+	0	0.0	0	0.0	-	-	-	-	-	-
All ages	0	0.0	0	0.0	29.1	0.25	-	-	-	-
Total	0	0.0	0	0.0	29.1	0.25	-	-	-	-

Table 54b FSE - PEAS - AESE   Diphtheria - Myocarditis

Age group (years)	Incidence 1990 Number ('000s)	Rate (per 100 000)	Prevalence 1990 Number ('000s)	Rate (per 100 000)	Avg. age at onset (years)	Average duration (years)	Deaths 1990 Number ('000s)	Rate (per 100 000)	Deaths 2000 (Projected) Number ('000s)	Rate (per 100 000)
Males										
0-4	0	0.0	0	0.0	0.5	0.25	-	-	-	-
5-14	0	0.1	0	0.0	10.0	0.25	-	-	-	-
15-44	0	0.1	0	0.0	35.0	0.25	-	-	-	-
45-59	0	0.0	0	0.0	55.0	0.25	-	-	-	-
60+	0	0.0	0	0.0	-	-	-	-	-	-
All ages	0	0.1	0	0.0	28.9	0.25	-	-	-	-
Females										
0-4	0	0.0	0	0.0	0.5	0.25	-	-	-	-
5-14	0	0.1	0	0.0	10.0	0.25	-	-	-	-
15-44	0	0.1	0	0.0	35.0	0.25	-	-	-	-
45-59	0	0.0	0	0.0	55.0	0.25	-	-	-	-
60+	0	0.0	0	0.0	-	-	-	-	-	-
All ages	0	0.0	0	0.0	28.9	0.25	-	-	-	-
Total	0	0.1	0	0.0	28.9	0.25	-	-	-	-

Table 54c India - India - Inde   Diphtheria - Myocarditis

Age group (years)	Incidence 1990 Number ('000s)	Rate (per 100 000)	Prevalence 1990 Number ('000s)	Rate (per 100 000)	Avg. age at onset (years)	Average duration (years)	Deaths 1990 Number ('000s)	Rate (per 100 000)	Deaths 2000 (Projected) Number ('000s)	Rate (per 100 000)
Males										
0-4	1	1.6	0	0.4	0.5	0.25	-	-	-	-
5-14	1	0.9	0	0.2	10.0	0.25	-	-	-	-
15-44	0	0.1	0	0.0	35.0	0.25	-	-	-	-
45-59	0	0.1	0	0.0	55.0	0.25	-	-	-	-
60+	0	0.0	0	0.0	-	-	-	-	-	-
All ages	2	0.5	1	0.1	9.5	0.25	-	-	-	-
Females										
0-4	1	1.6	0	0.4	0.5	0.25	-	-	-	-
5-14	1	0.9	0	0.2	10.0	0.25	-	-	-	-
15-44	0	0.1	0	0.0	35.0	0.25	-	-	-	-
45-59	0	0.1	0	0.0	55.0	0.25	-	-	-	-
60+	0	0.0	0	0.0	-	-	-	-	-	-
All ages	2	0.5	1	0.1	9.5	0.25	-	-	-	-
Total	4	0.5	1	0.1	9.5	0.25	-	-	-	-

For epidemiological sources see Galazka 1996a. For the methods used to estimate and project incidence, prevalence, and deaths see Murray and Lopez 1996a. See explanatory notes for definitions and caveats.

Table 54	Cuadro 54	Tableau 54
Diphtheria	**Difteria**	**Diphtérie**

Myocarditis	Miocarditis	Myocardite

Table 54d   China - China - Chine — Diphtheria - Myocarditis

Age group (years)	Incidence 1990 Number ('000s)	Rate (per 100 000)	Prevalence 1990 Number ('000s)	Rate (per 100 000)	Avg. age at onset (years)	Average duration (years)	Deaths 1990 Number ('000s)	Rate (per 100 000)	Deaths 2000 (Projected) Number ('000s)	Rate (per 100 000)
Males										
0-4	0	0.1	0	0.0	0.5	0.25	-	-	-	-
5-14	0	0.0	0	0.0	10.0	0.25	-	-	-	-
15-44	0	0.0	0	0.0	35.0	0.25	-	-	-	-
45-59	0	0.0	0	0.0	55.0	0.25	-	-	-	-
60+	0	0.0	0	0.0	-	-	-	-	-	-
All ages	0	0.0	0	0.0	9.4	0.25	-	-	-	-
Females										
0-4	0	0.1	0	0.0	0.5	0.25	-	-	-	-
5-14	0	0.0	0	0.0	10.0	0.25	-	-	-	-
15-44	0	0.0	0	0.0	35.0	0.25	-	-	-	-
45-59	0	0.0	0	0.0	55.0	0.25	-	-	-	-
60+	0	0.0	0	0.0	-	-	-	-	-	-
All ages	0	0.0	0	0.0	9.4	0.25	-	-	-	-
Total	0	0.0	0	0.0	9.4	0.25	-	-	-	-

Table 54e   OAI - OPAI - APAI — Diphtheria - Myocarditis

Age group (years)	Incidence 1990 Number ('000s)	Rate (per 100 000)	Prevalence 1990 Number ('000s)	Rate (per 100 000)	Avg. age at onset (years)	Average duration (years)	Deaths 1990 Number ('000s)	Rate (per 100 000)	Deaths 2000 (Projected) Number ('000s)	Rate (per 100 000)
Males										
0-4	1	1.3	0	0.3	0.5	0.25	-	-	-	-
5-14	0	0.6	0	0.1	10.0	0.25	-	-	-	-
15-44	0	0.1	0	0.0	35.0	0.25	-	-	-	-
45-59	0	0.0	0	0.0	55.0	0.25	-	-	-	-
60+	0	0.0	0	0.0	-	-	-	-	-	-
All ages	1	0.4	0	0.1	9.4	0.25	-	-	-	-
Females										
0-4	1	1.3	0	0.3	0.5	0.25	-	-	-	-
5-14	0	0.6	0	0.1	10.0	0.25	-	-	-	-
15-44	0	0.1	0	0.0	35.0	0.25	-	-	-	-
45-59	0	0.0	0	0.0	55.0	0.25	-	-	-	-
60+	0	0.0	0	0.0	-	-	-	-	-	-
All ages	1	0.3	0	0.1	9.4	0.25	-	-	-	-
Total	2	0.3	1	0.1	9.4	0.25	-	-	-	-

Table 54f   SSA - ASS - ASS — Diphtheria - Myocarditis

Age group (years)	Incidence 1990 Number ('000s)	Rate (per 100 000)	Prevalence 1990 Number ('000s)	Rate (per 100 000)	Avg. age at onset (years)	Average duration (years)	Deaths 1990 Number ('000s)	Rate (per 100 000)	Deaths 2000 (Projected) Number ('000s)	Rate (per 100 000)
Males										
0-4	0	0.9	0	0.2	0.5	0.25	-	-	-	-
5-14	0	0.6	0	0.1	10.0	0.25	-	-	-	-
15-44	0	0.1	0	0.0	35.0	0.25	-	-	-	-
45-59	0	0.0	0	0.0	55.0	0.25	-	-	-	-
60+	0	0.0	0	0.0	-	-	-	-	-	-
All ages	1	0.4	0	0.1	9.4	0.25	-	-	-	-
Females										
0-4	0	0.9	0	0.2	0.5	0.25	-	-	-	-
5-14	0	0.5	0	0.1	10.0	0.25	-	-	-	-
15-44	0	0.1	0	0.0	35.0	0.25	-	-	-	-
45-59	0	0.0	0	0.0	55.0	0.25	-	-	-	-
60+	0	0.0	0	0.0	-	-	-	-	-	-
All ages	1	0.4	0	0.1	9.4	0.25	-	-	-	-
Total	2	0.4	0	0.1	9.4	0.25	-	-	-	-

For epidemiological sources see Galazka 1996a. For the methods used to estimate and project incidence, prevalence, and deaths see Murray and Lopez 1996a. See explanatory notes for definitions and caveats.

Table 54
Diphtheria

Cuadro 54
Difteria

Tableau 54
Diphtérie

Myocarditis

Miocarditis

Myocardite

Table 54g — LAC - ALC - ALC — Diphtheria - Myocarditis

Age group (years)	Incidence 1990 Number ('000s)	Rate (per 100 000)	Prevalence 1990 Number ('000s)	Rate (per 100 000)	Avg. age at onset (years)	Average duration (years)	Deaths 1990 Number ('000s)	Rate (per 100 000)	Deaths 2000 (Projected) Number ('000s)	Rate (per 100 000)
Males										
0-4	0	0.4	0	0.1	0.5	0.25	-	-	-	-
5-14	0	0.2	0	0.0	10.0	0.25	-	-	-	-
15-44	0	0.0	0	0.0	35.0	0.25	-	-	-	-
45-59	0	0.0	0	0.0	55.0	0.25	-	-	-	-
60+	0	0.0	0	0.0	-	-	-	-	-	-
All ages	0	0.1	0	0.0	9.4	0.25	-	-	-	-
Females										
0-4	0	0.4	0	0.1	0.5	0.25	-	-	-	-
5-14	0	0.2	0	0.0	10.0	0.25	-	-	-	-
15-44	0	0.0	0	0.0	35.0	0.25	-	-	-	-
45-59	0	0.0	0	0.0	55.0	0.25	-	-	-	-
60+	0	0.0	0	0.0	-	-	-	-	-	-
All ages	0	0.1	0	0.0	9.4	0.25	-	-	-	-
Total	0	0.1	0	0.0	9.4	0.25	-	-	-	-

Table 54h — MEC - AOM - CMO — Diphtheria - Myocarditis

Age group (years)	Incidence 1990 Number ('000s)	Rate (per 100 000)	Prevalence 1990 Number ('000s)	Rate (per 100 000)	Avg. age at onset (years)	Average duration (years)	Deaths 1990 Number ('000s)	Rate (per 100 000)	Deaths 2000 (Projected) Number ('000s)	Rate (per 100 000)
Males										
0-4	0	0.7	0	0.2	0.5	0.25	-	-	-	-
5-14	0	0.4	0	0.1	10.0	0.25	-	-	-	-
15-44	0	0.1	0	0.0	35.0	0.25	-	-	-	-
45-59	0	0.0	0	0.0	55.0	0.25	-	-	-	-
60+	0	0.0	0	0.0	-	-	-	-	-	-
All ages	1	0.2	0	0.1	9.4	0.25	-	-	-	-
Females										
0-4	0	0.7	0	0.2	0.5	0.25	-	-	-	-
5-14	0	0.4	0	0.1	10.0	0.25	-	-	-	-
15-44	0	0.1	0	0.0	35.0	0.25	-	-	-	-
45-59	0	0.0	0	0.0	55.0	0.25	-	-	-	-
60+	0	0.0	0	0.0	-	-	-	-	-	-
All ages	1	0.2	0	0.1	9.4	0.25	-	-	-	-
Total	1	0.2	0	0.1	9.4	0.25	-	-	-	-

Table 54i — World - Mundo - Monde — Diphtheria - Myocarditis

Age group (years)	Incidence 1990 Number ('000s)	Rate (per 100 000)	Prevalence 1990 Number ('000s)	Rate (per 100 000)	Avg. age at onset (years)	Average duration (years)	Deaths 1990 Number ('000s)	Rate (per 100 000)	Deaths 2000 (Projected) Number ('000s)	Rate (per 100 000)
Males										
0-4	2	0.8	1	0.2	0.5	0.25	-	-	-	-
5-14	2	0.4	1	0.1	10.0	0.25	-	-	-	-
15-44	1	0.1	0	0.0	35.0	0.25	-	-	-	-
45-59	0	0.0	0	0.0	55.0	0.25	-	-	-	-
60+	0	0.0	0	0.0	-	-	-	-	-	-
All ages	5	0.2	1	0.1	9.8	0.25	-	-	-	-
Females										
0-4	2	0.7	1	0.2	0.5	0.25	-	-	-	-
5-14	2	0.4	1	0.1	10.0	0.25	-	-	-	-
15-44	1	0.1	0	0.0	35.0	0.25	-	-	-	-
45-59	0	0.0	0	0.0	55.0	0.25	-	-	-	-
60+	0	0.0	0	0.0	-	-	-	-	-	-
All ages	5	0.2	1	0.0	9.8	0.25	-	-	-	-
Total	11	0.2	3	0.1	9.8	0.25	-	-	-	-

For epidemiological sources see Galazka 1996a. For the methods used to estimate and project incidence, prevalence, and deaths see Murray and Lopez 1996a. See explanatory notes for definitions and caveats.

Table 55	Cuadro 55	Tableau 55
Measles	Sarampión	Rougeole
Episodes	Episodios	Episodes

Table 55a EME - PEMC - EMBE — Measles - Episodes

Age group (years)	Incidence 1990 Number ('000s)	Rate (per 100 000)	Prevalence 1990 Number ('000s)	Rate (per 100 000)	Avg. age at onset (years)	Average duration (years)	Deaths 1990 Number ('000s)	Rate (per 100 000)	Deaths 2000 (Projected) Number ('000s)	Rate (per 100 000)
Males										
0-4	1 615	6 119.9	62	235.4	2.5	0.04	0	0.1	0	0.1
5-14	220	412.7	8	15.9	10.0	0.04	0	0.0	0	0.0
15-44	18	10.0	1	0.4	35.0	0.04	0	0.0	0	0.0
45-59	7	10.0	0	0.4	55.0	0.04	0	0.0	0	0.0
60+	1	1.0	0	0.0	70.0	0.04	0	0.0	0	0.0
All ages	1 860	476.5	72	18.3	3.9	0.04	0	0.0	0	0.0
Females										
0-4	1 553	6 194.2	62	247.8	2.5	0.04	0	0.1	0	0.1
5-14	212	417.7	8	16.7	10.0	0.04	0	0.0	0	0.0
15-44	18	10.0	1	0.4	35.0	0.04	0	0.0	0	0.0
45-59	7	10.0	0	0.4	55.0	0.04	0	0.0	0	0.0
60+	1	1.0	0	0.0	70.0	0.04	0	0.0	0	0.0
All ages	1 790	439.4	72	17.6	3.9	0.04	0	0.0	0	0.0
Total	3 650	457.6	143	17.9	3.9	0.04	0	0.0	0	0.0

Table 55b FSE - PEAS - AESE — Measles - Episodes

Age group (years)	Incidence 1990 Number ('000s)	Rate (per 100 000)	Prevalence 1990 Number ('000s)	Rate (per 100 000)	Avg. age at onset (years)	Average duration (years)	Deaths 1990 Number ('000s)	Rate (per 100 000)	Deaths 2000 (Projected) Number ('000s)	Rate (per 100 000)
Males										
0-4	470	3 415.5	18	131.4	2.5	0.04	0	0.6	0	0.4
5-14	64	234.3	2	9.0	10.0	0.04	0	0.1	0	0.0
15-44	8	10.0	0	0.4	35.0	0.04	0	0.1	0	0.0
45-59	3	10.0	0	0.4	55.0	0.04	0	0.1	0	0.1
60+	0	1.0	0	0.0	70.0	0.04	0	0.1	0	0.1
All ages	545	329.4	21	12.7	4.1	0.04	0	0.1	0	0.1
Females										
0-4	452	3 440.1	18	137.6	2.5	0.04	0	0.5	0	0.4
5-14	62	233.2	2	9.3	10.0	0.04	0	0.1	0	0.0
15-44	7	10.0	0	0.4	35.0	0.04	0	0.0	0	0.0
45-59	3	10.0	0	0.4	55.0	0.04	0	0.1	0	0.0
60+	0	1.0	0	0.0	70.0	0.04	0	0.0	0	0.0
All ages	524	289.8	21	11.6	4.2	0.04	0	0.1	0	0.0
Total	1 069	308.7	42	12.1	4.2	0.04	0	0.1	0	0.1

Table 55c India - India - Inde — Measles - Episodes

Age group (years)	Incidence 1990 Number ('000s)	Rate (per 100 000)	Prevalence 1990 Number ('000s)	Rate (per 100 000)	Avg. age at onset (years)	Average duration (years)	Deaths 1990 Number ('000s)	Rate (per 100 000)	Deaths 2000 (Projected) Number ('000s)	Rate (per 100 000)
Males										
0-4	2 940	4 917.2	113	189.1	1.3	0.04	89	148.9	53	93.1
5-14	401	394.0	15	15.2	10.0	0.04	14	13.8	7	6.2
15-44	20	10.0	1	0.4	35.0	0.04	0	0.1	0	0.0
45-59	5	10.0	0	0.4	55.0	0.04	0	0.1	0	0.0
60+	0	1.0	0	0.0	70.0	0.04	0	0.1	0	0.1
All ages	3 366	766.0	129	29.5	2.6	0.04	103	23.5	60	11.7
Females										
0-4	2 827	4 987.5	113	199.5	1.3	0.04	88	155.6	50	93.4
5-14	385	404.6	15	16.2	10.0	0.04	14	15.2	7	6.6
15-44	18	10.0	1	0.4	35.0	0.04	0	0.1	0	0.0
45-59	5	10.0	0	0.4	55.0	0.04	0	0.1	0	0.0
60+	0	1.0	0	0.0	70.0	0.04	0	0.1	0	0.1
All ages	3 236	788.9	129	31.6	2.6	0.04	103	25.1	57	11.8
Total	6 601	777.1	259	30.5	2.6	0.04	206	24.3	117	11.8

For epidemiological sources see Clements and Hussey 1996. For the methods used to estimate and project incidence, prevalence, and deaths see Murray and Lopez 1996a. See explanatory notes for definitions and caveats.

Table 55　　　　　　　　　　**Cuadro 55**　　　　　　　　　**Tableau 55**
Measles　　　　　　　　　　**Sarampión**　　　　　　　　　**Rougeole**

Episodes　　　　　　　　　　Episodios　　　　　　　　　　Episodes

Table 55d　　　China - China - Chine　　　　　　　　　Measles - Episodes

Age group (years)	Incidence 1990 Number ('000s)	Rate (per 100 000)	Prevalence 1990 Number ('000s)	Rate (per 100 000)	Avg. age at onset (years)	Average duration (years)	Deaths 1990 Number ('000s)	Rate (per 100 000)	Deaths 2000 (Projected) Number ('000s)	Rate (per 100 000)
Males										
0-4	2 199	3 650.6	85	140.4	1.3	0.04	6	10.7	3	5.5
5-14	300	309.2	12	11.9	10.0	0.04	1	0.9	0	0.3
15-44	31	10.0	1	0.4	35.0	0.04	0	0.1	0	0.0
45-59	7	10.0	0	0.4	55.0	0.04	0	0.1	0	0.0
60+	0	1.0	0	0.0	70.0	0.04	0	0.1	0	0.1
All ages	2 538	433.6	98	16.7	2.9	0.04	8	1.3	4	0.6
Females										
0-4	2 115	3 649.4	85	146.0	1.3	0.04	6	10.7	3	5.3
5-14	288	319.0	12	12.8	10.0	0.04	1	0.9	0	0.3
15-44	28	10.0	1	0.4	35.0	0.04	0	0.1	0	0.0
45-59	6	10.0	0	0.4	55.0	0.04	0	0.1	0	0.0
60+	1	1.0	0	0.0	70.0	0.04	0	0.1	0	0.1
All ages	2 438	444.6	98	17.8	2.8	0.04	7	1.4	3	0.6
Total	4 976	438.9	195	17.2	2.8	0.04	15	1.3	7	0.6

Table 55e　　　OAI - OPAI - APAI　　　　　　　　　　　　Measles - Episodes

Age group (years)	Incidence 1990 Number ('000s)	Rate (per 100 000)	Prevalence 1990 Number ('000s)	Rate (per 100 000)	Avg. age at onset (years)	Average duration (years)	Deaths 1990 Number ('000s)	Rate (per 100 000)	Deaths 2000 (Projected) Number ('000s)	Rate (per 100 000)
Males										
0-4	2 421	5 531.0	93	212.7	1.3	0.04	52	118.2	34	76.1
5-14	330	392.8	13	15.1	10.0	0.04	8	9.3	4	4.6
15-44	16	10.0	1	0.4	35.0	0.04	0	0.1	0	0.0
45-59	3	10.0	0	0.4	55.0	0.04	0	0.1	0	0.1
60+	0	1.0	0	0.0	70.0	0.04	0	0.1	0	0.1
All ages	2 770	807.7	107	31.1	2.6	0.04	60	17.4	37	9.3
Females										
0-4	2 327	5 543.1	93	221.7	1.3	0.04	47	111.1	29	69.2
5-14	317	395.6	13	15.8	10.0	0.04	7	8.5	3	4.1
15-44	16	10.0	1	0.4	35.0	0.04	0	0.1	0	0.0
45-59	4	10.0	0	0.4	55.0	0.04	0	0.1	0	0.1
60+	0	1.0	0	0.0	70.0	0.04	0	0.1	0	0.1
All ages	2 664	784.7	107	31.4	2.6	0.04	54	15.8	33	8.1
Total	5 435	796.3	213	31.2	2.6	0.04	113	16.6	70	8.7

Table 55f　　　SSA - ASS - ASS　　　　　　　　　　　　Measles - Episodes

Age group (years)	Incidence 1990 Number ('000s)	Rate (per 100 000)	Prevalence 1990 Number ('000s)	Rate (per 100 000)	Avg. age at onset (years)	Average duration (years)	Deaths 1990 Number ('000s)	Rate (per 100 000)	Deaths 2000 (Projected) Number ('000s)	Rate (per 100 000)
Males										
0-4	5 829	12 276.4	224	472.2	1.3	0.04	257	540.7	256	389.2
5-14	795	1 131.4	31	43.5	10.0	0.04	43	61.3	31	32.9
15-44	10	10.0	0	0.4	35.0	0.04	0	0.1	0	0.0
45-59	2	10.0	0	0.4	55.0	0.04	0	0.1	0	0.1
60+	0	1.0	0	0.0	70.0	0.04	0	0.1	0	0.1
All ages	6 637	2 630.3	255	101.2	2.4	0.04	300	118.9	287	83.8
Females										
0-4	5 605	11 918.2	224	476.7	1.3	0.04	233	495.8	219	343.9
5-14	764	1 094.8	31	43.8	10.0	0.04	43	61.0	29	31.5
15-44	11	10.0	0	0.4	35.0	0.04	0	0.1	0	0.0
45-59	2	10.0	0	0.4	55.0	0.04	0	0.1	0	0.1
60+	0	1.0	0	0.0	70.0	0.04	0	0.1	0	0.1
All ages	6 382	2 474.3	255	99.0	2.4	0.04	276	106.9	248	71.2
Total	13 019	2 551.4	511	100.1	2.4	0.04	576	112.8	536	77.5

For epidemiological sources see Clements and Hussey 1996. For the methods used to estimate and project incidence, prevalence, and deaths see Murray and Lopez 1996a. See explanatory notes for definitions and caveats.

Table 55
Measles

Cuadro 55
Sarampión

Tableau 55
Rougeole

Episodes

Episodios

Episodes

Table 55g LAC - ALC - ALC — Measles - Episodes

Age group (years)	Incidence 1990 Number ('000s)	Rate (per 100 000)	Prevalence 1990 Number ('000s)	Rate (per 100 000)	Avg. age at onset (years)	Average duration (years)	Deaths 1990 Number ('000s)	Rate (per 100 000)	Deaths 2000 (Projected) Number ('000s)	Rate (per 100 000)
Males										
0-4	1 451	5 053.3	56	194.4	1.3	0.04	24	84.9	17	59.3
5-14	198	379.7	8	14.6	10.0	0.04	2	4.7	2	2.7
15-44	10	10.0	0	0.4	35.0	0.04	0	0.1	0	0.0
45-59	2	10.0	0	0.4	55.0	0.04	0	0.0	0	0.0
60+	0	1.0	0	0.0	70.0	0.04	0	0.0	0	0.0
All ages	1 662	750.0	64	28.8	2.6	0.04	27	12.1	19	7.1
Females										
0-4	1 396	5 042.4	56	201.7	1.3	0.04	22	78.5	15	53.5
5-14	190	375.0	8	15.0	10.0	0.04	3	5.3	2	3.0
15-44	10	10.0	0	0.4	35.0	0.04	0	0.2	0	0.1
45-59	2	10.0	0	0.4	55.0	0.04	0	0.0	0	0.0
60+	0	1.0	0	0.0	70.0	0.04	0	0.0	0	0.0
All ages	1 599	717.9	64	28.7	2.6	0.04	25	11.1	17	6.3
Total	3 261	733.9	128	28.8	2.6	0.04	52	11.6	36	6.7

Table 55h MEC - AOM - CMO — Measles - Episodes

Age group (years)	Incidence 1990 Number ('000s)	Rate (per 100 000)	Prevalence 1990 Number ('000s)	Rate (per 100 000)	Avg. age at onset (years)	Average duration (years)	Deaths 1990 Number ('000s)	Rate (per 100 000)	Deaths 2000 (Projected) Number ('000s)	Rate (per 100 000)
Males										
0-4	2 825	6 862.1	109	263.9	1.3	0.04	43	103.6	38	76.4
5-14	385	589.4	15	22.7	10.0	0.04	6	9.3	4	5.2
15-44	11	10.0	0	0.4	35.0	0.04	0	0.0	0	0.0
45-59	2	10.0	0	0.4	55.0	0.04	0	0.1	0	0.0
60+	0	1.0	0	0.0	70.0	0.04	0	0.1	0	0.1
All ages	3 223	1 257.2	124	48.4	2.5	0.04	49	19.0	43	12.7
Females										
0-4	2 716	6 835.1	109	273.4	1.3	0.04	41	103.2	35	73.7
5-14	370	597.3	15	23.9	10.0	0.04	6	9.7	4	5.2
15-44	11	10.0	0	0.4	35.0	0.04	0	0.1	0	0.0
45-59	2	10.0	0	0.4	55.0	0.04	0	0.1	0	0.0
60+	0	1.0	0	0.0	70.0	0.04	0	0.1	0	0.1
All ages	3 099	1 256.4	124	50.3	2.5	0.04	47	19.1	39	12.2
Total	6 323	1 256.8	248	49.3	2.5	0.04	96	19.1	82	12.5

Table 55i World - Mundo - Monde — Measles - Episodes

Age group (years)	Incidence 1990 Number ('000s)	Rate (per 100 000)	Prevalence 1990 Number ('000s)	Rate (per 100 000)	Avg. age at onset (years)	Average duration (years)	Deaths 1990 Number ('000s)	Rate (per 100 000)	Deaths 2000 (Projected) Number ('000s)	Rate (per 100 000)
Males										
0-4	19 750	6 147	760	236.4	1.4	0.04	471	146.6	402	116.1
5-14	2 693	489	104	18.8	10.0	0.04	74	13.5	48	7.6
15-44	125	10	5	0.4	35.0	0.04	1	0.1	0	0.0
45-59	31	10	1	0.4	55.0	0.04	0	0.1	0	0.0
60+	2	1	0	0.0	70.0	0.04	0	0.1	0	0.0
All ages	22 601	852	869	32.8	2.9	0.04	547	20.6	450	14.5
Females										
0-4	18 990	6 141	760	245.6	1.4	0.04	437	141.3	351	106.3
5-14	2 590	493	104	19.7	10.0	0.04	73	14.0	46	7.6
15-44	120	10	5	0.4	35.0	0.04	1	0.1	0	0.0
45-59	31	10	1	0.4	55.0	0.04	0	0.1	0	0.0
60+	3	1	0	0.0	70.0	0.04	0	0.1	0	0.0
All ages	21 733	832	869	33.3	2.9	0.04	512	19.6	398	13.0
Total	44 334	842	1 739	33.0	2.9	0.04	1 058	20.1	848	13.8

For epidemiological sources see Clements and Hussey 1996. For the methods used to estimate and project incidence, prevalence, and deaths see Murray and Lopez 1996a. See explanatory notes for definitions and caveats.

Table 56   **Cuadro 56**   **Tableau 56**
Tetanus   **Tétanos**   **Tétanos**

Episodes   Episodios   Episodes

Table 56a   EME - PEMC - EMBE   Tetanus - Episodes

Age group (years)	Incidence 1990 Number ('000s)	Rate (per 100 000)	Prevalence 1990 Number ('000s)	Rate (per 100 000)	Avg. age at onset (years)	Average duration (years)	Deaths 1990 Number ('000s)	Rate (per 100 000)	Deaths 2000 (Projected) Number ('000s)	Rate (per 100 000)
Males										
0-4	0	0.0	0	0.0	-	-	0	0.0	0	0.0
5-14	0	0.0	0	0.0	-	-	0	0.0	0	0.0
15-44	0	0.0	0	0.0	29.9	0.04	0	0.0	0	0.0
45-59	0	0.1	0	0.0	52.4	0.04	0	0.0	0	0.0
60+	0	0.4	0	0.0	71.1	0.04	0	0.1	0	0.1
All ages	0	0.1	0	0.0	64.0	0.04	0	0.0	0	0.0
Females										
0-4	0	0.0	0	0.0	-	-	0	0.0	0	0.0
5-14	0	0.0	0	0.0	-	-	0	0.0	0	0.0
15-44	0	0.0	0	0.0	30.0	0.04	0	0.0	0	0.0
45-59	0	0.1	0	0.0	52.4	0.04	0	0.0	0	0.0
60+	1	0.6	0	0.0	72.4	0.04	0	0.1	0	0.1
All ages	1	0.1	0	0.0	69.5	0.04	0	0.0	0	0.0
Total	1	0.1	0	0.0	67.5	0.04	0	0.0	0	0.0

Table 56b   FSE - PEAS - AESE   Tetanus - Episodes

Age group (years)	Incidence 1990 Number ('000s)	Rate (per 100 000)	Prevalence 1990 Number ('000s)	Rate (per 100 000)	Avg. age at onset (years)	Average duration (years)	Deaths 1990 Number ('000s)	Rate (per 100 000)	Deaths 2000 (Projected) Number ('000s)	Rate (per 100 000)
Males										
0-4	0	0.0	0	0.0	0.1	0.04	0	0.0	0	0.0
5-14	0	0.0	0	0.0	10.0	0.04	0	0.0	0	0.0
15-44	0	0.0	0	0.0	29.8	0.04	0	0.0	0	0.0
45-59	0	0.3	0	0.0	52.2	0.04	0	0.1	0	0.1
60+	0	0.7	0	0.0	70.0	0.04	0	0.2	0	0.2
All ages	0	0.2	0	0.0	58.9	0.04	0	0.0	0	0.0
Females										
0-4	0	0.0	0	0.0	0.1	0.04	0	0.0	0	0.0
5-14	0	0.0	0	0.0	10.0	0.04	0	0.0	0	0.0
15-44	0	0.0	0	0.0	29.9	0.04	0	0.0	0	0.0
45-59	0	0.3	0	0.0	52.4	0.04	0	0.1	0	0.1
60+	0	0.8	0	0.0	71.5	0.04	0	0.2	0	0.2
All ages	0	0.2	0	0.0	65.6	0.04	0	0.1	0	0.1
Total	1	0.2	0	0.0	63.0	0.04	0	0.1	0	0.1

Table 56c   India - India - Inde   Tetanus - Episodes

Age group (years)	Incidence 1990 Number ('000s)	Rate (per 100 000)	Prevalence 1990 Number ('000s)	Rate (per 100 000)	Avg. age at onset (years)	Average duration (years)	Deaths 1990 Number ('000s)	Rate (per 100 000)	Deaths 2000 (Projected) Number ('000s)	Rate (per 100 000)
Males										
0-4	96	160	4	6.2	0.1	0.04	77	128.2	45	80.2
5-14	20	20	1	0.8	10.0	0.04	8	7.8	4	3.5
15-44	33	17	1	0.6	29.8	0.04	13	6.6	7	2.7
45-59	9	18	0	0.7	52.3	0.04	3	7.3	2	3.4
60+	9	30	0	1.1	69.7	0.04	4	11.9	3	8.5
All ages	167	38	6	1.5	13.7	0.04	105	23.9	61	12.0
Females										
0-4	95	167	4	6.4	0.1	0.04	76	134.0	43	80.4
5-14	29	30	1	1.2	10.0	0.04	11	12.1	5	5.2
15-44	32	18	1	0.7	29.8	0.04	13	7.0	5	2.3
45-59	9	19	0	0.7	52.4	0.04	4	7.6	2	3.5
60+	8	29	0	1.1	70.1	0.04	3	11.7	3	8.2
All ages	173	42	7	1.6	13.3	0.04	107	26.1	59	12.3
Total	340	40	13	1.5	13.5	0.04	212	25.0	121	12.1

For epidemiological sources see Galazka et al. 1996c. For the methods used to estimate and project incidence, prevalence, and deaths see Murray and Lopez 1996a. See explanatory notes for definitions and caveats.

Table 56	Cuadro 56	Tableau 56
Tetanus	Tétanos	Tétanos
Episodes	Episodios	Episodes

Table 56d — China - China - Chine — Tetanus - Episodes

Age group (years)	Incidence 1990 Number ('000s)	Rate (per 100 000)	Prevalence 1990 Number ('000s)	Rate (per 100 000)	Avg. age at onset (years)	Average duration (years)	Deaths 1990 Number ('000s)	Rate (per 100 000)	Deaths 2000 (Projected) Number ('000s)	Rate (per 100 000)
Males										
0-4	10	16.2	0	0.6	0.1	0.04	8	12.9	4	6.7
5-14	1	1.3	0	0.1	10.0	0.04	1	0.5	0	0.2
15-44	3	0.9	0	0.0	29.9	0.04	1	0.3	0	0.1
45-59	1	0.9	0	0.0	52.3	0.04	0	0.4	0	0.1
60+	1	1.4	0	0.1	69.8	0.04	0	0.6	0	0.4
All ages	15	2.6	1	0.1	11.6	0.04	10	1.7	5	0.7
Females										
0-4	9	16.2	0	0.6	0.1	0.04	7	12.9	4	6.4
5-14	1	0.7	0	0.0	10.0	0.04	0	0.3	0	0.1
15-44	1	0.3	0	0.0	29.9	0.04	0	0.1	0	0.0
45-59	0	0.4	0	0.0	52.4	0.04	0	0.1	0	0.1
60+	0	0.4	0	0.0	70.6	0.04	0	0.2	0	0.1
All ages	11	2.1	0	0.1	5.6	0.04	8	1.5	4	0.6
Total	26	2.3	1	0.1	9.0	0.04	18	1.6	9	0.7

Table 56e — OAI - OPAI - APAI — Tetanus - Episodes

Age group (years)	Incidence 1990 Number ('000s)	Rate (per 100 000)	Prevalence 1990 Number ('000s)	Rate (per 100 000)	Avg. age at onset (years)	Average duration (years)	Deaths 1990 Number ('000s)	Rate (per 100 000)	Deaths 2000 (Projected) Number ('000s)	Rate (per 100 000)
Males										
0-4	32	74.2	1	2.9	0.1	0.04	26	59.4	17	38.2
5-14	9	11.1	1	0.4	10.0	0.04	4	4.4	2	2.2
15-44	14	8.5	1	0.3	29.7	0.04	5	3.4	3	1.6
45-59	4	11.1	0	0.4	52.3	0.04	2	4.5	1	2.2
60+	4	18.5	0	0.7	69.6	0.04	1	7.4	2	5.5
All ages	63	18.4	2	0.7	15.2	0.04	38	11.1	24	6.0
Females										
0-4	29	69.8	1	2.7	0.1	0.04	23	55.8	15	34.8
5-14	12	14.6	0	0.6	10.0	0.04	5	5.8	2	2.8
15-44	14	8.9	1	0.3	29.8	0.04	6	3.6	3	1.4
45-59	4	11.5	0	0.4	52.3	0.04	2	4.6	1	2.3
60+	4	16.2	0	0.6	70.3	0.04	1	6.5	2	5.0
All ages	63	18.5	2	0.7	16.1	0.04	37	10.9	22	5.6
Total	126	18.4	5	0.7	15.7	0.04	75	11.0	47	5.8

Table 56f — SSA - ASS - ASS — Tetanus - Episodes

Age group (years)	Incidence 1990 Number ('000s)	Rate (per 100 000)	Prevalence 1990 Number ('000s)	Rate (per 100 000)	Avg. age at onset (years)	Average duration (years)	Deaths 1990 Number ('000s)	Rate (per 100 000)	Deaths 2000 (Projected) Number ('000s)	Rate (per 100 000)
Males										
0-4	68	144	3	5.5	0.1	0.04	55	115.1	55	82.9
5-14	9	12	0	0.5	10.0	0.04	4	6.1	3	3.3
15-44	11	11	0	0.4	29.4	0.04	5	5.3	4	2.5
45-59	4	19	0	0.7	52.2	0.04	2	9.3	1	4.9
60+	4	37	0	1.4	69.2	0.04	2	18.4	2	13.3
All ages	95	38	4	1.5	9.2	0.04	68	27.0	64	18.8
Females										
0-4	62	132	2	5.1	0.1	0.04	50	105.6	47	73.2
5-14	10	15	0	0.6	10.0	0.04	5	7.4	4	3.8
15-44	12	12	0	0.5	29.5	0.04	6	5.9	3	2.4
45-59	3	15	0	0.6	52.2	0.04	2	7.5	1	3.9
60+	3	26	0	1.0	69.7	0.04	2	12.8	2	9.0
All ages	91	35	4	1.4	9.6	0.04	64	24.9	56	16.1
Total	187	37	7	1.4	9.4	0.04	133	26.0	121	17.5

For epidemiological sources see Galazka et al. 1996c. For the methods used to estimate and project incidence, prevalence, and deaths see Murray and Lopez 1996a. See explanatory notes for definitions and caveats.

Table 56	Cuadro 56	Tableau 56
Tetanus	Tétanos	Tétanos
Episodes	Episodios	Episodes

Table 56g   LAC - ALC - ALC   Tetanus - Episodes

Age group (years)	Incidence 1990 Number ('000s)	Rate (per 100 000)	Prevalence 1990 Number ('000s)	Rate (per 100 000)	Avg. age at onset (years)	Average duration (years)	Deaths 1990 Number ('000s)	Rate (per 100 000)	Deaths 2000 (Projected) Number ('000s)	Rate (per 100 000)
Males										
0-4	12	43.0	0	1.7	0.1	0.04	10	34.4	7	24.0
5-14	1	2.3	0	0.1	10.0	0.04	0	0.7	0	0.4
15-44	1	0.6	0	0.0	29.8	0.04	0	0.2	0	0.1
45-59	1	2.5	0	0.1	52.3	0.04	0	0.8	0	0.4
60+	1	5.1	0	0.2	70.3	0.04	0	1.5	0	1.2
All ages	15	7.0	1	0.3	7.3	0.04	11	4.9	8	2.9
Females										
0-4	11	39.7	0	1.5	0.1	0.04	9	31.8	6	21.6
5-14	1	1.0	0	0.0	10.0	0.04	0	0.3	0	0.2
15-44	1	1.0	0	0.0	29.9	0.04	0	0.3	0	0.1
45-59	1	2.6	0	0.1	52.4	0.04	0	0.8	0	0.4
60+	1	4.1	0	0.2	71.1	0.04	0	1.2	0	0.9
All ages	14	6.2	1	0.2	8.5	0.04	10	4.3	7	2.5
Total	29	6.6	1	0.3	7.8	0.04	20	4.6	14	2.7

Table 56h   MEC - AOM - CMO   Tetanus - Episodes

Age group (years)	Incidence 1990 Number ('000s)	Rate (per 100 000)	Prevalence 1990 Number ('000s)	Rate (per 100 000)	Avg. age at onset (years)	Average duration (years)	Deaths 1990 Number ('000s)	Rate (per 100 000)	Deaths 2000 (Projected) Number ('000s)	Rate (per 100 000)
Males										
0-4	48	117.4	2	4.5	0.1	0.04	39	93.9	35	69.3
5-14	5	7.9	0	0.3	10.0	0.04	2	3.2	1	1.8
15-44	1	1.2	0	0.0	29.8	0.04	1	0.5	0	0.2
45-59	1	4.1	0	0.2	52.3	0.04	0	1.7	0	0.9
60+	1	5.3	0	0.2	69.7	0.04	0	2.1	0	1.4
All ages	56	22.0	2	0.8	3.5	0.04	42	16.4	37	11.1
Females										
0-4	46	117.0	2	4.5	0.1	0.04	37	93.6	32	66.8
5-14	3	5.2	0	0.2	10.0	0.04	1	2.1	1	1.1
15-44	4	3.7	0	0.1	29.8	0.04	2	1.5	1	0.6
45-59	2	7.4	0	0.3	52.3	0.04	1	2.9	0	1.6
60+	1	3.5	0	0.1	70.4	0.04	0	1.4	0	0.9
All ages	56	22.6	2	0.9	5.0	0.04	41	16.6	34	10.6
Total	112	22.3	4	0.9	4.2	0.04	83	16.5	71	10.8

Table 56i   World - Mundo - Monde   Tetanus - Episodes

Age group (years)	Incidence 1990 Number ('000s)	Rate (per 100 000)	Prevalence 1990 Number ('000s)	Rate (per 100 000)	Avg. age at onset (years)	Average duration (years)	Deaths 1990 Number ('000s)	Rate (per 100 000)	Deaths 2000 (Projected) Number ('000s)	Rate (per 100 000)
Males										
0-4	267	83.1	10	3.2	0.1	0.04	214	66.5	162	46.9
5-14	45	8.2	2	0.3	10.0	0.04	19	3.4	11	1.7
15-44	63	5.0	2	0.2	29.7	0.04	26	2.1	14	1.0
45-59	19	6.0	1	0.2	52.3	0.04	8	2.5	5	1.2
60+	19	8.7	1	0.3	69.6	0.04	8	3.6	7	2.7
All ages	413	15.5	16	0.6	11.2	0.04	274	10.3	200	6.5
Females										
0-4	253	81.8	10	3.1	0.1	0.04	202	65.5	146	44.1
5-14	55	10.5	2	0.4	10.0	0.04	23	4.4	12	2.0
15-44	65	5.4	2	0.2	29.7	0.04	27	2.3	13	0.9
45-59	19	6.0	1	0.2	52.3	0.04	8	2.5	5	1.2
60+	18	6.5	1	0.3	70.2	0.04	7	2.7	5	2.1
All ages	409	15.7	16	0.6	11.5	0.04	267	10.2	183	6.0
Total	822	15.6	32	0.6	11.4	0.04	542	10.3	383	6.2

For epidemiological sources see Galazka et al. 1996c. For the methods used to estimate and project incidence, prevalence, and deaths see Murray and Lopez 1996a. See explanatory notes for definitions and caveats.

Table 57
Bacterial meningitis

Cuadro 57
Meninigitis bacteriana

Tableau 57
Méningite bactérienne

All forms - episodes

Todas las formas - episodios

Toutes les formes - épisodes

Table 57a EME - PEMC - EMBE — Bacterial meningitis - All forms - episodes

Age group (years)	Incidence 1990 Number ('000s)	Rate (per 100 000)	Prevalence 1990 Number ('000s)	Rate (per 100 000)	Avg. age at onset (years)	Average duration (years)	Deaths 1990 Number ('000s)	Rate (per 100 000)	Deaths 2000 (Projected) Number ('000s)	Rate (per 100 000)
Males										
0-4	12	43.7	1	3.6	2.5	0.08	1	3.1	1	2.1
5-14	2	4.0	0	0.3	10.0	0.08	0	0.2	0	0.1
15-44	1	0.7	0	0.1	29.9	0.08	0	0.2	0	0.1
45-59	0	0.6	0	0.0	52.4	0.08	0	0.5	0	0.3
60+	1	2.3	0	0.2	71.1	0.08	1	1.3	1	1.1
All ages	17	4.3	1	0.4	12.5	0.08	2	0.6	2	0.5
Females										
0-4	11	43.7	1	3.6	2.5	0.08	1	2.4	0	1.6
5-14	2	4.0	0	0.3	10.0	0.08	0	0.2	0	0.1
15-44	1	0.7	0	0.1	30.0	0.08	0	0.1	0	0.1
45-59	0	0.6	0	0.0	52.4	0.08	0	0.3	0	0.2
60+	2	2.3	0	0.2	72.4	0.08	1	1.1	1	0.9
All ages	17	4.1	1	0.3	15.0	0.08	2	0.5	2	0.4
Total	33	4.2	3	0.3	13.7	0.08	5	0.6	4	0.4

Table 57b FSE - PEAS - AESE — Bacterial meningitis - All forms - episodes

Age group (years)	Incidence 1990 Number ('000s)	Rate (per 100 000)	Prevalence 1990 Number ('000s)	Rate (per 100 000)	Avg. age at onset (years)	Average duration (years)	Deaths 1990 Number ('000s)	Rate (per 100 000)	Deaths 2000 (Projected) Number ('000s)	Rate (per 100 000)
Males										
0-4	10	69.7	1	5.7	2.5	0.08	2	11.5	1	8.7
5-14	2	6.2	0	0.5	10.0	0.08	0	0.3	0	0.2
15-44	2	3.2	0	0.3	29.8	0.08	1	0.7	0	0.4
45-59	1	4.0	0	0.3	52.2	0.08	1	2.0	1	1.3
60+	2	9.7	0	0.8	70.0	0.08	1	5.3	1	4.6
All ages	17	10.2	1	0.8	18.6	0.08	4	2.3	3	1.8
Females										
0-4	9	69.7	1	5.7	2.5	0.08	1	8.2	1	6.1
5-14	2	6.2	0	0.5	10.0	0.08	0	0.3	0	0.2
15-44	2	3.2	0	0.3	29.9	0.08	0	0.3	0	0.2
45-59	1	4.0	0	0.3	52.4	0.08	0	0.8	0	0.5
60+	4	9.7	0	0.8	71.5	0.08	1	2.4	1	2.0
All ages	18	9.9	1	0.8	23.8	0.08	3	1.4	2	1.0
Total	35	10.1	3	0.8	21.3	0.08	6	1.8	5	1.4

Table 57c India - India - Inde — Bacterial meningitis - All forms - episodes

Age group (years)	Incidence 1990 Number ('000s)	Rate (per 100 000)	Prevalence 1990 Number ('000s)	Rate (per 100 000)	Avg. age at onset (years)	Average duration (years)	Deaths 1990 Number ('000s)	Rate (per 100 000)	Deaths 2000 (Projected) Number ('000s)	Rate (per 100 000)
Males										
0-4	42	69.8	3	5.7	2.5	0.08	12	20.6	7	12.9
5-14	6	6.0	0	0.5	10.0	0.08	0	0.2	0	0.1
15-44	6	3.1	1	0.3	29.8	0.08	5	2.4	3	1.0
45-59	2	5.2	0	0.4	52.3	0.08	2	4.9	1	2.2
60+	3	9.8	0	0.1	69.7	0.08	3	9.9	2	6.3
All ages	59	13.5	5	1.1	8.7	0.08	23	5.2	14	2.6
Females										
0-4	40	69.8	3	5.7	2.5	0.08	12	21.3	7	12.8
5-14	6	6.0	0	0.5	10.0	0.08	0	0.2	0	0.1
15-44	6	3.1	0	0.3	29.8	0.08	4	2.2	2	0.7
45-59	2	5.2	0	0.4	52.4	0.08	2	4.9	1	2.2
60+	3	9.8	0	0.1	70.1	0.08	3	9.9	2	6.2
All ages	56	13.7	4	1.1	8.7	0.08	21	5.2	12	2.6
Total	116	13.6	9	1.1	8.7	0.08	44	5.2	26	2.6

For epidemiological sources see Schillinger et al. 1996. For the methods used to estimate and project incidence, prevalence, and deaths see Murray and Lopez 1996a. See explanatory notes for definitions and caveats.

Table 57	Cuadro 57	Tableau 57
Bacterial meningitis	**Meninigitis bacteriana**	**Méningite bactérienne**
All forms - episodes	Todas las formas - episodios	Toutes les formes - épisodes

Table 57d China - China - Chine — Bacterial meningitis - All forms - episodes

Age group (years)	Incidence 1990 Number ('000s)	Rate (per 100 000)	Prevalence 1990 Number ('000s)	Rate (per 100 000)	Avg. age at onset (years)	Average duration (years)	Deaths 1990 Number ('000s)	Rate (per 100 000)	Deaths 2000 (Projected) Number ('000s)	Rate (per 100 000)
Males										
0-4	42	69.3	3	5.7	2.5	0.08	7	11.4	3	5.9
5-14	5	5.7	0	0.5	10.0	0.08	0	0.1	0	0.0
15-44	9	3.0	1	0.2	29.9	0.08	6	2.1	3	0.8
45-59	4	5.2	0	0.4	52.3	0.08	3	4.4	2	1.7
60+	5	9.8	0	0.8	69.8	0.08	5	9.7	4	5.8
All ages	65	11.1	5	0.9	14.8	0.08	21	3.6	11	1.7
Females										
0-4	40	69.3	3	5.7	2.5	0.08	7	11.4	3	5.6
5-14	5	5.7	0	0.5	10.0	0.08	0	0.1	0	0.0
15-44	8	3.0	1	0.2	29.9	0.08	6	2.0	2	0.6
45-59	3	5.2	0	0.4	52.4	0.08	3	4.4	2	1.7
60+	5	9.8	0	0.8	70.6	0.08	5	9.7	4	5.9
All ages	62	11.3	5	0.9	15.1	0.08	20	3.7	11	1.7
Total	127	11.2	10	0.9	14.9	0.08	41	3.7	22	1.7

Table 57e OAI - OPAI - APAI — Bacterial meningitis - All forms - episodes

Age group (years)	Incidence 1990 Number ('000s)	Rate (per 100 000)	Prevalence 1990 Number ('000s)	Rate (per 100 000)	Avg. age at onset (years)	Average duration (years)	Deaths 1990 Number ('000s)	Rate (per 100 000)	Deaths 2000 (Projected) Number ('000s)	Rate (per 100 000)
Males										
0-4	30	69.7	3	5.7	2.5	0.08	6	13.3	4	8.6
5-14	5	5.5	0	0.5	10.0	0.08	0	0.1	0	0.1
15-44	4	2.5	0	0.2	29.7	0.08	3	1.7	2	0.8
45-59	2	5.4	0	0.4	52.3	0.08	2	5.1	1	2.6
60+	2	9.8	0	0.8	69.6	0.08	2	10.2	2	6.8
All ages	43	12.5	4	1.0	11.1	0.08	13	3.7	9	2.1
Females										
0-4	29	69.7	2	5.7	2.5	0.08	5	12.5	4	7.8
5-14	4	5.5	0	0.5	10.0	0.08	0	0.1	0	0.1
15-44	4	2.5	0	0.2	29.8	0.08	3	1.7	1	0.7
45-59	2	5.4	0	0.4	52.3	0.08	2	5.1	1	2.6
60+	2	9.8	0	0.8	70.3	0.08	2	8.2	2	5.7
All ages	42	12.3	3	1.0	11.8	0.08	12	3.5	8	1.9
Total	85	12.4	7	1.0	11.4	0.08	24	3.6	16	2.0

Table 57f SSA - ASS - ASS — Bacterial meningitis - All forms - episodes

Age group (years)	Incidence 1990 Number ('000s)	Rate (per 100 000)	Prevalence 1990 Number ('000s)	Rate (per 100 000)	Avg. age at onset (years)	Average duration (years)	Deaths 1990 Number ('000s)	Rate (per 100 000)	Deaths 2000 (Projected) Number ('000s)	Rate (per 100 000)
Males										
0-4	33	69.8	3	5.7	2.4	0.08	9	18.4	9	13.2
5-14	4	5.9	0	0.5	10.0	0.08	0	0.2	0	0.1
15-44	3	3.1	0	0.3	29.4	0.08	2	1.9	1	0.9
45-59	1	5.5	0	0.5	52.2	0.08	1	5.4	1	2.9
60+	1	9.7	0	0.8	69.2	0.08	1	10.0	1	6.5
All ages	43	16.9	4	1.4	8.1	0.08	13	5.1	12	3.4
Females										
0-4	33	69.8	3	5.7	2.4	0.08	8	17.4	8	12.1
5-14	4	5.9	0	0.5	10.0	0.08	0	0.2	0	0.1
15-44	3	3.1	0	0.3	29.5	0.08	3	2.4	1	0.9
45-59	1	5.5	0	0.5	52.2	0.08	1	5.5	1	2.8
60+	1	9.7	0	0.8	69.7	0.08	1	10.3	1	6.7
All ages	43	16.6	4	1.4	8.6	0.08	13	5.2	11	3.2
Total	85	16.7	7	1.4	8.3	0.08	26	5.1	23	3.3

For epidemiological sources see Schillinger et al. 1996. For the methods used to estimate and project incidence, prevalence, and deaths see Murray and Lopez 1996a. See explanatory notes for definitions and caveats.

Table 57
Bacterial meningitis

Cuadro 57
Meninigitis bacteriana

Tableau 57
Méningite bactérienne

All forms - episodes

Todas las formas - episodios

Toutes les formes - épisodes

Table 57g　　　LAC - ALC - ALC　　　　Bacterial meningitis - All forms - episodes

Age group (years)	Incidence 1990 Number ('000s)	Rate (per 100 000)	Prevalence 1990 Number ('000s)	Rate (per 100 000)	Avg. age at onset (years)	Average duration (years)	Deaths 1990 Number ('000s)	Rate (per 100 000)	Deaths 2000 (Projected) Number ('000s)	Rate (per 100 000)
Males										
0-4	20	69.0	2	5.7	2.5	0.08	3	10.7	2	7.5
5-14	3	6.0	0	0.5	10.0	0.08	0	0.1	0	0.1
15-44	3	3.1	0	0.3	29.8	0.08	2	1.5	1	0.8
45-59	1	5.3	0	0.4	52.3	0.08	1	4.2	1	2.3
60+	1	9.8	0	0.8	70.3	0.08	1	9.6	1	6.8
All ages	29	13.0	2	1.1	11.7	0.08	7	3.2	5	2.0
Females										
0-4	19	69.0	2	5.7	2.5	0.08	3	10.0	2	6.8
5-14	3	6.0	0	0.5	10.0	0.08	0	0.1	0	0.1
15-44	3	3.1	0	0.3	29.9	0.08	2	1.9	1	0.9
45-59	1	5.3	0	0.4	52.4	0.08	1	4.2	1	2.3
60+	2	9.8	0	0.8	71.1	0.08	2	9.6	2	6.8
All ages	28	12.7	2	1.0	12.6	0.08	7	3.3	5	2.0
Total	57	12.8	5	1.1	12.2	0.08	14	3.3	11	2.0

Table 57h　　　MEC - AOM - CMO　　　　Bacterial meningitis - All forms - episodes

Age group (years)	Incidence 1990 Number ('000s)	Rate (per 100 000)	Prevalence 1990 Number ('000s)	Rate (per 100 000)	Avg. age at onset (years)	Average duration (years)	Deaths 1990 Number ('000s)	Rate (per 100 000)	Deaths 2000 (Projected) Number ('000s)	Rate (per 100 000)
Males										
0-4	29	69.5	2	5.7	2.5	0.08	5	12.2	4	9.0
5-14	4	5.9	0	0.5	10.0	0.08	0	0.1	0	0.1
15-44	4	3.2	0	0.3	29.8	0.08	2	1.7	1	0.9
45-59	1	5.4	0	0.4	52.3	0.08	1	4.8	1	2.7
60+	1	9.7	0	0.8	69.7	0.08	1	9.6	1	6.5
All ages	39	15.1	3	1.2	9.7	0.08	9	3.7	8	2.4
Females										
0-4	28	69.5	2	5.7	2.5	0.08	5	12.2	4	8.7
5-14	4	5.9	0	0.5	10.0	0.08	0	0.1	0	0.1
15-44	3	3.2	0	0.3	29.8	0.08	2	1.6	1	0.7
45-59	1	5.4	0	0.4	52.3	0.08	1	4.8	1	2.6
60+	2	9.7	0	0.8	70.4	0.08	1	8.7	1	6.0
All ages	37	15.2	3	1.2	10.1	0.08	9	3.7	7	2.3
Total	76	15.1	6	1.2	9.9	0.08	18	3.7	15	2.3

Table 57i　　　World - Mundo - Monde　　　　Bacterial meningitis - All forms - episodes

Age group (years)	Incidence 1990 Number ('000s)	Rate (per 100 000)	Prevalence 1990 Number ('000s)	Rate (per 100 000)	Avg. age at onset (years)	Average duration (years)	Deaths 1990 Number ('000s)	Rate (per 100 000)	Deaths 2000 (Projected) Number ('000s)	Rate (per 100 000)
Males										
0-4	217	67.4	18	5.5	2.5	0.08	44	13.8	32	9.2
5-14	31	5.7	3	0.5	10.0	0.08	1	0.1	0	0.1
15-44	33	2.7	3	0.2	29.8	0.08	20	1.6	11	0.8
45-59	13	4.2	1	0.3	52.3	0.08	11	3.6	7	1.8
60+	17	7.7	1	0.5	69.9	0.08	15	7.0	13	4.8
All ages	311	11.7	25	1.0	11.4	0.08	92	3.5	64	2.1
Females										
0-4	209	67.5	17	5.5	2.5	0.08	41	13.4	28	8.5
5-14	30	5.7	2	0.5	10.0	0.08	1	0.2	0	0.1
15-44	32	2.6	3	0.2	29.8	0.08	19	1.6	9	0.6
45-59	13	4.1	1	0.3	52.4	0.08	11	3.4	7	1.7
60+	20	7.4	1	0.5	70.9	0.08	16	5.8	14	4.1
All ages	303	11.6	25	0.9	12.2	0.08	88	3.4	58	1.9
Total	614	11.7	50	0.9	11.8	0.08	180	3.4	122	2.0

For epidemiological sources see Schillinger et al. 1996. For the methods used to estimate and project incidence, prevalence, and deaths see Murray and Lopez 1996a. See explanatory notes for definitions and caveats.

Table 58
Bacterial meningitis
Streptococcus pneumoniae - episodes

Cuadro 58
Meninigitis bacteriana
Streptococcus pneumoniae - episodios

Tableau 58
Méningite bactérienne
Streptococcus pneumoniae - épisodes

Table 58a   EME - PEMC - EMBE   Bacterial meningitis - S. pneumoniae - episodes

Age group (years)	Incidence 1990 Number ('000s)	Rate (per 100 000)	Prevalence 1990 Number ('000s)	Rate (per 100 000)	Avg. age at onset (years)	Average duration (years)	Deaths 1990 Number ('000s)	Rate (per 100 000)	Deaths 2000 (Projected) Number ('000s)	Rate (per 100 000)
Males										
0-4	1	5.4	0	0.4	2.5	0.08	0	0.4	0	0.3
5-14	0	0.4	0	0.0	10.0	0.08	0	0.0	0	0.0
15-44	1	0.3	0	0.0	29.9	0.08	0	0.1	0	0.1
45-59	0	0.3	0	0.0	52.4	0.08	0	0.3	0	0.2
60+	1	2.1	0	0.2	71.1	0.08	1	1.2	1	1.0
All ages	4	0.9	0	0.1	33.6	0.08	1	0.3	1	0.2
Females										
0-4	1	5.4	0	0.4	2.5	0.08	0	0.3	0	0.2
5-14	0	0.4	0	0.0	10.0	0.08	0	0.0	0	0.0
15-44	1	0.3	0	0.0	30.0	0.08	0	0.1	0	0.0
45-59	0	0.3	0	0.0	52.4	0.08	0	0.2	0	0.1
60+	2	2.1	0	0.2	72.4	0.08	1	1.0	1	0.9
All ages	4	1.0	0	0.1	39.4	0.08	1	0.3	1	0.2
Total	8	1.0	1	0.1	36.7	0.08	2	0.3	2	0.2

Table 58b   FSE - PEAS - AESE   Bacterial meningitis - S. pneumoniae - episodes

Age group (years)	Incidence 1990 Number ('000s)	Rate (per 100 000)	Prevalence 1990 Number ('000s)	Rate (per 100 000)	Avg. age at onset (years)	Average duration (years)	Deaths 1990 Number ('000s)	Rate (per 100 000)	Deaths 2000 (Projected) Number ('000s)	Rate (per 100 000)
Males										
0-4	3	24.4	0	2.0	2.5	0.08	1	4.8	0	3.6
5-14	1	1.9	0	0.2	10.0	0.08	0	0.0	0	0.0
15-44	2	2.7	0	0.2	29.8	0.08	0	0.6	0	0.4
45-59	1	3.7	0	0.3	52.2	0.08	1	2.0	0	1.3
60+	2	9.4	0	0.8	70.0	0.08	1	5.2	1	4.6
All ages	9	5.4	1	0.4	29.8	0.08	3	1.7	2	1.3
Females										
0-4	3	24.4	0	2.0	2.5	0.08	0	3.4	0	2.5
5-14	1	1.9	0	0.2	10.0	0.08	0	0.0	0	0.0
15-44	2	2.7	0	0.2	29.9	0.08	0	0.3	0	0.2
45-59	1	3.7	0	0.3	52.4	0.08	0	0.8	0	0.5
60+	3	9.4	0	0.8	71.5	0.08	1	2.3	1	2.0
All ages	10	5.7	1	0.5	36.7	0.08	2	1.0	1	0.7
Total	19	5.5	2	0.5	33.5	0.08	5	1.3	4	1.0

Table 58c   India - India - Inde   Bacterial meningitis - S. pneumoniae - episodes

Age group (years)	Incidence 1990 Number ('000s)	Rate (per 100 000)	Prevalence 1990 Number ('000s)	Rate (per 100 000)	Avg. age at onset (years)	Average duration (years)	Deaths 1990 Number ('000s)	Rate (per 100 000)	Deaths 2000 (Projected) Number ('000s)	Rate (per 100 000)
Males										
0-4	15	24.4	1	2.0	2.5	0.08	5	9.2	3	5.7
5-14	2	1.8	0	0.1	10.0	0.08	0	0.0	0	0.0
15-44	5	2.6	0	0.2	29.8	0.08	5	2.3	2	1.0
45-59	2	4.7	0	0.4	52.3	0.08	2	4.8	1	2.2
60+	3	9.5	0	0.8	69.7	0.08	3	9.7	2	6.1
All ages	27	6.1	2	0.5	19.6	0.08	15	3.5	9	1.8
Females										
0-4	14	24.4	1	2.0	2.5	0.08	5	9.5	3	5.7
5-14	2	1.8	0	0.1	10.0	0.08	0	0.0	0	0.0
15-44	5	2.6	0	0.2	29.8	0.08	4	2.1	2	0.7
45-59	2	4.7	0	0.4	52.4	0.08	2	4.8	1	2.2
60+	3	9.5	0	0.8	70.1	0.08	3	9.7	2	6.1
All ages	25	6.1	2	0.5	19.8	0.08	14	3.5	8	1.7
Total	52	6.1	4	0.5	19.7	0.08	30	3.5	17	1.8

For epidemiological sources see Schillinger et al. 1996. For the methods used to estimate and project incidence, prevalence, and deaths see Murray and Lopez 1996a. See explanatory notes for definitions and caveats.

Table 58
Bacterial meningitis
Streptococcus pneumoniae -
episodes

Cuadro 58
Meninigitis bacteriana
Streptococcus pneumoniae -
episodios

Tableau 58
Méningite bactérienne
Streptococcus pneumoniae -
épisodes

Table 58d   China - China - Chine   Bacterial meningitis - S. pneumoniae - episodes

Age group (years)	Incidence 1990 Number ('000s)	Rate (per 100 000)	Prevalence 1990 Number ('000s)	Rate (per 100 000)	Avg. age at onset (years)	Average duration (years)	Deaths 1990 Number ('000s)	Rate (per 100 000)	Deaths 2000 (Projected) Number ('000s)	Rate (per 100 000)
Males										
0-4	15	24.3	1	2.0	2.5	0.08	3	4.8	1	2.5
5-14	2	1.7	0	0.1	10.0	0.08	0	0.0	0	0.0
15-44	8	2.5	1	0.2	29.9	0.08	6	2.0	2	0.8
45-59	3	4.8	0	0.4	52.3	0.08	3	4.4	2	1.7
60+	5	9.5	0	0.8	69.8	0.08	4	8.8	3	5.3
All ages	32	5.5	3	0.4	24.6	0.08	17	2.8	9	1.3
Females										
0-4	14	24.3	1	2.0	2.5	0.08	3	4.8	1	2.4
5-14	2	1.7	0	0.1	10.0	0.08	0	0.0	0	0.0
15-44	7	2.5	1	0.2	29.9	0.08	5	1.9	2	0.6
45-59	3	4.8	0	0.4	52.4	0.08	3	4.3	2	1.7
60+	5	9.5	0	0.8	70.6	0.08	5	8.8	3	5.4
All ages	31	5.6	3	0.5	25.1	0.08	16	2.8	8	1.3
Total	63	5.5	5	0.5	24.9	0.08	32	2.8	17	1.3

Table 58e   OAI - OPAI - APAI   Bacterial meningitis - S. pneumoniae - episodes

Age group (years)	Incidence 1990 Number ('000s)	Rate (per 100 000)	Prevalence 1990 Number ('000s)	Rate (per 100 000)	Avg. age at onset (years)	Average duration (years)	Deaths 1990 Number ('000s)	Rate (per 100 000)	Deaths 2000 (Projected) Number ('000s)	Rate (per 100 000)
Males										
0-4	11	24.4	1	2.0	2.5	0.08	3	5.7	2	3.7
5-14	1	1.4	0	0.1	10.0	0.08	0	0.0	0	0.0
15-44	3	2.0	0	0.2	29.7	0.08	3	1.7	2	0.8
45-59	2	4.9	0	0.4	52.3	0.08	2	5.1	1	2.5
60+	2	9.5	0	0.8	69.6	0.08	2	10.0	2	6.7
All ages	19	5.4	2	0.4	19.0	0.08	9	2.6	6	1.5
Females										
0-4	10	24.4	1	2.0	2.5	0.08	2	5.4	1	3.4
5-14	1	1.4	0	0.1	10.0	0.08	0	0.0	0	0.0
15-44	3	2.0	0	0.2	29.8	0.08	3	1.7	1	0.7
45-59	2	4.9	0	0.4	52.3	0.08	2	5.0	1	2.5
60+	2	9.5	0	0.8	70.3	0.08	2	8.0	2	5.6
All ages	18	5.4	2	0.4	20.2	0.08	8	2.5	6	1.4
Total	37	5.4	3	0.4	19.6	0.08	17	2.6	12	1.5

Table 58f   SSA - ASS - ASS   Bacterial meningitis - S. pneumoniae - episodes

Age group (years)	Incidence 1990 Number ('000s)	Rate (per 100 000)	Prevalence 1990 Number ('000s)	Rate (per 100 000)	Avg. age at onset (years)	Average duration (years)	Deaths 1990 Number ('000s)	Rate (per 100 000)	Deaths 2000 (Projected) Number ('000s)	Rate (per 100 000)
Males										
0-4	12	24.4	1	2.0	2.4	0.08	4	8.2	4	5.9
5-14	1	1.8	0	0.1	10.0	0.08	0	0.0	0	0.0
15-44	3	2.6	0	0.2	29.4	0.08	2	1.8	1	0.9
45-59	1	5.2	0	0.4	52.2	0.08	1	5.3	1	2.8
60+	1	9.4	0	0.8	69.2	0.08	1	9.7	1	6.4
All ages	18	7.0	1	0.6	13.8	0.08	8	3.1	7	2.1
Females										
0-4	11	24.4	1	2.0	2.4	0.08	4	7.7	3	5.3
5-14	1	1.8	0	0.1	10.0	0.08	0	0.0	0	0.0
15-44	3	2.6	0	0.2	29.5	0.08	2	2.3	1	0.9
45-59	1	5.2	0	0.4	52.2	0.08	1	5.4	1	2.8
60+	1	9.4	0	0.8	69.7	0.08	1	10.0	1	6.5
All ages	18	6.9	1	0.6	14.8	0.08	9	3.3	7	2.0
Total	35	6.9	3	0.6	14.3	0.08	16	3.2	14	2.1

For epidemiological sources see Schillinger et al. 1996. For the methods used to estimate and project incidence, prevalence, and deaths see Murray and Lopez 1996a. See explanatory notes for definitions and caveats.

Table 58
Bacterial meningitis
Streptococcus pneumoniae -
episodes

Cuadro 58
Meninigitis bacteriana
Streptococcus pneumoniae -
episodios

Tableau 58
Méningite bactérienne
Streptococcus pneumoniae -
épisodes

Table 58g   LAC - ALC - ALC   Bacterial meningitis - S. pneumoniae - episodes

Age group (years)	Incidence 1990 Number ('000s)	Rate (per 100 000)	Prevalence 1990 Number ('000s)	Rate (per 100 000)	Avg. age at onset (years)	Average duration (years)	Deaths 1990 Number ('000s)	Rate (per 100 000)	Deaths 2000 (Projected) Number ('000s)	Rate (per 100 000)
Males										
0-4	7	24.1	1	2.0	2.5	0.08	1	4.5	1	3.1
5-14	1	1.8	0	0.1	10.0	0.08	0	0.0	0	0.0
15-44	3	2.6	0	0.2	29.8	0.08	2	1.8	1	1.0
45-59	1	4.9	0	0.4	52.3	0.08	1	4.1	1	2.3
60+	1	9.5	0	0.8	70.3	0.08	1	9.5	1	6.7
All ages	13	5.9	1	0.5	19.9	0.08	5	2.5	4	1.6
Females										
0-4	7	24.1	1	2.0	2.5	0.08	1	4.5	1	3.1
5-14	1	1.8	0	0.1	10.0	0.08	0	0.0	0	0.0
15-44	3	2.6	0	0.2	29.9	0.08	2	1.8	1	0.9
45-59	1	4.9	0	0.4	52.4	0.08	1	4.1	1	2.3
60+	2	9.5	0	0.8	71.1	0.08	2	9.5	2	6.7
All ages	13	5.8	1	0.5	21.4	0.08	6	2.6	4	1.6
Total	26	5.9	2	0.5	20.6	0.08	11	2.5	8	1.6

Table 58h   MEC - AOM - CMO   Bacterial meningitis - S. pneumoniae - episodes

Age group (years)	Incidence 1990 Number ('000s)	Rate (per 100 000)	Prevalence 1990 Number ('000s)	Rate (per 100 000)	Avg. age at onset (years)	Average duration (years)	Deaths 1990 Number ('000s)	Rate (per 100 000)	Deaths 2000 (Projected) Number ('000s)	Rate (per 100 000)
Males										
0-4	10	24.3	1	2.0	2.5	0.08	2	5.2	2	3.8
5-14	1	1.8	0	0.1	10.0	0.08	0	0.0	0	0.0
15-44	3	2.6	0	0.2	29.8	0.08	2	2.1	2	1.1
45-59	1	5.0	0	0.4	52.3	0.08	1	4.8	1	2.7
60+	1	9.4	0	0.8	69.7	0.08	1	9.5	1	6.4
All ages	17	6.5	1	0.5	16.5	0.08	7	2.7	6	1.7
Females										
0-4	10	24.3	1	2.0	2.5	0.08	2	5.2	2	3.7
5-14	1	1.8	0	0.1	10.0	0.08	0	0.0	0	0.0
15-44	3	2.6	0	0.2	29.8	0.08	2	2.1	1	0.9
45-59	1	5.0	0	0.4	52.3	0.08	1	4.8	1	2.6
60+	1	9.4	0	0.8	70.4	0.08	1	9.4	1	6.4
All ages	16	6.5	1	0.5	17.3	0.08	7	2.8	5	1.7
Total	33	6.5	3	0.5	16.9	0.08	14	2.7	11	1.7

Table 58i   World - Mundo - Monde   Bacterial meningitis - S. pneumoniae - episodes

Age group (years)	Incidence 1990 Number ('000s)	Rate (per 100 000)	Prevalence 1990 Number ('000s)	Rate (per 100 000)	Avg. age at onset (years)	Average duration (years)	Deaths 1990 Number ('000s)	Rate (per 100 000)	Deaths 2000 (Projected) Number ('000s)	Rate (per 100 000)
Males										
0-4	73	22.8	6	1.9	2.5	0.08	19	5.9	14	3.9
5-14	9	1.6	1	0.1	10.0	0.08	0	0.0	0	0.0
15-44	27	2.1	2	0.2	29.8	0.08	19	1.6	10	0.7
45-59	12	3.8	1	0.3	52.3	0.08	11	3.5	7	1.7
60+	16	7.4	1	0.6	69.9	0.08	15	6.7	13	4.6
All ages	137	5.2	11	0.4	20.6	0.08	64	2.4	44	1.4
Females										
0-4	71	22.8	6	1.9	2.5	0.08	18	5.7	12	3.7
5-14	8	1.6	1	0.1	10.0	0.08	0	0.0	0	0.0
15-44	26	2.1	2	0.2	29.8	0.08	18	1.5	8	0.6
45-59	12	3.7	1	0.3	52.4	0.08	10	3.3	7	1.6
60+	19	7.2	1	0.6	70.8	0.08	15	5.6	13	3.9
All ages	135	5.2	11	0.4	22.1	0.08	61	2.4	41	1.3
Total	272	5.2	22	0.4	21.4	0.08	126	2.4	85	1.4

For epidemiological sources see Schillinger et al. 1996. For the methods used to estimate and project incidence, prevalence, and deaths see Murray and Lopez 1996a. See explanatory notes for definitions and caveats.

Table 59
Bacterial meningitis

Cuadro 59
Meninigitis bacteriana

Tableau 59
Méningite bactérienne

Haemophilus influenzae - episodes   Haemophilus influenzae - episodios   Haemophilus influenzae - épisodes

Table 59a — EME - PEMC - EMBE — Bacterial meningitis - H. influenzae - episodes

Age group (years)	Incidence 1990 Number ('000s)	Rate (per 100 000)	Prevalence 1990 Number ('000s)	Rate (per 100 000)	Avg. age at onset (years)	Average duration (years)	Deaths 1990 Number ('000s)	Rate (per 100 000)	Deaths 2000 (Projected) Number ('000s)	Rate (per 100 000)
Males										
0-4	9	33.2	1	2.7	2.5	0.08	0	1.1	0	0.8
5-14	2	2.9	0	0.2	10.0	0.08	0	0.0	0	0.0
15-44	0	0.1	0	0.0	29.9	0.08	0	0.0	0	0.0
45-59	0	0.1	0	0.0	52.4	0.08	0	0.0	0	0.0
60+	0	0.1	0	0.0	71.1	0.08	0	0.0	0	0.0
All ages	11	2.7	1	0.2	4.8	0.08	0	0.1	0	0.1
Females										
0-4	8	33.2	1	2.7	2.5	0.08	0	0.9	0	0.6
5-14	1	2.9	0	0.2	10.0	0.08	0	0.0	0	0.0
15-44	0	0.1	0	0.0	30.0	0.08	0	0.0	0	0.0
45-59	0	0.1	0	0.0	52.4	0.08	0	0.0	0	0.0
60+	0	0.1	0	0.0	72.4	0.08	0	0.0	0	0.0
All ages	10	2.5	1	0.2	5.1	0.08	0	0.1	0	0.0
Total	21	2.6	2	0.2	5.0	0.08	1	0.1	0	0.1

Table 59b — FSE - PEAS - AESE — Bacterial meningitis - H. influenzae - episodes

Age group (years)	Incidence 1990 Number ('000s)	Rate (per 100 000)	Prevalence 1990 Number ('000s)	Rate (per 100 000)	Avg. age at onset (years)	Average duration (years)	Deaths 1990 Number ('000s)	Rate (per 100 000)	Deaths 2000 (Projected) Number ('000s)	Rate (per 100 000)
Males										
0-4	5	37.8	0	3.1	2.5	0.08	1	4.6	0	3.5
5-14	1	3.2	0	0.3	10.0	0.08	0	0.0	0	0.0
15-44	0	0.1	0	0.0	29.8	0.08	0	0.0	0	0.0
45-59	0	0.1	0	0.0	52.2	0.08	0	0.0	0	0.0
60+	0	0.1	0	0.0	70.0	0.08	0	0.0	0	0.0
All ages	6	3.8	1	0.3	4.5	0.08	1	0.4	1	0.3
Females										
0-4	5	37.8	0	3.1	2.5	0.08	0	3.3	0	2.4
5-14	1	3.2	0	0.3	10.0	0.08	0	0.0	0	0.0
15-44	0	0.1	0	0.0	29.9	0.08	0	0.0	0	0.0
45-59	0	0.1	0	0.0	52.4	0.08	0	0.0	0	0.0
60+	0	0.1	0	0.0	71.5	0.08	0	0.0	0	0.0
All ages	6	3.3	1	0.3	4.8	0.08	0	0.2	0	0.2
Total	12	3.5	1	0.3	4.6	0.08	1	0.3	1	0.2

Table 59c — India - India - Inde — Bacterial meningitis - H. influenzae - episodes

Age group (years)	Incidence 1990 Number ('000s)	Rate (per 100 000)	Prevalence 1990 Number ('000s)	Rate (per 100 000)	Avg. age at onset (years)	Average duration (years)	Deaths 1990 Number ('000s)	Rate (per 100 000)	Deaths 2000 (Projected) Number ('000s)	Rate (per 100 000)
Males										
0-4	23	37.9	2	3.1	2.5	0.08	6	9.6	3	6.0
5-14	3	3.2	0	0.3	10.0	0.08	0	0.0	0	0.0
15-44	0	0.1	0	0.0	29.8	0.08	0	0.0	0	0.0
45-59	0	0.1	0	0.0	52.3	0.08	0	0.0	0	0.0
60+	0	0.2	0	0.0	69.7	0.08	0	0.2	0	0.1
All ages	26	6.0	2	0.5	3.9	0.08	6	1.3	3	0.7
Females										
0-4	21	37.9	2	3.1	2.5	0.08	6	9.9	3	6.0
5-14	3	3.2	0	0.3	10.0	0.08	0	0.0	0	0.0
15-44	0	0.1	0	0.0	29.8	0.08	0	0.0	0	0.0
45-59	0	0.1	0	0.0	52.4	0.08	0	0.0	0	0.0
60+	0	0.2	0	0.0	70.1	0.08	0	0.2	0	0.1
All ages	25	6.1	2	0.5	3.9	0.08	6	1.4	3	0.7
Total	51	6.0	4	0.5	3.9	0.08	11	1.3	7	0.7

For epidemiological sources see Schillinger et al. 1996. For the methods used to estimate and project incidence, prevalence, and deaths see Murray and Lopez 1996a. See explanatory notes for definitions and caveats.

Table 59   Cuadro 59   Tableau 59
Bacterial meningitis   **Meninigitis bacteriana**   **Méningite bactérienne**

Haemophilus influenzae - episodes   Haemophilus influenzae - episodios   Haemophilus influenzae - épisodes

Table 59d   China - China - Chine   Bacterial meningitis - H. influenzae - episodes

Age group (years)	Incidence 1990 Number ('000s)	Rate (per 100 000)	Prevalence 1990 Number ('000s)	Rate (per 100 000)	Avg. age at onset (years)	Average duration (years)	Deaths 1990 Number ('000s)	Rate (per 100 000)	Deaths 2000 (Projected) Number ('000s)	Rate (per 100 000)
Males										
0-4	23	37.6	2	3.1	2.5	0.08	3	4.8	*1*	*2.5*
5-14	3	3.2	0	0.3	10.0	0.08	0	0.0	*0*	*0.0*
15-44	0	0.1	0	0.0	29.9	0.08	0	0.0	*0*	*0.0*
45-59	0	0.1	0	0.0	52.3	0.08	0	0.0	*0*	*0.0*
60+	0	0.2	0	0.0	69.8	0.08	0	0.1	*0*	*0.1*
All ages	26	4.5	2	0.4	4.1	0.08	3	0.5	*2*	*0.2*
Females										
0-4	22	37.6	2	3.1	2.5	0.08	3	4.8	*1*	*2.4*
5-14	3	3.2	0	0.3	10.0	0.08	0	0.0	*0*	*0.0*
15-44	0	0.1	0	0.0	29.9	0.08	0	0.0	*0*	*0.0*
45-59	0	0.1	0	0.0	52.4	0.08	0	0.0	*0*	*0.0*
60+	0	0.2	0	0.0	70.6	0.08	0	0.1	*0*	*0.1*
All ages	25	4.6	2	0.4	4.0	0.08	3	0.5	*1*	*0.2*
Total	51	4.5	4	0.4	4.0	0.08	6	0.5	*3*	*0.2*

Table 59e   OAI - OPAI - APAI   Bacterial meningitis - H. influenzae - episodes

Age group (years)	Incidence 1990 Number ('000s)	Rate (per 100 000)	Prevalence 1990 Number ('000s)	Rate (per 100 000)	Avg. age at onset (years)	Average duration (years)	Deaths 1990 Number ('000s)	Rate (per 100 000)	Deaths 2000 (Projected) Number ('000s)	Number ('000s)
Males										
0-4	17	37.8	1	3.1	2.5	0.08	3	5.8	*2*	*3.7*
5-14	3	3.2	0	0.3	10.0	0.08	0	0.0	*0*	*0.0*
15-44	0	0.1	0	0.0	29.7	0.08	0	0.0	*0*	*0.0*
45-59	0	0.2	0	0.0	52.3	0.08	0	0.0	*0*	*0.0*
60+	0	0.2	0	0.0	69.6	0.08	0	0.1	*0*	*0.1*
All ages	19	5.7	2	0.5	4.0	0.08	3	0.7	*2*	*0.4*
Females										
0-4	16	37.8	1	3.1	2.5	0.08	2	5.4	*1*	*3.4*
5-14	3	3.2	0	0.3	10.0	0.08	0	0.0	*0*	*0.0*
15-44	0	0.1	0	0.0	29.8	0.08	0	0.0	*0*	*0.0*
45-59	0	0.2	0	0.0	52.3	0.08	0	0.0	*0*	*0.0*
60+	0	0.2	0	0.0	70.3	0.08	0	0.1	*0*	*0.1*
All ages	19	5.5	2	0.5	4.0	0.08	2	0.7	*2*	*0.4*
Total	38	5.6	3	0.5	4.0	0.08	5	0.7	*3*	*0.4*

Table 59f   SSA - ASS - ASS   Bacterial meningitis - H. influenzae - episodes

Age group (years)	Incidence 1990 Number ('000s)	Rate (per 100 000)	Prevalence 1990 Number ('000s)	Rate (per 100 000)	Avg. age at onset (years)	Average duration (years)	Deaths 1990 Number ('000s)	Rate (per 100 000)	Deaths 2000 (Projected) Number ('000s)	Number ('000s)
Males										
0-4	18	37.9	1	3.1	2.4	0.08	4	8.5	*4*	*6.1*
5-14	2	3.2	0	0.3	10.0	0.08	0	0.0	*0*	*0.0*
15-44	0	0.0	0	0.0	29.4	0.08	0	0.0	*0*	*0.0*
45-59	0	0.0	0	0.0	52.2	0.08	0	0.0	*0*	*0.0*
60+	0	0.1	0	0.0	69.2	0.08	0	0.2	*0*	*0.1*
All ages	20	8.1	2	0.7	3.4	0.08	4	1.6	*4*	*1.1*
Females										
0-4	18	37.9	1	3.1	2.4	0.08	4	8.0	*4*	*5.6*
5-14	2	3.2	0	0.3	10.0	0.08	0	0.0	*0*	*0.0*
15-44	0	0.0	0	0.0	29.5	0.08	0	0.0	*0*	*0.0*
45-59	0	0.0	0	0.0	52.2	0.08	0	0.0	*0*	*0.0*
60+	0	0.1	0	0.0	69.7	0.08	0	0.2	*0*	*0.1*
All ages	20	7.8	2	0.6	3.4	0.08	4	1.5	*3*	*0.9*
Total	40	7.9	3	0.7	3.4	0.08	8	1.5	*7*	*1.0*

For epidemiological sources see Schillinger et al. 1996. For the methods used to estimate and project incidence, prevalence, and deaths see Murray and Lopez 1996a. See explanatory notes for definitions and caveats.

Table 59
Bacterial meningitis

Cuadro 59
Meninigitis bacteriana

Tableau 59
Méningite bactérienne

Haemophilus influenzae - episodes   Haemophilus influenzae - episodios   Haemophilus influenzae - épisodes

Table 59g   LAC - ALC - ALC   Bacterial meningitis - H. influenzae - episodes

Age group (years)	Incidence 1990 Number ('000s)	Rate (per 100 000)	Prevalence 1990 Number ('000s)	Rate (per 100 000)	Avg. age at onset (years)	Average duration (years)	Deaths 1990 Number ('000s)	Rate (per 100 000)	Deaths 2000 (Projected) Number ('000s)	Rate (per 100 000)
Males										
0-4	11	37.4	1	3.1	2.5	0.08	1	4.5	1	3.1
5-14	2	3.2	0	0.3	10.0	0.08	0	0.0	0	0.0
15-44	0	0.1	0	0.0	29.8	0.08	0	0.0	0	0.0
45-59	0	0.2	0	0.0	52.3	0.08	0	0.0	0	0.0
60+	0	0.1	0	0.0	70.3	0.08	0	0.1	0	0.1
All ages	13	5.7	1	0.5	4.0	0.08	1	0.6	1	0.4
Females										
0-4	10	37.4	1	3.1	2.5	0.08	1	4.1	1	2.8
5-14	2	3.2	0	0.3	10.0	0.08	0	0.0	0	0.0
15-44	0	0.1	0	0.0	29.9	0.08	0	0.0	0	0.0
45-59	0	0.2	0	0.0	52.4	0.08	0	0.0	0	0.0
60+	0	0.1	0	0.0	71.1	0.08	0	0.1	0	0.1
All ages	12	5.5	1	0.4	4.0	0.08	1	0.5	1	0.3
Total	25	5.6	2	0.5	4.0	0.08	2	0.6	2	0.3

Table 59h   MEC - AOM - CMO   Bacterial meningitis - H. influenzae - episodes

Age group (years)	Incidence 1990 Number ('000s)	Rate (per 100 000)	Prevalence 1990 Number ('000s)	Rate (per 100 000)	Avg. age at onset (years)	Average duration (years)	Deaths 1990 Number ('000s)	Rate (per 100 000)	Deaths 2000 (Projected) Number ('000s)	Rate (per 100 000)
Males										
0-4	16	37.7	1	3.1	2.5	0.08	2	5.2	2	3.8
5-14	2	3.2	0	0.3	10.0	0.08	0	0.0	0	0.0
15-44	0	0.1	0	0.0	29.8	0.08	0	0.0	0	0.0
45-59	0	0.2	0	0.0	52.3	0.08	0	0.0	0	0.0
60+	0	0.1	0	0.0	69.7	0.08	0	0.1	0	0.1
All ages	18	6.9	1	0.6	3.7	0.08	2	0.8	2	0.5
Females										
0-4	15	37.7	1	3.1	2.5	0.08	2	5.2	2	3.7
5-14	2	3.2	0	0.3	10.0	0.08	0	0.0	0	0.0
15-44	0	0.1	0	0.0	29.8	0.08	0	0.0	0	0.0
45-59	0	0.2	0	0.0	52.3	0.08	0	0.0	0	0.0
60+	0	0.1	0	0.0	70.4	0.08	0	0.1	0	0.1
All ages	17	7.0	1	0.6	3.7	0.08	2	0.8	2	0.5
Total	35	6.9	3	0.6	3.7	0.08	4	0.8	3	0.5

Table 59i   World - Mundo - Monde   Bacterial meningitis - H. influenzae - episodes

Age group (years)	Incidence 1990 Number ('000s)	Rate (per 100 000)	Prevalence 1990 Number ('000s)	Rate (per 100 000)	Avg. age at onset (years)	Average duration (years)	Deaths 1990 Number ('000s)	Rate (per 100 000)	Deaths 2000 (Projected) Number ('000s)	Rate (per 100 000)
Males										
0-4	120	37.4	10	3.1	2.5	0.08	20	6.1	14	4.1
5-14	18	3.2	1	0.3	10.0	0.08	0	0.0	0	0.0
15-44	1	0.1	0	0.0	29.8	0.08	0	0.0	0	0.0
45-59	0	0.1	0	0.0	52.3	0.08	0	0.0	0	0.0
60+	0	0.1	0	0.0	70.1	0.08	0	0.1	0	0.1
All ages	139	5.3	11	0.4	3.9	0.08	20	0.7	14	0.4
Females										
0-4	116	37.4	10	3.1	2.5	0.08	18	5.9	13	3.8
5-14	17	3.2	1	0.3	10.0	0.08	0	0.0	0	0.0
15-44	1	0.1	0	0.0	29.9	0.08	0	0.0	0	0.0
45-59	0	0.1	0	0.0	52.4	0.08	0	0.0	0	0.0
60+	0	0.1	0	0.0	71.1	0.08	0	0.1	0	0.0
All ages	134	5.1	11	0.4	4.0	0.08	19	0.7	12	0.4
Total	274	5.2	22	0.4	4.0	0.08	38	0.7	26	0.4

For epidemiological sources see Schillinger et al. 1996. For the methods used to estimate and project incidence, prevalence, and deaths see Murray and Lopez 1996a. See explanatory notes for definitions and caveats.

Table 60
Bacterial meningitis

Cuadro 60
Meninigitis bacteriana

Tableau 60
Méningite bactérienne

Neisseria meningitidis - episodes   Neisseria meningitidis - episodios   Neisseria meningitidis - épisodes

Table 60a   EME - PEMC - EMBE   Bacterial meningitis - N. meningitidis - episodes

Age group (years)	Incidence 1990 Number ('000s)	Rate (per 100 000)	Prevalence 1990 Number ('000s)	Rate (per 100 000)	Avg. age at onset (years)	Average duration (years)	Deaths 1990 Number ('000s)	Rate (per 100 000)	Deaths 2000 (Projected) Number ('000s)	Rate (per 100 000)
Males										
0-4	1	5.1	0	0.4	2.5	0.08	0	0.9	0	0.6
5-14	0	0.7	0	0.1	10.0	0.08	0	0.1	0	0.1
15-44	1	0.3	0	0.0	29.9	0.08	0	0.1	0	0.0
45-59	0	0.2	0	0.0	52.4	0.08	0	0.1	0	0.1
60+	0	0.1	0	0.0	71.1	0.08	0	0.0	0	0.0
All ages	2	0.6	0	0.1	13.9	0.08	1	0.1	0	0.1
Females										
0-4	1	5.1	0	0.4	2.5	0.08	0	0.7	0	0.5
5-14	0	0.7	0	0.1	10.0	0.08	0	0.1	0	0.1
15-44	1	0.3	0	0.0	30.0	0.08	0	0.0	0	0.0
45-59	0	0.2	0	0.0	52.4	0.08	0	0.1	0	0.0
60+	0	0.1	0	0.0	72.4	0.08	0	0.0	0	0.0
All ages	2	0.6	0	0.0	14.8	0.08	0	0.1	0	0.1
Total	5	0.6	0	0.1	14.4	0.08	1	0.1	1	0.1

Table 60b   FSE - PEAS - AESE   Bacterial meningitis - N. meningitidis - episodes

Age group (years)	Incidence 1990 Number ('000s)	Rate (per 100 000)	Prevalence 1990 Number ('000s)	Rate (per 100 000)	Avg. age at onset (years)	Average duration (years)	Deaths 1990 Number ('000s)	Rate (per 100 000)	Deaths 2000 (Projected) Number ('000s)	Rate (per 100 000)
Males										
0-4	1	7.5	0	0.6	2.5	0.08	0	1.2	0	0.9
5-14	0	1.0	0	0.1	10.0	0.08	0	0.2	0	0.1
15-44	0	0.5	0	0.0	29.8	0.08	0	0.0	0	0.0
45-59	0	0.2	0	0.0	52.2	0.08	0	0.0	0	0.0
60+	0	0.1	0	0.0	70.0	0.08	0	0.0	0	0.0
All ages	2	1.1	0	0.1	12.0	0.08	0	0.2	0	0.1
Females										
0-4	1	7.5	0	0.6	2.5	0.08	0	0.9	0	0.7
5-14	0	1.0	0	0.1	10.0	0.08	0	0.2	0	0.1
15-44	0	0.5	0	0.0	29.9	0.08	0	0.0	0	0.0
45-59	0	0.2	0	0.0	52.4	0.08	0	0.0	0	0.0
60+	0	0.1	0	0.0	71.5	0.08	0	0.0	0	0.0
All ages	2	0.9	0	0.1	13.3	0.08	0	0.1	0	0.1
Total	3	1.0	0	0.1	12.6	0.08	0	0.1	0	0.1

Table 60c   India - India - Inde   Bacterial meningitis - N. meningitidis - episodes

Age group (years)	Incidence 1990 Number ('000s)	Rate (per 100 000)	Prevalence 1990 Number ('000s)	Rate (per 100 000)	Avg. age at onset (years)	Average duration (years)	Deaths 1990 Number ('000s)	Rate (per 100 000)	Deaths 2000 (Projected) Number ('000s)	Rate (per 100 000)
Males										
0-4	4	7.5	0	0.6	2.5	0.08	1	1.1	0	0.7
5-14	1	0.9	0	0.1	10.0	0.08	0	0.1	0	0.0
15-44	1	0.5	0	0.0	29.8	0.08	0	0.1	0	0.0
45-59	0	0.3	0	0.0	52.3	0.08	0	0.0	0	0.0
60+	0	0.2	0	0.0	69.7	0.08	0	0.1	0	0.0
All ages	7	1.5	1	0.1	9.0	0.08	1	0.2	1	0.1
Females										
0-4	4	7.5	0	0.6	2.5	0.08	1	1.1	0	0.7
5-14	1	0.9	0	0.1	10.0	0.08	0	0.1	0	0.0
15-44	1	0.5	0	0.0	29.8	0.08	0	0.0	0	0.0
45-59	0	0.3	0	0.0	52.4	0.08	0	0.0	0	0.0
60+	0	0.2	0	0.0	70.1	0.08	0	0.1	0	0.0
All ages	6	1.5	1	0.1	8.9	0.08	1	0.2	0	0.1
Total	13	1.5	1	0.1	9.0	0.08	2	0.2	1	0.1

For epidemiological sources see Schillinger et al. 1996. For the methods used to estimate and project incidence, prevalence, and deaths see Murray and Lopez 1996a. See explanatory notes for definitions and caveats.

Table 60
Bacterial meningitis

Cuadro 60
Meninigitis bacteriana

Tableau 60
Méningite bactérienne

Neisseria meningitidis - episodes

Neisseria meningitidis - episodios

Neisseria meningitidis - épisodes

Table 60d — China - China - Chine — Bacterial meningitis - N. meningitidis - episodes

Age group (years)	Incidence 1990 Number ('000s)	Rate (per 100 000)	Prevalence 1990 Number ('000s)	Rate (per 100 000)	Avg. age at onset (years)	Average duration (years)	Deaths 1990 Number ('000s)	Rate (per 100 000)	Deaths 2000 (Projected) Number ('000s)	Rate (per 100 000)
Males										
0-4	4	7.4	0	0.6	2.5	0.08	1	1.0	0	0.5
5-14	1	0.8	0	0.1	10.0	0.08	0	0.1	0	0.0
15-44	1	0.4	0	0.0	29.9	0.08	0	0.0	0	0.0
45-59	0	0.3	0	0.0	52.3	0.08	0	0.0	0	0.0
60+	0	0.2	0	0.0	69.8	0.08	0	0.5	0	0.3
All ages	7	1.1	1	0.1	10.4	0.08	1	0.2	1	0.1
Females										
0-4	4	7.4	0	0.6	2.5	0.08	1	1.0	0	0.5
5-14	1	0.8	0	0.1	10.0	0.08	0	0.1	0	0.0
15-44	1	0.4	0	0.0	29.9	0.08	0	0.0	0	0.0
45-59	0	0.3	0	0.0	52.4	0.08	0	0.0	0	0.0
60+	0	0.2	0	0.0	70.6	0.08	0	0.5	0	0.3
All ages	6	1.2	1	0.1	10.3	0.08	1	0.2	1	0.1
Total	13	1.2	1	0.1	10.4	0.08	2	0.2	1	0.1

Table 60e — OAI - OPAI - APAI — Bacterial meningitis - N. meningitidis - episodes

Age group (years)	Incidence 1990 Number ('000s)	Rate (per 100 000)	Prevalence 1990 Number ('000s)	Rate (per 100 000)	Avg. age at onset (years)	Average duration (years)	Deaths 1990 Number ('000s)	Rate (per 100 000)	Deaths 2000 (Projected) Number ('000s)	Rate (per 100 000)
Males										
0-4	3	7.5	0	0.6	2.5	0.08	0	1.0	0	0.7
5-14	1	0.9	0	0.1	10.0	0.08	0	0.1	0	0.0
15-44	1	0.5	0	0.0	29.7	0.08	0	0.0	0	0.0
45-59	0	0.3	0	0.0	52.3	0.08	0	0.0	0	0.0
60+	0	0.2	0	0.0	69.6	0.08	0	0.1	0	0.0
All ages	5	1.4	0	0.1	9.2	0.08	1	0.2	0	0.1
Females										
0-4	3	7.5	0	0.6	2.5	0.08	0	1.0	0	0.6
5-14	1	0.9	0	0.1	10.0	0.08	0	0.1	0	0.0
15-44	1	0.5	0	0.0	29.8	0.08	0	0.0	0	0.0
45-59	0	0.3	0	0.0	52.3	0.08	0	0.0	0	0.0
60+	0	0.2	0	0.0	70.3	0.08	0	0.0	0	0.0
All ages	5	1.4	0	0.1	9.5	0.08	1	0.2	0	0.1
Total	10	1.4	1	0.1	9.4	0.08	1	0.2	1	0.1

Table 60f — SSA - ASS - ASS — Bacterial meningitis - N. meningitidis - episodes

Age group (years)	Incidence 1990 Number ('000s)	Rate (per 100 000)	Prevalence 1990 Number ('000s)	Rate (per 100 000)	Avg. age at onset (years)	Average duration (years)	Deaths 1990 Number ('000s)	Rate (per 100 000)	Deaths 2000 (Projected) Number ('000s)	Rate (per 100 000)
Males										
0-4	4	7.5	0	0.6	2.4	0.08	0	1.0	0	0.7
5-14	1	0.9	0	0.1	10.0	0.08	0	0.1	0	0.0
15-44	1	0.5	0	0.0	29.4	0.08	0	0.0	0	0.0
45-59	0	0.3	0	0.0	52.2	0.08	0	0.0	0	0.0
60+	0	0.1	0	0.0	69.2	0.08	0	0.1	0	0.0
All ages	5	1.9	0	0.2	7.2	0.08	1	0.2	1	0.2
Females										
0-4	4	7.5	0	0.6	2.4	0.08	0	0.9	0	0.7
5-14	1	0.9	0	0.1	10.0	0.08	0	0.1	0	0.0
15-44	1	0.5	0	0.0	29.5	0.08	0	0.1	0	0.0
45-59	0	0.3	0	0.0	52.2	0.08	0	0.0	0	0.0
60+	0	0.1	0	0.0	69.7	0.08	0	0.1	0	0.0
All ages	5	1.8	0	0.2	7.4	0.08	1	0.2	0	0.1
Total	10	1.9	1	0.2	7.3	0.08	1	0.2	1	0.1

For epidemiological sources see Schillinger et al. 1996. For the methods used to estimate and project incidence, prevalence, and deaths see Murray and Lopez 1996a. See explanatory notes for definitions and caveats.

Table 60
Bacterial meningitis

Cuadro 60
Meninigitis bacteriana

Tableau 60
Méningite bactérienne

Neisseria meningitidis - episodes Neisseria meningitidis - episodios Neisseria meningitidis - épisodes

Table 60g LAC - ALC - ALC Bacterial meningitis - N. meningitidis - episodes

Age group (years)	Incidence 1990 Number ('000s)	Rate (per 100 000)	Prevalence 1990 Number ('000s)	Rate (per 100 000)	Avg. age at onset (years)	Average duration (years)	Deaths 1990 Number ('000s)	Rate (per 100 000)	Deaths 2000 (Projected) Number ('000s)	Rate (per 100 000)
Males										
0-4	2	7.4	0	0.6	2.5	0.08	0	1.0	0	0.7
5-14	0	0.9	0	0.1	10.0	0.08	0	0.1	0	0.0
15-44	0	0.5	0	0.0	29.8	0.08	0	0.0	0	0.0
45-59	0	0.3	0	0.0	52.3	0.08	0	0.0	0	0.0
60+	0	0.1	0	0.0	70.3	0.08	0	0.0	0	0.0
All ages	3	1.4	0	0.1	9.3	0.08	0	0.2	0	0.1
Females										
0-4	2	7.4	0	0.6	2.5	0.08	0	1.0	0	0.7
5-14	0	0.9	0	0.1	10.0	0.08	0	0.1	0	0.0
15-44	0	0.5	0	0.0	29.9	0.08	0	0.1	0	0.0
45-59	0	0.3	0	0.0	52.4	0.08	0	0.0	0	0.0
60+	0	0.1	0	0.0	71.1	0.08	0	0.0	0	0.0
All ages	3	1.4	0	0.1	9.6	0.08	0	0.2	0	0.1
Total	6	1.4	1	0.1	9.4	0.08	1	0.2	1	0.1

Table 60h MEC - AOM - CMO Bacterial meningitis - N. meningitidis - episodes

Age group (years)	Incidence 1990 Number ('000s)	Rate (per 100 000)	Prevalence 1990 Number ('000s)	Rate (per 100 000)	Avg. age at onset (years)	Average duration (years)	Deaths 1990 Number ('000s)	Rate (per 100 000)	Deaths 2000 (Projected) Number ('000s)	Number ('000s)
Males										
0-4	3	7.5	0	0.6	2.5	0.08	0	1.0	0	0.8
5-14	1	0.9	0	0.1	10.0	0.08	0	0.1	0	0.0
15-44	1	0.5	0	0.0	29.8	0.08	0	0.0	0	0.0
45-59	0	0.3	0	0.0	52.3	0.08	0	0.0	0	0.0
60+	0	0.1	0	0.0	69.7	0.08	0	0.0	0	0.0
All ages	4	1.7	0	0.1	8.1	0.08	1	0.2	0	0.1
Females										
0-4	3	7.5	0	0.6	2.5	0.08	0	1.0	0	0.7
5-14	1	0.9	0	0.1	10.0	0.08	0	0.1	0	0.0
15-44	1	0.5	0	0.0	29.8	0.08	0	0.0	0	0.0
45-59	0	0.3	0	0.0	52.3	0.08	0	0.0	0	0.0
60+	0	0.1	0	0.0	70.4	0.08	0	0.0	0	0.0
All ages	4	1.7	0	0.1	8.1	0.08	1	0.2	0	0.1
Total	8	1.7	1	0.1	8.1	0.08	1	0.2	1	0.1

Table 60i World - Mundo - Monde Bacterial meningitis - N. meningitidis - episodes

Age group (years)	Incidence 1990 Number ('000s)	Rate (per 100 000)	Prevalence 1990 Number ('000s)	Rate (per 100 000)	Avg. age at onset (years)	Average duration (years)	Deaths 1990 Number ('000s)	Rate (per 100 000)	Deaths 2000 (Projected) Number ('000s)	Number ('000s)
Males										
0-4	23	7.3	2	0.6	2.5	0.08	3	1.0	2	0.7
5-14	5	0.9	0	0.1	10.0	0.08	0	0.1	0	0.0
15-44	5	0.4	0	0.0	29.8	0.08	1	0.0	0	0.0
45-59	1	0.3	0	0.0	52.3	0.08	0	0.1	0	0.0
60+	0	0.1	0	0.0	70.0	0.08	0	0.1	0	0.1
All ages	35	1.3	3	0.1	9.5	0.08	5	0.2	3	0.1
Females										
0-4	23	7.3	2	0.6	2.5	0.08	3	1.0	2	0.6
5-14	5	0.9	0	0.1	10.0	0.08	0	0.1	0	0.0
15-44	5	0.4	0	0.0	29.8	0.08	1	0.0	0	0.0
45-59	1	0.3	0	0.0	52.4	0.08	0	0.0	0	0.0
60+	0	0.1	0	0.0	71.0	0.08	0	0.1	0	0.1
All ages	33	1.3	3	0.1	9.6	0.08	4	0.2	3	0.1
Total	68	1.3	6	0.1	9.6	0.08	9	0.2	6	0.1

For epidemiological sources see Schillinger et al. 1996. For the methods used to estimate and project incidence, prevalence, and deaths see Murray and Lopez 1996a. See explanatory notes for definitions and caveats.

Table 61	Cuadro 61	Tableau 61
Bacterial meningitis	**Meninigitis bacteriana**	**Méningite bactérienne**
Meningococcaemia	Meningococcemia	Méningococcémie
without meningitis	sin meningitis	sans méningite

Table 61a   EME - PEMC - EMBE   Bacterial meningitis - Meningococcaemia without meningitis

Age group (years)	Incidence 1990 Number ('000s)	Rate (per 100 000)	Prevalence 1990 Number ('000s)	Rate (per 100 000)	Avg. age at onset (years)	Average duration (years)	Deaths 1990 Number ('000s)	Rate (per 100 000)	Deaths 2000 (Projected) Number ('000s)	Rate (per 100 000)
Males										
0-4	1	3.7	0	0.3	2.5	0.08	0	0.7	0	0.5
5-14	0	0.5	0	0.0	10.0	0.08	0	0.1	0	0.0
15-44	0	0.2	0	0.0	29.9	0.08	0	0.0	0	0.0
45-59	0	0.1	0	0.0	52.4	0.08	0	0.1	0	0.0
60+	0	0.1	0	0.0	71.1	0.08	0	0.0	0	0.0
All ages	2	0.5	0	0.0	13.9	0.08	0	0.1	0	0.1
Females										
0-4	1	3.7	0	0.3	2.5	0.08	0	0.5	0	0.3
5-14	0	0.5	0	0.0	10.0	0.08	0	0.1	0	0.1
15-44	0	0.2	0	0.0	30.0	0.08	0	0.0	0	0.0
45-59	0	0.1	0	0.0	52.4	0.08	0	0.0	0	0.0
60+	0	0.1	0	0.0	72.4	0.08	0	0.0	0	0.0
All ages	2	0.4	0	0.0	14.8	0.08	0	0.1	0	0.1
Total	4	0.4	0	0.0	14.4	0.08	1	0.1	1	0.1

Table 61b   FSE - PEAS - AESE   Bacterial meningitis - Meningococcaemia without meningitis

Age group (years)	Incidence 1990 Number ('000s)	Rate (per 100 000)	Prevalence 1990 Number ('000s)	Rate (per 100 000)	Avg. age at onset (years)	Average duration (years)	Deaths 1990 Number ('000s)	Rate (per 100 000)	Deaths 2000 (Projected) Number ('000s)	Rate (per 100 000)
Males										
0-4	1	5.4	0	0.5	2.5	0.08	0	0.9	0	0.7
5-14	0	0.7	0	0.1	10.0	0.08	0	0.1	0	0.1
15-44	0	0.3	0	0.0	29.8	0.08	0	0.0	0	0.0
45-59	0	0.2	0	0.0	52.2	0.08	0	0.0	0	0.0
60+	0	0.1	0	0.0	70.0	0.08	0	0.0	0	0.0
All ages	1	0.8	0	0.1	12.0	0.08	0	0.1	0	0.1
Females										
0-4	1	5.4	0	0.5	2.5	0.08	0	0.6	0	0.5
5-14	0	0.7	0	0.1	10.0	0.08	0	0.1	0	0.1
15-44	0	0.3	0	0.0	29.9	0.08	0	0.0	0	0.0
45-59	0	0.2	0	0.0	52.4	0.08	0	0.0	0	0.0
60+	0	0.1	0	0.0	71.5	0.08	0	0.0	0	0.0
All ages	1	0.7	0	0.1	13.3	0.08	0	0.1	0	0.1
Total	3	0.7	0	0.1	12.6	0.08	0	0.1	0	0.1

Table 61c   India - India - Inde   Bacterial meningitis - Meningococcaemia without meningitis

Age group (years)	Incidence 1990 Number ('000s)	Rate (per 100 000)	Prevalence 1990 Number ('000s)	Rate (per 100 000)	Avg. age at onset (years)	Average duration (years)	Deaths 1990 Number ('000s)	Rate (per 100 000)	Deaths 2000 (Projected) Number ('000s)	Rate (per 100 000)
Males										
0-4	3	5.4	0	0.5	2.5	0.08	0	0.8	0	0.5
5-14	1	0.7	0	0.1	10.0	0.08	0	0.1	0	0.0
15-44	1	0.3	0	0.0	29.8	0.08	0	0.0	0	0.0
45-59	0	0.2	0	0.0	52.3	0.08	0	0.0	0	0.0
60+	0	0.1	0	0.0	69.7	0.08	0	0.0	0	0.0
All ages	5	1.1	0	0.1	9.0	0.08	1	0.1	0	0.1
Females										
0-4	3	5.4	0	0.5	2.5	0.08	0	0.8	0	0.5
5-14	1	0.7	0	0.1	10.0	0.08	0	0.1	0	0.0
15-44	1	0.3	0	0.0	29.8	0.08	0	0.0	0	0.0
45-59	0	0.2	0	0.0	52.4	0.08	0	0.0	0	0.0
60+	0	0.1	0	0.0	70.1	0.08	0	0.0	0	0.0
All ages	4	1.1	0	0.1	8.9	0.08	1	0.1	0	0.1
Total	9	1.1	1	0.1	9.0	0.08	1	0.1	1	0.1

For epidemiological sources see Schillinger et al. 1996. For the methods used to estimate and project incidence, prevalence, and deaths see Murray and Lopez 1996a. See explanatory notes for definitions and caveats.

Table 61 **Cuadro 61** **Tableau 61**
Bacterial meningitis **Meninigitis bacteriana** **Méningite bactérienne**
Meningococcaemia Meningococcemia Méningococcémie
without meningitis sin meningitis sans méningite

Table 61d   China - China - Chine   Bacterial meningitis - Meningococcaemia without meningitis

Age group (years)	Incidence 1990 Number ('000s)	Rate (per 100 000)	Prevalence 1990 Number ('000s)	Rate (per 100 000)	Avg. age at onset (years)	Average duration (years)	Deaths 1990 Number ('000s)	Rate (per 100 000)	Deaths 2000 (Projected) Number ('000s)	Rate (per 100 000)
Males										
0-4	3	5.4	0	0.4	2.5	0.08	0	0.7	*0*	*0.4*
5-14	1	0.6	0	0.0	10.0	0.08	0	0.0	*0*	*0.0*
15-44	1	0.3	0	0.0	29.9	0.08	0	0.0	*0*	*0.0*
45-59	0	0.2	0	0.0	52.3	0.08	0	0.0	*0*	*0.0*
60+	0	0.1	0	0.0	69.8	0.08	0	0.3	*0*	*0.2*
All ages	5	0.8	0	0.1	10.4	0.08	1	0.1	*0*	*0.1*
Females										
0-4	3	5.4	0	0.4	2.5	0.08	0	0.7	*0*	*0.4*
5-14	1	0.6	0	0.0	10.0	0.08	0	0.0	*0*	*0.0*
15-44	1	0.3	0	0.0	29.9	0.08	0	0.0	*0*	*0.0*
45-59	0	0.2	0	0.0	52.4	0.08	0	0.0	*0*	*0.0*
60+	0	0.1	0	0.0	70.6	0.08	0	0.3	*0*	*0.2*
All ages	5	0.8	0	0.1	10.3	0.08	1	0.1	*0*	*0.1*
Total	9	0.8	1	0.1	10.4	0.08	2	0.1	*1*	*0.1*

Table 61e   OAI - OPAI - APAI   Bacterial meningitis - Meningococcaemia without meningitis

Age group (years)	Incidence 1990 Number ('000s)	Rate (per 100 000)	Prevalence 1990 Number ('000s)	Rate (per 100 000)	Avg. age at onset (years)	Average duration (years)	Deaths 1990 Number ('000s)	Rate (per 100 000)	Deaths 2000 (Projected) Number ('000s)	Rate (per 100 000)
Males										
0-4	2	5.4	0	0.5	2.5	0.08	0	0.8	*0*	*0.5*
5-14	1	0.7	0	0.1	10.0	0.08	0	0.1	*0*	*0.0*
15-44	1	0.3	0	0.0	29.7	0.08	0	0.0	*0*	*0.0*
45-59	0	0.2	0	0.0	52.3	0.08	0	0.0	*0*	*0.0*
60+	0	0.1	0	0.0	69.6	0.08	0	0.0	*0*	*0.0*
All ages	4	1.0	0	0.1	9.2	0.08	0	0.1	*0*	*0.1*
Females										
0-4	2	5.4	0	0.5	2.5	0.08	0	0.7	*0*	*0.4*
5-14	1	0.7	0	0.1	10.0	0.08	0	0.1	*0*	*0.0*
15-44	1	0.3	0	0.0	29.8	0.08	0	0.0	*0*	*0.0*
45-59	0	0.2	0	0.0	52.3	0.08	0	0.0	*0*	*0.0*
60+	0	0.1	0	0.0	70.3	0.08	0	0.0	*0*	*0.0*
All ages	3	1.0	0	0.1	9.5	0.08	0	0.1	*0*	*0.1*
Total	7	1.0	1	0.1	9.4	0.08	1	0.1	*1*	*0.1*

Table 61f   SSA - ASS - ASS   Bacterial meningitis - Meningococcaemia without meningitis

Age group (years)	Incidence 1990 Number ('000s)	Rate (per 100 000)	Prevalence 1990 Number ('000s)	Rate (per 100 000)	Avg. age at onset (years)	Average duration (years)	Deaths 1990 Number ('000s)	Rate (per 100 000)	Deaths 2000 (Projected) Number ('000s)	Rate (per 100 000)
Males										
0-4	3	5.4	0	0.5	2.4	0.08	0	0.7	*0*	*0.5*
5-14	0	0.6	0	0.1	10.0	0.08	0	0.1	*0*	*0.0*
15-44	0	0.4	0	0.0	29.4	0.08	0	0.0	*0*	*0.0*
45-59	0	0.2	0	0.0	52.2	0.08	0	0.0	*0*	*0.0*
60+	0	0.1	0	0.0	69.2	0.08	0	0.0	*0*	*0.0*
All ages	3	1.4	0	0.1	7.2	0.08	0	0.2	*0*	*0.1*
Females										
0-4	3	5.4	0	0.5	2.4	0.08	0	0.7	*0*	*0.5*
5-14	0	0.6	0	0.1	10.0	0.08	0	0.1	*0*	*0.0*
15-44	0	0.4	0	0.0	29.5	0.08	0	0.0	*0*	*0.0*
45-59	0	0.2	0	0.0	52.2	0.08	0	0.0	*0*	*0.0*
60+	0	0.1	0	0.0	69.7	0.08	0	0.0	*0*	*0.0*
All ages	3	1.3	0	0.1	7.4	0.08	0	0.2	*0*	*0.1*
Total	7	1.4	1	0.1	7.3	0.08	1	0.2	*1*	*0.1*

For epidemiological sources see Schillinger et al. 1996. For the methods used to estimate and project incidence, prevalence, and deaths see Murray and Lopez 1996a. See explanatory notes for definitions and caveats.

Table 61
Bacterial meningitis
Meningococcaemia
without meningitis

Cuadro 61
Meninigitis bacteriana
Meningococcemia
sin meningitis

Tableau 61
Méningite bactérienne
Méningococcémie
sans méningite

| Table 61g | LAC - ALC - ALC | | | | | Bacterial meningitis - Meningococcaemia without meningitis | | | | |

Age group (years)	Incidence 1990 Number ('000s)	Rate (per 100 000)	Prevalence 1990 Number ('000s)	Rate (per 100 000)	Avg. age at onset (years)	Average duration (years)	Deaths 1990 Number ('000s)	Rate (per 100 000)	Deaths 2000 (Projected) Number ('000s)	Rate (per 100 000)
Males										
0-4	2	5.4	0	0.4	2.5	0.08	0	0.8	0	0.5
5-14	0	0.7	0	0.1	10.0	0.08	0	0.0	0	0.0
15-44	0	0.3	0	0.0	29.8	0.08	0	0.0	0	0.0
45-59	0	0.2	0	0.0	52.3	0.08	0	0.0	0	0.0
60+	0	0.1	0	0.0	70.3	0.08	0	0.0	0	0.0
All ages	2	1.0	0	0.1	9.3	0.08	0	0.1	0	0.1
Females										
0-4	1	5.4	0	0.4	2.5	0.08	0	0.7	0	0.5
5-14	0	0.7	0	0.1	10.0	0.08	0	0.0	0	0.0
15-44	0	0.3	0	0.0	29.9	0.08	0	0.0	0	0.0
45-59	0	0.2	0	0.0	52.4	0.08	0	0.0	0	0.0
60+	0	0.1	0	0.0	71.1	0.08	0	0.0	0	0.0
All ages	2	1.0	0	0.1	9.6	0.08	0	0.1	0	0.1
Total	5	1.0	0	0.1	9.4	0.08	1	0.1	0	0.1

| Table 61h | MEC - AOM - CMO | | | | | Bacterial meningitis - Meningococcaemia without meningitis | | | | |

Age group (years)	Incidence 1990 Number ('000s)	Rate (per 100 000)	Prevalence 1990 Number ('000s)	Rate (per 100 000)	Avg. age at onset (years)	Average duration (years)	Deaths 1990 Number ('000s)	Rate (per 100 000)	Deaths 2000 (Projected) Number ('000s)	Rate (per 100 000)
Males										
0-4	2	5.4	0	0.5	2.5	0.08	0	0.8	0	0.6
5-14	0	0.7	0	0.1	10.0	0.08	0	0.1	0	0.0
15-44	0	0.3	0	0.0	29.8	0.08	0	0.0	0	0.0
45-59	0	0.2	0	0.0	52.3	0.08	0	0.0	0	0.0
60+	0	0.1	0	0.0	69.7	0.08	0	0.0	0	0.0
All ages	3	1.2	0	0.1	8.1	0.08	0	0.2	0	0.1
Females										
0-4	2	5.4	0	0.5	2.5	0.08	0	0.8	0	0.5
5-14	0	0.7	0	0.1	10.0	0.08	0	0.1	0	0.0
15-44	0	0.3	0	0.0	29.8	0.08	0	0.0	0	0.0
45-59	0	0.2	0	0.0	52.3	0.08	0	0.0	0	0.0
60+	0	0.1	0	0.0	70.4	0.08	0	0.0	0	0.0
All ages	3	1.2	0	0.1	8.1	0.08	0	0.2	0	0.1
Total	6	1.2	1	0.1	8.1	0.08	1	0.2	1	0.1

| Table 61i | World - Mundo - Monde | | | | | Bacterial meningitis - Meningococcaemia without meningitis | | | | |

Age group (years)	Incidence 1990 Number ('000s)	Rate (per 100 000)	Prevalence 1990 Number ('000s)	Rate (per 100 000)	Avg. age at onset (years)	Average duration (years)	Deaths 1990 Number ('000s)	Rate (per 100 000)	Deaths 2000 (Projected) Number ('000s)	Rate (per 100 000)
Males										
0-4	17	5.3	1	0.4	2.5	0.08	2	0.7	2	0.5
5-14	4	0.6	0	0.1	10.0	0.08	0	0.1	0	0.0
15-44	4	0.3	0	0.0	29.8	0.08	0	0.0	0	0.0
45-59	1	0.2	0	0.0	52.3	0.08	0	0.0	0	0.0
60+	0	0.1	0	0.0	70.0	0.08	0	0.1	0	0.1
All ages	25	0.9	2	0.1	9.5	0.08	4	0.1	2	0.1
Females										
0-4	16	5.3	1	0.4	2.5	0.08	2	0.7	2	0.5
5-14	3	0.6	0	0.1	10.0	0.08	0	0.1	0	0.0
15-44	4	0.3	0	0.0	29.8	0.08	0	0.0	0	0.0
45-59	1	0.2	0	0.0	52.4	0.08	0	0.0	0	0.0
60+	0	0.1	0	0.0	71.0	0.08	0	0.1	0	0.1
All ages	24	0.9	2	0.1	9.6	0.08	3	0.1	2	0.1
Total	49	0.9	4	0.1	9.6	0.08	7	0.1	5	0.1

For epidemiological sources see Schillinger et al. 1996. For the methods used to estimate and project incidence, prevalence, and deaths see Murray and Lopez 1996a. See explanatory notes for definitions and caveats.

Table 62	Cuadro 62	Tableau 62
Bacterial meningitis	**Meninigitis bacteriana**	**Méningite bactérienne**
Deafness	Sordera	Surdité

Table 62a — EME - PEMC - EMBE — Bacterial meningitis - Deafness

Age group (years)	Incidence 1990 Number ('000s)	Rate (per 100 000)	Prevalence 1990 Number ('000s)	Rate (per 100 000)	Avg. age at onset (years)	Average duration (years)	Deaths 1990 Number ('000s)	Rate (per 100 000)	Deaths 2000 (Projected) Number ('000s)	Rate (per 100 000)
Males										
0-4	2	6.6	4	16	2.5	70.2	0	0	0	0
5-14	0	0.6	19	36	10.0	63.6	0	0	0	0
15-44	0	0.1	74	40	29.9	44.7	0	0	0	0
45-59	0	0.1	28	42	52.4	24.5	0	0	0	0
60+	0	0.4	28	47	71.1	11.3	0	0	0	0
All ages	3	0.6	154	39	12.5	61.4	0	0	0	0
Females										
0-4	2	6.6	4	16	2.5	76.1	0	0	0	0
5-14	0	0.6	18	36	10.0	69.5	0	0	0	0
15-44	0	0.1	72	40	30.0	50.0	0	0	0	0
45-59	0	0.1	29	42	52.4	28.8	0	0	0	0
60+	0	0.4	40	47	71.1	12.7	0	0	0	0
All ages	2	0.6	163	40	14.8	64.7	0	0	0	0
Total	5	0.6	317	40	13.6	63.1	0	0	0	0

Table 62b — FSE - PEAS - AESE — Bacterial meningitis - Deafness

Age group (years)	Incidence 1990 Number ('000s)	Rate (per 100 000)	Prevalence 1990 Number ('000s)	Rate (per 100 000)	Avg. age at onset (years)	Average duration (years)	Deaths 1990 Number ('000s)	Rate (per 100 000)	Deaths 2000 (Projected) Number ('000s)	Rate (per 100 000)
Males										
0-4	1	10.5	4	26	2.5	63.5	0	0	0	0
5-14	0	0.9	15	57	10.0	57.3	0	0	0	0
15-44	0	0.5	52	68	29.8	39.2	0	0	0	0
45-59	0	0.6	22	80	52.2	20.8	0	0	0	0
60+	0	1.5	21	99	70.0	10.1	0	0	0	0
All ages	3	1.5	114	69	18.6	50.2	0	0	0	0
Females										
0-4	1	10.5	3	26	2.5	72.4	0	0	0	0
5-14	0	0.9	15	57	10.0	66.0	0	0	0	0
15-44	0	0.5	51	68	29.9	46.8	0	0	0	0
45-59	0	0.6	24	80	52.4	26.1	0	0	0	0
60+	1	1.5	37	102	71.5	11.8	0	0	0	0
All ages	3	1.5	131	72	23.8	53.3	0	0	0	0
Total	5	1.5	244	71	21.3	51.8	0	0	0	0

Table 62c — India - India - Inde — Bacterial meningitis - Deafness

Age group (years)	Incidence 1990 Number ('000s)	Rate (per 100 000)	Prevalence 1990 Number ('000s)	Rate (per 100 000)	Avg. age at onset (years)	Average duration (years)	Deaths 1990 Number ('000s)	Rate (per 100 000)	Deaths 2000 (Projected) Number ('000s)	Rate (per 100 000)
Males										
0-4	5	8.2	12	20	2.5	59.9	0	0	0	0
5-14	1	0.7	45	44	10.0	57.4	0	0	0	0
15-44	1	0.4	107	53	29.8	39.9	0	0	0	0
45-59	0	0.6	30	63	52.3	21.0	0	0	0	0
60+	0	1.2	21	69	69.7	9.7	0	0	0	0
All ages	7	1.6	215	49	8.7	55.5	0	0	0	0
Females										
0-4	5	8.2	11	20	2.5	60.8	0	0	0	0
5-14	1	0.7	42	44	10.0	59.1	0	0	0	0
15-44	1	0.4	98	53	29.8	41.7	0	0	0	0
45-59	0	0.6	29	64	52.4	22.5	0	0	0	0
60+	0	1.2	20	69	70.1	10.2	0	0	0	0
All ages	7	1.6	201	49	8.7	56.7	0	0	0	0
Total	14	1.6	416	49	8.7	56.1	0	0	0	0

For epidemiological sources see Schillinger et al. 1996. For the methods used to estimate and project incidence, prevalence, and deaths see Murray and Lopez 1996a. See explanatory notes for definitions and caveats.

Table 62	Cuadro 62	Tableau 62
Bacterial meningitis	**Meninigitis bacteriana**	**Méningite bactérienne**
Deafness	Sordera	Surdité

Table 62d   China - China - Chine   Bacterial meningitis - Deafness

Age group (years)	Incidence 1990 Number ('000s)	Rate (per 100 000)	Prevalence 1990 Number ('000s)	Rate (per 100 000)	Avg. age at onset (years)	Average duration (years)	Deaths 1990 Number ('000s)	Rate (per 100 000)	Deaths 2000 (Projected) Number ('000s)	Rate (per 100 000)
Males										
0-4	5	8.2	12	20	2.5	65.5	0	0	0	0
5-14	1	0.7	43	44	10.0	59.9	0	0	0	0
15-44	1	0.3	161	53	29.9	41.2	0	0	0	0
45-59	0	0.6	45	62	52.3	21.4	0	0	0	0
60+	1	1.2	38	78	69.8	9.9	0	0	0	0
All ages	8	1.3	300	51	14.8	55.0	0	0	0	0
Females										
0-4	5	8.2	12	20	2.5	68.5	0	0	0	0
5-14	1	0.7	40	44	10.0	63.2	0	0	0	0
15-44	1	0.3	149	53	29.9	44.2	0	0	0	0
45-59	0	0.6	40	62	52.4	23.8	0	0	0	0
60+	1	1.2	41	79	70.6	10.8	0	0	0	0
All ages	7	1.3	282	51	15.1	57.0	0	0	0	0
Total	15	1.3	582	51	14.9	56.3	0	0	0	0

Table 62e   OAI - OPAI - APAI   Bacterial meningitis - Deafness

Age group (years)	Incidence 1990 Number ('000s)	Rate (per 100 000)	Prevalence 1990 Number ('000s)	Rate (per 100 000)	Avg. age at onset (years)	Average duration (years)	Deaths 1990 Number ('000s)	Rate (per 100 000)	Deaths 2000 (Projected) Number ('000s)	Rate (per 100 000)
Males										
0-4	4	8.2	9	20	2.5	59.8	0	0	0	0
5-14	1	0.7	37	44	10.0	56.2	0	0	0	0
15-44	0	0.3	83	52	29.7	38.8	0	0	0	0
45-59	0	0.6	21	61	52.3	20.3	0	0	0	0
60+	0	1.2	16	77	69.6	9.7	0	0	0	0
All ages	5	1.5	166	48	11.1	53.5	0	0	0	0
Females										
0-4	3	8.2	9	20	2.5	63.2	0	0	0	0
5-14	1	0.7	35	44	10.0	59.2	0	0	0	0
15-44	0	0.3	83	52	29.8	41.4	0	0	0	0
45-59	0	0.6	21	61	52.3	22.4	0	0	0	0
60+	0	1.2	18	78	70.3	10.5	0	0	0	0
All ages	5	1.5	166	49	11.8	56.0	0	0	0	0
Total	10	1.5	331	49	11.4	54.7	0	0	0	0

Table 62f   SSA - ASS - ASS   Bacterial meningitis - Deafness

Age group (years)	Incidence 1990 Number ('000s)	Rate (per 100 000)	Prevalence 1990 Number ('000s)	Rate (per 100 000)	Avg. age at onset (years)	Average duration (years)	Deaths 1990 Number ('000s)	Rate (per 100 000)	Deaths 2000 (Projected) Number ('000s)	Rate (per 100 000)
Males										
0-4	4	8.2	9	20	2.4	48.7	0	0	0	0
5-14	0	0.7	31	45	10.0	49.2	0	0	0	0
15-44	0	0.4	55	53	29.4	35.0	0	0	0	0
45-59	0	0.6	13	64	52.2	19.1	0	0	0	0
60+	0	1.1	8	79	69.2	9.3	0	0	0	0
All ages	5	2.0	117	47	8.1	46.0	0	0	0	0
Females										
0-4	4	8.2	9	20	2.4	51.9	0	0	0	0
5-14	0	0.7	31	44	10.0	51.9	0	0	0	0
15-44	0	0.4	57	53	29.5	37.2	0	0	0	0
45-59	0	0.6	14	64	52.2	20.5	0	0	0	0
60+	0	1.1	10	80	69.7	9.8	0	0	0	0
All ages	5	2.0	121	47	8.6	48.7	0	0	0	0
Total	10	2.0	239	47	8.3	47.3	0	0	0	0

For epidemiological sources see Schillinger et al. 1996. For the methods used to estimate and project incidence, prevalence, and deaths see Murray and Lopez 1996a. See explanatory notes for definitions and caveats.

Table 62	Cuadro 62	Tableau 62
Bacterial meningitis	**Meninigitis bacteriana**	**Méningite bactérienne**
Deafness	Sordera	Surdité

Table 62g — LAC - ALC - ALC — Bacterial meningitis - Deafness

Age group (years)	Incidence 1990 Number ('000s)	Rate (per 100 000)	Prevalence 1990 Number ('000s)	Rate (per 100 000)	Avg. age at onset (years)	Average duration (years)	Deaths 1990 Number ('000s)	Rate (per 100 000)	Deaths 2000 (Projected) Number ('000s)	Rate (per 100 000)
Males										
0-4	2	8.1	6	20	2.5	63.9	0	0	0	0
5-14	0	0.7	23	44	10.0	59.3	0	0	0	0
15-44	0	0.4	55	53	29.8	41.4	0	0	0	0
45-59	0	0.6	14	63	52.3	22.3	0	0	0	0
60+	0	1.2	11	80	70.3	10.4	0	0	0	0
All ages	3	1.5	110	49	11.7	56.5	0	0	0	0
Females										
0-4	2	8.1	6	20	2.5	67.9	0	0	0	0
5-14	0	0.7	22	44	10.0	63.0	0	0	0	0
15-44	0	0.4	55	53	29.9	44.6	0	0	0	0
45-59	0	0.6	15	63	52.4	24.8	0	0	0	0
60+	0	1.2	14	81	71.1	11.3	0	0	0	0
All ages	3	1.5	112	50	12.6	59.5	0	0	0	0
Total	7	1.5	221	50	12.2	58.0	0	0	0	0

Table 62h — MEC - AOM - CMO — Bacterial meningitis - Deafness

Age group (years)	Incidence 1990 Number ('000s)	Rate (per 100 000)	Prevalence 1990 Number ('000s)	Rate (per 100 000)	Avg. age at onset (years)	Average duration (years)	Deaths 1990 Number ('000s)	Rate (per 100 000)	Deaths 2000 (Projected) Number ('000s)	Rate (per 100 000)
Males										
0-4	3	8.2	8	20	2.5	61.1	0	0	0	0
5-14	0	0.7	29	44	10.0	58.1	0	0	0	0
15-44	0	0.4	61	53	29.8	40.0	0	0	0	0
45-59	0	0.6	14	64	52.3	20.8	0	0	0	0
60+	0	1.2	11	80	69.7	9.8	0	0	0	0
All ages	5	1.8	123	48	9.7	55.8	0	0	0	0
Females										
0-4	3	8.2	8	20	2.5	63.7	0	0	0	0
5-14	0	0.7	27	44	10.0	60.9	0	0	0	0
15-44	0	0.4	57	53	29.8	42.6	0	0	0	0
45-59	0	0.6	14	64	52.3	22.9	0	0	0	0
60+	0	1.2	12	81	70.4	10.6	0	0	0	0
All ages	4	1.8	119	48	10.1	58.0	0	0	0	0
Total	9	1.8	242	48	9.9	56.9	0	0	0	0

Table 62i — World - Mundo - Monde — Bacterial meningitis - Deafness

Age group (years)	Incidence 1990 Number ('000s)	Rate (per 100 000)	Prevalence 1990 Number ('000s)	Rate (per 100 000)	Avg. age at onset (years)	Average duration (years)	Deaths 1990 Number ('000s)	Rate (per 100 000)	Deaths 2000 (Projected) Number ('000s)	Rate (per 100 000)
Males										
0-4	26	8.2	65	20	2.5	60.7	0	0	0	0
5-14	4	0.7	243	44	10.0	57.4	0	0	0	0
15-44	4	0.3	649	52	29.8	40.0	0	0	0	0
45-59	2	0.5	187	60	52.3	21.0	0	0	0	0
60+	2	1.0	154	71	70.0	10.1	0	0	0	0
All ages	38	1.4	1 298	49	11.5	54.0	0	0	0	0
Females										
0-4	25	8.2	62	20	2.5	63.9	0	0	0	0
5-14	4	0.7	232	44	10.0	60.8	0	0	0	0
15-44	4	0.3	622	52	29.8	43.1	0	0	0	0
45-59	2	0.5	187	60	52.4	23.5	0	0	0	0
60+	3	0.9	192	71	70.8	11.2	0	0	0	0
All ages	37	1.4	1 295	50	12.4	56.4	0	0	0	0
Total	75	1.4	2 592	49	12.0	55.2	0	0	0	0

For epidemiological sources see Schillinger et al. 1996. For the methods used to estimate and project incidence, prevalence, and deaths see Murray and Lopez 1996a. See explanatory notes for definitions and caveats.

Table 63	Cuadro 63	Tableau 63
Bacterial meningitis	**Meninigitis bacteriana**	**Méningite bactérienne**
Seizure disorder	Trastorno convulsivo	Atteintes convulsives

Table 63a EME - PEMC - EMBE Bacterial meningitis - Seizure disorder

Age group (years)	Incidence 1990 Number ('000s)	Rate (per 100 000)	Prevalence 1990 Number ('000s)	Rate (per 100 000)	Avg. age at onset (years)	Average duration (years)	Deaths 1990 Number ('000s)	Rate (per 100 000)	Deaths 2000 (Projected) Number ('000s)	Rate (per 100 000)
Males										
0-4	1	2.5	2	6.3	2.5	70.2	0	0	0	0
5-14	0	0.2	7	13.8	10.0	63.6	0	0	0	0
15-44	0	0.0	29	15.5	29.9	44.7	0	0	0	0
45-59	0	0.0	11	16.4	52.4	24.5	0	0	0	0
60+	0	0.1	11	18.1	71.1	11.3	0	0	0	0
All ages	1	0.2	59	15.2	12.5	61.4	0	0	0	0
Females										
0-4	1	2.5	2	6.3	2.5	76.1	0	0	0	0
5-14	0	0.2	7	13.8	10.0	69.5	0	0	0	0
15-44	0	0.0	28	15.5	30.0	50.0	0	0	0	0
45-59	0	0.0	11	16.4	52.4	28.8	0	0	0	0
60+	0	0.1	15	18.3	72.4	12.7	0	0	0	0
All ages	1	0.2	63	15.5	15.0	64.7	0	0	0	0
Total	2	0.2	122	15.3	13.7	63.1	0	0	0	0

Table 63b FSE - PEAS - AESE Bacterial meningitis - Seizure disorder

Age group (years)	Incidence 1990 Number ('000s)	Rate (per 100 000)	Prevalence 1990 Number ('000s)	Rate (per 100 000)	Avg. age at onset (years)	Average duration (years)	Deaths 1990 Number ('000s)	Rate (per 100 000)	Deaths 2000 (Projected) Number ('000s)	Rate (per 100 000)
Males										
0-4	1	4.0	1	10	2.5	63.5	0	0	0	0
5-14	0	0.4	6	22	10.0	57.3	0	0	0	0
15-44	0	0.2	20	26	29.8	39.2	0	0	0	0
45-59	0	0.2	8	31	52.2	20.8	0	0	0	0
60+	0	0.6	8	38	70.0	10.1	0	0	0	0
All ages	1	0.6	44	27	18.6	50.2	0	0	0	0
Females										
0-4	1	4.0	1	10	2.5	72.4	0	0	0	0
5-14	0	0.4	6	22	10.0	66.0	0	0	0	0
15-44	0	0.2	20	27	29.9	46.8	0	0	0	0
45-59	0	0.2	9	31	52.4	26.1	0	0	0	0
60+	0	0.6	14	39	71.5	11.8	0	0	0	0
All ages	1	0.6	51	28	23.8	53.3	0	0	0	0
Total	2	0.6	95	27	21.3	51.8	0	0	0	0

Table 63c India - India - Inde Bacterial meningitis - Seizure disorder

Age group (years)	Incidence 1990 Number ('000s)	Rate (per 100 000)	Prevalence 1990 Number ('000s)	Rate (per 100 000)	Avg. age at onset (years)	Average duration (years)	Deaths 1990 Number ('000s)	Rate (per 100 000)	Deaths 2000 (Projected) Number ('000s)	Rate (per 100 000)
Males										
0-4	3	4.5	7	11	2.5	59.9	0	0	0	0
5-14	0	0.4	25	24	10.0	57.4	0	0	0	0
15-44	0	0.2	59	29	29.8	39.9	0	0	0	0
45-59	0	0.3	17	35	52.3	21.0	0	0	0	0
60+	0	0.6	11	38	69.7	9.7	0	0	0	0
All ages	4	0.9	118	27	8.7	55.5	0	0	0	0
Females										
0-4	3	4.5	6	11	2.5	60.8	0	0	0	0
5-14	0	0.4	23	24	10.0	59.1	0	0	0	0
15-44	0	0.2	54	29	29.8	41.7	0	0	0	0
45-59	0	0.3	16	35	52.4	22.5	0	0	0	0
60+	0	0.6	11	38	70.1	10.2	0	0	0	0
All ages	4	0.9	111	27	8.7	56.7	0	0	0	0
Total	8	0.9	229	27	8.7	56.1	0	0	0	0

For epidemiological sources see Schillinger et al. 1996. For the methods used to estimate and project incidence, prevalence, and deaths see Murray and Lopez 1996a. See explanatory notes for definitions and caveats.

Table 63   **Cuadro 63**   **Tableau 63**
Bacterial meningitis   **Meninigitis bacteriana**   **Méningite bactérienne**

Seizure disorder   Trastorno convulsivo   Atteintes convulsives

Table 63d   China - China - Chine   Bacterial meningitis - Seizure disorder

Age group (years)	Incidence 1990 Number ('000s)	Rate (per 100 000)	Prevalence 1990 Number ('000s)	Rate (per 100 000)	Avg. age at onset (years)	Average duration (years)	Deaths 1990 Number ('000s)	Rate (per 100 000)	Deaths 2000 (Projected) Number ('000s)	Rate (per 100 000)
Males										
0-4	3	4.5	7	11	2.5	65.5	0	0	0	0
5-14	0	0.4	24	24	10.0	59.9	0	0	0	0
15-44	1	0.2	89	29	29.9	41.2	0	0	0	0
45-59	0	0.3	25	34	52.3	21.4	0	0	0	0
60+	0	0.6	21	43	69.8	9.9	0	0	0	0
All ages	4	0.7	165	28	14.8	55.0	0	0	0	0
Females										
0-4	3	4.5	6	11	2.5	68.5	0	0	0	0
5-14	0	0.4	22	24	10.0	63.2	0	0	0	0
15-44	1	0.2	82	29	29.9	44.2	0	0	0	0
45-59	0	0.3	22	34	52.4	23.8	0	0	0	0
60+	0	0.6	23	44	70.6	10.8	0	0	0	0
All ages	4	0.7	155	28	15.1	57.6	0	0	0	0
Total	8	0.7	321	28	14.9	56.3	0	0	0	0

Table 63e   OAI - OPAI - APAI   Bacterial meningitis - Seizure disorder

Age group (years)	Incidence 1990 Number ('000s)	Rate (per 100 000)	Prevalence 1990 Number ('000s)	Rate (per 100 000)	Avg. age at onset (years)	Average duration (years)	Deaths 1990 Number ('000s)	Rate (per 100 000)	Deaths 2000 (Projected) Number ('000s)	Rate (per 100 000)
Males										
0-4	2	4.5	5	11	2.5	59.8	0	0	0	0
5-14	0	0.4	20	24	10.0	56.2	0	0	0	0
15-44	0	0.2	46	28	29.7	38.8	0	0	0	0
45-59	0	0.3	11	33	52.3	20.3	0	0	0	0
60+	0	0.6	9	42	69.6	9.7	0	0	0	0
All ages	3	0.8	91	27	11.1	53.5	0	0	0	0
Females										
0-4	2	4.5	5	11	2.5	63.2	0	0	0	0
5-14	0	0.4	20	24	10.0	59.2	0	0	0	0
15-44	0	0.2	45	28	29.8	41.4	0	0	0	0
45-59	0	0.3	12	34	52.3	22.4	0	0	0	0
60+	0	0.6	10	43	70.3	10.5	0	0	0	0
All ages	3	0.8	91	27	11.8	56.0	0	0	0	0
Total	6	0.8	182	27	11.4	54.7	0	0	0	0

Table 63f   SSA - ASS - ASS   Bacterial meningitis - Seizure disorder

Age group (years)	Incidence 1990 Number ('000s)	Rate (per 100 000)	Prevalence 1990 Number ('000s)	Rate (per 100 000)	Avg. age at onset (years)	Average duration (years)	Deaths 1990 Number ('000s)	Rate (per 100 000)	Deaths 2000 (Projected) Number ('000s)	Rate (per 100 000)
Males										
0-4	2	4.5	5	11	2.4	48.7	0	0	0	0
5-14	0	0.4	17	24	10.0	49.2	0	0	0	0
15-44	0	0.2	30	29	29.4	35.0	0	0	0	0
45-59	0	0.4	7	35	52.2	19.1	0	0	0	0
60+	0	0.6	5	44	69.2	9.3	0	0	0	0
All ages	3	1.1	64	26	8.1	46.0	0	0	0	0
Females										
0-4	2	4.5	5	11	2.4	51.9	0	0	0	0
5-14	0	0.4	17	24	10.0	51.9	0	0	0	0
15-44	0	0.2	31	29	29.5	37.2	0	0	0	0
45-59	0	0.4	8	35	52.2	20.5	0	0	0	0
60+	0	0.6	6	44	69.7	9.8	0	0	0	0
All ages	3	1.1	67	26	8.6	48.7	0	0	0	0
Total	6	1.1	131	26	8.3	47.3	0	0	0	0

For epidemiological sources see Schillinger et al. 1996. For the methods used to estimate and project incidence, prevalence, and deaths see Murray and Lopez 1996a. See explanatory notes for definitions and caveats.

Table 63 Bacterial meningitis	Cuadro 63 Meninigitis bacteriana	Tableau 63 Méningite bactérienne
Seizure disorder	Trastorno convulsivo	Atteintes convulsives

Table 63g   LAC - ALC - ALC   Bacterial meningitis - Seizure disorder

Age group (years)	Incidence 1990 Number ('000s)	Rate (per 100 000)	Prevalence 1990 Number ('000s)	Rate (per 100 000)	Avg. age at onset (years)	Average duration (years)	Deaths 1990 Number ('000s)	Rate (per 100 000)	Deaths 2000 (Projected) Number ('000s)	Rate (per 100 000)
Males										
0-4	1	4.5	3	11	2.5	63.9	0	0	0	0
5-14	0	0.4	13	24	10.0	59.3	0	0	0	0
15-44	0	0.2	30	29	29.8	41.4	0	0	0	0
45-59	0	0.3	8	35	52.3	22.3	0	0	0	0
60+	0	0.6	6	44	70.3	10.4	0	0	0	0
All ages	2	0.8	60	27	11.7	56.5	0	0	0	0
Females										
0-4	1	4.5	3	11	2.5	67.9	0	0	0	0
5-14	0	0.4	12	24	10.0	63.0	0	0	0	0
15-44	0	0.2	30	29	29.9	44.6	0	0	0	0
45-59	0	0.3	8	35	52.4	24.8	0	0	0	0
60+	0	0.6	7	45	71.1	11.3	0	0	0	0
All ages	2	0.8	61	28	12.6	59.5	0	0	0	0
Total	4	0.8	122	27	12.2	58.0	0	0	0	0

Table 63h   MEC - AOM - CMO   Bacterial meningitis - Seizure disorder

Age group (years)	Incidence 1990 Number ('000s)	Rate (per 100 000)	Prevalence 1990 Number ('000s)	Rate (per 100 000)	Avg. age at onset (years)	Average duration (years)	Deaths 1990 Number ('000s)	Rate (per 100 000)	Deaths 2000 (Projected) Number ('000s)	Rate (per 100 000)
Males										
0-4	2	4.5	5	11	2.5	61.1	0	0	0	0
5-14	0	0.4	16	24	10.0	58.1	0	0	0	0
15-44	0	0.2	34	30	29.8	40.0	0	0	0	0
45-59	0	0.4	8	35	52.3	20.8	0	0	0	0
60+	0	0.6	6	44	69.7	9.8	0	0	0	0
All ages	3	1.0	68	27	9.7	55.8	0	0	0	0
Females										
0-4	2	4.5	4	11	2.5	63.7	0	0	0	0
5-14	0	0.4	15	24	10.0	60.9	0	0	0	0
15-44	0	0.2	32	30	29.8	42.6	0	0	0	0
45-59	0	0.4	8	35	52.3	22.9	0	0	0	0
60+	0	0.6	7	45	70.4	10.6	0	0	0	0
All ages	2	1.0	66	27	10.1	58.0	0	0	0	0
Total	5	1.0	134	27	9.9	56.9	0	0	0	0

Table 63i   World - Mundo - Monde   Bacterial meningitis - Seizure disorder

Age group (years)	Incidence 1990 Number ('000s)	Rate (per 100 000)	Prevalence 1990 Number ('000s)	Rate (per 100 000)	Avg. age at onset (years)	Average duration (years)	Deaths 1990 Number ('000s)	Rate (per 100 000)	Deaths 2000 (Projected) Number ('000s)	Rate (per 100 000)
Males										
0-4	14	4.3	34	11	2.5	60.4	0	0	0	0
5-14	2	0.4	128	23	10.0	57.2	0	0	0	0
15-44	2	0.2	337	27	29.8	39.9	0	0	0	0
45-59	1	0.3	95	30	52.3	21.0	0	0	0	0
60+	1	0.5	77	35	69.9	10.0	0	0	0	0
All ages	20	0.8	671	25	11.3	53.9	0	0	0	0
Females										
0-4	13	4.3	33	11	2.5	63.5	0	0	0	0
5-14	2	0.4	122	23	10.0	60.4	0	0	0	0
15-44	2	0.2	322	27	29.8	42.9	0	0	0	0
45-59	1	0.3	94	30	52.4	23.4	0	0	0	0
60+	1	0.5	93	35	70.9	11.1	0	0	0	0
All ages	19	0.7	665	25	12.1	56.3	0	0	0	0
Total	39	0.7	1 336	25	11.7	55.1	0	0	0	0

For epidemiological sources see Schillinger et al. 1996. For the methods used to estimate and project incidence, prevalence, and deaths see Murray and Lopez 1996a. See explanatory notes for definitions and caveats.

Table 64
Bacterial meningitis

Cuadro 64
Meninigitis bacteriana

Tableau 64
Méningite bactérienne

Motor deficit

Déficit motriz

Déficit moteur

Table 64a EME - PEMC - EMBE Bacterial meningitis - Motor deficit

Age group (years)	Incidence 1990 Number ('000s)	Rate (per 100 000)	Prevalence 1990 Number ('000s)	Rate (per 100 000)	Avg. age at onset (years)	Average duration (years)	Deaths 1990 Number ('000s)	Rate (per 100 000)	Deaths 2000 (Projected) Number ('000s)	Rate (per 100 000)
Males										
0-4	1	2.6	2	6.5	2.5	70.2	0	0	0	0
5-14	0	0.2	8	14.3	10.0	63.6	0	0	0	0
15-44	0	0.0	30	16.1	29.9	44.7	0	0	0	0
45-59	0	0.0	11	17.0	52.4	24.5	0	0	0	0
60+	0	0.1	11	18.8	71.1	11.3	0	0	0	0
All ages	1	0.3	61	15.7	12.5	61.4	0	0	0	0
Females										
0-4	1	2.6	2	6.5	2.5	76.1	0	0	0	0
5-14	0	0.2	7	14.3	10.0	69.5	0	0	0	0
15-44	0	0.0	29	16.1	30.0	50.0	0	0	0	0
45-59	0	0.0	11	17.0	52.4	28.8	0	0	0	0
60+	0	0.1	16	19.0	72.4	12.7	0	0	0	0
All ages	1	0.2	65	16.0	15.0	64.7	0	0	0	0
Total	2	0.3	127	15.9	13.7	63.1	0	0	0	0

Table 64b FSE - PEAS - AESE Bacterial meningitis - Motor deficit

Age group (years)	Incidence 1990 Number ('000s)	Rate (per 100 000)	Prevalence 1990 Number ('000s)	Rate (per 100 000)	Avg. age at onset (years)	Average duration (years)	Deaths 1990 Number ('000s)	Rate (per 100 000)	Deaths 2000 (Projected) Number ('000s)	Rate (per 100 000)
Males										
0-4	1	4.2	1	10	2.5	63.5	0	0	0	0
5-14	0	0.4	6	23	10.0	57.3	0	0	0	0
15-44	0	0.2	21	27	29.8	39.2	0	0	0	0
45-59	0	0.2	9	32	52.2	20.8	0	0	0	0
60+	0	0.6	8	40	70.0	10.1	0	0	0	0
All ages	1	0.6	45	27	18.6	50.2	0	0	0	0
Females										
0-4	1	4.2	1	10	2.5	72.4	0	0	0	0
5-14	0	0.4	6	23	10.0	66.0	0	0	0	0
15-44	0	0.2	20	27	29.9	46.8	0	0	0	0
45-59	0	0.2	10	32	52.4	26.1	0	0	0	0
60+	0	0.6	15	40	71.5	11.8	0	0	0	0
All ages	1	0.6	52	29	23.8	53.3	0	0	0	0
Total	2	0.6	98	28	21.3	51.8	0	0	0	0

Table 64c India - India - Inde Bacterial meningitis - Motor deficit

Age group (years)	Incidence 1990 Number ('000s)	Rate (per 100 000)	Prevalence 1990 Number ('000s)	Rate (per 100 000)	Avg. age at onset (years)	Average duration (years)	Deaths 1990 Number ('000s)	Rate (per 100 000)	Deaths 2000 (Projected) Number ('000s)	Rate (per 100 000)
Males										
0-4	2	4.0	6	10	2.5	59.9	0	0	0	0
5-14	0	0.3	22	22	10.0	57.4	0	0	0	0
15-44	0	0.2	53	26	29.8	39.9	0	0	0	0
45-59	0	0.3	15	31	52.3	21.0	0	0	0	0
60+	0	0.6	10	34	69.7	9.7	0	0	0	0
All ages	3	0.8	106	24	8.7	55.5	0	0	0	0
Females										
0-4	2	4.0	6	10	2.5	60.8	0	0	0	0
5-14	0	0.3	21	22	10.0	59.1	0	0	0	0
15-44	0	0.2	48	26	29.8	41.7	0	0	0	0
45-59	0	0.3	14	31	52.4	22.5	0	0	0	0
60+	0	0.6	10	34	70.1	10.2	0	0	0	0
All ages	3	0.8	99	24	8.7	56.7	0	0	0	0
Total	7	0.8	205	24	8.7	56.1	0	0	0	0

For epidemiological sources see Schillinger et al. 1996. For the methods used to estimate and project incidence, prevalence, and deaths see Murray and Lopez 1996a. See explanatory notes for definitions and caveats.

Table 64 | **Cuadro 64** | **Tableau 64**
Bacterial meningitis | **Meninigitis bacteriana** | **Méningite bactérienne**

Motor deficit | Déficit motriz | Déficit moteur

Table 64d   China - China - Chine   Bacterial meningitis - Motor deficit

Age group (years)	Incidence 1990 Number ('000s)	Rate (per 100 000)	Prevalence 1990 Number ('000s)	Rate (per 100 000)	Avg. age at onset (years)	Average duration (years)	Deaths 1990 Number ('000s)	Rate (per 100 000)	Deaths 2000 (Projected) Number ('000s)	Rate (per 100 000)
Males										
0-4	2	4.0	6	10	2.5	65.5	0	0	0	0
5-14	0	0.3	21	22	10.0	59.9	0	0	0	0
15-44	1	0.2	79	26	29.9	41.2	0	0	0	0
45-59	0	0.3	22	31	52.3	21.4	0	0	0	0
60+	0	0.6	19	38	69.8	9.9	0	0	0	0
All ages	4	0.6	147	25	14.8	55.0	0	0	0	0
Females										
0-4	2	4.0	6	10	2.5	68.5	0	0	0	0
5-14	0	0.3	20	22	10.0	63.2	0	0	0	0
15-44	0	0.2	73	26	29.9	44.2	0	0	0	0
45-59	0	0.3	20	31	52.4	23.8	0	0	0	0
60+	0	0.6	20	39	70.6	10.8	0	0	0	0
All ages	4	0.7	139	25	15.1	57.6	0	0	0	0
Total	7	0.6	286	25	14.9	56.3	0	0	0	0

Table 64e   OAI - OPAI - APAI   Bacterial meningitis - Motor deficit

Age group (years)	Incidence 1990 Number ('000s)	Rate (per 100 000)	Prevalence 1990 Number ('000s)	Rate (per 100 000)	Avg. age at onset (years)	Average duration (years)	Deaths 1990 Number ('000s)	Rate (per 100 000)	Deaths 2000 (Projected) Number ('000s)	Rate (per 100 000)
Males										
0-4	2	4.0	5	11	2.5	59.8	0	0	0	0
5-14	0	0.3	20	23	10.0	56.2	0	0	0	0
15-44	0	0.1	44	27	29.7	38.8	0	0	0	0
45-59	0	0.3	11	32	52.3	20.3	0	0	0	0
60+	0	0.6	8	40	69.6	9.7	0	0	0	0
All ages	2	0.7	87	25	11.1	53.5	0	0	0	0
Females										
0-4	2	4.0	5	11	2.5	63.2	0	0	0	0
5-14	0	0.3	19	23	10.0	59.2	0	0	0	0
15-44	0	0.1	44	27	29.8	41.4	0	0	0	0
45-59	0	0.3	11	32	52.3	22.4	0	0	0	0
60+	0	0.6	9	40	70.3	10.5	0	0	0	0
All ages	2	0.7	87	26	11.8	56.0	0	0	0	0
Total	5	0.7	175	26	11.4	54.7	0	0	0	0

Table 64f   SSA - ASS - ASS   Bacterial meningitis - Motor deficit

Age group (years)	Incidence 1990 Number ('000s)	Rate (per 100 000)	Prevalence 1990 Number ('000s)	Rate (per 100 000)	Avg. age at onset (years)	Average duration (years)	Deaths 1990 Number ('000s)	Rate (per 100 000)	Deaths 2000 (Projected) Number ('000s)	Rate (per 100 000)
Males										
0-4	2	4.0	5	10	2.4	48.7	0	0	0	0
5-14	0	0.3	15	22	10.0	49.2	0	0	0	0
15-44	0	0.2	27	26	29.4	35.0	0	0	0	0
45-59	0	0.3	6	31	52.2	19.1	0	0	0	0
60+	0	0.6	4	39	69.2	9.3	0	0	0	0
All ages	2	1.0	58	23	8.1	46.0	0	0	0	0
Females										
0-4	2	4.0	5	10	2.4	51.9	0	0	0	0
5-14	0	0.3	15	22	10.0	51.9	0	0	0	0
15-44	0	0.2	28	26	29.5	37.2	0	0	0	0
45-59	0	0.3	7	31	52.2	20.5	0	0	0	0
60+	0	0.6	5	39	69.7	9.8	0	0	0	0
All ages	2	1.0	60	23	8.6	48.7	0	0	0	0
Total	5	1.0	117	23	8.3	47.3	0	0	0	0

For epidemiological sources see Schillinger et al. 1996. For the methods used to estimate and project incidence, prevalence, and deaths see Murray and Lopez 1996a. See explanatory notes for definitions and caveats.

Table 64	Cuadro 64	Tableau 64
Bacterial meningitis	Meninigitis bacteriana	Méningite bactérienne

Motor deficit | Déficit motriz | Déficit moteur

Table 64g LAC - ALC - ALC — Bacterial meningitis - Motor deficit

Age group (years)	Incidence 1990 Number ('000s)	Rate (per 100 000)	Prevalence 1990 Number ('000s)	Rate (per 100 000)	Avg. age at onset (years)	Average duration (years)	Deaths 1990 Number ('000s)	Rate (per 100 000)	Deaths 2000 (Projected) Number ('000s)	Rate (per 100 000)
Males										
0-4	1	4.0	3	10	2.5	63.9	0	0	0	0
5-14	0	0.3	11	22	10.0	59.3	0	0	0	0
15-44	0	0.2	27	26	29.8	41.4	0	0	0	0
45-59	0	0.3	7	31	52.3	22.3	0	0	0	0
60+	0	0.6	6	39	70.3	10.4	0	0	0	0
All ages	2	0.8	54	24	11.7	56.5	0	0	0	0
Females										
0-4	1	4.0	3	10	2.5	67.9	0	0	0	0
5-14	0	0.3	11	22	10.0	63.0	0	0	0	0
15-44	0	0.2	27	26	29.9	44.6	0	0	0	0
45-59	0	0.3	7	31	52.4	24.8	0	0	0	0
60+	0	0.6	7	40	71.1	11.3	0	0	0	0
All ages	2	0.7	55	25	12.6	59.5	0	0	0	0
Total	3	0.7	109	24	12.2	58.0	0	0	0	0

Table 64h MEC - AOM - CMO — Bacterial meningitis - Motor deficit

Age group (years)	Incidence 1990 Number ('000s)	Rate (per 100 000)	Prevalence 1990 Number ('000s)	Rate (per 100 000)	Avg. age at onset (years)	Average duration (years)	Deaths 1990 Number ('000s)	Rate (per 100 000)	Deaths 2000 (Projected) Number ('000s)	Rate (per 100 000)
Males										
0-4	2	4.0	4	10	2.5	61.1	0	0	0	0
5-14	0	0.3	14	22	10.0	58.1	0	0	0	0
15-44	0	0.2	30	26	29.8	40.0	0	0	0	0
45-59	0	0.3	7	31	52.3	20.8	0	0	0	0
60+	0	0.6	5	39	69.7	9.8	0	0	0	0
All ages	2	0.9	60	24	9.7	55.8	0	0	0	0
Females										
0-4	2	4.0	4	10	2.5	63.7	0	0	0	0
5-14	0	0.3	13	22	10.0	60.9	0	0	0	0
15-44	0	0.2	28	26	29.8	42.6	0	0	0	0
45-59	0	0.3	7	31	52.3	22.9	0	0	0	0
60+	0	0.6	6	40	70.4	10.6	0	0	0	0
All ages	2	0.9	58	24	10.1	58.0	0	0	0	0
Total	4	0.9	119	24	9.9	56.9	0	0	0	0

Table 64i World - Mundo - Monde — Bacterial meningitis - Motor deficit

Age group (years)	Incidence 1990 Number ('000s)	Rate (per 100 000)	Prevalence 1990 Number ('000s)	Rate (per 100 000)	Avg. age at onset (years)	Average duration (years)	Deaths 1990 Number ('000s)	Rate (per 100 000)	Deaths 2000 (Projected) Number ('000s)	Rate (per 100 000)
Males										
0-4	13	3.9	31	10	2.5	60.5	0	0	0	0
5-14	2	0.3	118	21	10.0	57.3	0	0	0	0
15-44	2	0.2	310	25	29.8	39.9	0	0	0	0
45-59	1	0.2	88	28	52.3	21.0	0	0	0	0
60+	1	0.5	72	33	69.9	10.0	0	0	0	0
All ages	18	0.7	619	23	11.4	54.0	0	0	0	0
Females										
0-4	12	3.9	30	10	2.5	63.6	0	0	0	0
5-14	2	0.3	112	21	10.0	60.5	0	0	0	0
15-44	2	0.2	297	25	29.8	43.0	0	0	0	0
45-59	1	0.2	87	28	52.4	23.4	0	0	0	0
60+	1	0.4	88	33	70.9	11.1	0	0	0	0
All ages	18	0.7	615	24	12.2	56.3	0	0	0	0
Total	36	0.7	1 234	23	11.8	55.1	0	0	0	0

For epidemiological sources see Schillinger et al. 1996. For the methods used to estimate and project incidence, prevalence, and deaths see Murray and Lopez 1996a. See explanatory notes for definitions and caveats.

Table 65	Cuadro 65	Tableau 65
Bacterial meningitis	**Meninigitis bacteriana**	**Méningite bactérienne**
Mental retardation	Retraso mental	Retard mental

Table 65a EME - PEMC - EMBE — Bacterial meningitis - Mental retardation

Age group (years)	Incidence 1990 Number ('000s)	Rate (per 100 000)	Prevalence 1990 Number ('000s)	Rate (per 100 000)	Avg. age at onset (years)	Average duration (years)	Deaths 1990 Number ('000s)	Rate (per 100 000)	Deaths 2000 (Projected) Number ('000s)	Rate (per 100 000)
Males										
0-4	1	3.0	2	7.4	2.5	70.2	0	0	0	0
5-14	0	0.3	9	16.2	10.0	63.6	0	0	0	0
15-44	0	0.0	34	18.2	29.9	44.7	0	0	0	0
45-59	0	0.0	13	19.2	52.4	24.5	0	0	0	0
60+	0	0.2	13	21.3	71.1	11.3	0	0	0	0
All ages	1	0.3	70	17.8	12.5	61.4	0	0	0	0
Females										
0-4	1	3.0	2	7.4	2.5	76.1	0	0	0	0
5-14	0	0.3	8	16.2	10.0	69.5	0	0	0	0
15-44	0	0.0	33	18.2	30.0	50.0	0	0	0	0
45-59	0	0.0	13	19.2	52.4	28.8	0	0	0	0
60+	0	0.2	18	21.5	72.4	12.7	0	0	0	0
All ages	1	0.3	74	18.1	15.0	64.7	0	0	0	0
Total	2	0.3	144	18.0	13.7	63.1	0	0	0	0

Table 65b FSE - PEAS - AESE — Bacterial meningitis - Mental retardation

Age group (years)	Incidence 1990 Number ('000s)	Rate (per 100 000)	Prevalence 1990 Number ('000s)	Rate (per 100 000)	Avg. age at onset (years)	Average duration (years)	Deaths 1990 Number ('000s)	Rate (per 100 000)	Deaths 2000 (Projected) Number ('000s)	Rate (per 100 000)
Males										
0-4	1	4.7	2	12	2.5	63.5	0	0	0	0
5-14	0	0.4	7	26	10.0	57.3	0	0	0	0
15-44	0	0.2	24	31	29.8	39.2	0	0	0	0
45-59	0	0.3	10	36	52.2	20.8	0	0	0	0
60+	0	0.7	9	45	70.0	10.1	0	0	0	0
All ages	1	0.7	52	31	18.6	50.2	0	0	0	0
Females										
0-4	1	4.7	2	12	2.5	72.4	0	0	0	0
5-14	0	0.4	7	26	10.0	66.0	0	0	0	0
15-44	0	0.2	23	31	29.9	46.8	0	0	0	0
45-59	0	0.3	11	36	52.4	26.1	0	0	0	0
60+	0	0.7	17	46	71.5	11.8	0	0	0	0
All ages	1	0.7	59	33	23.8	53.3	0	0	0	0
Total	2	0.7	111	32	21.3	51.8	0	0	0	0

Table 65c India - India - Inde — Bacterial meningitis - Mental retardation

Age group (years)	Incidence 1990 Number ('000s)	Rate (per 100 000)	Prevalence 1990 Number ('000s)	Rate (per 100 000)	Avg. age at onset (years)	Average duration (years)	Deaths 1990 Number ('000s)	Rate (per 100 000)	Deaths 2000 (Projected) Number ('000s)	Rate (per 100 000)
Males										
0-4	3	5.3	8	13	2.5	59.9	0	0	0	0
5-14	0	0.5	29	29	10.0	57.4	0	0	0	0
15-44	0	0.2	69	34	29.8	39.9	0	0	0	0
45-59	0	0.4	19	41	52.3	21.0	0	0	0	0
60+	0	0.7	13	44	69.7	9.7	0	0	0	0
All ages	5	1.0	139	32	8.7	55.5	0	0	0	0
Females										
0-4	3	5.3	7	13	2.5	60.8	0	0	0	0
5-14	0	0.5	27	29	10.0	59.1	0	0	0	0
15-44	0	0.2	63	34	29.8	41.7	0	0	0	0
45-59	0	0.4	19	41	52.4	22.5	0	0	0	0
60+	0	0.7	13	44	70.1	10.2	0	0	0	0
All ages	4	1.0	129	32	8.7	56.7	0	0	0	0
Total	9	1.0	268	32	8.7	56.1	0	0	0	0

For epidemiological sources see Schillinger et al. 1996. For the methods used to estimate and project incidence, prevalence, and deaths see Murray and Lopez 1996a. See explanatory notes for definitions and caveats.

Table 65
Bacterial meningitis

Cuadro 65
Meninigitis bacteriana

Tableau 65
Méningite bactérienne

Mental retardation

Retraso mental

Retard mental

Table 65d China - China - Chine

Bacterial meningitis - Mental retardation

Age group (years)	Incidence 1990 Number ('000s)	Rate (per 100 000)	Prevalence 1990 Number ('000s)	Rate (per 100 000)	Avg. age at onset (years)	Average duration (years)	Deaths 1990 Number ('000s)	Rate (per 100 000)	Deaths 2000 (Projected) Number ('000s)	Rate (per 100 000)
Males										
0-4	3	5.3	8	13	2.5	65.5	0	0	0	0
5-14	0	0.4	28	28	10.0	59.9	0	0	0	0
15-44	1	0.2	103	34	29.9	41.2	0	0	0	0
45-59	0	0.4	29	40	52.3	21.4	0	0	0	0
60+	0	0.7	25	50	69.8	9.9	0	0	0	0
All ages	5	0.8	193	33	14.8	55.0	0	0	0	0
Females										
0-4	3	5.3	8	13	2.5	68.5	0	0	0	0
5-14	0	0.4	26	28	10.0	63.2	0	0	0	0
15-44	1	0.2	96	34	29.9	44.2	0	0	0	0
45-59	0	0.4	26	40	52.4	23.8	0	0	0	0
60+	0	0.7	26	51	70.6	10.8	0	0	0	0
All ages	5	0.9	181	33	15.1	57.6	0	0	0	0
Total	10	0.9	374	33	14.9	56.3	0	0	0	0

Table 65e OAI - OPAI - APAI

Bacterial meningitis - Mental retardation

Age group (years)	Incidence 1990 Number ('000s)	Rate (per 100 000)	Prevalence 1990 Number ('000s)	Rate (per 100 000)	Avg. age at onset (years)	Average duration (years)	Deaths 1990 Number ('000s)	Rate (per 100 000)	Deaths 2000 (Projected) Number ('000s)	Rate (per 100 000)
Males										
0-4	2	5.3	6	13	2.5	59.8	0	0	0	0
5-14	0	0.4	24	28	10.0	56.2	0	0	0	0
15-44	0	0.2	54	33	29.7	38.8	0	0	0	0
45-59	0	0.4	13	39	52.3	20.3	0	0	0	0
60+	0	0.7	10	50	69.6	9.7	0	0	0	0
All ages	3	1.0	107	31	11.1	53.5	0	0	0	0
Females										
0-4	2	5.3	5	13	2.5	63.2	0	0	0	0
5-14	0	0.4	23	28	10.0	59.2	0	0	0	0
15-44	0	0.2	53	33	29.8	41.4	0	0	0	0
45-59	0	0.4	14	39	52.3	22.4	0	0	0	0
60+	0	0.7	11	50	70.3	10.5	0	0	0	0
All ages	3	0.9	107	31	11.8	56.0	0	0	0	0
Total	6	0.9	213	31	11.4	54.7	0	0	0	0

Table 65f SSA - ASS - ASS

Bacterial meningitis - Mental retardation

Age group (years)	Incidence 1990 Number ('000s)	Rate (per 100 000)	Prevalence 1990 Number ('000s)	Rate (per 100 000)	Avg. age at onset (years)	Average duration (years)	Deaths 1990 Number ('000s)	Rate (per 100 000)	Deaths 2000 (Projected) Number ('000s)	Rate (per 100 000)
Males										
0-4	3	5.3	6	13	2.4	48.7	0	0	0	0
5-14	0	0.4	20	29	10.0	49.2	0	0	0	0
15-44	0	0.2	36	34	29.4	35.0	0	0	0	0
45-59	0	0.4	8	41	52.2	19.1	0	0	0	0
60+	0	0.7	5	51	69.2	9.3	0	0	0	0
All ages	3	1.3	76	30	8.1	46.0	0	0	0	0
Females										
0-4	2	5.3	6	13	2.4	51.9	0	0	0	0
5-14	0	0.4	20	29	10.0	51.9	0	0	0	0
15-44	0	0.2	37	34	29.5	37.2	0	0	0	0
45-59	0	0.4	9	41	52.2	20.5	0	0	0	0
60+	0	0.7	7	52	69.7	9.8	0	0	0	0
All ages	3	1.3	78	30	8.6	48.7	0	0	0	0
Total	6	1.3	154	30	8.3	47.3	0	0	0	0

For epidemiological sources see Schillinger et al. 1996. For the methods used to estimate and project incidence, prevalence, and deaths see Murray and Lopez 1996a. See explanatory notes for definitions and caveats.

Table 65
Bacterial meningitis

Cuadro 65
Meninigitis bacteriana

Tableau 65
Méningite bactérienne

Mental retardation

Retraso mental

Retard mental

Table 65g	LAC - ALC - ALC									Bacterial meningitis - Mental retardation	
Age group (years)	Incidence 1990		Prevalence 1990		Avg. age at onset (years)	Average duration (years)	Deaths 1990		Deaths 2000 (Projected)		
	Number ('000s)	Rate (per 100 000)	Number ('000s)	Rate (per 100 000)			Number ('000s)	Rate (per 100 000)	Number ('000s)	Rate (per 100 000)	
Males											
0-4	2	5.2	4	13	2.5	63.9	0	0	0	0	
5-14	0	0.5	15	28	10.0	59.3	0	0	0	0	
15-44	0	0.2	36	34	29.8	41.4	0	0	0	0	
45-59	0	0.4	9	41	52.3	22.3	0	0	0	0	
60+	0	0.7	7	51	70.3	10.4	0	0	0	0	
All ages	2	1.0	70	32	11.7	56.5	0	0	0	0	
Females											
0-4	1	5.2	4	13	2.5	67.9	0	0	0	0	
5-14	0	0.5	14	28	10.0	63.0	0	0	0	0	
15-44	0	0.2	36	34	29.9	44.6	0	0	0	0	
45-59	0	0.4	10	41	52.4	24.8	0	0	0	0	
60+	0	0.7	9	52	71.1	11.3	0	0	0	0	
All ages	2	1.0	72	32	12.6	59.5	0	0	0	0	
Total	4	1.0	142	32	12.2	58.0	0	0	0	0	

Table 65h	MEC - AOM - CMO									Bacterial meningitis - Mental retardation	
Age group (years)	Incidence 1990		Prevalence 1990		Avg. age at onset (years)	Average duration (years)	Deaths 1990		Deaths 2000 (Projected)		
	Number ('000s)	Rate (per 100 000)	Number ('000s)	Rate (per 100 000)			Number ('000s)	Rate (per 100 000)	Number ('000s)	Rate (per 100 000)	
Males											
0-4	2	5.3	5	13	2.5	61.1	0	0	0	0	
5-14	0	0.5	19	29	10.0	58.1	0	0	0	0	
15-44	0	0.2	39	34	29.8	40.0	0	0	0	0	
45-59	0	0.4	9	41	52.3	20.8	0	0	0	0	
60+	0	0.7	7	51	69.7	9.8	0	0	0	0	
All ages	3	1.1	79	31	9.7	55.8	0	0	0	0	
Females											
0-4	2	5.3	5	13	2.5	63.7	0	0	0	0	
5-14	0	0.5	18	29	10.0	60.9	0	0	0	0	
15-44	0	0.2	37	34	29.8	42.6	0	0	0	0	
45-59	0	0.4	9	41	52.3	22.9	0	0	0	0	
60+	0	0.7	8	52	70.4	10.6	0	0	0	0	
All ages	3	1.2	77	31	10.1	58.0	0	0	0	0	
Total	6	1.1	156	31	9.9	56.9	0	0	0	0	

Table 65i	World - Mundo - Monde									Bacterial meningitis - Mental retardation	
Age group (years)	Incidence 1990		Prevalence 1990		Avg. age at onset (years)	Average duration (years)	Deaths 1990		Deaths 2000 (Projected)		
	Number ('000s)	Rate (per 100 000)	Number ('000s)	Rate (per 100 000)			Number ('000s)	Rate (per 100 000)	Number ('000s)	Rate (per 100 000)	
Males											
0-4	16	5.1	40	12	2.5	60.4	0	0	0	0	
5-14	2	0.4	150	27	10.0	57.2	0	0	0	0	
15-44	2	0.2	394	31	29.8	39.9	0	0	0	0	
45-59	1	0.3	111	36	52.3	21.0	0	0	0	0	
60+	1	0.6	90	41	69.9	10.0	0	0	0	0	
All ages	23	0.9	784	30	11.3	53.9	0	0	0	0	
Females											
0-4	16	5.1	39	12	2.5	63.5	0	0	0	0	
5-14	2	0.4	143	27	10.0	60.4	0	0	0	0	
15-44	2	0.2	377	31	29.8	42.9	0	0	0	0	
45-59	1	0.3	110	35	52.4	23.4	0	0	0	0	
60+	1	0.5	109	40	70.9	11.1	0	0	0	0	
All ages	23	0.9	777	30	12.1	56.3	0	0	0	0	
Total	46	0.9	1 562	30	11.7	55.1	0	0	0	0	

For epidemiological sources see Schillinger et al. 1996. For the methods used to estimate and project incidence, prevalence, and deaths see Murray and Lopez 1996a. See explanatory notes for definitions and caveats.

Table 66
Hepatitis B and hepatitis C

Cuadro 66
Hepatitis B y hepatitis C

Tableau 66
Hépatite B et hépatite C

Episodes

Episodios

Episodes

Table 66a	EME - PEMC - EMBE								Hepatitis B and hepatitis C - Episodes	
Age group (years)	Incidence 1990		Prevalence 1990		Avg. age at onset (years)	Average duration (years)	Deaths 1990		Deaths 2000 (Projected)	
	Number ('000s)	Rate (per 100 000)	Number ('000s)	Rate (per 100 000)			Number ('000s)	Rate (per 100 000)	Number ('000s)	Rate (per 100 000)
Males										
0-4	1	5.3	0	0.9	2.5	0.17	0	0.1	0	0.1
5-14	1	1.3	0	0.2	10.0	0.17	0	0.0	0	0.0
15-44	25	13.6	4	2.3	29.9	0.17	1	0.3	0	0.2
45-59	27	40.7	4	6.8	52.4	0.17	1	0.9	0	0.5
60+	51	84.8	9	14.1	71.1	0.17	1	1.8	1	1.5
All ages	105	27.0	18	4.5	55.2	0.17	2	0.6	2	0.4
Females										
0-4	1	5.0	0	0.8	2.5	0.17	0	0.1	0	0.1
5-14	1	1.1	0	0.2	10.0	0.17	0	0.0	0	0.0
15-44	14	7.8	2	1.3	30.0	0.17	0	0.2	0	0.1
45-59	13	18.8	2	3.1	52.4	0.17	0	0.4	0	0.3
60+	44	51.6	7	8.6	72.4	0.17	1	1.1	1	0.9
All ages	72	17.7	12	3.0	59.0	0.17	2	0.4	1	0.3
Total	177	22.2	30	3.7	56.8	0.17	4	0.5	3	0.4

Table 66b	FSE - PEAS - AESE								Hepatitis B and hepatitis C - Episodes	
Age group (years)	Incidence 1990		Prevalence 1990		Avg. age at onset (years)	Average duration (years)	Deaths 1990		Deaths 2000 (Projected)	
	Number ('000s)	Rate (per 100 000)	Number ('000s)	Rate (per 100 000)			Number ('000s)	Rate (per 100 000)	Number ('000s)	Rate (per 100 000)
Males										
0-4	10	71.9	2	12.0	2.5	0.17	0	1.5	0	1.1
5-14	2	8.2	0	1.4	10.0	0.17	0	0.2	0	0.1
15-44	9	12.1	2	2.0	29.8	0.17	0	0.3	0	0.2
45-59	7	26.3	1	4.4	52.2	0.17	0	0.6	0	0.4
60+	14	66.3	2	11.1	70.0	0.17	0	1.4	0	1.2
All ages	42	25.6	7	4.3	39.3	0.17	1	0.5	1	0.4
Females										
0-4	8	58.2	1	9.7	2.5	0.17	0	1.2	0	0.9
5-14	1	4.8	0	0.8	10.0	0.17	0	0.1	0	0.1
15-44	11	14.2	2	2.4	29.9	0.17	0	0.3	0	0.2
45-59	4	14.8	1	2.5	52.4	0.17	0	0.3	0	0.2
60+	11	30.8	2	5.1	71.5	0.17	0	0.7	0	0.5
All ages	35	19.4	6	3.2	39.3	0.17	1	0.4	1	0.3
Total	78	22.4	13	3.7	39.3	0.17	2	0.5	1	0.4

Table 66c	India - India - Inde								Hepatitis B and hepatitis C - Episodes	
Age group (years)	Incidence 1990		Prevalence 1990		Avg. age at onset (years)	Average duration (years)	Deaths 1990		Deaths 2000 (Projected)	
	Number ('000s)	Rate (per 100 000)	Number ('000s)	Rate (per 100 000)			Number ('000s)	Rate (per 100 000)	Number ('000s)	Rate (per 100 000)
Males										
0-4	21	34	3	5.7	2.5	0.17	1	2.2	1	1.4
5-14	10	10	2	1.6	10.0	0.17	1	0.7	0	0.3
15-44	38	19	6	3.2	29.8	0.17	2	1.2	1	0.5
45-59	34	71	6	11.8	52.3	0.17	2	4.6	1	2.1
60+	47	158	8	26.3	69.7	0.17	3	10.3	3	7.2
All ages	149	34	25	5.7	42.3	0.17	10	2.2	6	1.2
Females										
0-4	16	29	3	4.8	2.5	0.17	1	1.9	1	1.1
5-14	9	10	2	1.6	10.0	0.17	1	0.8	0	0.3
15-44	34	19	6	3.1	29.8	0.17	2	1.1	1	0.4
45-59	16	34	3	5.7	52.4	0.17	1	2.2	1	1.0
60+	42	144	7	24.0	70.1	0.17	3	9.4	3	6.6
All ages	117	29	20	4.8	41.7	0.17	8	1.8	5	1.0
Total	266	31	44	5.2	42.1	0.17	17	2.0	11	1.1

For epidemiological sources see Kane et al. 1996. For the methods used to estimate and project incidence, prevalence, and deaths see Murray and Lopez 1996a. See explanatory notes for definitions and caveats.

Table 66
Hepatitis B and hepatitis C

Cuadro 66
Hepatitis B y hepatitis C

Tableau 66
Hépatite B et hépatite C

Episodes

Episodios

Episodes

Table 66d	China - China - Chine								Hepatitis B and hepatitis C - Episodes	
Age group (years)	Incidence 1990		Prevalence 1990		Avg. age at onset (years)	Average duration (years)	Deaths 1990		Deaths 2000 (Projected)	
	Number ('000s)	Rate (per 100 000)	Number ('000s)	Rate (per 100 000)			Number ('000s)	Rate (per 100 000)	Number ('000s)	Rate (per 100 000)
Males										
0-4	30	49.2	5	8.2	2.5	0.17	2	3.1	*1*	*1.6*
5-14	3	2.8	0	0.5	10.0	0.17	0	0.3	*0*	*0.1*
15-44	117	38.3	20	6.4	29.9	0.17	8	2.5	*3*	*0.9*
45-59	114	157.1	19	26.2	52.3	0.17	7	10.0	*4*	*3.9*
60+	88	180.5	15	30.1	69.8	0.17	6	11.5	*5*	*8.3*
All ages	352	60.2	59	10.0	44.7	0.17	23	3.9	*13*	*1.9*
Females										
0-4	24	42.1	4	7.0	2.5	0.17	2	2.6	*1*	*1.3*
5-14	7	8.3	1	1.4	10.0	0.17	0	0.3	*0*	*0.1*
15-44	39	13.7	6	2.3	29.9	0.17	2	0.8	*1*	*0.2*
45-59	22	34.7	4	5.8	52.4	0.17	1	2.2	*1*	*0.9*
60+	93	179.5	15	29.9	70.6	0.17	6	11.5	*5*	*7.5*
All ages	186	33.9	31	5.6	48.5	0.17	12	2.1	*7*	*1.1*
Total	538	47.5	90	7.9	46.0	0.17	34	3.0	*20*	*1.6*

Table 66e	OAI - OPAI - APAI								Hepatitis B and hepatitis C - Episodes	
Age group (years)	Incidence 1990		Prevalence 1990		Avg. age at onset (years)	Average duration (years)	Deaths 1990		Deaths 2000 (Projected)	
	Number ('000s)	Rate (per 100 000)	Number ('000s)	Rate (per 100 000)			Number ('000s)	Rate (per 100 000)	Number ('000s)	Rate (per 100 000)
Males										
0-4	24	55	4	9.2	2.5	0.17	2	3.5	*1*	*2.3*
5-14	12	14	2	2.3	10.0	0.17	1	1.0	*0*	*0.5*
15-44	45	28	7	4.6	29.7	0.17	2	1.5	*1*	*0.7*
45-59	39	115	7	19.2	52.3	0.17	3	7.6	*2*	*3.8*
60+	55	272	9	45.3	69.6	0.17	4	18.3	*4*	*13.5*
All ages	175	51	29	8.5	42.2	0.17	11	3.2	*8*	*2.1*
Females										
0-4	19	46	3	7.6	2.5	0.17	1	2.7	*1*	*1.7*
5-14	11	14	2	2.3	10.0	0.17	1	0.9	*0*	*0.4*
15-44	40	25	7	4.2	29.8	0.17	2	1.2	*1*	*0.5*
45-59	18	53	3	8.8	52.3	0.17	1	3.4	*1*	*1.7*
60+	49	215	8	35.8	70.3	0.17	3	12.5	*3*	*9.6*
All ages	137	40	23	6.7	41.8	0.17	8	2.3	*6*	*1.5*
Total	312	46	52	7.6	42.0	0.17	19	2.8	*14*	*1.8*

Table 66f	SSA - ASS - ASS								Hepatitis B and hepatitis C - Episodes	
Age group (years)	Incidence 1990		Prevalence 1990		Avg. age at onset (years)	Average duration (years)	Deaths 1990		Deaths 2000 (Projected)	
	Number ('000s)	Rate (per 100 000)	Number ('000s)	Rate (per 100 000)			Number ('000s)	Rate (per 100 000)	Number ('000s)	Rate (per 100 000)
Males										
0-4	19	40	3	6.6	2.4	0.17	1	2.4	*1*	*1.7*
5-14	9	13	2	2.2	10.0	0.17	1	1.0	*0*	*0.5*
15-44	35	34	6	5.6	29.4	0.17	2	1.7	*1*	*0.8*
45-59	31	152	5	25.3	52.2	0.17	2	10.0	*1*	*5.3*
60+	43	410	7	68.4	69.2	0.17	3	27.2	*3*	*19.4*
All ages	137	54	23	9.1	42.0	0.17	8	3.3	*7*	*2.0*
Females										
0-4	15	32	3	5.3	2.4	0.17	1	1.8	*1*	*1.3*
5-14	9	12	1	2.1	10.0	0.17	1	0.9	*0*	*0.5*
15-44	31	29	5	4.9	29.5	0.17	2	1.8	*1*	*0.7*
45-59	14	66	2	10.9	52.2	0.17	1	4.3	*1*	*2.2*
60+	38	300	6	50.0	69.7	0.17	3	20.4	*3*	*14.3*
All ages	108	42	18	7.0	41.5	0.17	7	2.7	*5*	*1.6*
Total	245	48	41	8.0	41.8	0.17	15	3.0	*12*	*1.8*

For epidemiological sources see Kane et al. 1996. For the methods used to estimate and project incidence, prevalence, and deaths see Murray and Lopez 1996a. See explanatory notes for definitions and caveats.

Table 66
Hepatitis B and hepatitis C

Cuadro 66
Hepatitis B y hepatitis C

Tableau 66
Hépatite B et hépatite C

Episodes

Episodios

Episodes

Table 66g   LAC - ALC - ALC   Hepatitis B and hepatitis C - Episodes

Age group (years)	Incidence 1990 Number ('000s)	Rate (per 100 000)	Prevalence 1990 Number ('000s)	Rate (per 100 000)	Avg. age at onset (years)	Average duration (years)	Deaths 1990 Number ('000s)	Rate (per 100 000)	Deaths 2000 (Projected) Number ('000s)	Rate (per 100 000)
Males										
0-4	9	30.6	1	5.1	2.5	0.17	1	2.0	0	1.4
5-14	8	16.0	1	2.7	10.0	0.17	0	0.8	0	0.4
15-44	7	6.7	1	1.1	29.8	0.17	0	0.4	0	0.2
45-59	4	16.0	1	2.7	52.3	0.17	0	1.0	0	0.6
60+	5	37.1	1	6.2	70.3	0.17	0	2.4	0	1.8
All ages	33	14.9	6	2.5	26.4	0.17	2	0.9	1	0.5
Females										
0-4	7	25.4	1	4.2	2.5	0.17	0	1.5	0	1.0
5-14	8	15.7	1	2.6	10.0	0.17	0	0.9	0	0.5
15-44	17	15.9	3	2.6	29.9	0.17	1	1.0	1	0.4
45-59	5	21.0	1	3.5	52.4	0.17	0	1.3	0	0.7
60+	5	27.1	1	4.5	71.1	0.17	0	1.7	0	1.3
All ages	41	18.4	7	3.1	28.6	0.17	2	1.1	2	0.6
Total	74	16.7	12	2.8	27.6	0.17	4	1.0	3	0.6

Table 66h   MEC - AOM - CMO   Hepatitis B and hepatitis C - Episodes

Age group (years)	Incidence 1990 Number ('000s)	Rate (per 100 000)	Prevalence 1990 Number ('000s)	Rate (per 100 000)	Avg. age at onset (years)	Average duration (years)	Deaths 1990 Number ('000s)	Rate (per 100 000)	Deaths 2000 (Projected) Number ('000s)	Rate (per 100 000)
Males										
0-4	17	41	3	6.8	2.5	0.17	1	2.6	1	1.9
5-14	8	13	1	2.1	10.0	0.17	1	0.8	0	0.5
15-44	31	27	5	4.6	29.8	0.17	1	1.3	1	0.7
45-59	27	123	5	20.5	52.3	0.17	2	7.8	1	4.4
60+	38	281	6	46.9	69.7	0.17	2	17.8	2	13.2
All ages	122	48	20	7.9	42.3	0.17	7	2.8	6	1.9
Females										
0-4	13	34	2	5.6	2.5	0.17	1	2.2	1	1.5
5-14	8	12	1	2.1	10.0	0.17	1	0.8	0	0.5
15-44	28	26	5	4.3	29.8	0.17	1	1.2	1	0.5
45-59	13	58	2	9.6	52.3	0.17	1	3.7	1	2.0
60+	34	220	6	36.7	70.4	0.17	2	13.1	2	9.8
All ages	96	39	16	6.5	41.8	0.17	6	2.2	5	1.4
Total	218	43	36	7.2	42.1	0.17	13	2.5	11	1.6

Table 66i   World - Mundo - Monde   Hepatitis B and hepatitis C - Episodes

Age group (years)	Incidence 1990 Number ('000s)	Rate (per 100 000)	Prevalence 1990 Number ('000s)	Rate (per 100 000)	Avg. age at onset (years)	Average duration (years)	Deaths 1990 Number ('000s)	Rate (per 100 000)	Deaths 2000 (Projected) Number ('000s)	Rate (per 100 000)
Males										
0-4	130	41	22	6.8	2.5	0.17	8	2.4	5	1.6
5-14	53	10	9	1.6	10.0	0.17	4	0.6	2	0.3
15-44	308	25	51	4.1	29.8	0.17	17	1.3	8	0.6
45-59	283	91	47	15.1	52.3	0.17	17	5.4	10	2.5
60+	342	156	57	26.1	69.9	0.17	19	8.9	18	6.7
All ages	1 116	42	186	7.0	43.7	0.17	64	2.4	44	1.4
Females										
0-4	104	34	17	5.6	2.5	0.17	6	2.0	4	1.2
5-14	54	10	9	1.7	10.0	0.17	3	0.6	2	0.3
15-44	213	18	36	3.0	29.8	0.17	11	0.9	5	0.4
45-59	106	34	18	5.7	52.3	0.17	6	2.0	4	1.0
60+	315	117	52	19.5	70.6	0.17	18	6.5	17	4.9
All ages	792	30	132	5.1	44.1	0.17	44	1.7	32	1.0
Total	1 908	36	318	6.0	43.8	0.17	108	2.1	76	1.2

For epidemiological sources see Kane et al. 1996. For the methods used to estimate and project incidence, prevalence, and deaths see Murray and Lopez 1996a. See explanatory notes for definitions and caveats.

Table 67
Hepatitis B

Cuadro 67
Hepatitis B

Tableau 67
Hépatite B

Cirrhosis - symptomatic cases

Cirrosis - casos sintomáticos

Cirrhose - cas symptomatiques

Table 67a **EME - PEMC - EMBE** Hepatitis B - Cirrhosis - symptomatic cases

Age group (years)	Incidence 1990 Number ('000s)	Rate (per 100 000)	Prevalence 1990 Number ('000s)	Rate (per 100 000)	Avg. age at onset (years)	Average duration (years)	Deaths 1990 Number ('000s)	Rate (per 100 000)	Deaths 2000 (Projected) Number ('000s)	Rate (per 100 000)
Males										
0-4	0	6.0	0	0.2	2.5	10.3	0	0.0	0	0.0
5-14	0	0.0	0	0.2	-	-	0	0.0	0	0.0
15-44	2	1.2	15	8.4	29.9	10.0	1	0.8	1	0.8
45-59	8	11.5	41	62.3	52.4	8.8	4	5.9	5	6.2
60+	7	11.3	66	108.6	71.0	6.0	6	10.2	7	10.3
All ages	17	4.3	123	31.4	57.0	7.8	12	3.0	14	3.3
Females										
0-4	0	0.1	0	0.1	2.5	10.4	0	0.0	0	0.0
5-14	0	0.0	0	0.2	-	-	0	0.0	0	0.0
15-44	1	0.4	6	3.1	30.0	10.2	1	0.3	1	0.3
45-59	3	3.9	15	21.4	52.4	9.3	1	2.0	2	2.0
60+	5	6.0	43	50.8	72.4	6.5	4	4.7	4	4.4
All ages	9	2.1	63	15.5	62.1	7.7	6	1.4	6	1.5
Total	25	3.2	186	23.3	58.7	7.8	17	2.2	20	2.4

Table 67b **FSE - PEAS - AESE** Hepatitis B - Cirrhosis - symptomatic cases

Age group (years)	Incidence 1990 Number ('000s)	Rate (per 100 000)	Prevalence 1990 Number ('000s)	Rate (per 100 000)	Avg. age at onset (years)	Average duration (years)	Deaths 1990 Number ('000s)	Rate (per 100 000)	Deaths 2000 (Projected) Number ('000s)	Rate (per 100 000)
Males										
0-4	0	0.8	0	1.6	2.5	10.2	0	0.2	0	0.1
5-14	0	0.0	1	1.9	-	-	0	0.0	0	0.0
15-44	3	3.4	18	24.0	29.8	9.7	2	2.3	1	1.9
45-59	10	36.4	52	192.6	52.2	8.1	5	18.3	6	19.8
60+	7	33.2	68	326.6	69.9	5.6	6	30.3	8	32.8
All ages	19	11.8	140	84.4	55.3	7.5	13	7.9	16	9.3
Females										
0-4	0	0.6	0	1.3	2.5	10.3	0	0.1	0	0.1
5-14	0	0.0	0	1.5	-	-	0	0.1	0	0.0
15-44	1	1.2	7	9.0	29.9	10.1	1	0.9	1	0.7
45-59	4	13.7	22	73.2	52.4	9.0	2	6.9	2	6.6
60+	6	16.8	54	149.5	71.5	6.2	5	13.5	5	13.1
All ages	11	6.2	84	46.3	60.6	7.6	8	4.2	8	4.4
Total	31	8.9	223	64.5	57.2	7.5	21	6.0	24	6.8

Table 67c **India - India - Inde** Hepatitis B - Cirrhosis - symptomatic cases

Age group (years)	Incidence 1990 Number ('000s)	Rate (per 100 000)	Prevalence 1990 Number ('000s)	Rate (per 100 000)	Avg. age at onset (years)	Average duration (years)	Deaths 1990 Number ('000s)	Rate (per 100 000)	Deaths 2000 (Projected) Number ('000s)	Rate (per 100 000)
Males										
0-4	3	5.6	7	12	2.5	9.5	1	1.1	0	0.7
5-14	0	0.0	14	14	-	-	0	0.5	0	0.2
15-44	18	8.7	129	64	29.9	9.8	12	5.9	10	4.2
45-59	40	83.6	217	455	52.3	8.3	20	42.9	23	38.6
60+	20	68.8	213	715	69.6	5.6	20	68.4	24	66.3
All ages	81	18.5	579	132	49.8	8.0	54	12.2	58	11.4
Females										
0-4	4	7.7	9	16	2.5	9.4	1	1.4	1	0.9
5-14	0	0.0	19	19	-	-	1	1.0	1	0.6
15-44	6	3.5	52	29	29.8	9.9	5	2.7	4	1.7
45-59	14	30.3	77	168	52.4	8.6	7	15.8	7	12.3
60+	8	29.1	82	282	70.0	5.7	8	26.9	10	25.2
All ages	33	8.1	239	58	45.9	8.2	22	5.3	22	4.5
Total	114	13.5	818	96	48.6	8.1	76	8.9	80	8.1

For epidemiological sources see Kane et al. 1996. For the methods used to estimate and project incidence, prevalence, and deaths see Murray and Lopez 1996a. See explanatory notes for definitions and caveats.

Table 67	Cuadro 67	Tableau 67
Hepatitis B	Hepatitis B	Hépatite B
Cirrhosis - symptomatic cases	Cirrosis - casos sintomáticos	Cirrhose - cas symptomatiques

Table 67d   China - China - Chine   Hepatitis B - Cirrhosis - symptomatic cases

Age group (years)	Incidence 1990 Number ('000s)	Rate (per 100 000)	Prevalence 1990 Number ('000s)	Rate (per 100 000)	Avg. age at onset (years)	Average duration (years)	Deaths 1990 Number ('000s)	Rate (per 100 000)	Deaths 2000 (Projected) Number ('000s)	Rate (per 100 000)
Males										
0-4	5	9.0	12	19.3	2.5	10.2	1	2.1	1	1.1
5-14	0	0.0	22	23.0	-	-	0	0.5	0	0.2
15-44	29	9.6	220	71.9	29.9	9.9	21	6.8	18	5.6
45-59	53	73.3	296	407.3	52.3	8.4	28	38.5	32	33.0
60+	54	110.5	443	904.6	69.7	5.6	42	86.0	49	81.4
All ages	142	24.3	993	169.7	52.4	7.7	93	15.8	100	15.3
Females										
0-4	2	3.6	4	7.5	2.5	9.9	0	0.7	0	0.4
5-14	0	0.0	8	9.0	10.0	10.4	0	0.5	0	0.3
15-44	9	3.1	67	23.7	29.9	10.0	6	2.2	5	1.6
45-59	26	39.6	136	211.6	52.4	8.8	13	19.9	14	14.8
60+	38	73.0	296	573.1	70.6	5.9	28	53.9	31	48.7
All ages	74	13.5	512	93.4	57.6	7.5	48	8.7	50	8.0
Total	216	19.1	1 505	132.8	54.2	7.6	140	12.4	150	11.7

Table 67e   OAI - OPAI - APAI   Hepatitis B - Cirrhosis - symptomatic cases

Age group (years)	Incidence 1990 Number ('000s)	Rate (per 100 000)	Prevalence 1990 Number ('000s)	Rate (per 100 000)	Avg. age at onset (years)	Average duration (years)	Deaths 1990 Number ('000s)	Rate (per 100 000)	Deaths 2000 (Projected) Number ('000s)	Rate (per 100 000)
Males										
0-4	3	7.9	7	16	2.5	9.6	1	1.6	0	1.0
5-14	0	0.0	17	20	-	-	1	1.0	0	0.6
15-44	19	11.8	140	87	29.9	9.7	13	8.2	14	6.7
45-59	51	148.9	269	789	52.3	8.1	26	75.1	32	70.0
60+	26	130.5	266	1 316	69.5	5.5	26	128.2	34	122.5
All ages	100	29.1	699	204	50.9	7.8	66	19.4	81	19.9
Females										
0-4	2	5.6	5	12	2.5	9.7	0	1.1	0	0.7
5-14	0	0.0	11	14	-	-	1	1.0	0	0.6
15-44	4	2.6	33	21	29.8	9.8	3	2.2	3	1.7
45-59	16	45.0	82	234	52.4	8.5	8	22.4	9	18.6
60+	17	73.2	134	590	70.3	5.8	13	57.0	17	51.1
All ages	39	11.4	265	78	54.6	7.6	25	7.5	30	7.3
Total	139	20.3	964	141	51.9	7.7	92	13.5	110	13.6

Table 67f   SSA - ASS - ASS   Hepatitis B - Cirrhosis - symptomatic cases

Age group (years)	Incidence 1990 Number ('000s)	Rate (per 100 000)	Prevalence 1990 Number ('000s)	Rate (per 100 000)	Avg. age at onset (years)	Average duration (years)	Deaths 1990 Number ('000s)	Rate (per 100 000)	Deaths 2000 (Projected) Number ('000s)	Rate (per 100 000)
Males										
0-4	0	0.0	0	0.0	-	-	0	0.0	0	0.0
5-14	1	1.8	5	6.9	10.0	9.8	0	0.7	0	0.4
15-44	5	4.7	38	36.7	29.4	9.3	4	3.7	4	2.7
45-59	9	43.3	48	234.4	52.2	7.9	5	22.4	5	20.6
60+	7	64.8	55	526.3	69.2	5.4	5	50.4	7	47.3
All ages	22	8.6	146	57.8	49.9	7.5	14	5.6	16	4.8
Females										
0-4	0	0.0	0	0.0	-	-	0	0.0	0	0.0
5-14	1	1.0	3	3.7	10.0	9.9	0	0.4	0	0.2
15-44	2	2.0	17	16.1	29.5	9.5	1	1.0	1	0.7
45-59	4	16.2	20	89.3	52.3	8.2	2	8.5	2	7.0
60+	4	32.0	31	241.3	69.7	5.6	3	23.0	4	20.1
All ages	10	4.1	70	27.2	51.6	7.5	6	2.4	7	1.9
Total	32	6.3	216	42.3	50.5	7.5	20	4.0	23	3.4

For epidemiological sources see Kane et al. 1996. For the methods used to estimate and project incidence, prevalence, and deaths see Murray and Lopez 1996a. See explanatory notes for definitions and caveats.

Table 67 | **Cuadro 67** | **Tableau 67**
Hepatitis B | **Hepatitis B** | **Hépatite B**

Cirrhosis - symptomatic cases | Cirrosis - casos sintomáticos | Cirrhose - cas symptomatiques

Table 67g   LAC - ALC - ALC   Hepatitis B - Cirrhosis - symptomatic cases

Age group (years)	Incidence 1990 Number ('000s)	Rate (per 100 000)	Prevalence 1990 Number ('000s)	Rate (per 100 000)	Avg. age at onset (years)	Average duration (years)	Deaths 1990 Number ('000s)	Rate (per 100 000)	Deaths 2000 (Projected) Number ('000s)	Rate (per 100 000)
Males										
0-4	0	1.0	1	2.1	2.5	9.8	0	0.2	0	0.1
5-14	0	0.0	1	2.5	-	-	0	0.1	0	0.1
15-44	3	3.3	24	23.4	29.8	9.8	2	2.3	3	2.0
45-59	6	29.0	35	159.3	52.3	8.5	3	15.0	5	14.7
60+	3	20.8	33	230.3	70.3	5.8	3	21.9	4	21.5
All ages	13	5.9	95	42.7	49.4	8.3	9	4.0	11	4.3
Females										
0-4	0	0.8	0	1.8	2.5	9.9	0	0.2	0	0.1
5-14	0	0.0	1	2.1	-	-	0	0.1	0	0.1
15-44	1	1.0	8	7.2	29.9	10.0	1	0.7	1	0.6
45-59	2	9.0	12	49.5	52.4	8.9	1	4.7	1	4.1
60+	2	11.2	17	99.4	71.1	6.1	2	9.4	2	8.7
All ages	5	2.3	37	16.8	52.7	8.1	3	1.6	4	1.6
Total	18	4.1	132	29.7	50.4	8.2	12	2.8	16	2.9

Table 67h   MEC - AOM - CMO   Hepatitis B - Cirrhosis - symptomatic cases

Age group (years)	Incidence 1990 Number ('000s)	Rate (per 100 000)	Prevalence 1990 Number ('000s)	Rate (per 100 000)	Avg. age at onset (years)	Average duration (years)	Deaths 1990 Number ('000s)	Rate (per 100 000)	Deaths 2000 (Projected) Number ('000s)	Rate (per 100 000)
Males										
0-4	1	2.2	2	4.5	2.5	9.6	0	0.4	0	0.3
5-14	0	0.6	5	7.7	10.0	10.3	0	0.7	0	0.4
15-44	3	2.7	24	21.3	29.9	9.8	2	2.0	2	1.6
45-59	8	38.0	45	199.7	52.3	8.2	4	18.7	6	17.7
60+	7	51.6	59	434.9	69.7	5.6	6	41.3	7	39.7
All ages	20	7.8	135	52.7	51.9	7.6	13	5.0	16	4.8
Females										
0-4	1	1.7	1	3.4	2.5	9.6	0	0.3	0	0.2
5-14	2	2.9	9	15.1	10.0	10.3	1	1.4	1	0.9
15-44	1	1.0	15	14.1	29.9	9.9	1	1.4	1	1.0
45-59	6	24.8	28	127.4	52.4	8.6	3	11.9	3	10.1
60+	6	40.1	50	323.6	70.4	5.8	5	30.5	6	27.7
All ages	15	6.2	104	42.3	51.0	7.8	10	4.0	11	3.5
Total	35	7.0	239	47.6	51.5	7.7	23	4.5	27	4.1

Table 67i   World - Mundo - Monde   Hepatitis B - Cirrhosis - symptomatic cases

Age group (years)	Incidence 1990 Number ('000s)	Rate (per 100 000)	Prevalence 1990 Number ('000s)	Rate (per 100 000)	Avg. age at onset (years)	Average duration (years)	Deaths 1990 Number ('000s)	Rate (per 100 000)	Deaths 2000 (Projected) Number ('000s)	Rate (per 100 000)
Males										
0-4	14	4.2	28	8.9	2.5	9.8	3	0.9	2	0.5
5-14	2	0.3	65	11.8	10.0	9.9	3	0.5	2	0.3
15-44	82	6.6	609	48.7	29.9	9.8	58	4.6	53	3.7
45-59	185	59.2	1 003	321.0	52.3	8.3	95	30.4	114	28.3
60+	132	60.1	1 203	549.9	69.7	5.6	115	52.5	142	51.6
All ages	414	15.6	2 909	109.6	51.6	7.8	273	10.3	313	10.1
Females										
0-4	10	3.2	20	6.6	2.5	9.6	2	0.6	1	0.4
5-14	2	0.5	51	9.8	10.0	10.2	3	0.7	2	0.4
15-44	25	2.1	205	17.1	29.8	9.9	19	1.6	16	1.2
45-59	73	23.5	392	126.0	52.4	8.7	37	11.9	40	9.8
60+	86	31.9	706	262.3	70.6	5.9	67	24.8	79	23.4
All ages	197	7.5	1 375	52.6	54.4	7.7	128	4.9	138	4.5
Total	611	11.6	4 284	81.3	52.5	7.7	401	7.6	451	7.3

For epidemiological sources see Kane et al. 1996. For the methods used to estimate and project incidence, prevalence, and deaths see Murray and Lopez 1996a. See explanatory notes for definitions and caveats.

Table 68	Cuadro 68	Tableau 68
Hepatitis B	Hepatitis B	Hépatite B

Hepatoma	Hepatoma	Hépatome

Table 68a EME - PEMC - EMBE   Hepatitis B - Hepatoma

Age group (years)	Incidence 1990 Number ('000s)	Rate (per 100 000)	Prevalence 1990 Number ('000s)	Rate (per 100 000)	Avg. age at onset (years)	Average duration (years)	Deaths 1990 Number ('000s)	Rate (per 100 000)	Deaths 2000 (Projected) Number ('000s)	Rate (per 100 000)
Males										
0-4	0	0.1	0	0.1	2.5	4.11	0	0.0	0	0.0
5-14	0	0.0	0	0.1	10.0	4.11	0	0.0	0	0.0
15-44	0	0.1	1	0.3	29.9	2.92	0	0.1	0	0.1
45-59	1	2.2	4	6.4	52.4	2.88	1	1.6	1	1.5
60+	3	5.0	5	7.8	71.1	1.56	3	4.7	3	4.4
All ages	5	1.2	10	2.5	63.2	2.05	4	1.0	5	1.1
Females										
0-4	0	0.1	0	0.1	2.5	4.48	0	0.0	0	0.0
5-14	0	0.0	0	0.1	10.0	4.48	0	0.0	0	0.0
15-44	0	0.0	0	0.0	30.0	1.45	0	0.0	0	0.0
45-59	0	0.3	0	0.6	52.4	1.91	0	0.3	0	0.2
60+	1	1.6	1	1.1	72.4	0.72	1	1.6	1	1.5
All ages	2	0.4	2	0.4	67.6	0.96	2	0.4	2	0.4
Total	6	0.8	11	1.4	64.3	1.77	6	0.7	6	0.7

Table 68b FSE - PEAS - AESE   Hepatitis B - Hepatoma

Age group (years)	Incidence 1990 Number ('000s)	Rate (per 100 000)	Prevalence 1990 Number ('000s)	Rate (per 100 000)	Avg. age at onset (years)	Average duration (years)	Deaths 1990 Number ('000s)	Rate (per 100 000)	Deaths 2000 (Projected) Number ('000s)	Rate (per 100 000)
Males										
0-4	0	0.2	0	0.3	2.5	3.69	0	0.1	0	0.1
5-14	0	0.1	0	0.2	10.0	3.69	0	0.0	0	0.0
15-44	0	0.4	1	1.0	29.8	2.66	0	0.3	0	0.3
45-59	2	5.8	4	15.2	52.2	2.63	1	4.4	2	5.5
60+	3	14.6	4	21.4	70.0	1.47	3	14.0	4	15.7
All ages	5	3.0	9	5.7	61.5	1.92	4	2.7	6	3.5
Females										
0-4	0	0.2	0	0.3	2.5	4.00	0	0.1	0	0.1
5-14	0	0.1	0	0.3	10.0	4.00	0	0.0	0	0.0
15-44	0	0.2	0	0.2	29.9	1.36	0	0.2	0	0.2
45-59	1	2.2	1	3.9	52.4	1.78	1	2.0	1	1.9
60+	3	8.5	2	6.2	71.5	0.72	3	8.5	3	8.4
All ages	4	2.2	4	2.0	66.3	0.95	4	2.1	4	2.3
Total	9	2.6	13	3.8	63.6	1.49	8	2.4	10	2.8

Table 68c India - India - Inde   Hepatitis B - Hepatoma

Age group (years)	Incidence 1990 Number ('000s)	Rate (per 100 000)	Prevalence 1990 Number ('000s)	Rate (per 100 000)	Avg. age at onset (years)	Average duration (years)	Deaths 1990 Number ('000s)	Rate (per 100 000)	Deaths 2000 (Projected) Number ('000s)	Rate (per 100 000)
Males										
0-4	0	0.0	0	0.0	2.5	2.28	0	0.0	0	0.0
5-14	0	0.0	0	0.1	10.0	2.28	0	0.0	0	0.0
15-44	0	0.2	1	0.3	29.8	1.76	0	0.2	0	0.2
45-59	1	2.3	2	4.1	52.3	1.74	1	2.2	1	2.3
60+	2	5.6	2	6.2	69.7	1.10	2	5.5	2	6.1
All ages	3	0.7	4	1.0	58.5	1.41	3	0.7	4	0.8
Females										
0-4	0	0.0	0	0.0	2.5	2.43	0	0.0	0	0.0
5-14	0	0.0	0	0.0	10.0	2.43	0	0.0	0	0.0
15-44	0	0.1	0	0.1	29.8	1.04	0	0.1	0	0.1
45-59	0	0.9	1	1.2	52.4	1.28	0	0.9	1	0.9
60+	1	2.8	1	2.0	70.1	0.72	1	2.8	1	2.9
All ages	1	0.3	1	0.3	59.4	0.95	1	0.3	2	0.4
Total	5	0.5	6	0.7	58.8	1.27	4	0.5	6	0.6

For epidemiological sources see Kane et al. 1996. For the methods used to estimate and project incidence, prevalence, and deaths see Murray and Lopez 1996a. See explanatory notes for definitions and caveats.

Table 68	Cuadro 68	Tableau 68
Hepatitis B	**Hepatitis B**	**Hépatite B**

Hepatoma	Hepatoma	Hépatome

Table 68d   China - China - Chine   Hepatitis B - Hepatoma

Age group (years)	Incidence 1990 Number ('000s)	Rate (per 100 000)	Prevalence 1990 Number ('000s)	Rate (per 100 000)	Avg. age at onset (years)	Average duration (years)	Deaths 1990 Number ('000s)	Rate (per 100 000)	Deaths 2000 (Projected) Number ('000s)	Rate (per 100 000)
Males										
0-4	0	0.4	0	0.4	2.5	3.01	0	0.2	0	0.3
5-14	1	0.7	2	2.0	10.0	3.01	0	0.5	1	0.5
15-44	38	12.4	85	27.7	29.9	2.24	32	10.5	47	14.8
45-59	63	86.1	138	190.3	52.3	2.21	54	73.7	86	88.0
60+	64	130.4	83	169.5	69.8	1.30	62	127.4	91	150.1
All ages	165	28.2	308	52.7	53.7	1.87	149	25.4	225	34.2
Females										
0-4	0	0.4	0	0.6	2.5	3.25	0	0.3	0	0.3
5-14	1	0.8	2	2.6	10.0	3.25	0	0.5	1	0.4
15-44	8	2.8	10	3.4	29.9	1.22	8	2.7	10	3.4
45-59	17	25.9	26	40.1	52.4	1.55	16	24.7	23	25.7
60+	32	61.6	23	44.5	70.6	0.72	32	61.5	44	68.7
All ages	57	10.5	61	11.2	58.6	1.07	56	10.2	79	12.6
Total	223	19.6	370	32.6	55.0	1.66	205	18.1	303	23.7

Table 68e   OAI - OPAI - APAI   Hepatitis B - Hepatoma

Age group (years)	Incidence 1990 Number ('000s)	Rate (per 100 000)	Prevalence 1990 Number ('000s)	Rate (per 100 000)	Avg. age at onset (years)	Average duration (years)	Deaths 1990 Number ('000s)	Rate (per 100 000)	Deaths 2000 (Projected) Number ('000s)	Rate (per 100 000)
Males										
0-4	0	0.6	0	0.7	2.5	2.79	0	0.4	0	0.4
5-14	1	0.7	2	2.0	10.0	2.79	0	0.5	0	0.5
15-44	5	3.3	11	6.8	29.7	2.10	5	2.9	6	3.2
45-59	16	46.6	33	96.4	52.3	2.07	14	41.0	20	43.1
60+	15	75.5	19	93.8	69.6	1.24	15	74.0	22	79.2
All ages	37	10.9	65	18.9	55.2	1.75	34	10.0	49	12.1
Females										
0-4	0	0.5	0	0.6	2.5	3.00	0	0.4	0	0.4
5-14	0	0.4	1	1.3	10.0	3.00	0	0.3	0	0.3
15-44	1	0.8	1	0.9	29.8	1.17	1	0.7	2	0.8
45-59	3	9.8	5	14.4	52.3	1.47	3	9.4	4	9.0
60+	8	33.5	5	24.2	70.3	0.72	8	33.5	11	33.5
All ages	13	3.8	13	3.9	58.9	1.07	12	3.7	17	4.2
Total	50	7.3	78	11.4	56.1	1.58	47	6.8	66	8.1

Table 68f   SSA - ASS - ASS   Hepatitis B - Hepatoma

Age group (years)	Incidence 1990 Number ('000s)	Rate (per 100 000)	Prevalence 1990 Number ('000s)	Rate (per 100 000)	Avg. age at onset (years)	Average duration (years)	Deaths 1990 Number ('000s)	Rate (per 100 000)	Deaths 2000 (Projected) Number ('000s)	Rate (per 100 000)
Males										
0-4	0	0.1	0	0.1	2.4	1.96	0	0.1	0	0.1
5-14	0	0.3	0	0.5	10.0	1.96	0	0.2	0	0.2
15-44	7	7.0	11	10.8	29.4	1.55	7	6.6	10	6.7
45-59	10	49.4	15	75.8	52.2	1.54	10	47.2	12	45.9
60+	8	76.0	8	76.4	69.2	1.01	8	75.4	11	78.4
All ages	25	10.1	35	13.9	50.6	1.38	25	9.8	33	9.7
Females										
0-4	0	0.2	0	0.1	2.4	2.08	0	0.1	0	0.1
5-14	0	0.3	0	0.6	10.0	2.08	0	0.3	0	0.2
15-44	2	1.9	2	1.8	29.5	0.95	1	1.2	2	1.1
45-59	3	13.2	3	15.3	52.2	1.16	3	13.1	4	12.1
60+	5	37.3	3	27.0	69.7	0.72	5	37.2	6	35.5
All ages	10	3.9	9	3.6	54.6	0.94	9	3.5	12	3.3
Total	35	7.0	44	8.7	51.8	1.25	34	6.6	45	6.5

For epidemiological sources see Kane et al. 1996. For the methods used to estimate and project incidence, prevalence, and deaths see Murray and Lopez 1996a. See explanatory notes for definitions and caveats.

Table 68   **Cuadro 68**   **Tableau 68**
Hepatitis B   **Hepatitis B**   **Hépatite B**

Hepatoma   Hepatoma   Hépatome

Table 68g   LAC - ALC - ALC   Hepatitis B - Hepatoma

Age group (years)	Incidence 1990 Number ('000s)	Rate (per 100 000)	Prevalence 1990 Number ('000s)	Rate (per 100 000)	Avg. age at onset (years)	Average duration (years)	Deaths 1990 Number ('000s)	Rate (per 100 000)	Deaths 2000 (Projected) Number ('000s)	Rate (per 100 000)
Males										
0-4	0	0.0	0	0.0	2.5	3.22	0	0.0	0	0.0
5-14	0	0.0	0	0.1	10.0	3.22	0	0.0	0	0.0
15-44	0	0.1	0	0.1	29.8	2.37	0	0.0	0	0.1
45-59	0	0.7	0	1.6	52.3	2.34	0	0.6	0	0.6
60+	0	2.4	0	3.3	70.3	1.35	0	2.4	0	2.5
All ages	1	0.3	1	0.5	59.0	1.79	1	0.2	1	0.3
Females										
0-4	0	0.0	0	0.0	2.5	3.48	0	0.0	0	0.0
5-14	0	0.0	0	0.1	10.0	3.48	0	0.0	0	0.0
15-44	0	0.0	0	0.0	29.9	1.26	0	0.0	0	0.0
45-59	0	0.5	0	0.8	52.4	1.62	0	0.5	0	0.4
60+	0	2.6	0	1.8	71.1	0.72	0	2.6	1	2.6
All ages	1	0.3	1	0.3	63.5	1.00	1	0.3	1	0.3
Total	1	0.3	2	0.4	61.2	1.39	1	0.2	2	0.3

Table 68h   MEC - AOM - CMO   Hepatitis B - Hepatoma

Age group (years)	Incidence 1990 Number ('000s)	Rate (per 100 000)	Prevalence 1990 Number ('000s)	Rate (per 100 000)	Avg. age at onset (years)	Average duration (years)	Deaths 1990 Number ('000s)	Rate (per 100 000)	Deaths 2000 (Projected) Number ('000s)	Rate (per 100 000)
Males										
0-4	0	0.0	0	0.1	2.5	2.79	0	0.0	0	0.0
5-14	0	0.1	0	0.3	10.0	2.79	0	0.1	0	0.1
15-44	0	0.3	1	0.7	29.8	2.10	0	0.3	0	0.3
45-59	1	5.0	2	10.3	52.3	2.07	1	4.4	1	4.3
60+	1	9.6	2	12.0	69.7	1.24	1	9.5	2	9.3
All ages	3	1.1	5	1.9	55.9	1.72	3	1.0	4	1.1
Females										
0-4	0	0.1	0	0.1	2.5	3.00	0	0.0	0	0.0
5-14	0	0.1	0	0.4	10.0	3.00	0	0.1	0	0.1
15-44	0	0.2	0	0.2	29.8	1.17	0	0.2	0	0.2
45-59	0	2.2	1	3.3	52.3	1.47	0	2.2	1	1.9
60+	1	6.4	1	4.6	70.4	0.72	1	6.3	1	5.7
All ages	2	0.7	2	0.8	57.9	1.10	2	0.7	2	0.7
Total	5	0.9	7	1.4	56.7	1.49	4	0.9	6	0.9

Table 68i   World - Mundo - Monde   Hepatitis B - Hepatoma

Age group (years)	Incidence 1990 Number ('000s)	Rate (per 100 000)	Prevalence 1990 Number ('000s)	Rate (per 100 000)	Avg. age at onset (years)	Average duration (years)	Deaths 1990 Number ('000s)	Rate (per 100 000)	Deaths 2000 (Projected) Number ('000s)	Rate (per 100 000)
Males										
0-4	1	0.2	1	0.2	2.5	2.86	0	0.1	0	0.1
5-14	2	0.3	4	0.8	10.0	2.80	1	0.2	1	0.2
15-44	52	4.1	110	8.8	29.8	2.13	45	3.6	65	4.5
45-59	94	30.1	200	63.9	52.3	2.13	82	26.1	124	30.7
60+	97	44.1	123	56.3	69.8	1.28	94	43.1	134	48.6
All ages	244	9.2	438	16.5	54.0	1.80	222	8.4	324	10.5
Females										
0-4	1	0.2	1	0.2	2.5	3.07	0	0.1	0	0.1
5-14	1	0.3	4	0.8	10.0	3.02	1	0.2	1	0.2
15-44	12	1.0	14	1.1	29.8	1.17	11	0.9	14	1.0
45-59	25	8.0	37	12.0	52.4	1.49	24	7.7	33	8.3
60+	51	18.9	37	13.6	70.6	0.72	51	18.9	69	20.5
All ages	90	3.4	93	3.5	58.7	1.05	87	3.3	118	3.8
Total	334	6.3	530	10.1	55.3	1.60	309	5.9	442	7.2

For epidemiological sources see Kane et al. 1996. For the methods used to estimate and project incidence, prevalence, and deaths see Murray and Lopez 1996a. See explanatory notes for definitions and caveats.

Table 69	Cuadro 69	Tableau 69
Malaria	Paludismo	Paludisme
Episodes	Episodios	Episodes

Table 69a — EME - PEMC - EMBE — Malaria - Episodes

Age group (years)	Incidence 1990 Number ('000s)	Rate (per 100 000)	Prevalence 1990 Number ('000s)	Rate (per 100 000)	Avg. age at onset (years)	Average duration (years)	Deaths 1990 Number ('000s)	Rate (per 100 000)	Deaths 2000 (Projected) Number ('000s)	Rate (per 100 000)
Males										
0-4	0	0	0	0	-	-	0	0	0	0
5-14	0	0	0	0	-	-	0	0	0	0
15-44	0	0	0	0	-	-	0	0	0	0
45-59	0	0	0	0	-	-	0	0	0	0
60+	0	0	0	0	-	-	0	0	0	0
All ages	0	0	0	0	-	-	0	0	0	0
Females										
0-4	0	0	0	0	-	-	0	0	0	0
5-14	0	0	0	0	-	-	0	0	0	0
15-44	0	0	0	0	-	-	0	0	0	0
45-59	0	0	0	0	-	-	0	0	0	0
60+	0	0	0	0	-	-	0	0	0	0
All ages	0	0	0	0	-	-	0	0	0	0
Total	0	0	0	0	-	-	0	0	0	0

Table 69b — FSE - PEAS - AESE — Malaria - Episodes

Age group (years)	Incidence 1990 Number ('000s)	Rate (per 100 000)	Prevalence 1990 Number ('000s)	Rate (per 100 000)	Avg. age at onset (years)	Average duration (years)	Deaths 1990 Number ('000s)	Rate (per 100 000)	Deaths 2000 (Projected) Number ('000s)	Rate (per 100 000)
Males										
0-4	0	0	0	0	-	-	0	0	0	0
5-14	0	0	0	0	-	-	0	0	0	0
15-44	0	0	0	0	-	-	0	0	0	0
45-59	0	0	0	0	-	-	0	0	0	0
60+	0	0	0	0	-	-	0	0	0	0
All ages	0	0	0	0	-	-	0	0	0	0
Females										
0-4	0	0	0	0	-	-	0	0	0	0
5-14	0	0	0	0	-	-	0	0	0	0
15-44	0	0	0	0	-	-	0	0	0	0
45-59	0	0	0	0	-	-	0	0	0	0
60+	0	0	0	0	-	-	0	0	0	0
All ages	0	0	0	0	-	-	0	0	0	0
Total	0	0	0	0	-	-	0	0	0	0

Table 69c — India - India - Inde — Malaria - Episodes

Age group (years)	Incidence 1990 Number ('000s)	Rate (per 100 000)	Prevalence 1990 Number ('000s)	Rate (per 100 000)	Avg. age at onset (years)	Average duration (years)	Deaths 1990 Number ('000s)	Rate (per 100 000)	Deaths 2000 (Projected) Number ('000s)	Rate (per 100 000)
Males										
0-4	469	785	4	6.5	2.5	0.01	3	5.2	2	3.2
5-14	799	785	7	6.5	10.0	0.01	3	3.1	2	1.4
15-44	1 574	785	13	6.5	29.8	0.01	5	2.6	3	1.1
45-59	373	785	3	6.5	52.3	0.01	1	2.9	1	1.3
60+	233	785	2	6.5	69.7	0.01	1	3.4	1	2.4
All ages	3 449	785	28	6.5	26.6	0.01	14	3.2	8	1.5
Females										
0-4	445	785	4	6.5	2.5	0.01	3	4.7	2	2.8
5-14	748	785	6	6.5	10.0	0.01	4	3.9	2	1.7
15-44	1 438	785	12	6.5	29.8	0.01	4	2.3	2	0.8
45-59	361	785	3	6.5	52.4	0.01	1	2.4	1	1.1
60+	227	785	2	6.5	70.1	0.01	1	2.6	1	1.9
All ages	3 219	785	26	6.5	26.8	0.01	12	3.0	6	1.3
Total	6 668	785	55	6.5	26.7	0.01	26	3.1	14	1.4

For epidemiological sources see Najera et al. 1996. For the methods used to estimate and project incidence, prevalence, and deaths see Murray and Lopez 1996a. See explanatory notes for definitions and caveats.

Table 69	Cuadro 69	Tableau 69
Malaria	Paludismo	Paludisme
Episodes	Episodios	Episodes

Table 69d　　China - China - Chine　　　　　　　　　　Malaria - Episodes

Age group (years)	Incidence 1990 Number ('000s)	Rate (per 100 000)	Prevalence 1990 Number ('000s)	Rate (per 100 000)	Avg. age at onset (years)	Average duration (years)	Deaths 1990 Number ('000s)	Rate (per 100 000)	Deaths 2000 (Projected) Number ('000s)	Rate (per 100 000)
Males										
0-4	13	21	0	0.2	2.5	0.01	0	0	0	0
5-14	20	21	0	0.2	10.0	0.01	0	0	0	0
15-44	64	21	1	0.2	29.9	0.01	0	0	0	0
45-59	15	21	0	0.2	52.3	0.01	0	0	0	0
60+	10	21	0	0.2	69.8	0.01	0	0	0	0
All ages	123	21	1	0.2	29.9	0.01	0	0	0	0
Females										
0-4	12	21	0	0.2	2.5	0.01	0	0	0	0
5-14	19	21	0	0.2	10.0	0.01	0	0	0	0
15-44	60	21	0	0.2	29.9	0.01	0	0	0	0
45-59	14	21	0	0.2	52.4	0.01	0	0	0	0
60+	11	21	0	0.2	70.6	0.01	0	0	0	0
All ages	115	21	1	0.2	30.2	0.01	0	0	0	0
Total	238	21	2	0.2	30.0	0.01	0	0	0	0

Table 69e　　OAI - OPAI - APAI　　　　　　　　　　Malaria - Episodes

Age group (years)	Incidence 1990 Number ('000s)	Rate (per 100 000)	Prevalence 1990 Number ('000s)	Rate (per 100 000)	Avg. age at onset (years)	Average duration (years)	Deaths 1990 Number ('000s)	Rate (per 100 000)	Deaths 2000 (Projected) Number ('000s)	Rate (per 100 000)
Males										
0-4	862	1 970	7	16	2.5	0.01	5	12.4	4	8.0
5-14	1 655	1 970	14	16	10.0	0.01	12	13.7	6	6.7
15-44	3 168	1 970	26	16	29.7	0.01	17	10.5	10	4.7
45-59	673	1 970	6	16	52.3	0.01	4	12.8	3	6.4
60+	398	1 970	3	16	69.6	0.01	3	13.1	2	8.8
All ages	6 756	1 970	56	16	26.0	0.01	41	11.9	24	5.9
Females										
0-4	827	1 970	7	16	2.5	0.01	5	11.6	3	7.2
5-14	1 580	1 970	13	16	10.0	0.01	10	12.5	5	6.0
15-44	3 144	1 970	26	16	29.8	0.01	15	9.3	7	3.5
45-59	691	1 970	6	16	52.3	0.01	4	12.7	3	6.4
60+	446	1 970	4	16	70.3	0.01	2	10.6	2	7.4
All ages	6 689	1 970	55	16	26.8	0.01	37	10.8	20	5.1
Total	13 446	1 970	111	16	26.4	0.01	77	11.4	44	5.5

Table 69f　　SSA - ASS - ASS　　　　　　　　　　Malaria - Episodes

Age group (years)	Incidence 1990 Number ('000s)	Rate (per 100 000)	Prevalence 1990 Number ('000s)	Rate (per 100 000)	Avg. age at onset (years)	Average duration (years)	Deaths 1990 Number ('000s)	Rate (per 100 000)	Deaths 2000 (Projected) Number ('000s)	Rate (per 100 000)
Males										
0-4	56 981	120 000	781	1 644	1.5	0.01	325	685	325	493
5-14	12 295	17 500	168	240	10.0	0.01	29	41	21	22
15-44	18 159	17 500	249	240	29.4	0.01	27	26	18	12
45-59	3 554	17 500	49	240	52.2	0.01	7	36	5	19
60+	1 839	17 500	25	240	69.2	0.01	4	36	3	24
All ages	92 827	36 789	1 272	504	11.4	0.01	392	155	372	108
Females										
0-4	56 436	120 000	773	1 644	1.5	0.01	263	559	247	388
5-14	12 218	17 500	167	240	10.0	0.01	29	42	20	22
15-44	18 595	17 500	255	240	29.5	0.01	35	33	19	13
45-59	3 870	17 500	53	240	52.2	0.01	8	36	5	19
60+	2 228	17 500	31	240	69.7	0.01	4	37	4	24
All ages	93 347	36 188	1 279	496	11.9	0.01	340	132	296	85
Total	186 175	36 485	2 550	500	11.6	0.01	732	143	668	97

For epidemiological sources see Najera et al. 1996. For the methods used to estimate and project incidence, prevalence, and deaths see Murray and Lopez 1996a. See explanatory notes for definitions and caveats.

Table 69   **Cuadro 69**   **Tableau 69**
Malaria   **Paludismo**   **Paludisme**

Episodes   Episodios   Episodes

Table 69g   LAC - ALC - ALC   Malaria - Episodes

Age group (years)	Incidence 1990 Number ('000s)	Rate (per 100 000)	Prevalence 1990 Number ('000s)	Rate (per 100 000)	Avg. age at onset (years)	Average duration (years)	Deaths 1990 Number ('000s)	Rate (per 100 000)	Deaths 2000 (Projected) Number ('000s)	Rate (per 100 000)
Males										
0-4	284	990	2	8.1	2.5	0.01	1	3.4	1	2.4
5-14	516	990	4	8.1	10.0	0.01	1	2.5	1	1.4
15-44	1 032	990	8	8.1	29.8	0.01	3	2.9	2	1.5
45-59	220	990	2	8.1	52.3	0.01	1	3.4	1	1.9
60+	141	990	1	8.1	70.3	0.01	0	3.4	0	2.4
All ages	2 194	990	18	8.1	26.5	0.01	7	3.0	4	1.7
Females										
0-4	274	990	2	8.1	2.5	0.01	1	3.1	1	2.1
5-14	502	990	4	8.1	10.0	0.01	1	2.9	1	1.6
15-44	1 030	990	8	8.1	29.9	0.01	3	3.3	2	1.5
45-59	231	990	2	8.1	52.4	0.01	1	3.4	1	1.9
60+	167	990	1	8.1	71.1	0.01	1	3.4	1	2.4
All ages	2 205	990	18	8.1	27.4	0.01	7	3.2	5	1.7
Total	4 399	990	36	8.1	26.9	0.01	14	3.1	9	1.7

Table 69h   MEC - AOM - CMO   Malaria - Episodes

Age group (years)	Incidence 1990 Number ('000s)	Rate (per 100 000)	Prevalence 1990 Number ('000s)	Rate (per 100 000)	Avg. age at onset (years)	Average duration (years)	Deaths 1990 Number ('000s)	Rate (per 100 000)	Deaths 2000 (Projected) Number ('000s)	Rate (per 100 000)
Males										
0-4	231	560	2	4.6	2.5	0.01	1	1.5	1	1.1
5-14	366	560	3	4.6	10.0	0.01	1	1.6	1	0.9
15-44	638	560	5	4.6	29.8	0.01	1	1.1	1	0.5
45-59	125	560	1	4.6	52.3	0.01	0	1.5	0	0.9
60+	76	560	1	4.6	69.7	0.01	0	1.5	0	1.0
All ages	1 436	560	12	4.6	24.5	0.01	3	1.3	3	0.8
Females										
0-4	223	560	2	4.6	2.5	0.01	1	1.5	1	1.1
5-14	347	560	3	4.6	10.0	0.01	1	1.6	1	0.9
15-44	600	560	5	4.6	29.8	0.01	1	1.1	1	0.5
45-59	125	560	1	4.6	52.3	0.01	0	1.5	0	0.8
60+	87	560	1	4.6	70.4	0.01	0	1.4	0	1.0
All ages	1 381	560	11	4.6	25.0	0.01	3	1.4	2	0.7
Total	2 817	560	23	4.6	24.7	0.01	7	1.4	5	0.8

Table 69i   World - Mundo - Monde   Malaria - Episodes

Age group (years)	Incidence 1990 Number ('000s)	Rate (per 100 000)	Prevalence 1990 Number ('000s)	Rate (per 100 000)	Avg. age at onset (years)	Average duration (years)	Deaths 1990 Number ('000s)	Rate (per 100 000)	Deaths 2000 (Projected) Number ('000s)	Rate (per 100 000)
Males										
0-4	58 840	18 313	796	248	1.5	0.01	335	104.4	331	95.8
5-14	15 652	2 840	196	36	10.0	0.01	46	8.3	29	4.7
15-44	24 636	1 971	302	24	29.5	0.01	53	4.3	33	2.3
45-59	4 960	1 588	60	19	52.2	0.01	14	4.5	10	2.4
60+	2 698	1 233	32	15	69.4	0.01	8	3.7	7	2.7
All ages	106 785	4 024	1 386	52	13.3	0.01	457	17.2	411	13.3
Females										
0-4	58 217	18 825	788	255	1.5	0.01	272	88.0	253	76.4
5-14	15 415	2 933	194	37	10.0	0.01	46	8.7	29	4.7
15-44	24 868	2 075	306	26	29.6	0.01	58	4.9	30	2.2
45-59	5 292	1 701	65	21	52.2	0.01	15	4.7	10	2.5
60+	3 165	1 176	38	14	69.9	0.01	9	3.2	8	2.4
All ages	106 957	4 092	1 391	53	13.8	0.01	400	15.3	330	10.8
Total	213 743	4 058	2 777	53	13.5	0.01	856	16.3	740	12.0

For epidemiological sources see Najera et al. 1996. For the methods used to estimate and project incidence, prevalence, and deaths see Murray and Lopez 1996a. See explanatory notes for definitions and caveats.

Table 70	Cuadro 70	Tableau 70
Malaria	**Paludismo**	**Paludisme**
Anaemia	Anemia	Anémie

Table 70a   EME - PEMC - EMBE   Malaria - Anaemia

Age group (years)	Incidence 1990 Number ('000s)	Rate (per 100 000)	Prevalence 1990 Number ('000s)	Rate (per 100 000)	Avg. age at onset (years)	Average duration (years)	Deaths 1990 Number ('000s)	Rate (per 100 000)	Deaths 2000 (Projected) Number ('000s)	Rate (per 100 000)
Males										
0-4	-	-	0	0	-	-	0	0	0	0
5-14	-	-	0	0	-	-	0	0	0	0
15-44	-	-	0	0	-	-	0	0	0	0
45-59	-	-	0	0	-	-	0	0	0	0
60+	-	-	0	0	-	-	0	0	0	0
All ages	-	-	0	0	-	-	0	0	0	0
Females										
0-4	-	-	0	0	-	-	0	0	0	0
5-14	-	-	0	0	-	-	0	0	0	0
15-44	-	-	0	0	-	-	0	0	0	0
45-59	-	-	0	0	-	-	0	0	0	0
60+	-	-	0	0	-	-	0	0	0	0
All ages	-	-	0	0	-	-	0	0	0	0
Total	-	-	0	0	-	-	0	0	0	0

Table 70b   FSE - PEAS - AESE   Malaria - Anaemia

Age group (years)	Incidence 1990 Number ('000s)	Rate (per 100 000)	Prevalence 1990 Number ('000s)	Rate (per 100 000)	Avg. age at onset (years)	Average duration (years)	Deaths 1990 Number ('000s)	Rate (per 100 000)	Deaths 2000 (Projected) Number ('000s)	Rate (per 100 000)
Males										
0-4	-	-	0	0	-	-	0	0	0	0
5-14	-	-	0	0	-	-	0	0	0	0
15-44	-	-	0	0	-	-	0	0	0	0
45-59	-	-	0	0	-	-	0	0	0	0
60+	-	-	0	0	-	-	0	0	0	0
All ages	-	-	0	0	-	-	0	0	0	0
Females										
0-4	-	-	0	0	-	-	0	0	0	0
5-14	-	-	0	0	-	-	0	0	0	0
15-44	-	-	0	0	-	-	0	0	0	0
45-59	-	-	0	0	-	-	0	0	0	0
60+	-	-	0	0	-	-	0	0	0	0
All ages	-	-	0	0	-	-	0	0	0	0
Total	-	-	0	0	-	-	0	0	0	0

Table 70c   India - India - Inde   Malaria - Anaemia

Age group (years)	Incidence 1990 Number ('000s)	Rate (per 100 000)	Prevalence 1990 Number ('000s)	Rate (per 100 000)	Avg. age at onset (years)	Average duration (years)	Deaths 1990 Number ('000s)	Rate (per 100 000)	Deaths 2000 (Projected) Number ('000s)	Rate (per 100 000)
Males										
0-4	-	-	7 175	12 000	-	-	0	0	0	0
5-14	-	-	6 105	6 000	-	-	0	0	0	0
15-44	-	-	4 011	2 000	-	-	0	0	0	0
45-59	-	-	951	2 000	-	-	0	0	0	0
60+	-	-	595	2 000	-	-	0	0	0	0
All ages	-	-	18 837	4 287	-	-	0	0	0	0
Females										
0-4	-	-	6 801	12 000	-	-	0	0	0	0
5-14	-	-	5 716	6 000	-	-	0	0	0	0
15-44	-	-	3 665	2 000	-	-	0	0	0	0
45-59	-	-	920	2 000	-	-	0	0	0	0
60+	-	-	578	2 000	-	-	0	0	0	0
All ages	-	-	17 681	4 311	-	-	0	0	0	0
Total	-	-	36 518	4 299	-	-	0	0	0	0

For epidemiological sources see Najera et al. 1996. For the methods used to estimate and project incidence, prevalence, and deaths see Murray and Lopez 1996a. See explanatory notes for definitions and caveats.

Table 70
Malaria

Cuadro 70
Paludismo

Tableau 70
Paludisme

Anaemia

Anemia

Anémie

Table 70d   China - China - Chine

Malaria - Anaemia

Age group (years)	Incidence 1990 Number ('000s)	Rate (per 100 000)	Prevalence 1990 Number ('000s)	Rate (per 100 000)	Avg. age at onset (years)	Average duration (years)	Deaths 1990 Number ('000s)	Rate (per 100 000)	Deaths 2000 (Projected) Number ('000s)	Rate (per 100 000)
Males										
0-4	-	-	723	1 200	-	-	0	0	0	0
5-14	-	-	582	600	-	-	0	0	0	0
15-44	-	-	613	200	-	-	0	0	0	0
45-59	-	-	145	200	-	-	0	0	0	0
60+	-	-	98	200	-	-	0	0	0	0
All ages	-	-	2 161	369	-	-	0	0	0	0
Females										
0-4	-	-	695	1 200	-	-	0	0	0	0
5-14	-	-	542	600	-	-	0	0	0	0
15-44	-	-	568	200	-	-	0	0	0	0
45-59	-	-	129	200	-	-	0	0	0	0
60+	-	-	103	200	-	-	0	0	0	0
All ages	-	-	2 038	372	-	-	0	0	0	0
Total	-	-	4 199	370	-	-	0	0	0	0

Table 70e   OAI - OPAI - APAI

Malaria - Anaemia

Age group (years)	Incidence 1990 Number ('000s)	Rate (per 100 000)	Prevalence 1990 Number ('000s)	Rate (per 100 000)	Avg. age at onset (years)	Average duration (years)	Deaths 1990 Number ('000s)	Rate (per 100 000)	Deaths 2000 (Projected) Number ('000s)	Rate (per 100 000)
Males										
0-4	-	-	3 063	7 000	-	-	0	0	0	0
5-14	-	-	3 361	4 000	-	-	0	0	0	0
15-44	-	-	1 930	1 200	-	-	0	0	0	0
45-59	-	-	410	1 200	-	-	0	0	0	0
60+	-	-	242	1 200	-	-	0	0	0	0
All ages	-	-	9 007	2 626	-	-	0	0	0	0
Females										
0-4	-	-	2 939	7 000	-	-	0	0	0	0
5-14	-	-	3 209	4 000	-	-	0	0	0	0
15-44	-	-	1 915	1 200	-	-	0	0	0	0
45-59	-	-	421	1 200	-	-	0	0	0	0
60+	-	-	272	1 200	-	-	0	0	0	0
All ages	-	-	8 756	2 579	-	-	0	0	0	0
Total	-	-	17 763	2 602	-	-	0	0	0	0

Table 70f   SSA - ASS - ASS

Malaria - Anaemia

Age group (years)	Incidence 1990 Number ('000s)	Rate (per 100 000)	Prevalence 1990 Number ('000s)	Rate (per 100 000)	Avg. age at onset (years)	Average duration (years)	Deaths 1990 Number ('000s)	Rate (per 100 000)	Deaths 2000 (Projected) Number ('000s)	Rate (per 100 000)
Males										
0-4	-	-	4 274	9 000	-	-	0	0	0	0
5-14	-	-	2 810	4 000	-	-	0	0	0	0
15-44	-	-	2 075	2 000	-	-	0	0	0	0
45-59	-	-	406	2 000	-	-	0	0	0	0
60+	-	-	210	2 000	-	-	0	0	0	0
All ages	-	-	9 775	3 874	-	-	0	0	0	0
Females										
0-4	-	-	4 233	9 000	-	-	0	0	0	0
5-14	-	-	2 793	4 000	-	-	0	0	0	0
15-44	-	-	1 594	1 500	-	-	0	0	0	0
45-59	-	-	332	1 500	-	-	0	0	0	0
60+	-	-	255	2 000	-	-	0	0	0	0
All ages	-	-	9 206	3 569	-	-	0	0	0	0
Total	-	-	18 981	3 720	-	-	0	0	0	0

For epidemiological sources see Najera et al. 1996. For the methods used to estimate and project incidence, prevalence, and deaths see Murray and Lopez 1996a. See explanatory notes for definitions and caveats.

Table 70
Malaria

Cuadro 70
Paludismo

Tableau 70
Paludisme

Anaemia

Anemia

Anémie

Table 70g   LAC - ALC - ALC

Malaria - Anaemia

Age group (years)	Incidence 1990 Number ('000s)	Rate (per 100 000)	Prevalence 1990 Number ('000s)	Rate (per 100 000)	Avg. age at onset (years)	Average duration (years)	Deaths 1990 Number ('000s)	Rate (per 100 000)	Deaths 2000 (Projected) Number ('000s)	Rate (per 100 000)
Males										
0-4	-	-	862	3 000	-	-	0	0	0	0
5-14	-	-	782	1 500	-	-	0	0	0	0
15-44	-	-	521	500	-	-	0	0	0	0
45-59	-	-	111	500	-	-	0	0	0	0
60+	-	-	71	500	-	-	0	0	0	0
All ages	-	-	2 347	1 059	-	-	0	0	0	0
Females										
0-4	-	-	830	3 000	-	-	0	0	0	0
5-14	-	-	761	1 500	-	-	0	0	0	0
15-44	-	-	520	500	-	-	0	0	0	0
45-59	-	-	117	500	-	-	0	0	0	0
60+	-	-	84	500	-	-	0	0	0	0
All ages	-	-	2 313	1 039	-	-	0	0	0	0
Total	-	-	4 660	1 049	-	-	0	0	0	0

Table 70h   MEC - AOM - CMO

Malaria - Anaemia

Age group (years)	Incidence 1990 Number ('000s)	Rate (per 100 000)	Prevalence 1990 Number ('000s)	Rate (per 100 000)	Avg. age at onset (years)	Average duration (years)	Deaths 1990 Number ('000s)	Rate (per 100 000)	Deaths 2000 (Projected) Number ('000s)	Rate (per 100 000)
Males										
0-4	-	-	2 881	7 000	-	-	0	0	0	0
5-14	-	-	2 614	4 000	-	-	0	0	0	0
15-44	-	-	1 595	1 400	-	-	0	0	0	0
45-59	-	-	313	1 400	-	-	0	0	0	0
60+	-	-	191	1 400	-	-	0	0	0	0
All ages	-	-	7 593	2 962	-	-	0	0	0	0
Females										
0-4	-	-	2 781	7 000	-	-	0	0	0	0
5-14	-	-	2 480	4 000	-	-	0	0	0	0
15-44	-	-	1 501	1 400	-	-	0	0	0	0
45-59	-	-	312	1 400	-	-	0	0	0	0
60+	-	-	216	1 400	-	-	0	0	0	0
All ages	-	-	7 291	2 955	-	-	0	0	0	0
Total	-	-	14 884	2 959	-	-	0	0	0	0

Table 70i   World - Mundo - Monde

Malaria - Anaemia

Age group (years)	Incidence 1990 Number ('000s)	Rate (per 100 000)	Prevalence 1990 Number ('000s)	Rate (per 100 000)	Avg. age at onset (years)	Average duration (years)	Deaths 1990 Number ('000s)	Rate (per 100 000)	Deaths 2000 (Projected) Number ('000s)	Rate (per 100 000)
Males										
0-4	-	-	18 977	5 906	-	-	0	0	0	0
5-14	-	-	16 254	2 949	-	-	0	0	0	0
15-44	-	-	10 744	860	-	-	0	0	0	0
45-59	-	-	2 336	748	-	-	0	0	0	0
60+	-	-	1 408	643	-	-	0	0	0	0
All ages	-	-	49 721	1 874	-	-	0	0	0	0
Females										
0-4	-	-	18 280	5 911	-	-	0	0	0	0
5-14	-	-	15 501	2 950	-	-	0	0	0	0
15-44	-	-	9 764	815	-	-	0	0	0	0
45-59	-	-	2 231	717	-	-	0	0	0	0
60+	-	-	1 509	560	-	-	0	0	0	0
All ages	-	-	47 284	1 809	-	-	0	0	0	0
Total	-	-	97 005	1 842	-	-	0	0	0	0

For epidemiological sources see Najera et al. 1996. For the methods used to estimate and project incidence, prevalence, and deaths see Murray and Lopez 1996a. See explanatory notes for definitions and caveats.

Table 71   **Cuadro 71**   **Tableau 71**
Malaria   **Paludismo**   **Paludisme**

Neurological sequelae   Secuelas neurológicas   Séquelles neurologiques

Table 71a   EME - PEMC - EMBE   Malaria - Neurological sequelae

Age group (years)	Incidence 1990 Number ('000s)	Rate (per 100 000)	Prevalence 1990 Number ('000s)	Rate (per 100 000)	Avg. age at onset (years)	Average duration (years)	Deaths 1990 Number ('000s)	Rate (per 100 000)	Deaths 2000 (Projected) Number ('000s)	Rate (per 100 000)
Males										
0-4	0	0	0	0	-	-	0	0	0	0
5-14	0	0	0	0	-	-	0	0	0	0
15-44	0	0	0	0	-	-	0	0	0	0
45-59	0	0	0	0	-	-	0	0	0	0
60+	0	0	0	0	-	-	0	0	0	0
All ages	0	0	0	0	-	-	0	0	0	0
Females										
0-4	0	0	0	0	-	-	0	0	0	0
5-14	0	0	0	0	-	-	0	0	0	0
15-44	0	0	0	0	-	-	0	0	0	0
45-59	0	0	0	0	-	-	0	0	0	0
60+	0	0	0	0	-	-	0	0	0	0
All ages	0	0	0	0	-	-	0	0	0	0
Total	0	0	0	0	-	-	0	0	0	0

Table 71b   FSE - PEAS - AESE   Malaria - Neurological sequelae

Age group (years)	Incidence 1990 Number ('000s)	Rate (per 100 000)	Prevalence 1990 Number ('000s)	Rate (per 100 000)	Avg. age at onset (years)	Average duration (years)	Deaths 1990 Number ('000s)	Rate (per 100 000)	Deaths 2000 (Projected) Number ('000s)	Rate (per 100 000)
Males										
0-4	0	0	0	0	-	-	0	0	0	0
5-14	0	0	0	0	-	-	0	0	0	0
15-44	0	0	0	0	-	-	0	0	0	0
45-59	0	0	0	0	-	-	0	0	0	0
60+	0	0	0	0	-	-	0	0	0	0
All ages	0	0	0	0	-	-	0	0	0	0
Females										
0-4	0	0	0	0	-	-	0	0	0	0
5-14	0	0	0	0	-	-	0	0	0	0
15-44	0	0	0	0	-	-	0	0	0	0
45-59	0	0	0	0	-	-	0	0	0	0
60+	0	0	0	0	-	-	0	0	0	0
All ages	0	0	0	0	-	-	0	0	0	0
Total	0	0	0	0	-	-	0	0	0	0

Table 71c   India - India - Inde   Malaria - Neurological sequelae

Age group (years)	Incidence 1990 Number ('000s)	Rate (per 100 000)	Prevalence 1990 Number ('000s)	Rate (per 100 000)	Avg. age at onset (years)	Average duration (years)	Deaths 1990 Number ('000s)	Rate (per 100 000)	Deaths 2000 (Projected) Number ('000s)	Rate (per 100 000)
Males										
0-4	0	0.4	1	1.0	2.5	48.0	0	0	0	0
5-14	0	0.0	2	1.9	-	-	0	0	0	0
15-44	0	0.0	4	1.8	-	-	0	0	0	0
45-59	0	0.0	1	1.6	-	-	0	0	0	0
60+	0	0.0	0	1.0	-	-	0	0	0	0
All ages	0	0.1	7	1.6	2.5	48.0	0	0	0	0
Females										
0-4	0	0.4	1	1.0	2.5	48.5	0	0	0	0
5-14	0	0.0	2	1.9	-	-	0	0	0	0
15-44	0	0.0	3	1.8	-	-	0	0	0	0
45-59	0	0.0	1	1.6	-	-	0	0	0	0
60+	0	0.0	0	1.1	-	-	0	0	0	0
All ages	0	0.1	7	1.6	2.5	48.5	0	0	0	0
Total	0	0.1	14	1.6	2.5	48.2	0	0	0	0

For epidemiological sources see Najera et al. 1996. For the methods used to estimate and project incidence, prevalence, and deaths see Murray and Lopez 1996a. See explanatory notes for definitions and caveats.

Table 71   **Cuadro 71**   **Tableau 71**
Malaria   **Paludismo**   **Paludisme**

Neurological sequelae   Secuelas neurológicas   Séquelles neurologiques

Table 71d   China - China - Chine   Malaria - Neurological sequelae

Age group (years)	Incidence 1990 Number ('000s)	Rate (per 100 000)	Prevalence 1990 Number ('000s)	Rate (per 100 000)	Avg. age at onset (years)	Average duration (years)	Deaths 1990 Number ('000s)	Rate (per 100 000)	Deaths 2000 (Projected) Number ('000s)	Rate (per 100 000)
Males										
0-4	0	0	0	0	2.5	56.7	0	0	0	0
5-14	0	0	0	0	-	-	0	0	0	0
15-44	0	0	0	0	-	-	0	0	0	0
45-59	0	0	0	0	-	-	0	0	0	0
60+	0	0	0	0	-	-	0	0	0	0
All ages	0	0	0	0	2.5	56.7	0	0	0	0
Females										
0-4	0	0	0	0	2.5	59.8	0	0	0	0
5-14	0	0	0	0	-	-	0	0	0	0
15-44	0	0	0	0	-	-	0	0	0	0
45-59	0	0	0	0	-	-	0	0	0	0
60+	0	0	0	0	-	-	0	0	0	0
All ages	0	0	0	0	2.5	59.8	0	0	0	0
Total	0	0	0	0	2.5	58.2	0	0	0	0

Table 71e   OAI - OPAI - APAI   Malaria - Neurological sequelae

Age group (years)	Incidence 1990 Number ('000s)	Rate (per 100 000)	Prevalence 1990 Number ('000s)	Rate (per 100 000)	Avg. age at onset (years)	Average duration (years)	Deaths 1990 Number ('000s)	Rate (per 100 000)	Deaths 2000 (Projected) Number ('000s)	Rate (per 100 000)
Males										
0-4	1	1.9	2	4.4	2.5	48.4	0	0	0	0
5-14	0	0.0	7	8.7	-	-	0	0	0	0
15-44	0	0.0	13	8.3	-	-	0	0	0	0
45-59	0	0.0	2	7.1	-	-	0	0	0	0
60+	0	0.0	1	4.3	-	-	0	0	0	0
All ages	1	0.2	26	7.6	2.5	48.4	0	0	0	0
Females										
0-4	1	1.9	2	4.5	2.5	52.2	0	0	0	0
5-14	0	0.0	7	8.8	-	-	0	0	0	0
15-44	0	0.0	13	8.4	-	-	0	0	0	0
45-59	0	0.0	3	7.5	-	-	0	0	0	0
60+	0	0.0	1	4.8	-	-	0	0	0	0
All ages	1	0.2	26	7.7	2.5	52.2	0	0	0	0
Total	2	0.2	52	7.6	2.5	50.3	0	0	0	0

Table 71f   SSA - ASS - ASS   Malaria - Neurological sequelae

Age group (years)	Incidence 1990 Number ('000s)	Rate (per 100 000)	Prevalence 1990 Number ('000s)	Rate (per 100 000)	Avg. age at onset (years)	Average duration (years)	Deaths 1990 Number ('000s)	Rate (per 100 000)	Deaths 2000 (Projected) Number ('000s)	Rate (per 100 000)
Males										
0-4	78	164	176	371	1.5	33.8	0	0	0	0
5-14	0	0	501	714	-	-	0	0	0	0
15-44	0	0	663	639	-	-	0	0	0	0
45-59	0	0	104	513	-	-	0	0	0	0
60+	0	0	33	311	-	-	0	0	0	0
All ages	78	31	1 477	585	1.5	33.8	0	0	0	0
Females										
0-4	77	164	172	365	1.5	37.1	0	0	0	0
5-14	0	0	490	701	-	-	0	0	0	0
15-44	0	0	656	617	-	-	0	0	0	0
45-59	0	0	105	474	-	-	0	0	0	0
60+	0	0	34	270	-	-	0	0	0	0
All ages	77	30	1 456	565	1.5	37.1	0	0	0	0
Total	155	30	2 933	575	1.5	35.4	0	0	0	0

For epidemiological sources see Najera et al. 1996. For the methods used to estimate and project incidence, prevalence, and deaths see Murray and Lopez 1996a. See explanatory notes for definitions and caveats.

Table 71 **Cuadro 71** **Tableau 71**
Malaria **Paludismo** **Paludisme**

Neurological sequelae Secuelas neurológicas Séquelles neurologiques

Table 71g LAC - ALC - ALC Malaria - Neurological sequelae

Age group (years)	Incidence 1990 Number ('000s)	Rate (per 100 000)	Prevalence 1990 Number ('000s)	Rate (per 100 000)	Avg. age at onset (years)	Average duration (years)	Deaths 1990 Number ('000s)	Rate (per 100 000)	Deaths 2000 (Projected) Number ('000s)	Rate (per 100 000)
Males										
0-4	0	0.4	0	1.1	2.5	53.3	0	0	0	0
5-14	0	0.0	1	2.1	-	-	0	0	0	0
15-44	0	0.0	2	2.1	-	-	0	0	0	0
45-59	0	0.0	0	1.8	-	-	0	0	0	0
60+	0	0.0	0	1.2	-	-	0	0	0	0
All ages	0	0.1	4	1.9	2.5	53.3	0	0	0	0
Females										
0-4	0	0.4	0	1.1	2.5	58.2	0	0	0	0
5-14	0	0.0	1	2.2	-	-	0	0	0	0
15-44	0	0.0	2	2.1	-	-	0	0	0	0
45-59	0	0.0	0	1.9	-	-	0	0	0	0
60+	0	0.0	0	1.3	-	-	0	0	0	0
All ages	0	0.1	4	1.9	2.5	58.2	0	0	0	0
Total	0	0.1	8	1.9	2.5	55.7	0	0	0	0

Table 71h MEC - AOM - CMO Malaria - Neurological sequelae

Age group (years)	Incidence 1990 Number ('000s)	Rate (per 100 000)	Prevalence 1990 Number ('000s)	Rate (per 100 000)	Avg. age at onset (years)	Average duration (years)	Deaths 1990 Number ('000s)	Rate (per 100 000)	Deaths 2000 (Projected) Number ('000s)	Rate (per 100 000)
Males										
0-4	0	0.2	0	0.5	2.5	49.9	0	0	0	0
5-14	0	0.0	1	1.1	-	-	0	0	0	0
15-44	0	0.0	1	1.0	-	-	0	0	0	0
45-59	0	0.0	0	0.9	-	-	0	0	0	0
60+	0	0.0	0	0.6	-	-	0	0	0	0
All ages	0	0.0	2	0.9	2.5	49.9	0	0	0	0
Females										
0-4	0	0.2	0	0.5	2.5	52.5	0	0	0	0
5-14	0	0.0	1	1.1	-	-	0	0	0	0
15-44	0	0.0	1	1.0	-	-	0	0	0	0
45-59	0	0.0	0	0.9	-	-	0	0	0	0
60+	0	0.0	0	0.6	-	-	0	0	0	0
All ages	0	0.0	2	0.9	2.5	52.5	0	0	0	0
Total	0	0.0	5	0.9	2.5	51.1	0	0	0	0

Table 71i World - Mundo - Monde Malaria - Neurological sequelae

Age group (years)	Incidence 1990 Number ('000s)	Rate (per 100 000)	Prevalence 1990 Number ('000s)	Rate (per 100 000)	Avg. age at onset (years)	Average duration (years)	Deaths 1990 Number ('000s)	Rate (per 100 000)	Deaths 2000 (Projected) Number ('000s)	Rate (per 100 000)
Males										
0-4	79	24.6	179	56	2.4	50.6	0	0	0	0
5-14	0	0.0	512	93	-	-	0	0	0	0
15-44	0	0.0	683	55	-	-	0	0	0	0
45-59	0	0.0	108	35	-	-	0	0	0	0
60+	0	0.0	34	16	-	-	0	0	0	0
All ages	79	3.0	1 517	57	2.4	50.6	0	0	0	0
Females										
0-4	78	25.3	175	57	2.3	53.7	0	0	0	0
5-14	0	0.0	500	95	-	-	0	0	0	0
15-44	0	0.0	676	56	-	-	0	0	0	0
45-59	0	0.0	109	35	-	-	0	0	0	0
60+	0	0.0	36	13	-	-	0	0	0	0
All ages	78	3.0	1 496	57	2.3	53.7	0	0	0	0
Total	157	3.0	3 012	57	2.4	52.2	0	0	0	0

For epidemiological sources see Najera et al. 1996. For the methods used to estimate and project incidence, prevalence, and deaths see Murray and Lopez 1996a. See explanatory notes for definitions and caveats.

Table 72
Trypanosomiasis

Cuadro 72
Tripanosomiasis

Tableau 72
Trypanosomiase

Episodes

Episodios

Episodes

Table 72a   EME - PEMC - EMBE   Trypanosomiasis - Episodes

Age group (years)	Incidence 1990 Number ('000s)	Rate (per 100 000)	Prevalence 1990 Number ('000s)	Rate (per 100 000)	Avg. age at onset (years)	Average duration (years)	Deaths 1990 Number ('000s)	Rate (per 100 000)	Deaths 2000 (Projected) Number ('000s)	Rate (per 100 000)
Males										
0-4	0	0	0	0	-	-	0	0	0	0
5-14	0	0	0	0	-	-	0	0	0	0
15-44	0	0	0	0	-	-	0	0	0	0
45-59	0	0	0	0	-	-	0	0	0	0
60+	0	0	0	0	-	-	0	0	0	0
All ages	0	0	0	0	-	-	0	0	0	0
Females										
0-4	0	0	0	0	-	-	0	0	0	0
5-14	0	0	0	0	-	-	0	0	0	0
15-44	0	0	0	0	-	-	0	0	0	0
45-59	0	0	0	0	-	-	0	0	0	0
60+	0	0	0	0	-	-	0	0	0	0
All ages	0	0	0	0	-	-	0	0	0	0
Total	0	0	0	0	-	-	0	0	0	0

Table 72b   FSE - PEAS - AESE   Trypanosomiasis - Episodes

Age group (years)	Incidence 1990 Number ('000s)	Rate (per 100 000)	Prevalence 1990 Number ('000s)	Rate (per 100 000)	Avg. age at onset (years)	Average duration (years)	Deaths 1990 Number ('000s)	Rate (per 100 000)	Deaths 2000 (Projected) Number ('000s)	Rate (per 100 000)
Males										
0-4	0	0	0	0	-	-	0	0	0	0
5-14	0	0	0	0	-	-	0	0	0	0
15-44	0	0	0	0	-	-	0	0	0	0
45-59	0	0	0	0	-	-	0	0	0	0
60+	0	0	0	0	-	-	0	0	0	0
All ages	0	0	0	0	-	-	0	0	0	0
Females										
0-4	0	0	0	0	-	-	0	0	0	0
5-14	0	0	0	0	-	-	0	0	0	0
15-44	0	0	0	0	-	-	0	0	0	0
45-59	0	0	0	0	-	-	0	0	0	0
60+	0	0	0	0	-	-	0	0	0	0
All ages	0	0	0	0	-	-	0	0	0	0
Total	0	0	0	0	-	-	0	0	0	0

Table 72c   India - India - Inde   Trypanosomiasis - Episodes

Age group (years)	Incidence 1990 Number ('000s)	Rate (per 100 000)	Prevalence 1990 Number ('000s)	Rate (per 100 000)	Avg. age at onset (years)	Average duration (years)	Deaths 1990 Number ('000s)	Rate (per 100 000)	Deaths 2000 (Projected) Number ('000s)	Rate (per 100 000)
Males										
0-4	0	0	0	0	-	-	0	0	0	0
5-14	0	0	0	0	-	-	0	0	0	0
15-44	0	0	0	0	-	-	0	0	0	0
45-59	0	0	0	0	-	-	0	0	0	0
60+	0	0	0	0	-	-	0	0	0	0
All ages	0	0	0	0	-	-	0	0	0	0
Females										
0-4	0	0	0	0	-	-	0	0	0	0
5-14	0	0	0	0	-	-	0	0	0	0
15-44	0	0	0	0	-	-	0	0	0	0
45-59	0	0	0	0	-	-	0	0	0	0
60+	0	0	0	0	-	-	0	0	0	0
All ages	0	0	0	0	-	-	0	0	0	0
Total	0	0	0	0	-	-	0	0	0	0

For the methods used to estimate and project incidence, prevalence, and deaths see Murray and Lopez 1996a. See explanatory notes for definitions and caveats.

Table 72
Trypanosomiasis

Cuadro 72
Tripanosomiasis

Tableau 72
Trypanosomiase

Episodes

Episodios

Episodes

Table 72d   China - China - Chine   Trypanosomiasis - Episodes

Age group (years)	Incidence 1990 Number ('000s)	Rate (per 100 000)	Prevalence 1990 Number ('000s)	Rate (per 100 000)	Avg. age at onset (years)	Average duration (years)	Deaths 1990 Number ('000s)	Rate (per 100 000)	Deaths 2000 (Projected) Number ('000s)	Rate (per 100 000)
Males										
0-4	0	0	0	0	-	-	0	0	0	0
5-14	0	0	0	0	-	-	0	0	0	0
15-44	0	0	0	0	-	-	0	0	0	0
45-59	0	0	0	0	-	-	0	0	0	0
60+	0	0	0	0	-	-	0	0	0	0
All ages	0	0	0	0	-	-	0	0	0	0
Females										
0-4	0	0	0	0	-	-	0	0	0	0
5-14	0	0	0	0	-	-	0	0	0	0
15-44	0	0	0	0	-	-	0	0	0	0
45-59	0	0	0	0	-	-	0	0	0	0
60+	0	0	0	0	-	-	0	0	0	0
All ages	0	0	0	0	-	-	0	0	0	0
Total	0	0	0	0	-	-	0	0	0	0

Table 72e   OAI - OPAI - APAI   Trypanosomiasis - Episodes

Age group (years)	Incidence 1990 Number ('000s)	Rate (per 100 000)	Prevalence 1990 Number ('000s)	Rate (per 100 000)	Avg. age at onset (years)	Average duration (years)	Deaths 1990 Number ('000s)	Rate (per 100 000)	Deaths 2000 (Projected) Number ('000s)	Rate (per 100 000)
Males										
0-4	0	0	0	0	-	-	0	0	0	0
5-14	0	0	0	0	-	-	0	0	0	0
15-44	0	0	0	0	-	-	0	0	0	0
45-59	0	0	0	0	-	-	0	0	0	0
60+	0	0	0	0	-	-	0	0	0	0
All ages	0	0	0	0	-	-	0	0	0	0
Females										
0-4	0	0	0	0	-	-	0	0	0	0
5-14	0	0	0	0	-	-	0	0	0	0
15-44	0	0	0	0	-	-	0	0	0	0
45-59	0	0	0	0	-	-	0	0	0	0
60+	0	0	0	0	-	-	0	0	0	0
All ages	0	0	0	0	-	-	0	0	0	0
Total	0	0	0	0	-	-	0	0	0	0

Table 72f   SSA - ASS - ASS   Trypanosomiasis - Episodes

Age group (years)	Incidence 1990 Number ('000s)	Rate (per 100 000)	Prevalence 1990 Number ('000s)	Rate (per 100 000)	Avg. age at onset (years)	Average duration (years)	Deaths 1990 Number ('000s)	Rate (per 100 000)	Deaths 2000 (Projected) Number ('000s)	Rate (per 100 000)
Males										
0-4	2	3.8	3	7.3	2.4	5.0	0	1.0	0	0.7
5-14	8	12.0	28	39.9	10.0	5.0	6	9.2	5	4.9
15-44	14	13.9	72	69.8	29.4	5.0	10	9.6	7	4.7
45-59	6	29.5	25	122.3	52.2	5.0	5	25.4	4	13.5
60+	1	11.4	13	121.5	69.2	5.0	1	14.0	1	9.1
All ages	32	12.6	142	56.1	28.6	5.0	24	9.3	17	4.8
Females										
0-4	4	7.7	7	14.7	2.4	5.0	1	2.0	1	1.4
5-14	7	10.3	29	41.0	10.0	5.0	7	9.8	5	5.0
15-44	13	12.4	66	62.2	29.5	5.0	12	10.9	6	4.4
45-59	4	16.3	16	74.4	52.2	5.0	4	16.0	2	8.3
60+	1	4.7	7	56.4	69.7	5.0	1	7.1	1	4.3
All ages	28	10.9	125	48.6	24.8	5.0	24	9.2	15	4.3
Total	60	11.8	267	52.3	26.8	5.0	47	9.3	32	4.6

For the methods used to estimate and project incidence, prevalence, and deaths see Murray and Lopez 1996a. See explanatory notes for definitions and caveats.

Table 72
Trypanosomiasis

Cuadro 72
Tripanosomiasis

Tableau 72
Trypanosomiase

Episodes

Episodios

Episodes

Table 72g   LAC - ALC - ALC   Trypanosomiasis - Episodes

Age group (years)	Incidence 1990 Number ('000s)	Rate (per 100 000)	Prevalence 1990 Number ('000s)	Rate (per 100 000)	Avg. age at onset (years)	Average duration (years)	Deaths 1990 Number ('000s)	Rate (per 100 000)	Deaths 2000 (Projected) Number ('000s)	Rate (per 100 000)
Males										
0-4	0	0	0	0	-	-	0	0	0	0
5-14	0	0	0	0	-	-	0	0	0	0
15-44	0	0	0	0	-	-	0	0	0	0
45-59	0	0	0	0	-	-	0	0	0	0
60+	0	0	0	0	-	-	0	0	0	0
All ages	0	0	0	0	-	-	0	0	0	0
Females										
0-4	0	0	0	0	-	-	0	0	0	0
5-14	0	0	0	0	-	-	0	0	0	0
15-44	0	0	0	0	-	-	0	0	0	0
45-59	0	0	0	0	-	-	0	0	0	0
60+	0	0	0	0	-	-	0	0	0	0
All ages	0	0	0	0	-	-	0	0	0	0
Total	0	0	0	0	-	-	0	0	0	0

Table 72h   MEC - AOM - CMO   Trypanosomiasis - Episodes

Age group (years)	Incidence 1990 Number ('000s)	Rate (per 100 000)	Prevalence 1990 Number ('000s)	Rate (per 100 000)	Avg. age at onset (years)	Average duration (years)	Deaths 1990 Number ('000s)	Rate (per 100 000)	Deaths 2000 (Projected) Number ('000s)	Rate (per 100 000)
Males										
0-4	0	0	0	0	-	-	0	0	0	0
5-14	0	0	0	0	-	-	0	0	0	0
15-44	0	0	0	0	-	-	0	0	0	0
45-59	0	0	0	0	-	-	0	0	0	0
60+	0	0	0	0	-	-	0	0	0	0
All ages	0	0	0	0	-	-	0	0	0	0
Females										
0-4	0	0	0	0	-	-	0	0	0	0
5-14	0	0	0	0	-	-	0	0	0	0
15-44	0	0	0	0	-	-	0	0	0	0
45-59	0	0	0	0	-	-	0	0	0	0
60+	0	0	0	0	-	-	0	0	0	0
All ages	0	0	0	0	-	-	0	0	0	0
Total	0	0	0	0	-	-	0	0	0	0

Table 72i   World - Mundo - Monde   Trypanosomiasis - Episodes

Age group (years)	Incidence 1990 Number ('000s)	Rate (per 100 000)	Prevalence 1990 Number ('000s)	Rate (per 100 000)	Avg. age at onset (years)	Average duration (years)	Deaths 1990 Number ('000s)	Rate (per 100 000)	Deaths 2000 (Projected) Number ('000s)	Rate (per 100 000)
Males										
0-4	2	0.6	3	1.1	2.4	5.0	0	0.1	0	0.1
5-14	8	1.5	28	5.1	10.0	5.0	6	1.2	5	0.7
15-44	14	1.2	72	5.8	29.4	5.0	10	0.8	7	0.5
45-59	6	1.9	25	8.0	52.2	5.0	5	1.7	4	0.9
60+	1	0.5	13	5.8	69.2	5.0	1	0.7	1	0.5
All ages	32	1.2	142	5.3	28.6	5.0	24	0.9	17	0.5
Females										
0-4	4	1.2	7	2.2	2.4	5.0	1	0.3	1	0.3
5-14	7	1.4	29	5.4	10.0	5.0	7	1.3	5	0.8
15-44	13	1.1	66	5.5	29.5	5.0	12	1.0	6	0.5
45-59	4	1.2	16	5.3	52.2	5.0	4	1.1	2	0.6
60+	1	0.2	7	2.7	69.7	5.0	1	0.3	1	0.2
All ages	28	1.1	125	4.8	24.8	5.0	24	0.9	15	0.5
Total	60	1.1	267	5.1	26.8	5.0	47	0.9	32	0.5

For the methods used to estimate and project incidence, prevalence, and deaths see Murray and Lopez 1996a. See explanatory notes for definitions and caveats.

Table 73   **Cuadro 73**   **Tableau 73**
Chagas disease   **Enfermedad de Chagas**   **Maladie de Chagas**

Infection   Infección   Infection

Table 73a   EME - PEMC - EMBE   Chagas disease - Infection

Age group (years)	Incidence 1990 Number ('000s)	Rate (per 100 000)	Prevalence 1990 Number ('000s)	Rate (per 100 000)	Avg. age at onset (years)	Average duration (years)	Deaths 1990 Number ('000s)	Rate (per 100 000)	Deaths 2000 (Projected) Number ('000s)	Rate (per 100 000)
Males										
0-4	0	0	0	0	-	-	0	0	0	0
5-14	0	0	0	0	-	-	0	0	0	0
15-44	0	0	0	0	-	-	0	0	0	0
45-59	0	0	0	0	-	-	0	0	0	0
60+	0	0	0	0	-	-	0	0	0	0
All ages	0	0	0	0	-	-	0	0	0	0
Females										
0-4	0	0	0	0	-	-	0	0	0	0
5-14	0	0	0	0	-	-	0	0	0	0
15-44	0	0	0	0	-	-	0	0	0	0
45-59	0	0	0	0	-	-	0	0	0	0
60+	0	0	0	0	-	-	0	0	0	0
All ages	0	0	0	U	-	-	0	0	0	0
Total	0	0	0	0	-	-	0	0	0	0

Table 73b   FSE - PEAS - AESE   Chagas disease - Infection

Age group (years)	Incidence 1990 Number ('000s)	Rate (per 100 000)	Prevalence 1990 Number ('000s)	Rate (per 100 000)	Avg. age at onset (years)	Average duration (years)	Deaths 1990 Number ('000s)	Rate (per 100 000)	Deaths 2000 (Projected) Number ('000s)	Rate (per 100 000)
Males										
0-4	0	0	0	0	-	-	0	0	0	0
5-14	0	0	0	0	-	-	0	0	0	0
15-44	0	0	0	0	-	-	0	0	0	0
45-59	0	0	0	0	-	-	0	0	0	0
60+	0	0	0	0	-	-	0	0	0	0
All ages	0	0	0	0	-	-	0	0	0	0
Females										
0-4	0	0	0	0	-	-	0	0	0	0
5-14	0	0	0	0	-	-	0	0	0	0
15-44	0	0	0	0	-	-	0	0	0	0
45-59	0	0	0	0	-	-	0	0	0	0
60+	0	0	0	0	-	-	0	0	0	0
All ages	0	0	0	0	-	-	0	0	0	0
Total	0	0	0	0	-	-	0	0	0	0

Table 73c   India - India - Inde   Chagas disease - Infection

Age group (years)	Incidence 1990 Number ('000s)	Rate (per 100 000)	Prevalence 1990 Number ('000s)	Rate (per 100 000)	Avg. age at onset (years)	Average duration (years)	Deaths 1990 Number ('000s)	Rate (per 100 000)	Deaths 2000 (Projected) Number ('000s)	Rate (per 100 000)
Males										
0-4	0	0	0	0	-	-	0	0	0	0
5-14	0	0	0	0	-	-	0	0	0	0
15-44	0	0	0	0	-	-	0	0	0	0
45-59	0	0	0	0	-	-	0	0	0	0
60+	0	0	0	0	-	-	0	0	0	0
All ages	0	0	0	0	-	-	0	0	0	0
Females										
0-4	0	0	0	0	-	-	0	0	0	0
5-14	0	0	0	0	-	-	0	0	0	0
15-44	0	0	0	0	-	-	0	0	0	0
45-59	0	0	0	0	-	-	0	0	0	0
60+	0	0	0	0	-	-	0	0	0	0
All ages	0	0	0	0	-	-	0	0	0	0
Total	0	0	0	0	-	-	0	0	0	0

For epidemiological sources see Moncayo and Myoshi 1996. For the methods used to estimate and project incidence, prevalence, and deaths see Murray and Lopez 1996a. See explanatory notes for definitions and caveats.

Table 73
Chagas disease

Cuadro 73
Enfermedad de Chagas

Tableau 73
Maladie de Chagas

Infection

Infección

Infection

Table 73d China - China - Chine   Chagas disease - Infection

Age group (years)	Incidence 1990 Number ('000s)	Rate (per 100 000)	Prevalence 1990 Number ('000s)	Rate (per 100 000)	Avg. age at onset (years)	Average duration (years)	Deaths 1990 Number ('000s)	Rate (per 100 000)	Deaths 2000 (Projected) Number ('000s)	Rate (per 100 000)
Males										
0-4	0	0	0	0	-	-	0	0	0	0
5-14	0	0	0	0	-	-	0	0	0	0
15-44	0	0	0	0	-	-	0	0	0	0
45-59	0	0	0	0	-	-	0	0	0	0
60+	0	0	0	0	-	-	0	0	0	0
All ages	0	0	0	0	-	-	0	0	0	0
Females										
0-4	0	0	0	0	-	-	0	0	0	0
5-14	0	0	0	0	-	-	0	0	0	0
15-44	0	0	0	0	-	-	0	0	0	0
45-59	0	0	0	0	-	-	0	0	0	0
60+	0	0	0	0	-	-	0	0	0	0
All ages	0	0	0	0	-	-	0	0	0	0
Total	0	0	0	0	-	-	0	0	0	0

Table 73e OAI - OPAI - APAI   Chagas disease - Infection

Age group (years)	Incidence 1990 Number ('000s)	Rate (per 100 000)	Prevalence 1990 Number ('000s)	Rate (per 100 000)	Avg. age at onset (years)	Average duration (years)	Deaths 1990 Number ('000s)	Rate (per 100 000)	Deaths 2000 (Projected) Number ('000s)	Rate (per 100 000)
Males										
0-4	0	0	0	0	-	-	0	0	0	0
5-14	0	0	0	0	-	-	0	0	0	0
15-44	0	0	0	0	-	-	0	0	0	0
45-59	0	0	0	0	-	-	0	0	0	0
60+	0	0	0	0	-	-	0	0	0	0
All ages	0	0	0	0	-	-	0	0	0	0
Females										
0-4	0	0	0	0	-	-	0	0	0	0
5-14	0	0	0	0	-	-	0	0	0	0
15-44	0	0	0	0	-	-	0	0	0	0
45-59	0	0	0	0	-	-	0	0	0	0
60+	0	0	0	0	-	-	0	0	0	0
All ages	0	0	0	0	-	-	0	0	0	0
Total	0	0	0	0	-	-	0	0	0	0

Table 73f SSA - ASS - ASS   Chagas disease - Infection

Age group (years)	Incidence 1990 Number ('000s)	Rate (per 100 000)	Prevalence 1990 Number ('000s)	Rate (per 100 000)	Avg. age at onset (years)	Average duration (years)	Deaths 1990 Number ('000s)	Rate (per 100 000)	Deaths 2000 (Projected) Number ('000s)	Rate (per 100 000)
Males										
0-4	0	0	0	0	-	-	0	0	0	0
5-14	0	0	0	0	-	-	0	0	0	0
15-44	0	0	0	0	-	-	0	0	0	0
45-59	0	0	0	0	-	-	0	0	0	0
60+	0	0	0	0	-	-	0	0	0	0
All ages	0	0	0	0	-	-	0	0	0	0
Females										
0-4	0	0	0	0	-	-	0	0	0	0
5-14	0	0	0	0	-	-	0	0	0	0
15-44	0	0	0	0	-	-	0	0	0	0
45-59	0	0	0	0	-	-	0	0	0	0
60+	0	0	0	0	-	-	0	0	0	0
All ages	0	0	0	0	-	-	0	0	0	0
Total	0	0	0	0	-	-	0	0	0	0

For epidemiological sources see Moncayo and Myoshi 1996. For the methods used to estimate and project incidence, prevalence, and deaths see Murray and Lopez 1996a. See explanatory notes for definitions and caveats.

Table 73
Chagas disease

Cuadro 73
Enfermedad de Chagas

Tableau 73
Maladie de Chagas

Infection

Infección

Infection

Table 73g — LAC - ALC - ALC — Chagas disease - Infection

Age group (years)	Incidence 1990 Number ('000s)	Rate (per 100 000)	Prevalence 1990 Number ('000s)	Rate (per 100 000)	Avg. age at onset (years)	Average duration (years)	Deaths 1990 Number ('000s)	Rate (per 100 000)	Deaths 2000 (Projected) Number ('000s)	Rate (per 100 000)
Males										
0-4	162	564	331	1 153	2.5	29.9	0	0.1	0	0.1
5-14	122	234	1 624	3 116	10.0	36.3	0	0.1	0	0.1
15-44	90	86	4 498	4 313	29.7	27.2	2	2.1	1	1.1
45-59	9	38	920	4 135	52.3	16.7	3	14.0	2	7.9
60+	6	39	480	3 372	70.3	9.3	3	23.7	3	17.3
All ages	387	175	7 853	3 543	13.2	30.7	9	4.0	7	2.8
Females										
0-4	150	541	319	1 154	2.5	37.1	0	0.1	0	0.1
5-14	111	218	1 580	3 113	10.0	42.9	0	0.1	0	0.0
15-44	65	62	4 414	4 241	29.8	32.1	4	3.5	2	1.6
45-59	9	38	979	4 191	52.4	20.0	3	14.0	3	7.8
60+	6	39	641	3 809	71.1	10.3	3	18.9	3	13.5
All ages	341	153	7 933	3 562	12.7	37.1	10	4.6	8	2.9
Total	728	164	15 785	3 553	13.0	33.7	19	4.3	15	2.9

Table 73h — MEC - AOM - CMO — Chagas disease - Infection

Age group (years)	Incidence 1990 Number ('000s)	Rate (per 100 000)	Prevalence 1990 Number ('000s)	Rate (per 100 000)	Avg. age at onset (years)	Average duration (years)	Deaths 1990 Number ('000s)	Rate (per 100 000)	Deaths 2000 (Projected) Number ('000s)	Rate (per 100 000)
Males										
0-4	0	0	0	0	-	-	0	0	0	0
5-14	0	0	0	0	-	-	0	0	0	0
15-44	0	0	0	0	-	-	0	0	0	0
45-59	0	0	0	0	-	-	0	0	0	0
60+	0	0	0	0	-	-	0	0	0	0
All ages	0	0	0	0	-	-	0	0	0	0
Females										
0-4	0	0	0	0	-	-	0	0	0	0
5-14	0	0	0	0	-	-	0	0	0	0
15-44	0	0	0	0	-	-	0	0	0	0
45-59	0	0	0	0	-	-	0	0	0	0
60+	0	0	0	0	-	-	0	0	0	0
All ages	0	0	0	0	-	-	0	0	0	0
Total	0	0	0	0	-	-	0	0	0	0

Table 73i — World - Mundo - Monde — Chagas disease - Infection

Age group (years)	Incidence 1990 Number ('000s)	Rate (per 100 000)	Prevalence 1990 Number ('000s)	Rate (per 100 000)	Avg. age at onset (years)	Average duration (years)	Deaths 1990 Number ('000s)	Rate (per 100 000)	Deaths 2000 (Projected) Number ('000s)	Rate (per 100 000)
Males										
0-4	162	50.4	331	103	2.5	29.9	0	0.0	0	0.0
5-14	122	22.1	1 624	295	10.0	36.3	0	0.0	0	0.0
15-44	90	7.2	4 498	360	29.7	27.2	2	0.2	1	0.1
45-59	9	2.7	920	295	52.3	16.7	3	1.0	2	0.6
60+	6	2.5	480	219	70.3	9.3	3	1.5	3	1.2
All ages	387	14.6	7 853	296	13.2	30.7	9	0.3	7	0.2
Females										
0-4	150	48.4	319	103	2.5	37.1	0	0.0	0	0.0
5-14	111	21.0	1 580	301	10.0	42.9	0	0.0	0	0.0
15-44	65	5.4	4 414	368	29.8	32.1	4	0.3	2	0.1
45-59	9	2.9	979	315	52.4	20.0	3	1.1	3	0.6
60+	6	2.4	641	238	71.1	10.3	3	1.2	3	0.9
All ages	341	13.0	7 933	304	12.7	37.1	10	0.4	8	0.3
Total	728	13.8	15 785	300	13.0	33.7	19	0.4	15	0.2

For epidemiological sources see Moncayo and Myoshi 1996. For the methods used to estimate and project incidence, prevalence, and deaths see Murray and Lopez 1996a. See explanatory notes for definitions and caveats.

Table 74
Chagas disease
Cardiomyopathy without congestive
heart failure

Cuadro 74
Enfermedad de Chagas
Cardiomiopatía sin insuficiencia
cardiaca congestiva

Tableau 74
Maladie de Chagas
Cardiomyopathie sans insuffisance
cardiaque congestive

Table 74a   **EME - PEMC - EMBE**   Chagas disease - Cardiomyopathy without CHF

Age group (years)	Incidence 1990 Number ('000s)	Rate (per 100 000)	Prevalence 1990 Number ('000s)	Rate (per 100 000)	Avg. age at onset (years)	Average duration (years)	Deaths 1990 Number ('000s)	Rate (per 100 000)	Deaths 2000 (Projected) Number ('000s)	Rate (per 100 000)
Males										
0-4	0	0	0	0	-	-	-	-	-	-
5-14	0	0	0	0	-	-	-	-	-	-
15-44	0	0	0	0	-	-	-	-	-	-
45-59	0	0	0	0	-	-	-	-	-	-
60+	0	0	0	0	-	-	-	-	-	-
All ages	0	0	0	0	-	-	-	-	-	-
Females										
0-4	0	0	0	0	-	-	-	-	-	-
5-14	0	0	0	0	-	-	-	-	-	-
15-44	0	0	0	0	-	-	-	-	-	-
45-59	0	0	0	0	-	-	-	-	-	-
60+	0	0	0	0	-	-	-	-	-	-
All ages	0	0	0	0	-	-	-	-	-	-
Total	0	0	0	0	-	-	-	-	-	-

Table 74b   **FSE - PEAS - AESE**   Chagas disease - Cardiomyopathy without CHF

Age group (years)	Incidence 1990 Number ('000s)	Rate (per 100 000)	Prevalence 1990 Number ('000s)	Rate (per 100 000)	Avg. age at onset (years)	Average duration (years)	Deaths 1990 Number ('000s)	Rate (per 100 000)	Deaths 2000 (Projected) Number ('000s)	Rate (per 100 000)
Males										
0-4	0	0	0	0	-	-	-	-	-	-
5-14	0	0	0	0	-	-	-	-	-	-
15-44	0	0	0	0	-	-	-	-	-	-
45-59	0	0	0	0	-	-	-	-	-	-
60+	0	0	0	0	-	-	-	-	-	-
All ages	0	0	0	0	-	-	-	-	-	-
Females										
0-4	0	0	0	0	-	-	-	-	-	-
5-14	0	0	0	0	-	-	-	-	-	-
15-44	0	0	0	0	-	-	-	-	-	-
45-59	0	0	0	0	-	-	-	-	-	-
60+	0	0	0	0	-	-	-	-	-	-
All ages	0	0	0	0	-	-	-	-	-	-
Total	0	0	0	0	-	-	-	-	-	-

Table 74c   **India - India - Inde**   Chagas disease - Cardiomyopathy without CHF

Age group (years)	Incidence 1990 Number ('000s)	Rate (per 100 000)	Prevalence 1990 Number ('000s)	Rate (per 100 000)	Avg. age at onset (years)	Average duration (years)	Deaths 1990 Number ('000s)	Rate (per 100 000)	Deaths 2000 (Projected) Number ('000s)	Rate (per 100 000)
Males										
0-4	0	0	0	0	-	-	-	-	-	-
5-14	0	0	0	0	-	-	-	-	-	-
15-44	0	0	0	0	-	-	-	-	-	-
45-59	0	0	0	0	-	-	-	-	-	-
60+	0	0	0	0	-	-	-	-	-	-
All ages	0	0	0	0	-	-	-	-	-	-
Females										
0-4	0	0	0	0	-	-	-	-	-	-
5-14	0	0	0	0	-	-	-	-	-	-
15-44	0	0	0	0	-	-	-	-	-	-
45-59	0	0	0	0	-	-	-	-	-	-
60+	0	0	0	0	-	-	-	-	-	-
All ages	0	0	0	0	-	-	-	-	-	-
Total	0	0	0	0	-	-	-	-	-	-

For epidemiological sources see Moncayo and Myoshi 1996. For the methods used to estimate and project incidence,
prevalence, and deaths see Murray and Lopez 1996a. See explanatory notes for definitions and caveats.

Table 74
Chagas disease
Cardiomyopathy without congestive
heart failure

Cuadro 74
Enfermedad de Chagas
Cardiomiopatía sin insuficiencia
cardiaca congestiva

Tableau 74
Maladie de Chagas
Cardiomyopathie sans insuffisance
cardiaque congestive

Table 74d   China - China - Chine   Chagas disease - Cardiomyopathy without CHF

Age group (years)	Incidence 1990 Number ('000s)	Rate (per 100 000)	Prevalence 1990 Number ('000s)	Rate (per 100 000)	Avg. age at onset (years)	Average duration (years)	Deaths 1990 Number ('000s)	Rate (per 100 000)	Deaths 2000 (Projected) Number ('000s)	Rate (per 100 000)
Males										
0-4	0	0	0	0	-	-	-	-	-	-
5-14	0	0	0	0	-	-	-	-	-	-
15-44	0	0	0	0	-	-	-	-	-	-
45-59	0	0	0	0	-	-	-	-	-	-
60+	0	0	0	0	-	-	-	-	-	-
All ages	0	0	0	0	-	-	-	-	-	-
Females										
0-4	0	0	0	0	-	-	-	-	-	-
5-14	0	0	0	0	-	-	-	-	-	-
15-44	0	0	0	0	-	-	-	-	-	-
45-59	0	0	0	0	-	-	-	-	-	-
60+	0	0	0	0	-	-	-	-	-	-
All ages	0	0	0	0	-	-	-	-	-	-
Total	0	0	0	0	-	-	-	-	-	-

Table 74e   OAI - OPAI - APAI   Chagas disease - Cardiomyopathy without CHF

Age group (years)	Incidence 1990 Number ('000s)	Rate (per 100 000)	Prevalence 1990 Number ('000s)	Rate (per 100 000)	Avg. age at onset (years)	Average duration (years)	Deaths 1990 Number ('000s)	Rate (per 100 000)	Deaths 2000 (Projected) Number ('000s)	Rate (per 100 000)
Males										
0-4	0	0	0	0	-	-	-	-	-	-
5-14	0	0	0	0	-	-	-	-	-	-
15-44	0	0	0	0	-	-	-	-	-	-
45-59	0	0	0	0	-	-	-	-	-	-
60+	0	0	0	0	-	-	-	-	-	-
All ages	0	0	0	0	-	-	-	-	-	-
Females										
0-4	0	0	0	0	-	-	-	-	-	-
5-14	0	0	0	0	-	-	-	-	-	-
15-44	0	0	0	0	-	-	-	-	-	-
45-59	0	0	0	0	-	-	-	-	-	-
60+	0	0	0	0	-	-	-	-	-	-
All ages	0	0	0	0	-	-	-	-	-	-
Total	0	0	0	0	-	-	-	-	-	-

Table 74f   SSA - ASS - ASS   Chagas disease - Cardiomyopathy without CHF

Age group (years)	Incidence 1990 Number ('000s)	Rate (per 100 000)	Prevalence 1990 Number ('000s)	Rate (per 100 000)	Avg. age at onset (years)	Average duration (years)	Deaths 1990 Number ('000s)	Rate (per 100 000)	Deaths 2000 (Projected) Number ('000s)	Rate (per 100 000)
Males										
0-4	0	0	0	0	-	-	-	-	-	-
5-14	0	0	0	0	-	-	-	-	-	-
15-44	0	0	0	0	-	-	-	-	-	-
45-59	0	0	0	0	-	-	-	-	-	-
60+	0	0	0	0	-	-	-	-	-	-
All ages	0	0	0	0	-	-	-	-	-	-
Females										
0-4	0	0	0	0	-	-	-	-	-	-
5-14	0	0	0	0	-	-	-	-	-	-
15-44	0	0	0	0	-	-	-	-	-	-
45-59	0	0	0	0	-	-	-	-	-	-
60+	0	0	0	0	-	-	-	-	-	-
All ages	0	0	0	0	-	-	-	-	-	-
Total	0	0	0	0	-	-	-	-	-	-

For epidemiological sources see Moncayo and Myoshi 1996. For the methods used to estimate and project incidence, prevalence, and deaths see Murray and Lopez 1996a. See explanatory notes for definitions and caveats.

Table 74
Chagas disease
Cardiomyopathy without congestive
heart failure

Cuadro 74
Enfermedad de Chagas
Cardiomiopatía sin insuficiencia
cardiaca congestiva

Tableau 74
Maladie de Chagas
Cardiomyopathie sans insuffisance
cardiaque congestive

Table 74g	LAC - ALC - ALC						Chagas disease - Cardiomyopathy without CHF			
Age group (years)	Incidence 1990		Prevalence 1990		Avg. age at onset (years)	Average duration (years)	Deaths 1990		Deaths 2000 (Projected)	
	Number ('000s)	Rate (per 100 000)	Number ('000s)	Rate (per 100 000)			Number ('000s)	Rate (per 100 000)	Number ('000s)	Rate (per 100 000)
Males										
0-4	0	0	0	0	-	-	-	-	-	-
5-14	0	0	0	0	-	-	-	-	-	-
15-44	33	32	426	409	29.1	27.5	-	-	-	-
45-59	4	20	174	784	50.7	17.5	-	-	-	-
60+	0	0	87	611	70.3	9.3	-	-	-	-
All ages	37	17	688	310	31.7	26.3	-	-	-	-
Females										
0-4	0	0	0	0	-	-	-	-	-	-
5-14	0	0	0	0	-	-	-	-	-	-
15-44	31	30	420	403	29.8	32.1	-	-	-	-
45-59	4	19	189	808	52.4	20.0	-	-	-	-
60+	0	0	117	698	71.1	10.3	-	-	-	-
All ages	35	16	726	326	32.7	30.6	-	-	-	-
Total	73	16	1 414	318	32.2	28.4	-	-	-	-

Table 74h	MEC - AOM - CMO						Chagas disease - Cardiomyopathy without CHF			
Age group (years)	Incidence 1990		Prevalence 1990		Avg. age at onset (years)	Average duration (years)	Deaths 1990		Deaths 2000 (Projected)	
	Number ('000s)	Rate (per 100 000)	Number ('000s)	Rate (per 100 000)			Number ('000s)	Rate (per 100 000)	Number ('000s)	Rate (per 100 000)
Males										
0-4	0	0	0	0	-	-	-	-	-	-
5-14	0	0	0	0	-	-	-	-	-	-
15-44	0	0	0	0	-	-	-	-	-	-
45-59	0	0	0	0	-	-	-	-	-	-
60+	0	0	0	0	-	-	-	-	-	-
All ages	0	0	0	0	-	-	-	-	-	-
Females										
0-4	0	0	0	0	-	-	-	-	-	-
5-14	0	0	0	0	-	-	-	-	-	-
15-44	0	0	0	0	-	-	-	-	-	-
45-59	0	0	0	0	-	-	-	-	-	-
60+	0	0	0	0	-	-	-	-	-	-
All ages	0	0	0	0	-	-	-	-	-	-
Total	0	0	0	0	-	-	-	-	-	-

Table 74i	World - Mundo - Monde						Chagas disease - Cardiomyopathy without CHF			
Age group (years)	Incidence 1990		Prevalence 1990		Avg. age at onset (years)	Average duration (years)	Deaths 1990		Deaths 2000 (Projected)	
	Number ('000s)	Rate (per 100 000)	Number ('000s)	Rate (per 100 000)			Number ('000s)	Rate (per 100 000)	Number ('000s)	Rate (per 100 000)
Males										
0-4	0	0.0	0	0	-	-	-	-	-	-
5-14	0	0.0	0	0	-	-	-	-	-	-
15-44	33	2.6	426	34	29.1	27.5	-	-	-	-
45-59	4	1.4	174	56	50.7	17.5	-	-	-	-
60+	0	0.0	87	40	70.3	9.3	-	-	-	-
All ages	37	1.4	688	26	31.7	26.3	-	-	-	-
Females										
0-4	0	0.0	0	0	-	-	-	-	-	-
5-14	0	0.0	0	0	-	-	-	-	-	-
15-44	31	2.6	420	35	29.8	32.1	-	-	-	-
45-59	4	1.4	189	61	52.4	20.0	-	-	-	-
60+	0	0.0	117	44	71.1	10.3	-	-	-	-
All ages	35	1.3	726	28	32.7	30.6	-	-	-	-
Total	73	1.4	1 414	27	32.2	28.4	-	-	-	-

For epidemiological sources see Moncayo and Myoshi 1996. For the methods used to estimate and project incidence, prevalence, and deaths see Murray and Lopez 1996a. See explanatory notes for definitions and caveats.

Table 75
Chagas disease
Cardiomyopathy with congestive
heart failure

Cuadro 75
Enfermedad de Chagas
Cardiomiopatía con insuficiencia
cardiaca congestiva

Tableau 75
Maladie de Chagas
Cardiomyopathie avec insuffisance
cardiaque congestive

Table 75a   EME - PEMC - EMBE   Chagas disease - Cardiomyopathy with CHF

Age group (years)	Incidence 1990 Number ('000s)	Rate (per 100 000)	Prevalence 1990 Number ('000s)	Rate (per 100 000)	Avg. age at onset (years)	Average duration (years)	Deaths 1990 Number ('000s)	Rate (per 100 000)	Deaths 2000 (Projected) Number ('000s)	Rate (per 100 000)
Males										
0-4	0	0	0	0	-	-	-	-	-	-
5-14	0	0	0	0	-	-	-	-	-	-
15-44	0	0	0	0	-	-	-	-	-	-
45-59	0	0	0	0	-	-	-	-	-	-
60+	0	0	0	0	-	-	-	-	-	-
All ages	0	0	0	0	-	-	-	-	-	-
Females										
0-4	0	0	0	0	-	-	-	-	-	-
5-14	0	0	0	0	-	-	-	-	-	-
15-44	0	0	0	0	-	-	-	-	-	-
45-59	0	0	0	0	-	-	-	-	-	-
60+	0	0	0	0	-	-	-	-	-	-
All ages	0	0	0	0	-	-	-	-	-	-
Total	0	0	0	0	-	-	-	-	-	-

Table 75b   FSE - PEAS - AESE   Chagas disease - Cardiomyopathy with CHF

Age group (years)	Incidence 1990 Number ('000s)	Rate (per 100 000)	Prevalence 1990 Number ('000s)	Rate (per 100 000)	Avg. age at onset (years)	Average duration (years)	Deaths 1990 Number ('000s)	Rate (per 100 000)	Deaths 2000 (Projected) Number ('000s)	Rate (per 100 000)
Males										
0-4	0	0	0	0	-	-	-	-	-	-
5-14	0	0	0	0	-	-	-	-	-	-
15-44	0	0	0	0	-	-	-	-	-	-
45-59	0	0	0	0	-	-	-	-	-	-
60+	0	0	0	0	-	-	-	-	-	-
All ages	0	0	0	0	-	-	-	-	-	-
Females										
0-4	0	0	0	0	-	-	-	-	-	-
5-14	0	0	0	0	-	-	-	-	-	-
15-44	0	0	0	0	-	-	-	-	-	-
45-59	0	0	0	0	-	-	-	-	-	-
60+	0	0	0	0	-	-	-	-	-	-
All ages	0	0	0	0	-	-	-	-	-	-
Total	0	0	0	0	-	-	-	-	-	-

Table 75c   India - India - Inde   Chagas disease - Cardiomyopathy with CHF

Age group (years)	Incidence 1990 Number ('000s)	Rate (per 100 000)	Prevalence 1990 Number ('000s)	Rate (per 100 000)	Avg. age at onset (years)	Average duration (years)	Deaths 1990 Number ('000s)	Rate (per 100 000)	Deaths 2000 (Projected) Number ('000s)	Rate (per 100 000)
Males										
0-4	0	0	0	0	-	-	-	-	-	-
5-14	0	0	0	0	-	-	-	-	-	-
15-44	0	0	0	0	-	-	-	-	-	-
45-59	0	0	0	0	-	-	-	-	-	-
60+	0	0	0	0	-	-	-	-	-	-
All ages	0	0	0	0	-	-	-	-	-	-
Females										
0-4	0	0	0	0	-	-	-	-	-	-
5-14	0	0	0	0	-	-	-	-	-	-
15-44	0	0	0	0	-	-	-	-	-	-
45-59	0	0	0	0	-	-	-	-	-	-
60+	0	0	0	0	-	-	-	-	-	-
All ages	0	0	0	0	-	-	-	-	-	-
Total	0	0	0	0	-	-	-	-	-	-

For epidemiological sources see Moncayo and Myoshi 1996. For the methods used to estimate and project incidence, prevalence, and deaths see Murray and Lopez 1996a. See explanatory notes for definitions and caveats.

Table 75
Chagas disease
Cardiomyopathy with congestive
heart failure

Cuadro 75
Enfermedad de Chagas
Cardiomiopatía con insuficiencia
cardiaca congestiva

Tableau 75
Maladie de Chagas
Cardiomyopathie avec insuffisance
cardiaque congestive

Table 75d   **China - China - Chine**   Chagas disease - Cardiomyopathy with CHF

Age group (years)	Incidence 1990 Number ('000s)	Rate (per 100 000)	Prevalence 1990 Number ('000s)	Rate (per 100 000)	Avg. age at onset (years)	Average duration (years)	Deaths 1990 Number ('000s)	Rate (per 100 000)	Deaths 2000 (Projected) Number ('000s)	Rate (per 100 000)
Males										
0-4	0	0	0	0	-	-	-	-	-	-
5-14	0	0	0	0	-	-	-	-	-	-
15-44	0	0	0	0	-	-	-	-	-	-
45-59	0	0	0	0	-	-	-	-	-	-
60+	0	0	0	0	-	-	-	-	-	-
All ages	0	0	0	0	-	-	-	-	-	-
Females										
0-4	0	0	0	0	-	-	-	-	-	-
5-14	0	0	0	0	-	-	-	-	-	-
15-44	0	0	0	0	-	-	-	-	-	-
45-59	0	0	0	0	-	-	-	-	-	-
60+	0	0	0	0	-	-	-	-	-	-
All ages	0	0	0	0	-	-	-	-	-	-
Total	0	0	0	0	-	-	-	-	-	-

Table 75e   **OAI - OPAI - APAI**   Chagas disease - Cardiomyopathy with CHF

Age group (years)	Incidence 1990 Number ('000s)	Rate (per 100 000)	Prevalence 1990 Number ('000s)	Rate (per 100 000)	Avg. age at onset (years)	Average duration (years)	Deaths 1990 Number ('000s)	Rate (per 100 000)	Deaths 2000 (Projected) Number ('000s)	Rate (per 100 000)
Males										
0-4	0	0	0	0	-	-	-	-	-	-
5-14	0	0	0	0	-	-	-	-	-	-
15-44	0	0	0	0	-	-	-	-	-	-
45-59	0	0	0	0	-	-	-	-	-	-
60+	0	0	0	0	-	-	-	-	-	-
All ages	0	0	0	0	-	-	-	-	-	-
Females										
0-4	0	0	0	0	-	-	-	-	-	-
5-14	0	0	0	0	-	-	-	-	-	-
15-44	0	0	0	0	-	-	-	-	-	-
45-59	0	0	0	0	-	-	-	-	-	-
60+	0	0	0	0	-	-	-	-	-	-
All ages	0	0	0	0	-	-	-	-	-	-
Total	0	0	0	0	-	-	-	-	-	-

Table 75f   **SSA - ASS - ASS**   Chagas disease - Cardiomyopathy with CHF

Age group (years)	Incidence 1990 Number ('000s)	Rate (per 100 000)	Prevalence 1990 Number ('000s)	Rate (per 100 000)	Avg. age at onset (years)	Average duration (years)	Deaths 1990 Number ('000s)	Rate (per 100 000)	Deaths 2000 (Projected) Number ('000s)	Rate (per 100 000)
Males										
0-4	0	0	0	0	-	-	-	-	-	-
5-14	0	0	0	0	-	-	-	-	-	-
15-44	0	0	0	0	-	-	-	-	-	-
45-59	0	0	0	0	-	-	-	-	-	-
60+	0	0	0	0	-	-	-	-	-	-
All ages	0	0	0	0	-	-	-	-	-	-
Females										
0-4	0	0	0	0	-	-	-	-	-	-
5-14	0	0	0	0	-	-	-	-	-	-
15-44	0	0	0	0	-	-	-	-	-	-
45-59	0	0	0	0	-	-	-	-	-	-
60+	0	0	0	0	-	-	-	-	-	-
All ages	0	0	0	0	-	-	-	-	-	-
Total	0	0	0	0	-	-	-	-	-	-

For epidemiological sources see Moncayo and Myoshi 1996. For the methods used to estimate and project incidence, prevalence, and deaths see Murray and Lopez 1996a. See explanatory notes for definitions and caveats.

Table 75
Chagas disease
Cardiomyopathy with congestive heart failure

Cuadro 75
Enfermedad de Chagas
Cardiomiopatía con insuficiencia cardiaca congestiva

Tableau 75
Maladie de Chagas
Cardiomyopathie avec insuffisance cardiaque congestive

Table 75g LAC - ALC - ALC — Chagas disease - Cardiomyopathy with CHF

Age group (years)	Incidence 1990 Number ('000s)	Rate (per 100 000)	Prevalence 1990 Number ('000s)	Rate (per 100 000)	Avg. age at onset (years)	Average duration (years)	Deaths 1990 Number ('000s)	Rate (per 100 000)	Deaths 2000 (Projected) Number ('000s)	Rate (per 100 000)
Males										
0-4	0	0.0	0	0	-	-	-	-	-	-
5-14	0	0.0	0	0	-	-	-	-	-	-
15-44	6	6.0	83	80	28.7	27.7	-	-	-	-
45-59	1	3.4	31	139	50.9	17.4	-	-	-	-
60+	0	1.8	15	105	70.3	9.3	-	-	-	-
All ages	7	3.3	129	58	32.4	26.0	-	-	-	-
Females										
0-4	0	0.0	0	0	-	-	-	-	-	-
5-14	0	0.0	0	0	-	-	-	-	-	-
15-44	6	5.5	82	79	28.4	32.8	-	-	-	-
45-59	1	2.4	33	141	50.2	21.3	-	-	-	-
60+	0	1.2	20	118	71.1	10.3	-	-	-	-
All ages	7	2.9	135	60	31.6	31.1	-	-	-	-
Total	14	3.1	264	59	32.0	28.4	-	-	-	-

Table 75h MEC - AOM - CMO — Chagas disease - Cardiomyopathy with CHF

Age group (years)	Incidence 1990 Number ('000s)	Rate (per 100 000)	Prevalence 1990 Number ('000s)	Rate (per 100 000)	Avg. age at onset (years)	Average duration (years)	Deaths 1990 Number ('000s)	Rate (per 100 000)	Deaths 2000 (Projected) Number ('000s)	Rate (per 100 000)
Males										
0-4	0	0	0	0	-	-	-	-	-	-
5-14	0	0	0	0	-	-	-	-	-	-
15-44	0	0	0	0	-	-	-	-	-	-
45-59	0	0	0	0	-	-	-	-	-	-
60+	0	0	0	0	-	-	-	-	-	-
All ages	0	0	0	0	-	-	-	-	-	-
Females										
0-4	0	0	0	0	-	-	-	-	-	-
5-14	0	0	0	0	-	-	-	-	-	-
15-44	0	0	0	0	-	-	-	-	-	-
45-59	0	0	0	0	-	-	-	-	-	-
60+	0	0	0	0	-	-	-	-	-	-
All ages	0	0	0	0	-	-	-	-	-	-
Total	0	0	0	0	-	-	-	-	-	-

Table 75i World - Mundo - Monde — Chagas disease - Cardiomyopathy with CHF

Age group (years)	Incidence 1990 Number ('000s)	Rate (per 100 000)	Prevalence 1990 Number ('000s)	Rate (per 100 000)	Avg. age at onset (years)	Average duration (years)	Deaths 1990 Number ('000s)	Rate (per 100 000)	Deaths 2000 (Projected) Number ('000s)	Rate (per 100 000)
Males										
0-4	0	0.0	0	0.0	-	-	-	-	-	-
5-14	0	0.0	0	0.0	-	-	-	-	-	-
15-44	6	0.5	83	6.7	28.7	27.7	-	-	-	-
45-59	1	0.2	31	9.9	50.9	17.4	-	-	-	-
60+	0	0.1	15	6.8	70.3	9.3	-	-	-	-
All ages	7	0.3	129	4.9	32.4	26.0	-	-	-	-
Females										
0-4	0	0.0	0	0.0	-	-	-	-	-	-
5-14	0	0.0	0	0.0	-	-	-	-	-	-
15-44	6	0.5	82	6.8	28.4	32.8	-	-	-	-
45-59	1	0.2	33	10.6	50.2	21.3	-	-	-	-
60+	0	0.1	20	7.4	71.1	10.3	-	-	-	-
All ages	7	0.2	135	5.2	31.6	31.1	-	-	-	-
Total	14	0.3	264	5.0	32.0	28.4	-	-	-	-

For epidemiological sources see Moncayo and Myoshi 1996. For the methods used to estimate and project incidence, prevalence, and deaths see Murray and Lopez 1996a. See explanatory notes for definitions and caveats.

Table 76
Chagas disease

Cuadro 76
Enfermedad de Chagas

Tableau 76
Maladie de Chagas

Megaviscera

Megavícera

Mégaviscerose

Table 76a   EME - PEMC - EMBE   Chagas disease - Megaviscera

Age group (years)	Incidence 1990 Number ('000s)	Rate (per 100 000)	Prevalence 1990 Number ('000s)	Rate (per 100 000)	Avg. age at onset (years)	Average duration (years)	Deaths 1990 Number ('000s)	Rate (per 100 000)	Deaths 2000 (Projected) Number ('000s)	Rate (per 100 000)
Males										
0-4	0	0	0	0	-	-	-	-	-	-
5-14	0	0	0	0	-	-	-	-	-	-
15-44	0	0	0	0	-	-	-	-	-	-
45-59	0	0	0	0	-	-	-	-	-	-
60+	0	0	0	0	-	-	-	-	-	-
All ages	0	0	0	0	-	-	-	-	-	-
Females										
0-4	0	0	0	0	-	-	-	-	-	-
5-14	0	0	0	0	-	-	-	-	-	-
15-44	0	0	0	0	-	-	-	-	-	-
45-59	0	0	0	0	-	-	-	-	-	-
60+	0	0	0	0	-	-	-	-	-	-
All ages	0	0	0	0	-	-	-	-	-	-
Total	0	0	0	0	-	-	-	-	-	-

Table 76b   FSE - PEAS - AESE   Chagas disease - Megaviscera

Age group (years)	Incidence 1990 Number ('000s)	Rate (per 100 000)	Prevalence 1990 Number ('000s)	Rate (per 100 000)	Avg. age at onset (years)	Average duration (years)	Deaths 1990 Number ('000s)	Rate (per 100 000)	Deaths 2000 (Projected) Number ('000s)	Rate (per 100 000)
Males										
0-4	0	0	0	0	-	-	-	-	-	-
5-14	0	0	0	0	-	-	-	-	-	-
15-44	0	0	0	0	-	-	-	-	-	-
45-59	0	0	0	0	-	-	-	-	-	-
60+	0	0	0	0	-	-	-	-	-	-
All ages	0	0	0	0	-	-	-	-	-	-
Females										
0-4	0	0	0	0	-	-	-	-	-	-
5-14	0	0	0	0	-	-	-	-	-	-
15-44	0	0	0	0	-	-	-	-	-	-
45-59	0	0	0	0	-	-	-	-	-	-
60+	0	0	0	0	-	-	-	-	-	-
All ages	0	0	0	0	-	-	-	-	-	-
Total	0	0	0	0	-	-	-	-	-	-

Table 76c   India - India - Inde   Chagas disease - Megaviscera

Age group (years)	Incidence 1990 Number ('000s)	Rate (per 100 000)	Prevalence 1990 Number ('000s)	Rate (per 100 000)	Avg. age at onset (years)	Average duration (years)	Deaths 1990 Number ('000s)	Rate (per 100 000)	Deaths 2000 (Projected) Number ('000s)	Rate (per 100 000)
Males										
0-4	0	0	0	0	-	-	-	-	-	-
5-14	0	0	0	0	-	-	-	-	-	-
15-44	0	0	0	0	-	-	-	-	-	-
45-59	0	0	0	0	-	-	-	-	-	-
60+	0	0	0	0	-	-	-	-	-	-
All ages	0	0	0	0	-	-	-	-	-	-
Females										
0-4	0	0	0	0	-	-	-	-	-	-
5-14	0	0	0	0	-	-	-	-	-	-
15-44	0	0	0	0	-	-	-	-	-	-
45-59	0	0	0	0	-	-	-	-	-	-
60+	0	0	0	0	-	-	-	-	-	-
All ages	0	0	0	0	-	-	-	-	-	-
Total	0	0	0	0	-	-	-	-	-	-

For epidemiological sources see Moncayo and Myoshi 1996. For the methods used to estimate and project incidence, prevalence, and deaths see Murray and Lopez 1996a. See explanatory notes for definitions and caveats.

Table 76	Cuadro 76	Tableau 76
Chagas disease	**Enfermedad de Chagas**	**Maladie de Chagas**
Megaviscera	Megavícera	Mégaviscerose

Table 76d China - China - Chine   Chagas disease - Megaviscera

Age group (years)	Incidence 1990 Number ('000s)	Rate (per 100 000)	Prevalence 1990 Number ('000s)	Rate (per 100 000)	Avg. age at onset (years)	Average duration (years)	Deaths 1990 Number ('000s)	Rate (per 100 000)	Deaths 2000 (Projected) Number ('000s)	Rate (per 100 000)
Males										
0-4	0	0	0	0	-	-	-	-	-	-
5-14	0	0	0	0	-	-	-	-	-	-
15-44	0	0	0	0	-	-	-	-	-	-
45-59	0	0	0	0	-	-	-	-	-	-
60+	0	0	0	0	-	-	-	-	-	-
All ages	0	0	0	0	-	-	-	-	-	-
Females										
0-4	0	0	0	0	-	-	-	-	-	-
5-14	0	0	0	0	-	-	-	-	-	-
15-44	0	0	0	0	-	-	-	-	-	-
45-59	0	0	0	0	-	-	-	-	-	-
60+	0	0	0	0	-	-	-	-	-	-
All ages	0	0	0	0	-	-	*	-	-	-
Total	0	0	0	0	-	-	-	-	-	-

Table 76e OAI - OPAI - APAI   Chagas disease - Megaviscera

Age group (years)	Incidence 1990 Number ('000s)	Rate (per 100 000)	Prevalence 1990 Number ('000s)	Rate (per 100 000)	Avg. age at onset (years)	Average duration (years)	Deaths 1990 Number ('000s)	Rate (per 100 000)	Deaths 2000 (Projected) Number ('000s)	Rate (per 100 000)
Males										
0-4	0	0	0	0	-	-	-	-	-	-
5-14	0	0	0	0	-	-	-	-	-	-
15-44	0	0	0	0	-	-	-	-	-	-
45-59	0	0	0	0	-	-	-	-	-	-
60+	0	0	0	0	-	-	-	-	-	-
All ages	0	0	0	0	-	-	-	-	-	-
Females										
0-4	0	0	0	0	-	-	-	-	-	-
5-14	0	0	0	0	-	-	-	-	-	-
15-44	0	0	0	0	-	-	-	-	-	-
45-59	0	0	0	0	-	-	-	-	-	-
60+	0	0	0	0	-	-	-	-	-	-
All ages	0	0	0	0	-	-	-	-	-	-
Total	0	0	0	0	-	-	-	-	-	-

Table 76f SSA - ASS - ASS   Chagas disease - Megaviscera

Age group (years)	Incidence 1990 Number ('000s)	Rate (per 100 000)	Prevalence 1990 Number ('000s)	Rate (per 100 000)	Avg. age at onset (years)	Average duration (years)	Deaths 1990 Number ('000s)	Rate (per 100 000)	Deaths 2000 (Projected) Number ('000s)	Rate (per 100 000)
Males										
0-4	0	0	0	0	-	-	-	-	-	-
5-14	0	0	0	0	-	-	-	-	-	-
15-44	0	0	0	0	-	-	-	-	-	-
45-59	0	0	0	0	-	-	-	-	-	-
60+	0	0	0	0	-	-	-	-	-	-
All ages	0	0	0	0	-	-	-	-	-	-
Females										
0-4	0	0	0	0	-	-	-	-	-	-
5-14	0	0	0	0	-	-	-	-	-	-
15-44	0	0	0	0	-	-	-	-	-	-
45-59	0	0	0	0	-	-	-	-	-	-
60+	0	0	0	0	-	-	-	-	-	-
All ages	0	0	0	0	-	-	-	-	-	-
Total	0	0	0	0	-	-	-	-	-	-

For epidemiological sources see Moncayo and Myoshi 1996. For the methods used to estimate and project incidence, prevalence, and deaths see Murray and Lopez 1996a. See explanatory notes for definitions and caveats.

Table 76
Chagas disease

Cuadro 76
Enfermedad de Chagas

Tableau 76
Maladie de Chagas

Megaviscera

Megavícera

Mégaviscerose

Table 76g   LAC - ALC - ALC   Chagas disease - Megaviscera

Age group (years)	Incidence 1990 Number ('000s)	Rate (per 100 000)	Prevalence 1990 Number ('000s)	Rate (per 100 000)	Avg. age at onset (years)	Average duration (years)	Deaths 1990 Number ('000s)	Rate (per 100 000)	Deaths 2000 (Projected) Number ('000s)	Rate (per 100 000)
Males										
0-4	0	0.0	0	0	-	-	-	-	-	-
5-14	0	0.0	0	0	-	-	-	-	-	-
15-44	11	10.6	182	174	24.2	29.6	-	-	-	-
45-59	1	3.2	47	211	49.8	17.9	-	-	-	-
60+	0	2.2	21	147	70.3	9.3	-	-	-	-
All ages	12	5.4	249	113	26.9	28.4	-	-	-	-
Females										
0-4	0	0.0	0	0	-	-	-	-	-	-
5-14	0	0.0	0	0	-	-	-	-	-	-
15-44	10	9.7	179	172	23.9	35.1	-	-	-	-
45-59	0	1.6	50	215	47.5	22.8	-	-	-	-
60+	0	1.2	28	164	71.1	10.3	-	-	-	-
All ages	11	4.8	257	115	25.6	34.2	-	-	-	-
Total	23	5.1	506	114	26.3	31.1	-	-	-	-

Table 76h   MEC - AOM - CMO   Chagas disease - Megaviscera

Age group (years)	Incidence 1990 Number ('000s)	Rate (per 100 000)	Prevalence 1990 Number ('000s)	Rate (per 100 000)	Avg. age at onset (years)	Average duration (years)	Deaths 1990 Number ('000s)	Rate (per 100 000)	Deaths 2000 (Projected) Number ('000s)	Rate (per 100 000)
Males										
0-4	0	0	0	0	-	-	-	-	-	-
5-14	0	0	0	0	-	-	-	-	-	-
15-44	0	0	0	0	-	-	-	-	-	-
45-59	0	0	0	0	-	-	-	-	-	-
60+	0	0	0	0	-	-	-	-	-	-
All ages	0	0	0	0	-	-	-	-	-	-
Females										
0-4	0	0	0	0	-	-	-	-	-	-
5-14	0	0	0	0	-	-	-	-	-	-
15-44	0	0	0	0	-	-	-	-	-	-
45-59	0	0	0	0	-	-	-	-	-	-
60+	0	0	0	0	-	-	-	-	-	-
All ages	0	0	0	0	-	-	-	-	-	-
Total	0	0	0	0	-	-	-	-	-	-

Table 76i   World - Mundo - Monde   Chagas disease - Megaviscera

Age group (years)	Incidence 1990 Number ('000s)	Rate (per 100 000)	Prevalence 1990 Number ('000s)	Rate (per 100 000)	Avg. age at onset (years)	Average duration (years)	Deaths 1990 Number ('000s)	Rate (per 100 000)	Deaths 2000 (Projected) Number ('000s)	Rate (per 100 000)
Males										
0-4	0	0.0	0	0.0	-	-	-	-	-	-
5-14	0	0.0	0	0.0	-	-	-	-	-	-
15-44	11	0.9	182	14.5	24.2	29.6	-	-	-	-
45-59	1	0.2	47	15.0	49.8	17.9	-	-	-	-
60+	0	0.1	21	9.5	70.3	9.3	-	-	-	-
All ages	12	0.5	249	9.4	26.9	28.4	-	-	-	-
Females										
0-4	0	0.0	0	0.0	-	-	-	-	-	-
5-14	0	0.0	0	0.0	-	-	-	-	-	-
15-44	10	0.8	179	15.0	23.9	35.1	-	-	-	-
45-59	0	0.1	50	16.1	47.5	22.8	-	-	-	-
60+	0	0.1	28	10.2	71.1	10.3	-	-	-	-
All ages	11	0.4	257	9.8	25.6	34.2	-	-	-	-
Total	23	0.4	506	9.6	26.3	31.1	-	-	-	-

For epidemiological sources see Moncayo and Myoshi 1996. For the methods used to estimate and project incidence, prevalence, and deaths see Murray and Lopez 1996a. See explanatory notes for definitions and caveats.

Table 77	Cuadro 77	Tableau 77
Schistosomiasis	Esquistosomiasis	Schistosomiase
Infection	Infección	Infection

Table 77a EME - PEMC - EMBE Schistosomiasis - Infection

Age group (years)	Incidence 1990 Number ('000s)	Rate (per 100 000)	Prevalence 1990 Number ('000s)	Rate (per 100 000)	Avg. age at onset (years)	Average duration (years)	Deaths 1990 Number ('000s)	Rate (per 100 000)	Deaths 2000 (Projected) Number ('000s)	Rate (per 100 000)
Males										
0-4	-	-	0	0	-	-	0	0	0	0
5-14	-	-	0	0	-	-	0	0	0	0
15-44	-	-	0	0	-	-	0	0	0	0
45-59	-	-	0	0	-	-	0	0	0	0
60+	-	-	0	0	-	-	0	0	0	0
All ages	-	-	0	0	-	-	0	0	0	0
Females										
0-4	-	-	0	0	-	-	0	0	0	0
5-14	-	-	0	0	-	-	0	0	0	0
15-44	-	-	0	0	-	-	0	0	0	0
45-59	-	-	0	0	-	-	0	0	0	0
60+	-	-	0	0	-	-	0	0	0	0
All ages	-	-	0	0	-	-	0	0	0	0
Total	-	-	0	0	-	-	0	0	0	0

Table 77b FSE - PEAS - AESE Schistosomiasis - Infection

Age group (years)	Incidence 1990 Number ('000s)	Rate (per 100 000)	Prevalence 1990 Number ('000s)	Rate (per 100 000)	Avg. age at onset (years)	Average duration (years)	Deaths 1990 Number ('000s)	Rate (per 100 000)	Deaths 2000 (Projected) Number ('000s)	Rate (per 100 000)
Males										
0-4	-	-	0	0	-	-	0	0	0	0
5-14	-	-	0	0	-	-	0	0	0	0
15-44	-	-	0	0	-	-	0	0	0	0
45-59	-	-	0	0	-	-	0	0	0	0
60+	-	-	0	0	-	-	0	0	0	0
All ages	-	-	0	0	-	-	0	0	0	0
Females										
0-4	-	-	0	0	-	-	0	0	0	0
5-14	-	-	0	0	-	-	0	0	0	0
15-44	-	-	0	0	-	-	0	0	0	0
45-59	-	-	0	0	-	-	0	0	0	0
60+	-	-	0	0	-	-	0	0	0	0
All ages	-	-	0	0	-	-	0	0	0	0
Total	-	-	0	0	-	-	0	0	0	0

Table 77c India - India - Inde Schistosomiasis - Infection

Age group (years)	Incidence 1990 Number ('000s)	Rate (per 100 000)	Prevalence 1990 Number ('000s)	Rate (per 100 000)	Avg. age at onset (years)	Average duration (years)	Deaths 1990 Number ('000s)	Rate (per 100 000)	Deaths 2000 (Projected) Number ('000s)	Rate (per 100 000)
Males										
0-4	-	-	0	0	-	-	0	0	0	0
5-14	-	-	0	0	-	-	0	0	0	0
15-44	-	-	0	0	-	-	0	0	0	0
45-59	-	-	0	0	-	-	0	0	0	0
60+	-	-	0	0	-	-	0	0	0	0
All ages	-	-	0	0	-	-	0	0	0	0
Females										
0-4	-	-	0	0	-	-	0	0	0	0
5-14	-	-	0	0	-	-	0	0	0	0
15-44	-	-	0	0	-	-	0	0	0	0
45-59	-	-	0	0	-	-	0	0	0	0
60+	-	-	0	0	-	-	0	0	0	0
All ages	-	-	0	0	-	-	0	0	0	0
Total	-	-	0	0	-	-	0	0	0	0

For epidemiological sources see Mott 1996. For the methods used to estimate and project incidence, prevalence, and deaths see Murray and Lopez 1996a. See explanatory notes for definitions and caveats.

Table 77	Cuadro 77	Tableau 77
Schistosomiasis	Esquistosomiasis	Schistosomiase
Infection	Infección	Infection

Table 77d   China - China - Chine   Schistosomiasis - Infection

Age group (years)	Incidence 1990 Number ('000s)	Rate (per 100 000)	Prevalence 1990 Number ('000s)	Rate (per 100 000)	Avg. age at onset (years)	Average duration (years)	Deaths 1990 Number ('000s)	Rate (per 100 000)	Deaths 2000 (Projected) Number ('000s)	Rate (per 100 000)
Males										
0-4	-	-	35	59	-	-	0	0.0	0	0.0
5-14	-	-	170	175	-	-	0	0.0	0	0.0
15-44	-	-	501	164	-	-	0	0.1	0	0.0
45-59	-	-	145	199	-	-	0	0.4	0	0.1
60+	-	-	96	196	-	-	0	0.8	0	0.5
All ages	-	-	947	162	-	-	1	0.1	1	0.1
Females										
0-4	-	-	21	36	-	-	0	0.0	0	0.0
5-14	-	-	99	110	-	-	0	0.0	0	0.0
15-44	-	-	293	103	-	-	0	0.0	0	0.0
45-59	-	-	84	131	-	-	0	0.2	0	0.1
60+	-	-	56	108	-	-	0	0.6	0	0.4
All ages	-	-	553	101	-	-	0	0.1	0	0.1
Total	-	-	1 500	132	-	-	1	0.1	1	0.1

Table 77e   OAI - OPAI - APAI   Schistosomiasis - Infection

Age group (years)	Incidence 1990 Number ('000s)	Rate (per 100 000)	Prevalence 1990 Number ('000s)	Rate (per 100 000)	Avg. age at onset (years)	Average duration (years)	Deaths 1990 Number ('000s)	Rate (per 100 000)	Deaths 2000 (Projected) Number ('000s)	Rate (per 100 000)
Males										
0-4	-	-	35	79	-	-	0	0.0	0	0.0
5-14	-	-	167	198	-	-	0	0.0	0	0.0
15-44	-	-	192	119	-	-	0	0.0	0	0.0
45-59	-	-	55	162	-	-	0	0.3	0	0.2
60+	-	-	37	182	-	-	0	0.8	0	0.5
All ages	-	-	485	141	-	-	0	0.1	0	0.1
Females										
0-4	-	-	26	61	-	-	0	0.0	0	0.0
5-14	-	-	124	154	-	-	0	0.0	0	0.0
15-44	-	-	146	91	-	-	0	0.0	0	0.0
45-59	-	-	42	120	-	-	0	0.2	0	0.1
60+	-	-	28	123	-	-	0	0.6	0	0.4
All ages	-	-	365	107	-	-	0	0.1	0	0.1
Total	-	-	850	125	-	-	1	0.1	0	0.1

Table 77f   SSA - ASS - ASS   Schistosomiasis - Infection

Age group (years)	Incidence 1990 Number ('000s)	Rate (per 100 000)	Prevalence 1990 Number ('000s)	Rate (per 100 000)	Avg. age at onset (years)	Average duration (years)	Deaths 1990 Number ('000s)	Rate (per 100 000)	Deaths 2000 (Projected) Number ('000s)	Rate (per 100 000)
Males										
0-4	-	-	11 148	23 478	-	-	0	0.0	0	0.0
5-14	-	-	45 013	64 068	-	-	0	0.4	0	0.2
15-44	-	-	39 991	38 540	-	-	1	0.8	1	0.4
45-59	-	-	7 652	37 682	-	-	1	2.7	0	1.4
60+	-	-	3 442	32 758	-	-	0	4.7	0	3.0
All ages	-	-	107 246	42 504	-	-	2	0.9	2	0.5
Females										
0-4	-	-	7 512	15 972	-	-	0	0.0	0	0.0
5-14	-	-	30 330	43 442	-	-	0	0.3	0	0.2
15-44	-	-	28 124	26 468	-	-	1	0.7	0	0.3
45-59	-	-	5 382	24 333	-	-	0	1.0	0	0.5
60+	-	-	2 421	19 017	-	-	0	1.5	0	1.1
All ages	-	-	73 769	28 598	-	-	1	0.5	1	0.3
Total	-	-	181 015	35 474	-	-	4	0.7	2	0.4

For epidemiological sources see Mott 1996. For the methods used to estimate and project incidence, prevalence, and deaths see Murray and Lopez 1996a. See explanatory notes for definitions and caveats.

Table 77
Schistosomiasis

Cuadro 77
Esquistosomiasis

Tableau 77
Schistosomiase

Infection

Infección

Infection

Table 77g LAC - ALC - ALC Schistosomiasis - Infection

Age group (years)	Incidence 1990 Number ('000s)	Rate (per 100 000)	Prevalence 1990 Number ('000s)	Rate (per 100 000)	Avg. age at onset (years)	Average duration (years)	Deaths 1990 Number ('000s)	Rate (per 100 000)	Deaths 2000 (Projected) Number ('000s)	Rate (per 100 000)
Males										
0-4	-	-	301	1 047	-	-	0	0.0	0	0.0
5-14	-	-	1 455	2 791	-	-	0	0.0	0	0.0
15-44	-	-	2 549	2 444	-	-	0	0.1	0	0.1
45-59	-	-	496	2 230	-	-	0	0.4	0	0.2
60+	-	-	199	1 398	-	-	0	0.3	0	0.2
All ages	-	-	5 000	2 256	-	-	0	0.1	0	0.1
Females										
0-4	-	-	340	1 230	-	-	0	0.0	0	0.0
5-14	-	-	1 646	3 244	-	-	0	0.0	0	0.0
15-44	-	-	2 289	2 199	-	-	0	0.1	0	0.0
45-59	-	-	446	1 908	-	-	0	0.3	0	0.2
60+	-	-	179	1 062	-	-	0	0.3	0	0.2
All ages	-	-	4 900	2 200	-	-	0	0.1	0	0.1
Total	-	-	9 900	2 228	-	-	1	0.1	0	0.1

Table 77h MEC - AOM - CMO Schistosomiasis - Infection

Age group (years)	Incidence 1990 Number ('000s)	Rate (per 100 000)	Prevalence 1990 Number ('000s)	Rate (per 100 000)	Avg. age at onset (years)	Average duration (years)	Deaths 1990 Number ('000s)	Rate (per 100 000)	Deaths 2000 (Projected) Number ('000s)	Rate (per 100 000)
Males										
0-4	-	-	630	1 531	-	-	0	0.0	0	0.0
5-14	-	-	3 048	4 664	-	-	0	0.3	0	0.2
15-44	-	-	4 038	3 545	-	-	1	0.5	0	0.3
45-59	-	-	786	3 519	-	-	0	1.7	0	0.9
60+	-	-	315	2 308	-	-	0	2.4	0	1.6
All ages	-	-	8 817	3 439	-	-	1	0.6	1	0.3
Females										
0-4	-	-	408	1 028	-	-	0	0.0	0	0.0
5-14	-	-	1 976	3 187	-	-	0	0.0	0	0.0
15-44	-	-	2 994	2 792	-	-	0	0.3	0	0.1
45-59	-	-	583	2 614	-	-	0	0.7	0	0.4
60+	-	-	234	1 512	-	-	0	0.8	0	0.5
All ages	-	-	6 194	2 511	-	-	1	0.3	0	0.1
Total	-	-	15 011	2 984	-	-	2	0.4	2	0.2

Table 77i World - Mundo - Monde Schistosomiasis - Infection

Age group (years)	Incidence 1990 Number ('000s)	Rate (per 100 000)	Prevalence 1990 Number ('000s)	Rate (per 100 000)	Avg. age at onset (years)	Average duration (years)	Deaths 1990 Number ('000s)	Rate (per 100 000)	Deaths 2000 (Projected) Number ('000s)	Rate (per 100 000)
Males										
0-4	-	-	12 149	3 781	-	-	0	0.0	0	0.0
5-14	-	-	49 852	9 044	-	-	1	0.1	0	0.1
15-44	-	-	47 271	3 782	-	-	2	0.1	1	0.1
45-59	-	-	9 135	2 924	-	-	1	0.4	1	0.2
60+	-	-	4 089	1 868	-	-	1	0.6	1	0.4
All ages	-	-	122 495	4 616	-	-	5	0.2	4	0.1
Females										
0-4	-	-	8 307	2 686	-	-	0	0.0	0	0.0
5-14	-	-	34 175	6 503	-	-	0	0.0	0	0.0
15-44	-	-	33 846	2 824	-	-	1	0.1	1	0.0
45-59	-	-	6 537	2 101	-	-	1	0.2	0	0.1
60+	-	-	2 917	1 084	-	-	1	0.3	1	0.2
All ages	-	-	85 781	3 282	-	-	3	0.1	2	0.1
Total	-	-	208 276	3 954	-	-	8	0.2	6	0.1

For epidemiological sources see Mott 1996. For the methods used to estimate and project incidence, prevalence, and deaths see Murray and Lopez 1996a. See explanatory notes for definitions and caveats.

Table 78   **Cuadro 78**   **Tableau 78**
Leishmaniasis   **Leishmaniasis**   **Leishmaniose**

Visceral   Visceral   Viscerale

Table 78a   EME - PEMC - EMBE   Leishmaniasis - Visceral

Age group (years)	Incidence 1990 Number ('000s)	Rate (per 100 000)	Prevalence 1990 Number ('000s)	Rate (per 100 000)	Avg. age at onset (years)	Average duration (years)	Deaths 1990 Number ('000s)	Rate (per 100 000)	Deaths 2000 (Projected) Number ('000s)	Rate (per 100 000)
Males										
0-4	0	0.3	0	0.6	2.5	5.0	0	0	0	0
5-14	0	0.1	0	0.6	10.0	5.1	0	0	0	0
15-44	0	0.1	1	0.4	29.9	5.0	0	0	0	0
45-59	0	0.1	0	0.4	52.4	4.6	0	0	0	0
60+	0	0.1	0	0.4	71.1	3.4	0	0	0	0
All ages	0	0.1	2	0.4	32.8	4.6	0	0	0	0
Females										
0-4	0	0.3	0	0.6	2.5	5.0	0	0	0	0
5-14	0	0.1	0	0.6	10.0	5.0	0	0	0	0
15-44	0	0.1	1	0.4	30.0	5.0	0	0	0	0
45-59	0	0.1	0	0.4	52.4	4.6	0	0	0	0
60+	0	0.1	0	0.4	72.4	3.5	0	0	0	0
All ages	0	0.1	2	0.4	36.6	4.6	0	0	0	0
Total	1	0.1	3	0.4	34.8	4.6	0	0	0	0

Table 78b   FSE - PEAS - AESE   Leishmaniasis - Visceral

Age group (years)	Incidence 1990 Number ('000s)	Rate (per 100 000)	Prevalence 1990 Number ('000s)	Rate (per 100 000)	Avg. age at onset (years)	Average duration (years)	Deaths 1990 Number ('000s)	Rate (per 100 000)	Deaths 2000 (Projected) Number ('000s)	Rate (per 100 000)
Males										
0-4	0	0	0	0	-	-	0	0	0	0
5-14	0	0	0	0	-	-	0	0	0	0
15-44	0	0	0	0	-	-	0	0	0	0
45-59	0	0	0	0	-	-	0	0	0	0
60+	0	0	0	0	-	-	0	0	0	0
All ages	0	0	0	0	-	-	0	0	0	0
Females										
0-4	0	0	0	0	-	-	0	0	0	0
5-14	0	0	0	0	-	-	0	0	0	0
15-44	0	0	0	0	-	-	0	0	0	0
45-59	0	0	0	0	-	-	0	0	0	0
60+	0	0	0	0	-	-	0	0	0	0
All ages	0	0	0	0	-	-	0	0	0	0
Total	0	0	0	0	-	-	0	0	0	0

Table 78c   India - India - Inde   Leishmaniasis - Visceral

Age group (years)	Incidence 1990 Number ('000s)	Rate (per 100 000)	Prevalence 1990 Number ('000s)	Rate (per 100 000)	Avg. age at onset (years)	Average duration (years)	Deaths 1990 Number ('000s)	Rate (per 100 000)	Deaths 2000 (Projected) Number ('000s)	Rate (per 100 000)
Males										
0-4	23	38.8	36	59	2.5	2.9	1	2.4	1	1.5
5-14	65	63.9	168	165	10.0	3.0	8	7.7	4	3.4
15-44	83	41.3	264	132	29.8	3.0	11	5.3	5	2.1
45-59	3	5.8	19	40	52.3	2.8	1	1.6	0	0.8
60+	3	9.1	7	24	69.7	2.3	1	1.9	0	1.2
All ages	177	40.2	494	112	19.9	3.0	21	4.8	11	2.1
Females										
0-4	16	27.7	24	42	2.5	2.9	1	1.7	1	1.0
5-14	43	45.6	112	118	10.0	3.0	6	5.9	3	2.5
15-44	54	29.5	172	94	29.8	3.0	6	3.5	3	1.1
45-59	2	4.2	13	28	52.4	2.9	1	1.2	0	0.5
60+	2	6.5	5	17	70.1	2.3	0	1.4	0	0.9
All ages	117	28.5	327	80	19.8	3.0	14	3.4	6	1.3
Total	294	34.6	821	97	19.9	3.0	35	4.1	17	1.7

For epidemiological sources see Desjeux 1996. For the methods used to estimate and project incidence, prevalence, and deaths see Murray and Lopez 1996a. See explanatory notes for definitions and caveats.

Table 78	Cuadro 78	Tableau 78
Leishmaniasis	Leishmaniasis	Leishmaniose

Visceral · Visceral · Viscerale

Table 78d China - China - Chine — Leishmaniasis - Visceral

Age group (years)	Incidence 1990 Number ('000s)	Rate (per 100 000)	Prevalence 1990 Number ('000s)	Rate (per 100 000)	Avg. age at onset (years)	Average duration (years)	Deaths 1990 Number ('000s)	Rate (per 100 000)	Deaths 2000 (Projected) Number ('000s)	Rate (per 100 000)
Males										
0-4	0	0.1	0	0.1	2.5	3.0	0	0	0	0
5-14	0	0.1	0	0.2	10.0	3.0	0	0	0	0
15-44	0	0.0	0	0.1	29.9	3.0	0	0	0	0
45-59	0	0.0	0	0.0	52.3	2.9	0	0	0	0
60+	0	0.0	0	0.0	69.8	2.3	0	0	0	0
All ages	0	0.0	1	0.1	18.2	3.0	0	0	0	0
Females										
0-4	0	0.1	0	0.1	2.5	3.0	0	0	0	0
5-14	0	0.1	0	0.1	10.0	3.0	0	0	0	0
15-44	0	0.0	0	0.0	29.9	3.0	0	0	0	0
45-59	0	0.0	0	0.0	52.4	2.9	0	0	0	0
60+	0	0.0	0	0.0	-	-	0	0	0	0
All ages	0	0.0	0	0.1	15.7	3.0	0	0	0	0
Total	0	0.0	1	0.1	17.3	3.0	0	0	0	0

Table 78e OAI - OPAI - APAI — Leishmaniasis - Visceral

Age group (years)	Incidence 1990 Number ('000s)	Rate (per 100 000)	Prevalence 1990 Number ('000s)	Rate (per 100 000)	Avg. age at onset (years)	Average duration (years)	Deaths 1990 Number ('000s)	Rate (per 100 000)	Deaths 2000 (Projected) Number ('000s)	Rate (per 100 000)
Males										
0-4	1	1.6	1	2.4	2.5	2.9	0	0.1	0	0.1
5-14	3	3.2	7	8.0	10.0	3.0	0	0.4	0	0.2
15-44	8	4.8	22	14.0	29.7	3.0	1	0.5	0	0.2
45-59	0	1.2	2	5.9	52.3	2.8	0	0.2	0	0.1
60+	0	0.9	1	2.7	69.6	2.3	0	0.2	0	0.2
All ages	12	3.4	33	9.6	25.0	3.0	1	0.4	1	0.2
Females										
0-4	0	1.1	1	1.7	2.5	2.9	0	0.1	0	0.0
5-14	2	2.2	4	5.5	10.0	3.0	0	0.2	0	0.1
15-44	5	3.2	15	9.5	29.8	3.0	0	0.3	0	0.1
45-59	0	0.8	1	3.9	52.3	2.9	0	0.2	0	0.1
60+	0	0.6	0	1.8	70.3	2.3	0	0.1	0	0.1
All ages	8	2.3	22	6.5	25.3	3.0	1	0.2	0	0.1
Total	19	2.8	55	8.0	25.1	3.0	2	0.3	1	0.1

Table 78f SSA - ASS - ASS — Leishmaniasis - Visceral

Age group (years)	Incidence 1990 Number ('000s)	Rate (per 100 000)	Prevalence 1990 Number ('000s)	Rate (per 100 000)	Avg. age at onset (years)	Average duration (years)	Deaths 1990 Number ('000s)	Rate (per 100 000)	Deaths 2000 (Projected) Number ('000s)	Rate (per 100 000)
Males										
0-4	4	8.9	8	16.2	2.4	4.7	0	0.6	0	0.4
5-14	26	36.6	84	119.3	10.0	5.1	3	4.9	2	2.6
15-44	20	19.5	119	114.9	29.4	5.0	3	2.7	2	1.3
45-59	0	0.4	10	49.3	52.2	4.3	0	1.5	0	0.8
60+	0	0.0	1	5.9	-	-	0	0.4	0	0.2
All ages	50	19.9	221	87.7	17.2	5.0	7	2.7	5	1.4
Females										
0-4	2	4.3	4	7.9	2.4	4.7	0	0.3	0	0.2
5-14	13	18.5	42	59.9	10.0	5.1	2	2.5	1	1.3
15-44	10	9.9	61	57.6	29.5	5.0	2	1.7	1	0.7
45-59	0	2.0	5	24.5	52.2	4.4	0	0.7	0	0.4
60+	0	0.0	0	2.8	-	-	0	0.2	0	0.1
All ages	26	10.0	113	43.6	18.0	5.0	4	1.5	2	0.7
Total	76	14.9	334	65.4	17.5	5.0	11	2.1	7	1.1

For epidemiological sources see Desjeux 1996. For the methods used to estimate and project incidence, prevalence, and deaths see Murray and Lopez 1996a. See explanatory notes for definitions and caveats.

Table 78	Cuadro 78	Tableau 78
Leishmaniasis	**Leishmaniasis**	**Leishmaniose**
Visceral	Visceral	Viscerale

Table 78g LAC - ALC - ALC — Leishmaniasis - Visceral

Age group (years)	Incidence 1990 Number ('000s)	Rate (per 100 000)	Prevalence 1990 Number ('000s)	Rate (per 100 000)	Avg. age at onset (years)	Average duration (years)	Deaths 1990 Number ('000s)	Rate (per 100 000)	Deaths 2000 (Projected) Number ('000s)	Rate (per 100 000)
Males										
0-4	3	9.8	4	15.2	2.5	2.9	0	0.6	*0*	*0.4*
5-14	1	1.5	5	10.2	10.0	3.0	0	0.3	*0*	*0.2*
15-44	0	0.3	1	1.4	29.8	3.0	0	0.1	*0*	*0.0*
45-59	0	0.0	0	0.2	-	-	0	0.0	*0*	*0.0*
60+	0	0.0	0	0.0	-	-	0	0.0	*0*	*0.0*
All ages	4	1.8	11	5.1	6.3	3.0	0	0.2	*0*	*0.1*
Females										
0-4	2	6.4	3	9.9	2.5	3.0	0	0.4	*0*	*0.2*
5-14	1	1.0	3	6.7	10.0	3.0	0	0.2	*0*	*0.1*
15-44	0	0.2	1	0.9	29.9	3.0	0	0.0	*0*	*0.0*
45-59	0	0.0	0	0.1	-	-	0	0.0	*0*	*0.0*
60+	0	0.0	0	0.0	-	-	0	0.0	*0*	*0.0*
All ages	3	1.1	7	3.2	6.4	3.0	0	0.1	*0*	*0.1*
Total	6	1.5	18	4.1	6.4	3.0	1	0.1	*0*	*0.1*

Table 78h MEC - AOM - CMO — Leishmaniasis - Visceral

Age group (years)	Incidence 1990 Number ('000s)	Rate (per 100 000)	Prevalence 1990 Number ('000s)	Rate (per 100 000)	Avg. age at onset (years)	Average duration (years)	Deaths 1990 Number ('000s)	Rate (per 100 000)	Deaths 2000 (Projected) Number ('000s)	Rate (per 100 000)
Males										
0-4	7	16.9	11	25.9	2.5	2.9	0	1.0	*0*	*0.8*
5-14	3	4.6	14	21.8	10.0	3.0	1	0.9	*0*	*0.5*
15-44	0	0.4	3	2.5	29.8	3.0	0	0.1	*0*	*0.0*
45-59	0	0.0	0	0.2	-	-	0	0.0	*0*	*0.0*
60+	0	0.0	0	0.0	-	-	0	0.0	*0*	*0.0*
All ages	10	4.0	28	10.8	5.7	2.9	1	0.4	*1*	*0.3*
Females										
0-4	5	11.8	7	18.1	2.5	2.9	0	0.7	*0*	*0.5*
5-14	2	3.2	9	15.1	10.0	3.0	0	0.7	*0*	*0.4*
15-44	0	0.3	2	1.7	29.8	3.0	0	0.1	*0*	*0.0*
45-59	0	0.0	0	0.2	-	-	0	0.0	*0*	*0.0*
60+	0	0.0	0	0.0	-	-	0	0.0	*0*	*0.0*
All ages	7	2.8	18	7.5	5.7	2.9	1	0.3	*1*	*0.2*
Total	17	3.4	46	9.2	5.7	2.9	2	0.4	*1*	*0.2*

Table 78i World - Mundo - Monde — Leishmaniasis - Visceral

Age group (years)	Incidence 1990 Number ('000s)	Rate (per 100 000)	Prevalence 1990 Number ('000s)	Rate (per 100 000)	Avg. age at onset (years)	Average duration (years)	Deaths 1990 Number ('000s)	Rate (per 100 000)	Deaths 2000 (Projected) Number ('000s)	Rate (per 100 000)
Males										
0-4	38	11.8	60	18.5	2.5	3.1	2	0.7	*2*	*0.5*
5-14	97	17.7	279	50.6	10.0	3.6	12	2.2	*7*	*1.1*
15-44	112	8.9	411	32.9	29.7	3.4	14	1.1	*8*	*0.5*
45-59	3	1.1	31	10.0	52.3	2.9	1	0.4	*1*	*0.2*
60+	3	1.4	8	3.9	69.7	2.3	1	0.3	*1*	*0.2*
All ages	253	9.5	789	29.8	18.8	3.4	31	1.2	*17*	*0.6*
Females										
0-4	25	8.0	39	12.4	2.5	3.0	2	0.5	*1*	*0.3*
5-14	61	11.6	172	32.7	10.0	3.5	8	1.5	*4*	*0.7*
15-44	70	5.9	252	21.1	29.8	3.3	9	0.7	*4*	*0.3*
45-59	3	0.9	20	6.5	52.4	3.2	1	0.2	*0*	*0.1*
60+	2	0.8	6	2.2	70.2	2.3	0	0.2	*0*	*0.1*
All ages	161	6.1	489	18.7	19.0	3.3	20	0.7	*10*	*0.3*
Total	414	7.9	1 278	24.3	18.9	3.4	50	1.0	*28*	*0.4*

For epidemiological sources see Desjeux 1996. For the methods used to estimate and project incidence, prevalence, and deaths see Murray and Lopez 1996a. See explanatory notes for definitions and caveats.

Table 79	Cuadro 79	Tableau 79
Leishmaniasis	Leishmaniasis	Leishmaniose
Cutaneous	Cutánea	Cutanée

Table 79a — EME - PEMC - EMBE — Leishmaniasis - Cutaneous

Age group (years)	Incidence 1990 Number ('000s)	Rate (per 100 000)	Prevalence 1990 Number ('000s)	Rate (per 100 000)	Avg. age at onset (years)	Average duration (years)	Deaths 1990 Number ('000s)	Rate (per 100 000)	Deaths 2000 (Projected) Number ('000s)	Rate (per 100 000)
Males										
0-4	0	0	0	0	-	-	0	0	0	0
5-14	0	0	0	0	-	-	0	0	0	0
15-44	0	0	0	0	-	-	0	0	0	0
45-59	0	0	0	0	-	-	0	0	0	0
60+	0	0	0	0	-	-	0	0	0	0
All ages	0	0	0	0	-	-	0	0	0	0
Females										
0-4	0	0	0	0	-	-	0	0	0	0
5-14	0	0	0	0	-	-	0	0	0	0
15-44	0	0	0	0	-	-	0	0	0	0
45-59	0	0	0	0	-	-	0	0	0	0
60+	0	0	0	0	-	-	0	0	0	0
All ages	0	0	0	0	-	-	0	0	0	0
Total	0	0	0	0	-	-	0	0	0	0

Table 79b — FSE - PEAS - AESE — Leishmaniasis - Cutaneous

Age group (years)	Incidence 1990 Number ('000s)	Rate (per 100 000)	Prevalence 1990 Number ('000s)	Rate (per 100 000)	Avg. age at onset (years)	Average duration (years)	Deaths 1990 Number ('000s)	Rate (per 100 000)	Deaths 2000 (Projected) Number ('000s)	Rate (per 100 000)
Males										
0-4	0	0	0	0	-	-	0	0	0	0
5-14	0	0	0	0	-	-	0	0	0	0
15-44	0	0	0	0	-	-	0	0	0	0
45-59	0	0	0	0	-	-	0	0	0	0
60+	0	0	0	0	-	-	0	0	0	0
All ages	0	0	0	0	-	-	0	0	0	0
Females										
0-4	0	0	0	0	-	-	0	0	0	0
5-14	0	0	0	0	-	-	0	0	0	0
15-44	0	0	0	0	-	-	0	0	0	0
45-59	0	0	0	0	-	-	0	0	0	0
60+	0	0	0	0	-	-	0	0	0	0
All ages	0	0	0	0	-	-	0	0	0	0
Total	0	0	0	0	-	-	0	0	0	0

Table 79c — India - India - Inde — Leishmaniasis - Cutaneous

Age group (years)	Incidence 1990 Number ('000s)	Rate (per 100 000)	Prevalence 1990 Number ('000s)	Rate (per 100 000)	Avg. age at onset (years)	Average duration (years)	Deaths 1990 Number ('000s)	Rate (per 100 000)	Deaths 2000 (Projected) Number ('000s)	Rate (per 100 000)
Males										
0-4	0	0	0	0	-	-	0	0	0	0
5-14	0	0	0	0	-	-	0	0	0	0
15-44	0	0	0	0	-	-	0	0	0	0
45-59	0	0	0	0	-	-	0	0	0	0
60+	0	0	0	0	-	-	0	0	0	0
All ages	0	0	0	0	-	-	0	0	0	0
Females										
0-4	0	0	0	0	-	-	0	0	0	0
5-14	0	0	0	0	-	-	0	0	0	0
15-44	0	0	0	0	-	-	0	0	0	0
45-59	0	0	0	0	-	-	0	0	0	0
60+	0	0	0	0	-	-	0	0	0	0
All ages	0	0	0	0	-	-	0	0	0	0
Total	0	0	0	0	-	-	0	0	0	0

For epidemiological sources see Desjeux 1996. For the methods used to estimate and project incidence, prevalence, and deaths see Murray and Lopez 1996a. See explanatory notes for definitions and caveats.

Table 79
Leishmaniasis

Cuadro 79
Leishmaniasis

Tableau 79
Leishmaniose

Cutaneous　　　　　　　　　　　　　Cutánea　　　　　　　　　　　　　Cutanée

Table 79d　　　China - China - Chine　　　　　　　　　　Leishmaniasis - Cutaneous

Age group (years)	Incidence 1990 Number ('000s)	Rate (per 100 000)	Prevalence 1990 Number ('000s)	Rate (per 100 000)	Avg. age at onset (years)	Average duration (years)	Deaths 1990 Number ('000s)	Rate (per 100 000)	Deaths 2000 (Projected) Number ('000s)	Rate (per 100 000)
Males										
0-4	0	0	0	0	-	-	0	0	0	0
5-14	0	0	0	0	-	-	0	0	0	0
15-44	0	0	0	0	-	-	0	0	0	0
45-59	0	0	0	0	-	-	0	0	0	0
60+	0	0	0	0	-	-	0	0	0	0
All ages	0	0	0	0	-	-	0	0	0	0
Females										
0-4	0	0	0	0	-	-	0	0	0	0
5-14	0	0	0	0	-	-	0	0	0	0
15-44	0	0	0	0	-	-	0	0	0	0
45-59	0	0	0	0	-	-	0	0	0	0
60+	0	0	0	0	-	-	0	0	0	0
All ages	0	0	0	0	-	-	0	0	0	0
Total	0	0	0	0	-	-	0	0	0	0

Table 79e　　　OAI - OPAI - APAI　　　　　　　　　　Leishmaniasis - Cutaneous

Age group (years)	Incidence 1990 Number ('000s)	Rate (per 100 000)	Prevalence 1990 Number ('000s)	Rate (per 100 000)	Avg. age at onset (years)	Average duration (years)	Deaths 1990 Number ('000s)	Rate (per 100 000)	Deaths 2000 (Projected) Number ('000s)	Rate (per 100 000)
Males										
0-4	0	0	0	0	-	-	0	0	0	0
5-14	0	0	0	0	-	-	0	0	0	0
15-44	0	0	0	0	-	-	0	0	0	0
45-59	0	0	0	0	-	-	0	0	0	0
60+	0	0	0	0	-	-	0	0	0	0
All ages	0	0	0	0	-	-	0	0	0	0
Females										
0-4	0	0	0	0	-	-	0	0	0	0
5-14	0	0	0	0	-	-	0	0	0	0
15-44	0	0	0	0	-	-	0	0	0	0
45-59	0	0	0	0	-	-	0	0	0	0
60+	0	0	0	0	-	-	0	0	0	0
All ages	0	0	0	0	-	-	0	0	0	0
Total	0	0	0	0	-	-	0	0	0	0

Table 79f　　　SSA - ASS - ASS　　　　　　　　　　Leishmaniasis - Cutaneous

Age group (years)	Incidence 1990 Number ('000s)	Rate (per 100 000)	Prevalence 1990 Number ('000s)	Rate (per 100 000)	Avg. age at onset (years)	Average duration (years)	Deaths 1990 Number ('000s)	Rate (per 100 000)	Deaths 2000 (Projected) Number ('000s)	Rate (per 100 000)
Males										
0-4	0	0.4	0	0.3	2.4	1.0	0	0	0	0
5-14	1	1.3	1	1.2	10.0	1.0	0	0	0	0
15-44	2	1.5	2	1.5	29.4	1.0	0	0	0	0
45-59	0	0.2	0	0.3	52.2	1.0	0	0	0	0
60+	0	0.5	0	0.5	69.2	1.0	0	0	0	0
All ages	3	1.1	3	1.0	22.3	1.0	0	0	0	0
Females										
0-4	0	0.3	0	0.3	2.4	1.0	0	0	0	0
5-14	1	1.0	1	1.0	10.0	1.0	0	0	0	0
15-44	1	1.2	1	1.2	29.5	1.0	0	0	0	0
45-59	0	0.1	0	0.2	52.2	1.0	0	0	0	0
60+	0	0.4	0	0.4	69.7	1.0	0	0	0	0
All ages	2	0.9	2	0.8	22.7	1.0	0	0	0	0
Total	5	1.0	5	0.9	22.5	1.0	0	0	0	0

For epidemiological sources see Desjeux 1996. For the methods used to estimate and project incidence, prevalence, and deaths see Murray and Lopez 1996a. See explanatory notes for definitions and caveats.

Table 79	Cuadro 79	Tableau 79
Leishmaniasis	**Leishmaniasis**	**Leishmaniose**
Cutaneous	Cutánea	Cutanée

Table 79g LAC - ALC - ALC Leishmaniasis - Cutaneous

Age group (years)	Incidence 1990 Number ('000s)	Rate (per 100 000)	Prevalence 1990 Number ('000s)	Rate (per 100 000)	Avg. age at onset (years)	Average duration (years)	Deaths 1990 Number ('000s)	Rate (per 100 000)	Deaths 2000 (Projected) Number ('000s)	Rate (per 100 000)
Males										
0-4	8	28.1	12	43	2.5	3.0	0	0	0	0
5-14	48	91.8	114	218	10.0	3.0	0	0	0	0
15-44	145	139.0	423	406	29.8	3.0	0	0	0	0
45-59	17	74.7	59	266	52.3	3.0	0	0	0	0
60+	6	39.7	20	138	70.3	3.0	0	0	0	0
All ages	223	100.7	628	283	27.3	3.0	0	0	0	0
Females										
0-4	2	6.9	3	11	2.5	3.0	0	0	0	0
5-14	11	22.5	27	53	10.0	3.0	0	0	0	0
15-44	35	34.0	103	99	29.8	3.0	0	0	0	0
45-59	4	18.2	15	65	52.4	3.0	0	0	0	0
60+	2	9.6	6	33	71.1	3.0	0	0	0	0
All ages	55	24.5	154	69	27.7	3.0	0	0	0	0
Total	278	62.5	782	176	27.4	3.0	0	0	0	0

Table 79h MEC - AOM - CMO Leishmaniasis - Cutaneous

Age group (years)	Incidence 1990 Number ('000s)	Rate (per 100 000)	Prevalence 1990 Number ('000s)	Rate (per 100 000)	Avg. age at onset (years)	Average duration (years)	Deaths 1990 Number ('000s)	Rate (per 100 000)	Deaths 2000 (Projected) Number ('000s)	Rate (per 100 000)
Males										
0-4	155	378	166	404	2.5	1.5	0	0	0	0
5-14	380	581	541	828	10.0	1.5	0	0	0	0
15-44	181	159	308	271	29.8	1.5	0	0	0	0
45-59	18	79	29	131	52.3	1.5	0	0	0	0
60+	11	83	17	124	69.7	1.5	0	0	0	0
All ages	745	291	1 062	414	15.2	1.5	0	0	0	0
Females										
0-4	105	263	112	281	2.5	1.5	0	0	0	0
5-14	251	405	358	577	10.0	1.5	0	0	0	0
15-44	119	111	203	189	29.8	1.5	0	0	0	0
45-59	12	55	20	91	52.3	1.5	0	0	0	0
60+	9	58	13	86	70.4	1.5	0	0	0	0
All ages	496	201	706	286	15.3	1.5	0	0	0	0
Total	1 241	247	1 768	351	15.2	1.5	0	0	0	0

Table 79i World - Mundo - Monde Leishmaniasis - Cutaneous

Age group (years)	Incidence 1990 Number ('000s)	Rate (per 100 000)	Prevalence 1990 Number ('000s)	Rate (per 100 000)	Avg. age at onset (years)	Average duration (years)	Deaths 1990 Number ('000s)	Rate (per 100 000)	Deaths 2000 (Projected) Number ('000s)	Rate (per 100 000)
Males										
0-4	164	50.9	179	55.6	2.5	1.6	0	0	0	0
5-14	428	77.7	655	118.9	10.0	1.7	0	0	0	0
15-44	328	26.2	733	58.6	29.8	2.2	0	0	0	0
45-59	34	11.0	89	28.3	52.3	2.2	0	0	0	0
60+	17	7.8	37	16.8	69.9	2.0	0	0	0	0
All ages	971	36.6	1 692	63.8	18.0	1.8	0	0	0	0
Females										
0-4	107	34.5	115	37.1	2.5	1.5	0	0	0	0
5-14	263	50.1	386	73.4	10.0	1.6	0	0	0	0
15-44	156	13.0	307	25.6	29.8	1.8	0	0	0	0
45-59	17	5.3	35	11.4	52.3	1.9	0	0	0	0
60+	11	3.9	19	7.0	70.5	1.7	0	0	0	0
All ages	553	21.1	862	33.0	16.6	1.6	0	0	0	0
Total	1 523	28.9	2 554	48.5	17.4	1.8	0	0	0	0

For epidemiological sources see Desjeux 1996. For the methods used to estimate and project incidence, prevalence, and deaths see Murray and Lopez 1996a. See explanatory notes for definitions and caveats.

Table 80
Lymphatic filariasis

Cuadro 80
Filariasis linfática

Tableau 80
Filariose lymphatique

Hydrocele > 15 cm   Hidrocele > 15 cm   Hydrocèle > 15 cm

Table 80a   EME - PEMC - EMBE   Lymphatic filariasis - Hydrocele > 15 cm

Age group (years)	Incidence 1990 Number ('000s)	Rate (per 100 000)	Prevalence 1990 Number ('000s)	Rate (per 100 000)	Avg. age at onset (years)	Average duration (years)	Deaths 1990 Number ('000s)	Rate (per 100 000)	Deaths 2000 (Projected) Number ('000s)	Rate (per 100 000)
Males										
0-4	0	0	0	0	-	-	0	0	0	0
5-14	0	0	0	0	-	-	0	0	0	0
15-44	0	0	0	0	-	-	0	0	0	0
45-59	0	0	0	0	-	-	0	0	0	0
60+	0	0	0	0	-	-	0	0	0	0
All ages	0	0	0	0	-	-	0	0	0	0
Females										
0-4	0	0	0	0	-	-	0	0	0	0
5-14	0	0	0	0	-	-	0	0	0	0
15-44	0	0	0	0	-	-	0	0	0	0
45-59	0	0	0	0	-	-	0	0	0	0
60+	0	0	0	0	-	-	0	0	0	0
All ages	0	0	0	0	-	-	0	0	0	0
Total	0	0	0	0	-	-	0	0	0	0

Table 80b   FSE - PEAS - AESE   Lymphatic filariasis - Hydrocele > 15 cm

Age group (years)	Incidence 1990 Number ('000s)	Rate (per 100 000)	Prevalence 1990 Number ('000s)	Rate (per 100 000)	Avg. age at onset (years)	Average duration (years)	Deaths 1990 Number ('000s)	Rate (per 100 000)	Deaths 2000 (Projected) Number ('000s)	Rate (per 100 000)
Males										
0-4	0	0	0	0	-	-	0	0	0	0
5-14	0	0	0	0	-	-	0	0	0	0
15-44	0	0	0	0	-	-	0	0	0	0
45-59	0	0	0	0	-	-	0	0	0	0
60+	0	0	0	0	-	-	0	0	0	0
All ages	0	0	0	0	-	-	0	0	0	0
Females										
0-4	0	0	0	0	-	-	0	0	0	0
5-14	0	0	0	0	-	-	0	0	0	0
15-44	0	0	0	0	-	-	0	0	0	0
45-59	0	0	0	0	-	-	0	0	0	0
60+	0	0	0	0	-	-	0	0	0	0
All ages	0	0	0	0	-	-	0	0	0	0
Total	0	0	0	0	-	-	0	0	0	0

Table 80c   India - India - Inde   Lymphatic filariasis - Hydrocele > 15 cm

Age group (years)	Incidence 1990 Number ('000s)	Rate (per 100 000)	Prevalence 1990 Number ('000s)	Rate (per 100 000)	Avg. age at onset (years)	Average duration (years)	Deaths 1990 Number ('000s)	Rate (per 100 000)	Deaths 2000 (Projected) Number ('000s)	Rate (per 100 000)
Males										
0-4	9	14	21	35	2.5	59.9	0	0	0	0
5-14	162	159	886	871	10.0	57.5	0	0	0	0
15-44	260	130	7 210	3 596	29.8	40.0	0	0	0	0
45-59	26	55	2 837	5 964	52.3	21.0	0	0	0	0
60+	6	19	1 956	6 570	69.7	9.7	0	0	0	0
All ages	463	105	12 910	2 938	24.1	45.0	0	0	0	0
Females										
0-4	0	0	0	0	-	-	0	0	0	0
5-14	0	0	0	0	-	-	0	0	0	0
15-44	0	0	0	0	-	-	0	0	0	0
45-59	0	0	0	0	-	-	0	0	0	0
60+	0	0	0	0	-	-	0	0	0	0
All ages	0	0	0	0	-	-	0	0	0	0
Total	463	54	12 910	1 520	24.1	45.0	0	0	0	0

For epidemiological sources see Michael and Bundy 1996. For the methods used to estimate and project incidence, prevalence, and deaths see Murray and Lopez 1996a. See explanatory notes for definitions and caveats.

Table 80	Cuadro 80	Tableau 80
Lymphatic filariasis	**Filariasis linfática**	**Filariose lymphatique**
Hydrocele > 15 cm	Hidrocele > 15 cm	Hydrocèle > 15 cm

Table 80d   China - China - Chine

Lymphatic filariasis - Hydrocele > 15 cm

Age group (years)	Incidence 1990 Number ('000s)	Rate (per 100 000)	Prevalence 1990 Number ('000s)	Rate (per 100 000)	Avg. age at onset (years)	Average duration (years)	Deaths 1990 Number ('000s)	Rate (per 100 000)	Deaths 2000 (Projected) Number ('000s)	Rate (per 100 000)
Males										
0-4	2	3.4	5	8.3	2.5	65.5	0	0	0	0
5-14	6	6.4	47	48.6	10.0	59.9	0	0	0	0
15-44	48	15.5	955	311.8	29.9	41.4	0	0	0	0
45-59	5	6.4	431	593.4	52.3	21.4	0	0	0	0
60+	2	4.8	337	688.8	69.8	9.9	0	0	0	0
All ages	63	10.7	1 776	303.5	30.2	41.3	0	0	0	0
Females										
0-4	0	0	0	0	-	-	0	0	0	0
5-14	0	0	0	0	-	-	0	0	0	0
15-44	0	0	0	0	-	-	0	0	0	0
45-59	0	0	0	0	-	-	0	0	0	0
60+	0	0	0	0	-	-	0	0	0	0
All ages	0	0	0	0	-	-	0	0	0	0
Total	63	5.5	1 776	156.7	30.2	41.3	0	0	0	0

Table 80e   OAI - OPAI - APAI

Lymphatic filariasis - Hydrocele > 15 cm

Age group (years)	Incidence 1990 Number ('000s)	Rate (per 100 000)	Prevalence 1990 Number ('000s)	Rate (per 100 000)	Avg. age at onset (years)	Average duration (years)	Deaths 1990 Number ('000s)	Rate (per 100 000)	Deaths 2000 (Projected) Number ('000s)	Rate (per 100 000)
Males										
0-4	2	4.7	5	11	2.5	59.8	0	0	0	0
5-14	24	28.5	139	166	10.0	56.2	0	0	0	0
15-44	45	28.2	1 164	724	29.7	38.8	0	0	0	0
45-59	5	14.8	430	1 261	52.3	20.3	0	0	0	0
60+	2	11.8	301	1 489	69.6	9.7	0	0	0	0
All ages	79	22.9	2 040	595	25.7	42.5	0	0	0	0
Females										
0-4	0	0	0	0	-	-	0	0	0	0
5-14	0	0	0	0	-	-	0	0	0	0
15-44	0	0	0	0	-	-	0	0	0	0
45-59	0	0	0	0	-	-	0	0	0	0
60+	0	0	0	0	-	-	0	0	0	0
All ages	0	0	0	0	-	-	0	0	0	0
Total	79	11.5	2 040	299	25.7	42.5	0	0	0	0

Table 80f   SSA - ASS - ASS

Lymphatic filariasis - Hydrocele > 15 cm

Age group (years)	Incidence 1990 Number ('000s)	Rate (per 100 000)	Prevalence 1990 Number ('000s)	Rate (per 100 000)	Avg. age at onset (years)	Average duration (years)	Deaths 1990 Number ('000s)	Rate (per 100 000)	Deaths 2000 (Projected) Number ('000s)	Rate (per 100 000)
Males										
0-4	14	30	34	72	2.4	48.7	0	0	0	0
5-14	128	183	745	1 061	9.9	49.3	0	0	0	0
15-44	279	269	6 120	5 898	29.2	35.2	0	0	0	0
45-59	27	134	2 232	10 989	52.1	19.1	0	0	0	0
60+	7	70	1 332	12 678	69.2	9.3	0	0	0	0
All ages	456	181	10 463	4 147	24.9	38.2	0	0	0	0
Females										
0-4	0	0	0	0	-	-	0	0	0	0
5-14	0	0	0	0	-	-	0	0	0	0
15-44	0	0	0	0	-	-	0	0	0	0
45-59	0	0	0	0	-	-	0	0	0	0
60+	0	0	0	0	-	-	0	0	0	0
All ages	0	0	0	0	-	-	0	0	0	0
Total	456	89	10 463	2 051	24.9	38.2	0	0	0	0

For epidemiological sources see Michael and Bundy 1996. For the methods used to estimate and project incidence, prevalence, and deaths see Murray and Lopez 1996a. See explanatory notes for definitions and caveats.

Table 80
Lymphatic filariasis

Cuadro 80
Filariasis linfática

Tableau 80
Filariose lymphatique

Hydrocele > 15 cm

Hidrocele > 15 cm

Hydrocèle > 15 cm

Table 80g LAC - ALC - ALC — Lymphatic filariasis - Hydrocele > 15 cm

Age group (years)	Incidence 1990 Number ('000s)	Rate (per 100 000)	Prevalence 1990 Number ('000s)	Rate (per 100 000)	Avg. age at onset (years)	Average duration (years)	Deaths 1990 Number ('000s)	Rate (per 100 000)	Deaths 2000 (Projected) Number ('000s)	Rate (per 100 000)
Males										
0-4	0	0.3	0	0.7	2.5	63.9	0	0	0	0
5-14	1	1.3	4	7.7	10.0	59.3	0	0	0	0
15-44	1	1.0	30	28.8	29.8	41.4	0	0	0	0
45-59	1	2.6	14	62.9	52.3	22.3	0	0	0	0
60+	0	0.3	12	85.4	70.3	10.4	0	0	0	0
All ages	2	1.1	60	27.3	29.5	42.0	0	0	0	0
Females										
0-4	0	0	0	0	-	-	0	0	0	0
5-14	0	0	0	0	-	-	0	0	0	0
15-44	0	0	0	0	-	-	0	0	0	0
45-59	0	0	0	0	-	-	0	0	0	0
60+	0	0	0	0	-	-	0	0	0	0
All ages	0	0	0	0	-	-	0	0	0	0
Total	2	0.5	60	13.6	29.5	42.0	0	0	0	0

Table 80h MEC - AOM - CMO — Lymphatic filariasis - Hydrocele > 15 cm

Age group (years)	Incidence 1990 Number ('000s)	Rate (per 100 000)	Prevalence 1990 Number ('000s)	Rate (per 100 000)	Avg. age at onset (years)	Average duration (years)	Deaths 1990 Number ('000s)	Rate (per 100 000)	Deaths 2000 (Projected) Number ('000s)	Rate (per 100 000)
Males										
0-4	0	0.1	0	0.2	2.5	61.1	0	0	0	0
5-14	0	0.2	1	1.6	10.0	58.1	0	0	0	0
15-44	2	1.9	36	31.6	29.8	40.0	0	0	0	0
45-59	0	0.8	15	67.0	52.3	20.8	0	0	0	0
60+	0	0.8	11	81.0	69.7	9.8	0	0	0	0
All ages	3	1.1	63	24.6	31.4	38.8	0	0	0	0
Females										
0-4	0	0	0	0	-	-	0	0	0	0
5-14	0	0	0	0	-	-	0	0	0	0
15-44	0	0	0	0	-	-	0	0	0	0
45-59	0	0	0	0	-	-	0	0	0	0
60+	0	0	0	0	-	-	0	0	0	0
All ages	0	0	0	0	-	-	0	0	0	0
Total	3	0.5	63	12.6	31.4	38.8	0	0	0	0

Table 80i World - Mundo - Monde — Lymphatic filariasis - Hydrocele > 15 cm

Age group (years)	Incidence 1990 Number ('000s)	Rate (per 100 000)	Prevalence 1990 Number ('000s)	Rate (per 100 000)	Avg. age at onset (years)	Average duration (years)	Deaths 1990 Number ('000s)	Rate (per 100 000)	Deaths 2000 (Projected) Number ('000s)	Rate (per 100 000)
Males										
0-4	27	8.4	66	20	2.4	54.4	0	0	0	0
5-14	321	58.2	1 823	331	10.0	54.1	0	0	0	0
15-44	636	50.9	15 515	1 241	29.5	37.9	0	0	0	0
45-59	64	20.4	5 959	1 908	52.2	20.2	0	0	0	0
60+	18	8.1	3 949	1 805	69.5	9.6	0	0	0	0
All ages	1 065	40.1	27 313	1 029	25.0	41.7	0	0	0	0
Females										
0-4	0	0	0	0	-	-	0	0	0	0
5-14	0	0	0	0	-	-	0	0	0	0
15-44	0	0	0	0	-	-	0	0	0	0
45-59	0	0	0	0	-	-	0	0	0	0
60+	0	0	0	0	-	-	0	0	0	0
All ages	0	0	0	0	-	-	0	0	0	0
Total	1 065	20.2	27 313	519	25.0	41.7	0	0	0	0

For epidemiological sources see Michael and Bundy 1996. For the methods used to estimate and project incidence, prevalence, and deaths see Murray and Lopez 1996a. See explanatory notes for definitions and caveats.

Table 81
Lymphatic filariasis

Cuadro 81
Filariasis linfática

Tableau 81
Filariose lymphatique

Bancroftian lymphoedema

Linfedema bancroftiano

Lymphoedème bancroftien

Table 81a — EME - PEMC - EMBE — Lymphatic filariasis - Bancroftian lymphoedema

Age group (years)	Incidence 1990 Number ('000s)	Rate (per 100 000)	Prevalence 1990 Number ('000s)	Rate (per 100 000)	Avg. age at onset (years)	Average duration (years)	Deaths 1990 Number ('000s)	Rate (per 100 000)	Deaths 2000 (Projected) Number ('000s)	Rate (per 100 000)
Males										
0-4	0	0	0	0	-	-	0	0	0	0
5-14	0	0	0	0	-	-	0	0	0	0
15-44	0	0	0	0	-	-	0	0	0	0
45-59	0	0	0	0	-	-	0	0	0	0
60+	0	0	0	0	-	-	0	0	0	0
All ages	0	0	0	0	-	-	0	0	0	0
Females										
0-4	0	0	0	0	-	-	0	0	0	0
5-14	0	0	0	0	-	-	0	0	0	0
15-44	0	0	0	0	-	-	0	0	0	0
45-59	0	0	0	0	-	-	0	0	0	0
60+	0	0	0	0	-	-	0	0	0	0
All ages	0	0	0	0	-	-	0	0	0	0
Total	0	0	0	0	-	-	0	0	0	0

Table 81b — FSE - PEAS - AESE — Lymphatic filariasis - Bancroftian lymphoedema

Age group (years)	Incidence 1990 Number ('000s)	Rate (per 100 000)	Prevalence 1990 Number ('000s)	Rate (per 100 000)	Avg. age at onset (years)	Average duration (years)	Deaths 1990 Number ('000s)	Rate (per 100 000)	Deaths 2000 (Projected) Number ('000s)	Rate (per 100 000)
Males										
0-4	0	0	0	0	-	-	0	0	0	0
5-14	0	0	0	0	-	-	0	0	0	0
15-44	0	0	0	0	-	-	0	0	0	0
45-59	0	0	0	0	-	-	0	0	0	0
60+	0	0	0	0	-	-	0	0	0	0
All ages	0	0	0	0	-	-	0	0	0	0
Females										
0-4	0	0	0	0	-	-	0	0	0	0
5-14	0	0	0	0	-	-	0	0	0	0
15-44	0	0	0	0	-	-	0	0	0	0
45-59	0	0	0	0	-	-	0	0	0	0
60+	0	0	0	0	-	-	0	0	0	0
All ages	0	0	0	0	-	-	0	0	0	0
Total	0	0	0	0	-	-	0	0	0	0

Table 81c — India - India - Inde — Lymphatic filariasis - Bancroftian lymphoedema

Age group (years)	Incidence 1990 Number ('000s)	Rate (per 100 000)	Prevalence 1990 Number ('000s)	Rate (per 100 000)	Avg. age at onset (years)	Average duration (years)	Deaths 1990 Number ('000s)	Rate (per 100 000)	Deaths 2000 (Projected) Number ('000s)	Rate (per 100 000)
Males										
0-4	8	13.0	19	32	2.5	59.9	0	0	0	0
5-14	19	18.4	159	157	10.0	57.4	0	0	0	0
15-44	59	29.4	1 371	684	29.7	39.9	0	0	0	0
45-59	11	22.7	617	1 297	52.3	21.0	0	0	0	0
60+	2	7.9	461	1 547	69.7	9.7	0	0	0	0
All ages	99	22.4	2 627	598	27.2	42.0	0	0	0	0
Females										
0-4	11	18.8	26	46	2.5	60.8	0	0	0	0
5-14	30	31.7	240	252	10.0	59.1	0	0	0	0
15-44	82	44.6	1 964	1 072	29.7	41.8	0	0	0	0
45-59	23	49.3	972	2 113	52.3	22.5	0	0	0	0
60+	6	22.4	786	2 716	70.1	10.2	0	0	0	0
All ages	152	37.0	3 988	972	29.0	42.3	0	0	0	0
Total	250	29.5	6 615	779	28.3	42.2	0	0	0	0

For epidemiological sources see Michael and Bundy 1996. For the methods used to estimate and project incidence, prevalence, and deaths see Murray and Lopez 1996a. See explanatory notes for definitions and caveats.

Table 81
Lymphatic filariasis

Cuadro 81
Filariasis linfática

Tableau 81
Filariose lymphatique

Bancroftian lymphoedema

Linfedema bancroftiano

Lymphoedème bancroftien

Table 81d		China - China - Chine					Lymphatic filariasis - Bancroftian lymphoedema		
Age group (years)	Incidence 1990		Prevalence 1990		Avg. age at onset (years)	Average duration (years)	Deaths 1990		Deaths 2000 (Projected)	
	Number ('000s)	Rate (per 100 000)	Number ('000s)	Rate (per 100 000)			Number ('000s)	Rate (per 100 000)	Number ('000s)	Rate (per 100 000)
Males										
0-4	0	0.1	0	0.3	2.5	65.5	0	0	0	0
5-14	0	0.3	2	2.1	10.0	59.9	0	0	0	0
15-44	2	0.5	34	11.1	29.9	41.2	0	0	0	0
45-59	0	0.1	14	19.9	52.3	21.4	0	0	0	0
60+	0	0.1	11	22.3	69.8	9.9	0	0	0	0
All ages	2	0.4	62	10.5	28.7	42.6	0	0	0	0
Females										
0-4	0	0.6	1	1.4	2.5	68.5	0	0	0	0
5-14	0	0.1	3	3.4	10.0	63.2	0	0	0	0
15-44	1	0.4	29	10.2	29.9	44.2	0	0	0	0
45-59	0	0.1	11	17.5	52.4	23.8	0	0	0	0
60+	0	0.1	10	19.7	70.6	10.8	0	0	0	0
All ages	2	0.3	54	9.9	26.1	47.7	0	0	0	0
Total	4	0.3	116	10.2	27.5	45.0	0	0	0	0

Table 81e		OAI - OPAI - APAI					Lymphatic filariasis - Bancroftian lymphoedema		
Age group (years)	Incidence 1990		Prevalence 1990		Avg. age at onset (years)	Average duration (years)	Deaths 1990		Deaths 2000 (Projected)	
	Number ('000s)	Rate (per 100 000)	Number ('000s)	Rate (per 100 000)			Number ('000s)	Rate (per 100 000)	Number ('000s)	Rate (per 100 000)
Males										
0-4	2	5.6	6	14	2.5	59.8	0	0	0	0
5-14	5	6.0	49	58	10.0	56.2	0	0	0	0
15-44	26	15.9	520	323	29.7	38.8	0	0	0	0
45-59	3	8.0	213	624	52.3	20.3	0	0	0	0
60+	1	4.0	146	724	69.6	9.7	0	0	0	0
All ages	37	10.7	934	272	27.7	40.6	0	0	0	0
Females										
0-4	3	7.8	8	19	2.5	63.2	0	0	0	0
5-14	6	7.8	62	78	10.0	59.2	0	0	0	0
15-44	20	12.5	481	302	29.8	41.5	0	0	0	0
45-59	3	9.9	198	565	52.3	22.4	0	0	0	0
60+	1	6.6	161	709	70.3	10.5	0	0	0	0
All ages	34	10.1	911	268	27.6	43.5	0	0	0	0
Total	71	10.4	1 845	270	27.7	42.0	0	0	0	0

Table 81f		SSA - ASS - ASS					Lymphatic filariasis - Bancroftian lymphoedema		
Age group (years)	Incidence 1990		Prevalence 1990		Avg. age at onset (years)	Average duration (years)	Deaths 1990		Deaths 2000 (Projected)	
	Number ('000s)	Rate (per 100 000)	Number ('000s)	Rate (per 100 000)			Number ('000s)	Rate (per 100 000)	Number ('000s)	Rate (per 100 000)
Males										
0-4	6	12.2	14	29.4	2.4	48.7	0	0	0	0
5-14	16	22.2	120	171.2	10.0	49.2	0	0	0	0
15-44	40	39.0	877	844.9	29.4	35.0	0	0	0	0
45-59	20	99.8	441	2 170.4	52.1	19.1	0	0	0	0
60+	1	8.7	318	3 029.5	69.2	9.3	0	0	0	0
All ages	83	32.9	1 770	701.5	29.9	34.5	0	0	0	0
Females										
0-4	19	41.4	47	100.1	2.4	51.9	0	0	0	0
5-14	29	41.0	286	410.2	10.0	51.9	0	0	0	0
15-44	48	45.5	1 357	1 277.1	29.4	37.2	0	0	0	0
45-59	33	150.3	680	3 075.7	52.2	20.5	0	0	0	0
60+	7	57.2	610	4 791.6	69.7	9.8	0	0	0	0
All ages	137	53.1	2 981	1 155.5	29.2	36.9	0	0	0	0
Total	220	43.1	4 751	931.0	29.4	36.0	0	0	0	0

For epidemiological sources see Michael and Bundy 1996. For the methods used to estimate and project incidence, prevalence, and deaths see Murray and Lopez 1996a. See explanatory notes for definitions and caveats.

Table 81	Cuadro 81	Tableau 81
Lymphatic filariasis	**Filariasis linfática**	**Filariose lymphatique**
Bancroftian lymphoedema	Linfedema bancroftiano	Lymphoedème bancroftien

Table 81g LAC - ALC - ALC Lymphatic filariasis - Bancroftian lymphoedema

Age group (years)	Incidence 1990 Number ('000s)	Rate (per 100 000)	Prevalence 1990 Number ('000s)	Rate (per 100 000)	Avg. age at onset (years)	Average duration (years)	Deaths 1990 Number ('000s)	Rate (per 100 000)	Deaths 2000 (Projected) Number ('000s)	Rate (per 100 000)
Males										
0-4	0	0.0	0	0.0	-	-	0	0	0	0
5-14	0	0.2	1	1.1	10.0	59.3	0	0	0	0
15-44	0	0.3	7	6.7	29.8	41.4	0	0	0	0
45-59	0	0.3	4	18.1	52.3	22.3	0	0	0	0
60+	0	0.2	4	27.0	70.3	10.4	0	0	0	0
All ages	1	0.2	15	7.0	30.7	41.1	0	0	0	0
Females										
0-4	0	0.3	0	0.7	2.5	67.9	0	0	0	0
5-14	0	0.1	1	2.1	10.0	63.0	0	0	0	0
15-44	0	0.3	7	6.7	29.9	44.6	0	0	0	0
45-59	0	0.9	4	17.5	52.4	24.8	0	0	0	0
60+	0	0.6	5	30.5	71.1	11.3	0	0	0	0
All ages	1	0.3	17	7.9	36.9	38.8	0	0	0	0
Total	1	0.3	33	7.4	34.3	39.8	0	0	0	0

Table 81h MEC - AOM - CMO Lymphatic filariasis - Bancroftian lymphoedema

Age group (years)	Incidence 1990 Number ('000s)	Rate (per 100 000)	Prevalence 1990 Number ('000s)	Rate (per 100 000)	Avg. age at onset (years)	Average duration (years)	Deaths 1990 Number ('000s)	Rate (per 100 000)	Deaths 2000 (Projected) Number ('000s)	Rate (per 100 000)
Males										
0-4	0	0.0	0	0.0	-	-	0	0	0	0
5-14	0	0.2	0	0.8	10.0	58.1	0	0	0	0
15-44	1	0.6	12	10.6	29.8	40.0	0	0	0	0
45-59	1	2.5	9	38.1	52.3	20.8	0	0	0	0
60+	0	0.0	8	57.5	69.7	9.8	0	0	0	0
All ages	1	0.5	29	11.3	37.7	33.4	0	0	0	0
Females										
0-4	0	0.2	0	0.4	2.5	63.7	0	0	0	0
5-14	0	0.2	1	1.8	10.0	60.9	0	0	0	0
15-44	1	0.6	12	11.3	29.8	42.6	0	0	0	0
45-59	0	1.1	6	28.2	52.3	22.9	0	0	0	0
60+	1	3.5	11	73.2	70.4	10.6	0	0	0	0
All ages	2	0.6	31	12.6	44.5	30.9	0	0	0	0
Total	3	0.6	60	11.9	41.4	32.0	0	0	0	0

Table 81i World - Mundo - Monde Lymphatic filariasis - Bancroftian lymphoedema

Age group (years)	Incidence 1990 Number ('000s)	Rate (per 100 000)	Prevalence 1990 Number ('000s)	Rate (per 100 000)	Avg. age at onset (years)	Average duration (years)	Deaths 1990 Number ('000s)	Rate (per 100 000)	Deaths 2000 (Projected) Number ('000s)	Rate (per 100 000)
Males										
0-4	16	5.0	39	12	2.5	52.7	0	0	0	0
5-14	40	7.2	332	60	10.0	56.9	0	0	0	0
15-44	128	10.2	2 820	226	29.8	39.3	0	0	0	0
45-59	35	11.0	1 298	415	52.3	20.1	0	0	0	0
60+	4	1.9	948	433	70.1	9.1	0	0	0	0
All ages	222	8.4	5 436	205	28.5	39.9	0	0	0	0
Females										
0-4	34	10.9	82	27	2.5	63.7	0	0	0	0
5-14	65	12.4	595	113	10.0	60.1	0	0	0	0
15-44	152	12.7	3 851	321	29.8	42.3	0	0	0	0
45-59	60	19.3	1 872	602	52.4	22.3	0	0	0	0
60+	16	5.9	1 583	588	71.2	9.6	0	0	0	0
All ages	327	12.5	7 983	305	29.2	42.8	0	0	0	0
Total	550	10.4	13 419	255	28.9	41.6	0	0	0	0

For epidemiological sources see Michael and Bundy 1996. For the methods used to estimate and project incidence, prevalence, and deaths see Murray and Lopez 1996a. See explanatory notes for definitions and caveats.

Table 82
Lymphatic filariasis

Cuadro 82
Filariasis linfática

Tableau 82
Filariose lymphatique

Brugian lymphoedema

Linfedema brugiano

Lymphoedème brugien

Table 82a — EME - PEMC - EMBE — Lymphatic filariasis - Brugian lymphoedema

Age group (years)	Incidence 1990 Number ('000s)	Incidence 1990 Rate (per 100 000)	Prevalence 1990 Number ('000s)	Prevalence 1990 Rate (per 100 000)	Avg. age at onset (years)	Average duration (years)	Deaths 1990 Number ('000s)	Deaths 1990 Rate (per 100 000)	Deaths 2000 (Projected) Number ('000s)	Deaths 2000 (Projected) Rate (per 100 000)
Males										
0-4	0	0	0	0	-	-	0	0	0	0
5-14	0	0	0	0	-	-	0	0	0	0
15-44	0	0	0	0	-	-	0	0	0	0
45-59	0	0	0	0	-	-	0	0	0	0
60+	0	0	0	0	-	-	0	0	0	0
All ages	0	0	0	0	-	-	0	0	0	0
Females										
0-4	0	0	0	0	-	-	0	0	0	0
5-14	0	0	0	0	-	-	0	0	0	0
15-44	0	0	0	0	-	-	0	0	0	0
45-59	0	0	0	0	-	-	0	0	0	0
60+	0	0	0	0	-	-	0	0	0	0
All ages	0	0	0	0	-	-	0	0	0	0
Total	0	0	0	0	-	-	0	0	0	0

Table 82b — FSE - PEAS - AESE — Lymphatic filariasis - Brugian lymphoedema

Age group (years)	Incidence 1990 Number ('000s)	Incidence 1990 Rate (per 100 000)	Prevalence 1990 Number ('000s)	Prevalence 1990 Rate (per 100 000)	Avg. age at onset (years)	Average duration (years)	Deaths 1990 Number ('000s)	Deaths 1990 Rate (per 100 000)	Deaths 2000 (Projected) Number ('000s)	Deaths 2000 (Projected) Rate (per 100 000)
Males										
0-4	0	0	0	0	-	-	0	0	0	0
5-14	0	0	0	0	-	-	0	0	0	0
15-44	0	0	0	0	-	-	0	0	0	0
45-59	0	0	0	0	-	-	0	0	0	0
60+	0	0	0	0	-	-	0	0	0	0
All ages	0	0	0	0	-	-	0	0	0	0
Females										
0-4	0	0	0	0	-	-	0	0	0	0
5-14	0	0	0	0	-	-	0	0	0	0
15-44	0	0	0	0	-	-	0	0	0	0
45-59	0	0	0	0	-	-	0	0	0	0
60+	0	0	0	0	-	-	0	0	0	0
All ages	0	0	0	0	-	-	0	0	0	0
Total	0	0	0	0	-	-	0	0	0	0

Table 82c — India - India - Inde — Lymphatic filariasis - Brugian lymphoedema

Age group (years)	Incidence 1990 Number ('000s)	Incidence 1990 Rate (per 100 000)	Prevalence 1990 Number ('000s)	Prevalence 1990 Rate (per 100 000)	Avg. age at onset (years)	Average duration (years)	Deaths 1990 Number ('000s)	Deaths 1990 Rate (per 100 000)	Deaths 2000 (Projected) Number ('000s)	Deaths 2000 (Projected) Rate (per 100 000)
Males										
0-4	1	1.2	2	3.0	2.5	59.9	0	0	0	0
5-14	3	3.0	22	21.2	10.0	57.4	0	0	0	0
15-44	10	4.7	213	106.3	29.7	39.9	0	0	0	0
45-59	11	23.9	168	353.5	52.3	21.0	0	0	0	0
60+	1	2.5	167	561.4	69.7	9.7	0	0	0	0
All ages	25	5.8	572	130.1	37.8	33.2	0	0	0	0
Females										
0-4	0	0.0	0	0.0	-	-	0	0	0	0
5-14	1	1.3	6	6.5	10.0	59.1	0	0	0	0
15-44	4	2.0	78	42.6	29.8	41.7	0	0	0	0
45-59	7	16.0	88	190.7	52.4	22.5	0	0	0	0
60+	2	6.0	108	372.9	70.1	10.2	0	0	0	0
All ages	14	3.4	280	68.2	44.9	29.2	0	0	0	0
Total	39	4.6	852	100.2	40.3	31.8	0	0	0	0

For epidemiological sources see Michael and Bundy 1996. For the methods used to estimate and project incidence, prevalence, and deaths see Murray and Lopez 1996a. See explanatory notes for definitions and caveats.

Table 82
Lymphatic filariasis

Brugian lymphoedema

Cuadro 82
Filariasis linfática

Linfedema brugiano

Tableau 82
Filariose lymphatique

Lymphoedème brugien

Table 82d China - China - Chine Lymphatic filariasis - Brugian lymphoedema

Age group (years)	Incidence 1990 Number ('000s)	Rate (per 100 000)	Prevalence 1990 Number ('000s)	Rate (per 100 000)	Avg. age at onset (years)	Average duration (years)	Deaths 1990 Number ('000s)	Rate (per 100 000)	Deaths 2000 (Projected) Number ('000s)	Rate (per 100 000)
Males										
0-4	0	0.7	1	1.7	2.5	65.5	0	0	0	0
5-14	2	2.0	13	13.5	10.0	59.9	0	0	0	0
15-44	13	4.2	262	85.6	29.9	41.2	0	0	0	0
45-59	0	0.6	111	153.1	52.3	21.4	0	0	0	0
60+	0	0.5	80	162.4	69.8	9.9	0	0	0	0
All ages	16	2.7	467	79.8	28.0	43.2	0	0	0	0
Females										
0-4	0	0.5	1	1.3	2.5	68.5	0	0	0	0
5-14	1	1.2	8	8.9	10.0	63.2	0	0	0	0
15-44	7	2.6	152	53.6	29.9	44.2	0	0	0	0
45-59	0	0.5	62	95.8	52.4	23.8	0	0	0	0
60+	0	0.3	53	102.4	70.6	10.8	0	0	0	0
All ages	9	1.7	276	50.2	27.9	46.1	0	0	0	0
Total	25	2.2	743	65.5	28.0	44.2	0	0	0	0

Table 82e OAI - OPAI - APAI Lymphatic filariasis - Brugian lymphoedema

Age group (years)	Incidence 1990 Number ('000s)	Rate (per 100 000)	Prevalence 1990 Number ('000s)	Rate (per 100 000)	Avg. age at onset (years)	Average duration (years)	Deaths 1990 Number ('000s)	Rate (per 100 000)	Deaths 2000 (Projected) Number ('000s)	Rate (per 100 000)
Males										
0-4	0	0.0	0	0.0	-	-	0	0	0	0
5-14	1	1.0	4	4.9	10.0	56.2	0	0	0	0
15-44	19	12.0	300	186.8	29.7	38.8	0	0	0	0
45-59	15	43.0	233	682.7	52.3	20.3	0	0	0	0
60+	2	11.0	226	1 119.9	69.6	9.7	0	0	0	0
All ages	37	10.8	764	222.7	40.6	30.1	0	0	0	0
Females										
0-4	0	0.0	0	0.0	-	-	0	0	0	0
5-14	0	0.5	2	2.5	10.0	59.2	0	0	0	0
15-44	8	5.2	130	81.5	29.8	41.5	0	0	0	0
45-59	13	35.7	148	422.7	52.3	22.4	0	0	0	0
60+	1	6.3	173	761.2	70.3	10.5	0	0	0	0
All ages	23	6.7	453	133.4	44.5	29.3	0	0	0	0
Total	60	8.7	1 217	178.3	42.1	29.8	0	0	0	0

Table 82f SSA - ASS - ASS Lymphatic filariasis - Brugian lymphoedema

Age group (years)	Incidence 1990 Number ('000s)	Rate (per 100 000)	Prevalence 1990 Number ('000s)	Rate (per 100 000)	Avg. age at onset (years)	Average duration (years)	Deaths 1990 Number ('000s)	Rate (per 100 000)	Deaths 2000 (Projected) Number ('000s)	Rate (per 100 000)
Males										
0-4	0	0	0	0	-	-	0	0	0	0
5-14	0	0	0	0	-	-	0	0	0	0
15-44	0	0	0	0	-	-	0	0	0	0
45-59	0	0	0	0	-	-	0	0	0	0
60+	0	0	0	0	-	-	0	0	0	0
All ages	0	0	0	0	-	-	0	0	0	0
Females										
0-4	0	0	0	0	-	-	0	0	0	0
5-14	0	0	0	0	-	-	0	0	0	0
15-44	0	0	0	0	-	-	0	0	0	0
45-59	0	0	0	0	-	-	0	0	0	0
60+	0	0	0	0	-	-	0	0	0	0
All ages	0	0	0	0	-	-	0	0	0	0
Total	0	0	0	0	-	-	0	0	0	0

For epidemiological sources see Michael and Bundy 1996. For the methods used to estimate and project incidence, prevalence, and deaths see Murray and Lopez 1996a. See explanatory notes for definitions and caveats.

Table 82
Lymphatic filariasis

Cuadro 82
Filariasis linfática

Tableau 82
Filariose lymphatique

Brugian lymphoedema

Linfedema brugiano

Lymphoedème brugien

Table 82g   **LAC - ALC - ALC**   Lymphatic filariasis - Brugian lymphoedema

Age group (years)	Incidence 1990 Number ('000s)	Rate (per 100 000)	Prevalence 1990 Number ('000s)	Rate (per 100 000)	Avg. age at onset (years)	Average duration (years)	Deaths 1990 Number ('000s)	Rate (per 100 000)	Deaths 2000 (Projected) Number ('000s)	Rate (per 100 000)
Males										
0-4	0	0	0	0	-	-	0	0	0	0
5-14	0	0	0	0	-	-	0	0	0	0
15-44	0	0	0	0	-	-	0	0	0	0
45-59	0	0	0	0	-	-	0	0	0	0
60+	0	0	0	0	-	-	0	0	0	0
All ages	0	0	0	0	-	-	0	0	0	0
Females										
0-4	0	0	0	0	-	-	0	0	0	0
5-14	0	0	0	0	-	-	0	0	0	0
15-44	0	0	0	0	-	-	0	0	0	0
45-59	0	0	0	0	-	-	0	0	0	0
60+	0	0	0	0	-	-	0	0	0	0
All ages	0	0	0	0	-	-	0	0	0	0
Total	0	0	0	0	-	-	0	0	0	0

Table 82h   **MEC - AOM - CMO**   Lymphatic filariasis - Brugian lymphoedema

Age group (years)	Incidence 1990 Number ('000s)	Rate (per 100 000)	Prevalence 1990 Number ('000s)	Rate (per 100 000)	Avg. age at onset (years)	Average duration (years)	Deaths 1990 Number ('000s)	Rate (per 100 000)	Deaths 2000 (Projected) Number ('000s)	Rate (per 100 000)
Males										
0-4	0	0	0	0	-	-	0	0	0	0
5-14	0	0	0	0	-	-	0	0	0	0
15-44	0	0	0	0	-	-	0	0	0	0
45-59	0	0	0	0	-	-	0	0	0	0
60+	0	0	0	0	-	-	0	0	0	0
All ages	0	0	0	0	-	-	0	0	0	0
Females										
0-4	0	0	0	0	-	-	0	0	0	0
5-14	0	0	0	0	-	-	0	0	0	0
15-44	0	0	0	0	-	-	0	0	0	0
45-59	0	0	0	0	-	-	0	0	0	0
60+	0	0	0	0	-	-	0	0	0	0
All ages	0	0	0	0	-	-	0	0	0	0
Total	0	0	0	0	-	-	0	0	0	0

Table 82i   **World - Mundo - Monde**   Lymphatic filariasis - Brugian lymphoedema

Age group (years)	Incidence 1990 Number ('000s)	Rate (per 100 000)	Prevalence 1990 Number ('000s)	Rate (per 100 000)	Avg. age at onset (years)	Average duration (years)	Deaths 1990 Number ('000s)	Rate (per 100 000)	Deaths 2000 (Projected) Number ('000s)	Rate (per 100 000)
Males										
0-4	1	0.4	3	0.9	2.5	61.9	0	0	0	0
5-14	6	1.1	39	7.0	10.0	58.1	0	0	0	0
15-44	42	3.3	776	62.1	29.8	39.8	0	0	0	0
45-59	26	8.5	512	164.1	52.3	20.6	0	0	0	0
60+	3	1.5	473	216.1	69.6	9.7	0	0	0	0
All ages	78	2.9	1 803	67.9	37.2	33.8	0	0	0	0
Females										
0-4	0	0.1	1	0.2	2.5	68.5	0	0	0	0
5-14	3	0.5	16	3.1	10.0	60.7	0	0	0	0
15-44	19	1.6	360	30.1	29.8	42.5	0	0	0	0
45-59	20	6.5	298	95.7	52.3	22.5	0	0	0	0
60+	3	1.2	333	123.8	70.2	10.3	0	0	0	0
All ages	46	1.8	1 008	38.6	41.3	32.6	0	0	0	0
Total	124	2.4	2 811	53.4	38.7	33.3	0	0	0	0

For epidemiological sources see Michael and Bundy 1996. For the methods used to estimate and project incidence, prevalence, and deaths see Murray and Lopez 1996a. See explanatory notes for definitions and caveats.

Table 83 / **Cuadro 83** / **Tableau 83**
Onchocerciasis / Oncocercosis / Onchocercose

Blindness / Ceguera / Cécité

Table 83a — EME - PEMC - EMBE — Onchocerciasis - Blindness

Age group (years)	Incidence 1990 Number ('000s)	Rate (per 100 000)	Prevalence 1990 Number ('000s)	Rate (per 100 000)	Avg. age at onset (years)	Average duration (years)	Deaths 1990 Number ('000s)	Rate (per 100 000)	Deaths 2000 (Projected) Number ('000s)	Rate (per 100 000)
Males										
0-4	0	0	0	0	-	-	0	0	0	0
5-14	0	0	0	0	-	-	0	0	0	0
15-44	0	0	0	0	-	-	0	0	0	0
45-59	0	0	0	0	-	-	0	0	0	0
60+	0	0	0	0	-	-	0	0	0	0
All ages	0	0	0	0	-	-	0	0	0	0
Females										
0-4	0	0	0	0	-	-	0	0	0	0
5-14	0	0	0	0	-	-	0	0	0	0
15-44	0	0	0	0	-	-	0	0	0	0
45-59	0	0	0	0	-	-	0	0	0	0
60+	0	0	0	0	-	-	0	0	0	0
All ages	0	0	0	0	-	-	0	0	0	0
Total	0	0	0	0	-	-	0	0	0	0

Table 83b — FSE - PEAS - AESE — Onchocerciasis - Blindness

Age group (years)	Incidence 1990 Number ('000s)	Rate (per 100 000)	Prevalence 1990 Number ('000s)	Rate (per 100 000)	Avg. age at onset (years)	Average duration (years)	Deaths 1990 Number ('000s)	Rate (per 100 000)	Deaths 2000 (Projected) Number ('000s)	Rate (per 100 000)
Males										
0-4	0	0	0	0	-	-	0	0	0	0
5-14	0	0	0	0	-	-	0	0	0	0
15-44	0	0	0	0	-	-	0	0	0	0
45-59	0	0	0	0	-	-	0	0	0	0
60+	0	0	0	0	-	-	0	0	0	0
All ages	0	0	0	0	-	-	0	0	0	0
Females										
0-4	0	0	0	0	-	-	0	0	0	0
5-14	0	0	0	0	-	-	0	0	0	0
15-44	0	0	0	0	-	-	0	0	0	0
45-59	0	0	0	0	-	-	0	0	0	0
60+	0	0	0	0	-	-	0	0	0	0
All ages	0	0	0	0	-	-	0	0	0	0
Total	0	0	0	0	-	-	0	0	0	0

Table 83c — India - India - Inde — Onchocerciasis - Blindness

Age group (years)	Incidence 1990 Number ('000s)	Rate (per 100 000)	Prevalence 1990 Number ('000s)	Rate (per 100 000)	Avg. age at onset (years)	Average duration (years)	Deaths 1990 Number ('000s)	Rate (per 100 000)	Deaths 2000 (Projected) Number ('000s)	Rate (per 100 000)
Males										
0-4	0	0	0	0	-	-	0	0	0	0
5-14	0	0	0	0	-	-	0	0	0	0
15-44	0	0	0	0	-	-	0	0	0	0
45-59	0	0	0	0	-	-	0	0	0	0
60+	0	0	0	0	-	-	0	0	0	0
All ages	0	0	0	0	-	-	0	0	0	0
Females										
0-4	0	0	0	0	-	-	0	0	0	0
5-14	0	0	0	0	-	-	0	0	0	0
15-44	0	0	0	0	-	-	0	0	0	0
45-59	0	0	0	0	-	-	0	0	0	0
60+	0	0	0	0	-	-	0	0	0	0
All ages	0	0	0	0	-	-	0	0	0	0
Total	0	0	0	0	-	-	0	0	0	0

For epidemiological sources see Remme 1996. For the methods used to estimate and project incidence, prevalence, and deaths see Murray and Lopez 1996a. See explanatory notes for definitions and caveats.

Table 83 — **Cuadro 83** — **Tableau 83**
Onchocerciasis — Oncocercosis — Onchocercose

Blindness — Ceguera — Cécité

Table 83d	China - China - Chine								Onchocerciasis - Blindness	

Age group (years)	Incidence 1990 Number ('000s)	Rate (per 100 000)	Prevalence 1990 Number ('000s)	Rate (per 100 000)	Avg. age at onset (years)	Average duration (years)	Deaths 1990 Number ('000s)	Rate (per 100 000)	Deaths 2000 (Projected) Number ('000s)	Rate (per 100 000)
Males										
0-4	0	0	0	0	-	-	0	0	0	0
5-14	0	0	0	0	-	-	0	0	0	0
15-44	0	0	0	0	-	-	0	0	0	0
45-59	0	0	0	0	-	-	0	0	0	0
60+	0	0	0	0	-	-	0	0	0	0
All ages	0	0	0	0	-	-	0	0	0	0
Females										
0-4	0	0	0	0	-	-	0	0	0	0
5-14	0	0	0	0	-	-	0	0	0	0
15-44	0	0	0	0	-	-	0	0	0	0
45-59	0	0	0	0	-	-	0	0	0	0
60+	0	0	0	0	-	-	0	0	0	0
All ages	0	0	0	0	-	-	0	0	0	0
Total	0	0	0	0	-	-	0	0	0	0

Table 83e	OAI - OPAI - APAI								Onchocerciasis - Blindness	

Age group (years)	Incidence 1990 Number ('000s)	Rate (per 100 000)	Prevalence 1990 Number ('000s)	Rate (per 100 000)	Avg. age at onset (years)	Average duration (years)	Deaths 1990 Number ('000s)	Rate (per 100 000)	Deaths 2000 (Projected) Number ('000s)	Rate (per 100 000)
Males										
0-4	0	0	0	0	-	-	0	0	0	0
5-14	0	0	0	0	-	-	0	0	0	0
15-44	0	0	0	0	-	-	0	0	0	0
45-59	0	0	0	0	-	-	0	0	0	0
60+	0	0	0	0	-	-	0	0	0	0
All ages	0	0	0	0	-	-	0	0	0	0
Females										
0-4	0	0	0	0	-	-	0	0	0	0
5-14	0	0	0	0	-	-	0	0	0	0
15-44	0	0	0	0	-	-	0	0	0	0
45-59	0	0	0	0	-	-	0	0	0	0
60+	0	0	0	0	-	-	0	0	0	0
All ages	0	0	0	0	-	-	0	0	0	0
Total	0	0	0	0	-	-	0	0	0	0

Table 83f	SSA - ASS - ASS								Onchocerciasis - Blindness	

Age group (years)	Incidence 1990 Number ('000s)	Rate (per 100 000)	Prevalence 1990 Number ('000s)	Rate (per 100 000)	Avg. age at onset (years)	Average duration (years)	Deaths 1990 Number ('000s)	Rate (per 100 000)	Deaths 2000 (Projected) Number ('000s)	Rate (per 100 000)
Males										
0-4	0	0.0	0	0.0	-	-	0	0	0	0
5-14	0	0.3	1	1.5	10.0	32.3	0	0	0	0
15-44	5	4.1	57	54.7	29.4	22.2	0	0	0	0
45-59	11	49.5	80	391.6	52.2	11.0	0	0	0	0
60+	12	81.2	76	722.6	69.2	4.8	0	0	0	0
All ages	27	10.9	213	84.5	55.2	10.4	0	0	0	0
Females										
0-4	0	0.0	0	0.0	-	-	0	0	0	0
5-14	0	0.2	1	1.0	10.0	35.0	0	0	0	0
15-44	3	2.6	38	35.6	29.5	24.4	0	0	0	0
45-59	7	28.3	53	239.7	52.3	12.4	0	0	0	0
60+	6	35.7	51	397.7	69.7	5.2	0	0	0	0
All ages	16	6.3	142	55.1	54.5	12.0	0	0	0	0
Total	44	8.5	355	69.6	54.9	11.0	0	0	0	0

For epidemiological sources see Remme 1996. For the methods used to estimate and project incidence, prevalence, and deaths see Murray and Lopez 1996a. See explanatory notes for definitions and caveats.

Table 83 | **Cuadro 83** | **Tableau 83**
Onchocerciasis | **Oncocercosis** | **Onchocercose**

Blindness | Ceguera | Cécité

Table 83g   LAC - ALC - ALC   Onchocerciasis - Blindness

Age group (years)	Incidence 1990 Number ('000s)	Rate (per 100 000)	Prevalence 1990 Number ('000s)	Rate (per 100 000)	Avg. age at onset (years)	Average duration (years)	Deaths 1990 Number ('000s)	Rate (per 100 000)	Deaths 2000 (Projected) Number ('000s)	Rate (per 100 000)
Males										
0-4	0	0.0	0	0.0	-	-	0	0	0	0
5-14	0	0.0	0	0.0	10.0	46.0	0	0	0	0
15-44	0	0.0	0	0.2	29.8	30.2	0	0	0	0
45-59	0	0.1	0	0.8	52.4	14.1	0	0	0	0
60+	0	0.1	0	1.0	70.3	5.7	0	0	0	0
All ages	0	0.0	1	0.2	49.6	17.3	0	0	0	0
Females										
0-4	0	0.0	0	0.0	-	-	0	0	0	0
5-14	0	0.0	0	0.0	10.0	50.4	0	0	0	0
15-44	0	0.0	0	0.2	29.9	33.7	0	0	0	0
45-59	0	0.1	0	0.7	52.4	16.7	0	0	0	0
60+	0	0.0	0	0.7	71.1	6.5	0	0	0	0
All ages	0	0.0	0	0.2	45.9	22.4	0	0	0	0
Total	0	0.0	1	0.2	48.1	19.3	0	0	0	0

Table 83h   MEC - AOM - CMO   Onchocerciasis - Blindness

Age group (years)	Incidence 1990 Number ('000s)	Rate (per 100 000)	Prevalence 1990 Number ('000s)	Rate (per 100 000)	Avg. age at onset (years)	Average duration (years)	Deaths 1990 Number ('000s)	Rate (per 100 000)	Deaths 2000 (Projected) Number ('000s)	Rate (per 100 000)
Males										
0-4	0	0	0	0	-	-	0	0	0	0
5-14	0	0	0	0	-	-	0	0	0	0
15-44	0	0	0	0	-	-	0	0	0	0
45-59	0	0	0	0	-	-	0	0	0	0
60+	0	0	0	0	-	-	0	0	0	0
All ages	0	0	0	0	-	-	0	0	0	0
Females										
0-4	0	0	0	0	-	-	0	0	0	0
5-14	0	0	0	0	-	-	0	0	0	0
15-44	0	0	0	0	-	-	0	0	0	0
45-59	0	0	0	0	-	-	0	0	0	0
60+	0	0	0	0	-	-	0	0	0	0
All ages	0	0	0	0	-	-	0	0	0	0
Total	0	0	0	0	-	-	0	0	0	0

Table 83i   World - Mundo - Monde   Onchocerciasis - Blindness

Age group (years)	Incidence 1990 Number ('000s)	Rate (per 100 000)	Prevalence 1990 Number ('000s)	Rate (per 100 000)	Avg. age at onset (years)	Average duration (years)	Deaths 1990 Number ('000s)	Rate (per 100 000)	Deaths 2000 (Projected) Number ('000s)	Rate (per 100 000)
Males										
0-4	0	0.0	0	0.0	-	-	0	0	0	0
5-14	0	0.0	1	0.2	10.0	32.3	0	0	0	0
15-44	5	0.4	57	4.6	29.4	22.2	0	0	0	0
45-59	11	3.6	80	25.5	52.2	11.0	0	0	0	0
60+	12	5.3	76	34.8	69.2	4.8	0	0	0	0
All ages	27	1.0	214	8.1	55.2	10.4	0	0	0	0
Females										
0-4	0	0.0	0	0.0	-	-	0	0	0	0
5-14	0	0.0	1	0.1	10.0	35.1	0	0	0	0
15-44	3	0.2	38	3.2	29.5	24.4	0	0	0	0
45-59	7	2.2	53	17.1	52.3	12.4	0	0	0	0
60+	6	2.3	51	18.8	69.7	5.2	0	0	0	0
All ages	16	0.6	143	5.5	54.5	12.0	0	0	0	0
Total	44	0.8	356	6.8	54.9	11.0	0	0	0	0

For epidemiological sources see Remme 1996. For the methods used to estimate and project incidence, prevalence, and deaths see Murray and Lopez 1996a. See explanatory notes for definitions and caveats.

Table 84
Onchocerciasis

Cuadro 84
Oncocercosis

Tableau 84
Onchocercose

Itching

Prurito

Prurit

Table 84a   **EME - PEMC - EMBE**   Onchocerciasis - Itching

Age group (years)	Incidence 1990 Number ('000s)	Rate (per 100 000)	Prevalence 1990 Number ('000s)	Rate (per 100 000)	Avg. age at onset (years)	Average duration (years)	Deaths 1990 Number ('000s)	Rate (per 100 000)	Deaths 2000 (Projected) Number ('000s)	Rate (per 100 000)
Males										
0-4	0	0	0	0	-	-	0	0	0	0
5-14	0	0	0	0	-	-	0	0	0	0
15-44	0	0	0	0	-	-	0	0	0	0
45-59	0	0	0	0	-	-	0	0	0	0
60+	0	0	0	0	-	-	0	0	0	0
All ages	0	0	0	0	-	-	0	0	0	0
Females										
0-4	0	0	0	0	-	-	0	0	0	0
5-14	0	0	0	0	-	-	0	0	0	0
15-44	0	0	0	0	-	-	0	0	0	0
45-59	0	0	0	0	-	-	0	0	0	0
60+	0	0	0	0	-	-	0	0	0	0
All ages	0	0	0	0	-	-	0	0	0	0
Total	0	0	0	0	-	-	0	0	0	0

Table 84b   **FSE - PEAS - AESE**   Onchocerciasis - Itching

Age group (years)	Incidence 1990 Number ('000s)	Rate (per 100 000)	Prevalence 1990 Number ('000s)	Rate (per 100 000)	Avg. age at onset (years)	Average duration (years)	Deaths 1990 Number ('000s)	Rate (per 100 000)	Deaths 2000 (Projected) Number ('000s)	Rate (per 100 000)
Males										
0-4	0	0	0	0	-	-	0	0	0	0
5-14	0	0	0	0	-	-	0	0	0	0
15-44	0	0	0	0	-	-	0	0	0	0
45-59	0	0	0	0	-	-	0	0	0	0
60+	0	0	0	0	-	-	0	0	0	0
All ages	0	0	0	0	-	-	0	0	0	0
Females										
0-4	0	0	0	0	-	-	0	0	0	0
5-14	0	0	0	0	-	-	0	0	0	0
15-44	0	0	0	0	-	-	0	0	0	0
45-59	0	0	0	0	-	-	0	0	0	0
60+	0	0	0	0	-	-	0	0	0	0
All ages	0	0	0	0	-	-	0	0	0	0
Total	0	0	0	0	-	-	0	0	0	0

Table 84c   **India - India - Inde**   Onchocerciasis - Itching

Age group (years)	Incidence 1990 Number ('000s)	Rate (per 100 000)	Prevalence 1990 Number ('000s)	Rate (per 100 000)	Avg. age at onset (years)	Average duration (years)	Deaths 1990 Number ('000s)	Rate (per 100 000)	Deaths 2000 (Projected) Number ('000s)	Rate (per 100 000)
Males										
0-4	0	0	0	0	-	-	0	0	0	0
5-14	0	0	0	0	-	-	0	0	0	0
15-44	0	0	0	0	-	-	0	0	0	0
45-59	0	0	0	0	-	-	0	0	0	0
60+	0	0	0	0	-	-	0	0	0	0
All ages	0	0	0	0	-	-	0	0	0	0
Females										
0-4	0	0	0	0	-	-	0	0	0	0
5-14	0	0	0	0	-	-	0	0	0	0
15-44	0	0	0	0	-	-	0	0	0	0
45-59	0	0	0	0	-	-	0	0	0	0
60+	0	0	0	0	-	-	0	0	0	0
All ages	0	0	0	0	-	-	0	0	0	0
Total	0	0	0	0	-	-	0	0	0	0

For epidemiological sources see Remme 1996. For the methods used to estimate and project incidence, prevalence, and deaths see Murray and Lopez 1996a. See explanatory notes for definitions and caveats.

Table 84	Cuadro 84	Tableau 84
Onchocerciasis	Oncocercosis	Onchocercose
Itching	Prurito	Prurit

Table 84d China - China - Chine — Onchocerciasis - Itching

Age group (years)	Incidence 1990 Number ('000s)	Rate (per 100 000)	Prevalence 1990 Number ('000s)	Rate (per 100 000)	Avg. age at onset (years)	Average duration (years)	Deaths 1990 Number ('000s)	Rate (per 100 000)	Deaths 2000 (Projected) Number ('000s)	Rate (per 100 000)
Males										
0-4	0	0	0	0	-	-	0	0	0	0
5-14	0	0	0	0	-	-	0	0	0	0
15-44	0	0	0	0	-	-	0	0	0	0
45-59	0	0	0	0	-	-	0	0	0	0
60+	0	0	0	0	-	-	0	0	0	0
All ages	0	0	0	0	-	-	0	0	0	0
Females										
0-4	0	0	0	0	-	-	0	0	0	0
5-14	0	0	0	0	-	-	0	0	0	0
15-44	0	0	0	0	-	-	0	0	0	0
45-59	0	0	0	0	-	-	0	0	0	0
60+	0	0	0	0	-	-	0	0	0	0
All ages	0	0	0	0	-	-	0	0	0	0
Total	0	0	0	0	-	-	0	0	0	0

Table 84e OAI - OPAI - APAI — Onchocerciasis - Itching

Age group (years)	Incidence 1990 Number ('000s)	Rate (per 100 000)	Prevalence 1990 Number ('000s)	Rate (per 100 000)	Avg. age at onset (years)	Average duration (years)	Deaths 1990 Number ('000s)	Rate (per 100 000)	Deaths 2000 (Projected) Number ('000s)	Rate (per 100 000)
Males										
0-4	0	0	0	0	-	-	0	0	0	0
5-14	0	0	0	0	-	-	0	0	0	0
15-44	0	0	0	0	-	-	0	0	0	0
45-59	0	0	0	0	-	-	0	0	0	0
60+	0	0	0	0	-	-	0	0	0	0
All ages	0	0	0	0	-	-	0	0	0	0
Females										
0-4	0	0	0	0	-	-	0	0	0	0
5-14	0	0	0	0	-	-	0	0	0	0
15-44	0	0	0	0	-	-	0	0	0	0
45-59	0	0	0	0	-	-	0	0	0	0
60+	0	0	0	0	-	-	0	0	0	0
All ages	0	0	0	0	-	-	0	0	0	0
Total	0	0	0	0	-	-	0	0	0	0

Table 84f SSA - ASS - ASS — Onchocerciasis - Itching

Age group (years)	Incidence 1990 Number ('000s)	Rate (per 100 000)	Prevalence 1990 Number ('000s)	Rate (per 100 000)	Avg. age at onset (years)	Average duration (years)	Deaths 1990 Number ('000s)	Rate (per 100 000)	Deaths 2000 (Projected) Number ('000s)	Rate (per 100 000)
Males										
0-4	42	87	74	157	2.4	4.5	0	0	0	0
5-14	201	287	656	934	10.0	5.0	0	0	0	0
15-44	335	323	1 683	1 622	29.4	5.0	0	0	0	0
45-59	123	605	525	2 584	52.2	5.0	0	0	0	0
60+	19	183	236	2 244	69.3	5.0	0	0	0	0
All ages	720	286	3 174	1 258	27.4	5.0	0	0	0	0
Females										
0-4	34	72	61	129	2.4	4.5	0	0	0	0
5-14	165	236	537	769	10.0	5.0	0	0	0	0
15-44	273	257	1 377	1 296	29.5	5.0	0	0	0	0
45-59	99	446	429	1 942	52.2	5.1	0	0	0	0
60+	16	126	193	1 515	69.7	4.9	0	0	0	0
All ages	586	227	2 597	1 007	27.4	5.0	0	0	0	0
Total	1 307	256	5 771	1 131	27.4	5.0	0	0	0	0

For epidemiological sources see Remme 1996. For the methods used to estimate and project incidence, prevalence, and deaths see Murray and Lopez 1996a. See explanatory notes for definitions and caveats.

Table 84
Onchocerciasis

Cuadro 84
Oncocercosis

Tableau 84
Onchocercose

Itching　　　　　　　　　　　　　Prurito　　　　　　　　　　　　　Prurit

Table 84g　　LAC - ALC - ALC　　　　　　　　　　　　　Onchocerciasis - Itching

Age group (years)	Incidence 1990 Number ('000s)	Rate (per 100 000)	Prevalence 1990 Number ('000s)	Rate (per 100 000)	Avg. age at onset (years)	Average duration (years)	Deaths 1990 Number ('000s)	Rate (per 100 000)	Deaths 2000 (Projected) Number ('000s)	Rate (per 100 000)
Males										
0-4	0	0.5	0	0.9	2.5	4.8	0	0	0	0
5-14	1	1.3	2	4.5	10.0	5.1	0	0	0	0
15-44	1	1.2	6	6.1	29.8	5.1	0	0	0	0
45-59	0	2.0	2	8.5	52.3	5.0	0	0	0	0
60+	0	0.4	1	5.5	70.3	4.9	0	0	0	0
All ages	3	1.2	12	5.3	27.7	5.0	0	0	0	0
Females										
0-4	0	0.4	0	0.8	2.5	4.9	0	0	0	0
5-14	1	1.1	2	3.8	10.0	5.0	0	0	0	0
15-44	1	1.0	5	5.0	29.9	4.9	0	0	0	0
45-59	0	1.6	2	6.6	52.4	5.0	0	0	0	0
60+	0	0.3	1	3.8	71.1	5.1	0	0	0	0
All ages	2	1.0	10	4.3	27.8	4.9	0	0	0	0
Total	5	1.1	21	4.8	27.7	5.0	0	0	0	0

Table 84h　　MEC - AOM - CMO　　　　　　　　　　　　　Onchocerciasis - Itching

Age group (years)	Incidence 1990 Number ('000s)	Rate (per 100 000)	Prevalence 1990 Number ('000s)	Rate (per 100 000)	Avg. age at onset (years)	Average duration (years)	Deaths 1990 Number ('000s)	Rate (per 100 000)	Deaths 2000 (Projected) Number ('000s)	Rate (per 100 000)
Males										
0-4	0	0.2	0	0.3	-	-	0	0	0	0
5-14	0	0.5	1	1.7	-	-	0	0	0	0
15-44	1	0.5	3	2.6	-	-	0	0	0	0
45-59	0	1.0	1	3.9	-	-	0	0	0	0
60+	0	0.2	0	2.7	-	-	0	0	0	0
All ages	1	0.5	5	2.1	-	-	0	0	0	0
Females										
0-4	0	0.1	0	0.3	-	-	0	0	0	0
5-14	0	0.4	1	1.5	-	-	0	0	0	0
15-44	0	0.5	2	2.3	-	-	0	0	0	0
45-59	0	0.8	1	3.2	-	-	0	0	0	0
60+	0	0.1	0	1.9	-	-	0	0	0	0
All ages	1	0.4	4	1.8	-	-	0	0	0	0
Total	2	0.5	10	2.0	-	-	0	0	0	0

Table 84i　　World - Mundo - Monde　　　　　　　　　　　　　Onchocerciasis - Itching

Age group (years)	Incidence 1990 Number ('000s)	Rate (per 100 000)	Prevalence 1990 Number ('000s)	Rate (per 100 000)	Avg. age at onset (years)	Average duration (years)	Deaths 1990 Number ('000s)	Rate (per 100 000)	Deaths 2000 (Projected) Number ('000s)	Rate (per 100 000)
Males										
0-4	42	13.0	75	23	2.4	4.5	0	0	0	0
5-14	202	36.7	660	120	10.0	5.0	0	0	0	0
15-44	337	27.0	1 692	135	29.4	5.0	0	0	0	0
45-59	123	39.5	528	169	52.2	5.0	0	0	0	0
60+	19	8.8	237	108	69.3	5.0	0	0	0	0
All ages	724	27.3	3 191	120	27.4	5.0	0	0	0	0
Females										
0-4	34	11.0	61	20	2.4	4.5	0	0	0	0
5-14	166	31.5	540	103	10.0	5.0	0	0	0	0
15-44	274	22.9	1 385	116	29.5	5.0	0	0	0	0
45-59	99	31.9	432	139	52.2	5.1	0	0	0	0
60+	16	6.0	194	72	69.7	4.9	0	0	0	0
All ages	589	22.5	2 611	100	27.4	5.0	0	0	0	0
Total	1 314	24.9	5 802	110	27.4	5.0	0	0	0	0

For epidemiological sources see Remme 1996. For the methods used to estimate and project incidence, prevalence, and deaths see Murray and Lopez 1996a. See explanatory notes for definitions and caveats.

Table 85
Onchocerciasis

Cuadro 85
Oncocercosis

Tableau 85
Onchocercose

Low vision

Disminución de la agudeza visual

Baisse de la vision

Table 85a	EME - PEMC - EMBE								Onchocerciasis - Low vision	
Age group (years)	Incidence 1990		Prevalence 1990		Avg. age at onset (years)	Average duration (years)	Deaths 1990		Deaths 2000 (Projected)	
	Number ('000s)	Rate (per 100 000)	Number ('000s)	Rate (per 100 000)			Number ('000s)	Rate (per 100 000)	Number ('000s)	Rate (per 100 000)
Males										
0-4	0	0	0	0	-	-	0	0	0	0
5-14	0	0	0	0	-	-	0	0	0	0
15-44	0	0	0	0	-	-	0	0	0	0
45-59	0	0	0	0	-	-	0	0	0	0
60+	0	0	0	0	-	-	0	0	0	0
All ages	0	0	0	0	-	-	0	0	0	0
Females										
0-4	0	0	0	0	-	-	0	0	0	0
5-14	0	0	0	0	-	-	0	0	0	0
15-44	0	0	0	0	-	-	0	0	0	0
45-59	0	0	0	0	-	-	0	0	0	0
60+	0	0	0	0	-	-	0	0	0	0
All ages	0	0	0	0	-	-	0	0	0	0
Total	0	0	0	0	-	-	0	0	0	0

Table 85b	FSE - PEAS - AESE								Onchocerciasis - Low vision	
Age group (years)	Incidence 1990		Prevalence 1990		Avg. age at onset (years)	Average duration (years)	Deaths 1990		Deaths 2000 (Projected)	
	Number ('000s)	Rate (per 100 000)	Number ('000s)	Rate (per 100 000)			Number ('000s)	Rate (per 100 000)	Number ('000s)	Rate (per 100 000)
Males										
0-4	0	0	0	0	-	-	0	0	0	0
5-14	0	0	0	0	-	-	0	0	0	0
15-44	0	0	0	0	-	-	0	0	0	0
45-59	0	0	0	0	-	-	0	0	0	0
60+	0	0	0	0	-	-	0	0	0	0
All ages	0	0	0	0	-	-	0	0	0	0
Females										
0-4	0	0	0	0	-	-	0	0	0	0
5-14	0	0	0	0	-	-	0	0	0	0
15-44	0	0	0	0	-	-	0	0	0	0
45-59	0	0	0	0	-	-	0	0	0	0
60+	0	0	0	0	-	-	0	0	0	0
All ages	0	0	0	0	-	-	0	0	0	0
Total	0	0	0	0	-	-	0	0	0	0

Table 85c	India - India - Inde								Onchocerciasis - Low vision	
Age group (years)	Incidence 1990		Prevalence 1990		Avg. age at onset (years)	Average duration (years)	Deaths 1990		Deaths 2000 (Projected)	
	Number ('000s)	Rate (per 100 000)	Number ('000s)	Rate (per 100 000)			Number ('000s)	Rate (per 100 000)	Number ('000s)	Rate (per 100 000)
Males										
0-4	0	0	0	0	-	-	0	0	0	0
5-14	0	0	0	0	-	-	0	0	0	0
15-44	0	0	0	0	-	-	0	0	0	0
45-59	0	0	0	0	-	-	0	0	0	0
60+	0	0	0	0	-	-	0	0	0	0
All ages	0	0	0	0	-	-	0	0	0	0
Females										
0-4	0	0	0	0	-	-	0	0	0	0
5-14	0	0	0	0	-	-	0	0	0	0
15-44	0	0	0	0	-	-	0	0	0	0
45-59	0	0	0	0	-	-	0	0	0	0
60+	0	0	0	0	-	-	0	0	0	0
All ages	0	0	0	0	-	-	0	0	0	0
Total	0	0	0	0	-	-	0	0	0	0

For epidemiological sources see Remme 1996. For the methods used to estimate and project incidence, prevalence, and deaths see Murray and Lopez 1996a. See explanatory notes for definitions and caveats.

Table 85	Cuadro 85	Tableau 85
Onchocerciasis	**Oncocercosis**	**Onchocercose**
Low vision	Disminución de la agudeza visual	Baisse de la vision

Table 85d — China - China - Chine — Onchocerciasis - Low vision

Age group (years)	Incidence 1990 Number ('000s)	Rate (per 100 000)	Prevalence 1990 Number ('000s)	Rate (per 100 000)	Avg. age at onset (years)	Average duration (years)	Deaths 1990 Number ('000s)	Rate (per 100 000)	Deaths 2000 (Projected) Number ('000s)	Rate (per 100 000)
Males										
0-4	0	0	0	0	-	-	0	0	0	0
5-14	0	0	0	0	-	-	0	0	0	0
15-44	0	0	0	0	-	-	0	0	0	0
45-59	0	0	0	0	-	-	0	0	0	0
60+	0	0	0	0	-	-	0	0	0	0
All ages	0	0	0	0	-	-	0	0	0	0
Females										
0-4	0	0	0	0	-	-	0	0	0	0
5-14	0	0	0	0	-	-	0	0	0	0
15-44	0	0	0	0	-	-	0	0	0	0
45-59	0	0	0	0	-	-	0	0	0	0
60+	0	0	0	0	-	-	0	0	0	0
All ages	0	0	0	0	-	-	0	0	0	0
Total	0	0	0	0	-	-	0	0	0	0

Table 85e — OAI - OPAI - APAI — Onchocerciasis - Low vision

Age group (years)	Incidence 1990 Number ('000s)	Rate (per 100 000)	Prevalence 1990 Number ('000s)	Rate (per 100 000)	Avg. age at onset (years)	Average duration (years)	Deaths 1990 Number ('000s)	Rate (per 100 000)	Deaths 2000 (Projected) Number ('000s)	Rate (per 100 000)
Males										
0-4	0	0	0	0	-	-	0	0	0	0
5-14	0	0	0	0	-	-	0	0	0	0
15-44	0	0	0	0	-	-	0	0	0	0
45-59	0	0	0	0	-	-	0	0	0	0
60+	0	0	0	0	-	-	0	0	0	0
All ages	0	0	0	0	-	-	0	0	0	0
Females										
0-4	0	0	0	0	-	-	0	0	0	0
5-14	0	0	0	0	-	-	0	0	0	0
15-44	0	0	0	0	-	-	0	0	0	0
45-59	0	0	0	0	-	-	0	0	0	0
60+	0	0	0	0	-	-	0	0	0	0
All ages	0	0	0	0	-	-	0	0	0	0
Total	0	0	0	0	-	-	0	0	0	0

Table 85f — SSA - ASS - ASS — Onchocerciasis - Low vision

Age group (years)	Incidence 1990 Number ('000s)	Rate (per 100 000)	Prevalence 1990 Number ('000s)	Rate (per 100 000)	Avg. age at onset (years)	Average duration (years)	Deaths 1990 Number ('000s)	Rate (per 100 000)	Deaths 2000 (Projected) Number ('000s)	Rate (per 100 000)
Males										
0-4	0	0.0	0	0.0	-	-	0	0	0	0
5-14	0	0.6	1	2.0	10.0	9.9	0	0	0	0
15-44	9	8.2	76	73.2	29.4	11.9	0	0	0	0
45-59	20	99.0	106	524.1	52.2	7.4	0	0	0	0
60+	13	122.7	102	969.7	69.2	5.0	0	0	0	0
All ages	42	16.6	286	113.2	52.3	7.6	0	0	0	0
Females										
0-4	0	0.0	0	0.0	-	-	0	0	0	0
5-14	0	0.4	1	1.3	10.0	10.0	0	0	0	0
15-44	6	5.3	51	47.6	29.5	12.2	0	0	0	0
45-59	13	59.7	71	320.8	52.2	8.1	0	0	0	0
60+	7	52.9	68	534.7	69.7	5.7	0	0	0	0
All ages	26	10.0	191	73.9	51.3	8.4	0	0	0	0
Total	68	13.3	476	93.3	51.9	7.9	0	0	0	0

For epidemiological sources see Remme 1996. For the methods used to estimate and project incidence, prevalence, and deaths see Murray and Lopez 1996a. See explanatory notes for definitions and caveats.

Table 85 | **Cuadro 85** | **Tableau 85**
Onchocerciasis | Oncocercosis | Onchocercose

Low vision | Disminución de la agudeza visual | Baisse de la vision

Table 85g LAC - ALC - ALC — Onchocerciasis - Low vision

Age group (years)	Incidence 1990 Number ('000s)	Rate (per 100 000)	Prevalence 1990 Number ('000s)	Rate (per 100 000)	Avg. age at onset (years)	Average duration (years)	Deaths 1990 Number ('000s)	Rate (per 100 000)	Deaths 2000 (Projected) Number ('000s)	Rate (per 100 000)
Males										
0-4	0	0.0	0	0.0	-	-	0	0	0	0
5-14	0	0.0	0	0.0	10.0	14.1	0	0	0	0
15-44	0	0.0	0	0.3	29.8	15.3	0	0	0	0
45-59	0	0.2	0	1.1	52.3	10.8	0	0	0	0
60+	0	0.1	0	1.4	70.3	7.0	0	0	0	0
All ages	0	0.0	1	0.3	44.4	12.1	0	0	0	0
Females										
0-4	0	0.0	0	0.0	-	-	0	0	0	0
5-14	0	0.0	0	0.0	10.0	13.1	0	0	0	0
15-44	0	0.0	0	0.2	29.9	16.8	0	0	0	0
45-59	0	0.1	0	0.9	52.4	14.0	0	0	0	0
60+	0	0.0	0	0.9	71.1	9.0	0	0	0	0
All ages	0	0.0	1	0.3	40.9	15.2	0	0	0	0
Total	0	0.0	1	0.3	43.0	13.4	0	0	0	0

Table 85h MEC - AOM - CMO — Onchocerciasis - Low vision

Age group (years)	Incidence 1990 Number ('000s)	Rate (per 100 000)	Prevalence 1990 Number ('000s)	Rate (per 100 000)	Avg. age at onset (years)	Average duration (years)	Deaths 1990 Number ('000s)	Rate (per 100 000)	Deaths 2000 (Projected) Number ('000s)	Rate (per 100 000)
Males										
0-4	0	0	0	0	-	-	0	0	0	0
5-14	0	0	0	0	-	-	0	0	0	0
15-44	0	0	0	0	-	-	0	0	0	0
45-59	0	0	0	0	-	-	0	0	0	0
60+	0	0	0	0	-	-	0	0	0	0
All ages	0	0	0	0	-	-	0	0	0	0
Females										
0-4	0	0	0	0	-	-	0	0	0	0
5-14	0	0	0	0	-	-	0	0	0	0
15-44	0	0	0	0	-	-	0	0	0	0
45-59	0	0	0	0	-	-	0	0	0	0
60+	0	0	0	0	-	-	0	0	0	0
All ages	0	0	0	0	-	-	0	0	0	0
Total	0	0	0	0	-	-	0	0	0	0

Table 85i World - Mundo - Monde — Onchocerciasis - Low vision

Age group (years)	Incidence 1990 Number ('000s)	Rate (per 100 000)	Prevalence 1990 Number ('000s)	Rate (per 100 000)	Avg. age at onset (years)	Average duration (years)	Deaths 1990 Number ('000s)	Rate (per 100 000)	Deaths 2000 (Projected) Number ('000s)	Rate (per 100 000)
Males										
0-4	0	0.0	0	0.0	-	-	0	0	0	0
5-14	0	0.1	1	0.3	10.0	9.9	0	0	0	0
15-44	9	0.7	76	6.1	29.4	12.0	0	0	0	0
45-59	20	6.4	107	34.2	52.2	7.4	0	0	0	0
60+	13	5.9	102	46.6	69.2	5.0	0	0	0	0
All ages	42	1.6	286	10.8	52.3	7.6	0	0	0	0
Females										
0-4	0	0.0	0	0.0	-	-	0	0	0	0
5-14	0	0.1	1	0.2	10.0	10.1	0	0	0	0
15-44	6	0.5	51	4.2	29.5	12.2	0	0	0	0
45-59	13	4.3	71	22.9	52.2	8.1	0	0	0	0
60+	7	2.5	68	25.3	69.7	5.7	0	0	0	0
All ages	26	1.0	191	7.3	51.3	8.4	0	0	0	0
Total	68	1.3	478	9.1	51.9	7.9	0	0	0	0

For epidemiological sources see Remme 1996. For the methods used to estimate and project incidence, prevalence, and deaths see Murray and Lopez 1996a. See explanatory notes for definitions and caveats.

Table 86   **Cuadro 86**   **Tableau 86**

Leprosy   **Lepra**   **Lèpre**

Cases   Casos   Cas

Table 86a   EME - PEMC - EMBE   Leprosy - Cases

Age group (years)	Incidence 1990 Number ('000s)	Rate (per 100 000)	Prevalence 1990 Number ('000s)	Rate (per 100 000)	Avg. age at onset (years)	Average duration (years)	Deaths 1990 Number ('000s)	Rate (per 100 000)	Deaths 2000 (Projected) Number ('000s)	Rate (per 100 000)
Males										
0-4	0	0.0	0	0.0	-	-	0	0	0	0
5-14	0	0.0	0	0.1	10.1	4.8	0	0	0	0
15-44	0	0.1	1	0.6	29.9	4.8	0	0	0	0
45-59	1	1.3	3	4.3	52.4	4.8	0	0	0	0
60+	0	0.0	1	1.8	-	-	0	0	0	0
All ages	1	0.3	5	1.3	46.8	4.8	0	0	0	0
Females										
0-4	0	0.0	0	0.0	-	-	0	0	0	0
5-14	0	0.0	0	0.1	10.1	4.8	0	0	0	0
15-44	0	0.1	1	0.6	30.0	4.8	0	0	0	0
45-59	1	1.3	3	4.3	52.5	4.9	0	0	0	0
60+	0	0.0	1	1.6	-	-	0	0	0	0
All ages	1	0.3	5	1.3	47.3	4.8	0	0	0	0
Total	2	0.3	10	1.3	47.0	4.8	0	0	0	0

Table 86b   FSE - PEAS - AESE   Leprosy - Cases

Age group (years)	Incidence 1990 Number ('000s)	Rate (per 100 000)	Prevalence 1990 Number ('000s)	Rate (per 100 000)	Avg. age at onset (years)	Average duration (years)	Deaths 1990 Number ('000s)	Rate (per 100 000)	Deaths 2000 (Projected) Number ('000s)	Rate (per 100 000)
Males										
0-4	0	0.0	0	0.0	-	-	0	0	0	0
5-14	0	0.0	0	0.0	-	-	0	0	0	0
15-44	0	0.0	0	0.0	-	-	0	0	0	0
45-59	0	1.3	1	4.3	52.3	4.6	0	0	0	0
60+	0	0.0	0	2.1	-	-	0	0	0	0
All ages	0	0.2	2	1.0	52.3	4.6	0	0	0	0
Females										
0-4	0	0.0	0	0.0	-	-	0	0	0	0
5-14	0	0.0	0	0.0	-	-	0	0	0	0
15-44	0	0.0	0	0.0	-	-	0	0	0	0
45-59	0	1.4	1	4.4	52.4	4.6	0	0	0	0
60+	0	0.0	1	1.6	-	-	0	0	0	0
All ages	0	0.2	2	1.1	52.4	4.6	0	0	0	0
Total	1	0.2	4	1.0	52.4	4.6	0	0	0	0

Table 86c   India - India - Inde   Leprosy - Cases

Age group (years)	Incidence 1990 Number ('000s)	Rate (per 100 000)	Prevalence 1990 Number ('000s)	Rate (per 100 000)	Avg. age at onset (years)	Average duration (years)	Deaths 1990 Number ('000s)	Rate (per 100 000)	Deaths 2000 (Projected) Number ('000s)	Rate (per 100 000)
Males										
0-4	3	5.2	6	10	2.5	4.8	0	0.0	0	0.0
5-14	40	39.0	121	119	10.0	4.8	0	0.0	0	0.0
15-44	75	37.3	366	182	29.8	4.8	0	0.0	0	0.0
45-59	19	41.0	89	187	52.3	4.8	0	0.3	0	0.1
60+	0	1.4	24	79	69.7	4.8	0	1.2	0	0.8
All ages	138	31.3	605	138	26.8	4.8	1	0.1	0	0.1
Females										
0-4	3	5.2	6	10	2.5	4.8	0	0.1	0	0.0
5-14	37	39.0	113	119	10.0	4.8	0	0.0	0	0.0
15-44	68	37.3	333	182	29.8	4.8	0	0.0	0	0.0
45-59	19	41.6	86	187	52.4	4.8	0	0.1	0	0.1
60+	1	2.5	23	80	70.1	4.8	0	0.7	0	0.4
All ages	128	31.3	561	137	27.0	4.8	0	0.1	0	0.1
Total	266	31.3	1 166	137	26.9	4.8	1	0.1	1	0.1

For epidemiological sources see Daumerie 1996. For the methods used to estimate and project incidence, prevalence, and deaths see Murray and Lopez 1996a. See explanatory notes for definitions and caveats.

Table 86
Leprosy

Cuadro 86
Lepra

Tableau 86
Lèpre

Cases

Casos

Cas

Table 86d China - China - Chine Leprosy - Cases

Age group (years)	Incidence 1990 Number ('000s)	Rate (per 100 000)	Prevalence 1990 Number ('000s)	Rate (per 100 000)	Avg. age at onset (years)	Average duration (years)	Deaths 1990 Number ('000s)	Rate (per 100 000)	Deaths 2000 (Projected) Number ('000s)	Rate (per 100 000)
Males										
0-4	0	0.1	0	0.2	2.5	2.7	0	0	0	0
5-14	1	1.3	3	2.7	10.0	2.7	0	0	0	0
15-44	3	0.9	8	2.5	29.9	2.7	0	0	0	0
45-59	1	1.0	2	2.7	52.4	2.7	0	0	0	0
60+	0	0.2	0	1.0	69.8	2.7	0	0	0	0
All ages	5	0.8	13	2.2	28.6	2.7	0	0	0	0
Females										
0-4	0	0.1	0	0.2	2.5	2.7	0	0	0	0
5-14	1	1.3	2	2.7	10.0	2.7	0	0	0	0
15-44	3	0.9	7	2.5	30.0	2.7	0	0	0	0
45-59	1	1.0	2	2.7	52.4	2.7	0	0	0	0
60+	0	0.2	1	1.0	70.6	2.7	0	0	0	0
All ages	5	0.8	12	2.2	28.7	2.7	0	0	0	0
Total	9	0.8	25	2.2	28.7	2.7	0	0	0	0

Table 86e OAI - OPAI - APAI Leprosy - Cases

Age group (years)	Incidence 1990 Number ('000s)	Rate (per 100 000)	Prevalence 1990 Number ('000s)	Rate (per 100 000)	Avg. age at onset (years)	Average duration (years)	Deaths 1990 Number ('000s)	Rate (per 100 000)	Deaths 2000 (Projected) Number ('000s)	Rate (per 100 000)
Males										
0-4	1	3.0	3	5.9	2.5	5.7	0	0.0	0	0.0
5-14	16	19.0	52	61.8	10.0	5.7	0	0.1	0	0.0
15-44	26	16.0	152	94.5	29.7	5.7	0	0.0	0	0.0
45-59	8	22.0	38	110.0	52.3	5.7	0	0.5	0	0.3
60+	0	0.0	12	58.3	-	-	0	0.9	0	0.6
All ages	50	14.7	256	74.6	26.1	5.7	0	0.1	0	0.1
Females										
0-4	1	3.0	2	5.9	2.5	5.7	0	0.4	0	0.3
5-14	15	19.0	50	61.7	10.0	5.7	0	0.0	0	0.0
15-44	26	16.0	151	94.5	29.8	5.7	0	0.0	0	0.0
45-59	8	22.0	38	108.9	52.3	5.7	0	0.2	0	0.1
60+	0	0.0	12	51.7	-	-	0	0.2	0	0.1
All ages	50	14.6	253	74.4	26.5	5.7	0	0.1	0	0.1
Total	100	14.7	509	74.5	26.3	5.7	1	0.1	1	0.1

Table 86f SSA - ASS - ASS Leprosy - Cases

Age group (years)	Incidence 1990 Number ('000s)	Rate (per 100 000)	Prevalence 1990 Number ('000s)	Rate (per 100 000)	Avg. age at onset (years)	Average duration (years)	Deaths 1990 Number ('000s)	Rate (per 100 000)	Deaths 2000 (Projected) Number ('000s)	Rate (per 100 000)
Males										
0-4	1	1.6	2	3.3	2.4	6.0	0	0.0	0	0.0
5-14	9	13.4	31	44.4	10.0	6.0	0	0.1	0	0.0
15-44	16	15.0	93	89.9	29.4	6.0	0	0.1	0	0.0
45-59	4	21.0	23	111.2	52.2	6.0	0	0.1	0	0.1
60+	0	0.0	7	68.0	-	-	0	0.1	0	0.0
All ages	30	11.9	156	61.8	25.9	6.0	0	0.1	0	0.0
Females										
0-4	1	1.6	2	3.3	2.4	6.0	0	0.0	0	0.0
5-14	9	13.4	31	44.2	10.0	6.0	0	0.0	0	0.0
15-44	16	15.0	96	89.9	29.5	6.0	0	0.1	0	0.0
45-59	5	22.0	25	111.0	52.2	6.0	0	0.2	0	0.1
60+	0	0.0	8	65.9	-	-	0	0.2	0	0.2
All ages	31	12.0	161	62.3	26.5	6.0	0	0.1	0	0.0
Total	61	11.9	317	62.1	26.2	6.0	0	0.1	0	0.0

For epidemiological sources see Daumerie 1996. For the methods used to estimate and project incidence, prevalence, and deaths see Murray and Lopez 1996a. See explanatory notes for definitions and caveats.

Table 86
Leprosy

Cuadro 86
Lepra

Tableau 86
Lèpre

Cases

Casos

Cas

Table 86g LAC - ALC - ALC   Leprosy - Cases

Age group (years)	Incidence 1990 Number ('000s)	Rate (per 100 000)	Prevalence 1990 Number ('000s)	Rate (per 100 000)	Avg. age at onset (years)	Average duration (years)	Deaths 1990 Number ('000s)	Rate (per 100 000)	Deaths 2000 (Projected) Number ('000s)	Rate (per 100 000)
Males										
0-4	1	3.1	2	6.1	2.5	5.7	0	0.0	0	0.0
5-14	11	20.5	35	66.4	10.0	5.7	0	0.0	0	0.0
15-44	17	16.5	102	97.9	29.8	5.7	0	0.0	0	0.0
45-59	5	22.5	25	111.5	52.3	5.7	0	0.4	0	0.2
60+	0	0.0	8	52.8	-	-	0	1.7	0	1.3
All ages	34	15.2	171	77.0	26.2	5.7	0	0.2	0	0.1
Females										
0-4	1	3.1	2	6.1	2.5	5.7	0	0.0	0	0.0
5-14	10	20.5	34	66.5	10.0	5.7	0	0.0	0	0.0
15-44	17	16.5	101	97.5	29.9	5.7	0	0.0	0	0.0
45-59	5	23.0	26	111.2	52.4	5.7	0	0.2	0	0.1
60+	0	0.0	8	47.3	-	-	0	0.9	0	0.6
All ages	34	15.2	171	76.7	26.7	5.7	0	0.1	0	0.1
Total	**68**	**15.2**	**342**	**76.9**	**26.4**	**5.7**	**1**	**0.1**	**1**	**0.1**

Table 86h MEC - AOM - CMO   Leprosy - Cases

Age group (years)	Incidence 1990 Number ('000s)	Rate (per 100 000)	Prevalence 1990 Number ('000s)	Rate (per 100 000)	Avg. age at onset (years)	Average duration (years)	Deaths 1990 Number ('000s)	Rate (per 100 000)	Deaths 2000 (Projected) Number ('000s)	Rate (per 100 000)
Males										
0-4	0	0.5	0	0.9	2.5	5.0	0	0.1	0	0.0
5-14	2	3.2	6	9.8	10.0	5.0	0	0.0	0	0.0
15-44	4	3.4	19	16.9	29.8	5.0	0	0.0	0	0.0
45-59	1	4.7	5	20.9	52.3	5.0	0	0.1	0	0.0
60+	0	0.0	1	9.3	-	-	0	0.2	0	0.1
All ages	7	2.8	32	12.5	26.6	5.0	0	0.0	0	0.0
Females										
0-4	0	0.5	0	0.9	2.5	5.0	0	0.0	0	0.0
5-14	2	3.2	6	9.8	10.0	5.0	0	0.0	0	0.0
15-44	4	3.4	18	16.9	29.8	5.0	0	0.0	0	0.0
45-59	1	4.8	5	20.9	52.3	5.0	0	0.0	0	0.0
60+	0	0.0	1	8.4	-	-	0	0.0	0	0.0
All ages	7	2.8	31	12.4	26.8	5.0	0	0.0	0	0.0
Total	**14**	**2.8**	**63**	**12.4**	**26.7**	**5.0**	**0**	**0.0**	**0**	**0.0**

Table 86i World - Mundo - Monde   Leprosy - Cases

Age group (years)	Incidence 1990 Number ('000s)	Rate (per 100 000)	Prevalence 1990 Number ('000s)	Rate (per 100 000)	Avg. age at onset (years)	Average duration (years)	Deaths 1990 Number ('000s)	Rate (per 100 000)	Deaths 2000 (Projected) Number ('000s)	Rate (per 100 000)
Males										
0-4	6	2.0	12	3.8	2.5	5.2	0	0.0	0	0.0
5-14	79	14.3	247	44.9	10.0	5.2	0	0.0	0	0.0
15-44	140	11.2	741	59.3	29.7	5.2	0	0.0	0	0.0
45-59	39	12.6	185	59.1	52.3	5.2	0	0.1	0	0.1
60+	1	0.2	53	24.4	69.7	4.5	1	0.4	1	0.3
All ages	265	10.0	1 239	46.7	26.6	5.2	2	0.1	1	0.0
Females										
0-4	6	2.0	12	3.8	2.5	5.2	0	0.1	0	0.0
5-14	75	14.3	236	44.9	10.0	5.2	0	0.0	0	0.0
15-44	133	11.1	707	59.0	29.8	5.2	0	0.0	0	0.0
45-59	40	12.9	185	59.6	52.4	5.2	0	0.1	0	0.0
60+	1	0.3	55	20.3	70.2	4.5	0	0.2	0	0.1
All ages	256	9.8	1 195	45.7	27.0	5.2	1	0.0	1	0.0
Total	**521**	**9.9**	**2 434**	**46.2**	**26.8**	**5.2**	**3**	**0.1**	**2**	**0.0**

For epidemiological sources see Daumerie 1996. For the methods used to estimate and project incidence, prevalence, and deaths see Murray and Lopez 1996a. See explanatory notes for definitions and caveats.

Table 87	Cuadro 87	Tableau 87
Leprosy	**Lepra**	**Lèpre**
Disabling leprosy	Lepra discapacitante	Lèpre avec incapacité

Table 87a — EME - PEMC - EMBE — Leprosy - Disabling leprosy

Age group (years)	Incidence 1990 Number ('000s)	Rate (per 100 000)	Prevalence 1990 Number ('000s)	Rate (per 100 000)	Avg. age at onset (years)	Average duration (years)	Deaths 1990 Number ('000s)	Rate (per 100 000)	Deaths 2000 (Projected) Number ('000s)	Rate (per 100 000)
Males										
0-4	0	0.0	0	0.0	-	-	-	-	-	-
5-14	0	0.0	0	0.0	10.0	63.6	-	-	-	-
15-44	0	0.0	1	0.3	29.9	44.7	-	-	-	-
45-59	0	0.2	1	2.0	52.4	24.5	-	-	-	-
60+	0	0.0	2	3.4	-	-	-	-	-	-
All ages	0	0.0	4	1.0	46.7	29.7	-	-	-	-
Females										
0-4	0	0.0	0	0.0	-	-	-	-	-	-
5-14	0	0.0	0	0.0	10.0	69.5	-	-	-	-
15-44	0	0.0	1	0.3	30.0	50.0	-	-	-	-
45-59	0	0.2	1	2.1	52.4	28.8	-	-	-	-
60+	0	0.0	3	3.6	-	-	-	-	-	-
All ages	0	0.0	5	1.2	47.1	33.8	-	-	-	-
Total	0	0.0	9	1.1	46.9	31.8	-	-	-	-

Table 87b — FSE - PEAS - AESE — Leprosy - Disabling leprosy

Age group (years)	Incidence 1990 Number ('000s)	Rate (per 100 000)	Prevalence 1990 Number ('000s)	Rate (per 100 000)	Avg. age at onset (years)	Average duration (years)	Deaths 1990 Number ('000s)	Rate (per 100 000)	Deaths 2000 (Projected) Number ('000s)	Rate (per 100 000)
Males										
0-4	0	0.0	0	0.0	-	-	-	-	-	-
5-14	0	0.0	0	0.0	-	-	-	-	-	-
15-44	0	0.0	0	0.0	-	-	-	-	-	-
45-59	0	0.2	0	1.4	52.4	20.8	-	-	-	-
60+	0	0.0	1	3.0	-	-	-	-	-	-
All ages	0	0.0	1	0.6	52.4	20.8	-	-	-	-
Females										
0-4	0	0.0	0	0.0	-	-	-	-	-	-
5-14	0	0.0	0	0.0	-	-	-	-	-	-
15-44	0	0.0	0	0.0	-	-	-	-	-	-
45-59	0	0.2	0	1.5	52.4	26.1	-	-	-	-
60+	0	0.0	1	3.1	-	-	-	-	-	-
All ages	0	0.0	2	0.9	52.4	26.1	-	-	-	-
Total	0	0.0	3	0.8	52.4	23.6	-	-	-	-

Table 87c — India - India - Inde — Leprosy - Disabling leprosy

Age group (years)	Incidence 1990 Number ('000s)	Rate (per 100 000)	Prevalence 1990 Number ('000s)	Rate (per 100 000)	Avg. age at onset (years)	Average duration (years)	Deaths 1990 Number ('000s)	Rate (per 100 000)	Deaths 2000 (Projected) Number ('000s)	Rate (per 100 000)
Males										
0-4	0	0.8	1	1.9	2.5	59.9	-	-	-	-
5-14	6	5.8	34	33.1	10.0	57.4	-	-	-	-
15-44	11	5.6	291	145.0	29.8	39.9	-	-	-	-
45-59	3	6.1	131	274.9	52.3	21.0	-	-	-	-
60+	0	0.2	96	324.1	69.7	9.7	-	-	-	-
All ages	21	4.7	553	125.8	26.8	42.6	-	-	-	-
Females										
0-4	0	0.8	1	1.9	2.5	60.8	-	-	-	-
5-14	6	5.8	32	33.1	10.0	59.1	-	-	-	-
15-44	10	5.6	266	145.0	29.8	41.7	-	-	-	-
45-59	3	6.2	127	275.9	52.4	22.5	-	-	-	-
60+	0	0.4	95	327.1	70.1	10.2	-	-	-	-
All ages	19	4.7	520	126.8	27.0	44.1	-	-	-	-
Total	40	4.7	1 073	126.3	26.9	43.4	-	-	-	-

For epidemiological sources see Daumerie 1996. For the methods used to estimate and project incidence, prevalence, and deaths see Murray and Lopez 1996a. See explanatory notes for definitions and caveats.

Table 87
Leprosy

Cuadro 87
Lepra

Tableau 87
Lèpre

Disabling leprosy

Lepra discapacitante

Lèpre avec incapacité

Table 87d   China - China - Chine

Leprosy - Disabling leprosy

Age group (years)	Incidence 1990 Number ('000s)	Rate (per 100 000)	Prevalence 1990 Number ('000s)	Rate (per 100 000)	Avg. age at onset (years)	Average duration (years)	Deaths 1990 Number ('000s)	Rate (per 100 000)	Deaths 2000 (Projected) Number ('000s)	Rate (per 100 000)
Males										
0-4	0	0.0	0	0.1	2.5	65.5	-	-	-	-
5-14	0	0.2	1	1.1	10.0	59.9	-	-	-	-
15-44	0	0.1	12	4.0	29.9	41.2	-	-	-	-
45-59	0	0.2	5	7.2	52.3	21.4	-	-	-	-
60+	0	0.0	4	8.6	69.8	9.9	-	-	-	-
All ages	1	0.1	23	3.9	28.6	42.7	-	-	-	-
Females										
0-4	0	0.0	0	0.1	2.5	68.5	-	-	-	-
5-14	0	0.2	1	1.1	10.0	63.2	-	-	-	-
15-44	0	0.1	11	4.0	29.9	44.2	-	-	-	-
45-59	0	0.2	5	7.2	52.4	23.8	-	-	-	-
60+	0	0.0	4	8.7	70.6	10.8	-	-	-	-
All ages	1	0.1	21	3.9	28.7	45.6	-	-	-	-
Total	1	0.1	44	3.9	28.6	44.1	-	-	-	-

Table 87e   OAI - OPAI - APAI

Leprosy - Disabling leprosy

Age group (years)	Incidence 1990 Number ('000s)	Rate (per 100 000)	Prevalence 1990 Number ('000s)	Rate (per 100 000)	Avg. age at onset (years)	Average duration (years)	Deaths 1990 Number ('000s)	Rate (per 100 000)	Deaths 2000 (Projected) Number ('000s)	Rate (per 100 000)
Males										
0-4	0	0.5	0	1.1	2.5	59.8	-	-	-	-
5-14	2	2.8	14	16.5	10.0	56.2	-	-	-	-
15-44	4	2.4	106	66.1	29.7	38.8	-	-	-	-
45-59	1	3.3	43	126.6	52.3	20.3	-	-	-	-
60+	0	0.0	31	152.0	-	-	-	-	-	-
All ages	8	2.2	195	56.7	26.1	42.1	-	-	-	-
Females										
0-4	0	0.5	0	1.1	2.5	63.2	-	-	-	-
5-14	2	2.8	13	16.5	10.0	59.2	-	-	-	-
15-44	4	2.4	106	66.2	29.8	41.5	-	-	-	-
45-59	1	3.3	44	126.8	52.3	22.4	-	-	-	-
60+	0	0.0	34	152.0	-	-	-	-	-	-
All ages	7	2.2	198	58.4	26.5	44.5	-	-	-	-
Total	15	2.2	393	57.6	26.3	43.3	-	-	-	-

Table 87f   SSA - ASS - ASS

Leprosy - Disabling leprosy

Age group (years)	Incidence 1990 Number ('000s)	Rate (per 100 000)	Prevalence 1990 Number ('000s)	Rate (per 100 000)	Avg. age at onset (years)	Average duration (years)	Deaths 1990 Number ('000s)	Rate (per 100 000)	Deaths 2000 (Projected) Number ('000s)	Rate (per 100 000)
Males										
0-4	0	0.2	0	0.6	2.4	48.7	-	-	-	-
5-14	1	2.0	8	11.2	10.0	49.2	-	-	-	-
15-44	2	2.2	56	53.7	29.4	35.0	-	-	-	-
45-59	1	3.1	23	111.3	52.2	19.1	-	-	-	-
60+	0	0.0	14	135.9	-	-	-	-	-	-
All ages	4	1.8	101	39.9	25.9	37.6	-	-	-	-
Females										
0-4	0	0.2	0	0.6	2.4	51.9	-	-	-	-
5-14	1	2.0	8	11.2	10.0	51.9	-	-	-	-
15-44	2	2.2	57	53.9	29.5	37.2	-	-	-	-
45-59	1	3.3	25	112.6	52.2	20.5	-	-	-	-
60+	0	0.0	18	138.1	-	-	-	-	-	-
All ages	5	1.8	108	41.8	26.5	39.4	-	-	-	-
Total	9	1.8	209	40.9	26.2	38.5	-	-	-	-

For epidemiological sources see Daumerie 1996. For the methods used to estimate and project incidence, prevalence, and deaths see Murray and Lopez 1996a. See explanatory notes for definitions and caveats.

Table 87	Cuadro 87	Tableau 87
Leprosy	Lepra	Lèpre

Disabling leprosy	Lepra discapacitante	Lèpre avec incapacité

Table 87g LAC - ALC - ALC — Leprosy - Disabling leprosy

Age group (years)	Incidence 1990 Number ('000s)	Rate (per 100 000)	Prevalence 1990 Number ('000s)	Rate (per 100 000)	Avg. age at onset (years)	Average duration (years)	Deaths 1990 Number ('000s)	Rate (per 100 000)	Deaths 2000 (Projected) Number ('000s)	Rate (per 100 000)
Males										
0-4	0	0.5	0	1.2	2.5	63.9	-	-	-	-
5-14	2	3.1	9	17.7	10.0	59.3	-	-	-	-
15-44	3	2.5	73	69.6	29.8	41.4	-	-	-	-
45-59	1	3.4	29	131.9	52.3	22.3	-	-	-	-
60+	0	0.0	22	157.7	-	-	-	-	-	-
All ages	5	2.3	134	60.5	26.2	44.9	-	-	-	-
Females										
0-4	0	0.5	0	1.2	2.5	67.9	-	-	-	-
5-14	2	3.1	9	17.7	10.0	63.0	-	-	-	-
15-44	3	2.5	73	69.8	29.8	44.6	-	-	-	-
45-59	1	3.4	31	132.6	52.4	24.8	-	-	-	-
60+	0	0.0	27	158.8	-	-	-	-	-	-
All ages	5	2.3	140	62.7	26.6	47.7	-	-	-	*
Total	10	2.3	274	61.6	26.4	46.3	-	-	-	-

Table 87h MEC - AOM - CMO — Leprosy - Disabling leprosy

Age group (years)	Incidence 1990 Number ('000s)	Rate (per 100 000)	Prevalence 1990 Number ('000s)	Rate (per 100 000)	Avg. age at onset (years)	Average duration (years)	Deaths 1990 Number ('000s)	Rate (per 100 000)	Deaths 2000 (Projected) Number ('000s)	Rate (per 100 000)
Males										
0-4	0	0.1	0	0.2	2.5	61.1	-	-	-	-
5-14	0	0.5	2	2.8	10.0	58.1	-	-	-	-
15-44	1	0.5	15	12.8	29.8	40.0	-	-	-	-
45-59	0	0.7	6	25.6	52.3	20.8	-	-	-	-
60+	0	0.0	4	31.1	-	-	-	-	-	-
All ages	1	0.4	26	10.3	26.6	43.1	-	-	-	-
Females										
0-4	0	0.1	0	0.2	2.5	63.7	-	-	-	-
5-14	0	0.5	2	2.8	10.0	60.9	-	-	-	-
15-44	1	0.5	14	12.8	29.8	42.6	-	-	-	-
45-59	0	0.7	6	25.8	52.3	22.9	-	-	-	-
60+	0	0.0	5	31.3	-	-	-	-	-	-
All ages	1	0.4	26	10.6	26.8	45.4	-	-	-	-
Total	2	0.4	52	10.4	26.7	44.2	-	-	-	-

Table 87i World - Mundo - Monde — Leprosy - Disabling leprosy

Age group (years)	Incidence 1990 Number ('000s)	Rate (per 100 000)	Prevalence 1990 Number ('000s)	Rate (per 100 000)	Avg. age at onset (years)	Average duration (years)	Deaths 1990 Number ('000s)	Rate (per 100 000)	Deaths 2000 (Projected) Number ('000s)	Rate (per 100 000)
Males										
0-4	1	0.3	2	0.7	2.5	59.2	-	-	-	-
5-14	12	2.2	68	12.3	10.0	56.5	-	-	-	-
15-44	21	1.7	553	44.2	29.7	39.4	-	-	-	-
45-59	6	1.9	239	76.4	52.3	20.9	-	-	-	-
60+	0	0.0	175	80.0	69.7	9.8	-	-	-	-
All ages	40	1.5	1 036	39.1	26.6	42.2	-	-	-	-
Females										
0-4	1	0.3	2	0.7	2.5	61.4	-	-	-	-
5-14	11	2.1	64	12.2	10.0	58.8	-	-	-	-
15-44	20	1.7	527	44.0	29.8	41.6	-	-	-	-
45-59	6	1.9	240	77.0	52.4	22.7	-	-	-	-
60+	0	0.0	187	69.4	70.2	10.2	-	-	-	-
All ages	38	1.5	1 020	39.0	27.0	44.1	-	-	-	-
Total	78	1.5	2 056	39.0	26.8	43.1	-	-	-	-

For epidemiological sources see Daumerie 1996. For the methods used to estimate and project incidence, prevalence, and deaths see Murray and Lopez 1996a. See explanatory notes for definitions and caveats.

Table 88
Dengue

Cuadro 88
Dengue

Tableau 88
Dengue

Dengue haemorrhagic fever

Fiebre del dengue hemorrágico

Fièvre hémorragique de la dengue

Table 88a — EME - PEMC - EMBE — Dengue - Dengue haemorrhagic fever

Age group (years)	Incidence 1990 Number ('000s)	Rate (per 100 000)	Prevalence 1990 Number ('000s)	Rate (per 100 000)	Avg. age at onset (years)	Average duration (years)	Deaths 1990 Number ('000s)	Rate (per 100 000)	Deaths 2000 (Projected) Number ('000s)	Rate (per 100 000)
Males										
0-4	0	0	0	0	-	-	0	0	0	0
5-14	0	0	0	0	-	-	0	0	0	0
15-44	0	0	0	0	-	-	0	0	0	0
45-59	0	0	0	0	-	-	0	0	0	0
60+	0	0	0	0	-	-	0	0	0	0
All ages	0	0	0	0	-	-	0	0	0	0
Females										
0-4	0	0	0	0	-	-	0	0	0	0
5-14	0	0	0	0	-	-	0	0	0	0
15-44	0	0	0	0	-	-	0	0	0	0
45-59	0	0	0	0	-	-	0	0	0	0
60+	0	0	0	0	-	-	0	0	0	0
All ages	0	0	0	0	-	-	0	0	0	0
Total	0	0	0	0	-	-	0	0	0	0

Table 88b — FSE - PEAS - AESE — Dengue - Dengue haemorrhagic fever

Age group (years)	Incidence 1990 Number ('000s)	Rate (per 100 000)	Prevalence 1990 Number ('000s)	Rate (per 100 000)	Avg. age at onset (years)	Average duration (years)	Deaths 1990 Number ('000s)	Rate (per 100 000)	Deaths 2000 (Projected) Number ('000s)	Rate (per 100 000)
Males										
0-4	0	0	0	0	-	-	0	0	0	0
5-14	0	0	0	0	-	-	0	0	0	0
15-44	0	0	0	0	-	-	0	0	0	0
45-59	0	0	0	0	-	-	0	0	0	0
60+	0	0	0	0	-	-	0	0	0	0
All ages	0	0	0	0	-	-	0	0	0	0
Females										
0-4	0	0	0	0	-	-	0	0	0	0
5-14	0	0	0	0	-	-	0	0	0	0
15-44	0	0	0	0	-	-	0	0	0	0
45-59	0	0	0	0	-	-	0	0	0	0
60+	0	0	0	0	-	-	0	0	0	0
All ages	0	0	0	0	-	-	0	0	0	0
Total	0	0	0	0	-	-	0	0	0	0

Table 88c — India - India - Inde — Dengue - Dengue haemorrhagic fever

Age group (years)	Incidence 1990 Number ('000s)	Rate (per 100 000)	Prevalence 1990 Number ('000s)	Rate (per 100 000)	Avg. age at onset (years)	Average duration (years)	Deaths 1990 Number ('000s)	Rate (per 100 000)	Deaths 2000 (Projected) Number ('000s)	Rate (per 100 000)
Males										
0-4	23	37.7	2	3.2	2.5	0.08	1	2.0	1	1.2
5-14	68	66.5	6	5.6	10.0	0.08	4	4.0	2	1.8
15-44	3	1.4	0	0.1	29.8	0.08	0	0.1	0	0.0
45-59	1	3.0	0	0.2	52.3	0.08	0	0.2	0	0.1
60+	0	1.6	0	0.1	69.7	0.08	0	0.1	0	0.1
All ages	95	21.6	8	1.8	9.7	0.08	6	1.3	3	0.6
Females										
0-4	26	37.7	2	3.1	2.5	0.08	1	2.5	1	1.5
5-14	77	66.5	5	5.5	10.0	0.08	5	5.3	2	2.3
15-44	3	1.4	0	0.1	29.8	0.08	0	0.1	0	0.0
45-59	2	3.0	0	0.2	52.4	0.08	0	0.2	0	0.1
60+	1	1.6	0	0.1	70.1	0.08	0	0.1	0	0.1
All ages	108	26.4	7	1.8	9.7	0.08	7	1.6	3	0.7
Total	203	23.9	15	1.8	9.7	0.08	12	1.4	6	0.6

For epidemiological sources see LeDuc et al. 1996. For the methods used to estimate and project incidence, prevalence, and deaths see Murray and Lopez 1996a. See explanatory notes for definitions and caveats.

Table 88	Cuadro 88	Tableau 88
Dengue	**Dengue**	**Dengue**
Dengue haemorrhagic fever	Fiebre del dengue hemorrágico	Fièvre hémorragique de la dengue

Table 88d   China - China - Chine   Dengue - Dengue haemorrhagic fever

Age group (years)	Incidence 1990 Number ('000s)	Rate (per 100 000)	Prevalence 1990 Number ('000s)	Rate (per 100 000)	Avg. age at onset (years)	Average duration (years)	Deaths 1990 Number ('000s)	Rate (per 100 000)	Deaths 2000 (Projected) Number ('000s)	Rate (per 100 000)
Males										
0-4	3	4.0	0	0.3	2.5	0.08	0	0.2	0	0.1
5-14	8	8.0	1	0.7	10.0	0.08	0	0.3	0	0.1
15-44	0	0.1	0	0.0	29.9	0.08	0	0.0	0	0.0
45-59	0	0.2	0	0.0	52.3	0.08	0	0.0	0	0.0
60+	0	0.1	0	0.0	69.8	0.08	0	0.0	0	0.0
All ages	11	1.8	1	0.1	9.8	0.08	0	0.1	0	0.0
Females										
0-4	3	5.0	0	0.4	2.5	0.08	0	0.2	0	0.1
5-14	9	10.0	1	0.8	10.0	0.08	0	0.3	0	0.1
15-44	0	0.1	0	0.0	29.9	0.08	0	0.0	0	0.0
45-59	0	0.3	0	0.0	52.4	0.08	0	0.0	0	0.0
60+	0	0.1	0	0.0	70.6	0.08	0	0.0	0	0.0
All ages	12	2.2	1	0.2	9.8	0.08	0	0.1	0	0.0
Total	23	2.0	2	0.2	9.8	0.08	1	0.1	0	0.0

Table 88e   OAI - OPAI - APAI   Dengue - Dengue haemorrhagic fever

Age group (years)	Incidence 1990 Number ('000s)	Rate (per 100 000)	Prevalence 1990 Number ('000s)	Rate (per 100 000)	Avg. age at onset (years)	Average duration (years)	Deaths 1990 Number ('000s)	Rate (per 100 000)	Deaths 2000 (Projected) Number ('000s)	Rate (per 100 000)
Males										
0-4	19	43.0	2	3.6	2.5	0.08	1	1.7	0	1.1
5-14	57	68.0	5	5.7	10.0	0.08	2	2.9	1	1.4
15-44	2	1.0	0	0.1	29.7	0.08	0	0.0	0	0.0
45-59	1	4.0	0	0.3	52.3	0.08	0	0.1	0	0.1
60+	0	2.0	0	0.2	69.6	0.08	0	0.1	0	0.1
All ages	80	23.3	7	1.9	9.7	0.08	3	1.0	2	0.4
Females										
0-4	23	55.0	2	4.6	2.5	0.08	1	2.0	1	1.2
5-14	69	86.0	6	7.2	10.0	0.08	3	3.4	1	1.6
15-44	3	2.0	0	0.2	29.8	0.08	0	0.1	0	0.0
45-59	1	4.0	0	0.3	52.3	0.08	0	0.2	0	0.1
60+	0	2.0	0	0.2	70.3	0.08	0	0.1	0	0.1
All ages	97	28.5	8	2.4	9.7	0.08	4	1.1	2	0.5
Total	177	25.9	15	2.2	9.7	0.08	7	1.0	4	0.5

Table 88f   SSA - ASS - ASS   Dengue - Dengue haemorrhagic fever

Age group (years)	Incidence 1990 Number ('000s)	Rate (per 100 000)	Prevalence 1990 Number ('000s)	Rate (per 100 000)	Avg. age at onset (years)	Average duration (years)	Deaths 1990 Number ('000s)	Rate (per 100 000)	Deaths 2000 (Projected) Number ('000s)	Rate (per 100 000)
Males										
0-4	1	2.3	0	0.2	2.4	0.08	0	0.1	0	0.1
5-14	3	4.6	0	0.4	10.0	0.08	0	0.3	0	0.1
15-44	0	0.1	0	0.0	29.4	0.08	0	0.0	0	0.0
45-59	0	0.3	0	0.0	52.2	0.08	0	0.0	0	0.0
60+	0	0.2	0	0.0	69.2	0.08	0	0.0	0	0.0
All ages	5	1.8	0	0.2	9.7	0.08	0	0.1	0	0.1
Females										
0-4	1	2.8	0	0.2	2.4	0.08	0	0.1	0	0.1
5-14	2	5.6	0	0.5	10.0	0.08	0	0.3	0	0.2
15-44	2	0.2	0	0.0	29.5	0.08	0	0.0	0	0.0
45-59	0	0.4	0	0.0	52.2	0.08	0	0.0	0	0.0
60+	0	0.3	0	0.0	69.7	0.08	0	0.0	0	0.0
All ages	6	2.2	0	0.2	23.2	0.08	0	0.1	0	0.1
Total	10	2.0	1	0.2	17.2	0.08	1	0.1	0	0.1

For epidemiological sources see LeDuc et al. 1996. For the methods used to estimate and project incidence, prevalence, and deaths see Murray and Lopez 1996a. See explanatory notes for definitions and caveats.

Table 88 **Cuadro 88** **Tableau 88**
Dengue **Dengue** **Dengue**

Dengue haemorrhagic fever   Fiebre del dengue hemorrágico   Fièvre hémorragique de la dengue

Table 88g   LAC - ALC - ALC   Dengue - Dengue haemorrhagic fever

Age group (years)	Incidence 1990 Number ('000s)	Rate (per 100 000)	Prevalence 1990 Number ('000s)	Rate (per 100 000)	Avg. age at onset (years)	Average duration (years)	Deaths 1990 Number ('000s)	Rate (per 100 000)	Deaths 2000 (Projected) Number ('000s)	Rate (per 100 000)
Males										
0-4	0	0.8	0	0.1	2.5	0.08	0	0	0	0
5-14	1	1.4	0	0.1	10.0	0.08	0	0	0	0
15-44	0	0.0	0	0.0	29.8	0.08	0	0	0	0
45-59	0	0.1	0	0.0	52.3	0.08	0	0	0	0
60+	0	0.0	0	0.0	70.3	0.08	0	0	0	0
All ages	1	0.4	0	0.0	9.8	0.08	0	0	0	0
Females										
0-4	0	1.0	0	0.1	2.5	0.08	0	0	0	0
5-14	1	1.6	0	0.2	10.0	0.08	0	0	0	0
15-44	0	0.0	0	0.0	29.9	0.08	0	0	0	0
45-59	0	0.1	0	0.0	52.4	0.08	0	0	0	0
60+	0	0.0	0	0.0	71.1	0.08	0	0	0	0
All ages	1	0.5	0	0.0	9.8	0.08	0	0	0	0
Total	2	0.5	0	0.0	9.8	0.08	0	0	0	0

Table 88h   MEC - AOM - CMO   Dengue - Dengue haemorrhagic fever

Age group (years)	Incidence 1990 Number ('000s)	Rate (per 100 000)	Prevalence 1990 Number ('000s)	Rate (per 100 000)	Avg. age at onset (years)	Average duration (years)	Deaths 1990 Number ('000s)	Rate (per 100 000)	Deaths 2000 (Projected) Number ('000s)	Rate (per 100 000)
Males										
0-4	0	0	0	0	-	-	0	0	0	0
5-14	0	0	0	0	-	-	0	0	0	0
15-44	0	0	0	0	-	-	0	0	0	0
45-59	0	0	0	0	-	-	0	0	0	0
60+	0	0	0	0	-	-	0	0	0	0
All ages	0	0	0	0	-	-	0	0	0	0
Females										
0-4	0	0	0	0	-	-	0	0	0	0
5-14	0	0	0	0	-	-	0	0	0	0
15-44	0	0	0	0	-	-	0	0	0	0
45-59	0	0	0	0	-	-	0	0	0	0
60+	0	0	0	0	-	-	0	0	0	0
All ages	0	0	0	0	-	-	0	0	0	0
Total	0	0	0	0	-	-	0	0	0	0

Table 88i   World - Mundo - Monde   Dengue - Dengue haemorrhagic fever

Age group (years)	Incidence 1990 Number ('000s)	Rate (per 100 000)	Prevalence 1990 Number ('000s)	Rate (per 100 000)	Avg. age at onset (years)	Average duration (years)	Deaths 1990 Number ('000s)	Rate (per 100 000)	Deaths 2000 (Projected) Number ('000s)	Rate (per 100 000)
Males										
0-4	45	14.1	4	1.2	2.5	0.08	2	0.6	1	0.4
5-14	136	24.7	11	2.1	10.0	0.08	7	1.3	3	0.5
15-44	6	0.5	0	0.0	29.8	0.08	0	0.0	0	0.0
45-59	3	0.9	0	0.1	52.3	0.08	0	0.0	0	0.0
60+	1	0.4	0	0.0	69.7	0.08	0	0.0	0	0.0
All ages	191	7.2	16	0.6	9.7	0.08	9	0.4	5	0.2
Females										
0-4	53	17.1	4	1.3	2.5	0.08	2	0.8	1	0.4
5-14	157	29.9	12	2.3	10.0	0.08	8	1.6	4	0.7
15-44	9	0.7	0	0.0	29.7	0.08	0	0.0	0	0.0
45-59	4	1.2	0	0.1	52.3	0.08	0	0.0	0	0.0
60+	1	0.5	0	0.0	70.1	0.08	0	0.0	0	0.0
All ages	224	8.6	17	0.7	10.1	0.08	11	0.4	6	0.2
Total	415	7.9	33	0.6	9.9	0.08	21	0.4	11	0.2

For epidemiological sources see LeDuc et al. 1996. For the methods used to estimate and project incidence, prevalence, and deaths see Murray and Lopez 1996a. See explanatory notes for definitions and caveats.

Table 89	Cuadro 89	Tableau 89
Japanese encephalitis	**Encefalitis japonesa**	**Encéphalite japonaise**
Episodes	Episodios	Episodes

Table 89a　　EME - PEMC - EMBE　　　　　　　　Japanese encephalitis - Episodes

Age group (years)	Incidence 1990 Number ('000s)	Rate (per 100 000)	Prevalence 1990 Number ('000s)	Rate (per 100 000)	Avg. age at onset (years)	Average duration (years)	Deaths 1990 Number ('000s)	Rate (per 100 000)	Deaths 2000 (Projected) Number ('000s)	Rate (per 100 000)
Males										
0-4	0	0.0	0	0.0	2.5	0.50	0	0	0	0
5-14	0	0.0	0	0.0	10.0	0.50	0	0	0	0
15-44	0	0.0	0	0.0	29.9	0.50	0	0	0	0
45-59	0	0.0	0	0.0	52.4	0.50	0	0	0	0
60+	0	0.0	0	0.0	71.1	0.50	0	0	0	0
All ages	0	0.0	0	0.0	50.5	0.50	0	0	0	0
Females										
0-4	0	0.0	0	0.0	-	-	0	0	0	0
5-14	0	0.0	0	0.0	10.0	0.50	0	0	0	0
15-44	0	0.0	0	0.0	30.0	0.50	0	0	0	0
45-59	0	0.0	0	0.0	52.4	0.50	0	0	0	0
60+	0	0.0	0	0.0	72.4	0.50	0	0	0	0
All ages	0	0.0	0	0.0	57.2	0.50	0	0	0	0
Total	0	0.0	0	0.0	54.0	0.50	0	0	0	0

Table 89b　　FSE - PEAS - AESE　　　　　　　　Japanese encephalitis - Episodes

Age group (years)	Incidence 1990 Number ('000s)	Rate (per 100 000)	Prevalence 1990 Number ('000s)	Rate (per 100 000)	Avg. age at onset (years)	Average duration (years)	Deaths 1990 Number ('000s)	Rate (per 100 000)	Deaths 2000 (Projected) Number ('000s)	Rate (per 100 000)
Males										
0-4	0	0.0	0	0.0	-	-	0	0	0	0
5-14	0	0.0	0	0.0	-	-	0	0	0	0
15-44	0	0.0	0	0.0	-	-	0	0	0	0
45-59	0	0.0	0	0.0	-	-	0	0	0	0
60+	0	0.0	0	0.0	-	-	0	0	0	0
All ages	0	0.0	0	0.0	-	-	0	0	0	0
Females										
0-4	0	0.0	0	0.0	-	-	0	0	0	0
5-14	0	0.0	0	0.0	-	-	0	0	0	0
15-44	0	0.0	0	0.0	-	-	0	0	0	0
45-59	0	0.0	0	0.0	-	-	0	0	0	0
60+	0	0.0	0	0.0	-	-	0	0	0	0
All ages	0	0.0	0	0.0	-	-	0	0	0	0
Total	0	0.0	0	0.0	-	-	0	0	0	0

Table 89c　　India - India - Inde　　　　　　　　Japanese encephalitis - Episodes

Age group (years)	Incidence 1990 Number ('000s)	Rate (per 100 000)	Prevalence 1990 Number ('000s)	Rate (per 100 000)	Avg. age at onset (years)	Average duration (years)	Deaths 1990 Number ('000s)	Rate (per 100 000)	Deaths 2000 (Projected) Number ('000s)	Rate (per 100 000)
Males										
0-4	2	2.5	1	1.2	2.5	0.50	0	0.4	0	0.3
5-14	1	0.9	0	0.5	10.0	0.50	0	0.1	0	0.1
15-44	0	0.1	0	0.1	29.8	0.50	0	0.0	0	0.0
45-59	0	0.1	0	0.0	52.3	0.50	0	0.0	0	0.0
60+	0	0.1	0	0.0	69.7	0.50	0	0.0	0	0.0
All ages	3	0.6	1	0.3	8.5	0.50	0	0.1	0	0.1
Females										
0-4	1	2.5	1	1.2	2.5	0.50	0	0.5	0	0.3
5-14	1	0.9	0	0.5	10.0	0.50	0	0.2	0	0.1
15-44	0	0.1	0	0.1	29.8	0.50	0	0.0	0	0.0
45-59	0	0.1	0	0.0	52.4	0.50	0	0.0	0	0.0
60+	0	0.1	0	0.0	70.1	0.50	0	0.0	0	0.0
All ages	3	0.6	1	0.3	8.5	0.50	1	0.1	0	0.1
Total	5	0.6	3	0.3	8.5	0.50	1	0.1	1	0.1

For epidemiological sources see Tsai 1996. For the methods used to estimate and project incidence, prevalence, and deaths see Murray and Lopez 1996a. See explanatory notes for definitions and caveats.

Table 89
Japanese encephalitis

Cuadro 89
Encefalitis japonesa

Tableau 89
Encéphalite japonaise

Episodes

Episodios

Episodes

Table 89d   China - China - Chine   Japanese encephalitis - Episodes

Age group (years)	Incidence 1990 Number ('000s)	Rate (per 100 000)	Prevalence 1990 Number ('000s)	Rate (per 100 000)	Avg. age at onset (years)	Average duration (years)	Deaths 1990 Number ('000s)	Rate (per 100 000)	Deaths 2000 (Projected) Number ('000s)	Rate (per 100 000)
Males										
0-4	11	18.8	5	8.7	2.5	0.50	1	1.1	0	0.6
5-14	7	6.8	4	3.7	10.0	0.50	0	0.4	0	0.2
15-44	2	0.5	1	0.3	29.9	0.50	0	0.1	0	0.0
45-59	0	0.4	0	0.2	52.3	0.50	0	0.1	0	0.0
60+	0	0.4	0	0.2	69.8	0.50	0	0.1	0	0.1
All ages	20	3.4	10	1.7	8.6	0.50	1	0.2	1	0.1
Females										
0-4	11	18.8	5	8.8	2.5	0.50	1	1.3	0	0.6
5-14	6	6.8	3	3.6	10.0	0.50	0	0.3	0	0.1
15-44	2	0.5	1	0.3	29.9	0.50	0	0.0	0	0.0
45-59	0	0.4	0	0.2	52.4	0.50	0	0.0	0	0.0
60+	0	0.4	0	0.2	70.6	0.50	0	0.1	0	0.0
All ages	19	3.5	9	1.7	8.5	0.50	1	0.2	1	0.1
Total	39	3.5	20	1.7	8.5	0.50	3	0.2	1	0.1

Table 89e   OAI - OPAI - APAI   Japanese encephalitis - Episodes

Age group (years)	Incidence 1990 Number ('000s)	Rate (per 100 000)	Prevalence 1990 Number ('000s)	Rate (per 100 000)	Avg. age at onset (years)	Average duration (years)	Deaths 1990 Number ('000s)	Rate (per 100 000)	Deaths 2000 (Projected) Number ('000s)	Rate (per 100 000)
Males										
0-4	4	9.1	2	4.2	2.5	0.50	0	0.9	0	0.6
5-14	2	2.7	1	1.5	10.0	0.50	0	0.3	0	0.1
15-44	1	0.4	0	0.2	29.7	0.50	0	0.0	0	0.0
45-59	0	0.3	0	0.1	52.3	0.50	0	0.1	0	0.0
60+	0	0.3	0	0.2	69.6	0.50	0	0.1	0	0.1
All ages	7	2.0	3	1.0	8.4	0.50	1	0.2	0	0.1
Females										
0-4	4	9.1	2	4.2	2.5	0.50	0	0.7	0	0.5
5-14	2	2.7	1	1.5	10.0	0.50	0	0.2	0	0.1
15-44	1	0.4	0	0.2	29.8	0.50	0	0.0	0	0.0
45-59	0	0.3	0	0.1	52.3	0.50	0	0.0	0	0.0
60+	0	0.3	0	0.2	70.3	0.50	0	0.1	0	0.0
All ages	7	2.0	3	1.0	8.6	0.50	1	0.2	0	0.1
Total	14	2.0	7	1.0	8.5	0.50	1	0.2	1	0.1

Table 89f   SSA - ASS - ASS   Japanese encephalitis - Episodes

Age group (years)	Incidence 1990 Number ('000s)	Rate (per 100 000)	Prevalence 1990 Number ('000s)	Rate (per 100 000)	Avg. age at onset (years)	Average duration (years)	Deaths 1990 Number ('000s)	Rate (per 100 000)	Deaths 2000 (Projected) Number ('000s)	Rate (per 100 000)
Males										
0-4	0	0	0	0	-	-	0	0	0	0
5-14	0	0	0	0	-	-	0	0	0	0
15-44	0	0	0	0	-	-	0	0	0	0
45-59	0	0	0	0	-	-	0	0	0	0
60+	0	0	0	0	-	-	0	0	0	0
All ages	0	0	0	0	-	-	0	0	0	0
Females										
0-4	0	0	0	0	-	-	0	0	0	0
5-14	0	0	0	0	-	-	0	0	0	0
15-44	0	0	0	0	-	-	0	0	0	0
45-59	0	0	0	0	-	-	0	0	0	0
60+	0	0	0	0	-	-	0	0	0	0
All ages	0	0	0	0	-	-	0	0	0	0
Total	0	0	0	0	-	-	0	0	0	0

For epidemiological sources see Tsai 1996. For the methods used to estimate and project incidence, prevalence, and deaths see Murray and Lopez 1996a. See explanatory notes for definitions and caveats.

Table 89	Cuadro 89	Tableau 89
Japanese encephalitis	Encefalitis japonesa	Encéphalite japonaise
Episodes	Episodios	Episodes

Table 89g   LAC - ALC - ALC — Japanese encephalitis - Episodes

Age group (years)	Incidence 1990 Number ('000s)	Rate (per 100 000)	Prevalence 1990 Number ('000s)	Rate (per 100 000)	Avg. age at onset (years)	Average duration (years)	Deaths 1990 Number ('000s)	Rate (per 100 000)	Deaths 2000 (Projected) Number ('000s)	Rate (per 100 000)
Males										
0-4	0	0	0	0	-	-	0	0	0	0
5-14	0	0	0	0	-	-	0	0	0	0
15-44	0	0	0	0	-	-	0	0	0	0
45-59	0	0	0	0	-	-	0	0	0	0
60+	0	0	0	0	-	-	0	0	0	0
All ages	0	0	0	0	-	-	0	0	0	0
Females										
0-4	0	0	0	0	-	-	0	0	0	0
5-14	0	0	0	0	-	-	0	0	0	0
15-44	0	0	0	0	-	-	0	0	0	0
45-59	0	0	0	0	-	-	0	0	0	0
60+	0	0	0	0	-	-	0	0	0	0
All ages	0	0	0	0	-	-	0	0	0	0
Total	0	0	0	0	-	-	0	0	0	0

Table 89h   MEC - AOM - CMO — Japanese encephalitis - Episodes

Age group (years)	Incidence 1990 Number ('000s)	Rate (per 100 000)	Prevalence 1990 Number ('000s)	Rate (per 100 000)	Avg. age at onset (years)	Average duration (years)	Deaths 1990 Number ('000s)	Rate (per 100 000)	Deaths 2000 (Projected) Number ('000s)	Rate (per 100 000)
Males										
0-4	0	0	0	0	-	-	0	0	0	0
5-14	0	0	0	0	-	-	0	0	0	0
15-44	0	0	0	0	-	-	0	0	0	0
45-59	0	0	0	0	-	-	0	0	0	0
60+	0	0	0	0	-	-	0	0	0	0
All ages	0	0	0	0	-	-	0	0	0	0
Females										
0-4	0	0	0	0	-	-	0	0	0	0
5-14	0	0	0	0	-	-	0	0	0	0
15-44	0	0	0	0	-	-	0	0	0	0
45-59	0	0	0	0	-	-	0	0	0	0
60+	0	0	0	0	-	-	0	0	0	0
All ages	0	0	0	0	-	-	0	0	0	0
Total	0	0	0	0	-	-	0	0	0	0

Table 89i   World - Mundo - Monde — Japanese encephalitis - Episodes

Age group (years)	Incidence 1990 Number ('000s)	Rate (per 100 000)	Prevalence 1990 Number ('000s)	Rate (per 100 000)	Avg. age at onset (years)	Average duration (years)	Deaths 1990 Number ('000s)	Rate (per 100 000)	Deaths 2000 (Projected) Number ('000s)	Rate (per 100 000)
Males										
0-4	17	5.2	8	2.4	2.5	0.50	1	0.4	1	0.2
5-14	10	1.8	5	1.0	10.0	0.50	1	0.1	0	0.1
15-44	2	0.2	1	0.1	29.8	0.50	0	0.0	0	0.0
45-59	0	0.1	0	0.1	52.3	0.50	0	0.0	0	0.0
60+	0	0.1	0	0.1	69.8	0.50	0	0.0	0	0.0
All ages	30	1.1	15	0.6	8.6	0.50	3	0.1	1	0.0
Females										
0-4	16	5.2	8	2.4	2.5	0.50	1	0.4	1	0.2
5-14	9	1.7	5	0.9	10.0	0.50	1	0.1	0	0.1
15-44	2	0.2	1	0.1	29.9	0.50	0	0.0	0	0.0
45-59	0	0.1	0	0.1	52.4	0.50	0	0.0	0	0.0
60+	0	0.1	0	0.1	70.6	0.50	0	0.0	0	0.0
All ages	28	1.1	14	0.5	8.6	0.50	2	0.1	1	0.0
Total	58	1.1	29	0.5	8.6	0.50	5	0.1	3	0.0

For epidemiological sources see Tsai 1996. For the methods used to estimate and project incidence, prevalence, and deaths see Murray and Lopez 1996a. See explanatory notes for definitions and caveats.

Table 90
Japanese encephalitis

Cuadro 90
Encefalitis japonesa

Tableau 90
Encéphalite japonaise

Cognitive impairment

Deficiencia cognocitiva

Déficience cognitive

Table 90a   EME - PEMC - EMBE   Japanese encephalitis - Cognitive impairment

Age group (years)	Incidence 1990 Number ('000s)	Rate (per 100 000)	Prevalence 1990 Number ('000s)	Rate (per 100 000)	Avg. age at onset (years)	Average duration (years)	Deaths 1990 Number ('000s)	Rate (per 100 000)	Deaths 2000 (Projected) Number ('000s)	Rate (per 100 000)
Males										
0-4	0	0.0	0	0.0	2.5	70.2	0	0	0	0
5-14	0	0.0	0	0.0	10.0	63.6	0	0	0	0
15-44	0	0.0	0	0.0	29.9	44.7	0	0	0	0
45-59	0	0.0	0	0.1	52.4	24.5	0	0	0	0
60+	0	0.0	0	0.1	71.1	11.3	0	0	0	0
All ages	0	0.0	0	0.0	50.6	27.7	0	0	0	0
Females										
0-4	0	0.0	0	0.0	2.5	76.1	0	0	0	0
5-14	0	0.0	0	0.0	10.0	69.5	0	0	0	0
15-44	0	0.0	0	0.0	30.0	50.0	0	0	0	0
45-59	0	0.0	0	0.1	52.4	28.8	0	0	0	0
60+	0	0.0	0	0.2	72.4	12.7	0	0	0	0
All ages	0	0.0	0	0.1	54.6	28.2	0	0	0	0
Total	0	0.0	0	0.1	52.8	28.0	0	0	0	0

Table 90b   FSE - PEAS - AESE   Japanese encephalitis - Cognitive impairment

Age group (years)	Incidence 1990 Number ('000s)	Rate (per 100 000)	Prevalence 1990 Number ('000s)	Rate (per 100 000)	Avg. age at onset (years)	Average duration (years)	Deaths 1990 Number ('000s)	Rate (per 100 000)	Deaths 2000 (Projected) Number ('000s)	Rate (per 100 000)
Males										
0-4	0	0	0	0	-	-	0	0	0	0
5-14	0	0	0	0	-	-	0	0	0	0
15-44	0	0	0	0	-	-	0	0	0	0
45-59	0	0	0	0	-	-	0	0	0	0
60+	0	0	0	0	-	-	0	0	0	0
All ages	0	0	0	0	-	-	0	0	0	0
Females										
0-4	0	0	0	0	-	-	0	0	0	0
5-14	0	0	0	0	-	-	0	0	0	0
15-44	0	0	0	0	-	-	0	0	0	0
45-59	0	0	0	0	-	-	0	0	0	0
60+	0	0	0	0	-	-	0	0	0	0
All ages	0	0	0	0	-	-	0	0	0	0
Total	0	0	0	0	-	-	0	0	0	0

Table 90c   India - India - Inde   Japanese encephalitis - Cognitive impairment

Age group (years)	Incidence 1990 Number ('000s)	Rate (per 100 000)	Prevalence 1990 Number ('000s)	Rate (per 100 000)	Avg. age at onset (years)	Average duration (years)	Deaths 1990 Number ('000s)	Rate (per 100 000)	Deaths 2000 (Projected) Number ('000s)	Rate (per 100 000)
Males										
0-4	0	0.8	1	1.9	2.5	59.9	0	0	0	0
5-14	0	0.3	5	5.1	10.0	57.4	0	0	0	0
15-44	0	0.0	14	6.8	29.8	39.9	0	0	0	0
45-59	0	0.0	4	7.5	52.3	21.0	0	0	0	0
60+	0	0.0	2	7.9	69.7	9.7	0	0	0	0
All ages	1	0.2	26	5.9	8.5	56.4	0	0	0	0
Females										
0-4	0	0.8	1	1.9	2.5	60.8	0	0	0	0
5-14	0	0.3	5	5.1	10.0	59.1	0	0	0	0
15-44	0	0.0	13	6.8	29.8	41.7	0	0	0	0
45-59	0	0.0	3	7.5	52.4	22.5	0	0	0	0
60+	0	0.0	2	7.9	70.1	10.2	0	0	0	0
All ages	1	0.2	24	5.9	8.5	57.7	0	0	0	0
Total	2	0.2	50	5.9	8.5	57.0	0	0	0	0

For epidemiological sources see Tsai 1996. For the methods used to estimate and project incidence, prevalence, and deaths see Murray and Lopez 1996a. See explanatory notes for definitions and caveats.

Table 90
Japanese encephalitis

Cuadro 90
Encefalitis japonesa

Tableau 90
Encéphalite japonaise

Cognitive impairment

Deficiencia cognocitiva

Déficience cognitive

Table 90d　　China - China - Chine　　Japanese encephalitis - Cognitive impairment

Age group (years)	Incidence 1990 Number ('000s)	Rate (per 100 000)	Prevalence 1990 Number ('000s)	Rate (per 100 000)	Avg. age at onset (years)	Average duration (years)	Deaths 1990 Number ('000s)	Rate (per 100 000)	Deaths 2000 (Projected) Number ('000s)	Rate (per 100 000)
Males										
0-4	3	5.6	8	14	2.5	65.5	0	0	0	0
5-14	2	2.0	37	38	10.0	59.9	0	0	0	0
15-44	1	0.2	156	51	29.9	41.2	0	0	0	0
45-59	0	0.1	39	54	52.3	21.4	0	0	0	0
60+	0	0.1	28	56	69.8	9.9	0	0	0	0
All ages	6	1.0	268	46	8.6	60.5	0	0	0	0
Females										
0-4	3	5.6	8	14	2.5	68.5	0	0	0	0
5-14	2	2.0	35	38	10.0	63.2	0	0	0	0
15-44	0	0.2	145	51	29.9	44.2	0	0	0	0
45-59	0	0.1	35	54	52.4	23.8	0	0	0	0
60+	0	0.1	29	56	70.6	10.8	0	0	0	0
All ages	6	1.0	251	46	8.5	63.6	0	0	0	0
Total	12	1.0	520	46	8.5	62.0	0	0	0	0

Table 90e　　OAI - OPAI - APAI　　Japanese encephalitis - Cognitive impairment

Age group (years)	Incidence 1990 Number ('000s)	Rate (per 100 000)	Prevalence 1990 Number ('000s)	Rate (per 100 000)	Avg. age at onset (years)	Average duration (years)	Deaths 1990 Number ('000s)	Rate (per 100 000)	Deaths 2000 (Projected) Number ('000s)	Rate (per 100 000)
Males										
0-4	1	2.7	3	6.7	2.5	59.8	0	0	0	0
5-14	1	0.8	15	17.6	10.0	56.2	0	0	0	0
15-44	0	0.1	37	23.2	29.7	38.8	0	0	0	0
45-59	0	0.1	9	25.4	52.3	20.3	0	0	0	0
60+	0	0.1	5	26.9	69.6	9.7	0	0	0	0
All ages	2	0.6	69	20.1	8.4	56.0	0	0	0	0
Females										
0-4	1	2.7	3	6.7	2.5	63.2	0	0	0	0
5-14	1	0.8	14	17.6	10.0	59.2	0	0	0	0
15-44	0	0.1	37	23.2	29.8	41.4	0	0	0	0
45-59	0	0.1	9	25.4	52.3	22.4	0	0	0	0
60+	0	0.1	6	26.9	70.3	10.5	0	0	0	0
All ages	2	0.6	69	20.3	8.6	59.0	0	0	0	0
Total	4	0.6	138	20.2	8.5	57.4	0	0	0	0

Table 90f　　SSA - ASS - ASS　　Japanese encephalitis - Cognitive impairment

Age group (years)	Incidence 1990 Number ('000s)	Rate (per 100 000)	Prevalence 1990 Number ('000s)	Rate (per 100 000)	Avg. age at onset (years)	Average duration (years)	Deaths 1990 Number ('000s)	Rate (per 100 000)	Deaths 2000 (Projected) Number ('000s)	Rate (per 100 000)
Males										
0-4	0	0	0	0	-	-	0	0	0	0
5-14	0	0	0	0	-	-	0	0	0	0
15-44	0	0	0	0	-	-	0	0	0	0
45-59	0	0	0	0	-	-	0	0	0	0
60+	0	0	0	0	-	-	0	0	0	0
All ages	0	0	0	0	-	-	0	0	0	0
Females										
0-4	0	0	0	0	-	-	0	0	0	0
5-14	0	0	0	0	-	-	0	0	0	0
15-44	0	0	0	0	-	-	0	0	0	0
45-59	0	0	0	0	-	-	0	0	0	0
60+	0	0	0	0	-	-	0	0	0	0
All ages	0	0	0	0	-	-	0	0	0	0
Total	0	0	0	0	-	-	0	0	0	0

For epidemiological sources see Tsai 1996. For the methods used to estimate and project incidence, prevalence, and deaths see Murray and Lopez 1996a. See explanatory notes for definitions and caveats.

Table 90
Japanese encephalitis

Cuadro 90
Encefalitis japonesa

Tableau 90
Encéphalite japonaise

Cognitive impairment

Deficiencia cognocitiva

Déficience cognitive

Table 90g   **LAC - ALC - ALC**   Japanese encephalitis - Cognitive impairment

Age group (years)	Incidence 1990 Number ('000s)	Rate (per 100 000)	Prevalence 1990 Number ('000s)	Rate (per 100 000)	Avg. age at onset (years)	Average duration (years)	Deaths 1990 Number ('000s)	Rate (per 100 000)	Deaths 2000 (Projected) Number ('000s)	Rate (per 100 000)
Males										
0-4	0	0	0	0	-	-	0	0	0	0
5-14	0	0	0	0	-	-	0	0	0	0
15-44	0	0	0	0	-	-	0	0	0	0
45-59	0	0	0	0	-	-	0	0	0	0
60+	0	0	0	0	-	-	0	0	0	0
All ages	0	0	0	0	-	-	0	0	0	0
Females										
0-4	0	0	0	0	-	-	0	0	0	0
5-14	0	0	0	0	-	-	0	0	0	0
15-44	0	0	0	0	-	-	0	0	0	0
45-59	0	0	0	0	-	-	0	0	0	0
60+	0	0	0	0	-	-	0	0	0	0
All ages	0	0	0	0	-	-	0	0	0	0
Total	0	0	0	0	-	-	0	0	0	0

Table 90h   **MEC - AOM - CMO**   Japanese encephalitis - Cognitive impairment

Age group (years)	Incidence 1990 Number ('000s)	Rate (per 100 000)	Prevalence 1990 Number ('000s)	Rate (per 100 000)	Avg. age at onset (years)	Average duration (years)	Deaths 1990 Number ('000s)	Rate (per 100 000)	Deaths 2000 (Projected) Number ('000s)	Rate (per 100 000)
Males										
0-4	0	0	0	0	-	-	0	0	0	0
5-14	0	0	0	0	-	-	0	0	0	0
15-44	0	0	0	0	-	-	0	0	0	0
45-59	0	0	0	0	-	-	0	0	0	0
60+	0	0	0	0	-	-	0	0	0	0
All ages	0	0	0	0	-	-	0	0	0	0
Females										
0-4	0	0	0	0	-	-	0	0	0	0
5-14	0	0	0	0	-	-	0	0	0	0
15-44	0	0	0	0	-	-	0	0	0	0
45-59	0	0	0	0	-	-	0	0	0	0
60+	0	0	0	0	-	-	0	0	0	0
All ages	0	0	0	0	-	-	0	0	0	0
Total	0	0	0	0	-	-	0	0	0	0

Table 90i   **World - Mundo - Monde**   Japanese encephalitis - Cognitive impairment

Age group (years)	Incidence 1990 Number ('000s)	Rate (per 100 000)	Prevalence 1990 Number ('000s)	Rate (per 100 000)	Avg. age at onset (years)	Average duration (years)	Deaths 1990 Number ('000s)	Rate (per 100 000)	Deaths 2000 (Projected) Number ('000s)	Rate (per 100 000)
Males										
0-4	5	1.6	12	3.9	2.5	63.7	0	0	0	0
5-14	3	0.5	57	10.4	10.0	58.8	0	0	0	0
15-44	1	0.1	207	16.6	29.8	40.6	0	0	0	0
45-59	0	0.0	52	16.5	52.3	21.2	0	0	0	0
60+	0	0.0	35	16.2	69.8	9.9	0	0	0	0
All ages	9	0.3	364	13.7	8.6	59.1	0	0	0	0
Females										
0-4	5	1.6	12	3.9	2.5	66.6	0	0	0	0
5-14	3	0.5	54	10.2	10.0	61.9	0	0	0	0
15-44	1	0.1	194	16.2	29.9	43.3	0	0	0	0
45-59	0	0.0	47	15.2	52.4	23.4	0	0	0	0
60+	0	0.0	38	14.0	70.6	10.7	0	0	0	0
All ages	8	0.3	345	13.2	8.6	62.0	0	0	0	0
Total	17	0.3	708	13.4	8.6	60.5	0	0	0	0

For epidemiological sources see Tsai 1996. For the methods used to estimate and project incidence, prevalence, and deaths see Murray and Lopez 1996a. See explanatory notes for definitions and caveats.

Table 91
Japanese encephalitis

Cuadro 91
Encefalitis japonesa

Tableau 91
Encéphalite japonaise

Neurological sequelae　　　Secuela neurológica　　　Séquelles neurologiques

Table 91a EME - PEMC - EMBE Japanese encephalitis - Neurological sequelae

Age group (years)	Incidence 1990 Number ('000s)	Rate (per 100 000)	Prevalence 1990 Number ('000s)	Rate (per 100 000)	Avg. age at onset (years)	Average duration (years)	Deaths 1990 Number ('000s)	Rate (per 100 000)	Deaths 2000 (Projected) Number ('000s)	Rate (per 100 000)
Males										
0-4	0	0	0	0.0	2.5	70.2	0	0	0	0
5-14	0	0	0	0.0	10.0	63.6	0	0	0	0
15-44	0	0	0	0.0	29.9	44.7	0	0	0	0
45-59	0	0	0	0.1	52.4	24.5	0	0	0	0
60+	0	0	0	0.2	71.1	11.3	0	0	0	0
All ages	0	0	0	0.1	50.5	27.8	0	0	0	0
Females										
0-4	0	0	0	0.0	2.5	76.1	0	0	0	0
5-14	0	0	0	0.0	10.0	69.5	0	0	0	0
15-44	0	0	0	0.0	30.0	50.0	0	0	0	0
45-59	0	0	0	0.1	52.4	28.8	0	0	0	0
60+	0	0	0	0.2	72.4	12.7	0	0	0	0
All ages	0	0	0	0.1	54.4	28.3	0	0	0	0
Total	0	0	1	0.1	52.6	28.1	0	0	0	0

Table 91b FSE - PEAS - AESE Japanese encephalitis - Neurological sequelae

Age group (years)	Incidence 1990 Number ('000s)	Rate (per 100 000)	Prevalence 1990 Number ('000s)	Rate (per 100 000)	Avg. age at onset (years)	Average duration (years)	Deaths 1990 Number ('000s)	Rate (per 100 000)	Deaths 2000 (Projected) Number ('000s)	Rate (per 100 000)
Males										
0-4	0	0	0	0	-	-	0	0	0	0
5-14	0	0	0	0	-	-	0	0	0	0
15-44	0	0	0	0	-	-	0	0	0	0
45-59	0	0	0	0	-	-	0	0	0	0
60+	0	0	0	0	-	-	0	0	0	0
All ages	0	0	0	0	-	-	0	0	0	0
Females										
0-4	0	0	0	0	-	-	0	0	0	0
5-14	0	0	0	0	-	-	0	0	0	0
15-44	0	0	0	0	-	-	0	0	0	0
45-59	0	0	0	0	-	-	0	0	0	0
60+	0	0	0	0	-	-	0	0	0	0
All ages	0	0	0	0	-	-	0	0	0	0
Total	0	0	0	0	-	-	0	0	0	0

Table 91c India - India - Inde Japanese encephalitis - Neurological sequelae

Age group (years)	Incidence 1990 Number ('000s)	Rate (per 100 000)	Prevalence 1990 Number ('000s)	Rate (per 100 000)	Avg. age at onset (years)	Average duration (years)	Deaths 1990 Number ('000s)	Rate (per 100 000)	Deaths 2000 (Projected) Number ('000s)	Rate (per 100 000)
Males										
0-4	1	1.0	1	2.5	2.5	59.9	0	0	0	0
5-14	0	0.3	7	6.7	10.0	57.4	0	0	0	0
15-44	0	0.0	18	9.1	29.8	39.9	0	0	0	0
45-59	0	0.0	5	10.0	52.3	21.0	0	0	0	0
60+	0	0.0	3	10.5	69.7	9.7	0	0	0	0
All ages	1	0.2	34	7.8	8.5	56.4	0	0	0	0
Females										
0-4	1	1.0	1	2.5	2.5	60.8	0	0	0	0
5-14	0	0.3	6	6.7	10.0	59.1	0	0	0	0
15-44	0	0.0	17	9.1	29.8	41.7	0	0	0	0
45-59	0	0.0	5	10.0	52.4	22.5	0	0	0	0
60+	0	0.0	3	10.5	70.1	10.2	0	0	0	0
All ages	1	0.2	32	7.8	8.5	57.7	0	0	0	0
Total	2	0.2	67	7.8	8.5	57.0	0	0	0	0

For epidemiological sources see Tsai 1996. For the methods used to estimate and project incidence, prevalence, and deaths see Murray and Lopez 1996a. See explanatory notes for definitions and caveats.

Table 91	Cuadro 91	Tableau 91
Japanese encephalitis	**Encefalitis japonesa**	**Encéphalite japonaise**
Neurological sequelae	Secuela neurológica	Séquelles neurologiques

Table 91d   China - China - Chine   Japanese encephalitis - Neurological sequelae

Age group (years)	Incidence 1990 Number ('000s)	Rate (per 100 000)	Prevalence 1990 Number ('000s)	Rate (per 100 000)	Avg. age at onset (years)	Average duration (years)	Deaths 1990 Number ('000s)	Rate (per 100 000)	Deaths 2000 (Projected) Number ('000s)	Rate (per 100 000)
Males										
0-4	5	7.5	11	19	2.5	65.5	0	0	0	0
5-14	3	2.7	50	51	10.0	59.9	0	0	0	0
15-44	1	0.2	208	68	29.9	41.2	0	0	0	0
45-59	0	0.1	53	72	52.3	21.4	0	0	0	0
60+	0	0.2	37	75	69.8	9.9	0	0	0	0
All ages	8	1.4	358	61	8.6	60.5	0	0	0	0
Females										
0-4	4	7.5	11	19	2.5	68.5	0	0	0	0
5-14	2	2.7	46	51	10.0	63.2	0	0	0	0
15-44	1	0.2	193	68	29.9	44.2	0	0	0	0
45-59	0	0.1	47	72	52.4	23.8	0	0	0	0
60+	0	0.2	39	75	70.6	10.8	0	0	0	0
All ages	8	1.4	335	61	8.5	63.6	0	0	0	0
Total	16	1.4	693	61	8.5	62.0	0	0	0	0

Table 91e   OAI - OPAI - APAI   Japanese encephalitis - Neurological sequelae

Age group (years)	Incidence 1990 Number ('000s)	Rate (per 100 000)	Prevalence 1990 Number ('000s)	Rate (per 100 000)	Avg. age at onset (years)	Average duration (years)	Deaths 1990 Number ('000s)	Rate (per 100 000)	Deaths 2000 (Projected) Number ('000s)	Rate (per 100 000)
Males										
0-4	2	3.6	4	8.9	2.5	59.8	0	0	0	0
5-14	1	1.1	20	23.4	10.0	56.2	0	0	0	0
15-44	0	0.1	50	30.9	29.7	38.8	0	0	0	0
45-59	0	0.1	12	33.8	52.3	20.3	0	0	0	0
60+	0	0.1	7	35.8	69.6	9.7	0	0	0	0
All ages	3	0.8	92	26.9	8.4	56.0	0	0	0	0
Females										
0-4	2	3.6	4	8.9	2.5	63.2	0	0	0	0
5-14	1	1.1	19	23.4	10.0	59.2	0	0	0	0
15-44	0	0.1	49	30.9	29.8	41.4	0	0	0	0
45-59	0	0.1	12	33.8	52.3	22.4	0	0	0	0
60+	0	0.1	8	35.9	70.3	10.5	0	0	0	0
All ages	3	0.8	92	27.1	8.6	59.0	0	0	0	0
Total	5	0.8	184	27.0	8.5	57.4	0	0	0	0

Table 91f   SSA - ASS - ASS   Japanese encephalitis - Neurological sequelae

Age group (years)	Incidence 1990 Number ('000s)	Rate (per 100 000)	Prevalence 1990 Number ('000s)	Rate (per 100 000)	Avg. age at onset (years)	Average duration (years)	Deaths 1990 Number ('000s)	Rate (per 100 000)	Deaths 2000 (Projected) Number ('000s)	Rate (per 100 000)
Males										
0-4	0	0	0	0	-	-	0	0	0	0
5-14	0	0	0	0	-	-	0	0	0	0
15-44	0	0	0	0	-	-	0	0	0	0
45-59	0	0	0	0	-	-	0	0	0	0
60+	0	0	0	0	-	-	0	0	0	0
All ages	0	0	0	0	-	-	0	0	0	0
Females										
0-4	0	0	0	0	-	-	0	0	0	0
5-14	0	0	0	0	-	-	0	0	0	0
15-44	0	0	0	0	-	-	0	0	0	0
45-59	0	0	0	0	-	-	0	0	0	0
60+	0	0	0	0	-	-	0	0	0	0
All ages	0	0	0	0	-	-	0	0	0	0
Total	0	0	0	0	-	-	0	0	0	0

For epidemiological sources see Tsai 1996. For the methods used to estimate and project incidence, prevalence, and deaths see Murray and Lopez 1996a. See explanatory notes for definitions and caveats.

Table 91
Japanese encephalitis

Cuadro 91
Encefalitis japonesa

Tableau 91
Encéphalite japonaise

Neurological sequelae

Secuela neurológica

Séquelles neurologiques

Table 91g LAC - ALC - ALC Japanese encephalitis - Neurological sequelae

Age group (years)	Incidence 1990 Number ('000s)	Rate (per 100 000)	Prevalence 1990 Number ('000s)	Rate (per 100 000)	Avg. age at onset (years)	Average duration (years)	Deaths 1990 Number ('000s)	Rate (per 100 000)	Deaths 2000 (Projected) Number ('000s)	Rate (per 100 000)
Males										
0-4	0	0	0	0	-	-	0	0	0	0
5-14	0	0	0	0	-	-	0	0	0	0
15-44	0	0	0	0	-	-	0	0	0	0
45-59	0	0	0	0	-	-	0	0	0	0
60+	0	0	0	0	-	-	0	0	0	0
All ages	0	0	0	0	-	-	0	0	0	0
Females										
0-4	0	0	0	0	-	-	0	0	0	0
5-14	0	0	0	0	-	-	0	0	0	0
15-44	0	0	0	0	-	-	0	0	0	0
45-59	0	0	0	0	-	-	0	0	0	0
60+	0	0	0	0	-	-	0	0	0	0
All ages	0	0	0	0	-	-	0	0	0	0
Total	0	0	0	0	-	-	0	0	0	0

Table 91h MEC - AOM - CMO Japanese encephalitis - Neurological sequelae

Age group (years)	Incidence 1990 Number ('000s)	Rate (per 100 000)	Prevalence 1990 Number ('000s)	Rate (per 100 000)	Avg. age at onset (years)	Average duration (years)	Deaths 1990 Number ('000s)	Rate (per 100 000)	Deaths 2000 (Projected) Number ('000s)	Rate (per 100 000)
Males										
0-4	0	0	0	0	-	-	0	0	0	0
5-14	0	0	0	0	-	-	0	0	0	0
15-44	0	0	0	0	-	-	0	0	0	0
45-59	0	0	0	0	-	-	0	0	0	0
60+	0	0	0	0	-	-	0	0	0	0
All ages	0	0	0	0	-	-	0	0	0	0
Females										
0-4	0	0	0	0	-	-	0	0	0	0
5-14	0	0	0	0	-	-	0	0	0	0
15-44	0	0	0	0	-	-	0	0	0	0
45-59	0	0	0	0	-	-	0	0	0	0
60+	0	0	0	0	-	-	0	0	0	0
All ages	0	0	0	0	-	-	0	0	0	0
Total	0	0	0	0	-	-	0	0	0	0

Table 91i World - Mundo - Monde Japanese encephalitis - Neurological sequelae

Age group (years)	Incidence 1990 Number ('000s)	Rate (per 100 000)	Prevalence 1990 Number ('000s)	Rate (per 100 000)	Avg. age at onset (years)	Average duration (years)	Deaths 1990 Number ('000s)	Rate (per 100 000)	Deaths 2000 (Projected) Number ('000s)	Rate (per 100 000)
Males										
0-4	7	2.1	17	5.2	2.5	63.7	0	0	0	0
5-14	4	0.7	76	13.8	10.0	58.8	0	0	0	0
15-44	1	0.1	276	22.1	29.8	40.6	0	0	0	0
45-59	0	0.1	69	22.1	52.3	21.2	0	0	0	0
60+	0	0.1	47	21.6	69.8	9.9	0	0	0	0
All ages	12	0.4	485	18.3	8.6	59.1	0	0	0	0
Females										
0-4	6	2.1	16	5.2	2.5	66.6	0	0	0	0
5-14	4	0.7	71	13.6	10.0	61.9	0	0	0	0
15-44	1	0.1	259	21.6	29.9	43.3	0	0	0	0
45-59	0	0.0	63	20.3	52.4	23.4	0	0	0	0
60+	0	0.0	50	18.6	70.6	10.7	0	0	0	0
All ages	11	0.4	460	17.6	8.6	62.0	0	0	0	0
Total	23	0.4	944	17.9	8.6	60.5	0	0	0	0

For epidemiological sources see Tsai 1996. For the methods used to estimate and project incidence, prevalence, and deaths see Murray and Lopez 1996a. See explanatory notes for definitions and caveats.

Table 92
Trachoma

Cuadro 92
Tracoma

Tableau 92
Trachome

Blindness

Ceguera

Cécité

Table 92a EME - PEMC - EMBE Trachoma - Blindness

Age group (years)	Incidence 1990 Number ('000s)	Rate (per 100 000)	Prevalence 1990 Number ('000s)	Rate (per 100 000)	Avg. age at onset (years)	Average duration (years)	Deaths 1990 Number ('000s)	Rate (per 100 000)	Deaths 2000 (Projected) Number ('000s)	Rate (per 100 000)
Males										
0-4	0	0	0	0	-	-	0	0	0	0
5-14	0	0	0	0	-	-	0	0	0	0
15-44	0	0	0	0	-	-	0	0	0	0
45-59	0	0	0	0	-	-	0	0	0	0
60+	0	0	0	0	-	-	0	0	0	0
All ages	0	0	0	0	-	-	0	0	0	0
Females										
0-4	0	0	0	0	-	-	0	0	0	0
5-14	0	0	0	0	-	-	0	0	0	0
15-44	0	0	0	0	-	-	0	0	0	0
45-59	0	0	0	0	-	-	0	0	0	0
60+	0	0	0	0	-	-	0	0	0	0
All ages	0	0	0	0	-	-	0	0	0	0
Total	0	0	0	0	-	-	0	0	0	0

Table 92b FSE - PEAS - AESE Trachoma - Blindness

Age group (years)	Incidence 1990 Number ('000s)	Rate (per 100 000)	Prevalence 1990 Number ('000s)	Rate (per 100 000)	Avg. age at onset (years)	Average duration (years)	Deaths 1990 Number ('000s)	Rate (per 100 000)	Deaths 2000 (Projected) Number ('000s)	Rate (per 100 000)
Males										
0-4	0	0	0	0	-	-	0	0	0	0
5-14	0	0	0	0	-	-	0	0	0	0
15-44	0	0	0	0	-	-	0	0	0	0
45-59	0	0	0	0	-	-	0	0	0	0
60+	0	0	0	0	-	-	0	0	0	0
All ages	0	0	0	0	-	-	0	0	0	0
Females										
0-4	0	0	0	0	-	-	0	0	0	0
5-14	0	0	0	0	-	-	0	0	0	0
15-44	0	0	0	0	-	-	0	0	0	0
45-59	0	0	0	0	-	-	0	0	0	0
60+	0	0	0	0	-	-	0	0	0	0
All ages	0	0	0	0	-	-	0	0	0	0
Total	0	0	0	0	-	-	0	0	0	0

Table 92c India - India - Inde Trachoma - Blindness

Age group (years)	Incidence 1990 Number ('000s)	Rate (per 100 000)	Prevalence 1990 Number ('000s)	Rate (per 100 000)	Avg. age at onset (years)	Average duration (years)	Deaths 1990 Number ('000s)	Rate (per 100 000)	Deaths 2000 (Projected) Number ('000s)	Rate (per 100 000)
Males										
0-4	0	0.0	0	0.0	-	-	0	0	0	0
5-14	0	0.0	0	0.0	-	-	0	0	0	0
15-44	0	0.0	1	0.6	29.8	28.8	0	0	0	0
45-59	0	0.6	2	5.1	52.3	13.2	0	0	0	0
60+	1	3.4	7	22.4	69.7	5.2	0	0	0	0
All ages	1	0.3	10	2.3	63.6	8.3	0	0	0	0
Females										
0-4	0	0.0	0	0.0	-	-	0	0	0	0
5-14	0	0.0	0	0.0	-	-	0	0	0	0
15-44	0	0.1	3	1.5	29.8	30.8	0	0	0	0
45-59	1	1.7	6	14.0	52.4	14.7	0	0	0	0
60+	3	8.8	18	63.1	70.1	5.5	0	0	0	0
All ages	4	0.9	28	6.7	64.0	9.0	0	0	0	0
Total	5	0.6	38	4.4	63.9	8.8	0	0	0	0

For epidemiological sources see Thylefors et al. 1996. For the methods used to estimate and project incidence, prevalence, and deaths see Murray and Lopez 1996a. See explanatory notes for definitions and caveats.

Table 92	Cuadro 92	Tableau 92
Trachoma	Tracoma	Trachome
Blindness	Ceguera	Cécité

Table 92d — China - China - Chine — Trachoma - Blindness

Age group (years)	Incidence 1990 Number ('000s)	Incidence 1990 Rate (per 100 000)	Prevalence 1990 Number ('000s)	Prevalence 1990 Rate (per 100 000)	Avg. age at onset (years)	Average duration (years)	Deaths 1990 Number ('000s)	Deaths 1990 Rate (per 100 000)	Deaths 2000 (Projected) Number ('000s)	Deaths 2000 (Projected) Rate (per 100 000)
Males										
0-4	0	0.0	0	0.0	-	-	0	0	0	0
5-14	0	0.0	0	0.0	-	-	0	0	0	0
15-44	1	0.3	15	5.0	29.9	31.1	0	0	0	0
45-59	4	5.3	32	44.6	52.3	13.6	0	0	0	0
60+	15	30.0	97	198.9	69.8	5.2	0	0	0	0
All ages	20	3.3	145	24.8	64.2	8.2	0	0	0	0
Females										
0-4	0	0.0	0	0.0	-	-	0	0	0	0
5-14	0	0.0	0	0.0	-	-	0	0	0	0
15-44	3	0.9	38	13.3	29.9	34.2	0	0	0	0
45-59	9	13.5	76	118.3	52.4	15.9	0	0	0	0
60+	35	68.5	276	534.0	70.6	6.0	0	0	0	0
All ages	47	8.5	390	71.1	65.0	9.4	0	0	0	0
Total	66	5.8	535	47.2	64.7	9.1	0	0	0	0

Table 92e — OAI - OPAI - APAI — Trachoma - Blindness

Age group (years)	Incidence 1990 Number ('000s)	Incidence 1990 Rate (per 100 000)	Prevalence 1990 Number ('000s)	Prevalence 1990 Rate (per 100 000)	Avg. age at onset (years)	Average duration (years)	Deaths 1990 Number ('000s)	Deaths 1990 Rate (per 100 000)	Deaths 2000 (Projected) Number ('000s)	Deaths 2000 (Projected) Rate (per 100 000)
Males										
0-4	0	0.0	0	0.0	-	-	0	0	0	0
5-14	0	0.0	0	0.0	-	-	0	0	0	0
15-44	0	0.1	2	1.4	29.7	27.4	0	0	0	0
45-59	1	1.6	4	12.4	52.3	12.3	0	0	0	0
60+	2	8.9	11	55.7	69.6	5.0	0	0	0	0
All ages	2	0.7	18	5.2	63.3	8.0	0	0	0	0
Females										
0-4	0	0.0	0	0.0	-	-	0	0	0	0
5-14	0	0.0	0	0.0	-	-	0	0	0	0
15-44	0	0.3	6	3.6	29.8	30.1	0	0	0	0
45-59	1	3.8	11	32.0	52.3	14.2	0	0	0	0
60+	5	20.0	33	143.7	70.3	5.6	0	0	0	0
All ages	6	1.8	50	14.6	63.8	9.1	0	0	0	0
Total	9	1.3	67	9.9	63.7	8.8	0	0	0	0

Table 92f — SSA - ASS - ASS — Trachoma - Blindness

Age group (years)	Incidence 1990 Number ('000s)	Incidence 1990 Rate (per 100 000)	Prevalence 1990 Number ('000s)	Prevalence 1990 Rate (per 100 000)	Avg. age at onset (years)	Average duration (years)	Deaths 1990 Number ('000s)	Deaths 1990 Rate (per 100 000)	Deaths 2000 (Projected) Number ('000s)	Deaths 2000 (Projected) Rate (per 100 000)
Males										
0-4	0	0.0	0	0	-	-	0	0	0	0
5-14	0	0.0	0	0	-	-	0	0	0	0
15-44	1	1.4	18	17	29.4	22.1	0	0	0	0
45-59	4	21.0	31	155	52.2	11.0	0	0	0	0
60+	12	114.4	72	681	69.2	4.7	0	0	0	0
All ages	18	7.0	121	48	62.0	7.6	0	0	0	0
Females										
0-4	0	0.0	0	0	-	-	0	0	0	0
5-14	0	0.0	0	0	-	-	0	0	0	0
15-44	4	3.3	46	43	29.5	24.3	0	0	0	0
45-59	11	49.8	86	389	52.2	12.4	0	0	0	0
60+	34	265.6	221	1 737	69.6	5.1	0	0	0	0
All ages	48	18.8	353	137	62.7	8.2	0	0	0	0
Total	66	12.9	473	93	62.5	8.0	0	0	0	0

For epidemiological sources see Thylefors et al. 1996. For the methods used to estimate and project incidence, prevalence, and deaths see Murray and Lopez 1996a. See explanatory notes for definitions and caveats.

Table 92 | **Cuadro 92** | **Tableau 92**
Trachoma | **Tracoma** | **Trachome**

Blindness | Ceguera | Cécité

Table 92g LAC - ALC - ALC   Trachoma - Blindness

Age group (years)	Incidence 1990 Number ('000s)	Rate (per 100 000)	Prevalence 1990 Number ('000s)	Rate (per 100 000)	Avg. age at onset (years)	Average duration (years)	Deaths 1990 Number ('000s)	Rate (per 100 000)	Deaths 2000 (Projected) Number ('000s)	Rate (per 100 000)
Males										
0-4	0	0	0	0	-	-	0	0	0	0
5-14	0	0	0	0	-	-	0	0	0	0
15-44	0	0	0	0	-	-	0	0	0	0
45-59	0	0	0	0	-	-	0	0	0	0
60+	0	0	0	0	-	-	0	0	0	0
All ages	0	0	0	0	-	-	0	0	0	0
Females										
0-4	0	0	0	0	-	-	0	0	0	0
5-14	0	0	0	0	-	-	0	0	0	0
15-44	0	0	0	0	-	-	0	0	0	0
45-59	0	0	0	0	-	-	0	0	0	0
60+	0	0	0	0	-	-	0	0	0	0
All ages	0	0	0	0	-	-	0	0	0	0
Total	0	0	0	0	-	-	0	0	0	0

Table 92h MEC - AOM - CMO   Trachoma - Blindness

Age group (years)	Incidence 1990 Number ('000s)	Rate (per 100 000)	Prevalence 1990 Number ('000s)	Rate (per 100 000)	Avg. age at onset (years)	Average duration (years)	Deaths 1990 Number ('000s)	Rate (per 100 000)	Deaths 2000 (Projected) Number ('000s)	Rate (per 100 000)
Males										
0-4	0	0.0	0	0	-	-	0	0	0	0
5-14	0	0.0	0	0	-	-	0	0	0	0
15-44	1	0.8	13	11	29.8	29.2	0	0	0	0
45-59	3	12.5	23	102	52.3	12.8	0	0	0	0
60+	10	69.8	62	451	69.7	5.1	0	0	0	0
All ages	13	5.2	97	38	63.3	8.4	0	0	0	0
Females										
0-4	0	0.0	0	0	-	-	0	0	0	0
5-14	0	0.0	0	0	-	-	0	0	0	0
15-44	2	2.0	31	29	29.8	31.8	0	0	0	0
45-59	7	30.4	58	258	52.3	14.8	0	0	0	0
60+	24	155.3	179	1 161	70.4	5.8	0	0	0	0
All ages	33	13.3	268	108	64.0	9.3	0	0	0	0
Total	46	9.2	365	73	63.8	9.1	0	0	0	0

Table 92i World - Mundo - Monde   Trachoma - Blindness

Age group (years)	Incidence 1990 Number ('000s)	Rate (per 100 000)	Prevalence 1990 Number ('000s)	Rate (per 100 000)	Avg. age at onset (years)	Average duration (years)	Deaths 1990 Number ('000s)	Rate (per 100 000)	Deaths 2000 (Projected) Number ('000s)	Rate (per 100 000)
Males										
0-4	0	0.0	0	0.0	-	-	0	0	0	0
5-14	0	0.0	0	0.0	-	-	0	0	0	0
15-44	4	0.3	49	3.9	29.7	26.9	0	0	0	0
45-59	12	3.8	93	29.8	52.3	12.4	0	0	0	0
60+	39	17.8	248	113.5	69.6	5.0	0	0	0	0
All ages	54	2.0	391	14.7	63.2	8.1	0	0	0	0
Females										
0-4	0	0.0	0	0.0	-	-	0	0	0	0
5-14	0	0.0	0	0.0	-	-	0	0	0	0
15-44	9	0.7	123	10.2	29.7	29.4	0	0	0	0
45-59	29	9.2	237	76.3	52.3	14.2	0	0	0	0
60+	100	37.2	727	270.1	70.2	5.6	0	0	0	0
All ages	138	5.3	1 087	41.6	63.9	8.9	0	0	0	0
Total	192	3.6	1 478	28.1	63.7	8.7	0	0	0	0

For epidemiological sources see Thylefors et al. 1996. For the methods used to estimate and project incidence, prevalence, and deaths see Murray and Lopez 1996a. See explanatory notes for definitions and caveats.

Table 93 / **Cuadro 93** / **Tableau 93**
Trachoma / **Tracoma** / **Trachome**

Low vision / Disminución de la agudeza visual / Baisse de la vision

Table 93a — EME - PEMC - EMBE — Trachoma - Low vision

Age group (years)	Incidence 1990 Number ('000s)	Rate (per 100 000)	Prevalence 1990 Number ('000s)	Rate (per 100 000)	Avg. age at onset (years)	Average duration (years)	Deaths 1990 Number ('000s)	Rate (per 100 000)	Deaths 2000 (Projected) Number ('000s)	Rate (per 100 000)
Males										
0-4	0	0	0	0	-	-	0	0	0	0
5-14	0	0	0	0	-	-	0	0	0	0
15-44	0	0	0	0	-	-	0	0	0	0
45-59	0	0	0	0	-	-	0	0	0	0
60+	0	0	0	0	-	-	0	0	0	0
All ages	0	0	0	0	-	-	0	0	0	0
Females										
0-4	0	0	0	0	-	-	0	0	0	0
5-14	0	0	0	0	-	-	0	0	0	0
15-44	0	0	0	0	-	-	0	0	0	0
45-59	0	0	0	0	-	-	0	0	0	0
60+	0	0	0	0	-	-	0	0	0	0
All ages	0	0	0	0	-	-	0	0	0	0
Total	0	0	0	0	-	-	0	0	0	0

Table 93b — FSE - PEAS - AESE — Trachoma - Low vision

Age group (years)	Incidence 1990 Number ('000s)	Rate (per 100 000)	Prevalence 1990 Number ('000s)	Rate (per 100 000)	Avg. age at onset (years)	Average duration (years)	Deaths 1990 Number ('000s)	Rate (per 100 000)	Deaths 2000 (Projected) Number ('000s)	Rate (per 100 000)
Males										
0-4	0	0	0	0	-	-	0	0	0	0
5-14	0	0	0	0	-	-	0	0	0	0
15-44	0	0	0	0	-	-	0	0	0	0
45-59	0	0	0	0	-	-	0	0	0	0
60+	0	0	0	0	-	-	0	0	0	0
All ages	0	0	0	0	-	-	0	0	0	0
Females										
0-4	0	0	0	0	-	-	0	0	0	0
5-14	0	0	0	0	-	-	0	0	0	0
15-44	0	0	0	0	-	-	0	0	0	0
45-59	0	0	0	0	-	-	0	0	0	0
60+	0	0	0	0	-	-	0	0	0	0
All ages	0	0	0	0	-	-	0	0	0	0
Total	0	0	0	0	-	-	0	0	0	0

Table 93c — India - India - Inde — Trachoma - Low vision

Age group (years)	Incidence 1990 Number ('000s)	Rate (per 100 000)	Prevalence 1990 Number ('000s)	Rate (per 100 000)	Avg. age at onset (years)	Average duration (years)	Deaths 1990 Number ('000s)	Rate (per 100 000)	Deaths 2000 (Projected) Number ('000s)	Rate (per 100 000)
Males										
0-4	0	0.0	0	0.0	-	-	0	0	0	0
5-14	0	0.0	0	0.0	-	-	0	0	0	0
15-44	0	0.1	1	0.7	29.8	12.2	0	0	0	0
45-59	1	1.1	3	5.9	52.3	7.3	0	0	0	0
60+	1	4.8	8	26.2	69.7	4.8	0	0	0	0
All ages	2	0.5	12	2.7	62.5	5.9	0	0	0	0
Females										
0-4	0	0.0	0	0.0	-	-	0	0	0	0
5-14	0	0.0	0	0.0	-	-	0	0	0	0
15-44	0	0.2	3	1.8	29.8	12.6	0	0	0	0
45-59	1	3.1	8	16.3	52.4	7.8	0	0	0	0
60+	4	12.5	21	72.5	70.1	5.1	0	0	0	0
All ages	5	1.3	32	7.8	62.7	6.3	0	0	0	0
Total	8	0.9	44	5.1	62.6	6.2	0	0	0	0

For epidemiological sources see Thylefors et al. 1996. For the methods used to estimate and project incidence, prevalence, and deaths see Murray and Lopez 1996a. See explanatory notes for definitions and caveats.

Table 93
Trachoma

Cuadro 93
Tracoma

Tableau 93
Trachome

Low vision

Disminución de la agudeza visual

Baisse de la vision

Table 93d	China - China - Chine								Trachoma - Low vision	
Age group (years)	Incidence 1990		Prevalence 1990		Avg. age at onset (years)	Average duration (years)	Deaths 1990		Deaths 2000 (Projected)	
	Number ('000s)	Rate (per 100 000)	Number ('000s)	Rate (per 100 000)			Number ('000s)	Rate (per 100 000)	Number ('000s)	Rate (per 100 000)
Males										
0-4	0	0.0	0	0.0	-	-	0	0	0	0
5-14	0	0.0	0	0.0	-	-	0	0	0	0
15-44	2	0.6	18	5.8	29.9	12.7	0	0	0	0
45-59	7	9.8	38	51.7	52.4	7.5	0	0	0	0
60+	21	42.2	113	229.7	69.8	4.8	0	0	0	0
All ages	30	5.1	168	28.7	63.0	5.9	0	0	0	0
Females										
0-4	0	0.0	0	0.0	-	-	0	0	0	0
5-14	0	0.0	0	0.0	-	-	0	0	0	0
15-44	5	1.7	43	15.3	30.0	13.1	0	0	0	0
45-59	13	20.0	71	110.6	52.4	8.3	0	0	0	0
60+	52	101.5	316	612.4	70.6	5.4	0	0	0	0
All ages	70	12.8	431	78.6	64.5	6.5	0	0	0	0
Total	100	8.8	599	52.8	64.0	6.3	0	0	0	0

Table 93e	OAI - OPAI - APAI								Trachoma - Low vision	
Age group (years)	Incidence 1990		Prevalence 1990		Avg. age at onset (years)	Average duration (years)	Deaths 1990		Deaths 2000 (Projected)	
	Number ('000s)	Rate (per 100 000)	Number ('000s)	Rate (per 100 000)			Number ('000s)	Rate (per 100 000)	Number ('000s)	Rate (per 100 000)
Males										
0-4	0	0.0	0	0.0	-	-	0	0	0	0
5-14	0	0.0	0	0.0	-	-	0	0	0	0
15-44	0	0.2	3	1.6	29.8	12.0	0	0	0	0
45-59	1	2.8	5	14.4	52.3	7.0	0	0	0	0
60+	3	12.4	13	63.9	69.6	4.5	0	0	0	0
All ages	4	1.1	20	5.9	62.1	5.8	0	0	0	0
Females										
0-4	0	0.0	0	0.0	-	-	0	0	0	0
5-14	0	0.0	0	0.0	-	-	0	0	0	0
15-44	1	0.5	7	4.2	29.8	12.4	0	0	0	0
45-59	2	7.1	13	37.6	52.4	7.8	0	0	0	0
60+	6	28.4	38	166.9	70.3	5.1	0	0	0	0
All ages	10	2.9	58	17.0	62.5	6.4	0	0	0	0
Total	13	2.0	78	11.4	62.4	6.2	0	0	0	0

Table 93f	SSA - ASS - ASS								Trachoma - Low vision	
Age group (years)	Incidence 1990		Prevalence 1990		Avg. age at onset (years)	Average duration (years)	Deaths 1990		Deaths 2000 (Projected)	
	Number ('000s)	Rate (per 100 000)	Number ('000s)	Rate (per 100 000)			Number ('000s)	Rate (per 100 000)	Number ('000s)	Rate (per 100 000)
Males										
0-4	0	0.0	0	0	-	-	0	0	0	0
5-14	0	0.0	0	0	-	-	0	0	0	0
15-44	2	2.4	20	20	29.4	10.8	0	0	0	0
45-59	7	36.6	36	177	52.2	6.5	0	0	0	0
60+	17	159.2	83	788	69.2	4.4	0	0	0	0
All ages	27	10.6	139	55	60.8	5.5	0	0	0	0
Females										
0-4	0	0.0	0	0	-	-	0	0	0	0
5-14	0	0.0	0	0	-	-	0	0	0	0
15-44	6	6.0	53	50	29.5	11.2	0	0	0	0
45-59	20	89.3	100	450	52.3	7.0	0	0	0	0
60+	47	373.0	255	2 000	69.7	4.7	0	0	0	0
All ages	74	28.5	407	158	61.6	5.9	0	0	0	0
Total	100	19.6	547	107	61.4	5.8	0	0	0	0

For epidemiological sources see Thylefors et al. 1996. For the methods used to estimate and project incidence, prevalence, and deaths see Murray and Lopez 1996a. See explanatory notes for definitions and caveats.

Table 93   **Cuadro 93**   **Tableau 93**
Trachoma   **Tracoma**   **Trachome**

Low vision   Disminución de la agudeza visual   Baisse de la vision

Table 93g   LAC - ALC - ALC   Trachoma - Low vision

Age group (years)	Incidence 1990 Number ('000s)	Rate (per 100 000)	Prevalence 1990 Number ('000s)	Rate (per 100 000)	Avg. age at onset (years)	Average duration (years)	Deaths 1990 Number ('000s)	Rate (per 100 000)	Deaths 2000 (Projected) Number ('000s)	Rate (per 100 000)
Males										
0-4	0	0	0	0	-	-	0	0	0	0
5-14	0	0	0	0	-	-	0	0	0	0
15-44	0	0	0	0	-	-	0	0	0	0
45-59	0	0	0	0	-	-	0	0	0	0
60+	0	0	0	0	-	-	0	0	0	0
All ages	0	0	0	0	-	-	0	0	0	0
Females										
0-4	0	0	0	0	-	-	0	0	0	0
5-14	0	0	0	0	-	-	0	0	0	0
15-44	0	0	0	0	-	-	0	0	0	0
45-59	0	0	0	0	-	-	0	0	0	0
60+	0	0	0	0	-	-	0	0	0	0
All ages	0	0	0	0	-	-	0	0	0	0
Total	0	0	0	0	-	-	0	0	0	0

Table 93h   MEC - AOM - CMO   Trachoma - Low vision

Age group (years)	Incidence 1990 Number ('000s)	Rate (per 100 000)	Prevalence 1990 Number ('000s)	Rate (per 100 000)	Avg. age at onset (years)	Average duration (years)	Deaths 1990 Number ('000s)	Rate (per 100 000)	Deaths 2000 (Projected) Number ('000s)	Rate (per 100 000)
Males										
0-4	0	0.0	0	0	-	-	0	0	0	0
5-14	0	0.0	0	0	-	-	0	0	0	0
15-44	2	1.5	15	13	29.9	12.3	0	0	0	0
45-59	5	22.8	26	118	52.3	7.2	0	0	0	0
60+	13	97.8	71	523	69.7	4.7	0	0	0	0
All ages	20	7.8	113	44	62.0	6.0	0	0	0	0
Females										
0-4	0	0.0	0	0	-	-	0	0	0	0
5-14	0	0.0	0	0	-	-	0	0	0	0
15-44	4	3.7	36	33	29.9	12.8	0	0	0	0
45-59	13	56.7	67	301	52.4	7.9	0	0	0	0
60+	34	221.7	207	1 337	70.4	5.3	0	0	0	0
All ages	51	20.6	309	125	62.8	6.5	0	0	0	0
Total	71	14.1	422	84	62.5	6.4	0	0	0	0

Table 93i   World - Mundo - Monde   Trachoma - Low vision

Age group (years)	Incidence 1990 Number ('000s)	Rate (per 100 000)	Prevalence 1990 Number ('000s)	Rate (per 100 000)	Avg. age at onset (years)	Average duration (years)	Deaths 1990 Number ('000s)	Rate (per 100 000)	Deaths 2000 (Projected) Number ('000s)	Rate (per 100 000)
Males										
0-4	0	0.0	0	0.0	-	-	0	0	0	0
5-14	0	0.0	0	0.0	-	-	0	0	0	0
15-44	7	0.5	57	4.5	29.7	11.8	0	0	0	0
45-59	21	6.8	108	34.4	52.3	7.0	0	0	0	0
60+	55	25.0	287	131.3	69.6	4.6	0	0	0	0
All ages	82	3.1	452	17.0	62.0	5.8	0	0	0	0
Females										
0-4	0	0.0	0	0.0	-	-	0	0	0	0
5-14	0	0.0	0	0.0	-	-	0	0	0	0
15-44	16	1.4	142	11.9	29.8	12.2	0	0	0	0
45-59	49	15.8	258	83.1	52.4	7.6	0	0	0	0
60+	144	53.6	836	310.6	70.2	5.1	0	0	0	0
All ages	210	8.0	1 237	47.3	62.9	6.3	0	0	0	0
Total	292	5.5	1 689	32.1	62.6	6.1	0	0	0	0

For epidemiological sources see Thylefors et al. 1996. For the methods used to estimate and project incidence, prevalence, and deaths see Murray and Lopez 1996a. See explanatory notes for definitions and caveats.

Table 94   **Cuadro 94**   **Tableau 94**
Ascariasis   **Ascaridiasis**   **Ascaridose**

High intensity infection   Infección de alta intensidad   Infection de forte intensité

Table 94a   EME - PEMC - EMBE — Ascariasis - High intensity infection

Age group (years)	Incidence 1990 Number ('000s)	Rate (per 100 000)	Prevalence 1990 Number ('000s)	Rate (per 100 000)	Avg. age at onset (years)	Average duration (years)	Deaths 1990 Number ('000s)	Rate (per 100 000)	Deaths 2000 (Projected) Number ('000s)	Rate (per 100 000)
Males										
0-4	-	-	0	0	-	-	-	-	-	-
5-14	-	-	0	0	-	-	-	-	-	-
15-44	-	-	0	0	-	-	-	-	-	-
45-59	-	-	0	0	-	-	-	-	-	-
60+	-	-	0	0	-	-	-	-	-	-
All ages	-	-	0	0	-	-	-	-	-	-
Females										
0-4	-	-	0	0	-	-	-	-	-	-
5-14	-	-	0	0	-	-	-	-	-	-
15-44	-	-	0	0	-	-	-	-	-	-
45-59	-	-	0	0	-	-	-	-	-	-
60+	-	-	0	0	-	-	-	-	-	-
All ages	-	-	0	0	-	-	-	-	-	-
Total	-	-	0	0	-	-	-	-	-	-

Table 94b   FSE - PEAS - AESE — Ascariasis - High intensity infection

Age group (years)	Incidence 1990 Number ('000s)	Rate (per 100 000)	Prevalence 1990 Number ('000s)	Rate (per 100 000)	Avg. age at onset (years)	Average duration (years)	Deaths 1990 Number ('000s)	Rate (per 100 000)	Deaths 2000 (Projected) Number ('000s)	Rate (per 100 000)
Males										
0-4	-	-	0	0	-	-	-	-	-	-
5-14	-	-	0	0	-	-	-	-	-	-
15-44	-	-	0	0	-	-	-	-	-	-
45-59	-	-	0	0	-	-	-	-	-	-
60+	-	-	0	0	-	-	-	-	-	-
All ages	-	-	0	0	-	-	-	-	-	-
Females										
0-4	-	-	0	0	-	-	-	-	-	-
5-14	-	-	0	0	-	-	-	-	-	-
15-44	-	-	0	0	-	-	-	-	-	-
45-59	-	-	0	0	-	.	-	-	-	-
60+	-	-	0	0	-	-	-	-	-	-
All ages	-	-	0	0	-	-	-	-	-	-
Total	-	-	0	0	-	-	-	-	-	-

Table 94c   India - India - Inde — Ascariasis - High intensity infection

Age group (years)	Incidence 1990 Number ('000s)	Rate (per 100 000)	Prevalence 1990 Number ('000s)	Rate (per 100 000)	Avg. age at onset (years)	Average duration (years)	Deaths 1990 Number ('000s)	Rate (per 100 000)	Deaths 2000 (Projected) Number ('000s)	Rate (per 100 000)
Males										
0-4	-	-	102	170	-	-	-	-	-	-
5-14	-	-	2 574	2 530	-	-	-	-	-	-
15-44	-	-	501	250	-	-	-	-	-	-
45-59	-	-	119	250	-	-	-	-	-	-
60+	-	-	74	250	-	-	-	-	-	-
All ages	-	-	3 371	767	-	-	-	-	-	-
Females										
0-4	-	-	96	170	-	-	-	-	-	-
5-14	-	-	2 410	2 530	-	-	-	-	-	-
15-44	-	-	458	250	-	-	-	-	-	-
45-59	-	-	115	250	-	-	-	-	-	-
60+	-	-	72	250	-	-	-	-	-	-
All ages	-	-	3 152	769	-	-	-	-	-	-
Total	-	-	6 523	768	-	-	-	-	-	-

For epidemiological sources see Bundy et al. 1996. See explanatory notes for definitions and caveats.

Table 94	Cuadro 94	Tableau 94
Ascariasis	**Ascaridiasis**	**Ascaridose**

High intensity infection | Infección de alta intensidad | Infection de forte intensité

Table 94d   China - China - Chine   Ascariasis - High intensity infection

Age group (years)	Incidence 1990 Number ('000s)	Rate (per 100 000)	Prevalence 1990 Number ('000s)	Rate (per 100 000)	Avg. age at onset (years)	Average duration (years)	Deaths 1990 Number ('000s)	Rate (per 100 000)	Deaths 2000 (Projected) Number ('000s)	Rate (per 100 000)
Males										
0-4	-	-	361	600	-	-	-	-	-	-
5-14	-	-	8 604	8 870	-	-	-	-	-	-
15-44	-	-	2 726	890	-	-	-	-	-	-
45-59	-	-	647	890	-	-	-	-	-	-
60+	-	-	436	890	-	-	-	-	-	-
All ages	-	-	12 774	2 183	-	-	-	-	-	-
Females										
0-4	-	-	348	600	-	-	-	-	-	-
5-14	-	-	8 019	8 870	-	-	-	-	-	-
15-44	-	-	2 528	890	-	-	-	-	-	-
45-59	-	-	573	890	-	-	-	-	-	-
60+	-	-	460	890	-	-	-	-	-	-
All ages	-	-	11 928	2 175	-	-	-	-	-	-
Total	-	-	24 701	2 179	-	-	-	-	-	-

Table 94e   OAI - OPAI - APAI   Ascariasis - High intensity infection

Age group (years)	Incidence 1990 Number ('000s)	Rate (per 100 000)	Prevalence 1990 Number ('000s)	Rate (per 100 000)	Avg. age at onset (years)	Average duration (years)	Deaths 1990 Number ('000s)	Rate (per 100 000)	Deaths 2000 (Projected) Number ('000s)	Rate (per 100 000)
Males										
0-4	-	-	236	540	-	-	-	-	-	-
5-14	-	-	6 597	7 850	-	-	-	-	-	-
15-44	-	-	1 238	770	-	-	-	-	-	-
45-59	-	-	263	770	-	-	-	-	-	-
60+	-	-	156	770	-	-	-	-	-	-
All ages	-	-	8 490	2 475	-	-	-	-	-	-
Females										
0-4	-	-	227	540	-	-	-	-	-	-
5-14	-	-	6 297	7 850	-	-	-	-	-	-
15-44	-	-	1 229	770	-	-	-	-	-	-
45-59	-	-	270	770	-	-	-	-	-	-
60+	-	-	174	770	-	-	-	-	-	-
All ages	-	-	8 197	2 414	-	-	-	-	-	-
Total	-	-	16 687	2 445	-	-	-	-	-	-

Table 94f   SSA - ASS - ASS   Ascariasis - High intensity infection

Age group (years)	Incidence 1990 Number ('000s)	Rate (per 100 000)	Prevalence 1990 Number ('000s)	Rate (per 100 000)	Avg. age at onset (years)	Average duration (years)	Deaths 1990 Number ('000s)	Rate (per 100 000)	Deaths 2000 (Projected) Number ('000s)	Rate (per 100 000)
Males										
0-4	-	-	57	120	-	-	-	-	-	-
5-14	-	-	1 208	1 720	-	-	-	-	-	-
15-44	-	-	176	170	-	-	-	-	-	-
45-59	-	-	35	170	-	-	-	-	-	-
60+	-	-	18	170	-	-	-	-	-	-
All ages	-	-	1 494	592	-	-	-	-	-	-
Females										
0-4	-	-	56	120	-	-	-	-	-	-
5-14	-	-	1 201	1 720	-	-	-	-	-	-
15-44	-	-	181	170	-	-	-	-	-	-
45-59	-	-	38	170	-	-	-	-	-	-
60+	-	-	22	170	-	-	-	-	-	-
All ages	-	-	1 497	580	-	-	-	-	-	-
Total	-	-	2 991	586	-	-	-	-	-	-

For epidemiological sources see Bundy et al. 1996. See explanatory notes for definitions and caveats.

Table 94	Cuadro 94	Tableau 94
Ascariasis	**Ascaridiasis**	**Ascaridose**

High intensity infection	Infección de alta intensidad	Infection de forte intensité

Table 94g LAC - ALC - ALC

Ascariasis - High intensity infection

Age group (years)	Incidence 1990 Number ('000s)	Rate (per 100 000)	Prevalence 1990 Number ('000s)	Rate (per 100 000)	Avg. age at onset (years)	Average duration (years)	Deaths 1990 Number ('000s)	Rate (per 100 000)	Deaths 2000 (Projected) Number ('000s)	Rate (per 100 000)
Males										
0-4	-	-	118	410	-	-	-	-	-	-
5-14	-	-	3 101	5 950	-	-	-	-	-	-
15-44	-	-	605	580	-	-	-	-	-	-
45-59	-	-	129	580	-	-	-	-	-	-
60+	-	-	83	580	-	-	-	-	-	-
All ages	-	-	4 036	1 821	-	-	-	-	-	-
Females										
0-4	-	-	113	410	-	-	-	-	-	-
5-14	-	-	3 019	5 950	-	-	-	-	-	-
15-44	-	-	604	580	-	-	-	-	-	-
45-59	-	-	135	580	-	-	-	-	-	-
60+	-	-	98	580	-	-	-	-	-	-
All ages	-	-	3 969	1 783	-	-	-	-	-	-
Total	-	-	8 005	1 802	-	-	-	-	-	-

Table 94h MEC - AOM - CMO

Ascariasis - High intensity infection

Age group (years)	Incidence 1990 Number ('000s)	Rate (per 100 000)	Prevalence 1990 Number ('000s)	Rate (per 100 000)	Avg. age at onset (years)	Average duration (years)	Deaths 1990 Number ('000s)	Rate (per 100 000)	Deaths 2000 (Projected) Number ('000s)	Rate (per 100 000)
Males										
0-4	-	-	49	120	-	-	-	-	-	-
5-14	-	-	1 186	1 815	-	-	-	-	-	-
15-44	-	-	205	180	-	-	-	-	-	-
45-59	-	-	40	180	-	-	-	-	-	-
60+	-	-	25	180	-	-	-	-	-	-
All ages	-	-	1 505	587	-	-	-	-	-	-
Females										
0-4	-	-	48	120	-	-	-	-	-	-
5-14	-	-	1 125	1 815	-	-	-	-	-	-
15-44	-	-	193	180	-	-	-	-	-	-
45-59	-	-	40	180	-	-	-	-	-	-
60+	-	-	28	180	-	-	-	-	-	-
All ages	-	-	1 434	581	-	-	-	-	-	-
Total	-	-	2 939	584	-	-	-	-	-	-

Table 94i World - Mundo - Monde

Ascariasis - High intensity infection

Age group (years)	Incidence 1990 Number ('000s)	Rate (per 100 000)	Prevalence 1990 Number ('000s)	Rate (per 100 000)	Avg. age at onset (years)	Average duration (years)	Deaths 1990 Number ('000s)	Rate (per 100 000)	Deaths 2000 (Projected) Number ('000s)	Rate (per 100 000)
Males										
0-4	-	-	924	287	-	-	-	-	-	-
5-14	-	-	23 270	4 222	-	-	-	-	-	-
15-44	-	-	5 452	436	-	-	-	-	-	-
45-59	-	-	1 232	395	-	-	-	-	-	-
60+	-	-	791	361	-	-	-	-	-	-
All ages	-	-	31 669	1 193	-	-	-	-	-	-
Females										
0-4	-	-	888	287	-	-	-	-	-	-
5-14	-	-	22 071	4 200	-	-	-	-	-	-
15-44	-	-	5 193	433	-	-	-	-	-	-
45-59	-	-	1 172	377	-	-	-	-	-	-
60+	-	-	854	317	-	-	-	-	-	-
All ages	-	-	30 177	1 155	-	-	-	-	-	-
Total	-	-	61 847	1 174	-	-	-	-	-	-

For epidemiological sources see Bundy et al. 1996. See explanatory notes for definitions and caveats.

Table 95 | **Cuadro 95** | **Tableau 95**
Ascariasis | **Ascaridiasis** | **Ascaridose**

Cotemporaneous cognitive deficit   Deficit cognocitivo contemporaneo   Deficit cognitif simultané

Table 95a   EME - PEMC - EMBE   Ascariasis - Cotemporaneous cognitive deficit

Age group (years)	Incidence 1990 Number ('000s)	Rate (per 100 000)	Prevalence 1990 Number ('000s)	Rate (per 100 000)	Avg. age at onset (years)	Average duration (years)	Deaths 1990 Number ('000s)	Rate (per 100 000)	Deaths 2000 (Projected) Number ('000s)	Rate (per 100 000)
Males										
0-4	0	0	0	0	-	-	0	0	0	0
5-14	0	0	0	0	-	-	0	0	0	0
15-44	0	0	0	0	-	-	0	0	0	0
45-59	0	0	0	0	-	-	0	0	0	0
60+	0	0	0	0	-	-	0	0	0	0
All ages	0	0	0	0	-	-	0	0	0	0
Females										
0-4	0	0	0	0	-	-	0	0	0	0
5-14	0	0	0	0	-	-	0	0	0	0
15-44	0	0	0	0	-	-	0	0	0	0
45-59	0	0	0	0	-	-	0	0	0	0
60+	0	0	0	0	-	-	0	0	0	0
All ages	0	0	0	0	-	-	0	0	0	0
Total	0	0	0	0	-	-	0	0	0	0

Table 95b   FSE - PEAS - AESE   Ascariasis - Cotemporaneous cognitive deficit

Age group (years)	Incidence 1990 Number ('000s)	Rate (per 100 000)	Prevalence 1990 Number ('000s)	Rate (per 100 000)	Avg. age at onset (years)	Average duration (years)	Deaths 1990 Number ('000s)	Rate (per 100 000)	Deaths 2000 (Projected) Number ('000s)	Rate (per 100 000)
Males										
0-4	0	0	0	0	-	-	0	0	0	0
5-14	0	0	0	0	-	-	0	0	0	0
15-44	0	0	0	0	-	-	0	0	0	0
45-59	0	0	0	0	-	-	0	0	0	0
60+	0	0	0	0	-	-	0	0	0	0
All ages	0	0	0	0	-	-	0	0	0	0
Females										
0-4	0	0	0	0	-	-	0	0	0	0
5-14	0	0	0	0	-	-	0	0	0	0
15-44	0	0	0	0	-	-	0	0	0	0
45-59	0	0	0	0	-	-	0	0	0	0
60+	0	0	0	0	-	-	0	0	0	0
All ages	0	0	0	0	-	-	0	0	0	0
Total	0	0	0	0	-	-	0	0	0	0

Table 95c   India - India - Inde   Ascariasis - Cotemporaneous cognitive deficit

Age group (years)	Incidence 1990 Number ('000s)	Rate (per 100 000)	Prevalence 1990 Number ('000s)	Rate (per 100 000)	Avg. age at onset (years)	Average duration (years)	Deaths 1990 Number ('000s)	Rate (per 100 000)	Deaths 2000 (Projected) Number ('000s)	Rate (per 100 000)
Males										
0-4	0	0	0	0	2.5	1.0	0	0	0	0
5-14	783	770	783	770	10.0	1.0	0	0	0	0
15-44	20	10	20	10	29.8	1.0	0	0	0	0
45-59	5	10	5	10	52.3	1.0	0	0	0	0
60+	3	10	3	10	69.7	1.0	0	0	0	0
All ages	811	185	811	185	11.0	1.0	0	0	0	0
Females										
0-4	0	0	0	0	2.5	1.0	0	0	0	0
5-14	734	770	734	770	10.0	1.0	0	0	0	0
15-44	18	10	18	10	29.8	1.0	0	0	0	0
45-59	5	10	5	10	52.4	1.0	0	0	0	0
60+	0	0	3	10	70.1	1.0	0	0	0	0
All ages	756	184	759	185	10.7	1.0	0	0	0	0
Total	1 568	185	1 571	185	10.9	1.0	0	0	0	0

For epidemiological sources see Bundy et al. 1996. See explanatory notes for definitions and caveats.

Table 95	Cuadro 95	Tableau 95
Ascariasis	**Ascaridiasis**	**Ascaridose**

Cotemporaneous cognitive deficit | Deficit cognocitivo contemporaneo | Deficit cognitif simultané

Table 95d China - China - Chine

Ascariasis - Cotemporaneous cognitive deficit

Age group (years)	Incidence 1990 Number ('000s)	Rate (per 100 000)	Prevalence 1990 Number ('000s)	Rate (per 100 000)	Avg. age at onset (years)	Average duration (years)	Deaths 1990 Number ('000s)	Rate (per 100 000)	Deaths 2000 (Projected) Number ('000s)	Rate (per 100 000)
Males										
0-4	12	20	12	20	2.5	1.0	0	0	0	0
5-14	2 726	2 810	2 726	2 810	10.0	1.0	0	0	0	0
15-44	123	40	123	40	29.9	1.0	0	0	0	0
45-59	29	40	29	40	52.3	1.0	0	0	0	0
60+	20	40	20	40	69.8	1.0	0	0	0	0
All ages	2 909	497	2 909	497	11.6	1.0	0	0	0	0
Females										
0-4	12	20	12	20	2.5	1.0	0	0	0	0
5-14	2 540	2 810	2 540	2 810	10.0	1.0	0	0	0	0
15-44	114	40	114	40	29.9	1.0	0	0	0	0
45-59	26	40	26	40	52.4	1.0	0	0	0	0
60+	21	40	21	40	70.6	1.0	0	0	0	0
All ages	2 712	494	2 712	494	11.7	1.0	0	0	0	0
Total	5 621	496	5 621	496	11.6	1.0	0	0	0	0

Table 95e OAI - OPAI - APAI

Ascariasis - Cotemporaneous cognitive deficit

Age group (years)	Incidence 1990 Number ('000s)	Rate (per 100 000)	Prevalence 1990 Number ('000s)	Rate (per 100 000)	Avg. age at onset (years)	Average duration (years)	Deaths 1990 Number ('000s)	Rate (per 100 000)	Deaths 2000 (Projected) Number ('000s)	Rate (per 100 000)
Males										
0-4	4	10	4	10	2.5	1.0	0	0	0	0
5-14	1 971	2 345	1 971	2 345	10.0	1.0	0	0	0	0
15-44	48	30	48	30	29.7	1.0	0	0	0	0
45-59	10	30	10	30	52.3	1.0	0	0	0	0
60+	6	30	6	30	69.6	1.0	0	0	0	0
All ages	2 039	595	2 039	595	10.8	1.0	0	0	0	0
Females										
0-4	4	10	4	10	2.4	1.0	0	0	0	0
5-14	1 881	2 345	1 881	2 345	10.0	1.0	0	0	0	0
15-44	48	30	48	30	29.4	1.0	0	0	0	0
45-59	11	30	11	30	52.2	1.0	0	0	0	0
60+	7	30	7	30	69.2	1.0	0	0	0	0
All ages	1 950	574	1 950	574	10.9	1.0	0	0	0	0
Total	3 990	585	3 990	585	10.9	1.0	0	0	0	0

Table 95f SSA - ASS - ASS

Ascariasis - Cotemporaneous cognitive deficit

Age group (years)	Incidence 1990 Number ('000s)	Rate (per 100 000)	Prevalence 1990 Number ('000s)	Rate (per 100 000)	Avg. age at onset (years)	Average duration (years)	Deaths 1990 Number ('000s)	Rate (per 100 000)	Deaths 2000 (Projected) Number ('000s)	Rate (per 100 000)
Males										
0-4	0	0	0	0	2.4	1.0	0	0	0	0
5-14	369	525	369	525	10.0	1.0	0	0	0	0
15-44	10	10	10	10	29.4	1.0	0	0	0	0
45-59	2	10	2	10	52.2	1.0	0	0	0	0
60+	1	10	1	10	69.2	1.0	0	0	0	0
All ages	382	152	382	152	10.9	1.0	0	0	0	0
Females										
0-4	0	0	0	0	2.4	1.0	0	0	0	0
5-14	367	525	367	525	10.0	1.0	0	0	0	0
15-44	11	10	11	10	29.5	1.0	0	0	0	0
45-59	2	10	2	10	52.2	1.0	0	0	0	0
60+	1	10	1	10	69.7	1.0	0	0	0	0
All ages	381	148	381	148	11.0	1.0	0	0	0	0
Total	763	150	763	150	11.0	1.0	0	0	0	0

For epidemiological sources see Bundy et al. 1996. See explanatory notes for definitions and caveats.

Table 95 — **Cuadro 95** — **Tableau 95**
Ascariasis — **Ascaridiasis** — **Ascaridose**

Cotemporaneous cognitive deficit — Deficit cognocitivo contemporaneo — Deficit cognitif simultané

Table 95g LAC - ALC - ALC — Ascariasis - Cotemporaneous cognitive deficit

Age group (years)	Incidence 1990 Number ('000s)	Rate (per 100 000)	Prevalence 1990 Number ('000s)	Rate (per 100 000)	Avg. age at onset (years)	Average duration (years)	Deaths 1990 Number ('000s)	Rate (per 100 000)	Deaths 2000 (Projected) Number ('000s)	Rate (per 100 000)
Males										
0-4	3	10	3	10	2.5	1.0	0	0	0	0
5-14	933	1 790	933	1 790	10.0	1.0	0	0	0	0
15-44	21	20	21	20	29.8	1.0	0	0	0	0
45-59	4	20	4	20	52.3	1.0	0	0	0	0
60+	3	20	3	20	70.3	1.0	0	0	0	0
All ages	964	435	964	435	10.8	1.0	0	0	0	0
Females										
0-4	3	10	3	10	2.5	1.0	0	0	0	0
5-14	908	1 790	908	1 790	10.0	1.0	0	0	0	0
15-44	21	20	21	20	29.9	1.0	0	0	0	0
45-59	5	20	5	20	52.4	1.0	0	0	0	0
60+	3	20	3	20	71.1	1.0	0	0	0	0
All ages	940	422	940	422	10.8	1.0	0	0	0	0
Total	1 904	429	1 904	429	10.8	1.0	0	0	0	0

Table 95h MEC - AOM - CMO — Ascariasis - Cotemporaneous cognitive deficit

Age group (years)	Incidence 1990 Number ('000s)	Rate (per 100 000)	Prevalence 1990 Number ('000s)	Rate (per 100 000)	Avg. age at onset (years)	Average duration (years)	Deaths 1990 Number ('000s)	Rate (per 100 000)	Deaths 2000 (Projected) Number ('000s)	Rate (per 100 000)
Males										
0-4	0	0	0	0	2.5	1.0	0	0	0	0
5-14	363	555	363	555	10.0	1.0	0	0	0	0
15-44	11	10	11	10	29.8	1.0	0	0	0	0
45-59	2	10	2	10	52.3	1.0	0	0	0	0
60+	1	10	1	10	69.7	1.0	0	0	0	0
All ages	378	147	378	147	11.1	1.0	0	0	0	0
Females										
0-4	0	0	0	0	2.5	1.0	0	0	0	0
5-14	344	555	344	555	10.0	1.0	0	0	0	0
15-44	11	10	11	10	29.8	1.0	0	0	0	0
45-59	2	10	2	10	52.3	1.0	0	0	0	0
60+	2	10	2	10	70.4	1.0	0	0	0	0
All ages	359	145	359	145	11.1	1.0	0	0	0	0
Total	736	146	736	146	11.1	1.0	0	0	0	0

Table 95i World - Mundo - Monde — Ascariasis - Cotemporaneous cognitive deficit

Age group (years)	Incidence 1990 Number ('000s)	Rate (per 100 000)	Prevalence 1990 Number ('000s)	Rate (per 100 000)	Avg. age at onset (years)	Average duration (years)	Deaths 1990 Number ('000s)	Rate (per 100 000)	Deaths 2000 (Projected) Number ('000s)	Rate (per 100 000)
Males										
0-4	19	6.0	19	6.0	2.5	1.0	0	0	0	0
5-14	7 144	1 296.1	7 144	1 296.1	10.0	1.0	0	0	0	0
15-44	233	18.7	233	18.7	29.8	1.0	0	0	0	0
45-59	53	16.9	53	16.9	52.3	1.0	0	0	0	0
60+	34	15.5	34	15.5	69.8	1.0	0	0	0	0
All ages	7 484	282.0	7 484	282.0	11.2	1.0	0	0	0	0
Females										
0-4	19	6.0	19	6.0	2.5	1.0	0	0	0	0
5-14	6 774	1 288.9	6 774	1 288.9	10.0	1.0	0	0	0	0
15-44	222	18.5	222	18.5	29.8	1.0	0	0	0	0
45-59	50	16.1	50	16.1	52.3	1.0	0	0	0	0
60+	34	12.5	37	13.6	70.3	1.0	0	0	0	0
All ages	7 098	271.6	7 101	271.7	11.2	1.0	0	0	0	0
Total	14 582	276.8	14 585	276.9	11.2	1.0	0	0	0	0

For epidemiological sources see Bundy et al. 1996. See explanatory notes for definitions and caveats.

Annex Table 2. **Cause groups, diseases and injuries, and sequelae included in the Global Burden of Disease Study**

GBD Classification Code	Cause group, disease, injury, or sequela
I	Communicable, maternal, perinatal, and nutritional conditions
IA	Infectious and parasitic diseases
IA1	Tuberculosis
IA1-1	HIV sero-negative cases
IA1-2	HIV sero-positive cases
IA2	Sexually transmitted diseases excluding HIV
IA2a	Syphilis
IA2a-1	Congenital syphilis
IA2a-2	Low birth weight
IA2a-3	Primary
IA2a-4	Secondary
IA2a-5	Tertiary – cardiovascular
IA2a-6	Tertiary – gummas
IA2a-7	Tertiary – neurologic
IA2b	Chlamydia
IA2b-1	Ophthalmia neonatorum
IA2b-2	Low birth weight
IA2b-3	Corneal scar – blindness
IA2b-4	Corneal scar – low vision
IA2b-5	Cervicitis
IA2b-6	Neonatal pneumonia
IA2b-7	Pelvic inflammatory disease
IA2b-8	Ectopic pregnancy
IA2b-9	Tubo-ovarian abscess
IA2b-10	Chronic pelvic pain
IA2b-11	Infertility
IA2b-12	Symptomatic urethritis
IA2b-13	Epididymitis
IA2b-14	Stricture
IA2c	Gonorrhoea
IA2c-1	Ophthalmia neonatorum
IA2c-2	Low birth weight
IA2c-3	Corneal scar – blindness
IA2c-4	Corneal scar – low vision
IA2c-5	Cervicitis
IA2c-6	Pelvic inflammatory disease
IA2c-7	Ectopic pregnancy
IA2c-8	Tubo-ovarian abscess
IA2c-9	Chronic pelvic pain
IA2c-10	Infertility
IA2c-11	Symptomatic urethritis
IA2c-12	Epididymitis
IA2c-13	Stricture
IA3	HIV
IA3-1	Cases
IA3-2	AIDS
IA4	Diarrhoeal diseases
IA4-1	Episodes

Annex Table 2, continued.

GBD Classification Code	Cause group, disease, injury, or sequela
IA5	Childhood-cluster diseases
IA5a	Pertussis
IA5a-1	Episodes
IA5a-2	Mental retardation
IA5b	Poliomyelitis
IA5b-1	Lameness
IA5c	Diphtheria
IA5c-1	Episodes
IA5c-2	Neurological complications
IA5c-3	Myocarditis
IA5d	Measles
IA5d-1	Episodes
IA5e	Tetanus
IA5e-1	Episodes
IA6	Bacterial meningitis and meningococcaemia
IA6-1	All forms – episodes
IA6-2	Streptococcus pneumoniae – episodes
IA6-3	Haemophilus influenzae – episodes
IA6-4	Neisseria meningitidis – episodes
IA6-5	Meningococcaemia without meningitis – episodes
IA6-6	Deafness
IA6-7	Seizure disorder
IA6-8	Motor deficit
IA6-9	Mental retardation
IA7	Hepatitis B and hepatitis C
IA7-1	Episodes
IA7-2	Cirrhosis of the liver – symptomatic cases
IA7-3	Hepatoma
IA8	Malaria
IA8-1	Episodes
IA8-2	Anaemia
IA8-3	Neurological sequelae
IA9	Tropical-cluster diseases
IA9a	Trypanosomiasis
IA9a-1	Episodes
IA9b	Chagas disease
IA9b-1	Infection
IA9b-2	Cardiomyopathy without congestive heart failure
IA9b-3	Cardiomyopathy with congestive heart failure
IA9b-4	Megaviscera
IA9c	Schistosomiasis
IA9c-1	Infection
IA9d	Leishmaniasis
IA9d-1	Visceral
IA9d-2	Cutaneous
IA9e	Lymphatic filariasis
IA9e-1	Hydrocele > 15 cm0
IA9e-2	Bancroftian lymphoedema
IA9e-3	Brugian lymphoedema
IA9f	Onchocerciasis
IA9f-1	Blindness

Table 96 / Cuadro 96 / Tableau 96
Ascariasis / Ascaridiasis / Ascaridose

Cognitive impairment — Deficiencia cognocitiva — Déficience cognitive

Table 96g — LAC - ALC - ALC — Ascariasis - Cognitive impairment

Age group (years)	Incidence 1990 Number ('000s)	Rate (per 100 000)	Prevalence 1990 Number ('000s)	Rate (per 100 000)	Avg. age at onset (years)	Average duration (years)	Deaths 1990 Number ('000s)	Rate (per 100 000)	Deaths 2000 (Projected) Number ('000s)	Rate (per 100 000)
Males										
0-4	3	12	9	30	2.5	62.2	0	0	0	0
5-14	92	177	508	975	10.0	59.4	0	0	0	0
15-44	0	0	1 910	1 832	-	-	0	0	0	0
45-59	0	0	408	1 832	-	-	0	0	0	0
60+	0	0	261	1 832	-	-	0	0	0	0
All ages	96	43	3 095	1 397	9.7	59.5	0	0	0	0
Females										
0-4	3	12	8	30	2.5	66.1	0	0	0	0
5-14	90	177	495	976	10.0	63.0	0	0	0	0
15-44	0	0	1 906	1 832	-	-	0	0	0	0
45-59	0	0	428	1 832	-	-	0	0	0	0
60+	0	0	308	1 832	-	-	0	0	0	0
All ages	93	42	3 146	1 413	9.7	63.1	0	0	0	0
Total	189	43	6 241	1 405	9.7	61.3	0	0	0	0

Table 96h — MEC - AOM - CMO — Ascariasis - Cognitive impairment

Age group (years)	Incidence 1990 Number ('000s)	Rate (per 100 000)	Prevalence 1990 Number ('000s)	Rate (per 100 000)	Avg. age at onset (years)	Average duration (years)	Deaths 1990 Number ('000s)	Rate (per 100 000)	Deaths 2000 (Projected) Number ('000s)	Rate (per 100 000)
Males										
0-4	2	4.0	4	10	2.5	59.6	0	0	0	0
5-14	35	53.8	194	297	10.0	58.1	0	0	0	0
15-44	0	0.0	636	558	-	-	0	0	0	0
45-59	0	0.0	125	558	-	-	0	0	0	0
60+	0	0.0	76	558	-	-	0	0	0	0
All ages	37	14.4	1 035	404	9.7	58.2	0	0	0	0
Females										
0-4	2	4.0	4	10	2.5	62.1	0	0	0	0
5-14	33	53.8	184	297	10.0	60.9	0	0	0	0
15-44	0	0.0	598	558	-	-	0	0	0	0
45-59	0	0.0	124	558	-	-	0	0	0	0
60+	0	0.0	86	558	-	-	0	0	0	0
All ages	35	14.2	997	404	9.7	60.9	0	0	0	0
Total	72	14.3	2 032	404	9.7	59.5	0	0	0	0

Table 96i — World - Mundo - Monde — Ascariasis - Cognitive impairment

Age group (years)	Incidence 1990 Number ('000s)	Rate (per 100 000)	Prevalence 1990 Number ('000s)	Rate (per 100 000)	Avg. age at onset (years)	Average duration (years)	Deaths 1990 Number ('000s)	Rate (per 100 000)	Deaths 2000 (Projected) Number ('000s)	Rate (per 100 000)
Males										
0-4	28	8.7	69	21	2.5	60.2	0	0	0	0
5-14	691	125.4	3 807	691	10.0	57.9	0	0	0	0
15-44	0	0.0	16 849	1 348	-	-	0	0	0	0
45-59	0	0.0	3 806	1 218	-	-	0	0	0	0
60+	0	0.0	2 441	1 115	-	-	0	0	0	0
All ages	719	27.1	26 971	1 016	9.7	58.0	0	0	0	0
Females										
0-4	27	8.7	66	21	2.5	63.1	0	0	0	0
5-14	656	124.8	3 612	687	10.0	60.8	0	0	0	0
15-44	0	0.0	16 055	1 339	-	-	0	0	0	0
45-59	0	0.0	3 622	1 164	-	-	0	0	0	0
60+	0	0.0	2 635	979	-	-	0	0	0	0
All ages	682	26.1	25 990	994	9.7	60.9	0	0	0	0
Total	1 402	26.6	52 961	1 005	9.7	59.4	0	0	0	0

For epidemiological sources see Bundy et al. 1996. See explanatory notes for definitions and caveats.

Table 97	Cuadro 97	Tableau 97
Ascariasis	Ascaridiasis	Ascaridose

Intestinal obstruction	Obstrucción intestinal	Obstruction intestinale

Table 97a EME - PEMC - EMBE — Ascariasis - Intestinal obstruction

Age group (years)	Incidence 1990 Number ('000s)	Rate (per 100 000)	Prevalence 1990 Number ('000s)	Rate (per 100 000)	Avg. age at onset (years)	Average duration (years)	Deaths 1990 Number ('000s)	Rate (per 100 000)	Deaths 2000 (Projected) Number ('000s)	Rate (per 100 000)
Males										
0-4	0	0	0	0	-	-	0	0	0	0
5-14	0	0	0	0	-	-	0	0	0	0
15-44	0	0	0	0	-	-	0	0	0	0
45-59	0	0	0	0	-	-	0	0	0	0
60+	0	0	0	0	-	-	0	0	0	0
All ages	0	0	0	0	-	-	0	0	0	0
Females										
0-4	0	0	0	0	-	-	0	0	0	0
5-14	0	0	0	0	-	-	0	0	0	0
15-44	0	0	0	0	-	-	0	0	0	0
45-59	0	0	0	0	-	-	0	0	0	0
60+	0	0	0	0	-	-	0	0	0	0
All ages	0	0	0	0	-	-	0	0	0	0
Total	0	0	0	0	-	-	0	0	0	0

Table 97b FSE - PEAS - AESE — Ascariasis - Intestinal obstruction

Age group (years)	Incidence 1990 Number ('000s)	Rate (per 100 000)	Prevalence 1990 Number ('000s)	Rate (per 100 000)	Avg. age at onset (years)	Average duration (years)	Deaths 1990 Number ('000s)	Rate (per 100 000)	Deaths 2000 (Projected) Number ('000s)	Rate (per 100 000)
Males										
0-4	0	0	0	0	-	-	0	0	0	0
5-14	0	0	0	0	-	-	0	0	0	0
15-44	0	0	0	0	-	-	0	0	0	0
45-59	0	0	0	0	-	-	0	0	0	0
60+	0	0	0	0	-	-	0	0	0	0
All ages	0	0	0	0	-	-	0	0	0	0
Females										
0-4	0	0	0	0	-	-	0	0	0	0
5-14	0	0	0	0	-	-	0	0	0	0
15-44	0	0	0	0	-	-	0	0	0	0
45-59	0	0	0	0	-	-	0	0	0	0
60+	0	0	0	0	-	-	0	0	0	0
All ages	0	0	0	0	-	-	0	0	0	0
Total	0	0	0	0	-	-	0	0	0	0

Table 97c India - India - Inde — Ascariasis - Intestinal obstruction

Age group (years)	Incidence 1990 Number ('000s)	Rate (per 100 000)	Prevalence 1990 Number ('000s)	Rate (per 100 000)	Avg. age at onset (years)	Average duration (years)	Deaths 1990 Number ('000s)	Rate (per 100 000)	Deaths 2000 (Projected) Number ('000s)	Rate (per 100 000)
Males										
0-4	0	0.0	0	0.0	-	-	0	0.0	0	0.0
5-14	39	38.5	2	2.2	10.0	0.06	1	0.7	0	0.3
15-44	1	0.5	0	0.0	29.8	0.06	0	0.0	0	0.0
45-59	0	0.5	0	0.0	52.3	0.06	0	0.0	0	0.0
60+	0	0.5	0	0.0	69.7	0.06	0	0.0	0	0.0
All ages	41	9.2	2	0.5	11.0	0.06	1	0.2	0	0.1
Females										
0-4	0	0.0	0	0.0	-	-	0	0.0	0	0.0
5-14	37	38.5	2	2.2	10.0	0.06	1	0.7	0	0.3
15-44	1	0.5	0	0.0	29.8	0.06	0	0.0	0	0.0
45-59	0	0.5	0	0.0	52.4	0.06	0	0.0	0	0.0
60+	0	0.5	0	0.0	70.1	0.06	0	0.0	0	0.0
All ages	38	9.3	2	0.5	11.0	0.06	1	0.2	0	0.1
Total	79	9.2	5	0.5	11.0	0.06	1	0.2	1	0.1

For epidemiological sources see Bundy et al. 1996. See explanatory notes for definitions and caveats.

Table 97 **Cuadro 97** **Tableau 97**
Ascariasis **Ascaridiasis** **Ascaridose**

Intestinal obstruction Obstrucción intestinal Obstruction intestinale

Table 97d China - China - Chine — Ascariasis - Intestinal obstruction

Age group (years)	Incidence 1990 Number ('000s)	Rate (per 100 000)	Prevalence 1990 Number ('000s)	Rate (per 100 000)	Avg. age at onset (years)	Average duration (years)	Deaths 1990 Number ('000s)	Rate (per 100 000)	Deaths 2000 (Projected) Number ('000s)	Rate (per 100 000)
Males										
0-4	1	1.0	0	0.1	2.5	0.06	0	0.0	0	0.0
5-14	136	140.5	8	8.1	10.0	0.06	2	2.0	1	0.7
15-44	6	2.0	0	0.1	29.9	0.06	0	0.0	0	0.0
45-59	1	2.0	0	0.1	52.3	0.06	0	0.0	0	0.0
60+	1	2.0	0	0.1	69.8	0.06	0	0.0	0	0.0
All ages	145	24.9	8	1.4	11.6	0.06	2	0.4	1	0.1
Females										
0-4	1	1.0	0	0.1	2.5	0.06	0	0.0	0	0.0
5-14	127	140.5	7	8.1	10.0	0.06	2	2.0	1	0.7
15-44	6	2.0	0	0.1	29.9	0.06	0	0.0	0	0.0
45-59	1	2.0	0	0.1	52.4	0.06	0	0.0	0	0.0
60+	1	2.0	0	0.1	70.6	0.06	0	0.0	0	0.0
All ages	136	24.7	8	1.4	11.7	0.06	2	0.4	1	0.1
Total	281	24.8	16	1.4	11.6	0.06	4	0.4	2	0.1

Table 97e OAI - OPAI - APAI — Ascariasis - Intestinal obstruction

Age group (years)	Incidence 1990 Number ('000s)	Rate (per 100 000)	Prevalence 1990 Number ('000s)	Rate (per 100 000)	Avg. age at onset (years)	Average duration (years)	Deaths 1990 Number ('000s)	Rate (per 100 000)	Deaths 2000 (Projected) Number ('000s)	Rate (per 100 000)
Males										
0-4	0	0.5	0	0.0	2.5	0.06	0	0.0	0	0.0
5-14	99	117.3	6	6.8	10.0	0.06	2	1.9	1	1.0
15-44	2	1.5	0	0.1	29.7	0.06	0	0.0	0	0.0
45-59	1	1.5	0	0.1	52.3	0.06	0	0.0	0	0.0
60+	0	1.5	0	0.1	69.6	0.06	0	0.0	0	0.0
All ages	102	29.7	6	1.7	10.8	0.06	2	0.5	1	0.2
Females										
0-4	0	0.5	0	0.0	2.4	0.06	0	0.0	0	0.0
5-14	94	117.3	5	6.8	10.0	0.06	1	1.8	1	0.9
15-44	2	1.5	0	0.1	29.4	0.06	0	0.0	0	0.0
45-59	1	1.5	0	0.1	52.2	0.06	0	0.0	0	0.0
60+	0	1.5	0	0.1	69.2	0.06	0	0.0	0	0.0
All ages	98	28.7	6	1.7	10.9	0.06	1	0.4	1	0.2
Total	199	29.2	12	1.7	10.9	0.06	3	0.5	2	0.2

Table 97f SSA - ASS - ASS — Ascariasis - Intestinal obstruction

Age group (years)	Incidence 1990 Number ('000s)	Rate (per 100 000)	Prevalence 1990 Number ('000s)	Rate (per 100 000)	Avg. age at onset (years)	Average duration (years)	Deaths 1990 Number ('000s)	Rate (per 100 000)	Deaths 2000 (Projected) Number ('000s)	Rate (per 100 000)
Males										
0-4	0	0.0	0	0.0	-	-	0	0.0	0	0.0
5-14	18	26.3	1	1.5	10.0	0.06	0	0.5	0	0.2
15-44	1	0.5	0	0.0	29.4	0.06	0	0.0	0	0.0
45-59	0	0.5	0	0.0	52.2	0.06	0	0.0	0	0.0
60+	0	0.5	0	0.0	69.2	0.06	0	0.0	0	0.0
All ages	19	7.6	1	0.4	10.9	0.06	0	0.1	0	0.1
Females										
0-4	0	0.0	0	0.0	-	-	0	0.0	0	0.0
5-14	18	26.3	1	1.5	10.0	0.06	0	0.5	0	0.2
15-44	1	0.5	0	0.0	29.5	0.06	0	0.0	0	0.0
45-59	0	0.5	0	0.0	52.2	0.06	0	0.0	0	0.0
60+	0	0.5	0	0.0	69.7	0.06	0	0.0	0	0.0
All ages	19	7.4	1	0.4	11.0	0.06	0	0.1	0	0.1
Total	38	7.5	2	0.4	11.0	0.06	1	0.1	0	0.1

For epidemiological sources see Bundy et al. 1996. See explanatory notes for definitions and caveats.

Table 97	Cuadro 97	Tableau 97
Ascariasis	Ascaridiasis	Ascaridose
Intestinal obstruction	Obstrucción intestinal	Obstruction intestinale

Table 97g LAC - ALC - ALC — Ascariasis - Intestinal obstruction

Age group (years)	Incidence 1990 Number ('000s)	Rate (per 100 000)	Prevalence 1990 Number ('000s)	Rate (per 100 000)	Avg. age at onset (years)	Average duration (years)	Deaths 1990 Number ('000s)	Rate (per 100 000)	Deaths 2000 (Projected) Number ('000s)	Rate (per 100 000)
Males										
0-4	0	0.5	0	0.0	2.5	0.06	0	0.0	0	0.0
5-14	47	89.5	3	5.2	10.0	0.06	1	1.0	0	0.6
15-44	1	1.0	0	0.1	29.8	0.06	0	0.0	0	0.0
45-59	0	1.0	0	0.1	52.3	0.06	0	0.0	0	0.0
60+	0	1.0	0	0.1	70.3	0.06	0	0.0	0	0.0
All ages	48	21.8	3	1.3	10.8	0.06	1	0.2	0	0.1
Females										
0-4	0	0.5	0	0.0	2.5	0.06	0	0.0	0	0.0
5-14	45	89.5	3	5.2	10.0	0.06	1	1.1	0	0.6
15-44	1	1.0	0	0.1	29.9	0.06	0	0.0	0	0.0
45-59	0	1.0	0	0.1	52.4	0.06	0	0.0	0	0.0
60+	0	1.0	0	0.1	71.1	0.06	0	0.0	0	0.0
All ages	47	21.1	3	1.2	10.8	0.06	1	0.3	0	0.1
Total	95	21.4	6	1.2	10.8	0.06	1	0.3	1	0.1

Table 97h MEC - AOM - CMO — Ascariasis - Intestinal obstruction

Age group (years)	Incidence 1990 Number ('000s)	Rate (per 100 000)	Prevalence 1990 Number ('000s)	Rate (per 100 000)	Avg. age at onset (years)	Average duration (years)	Deaths 1990 Number ('000s)	Rate (per 100 000)	Deaths 2000 (Projected) Number ('000s)	Rate (per 100 000)
Males										
0-4	0	0.0	0	0.0	-	-	0	0.0	0	0.0
5-14	18	27.8	1	1.6	10.0	0.06	0	0.4	0	0.2
15-44	1	0.5	0	0.0	29.8	0.06	0	0.0	0	0.0
45-59	0	0.5	0	0.0	52.3	0.06	0	0.0	0	0.0
60+	0	0.5	0	0.0	69.7	0.06	0	0.0	0	0.0
All ages	19	7.4	1	0.4	11.1	0.06	0	0.1	0	0.1
Females										
0-4	0	0.0	0	0.0	-	-	0	0.0	0	0.0
5-14	17	27.8	1	1.6	10.0	0.06	0	0.4	0	0.2
15-44	1	0.5	0	0.0	29.8	0.06	0	0.0	0	0.0
45-59	0	0.5	0	0.0	52.3	0.06	0	0.0	0	0.0
60+	0	0.5	0	0.0	70.4	0.06	0	0.0	0	0.0
All ages	18	7.3	1	0.4	11.1	0.06	0	0.1	0	0.1
Total	37	7.3	2	0.4	11.1	0.06	1	0.1	0	0.1

Table 97i World - Mundo - Monde — Ascariasis - Intestinal obstruction

Age group (years)	Incidence 1990 Number ('000s)	Rate (per 100 000)	Prevalence 1990 Number ('000s)	Rate (per 100 000)	Avg. age at onset (years)	Average duration (years)	Deaths 1990 Number ('000s)	Rate (per 100 000)	Deaths 2000 (Projected) Number ('000s)	Rate (per 100 000)
Males										
0-4	1	0.3	0	0.0	2.5	0.06	0	0.0	0	0.0
5-14	357	64.8	21	3.8	10.0	0.06	5	1.0	3	0.4
15-44	12	0.9	1	0.1	29.8	0.06	0	0.0	0	0.0
45-59	3	0.8	0	0.0	52.3	0.06	0	0.0	0	0.0
60+	2	0.8	0	0.0	69.8	0.06	0	0.0	0	0.0
All ages	374	14.1	22	0.8	11.2	0.06	6	0.2	3	0.1
Females										
0-4	1	0.3	0	0.0	2.5	0.06	0	0.0	0	0.0
5-14	339	64.4	20	3.7	10.0	0.06	5	1.0	3	0.4
15-44	11	0.9	1	0.1	29.8	0.06	0	0.0	0	0.0
45-59	3	0.8	0	0.0	52.3	0.06	0	0.0	0	0.0
60+	2	0.7	0	0.0	70.3	0.06	0	0.0	0	0.0
All ages	355	13.6	21	0.8	11.2	0.06	5	0.2	3	0.1
Total	729	13.8	42	0.8	11.2	0.06	11	0.2	6	0.1

For epidemiological sources see Bundy et al. 1996. See explanatory notes for definitions and caveats.

Table 98　　　　　　　　　　**Cuadro 98**　　　　　　　　　　**Tableau 98**
Trichuriasis　　　　　　　　　**Tricocefalosis**　　　　　　　　**Tricocéphalose**

High intensity infection　　　　　Infección de alta intensidad　　　　Infection de forte intensité

Table 98a　　　EME - PEMC - EMBE　　　　　　Trichuriasis - High intensity infection

Age group (years)	Incidence 1990 Number ('000s)	Rate (per 100 000)	Prevalence 1990 Number ('000s)	Rate (per 100 000)	Avg. age at onset (years)	Average duration (years)	Deaths 1990 Number ('000s)	Rate (per 100 000)	Deaths 2000 (Projected) Number ('000s)	Rate (per 100 000)
Males										
0-4	-	-	0	0	-	-	-	-	-	-
5-14	-	-	0	0	-	-	-	-	-	-
15-44	-	-	0	0	-	-	-	-	-	-
45-59	-	-	0	0	-	-	-	-	-	-
60+	-	-	0	0	-	-	-	-	-	-
All ages	-	-	0	0	-	-	-	-	-	-
Females										
0-4	-	-	0	0	-	-	-	-	-	-
5-14	-	-	0	0	-	-	-	-	-	-
15-44	-	-	0	0	-	-	-	-	-	-
45-59	-	-	0	0	-	-	-	-	-	-
60+	-	-	0	0	-	-	-	-	-	-
All ages	-	-	0	0	-	-	-	-	-	-
Total	-	-	0	0	-	-	-	-	-	-

Table 98b　　　FSE - PEAS - AESE　　　　　　Trichuriasis - High intensity infection

Age group (years)	Incidence 1990 Number ('000s)	Rate (per 100 000)	Prevalence 1990 Number ('000s)	Rate (per 100 000)	Avg. age at onset (years)	Average duration (years)	Deaths 1990 Number ('000s)	Rate (per 100 000)	Deaths 2000 (Projected) Number ('000s)	Rate (per 100 000)
Males										
0-4	-	-	0	0	-	-	-	-	-	-
5-14	-	-	0	0	-	-	-	-	-	-
15-44	-	-	0	0	-	-	-	-	-	-
45-59	-	-	0	0	-	-	-	-	-	-
60+	-	-	0	0	-	-	-	-	-	-
All ages	-	-	0	0	-	-	-	-	-	-
Females										
0-4	-	-	0	0	-	-	-	-	-	-
5-14	-	-	0	0	-	-	-	-	-	-
15-44	-	-	0	0	-	-	-	-	-	-
45-59	-	-	0	0	-	-	-	-	-	-
60+	-	-	0	0	-	-	-	-	-	-
All ages	-	-	0	0	-	-	-	-	-	-
Total	-	-	0	0	-	-	-	-	-	-

Table 98c　　　India - India - Inde　　　　　　Trichuriasis - High intensity infection

Age group (years)	Incidence 1990 Number ('000s)	Rate (per 100 000)	Prevalence 1990 Number ('000s)	Rate (per 100 000)	Avg. age at onset (years)	Average duration (years)	Deaths 1990 Number ('000s)	Rate (per 100 000)	Deaths 2000 (Projected) Number ('000s)	Rate (per 100 000)
Males										
0-4	-	-	0	0	-	-	-	-	-	-
5-14	-	-	1 262	1 240	-	-	-	-	-	-
15-44	-	-	201	100	-	-	-	-	-	-
45-59	-	-	48	100	-	-	-	-	-	-
60+	-	-	30	100	-	-	-	-	-	-
All ages	-	-	1 540	350	-	-	-	-	-	-
Females										
0-4	-	-	0	0	-	-	-	-	-	-
5-14	-	-	1 181	1 240	-	-	-	-	-	-
15-44	-	-	183	100	-	-	-	-	-	-
45-59	-	-	46	100	-	-	-	-	-	-
60+	-	-	29	100	-	-	-	-	-	-
All ages	-	-	1 439	351	-	-	-	-	-	-
Total	-	-	2 979	351	-	-	-	-	-	-

For epidemiological sources see Bundy et al. 1996. See explanatory notes for definitions and caveats.

Table 98
Trichuriasis

Cuadro 98
Tricocefalosis

Tableau 98
Tricocéphalose

High intensity infection

Infección de alta intensidad

Infection de forte intensité

Table 98d　　China - China - Chine　　　　　　Trichuriasis - High intensity infection

Age group (years)	Incidence 1990 Number ('000s)	Rate (per 100 000)	Prevalence 1990 Number ('000s)	Rate (per 100 000)	Avg. age at onset (years)	Average duration (years)	Deaths 1990 Number ('000s)	Rate (per 100 000)	Deaths 2000 (Projected) Number ('000s)	Rate (per 100 000)
Males										
0-4	-	-	6	10	-	-	-	-	-	-
5-14	-	-	6 281	6 475	-	-	-	-	-	-
15-44	-	-	1 746	570	-	-	-	-	-	-
45-59	-	-	414	570	-	-	-	-	-	-
60+	-	-	279	570	-	-	-	-	-	-
All ages	-	-	8 726	1 491	-	-	-	-	-	-
Females										
0-4	-	-	6	10	-	-	-	-	-	-
5-14	-	-	5 853	6 475	-	-	-	-	-	-
15-44	-	-	1 619	570	-	-	-	-	-	-
45-59	-	-	367	570	-	-	-	-	-	-
60+	-	-	294	570	-	-	-	-	-	-
All ages	-	-	8 140	1 484	-	-	-	-	-	-
Total	-	-	16 866	1 488	-	-	-	-	-	-

Table 98e　　OAI - OPAI - APAI　　　　　　Trichuriasis - High intensity infection

Age group (years)	Incidence 1990 Number ('000s)	Rate (per 100 000)	Prevalence 1990 Number ('000s)	Rate (per 100 000)	Avg. age at onset (years)	Average duration (years)	Deaths 1990 Number ('000s)	Rate (per 100 000)	Deaths 2000 (Projected) Number ('000s)	Rate (per 100 000)
Males										
0-4	-	-	9	20	-	-	-	-	-	-
5-14	-	-	6 765	8 050	-	-	-	-	-	-
15-44	-	-	1 045	650	-	-	-	-	-	-
45-59	-	-	222	650	-	-	-	-	-	-
60+	-	-	131	650	-	-	-	-	-	-
All ages	-	-	8 172	2 383	-	-	-	-	-	-
Females										
0-4	-	-	8	20	-	-	-	-	-	-
5-14	-	-	6 457	8 050	-	-	-	-	-	-
15-44	-	-	1 037	650	-	-	-	-	-	-
45-59	-	-	228	650	-	-	-	-	-	-
60+	-	-	147	650	-	-	-	-	-	-
All ages	-	-	7 879	2 320	-	-	-	-	-	-
Total	-	-	16 051	2 352	-	-	-	-	-	-

Table 98f　　SSA - ASS - ASS　　　　　　Trichuriasis - High intensity infection

Age group (years)	Incidence 1990 Number ('000s)	Rate (per 100 000)	Prevalence 1990 Number ('000s)	Rate (per 100 000)	Avg. age at onset (years)	Average duration (years)	Deaths 1990 Number ('000s)	Rate (per 100 000)	Deaths 2000 (Projected) Number ('000s)	Rate (per 100 000)
Males										
0-4	-	-	0	0	-	-	-	-	-	-
5-14	-	-	941	1 340	-	-	-	-	-	-
15-44	-	-	114	110	-	-	-	-	-	-
45-59	-	-	22	110	-	-	-	-	-	-
60+	-	-	12	110	-	-	-	-	-	-
All ages	-	-	1 089	432	-	-	-	-	-	-
Females										
0-4	-	-	0	0	-	-	-	-	-	-
5-14	-	-	936	1 340	-	-	-	-	-	-
15-44	-	-	117	110	-	-	-	-	-	-
45-59	-	-	24	110	-	-	-	-	-	-
60+	-	-	14	110	-	-	-	-	-	-
All ages	-	-	1 091	423	-	-	-	-	-	-
Total	-	-	2 180	427	-	-	-	-	-	-

For epidemiological sources see Bundy et al. 1996.　See explanatory notes for definitions and caveats.

Table 98   **Cuadro 98**   **Tableau 98**
Trichuriasis   **Tricocefalosis**   **Tricocéphalose**

High intensity infection   Infección de alta intensidad   Infection de forte intensité

Table 98g   LAC - ALC - ALC   Trichuriasis - High intensity infection

Age group (years)	Incidence 1990 Number ('000s)	Rate (per 100 000)	Prevalence 1990 Number ('000s)	Rate (per 100 000)	Avg. age at onset (years)	Average duration (years)	Deaths 1990 Number ('000s)	Rate (per 100 000)	Deaths 2000 (Projected) Number ('000s)	Rate (per 100 000)
Males										
0-4	-	-	3	10	-	-	-	-	-	-
5-14	-	-	3 021	5 795	-	-	-	-	-	-
15-44	-	-	490	470	-	-	-	-	-	-
45-59	-	-	105	470	-	-	-	-	-	-
60+	-	-	67	470	-	-	-	-	-	-
All ages	-	-	3 685	1 663	-	-	-	-	-	-
Females										
0-4	-	-	3	10	-	-	-	-	-	-
5-14	-	-	2 941	5 795	-	-	-	-	-	-
15-44	-	-	489	470	-	-	-	-	-	-
45-59	-	-	110	470	-	-	-	-	-	-
60+	-	-	79	470	-	-	-	-	-	-
All ages	-	-	3 621	1 626	-	-	-	-	-	-
Total	-	-	7 306	1 645	-	-	-	-	-	-

Table 98h   MEC - AOM - CMO   Trichuriasis - High intensity infection

Age group (years)	Incidence 1990 Number ('000s)	Rate (per 100 000)	Prevalence 1990 Number ('000s)	Rate (per 100 000)	Avg. age at onset (years)	Average duration (years)	Deaths 1990 Number ('000s)	Rate (per 100 000)	Deaths 2000 (Projected) Number ('000s)	Rate (per 100 000)
Males										
0-4	-	-	0	0.0	-	-	-	-	-	-
5-14	-	-	20	30.0	-	-	-	-	-	-
15-44	-	-	0	0.0	-	-	-	-	-	-
45-59	-	-	0	0.0	-	-	-	-	-	-
60+	-	-	0	0.0	-	-	-	-	-	-
All ages	-	-	20	7.6	-	-	-	-	-	-
Females										
0-4	-	-	0	0.0	-	-	-	-	-	-
5-14	-	-	19	30.0	-	-	-	-	-	-
15-44	-	-	0	0.0	-	-	-	-	-	-
45-59	-	-	0	0.0	-	-	-	-	-	-
60+	-	-	0	0.0	-	-	-	-	-	-
All ages	-	-	19	7.5	-	-	-	-	-	-
Total	-	-	38	7.6	-	-	-	-	-	-

Table 98i   World - Mundo - Monde   Trichuriasis - High intensity infection

Age group (years)	Incidence 1990 Number ('000s)	Rate (per 100 000)	Prevalence 1990 Number ('000s)	Rate (per 100 000)	Avg. age at onset (years)	Average duration (years)	Deaths 1990 Number ('000s)	Rate (per 100 000)	Deaths 2000 (Projected) Number ('000s)	Rate (per 100 000)
Males										
0-4	-	-	18	5.5	-	-	-	-	-	-
5-14	-	-	18 289	3 318.0	-	-	-	-	-	-
15-44	-	-	3 596	287.7	-	-	-	-	-	-
45-59	-	-	811	259.5	-	-	-	-	-	-
60+	-	-	519	237.0	-	-	-	-	-	-
All ages	-	-	23 232	875.5	-	-	-	-	-	-
Females										
0-4	-	-	17	5.5	-	-	-	-	-	-
5-14	-	-	17 387	3 308.4	-	-	-	-	-	-
15-44	-	-	3 446	287.5	-	-	-	-	-	-
45-59	-	-	775	249.2	-	-	-	-	-	-
60+	-	-	564	209.4	-	-	-	-	-	-
All ages	-	-	22 189	849.0	-	-	-	-	-	-
Total	-	-	45 421	862.3	-	-	-	-	-	-

For epidemiological sources see Bundy et al. 1996. See explanatory notes for definitions and caveats.

Table 99
Trichuriasis

Cuadro 99
Tricocefalosis

Tableau 99
Tricocéphalose

Cotemporaneous cognitive deficit Deficit cognocitivo contemporaneo Deficit cognitif simultané

Table 99a EME - PEMC - EMBE Trichuriasis - Cotemporaneous cognitive deficit

Age group (years)	Incidence 1990 Number ('000s)	Rate (per 100 000)	Prevalence 1990 Number ('000s)	Rate (per 100 000)	Avg. age at onset (years)	Average duration (years)	Deaths 1990 Number ('000s)	Rate (per 100 000)	Deaths 2000 (Projected) Number ('000s)	Rate (per 100 000)
Males										
0-4	-	-	0	0	-	-	0	0	0	0
5-14	-	-	0	0	-	-	0	0	0	0
15-44	-	-	0	0	-	-	0	0	0	0
45-59	-	-	0	0	-	-	0	0	0	0
60+	-	-	0	0	-	-	0	0	0	0
All ages	-	-	0	0	-	-	0	0	0	0
Females										
0-4	-	-	0	0	-	-	0	0	0	0
5-14	-	-	0	0	-	-	0	0	0	0
15-44	-	-	0	0	-	-	0	0	0	0
45-59	-	-	0	0	-	-	0	0	0	0
60+	-	-	0	0	-	-	0	0	0	0
All ages	-	-	0	0	-	-	0	0	0	0
Total	-	-	0	0	-	-	0	0	0	0

Table 99b FSE - PEAS - AESE Trichuriasis - Cotemporaneous cognitive deficit

Age group (years)	Incidence 1990 Number ('000s)	Rate (per 100 000)	Prevalence 1990 Number ('000s)	Rate (per 100 000)	Avg. age at onset (years)	Average duration (years)	Deaths 1990 Number ('000s)	Rate (per 100 000)	Deaths 2000 (Projected) Number ('000s)	Rate (per 100 000)
Males										
0-4	-	-	0	0	-	-	0	0	0	0
5-14	-	-	0	0	-	-	0	0	0	0
15-44	-	-	0	0	-	-	0	0	0	0
45-59	-	-	0	0	-	-	0	0	0	0
60+	-	-	0	0	-	-	0	0	0	0
All ages	-	-	0	0	-	-	0	0	0	0
Females										
0-4	-	-	0	0	-	-	0	0	0	0
5-14	-	-	0	0	-	-	0	0	0	0
15-44	-	-	0	0	-	-	0	0	0	0
45-59	-	-	0	0	-	-	0	0	0	0
60+	-	-	0	0	-	-	0	0	0	0
All ages	-	-	0	0	-	-	0	0	0	0
Total	-	-	0	0	-	-	0	0	0	0

Table 99c India - India - Inde Trichuriasis - Cotemporaneous cognitive deficit

Age group (years)	Incidence 1990 Number ('000s)	Rate (per 100 000)	Prevalence 1990 Number ('000s)	Rate (per 100 000)	Avg. age at onset (years)	Average duration (years)	Deaths 1990 Number ('000s)	Rate (per 100 000)	Deaths 2000 (Projected) Number ('000s)	Rate (per 100 000)
Males										
0-4	-	-	0	0	-	-	0	0	0	0
5-14	-	-	631	620	-	-	0	0	0	0
15-44	-	-	0	0	-	-	0	0	0	0
45-59	-	-	0	0	-	-	0	0	0	0
60+	-	-	0	0	-	-	0	0	0	0
All ages	-	-	631	144	-	-	0	0	0	0
Females										
0-4	-	-	0	0	-	-	0	0	0	0
5-14	-	-	591	620	-	-	0	0	0	0
15-44	-	-	0	0	-	-	0	0	0	0
45-59	-	-	0	0	-	-	0	0	0	0
60+	-	-	0	0	-	-	0	0	0	0
All ages	-	-	591	144	-	-	0	0	0	0
Total	-	-	1 221	144	-	-	0	0	0	0

For epidemiological sources see Bundy et al. 1996. See explanatory notes for definitions and caveats.

Table 99
Trichuriasis

Cuadro 99
Tricocefalosis

Tableau 99
Tricocéphalose

Cotemporaneous cognitive deficit   Deficit cognocitivo contemporaneo   Deficit cognitif simultané

Table 99d   China - China - Chine   Trichuriasis - Cotemporaneous cognitive deficit

Age group (years)	Incidence 1990 Number ('000s)	Rate (per 100 000)	Prevalence 1990 Number ('000s)	Rate (per 100 000)	Avg. age at onset (years)	Average duration (years)	Deaths 1990 Number ('000s)	Rate (per 100 000)	Deaths 2000 (Projected) Number ('000s)	Rate (per 100 000)
Males										
0-4	-	-	0	0	-	-	0	0	0	0
5-14	-	-	3 278	3 380	-	-	0	0	0	0
15-44	-	-	61	20	-	-	0	0	0	0
45-59	-	-	15	20	-	-	0	0	0	0
60+	-	-	10	20	-	-	0	0	0	0
All ages	-	-	3 364	575	-	-	0	0	0	0
Females										
0-4	-	-	0	0	-	-	0	0	0	0
5-14	-	-	3 056	3 380	-	-	0	0	0	0
15-44	-	-	57	20	-	-	0	0	0	0
45-59	-	-	13	20	-	-	0	0	0	0
60+	-	-	10	20	-	-	0	0	0	0
All ages	-	-	3 136	572	-	-	0	0	0	0
Total	-	-	6 500	573	-	-	0	0	0	0

Table 99e   OAI - OPAI - APAI   Trichuriasis - Cotemporaneous cognitive deficit

Age group (years)	Incidence 1990 Number ('000s)	Rate (per 100 000)	Prevalence 1990 Number ('000s)	Rate (per 100 000)	Avg. age at onset (years)	Average duration (years)	Deaths 1990 Number ('000s)	Rate (per 100 000)	Deaths 2000 (Projected) Number ('000s)	Rate (per 100 000)
Males										
0-4	-	-	0	0	-	-	0	0	0	0
5-14	-	-	3 344	3 980	-	-	0	0	0	0
15-44	-	-	32	20	-	-	0	0	0	0
45-59	-	-	7	20	-	-	0	0	0	0
60+	-	-	4	20	-	-	0	0	0	0
All ages	-	-	3 388	988	-	-	0	0	0	0
Females										
0-4	-	-	0	0	-	-	0	0	0	0
5-14	-	-	3 193	3 980	-	-	0	0	0	0
15-44	-	-	32	20	-	-	0	0	0	0
45-59	-	-	7	20	-	-	0	0	0	0
60+	-	-	5	20	-	-	0	0	0	0
All ages	-	-	3 236	953	-	-	0	0	0	0
Total	-	-	6 624	970	-	-	0	0	0	0

Table 99f   SSA - ASS - ASS   Trichuriasis - Cotemporaneous cognitive deficit

Age group (years)	Incidence 1990 Number ('000s)	Rate (per 100 000)	Prevalence 1990 Number ('000s)	Rate (per 100 000)	Avg. age at onset (years)	Average duration (years)	Deaths 1990 Number ('000s)	Rate (per 100 000)	Deaths 2000 (Projected) Number ('000s)	Rate (per 100 000)
Males										
0-4	-	-	0	0	-	-	0	0	0	0
5-14	-	-	478	680	-	-	0	0	0	0
15-44	-	-	0	0	-	-	0	0	0	0
45-59	-	-	0	0	-	-	0	0	0	0
60+	-	-	0	0	-	-	0	0	0	0
All ages	-	-	478	189	-	-	0	0	0	0
Females										
0-4	-	-	0	0	-	-	0	0	0	0
5-14	-	-	475	680	-	-	0	0	0	0
15-44	-	-	0	0	-	-	0	0	0	0
45-59	-	-	0	0	-	-	0	0	0	0
60+	-	-	0	0	-	-	0	0	0	0
All ages	-	-	475	184	-	-	0	0	0	0
Total	-	-	953	187	-	-	0	0	0	0

For epidemiological sources see Bundy et al. 1996. See explanatory notes for definitions and caveats.

Table 99
Trichuriasis

Cuadro 99
Tricocefalosis

Tableau 99
Tricocéphalose

Cotemporaneous cognitive deficit   Deficit cognocitivo contemporaneo   Deficit cognitif simultané

Table 99g		LAC - ALC - ALC									Trichuriasis - Cotemporaneous cognitive deficit
Age group (years)	Incidence 1990		Prevalence 1990		Avg. age at onset (years)	Average duration (years)	Deaths 1990		Deaths 2000 (Projected)	
	Number ('000s)	Rate (per 100 000)	Number ('000s)	Rate (per 100 000)			Number ('000s)	Rate (per 100 000)	Number ('000s)	Rate (per 100 000)
Males										
0-4	-	-	0	0	-	-	0	0	0	0
5-14	-	-	1 488	2 855	-	-	0	0	0	0
15-44	-	-	10	10	-	-	0	0	0	0
45-59	-	-	2	10	-	-	0	0	0	0
60+	-	-	1	10	-	-	0	0	0	0
All ages	-	-	1 502	678	-	-	0	0	0	0
Females										
0-4	-	-	0	0	-	-	0	0	0	0
5-14	-	-	1 449	2 855	-	-	0	0	0	0
15-44	-	-	10	10	-	-	0	0	0	0
45-59	-	-	2	10	-	-	0	0	0	0
60+	-	-	2	10	-	-	0	0	0	0
All ages	-	-	1 463	657	-	-	0	0	0	0
Total	-	-	2 965	667	-	-	0	0	0	0

Table 99h		MEC - AOM - CMO									Trichuriasis - Cotemporaneous cognitive deficit
Age group (years)	Incidence 1990		Prevalence 1990		Avg. age at onset (years)	Average duration (years)	Deaths 1990		Deaths 2000 (Projected)	
	Number ('000s)	Rate (per 100 000)	Number ('000s)	Rate (per 100 000)			Number ('000s)	Rate (per 100 000)	Number ('000s)	Rate (per 100 000)
Males										
0-4	-	-	0	0	-	-	0	0	0	0
5-14	-	-	0	0	-	-	0	0	0	0
15-44	-	-	0	0	-	-	0	0	0	0
45-59	-	-	0	0	-	-	0	0	0	0
60+	-	-	0	0	-	-	0	0	0	0
All ages	-	-	0	0	-	-	0	0	0	0
Females										
0-4	-	-	0	0	-	-	0	0	0	0
5-14	-	-	0	0	-	-	0	0	0	0
15-44	-	-	0	0	-	-	0	0	0	0
45-59	-	-	0	0	-	-	0	0	0	0
60+	-	-	0	0	-	-	0	0	0	0
All ages	-	-	0	0	-	-	0	0	0	0
Total	-	-	0	0	-	-	0	0	0	0

Table 99i		World - Mundo - Monde									Trichuriasis - Cotemporaneous cognitive deficit
Age group (years)	Incidence 1990		Prevalence 1990		Avg. age at onset (years)	Average duration (years)	Deaths 1990		Deaths 2000 (Projected)	
	Number ('000s)	Rate (per 100 000)	Number ('000s)	Rate (per 100 000)			Number ('000s)	Rate (per 100 000)	Number ('000s)	Rate (per 100 000)
Males										
0-4	-	-	0	0.0	-	-	0	0	0	0
5-14	-	-	9 220	1 672.7	-	-	0	0	0	0
15-44	-	-	104	8.3	-	-	0	0	0	0
45-59	-	-	24	7.6	-	-	0	0	0	0
60+	-	-	15	7.0	-	-	0	0	0	0
All ages	-	-	9 362	352.8	-	-	0	0	0	0
Females										
0-4	-	-	0	0.0	-	-	0	0	0	0
5-14	-	-	8 762	1 667.3	-	-	0	0	0	0
15-44	-	-	99	8.3	-	-	0	0	0	0
45-59	-	-	22	7.1	-	-	0	0	0	0
60+	-	-	17	6.1	-	-	0	0	0	0
All ages	-	-	8 900	340.5	-	-	0	0	0	0
Total	-	-	18 263	346.7	-	-	0	0	0	0

For epidemiological sources see Bundy et al. 1996. See explanatory notes for definitions and caveats.

Table 100
Trichuriasis

Cuadro 100
Tricocefalosis

Tableau 100
Tricocéphalose

Massive dysentery syndrome

Síndrome masivo de dysenteria

Syndrome dysentérique massif

Table 100a   EME - PEMC - EMBE   Trichuriasis - Massive dysentery syndrome

Age group (years)	Incidence 1990 Number ('000s)	Rate (per 100 000)	Prevalence 1990 Number ('000s)	Rate (per 100 000)	Avg. age at onset (years)	Average duration (years)	Deaths 1990 Number ('000s)	Rate (per 100 000)	Deaths 2000 (Projected) Number ('000s)	Rate (per 100 000)
Males										
0-4	0	0	0	0	-	-	0	0	0	0
5-14	0	0	0	0	-	-	0	0	0	0
15-44	0	0	0	0	-	-	0	0	0	0
45-59	0	0	0	0	-	-	0	0	0	0
60+	0	0	0	0	-	-	0	0	0	0
All ages	0	0	0	0	-	-	0	0	0	0
Females										
0-4	0	0	0	0	-	-	0	0	0	0
5-14	0	0	0	0	-	-	0	0	0	0
15-44	0	0	0	0	-	-	0	0	0	0
45-59	0	0	0	0	-	-	0	0	0	0
60+	0	0	0	0	-	-	0	0	0	0
All ages	0	0	0	0	-	-	0	0	0	0
Total	0	0	0	0	-	-	0	0	0	0

Table 100b   FSE - PEAS - AESE   Trichuriasis - Massive dysentery syndrome

Age group (years)	Incidence 1990 Number ('000s)	Rate (per 100 000)	Prevalence 1990 Number ('000s)	Rate (per 100 000)	Avg. age at onset (years)	Average duration (years)	Deaths 1990 Number ('000s)	Rate (per 100 000)	Deaths 2000 (Projected) Number ('000s)	Rate (per 100 000)
Males										
0-4	0	0	0	0	-	-	0	0	0	0
5-14	0	0	0	0	-	-	0	0	0	0
15-44	0	0	0	0	-	-	0	0	0	0
45-59	0	0	0	0	-	-	0	0	0	0
60+	0	0	0	0	-	-	0	0	0	0
All ages	0	0	0	0	-	-	0	0	0	0
Females										
0-4	0	0	0	0	-	-	0	0	0	0
5-14	0	0	0	0	-	-	0	0	0	0
15-44	0	0	0	0	-	-	0	0	0	0
45-59	0	0	0	0	-	-	0	0	0	0
60+	0	0	0	0	-	-	0	0	0	0
All ages	0	0	0	0	-	-	0	0	0	0
Total	0	0	0	0	-	-	0	0	0	0

Table 100c   India - India - Inde   Trichuriasis - Massive dysentery syndrome

Age group (years)	Incidence 1990 Number ('000s)	Rate (per 100 000)	Prevalence 1990 Number ('000s)	Rate (per 100 000)	Avg. age at onset (years)	Average duration (years)	Deaths 1990 Number ('000s)	Rate (per 100 000)	Deaths 2000 (Projected) Number ('000s)	Rate (per 100 000)
Males										
0-4	0	0	0	0	-	-	0	0.0	0	0.0
5-14	126	124	126	124	10.0	1.0	0	0.3	0	0.1
15-44	0	0	0	0	-	-	0	0.0	0	0.0
45-59	0	0	0	0	-	-	0	0.0	0	0.0
60+	0	0	0	0	-	-	0	0.0	0	0.0
All ages	126	29	126	29	10.0	1.0	0	0.1	0	0.0
Females										
0-4	0	0	0	0	-	-	0	0.0	0	0.0
5-14	118	124	118	124	10.0	1.0	0	0.3	0	0.1
15-44	0	0	0	0	-	-	0	0.0	0	0.0
45-59	0	0	0	0	-	-	0	0.0	0	0.0
60+	0	0	0	0	-	-	0	0.0	0	0.0
All ages	118	29	118	29	10.0	1.0	0	0.1	0	0.0
Total	244	29	244	29	10.0	1.0	1	0.1	0	0.0

For epidemiological sources see Bundy et al. 1996. See explanatory notes for definitions and caveats.

Table 100
Trichuriasis

Cuadro 100
Tricocefalosis

Tableau 100
Tricocéphalose

Massive dysentery syndrome

Síndrome masivo de dysenteria

Syndrome dysentérique massif

| Table 100d | China - China - Chine | | | | | | Trichuriasis - Massive dysentery syndrome | | | |

Age group (years)	Incidence 1990 Number ('000s)	Rate (per 100 000)	Prevalence 1990 Number ('000s)	Rate (per 100 000)	Avg. age at onset (years)	Average duration (years)	Deaths 1990 Number ('000s)	Rate (per 100 000)	Deaths 2000 (Projected) Number ('000s)	Rate (per 100 000)
Males										
0-4	0	0	0	0	-	-	0	0.0	0	0.0
5-14	656	676	656	676	10.0	1.0	1	1.3	1	0.5
15-44	0	0	0	0	-	-	0	0.0	0	0.0
45-59	0	0	0	0	-	-	0	0.0	0	0.0
60+	0	0	0	0	-	-	0	0.0	0	0.0
All ages	656	112	656	112	10.0	1.0	1	0.2	1	0.1
Females										
0-4	0	0	0	0	-	-	0	0.0	0	0.0
5-14	611	676	611	676	10.0	1.0	1	1.3	1	0.5
15-44	0	0	0	0	-	-	0	0.0	0	0.0
45-59	0	0	0	0	-	-	0	0.0	0	0.0
60+	0	0	0	0	-	-	0	0.0	0	0.0
All ages	611	111	611	111	10.0	1.0	1	0.2	1	0.1
Total	1 267	112	1 267	112	10.0	1.0	2	0.2	1	0.1

| Table 100e | OAI - OPAI - APAI | | | | | | Trichuriasis - Massive dysentery syndrome | | | |

Age group (years)	Incidence 1990 Number ('000s)	Rate (per 100 000)	Prevalence 1990 Number ('000s)	Rate (per 100 000)	Avg. age at onset (years)	Average duration (years)	Deaths 1990 Number ('000s)	Rate (per 100 000)	Deaths 2000 (Projected) Number ('000s)	Rate (per 100 000)
Males										
0-4	0	0	0	0	-	-	0	0.0	0	0.0
5-14	669	796	669	796	10.0	1.0	1	1.8	1	0.9
15-44	0	0	0	0	-	-	0	0.0	0	0.0
45-59	0	0	0	0	-	-	0	0.0	0	0.0
60+	0	0	0	0	-	-	0	0.0	0	0.0
All ages	669	195	669	195	10.0	1.0	1	0.4	1	0.2
Females										
0-4	0	0	0	0	-	-	0	0.0	0	0.0
5-14	639	796	639	796	10.0	1.0	1	1.6	1	0.8
15-44	0	0	0	0	-	-	0	0.0	0	0.0
45-59	0	0	0	0	-	-	0	0.0	0	0.0
60+	0	0	0	0	-	-	0	0.0	0	0.0
All ages	639	188	639	188	10.0	1.0	1	0.4	1	0.2
Total	1 307	192	1 307	192	10.0	1.0	3	0.4	1	0.2

| Table 100f | SSA - ASS - ASS | | | | | | Trichuriasis - Massive dysentery syndrome | | | |

Age group (years)	Incidence 1990 Number ('000s)	Rate (per 100 000)	Prevalence 1990 Number ('000s)	Rate (per 100 000)	Avg. age at onset (years)	Average duration (years)	Deaths 1990 Number ('000s)	Rate (per 100 000)	Deaths 2000 (Projected) Number ('000s)	Rate (per 100 000)
Males										
0-4	0	0	0	0	-	-	0	0.0	0	0.0
5-14	96	136	96	136	10.0	1.0	0	0.3	0	0.2
15-44	0	0	0	0	-	-	0	0.0	0	0.0
45-59	0	0	0	0	-	-	0	0.0	0	0.0
60+	0	0	0	0	-	-	0	0.0	0	0.0
All ages	96	38	96	38	10.0	1.0	0	0.1	0	0.0
Females										
0-4	0	0	0	0	-	-	0	0.0	0	0.0
5-14	95	136	95	136	10.0	1.0	0	0.3	0	0.2
15-44	0	0	0	0	-	-	0	0.0	0	0.0
45-59	0	0	0	0	-	-	0	0.0	0	0.0
60+	0	0	0	0	-	-	0	0.0	0	0.0
All ages	95	37	95	37	10.0	1.0	0	0.1	0	0.0
Total	191	37	191	37	10.0	1.0	0	0.1	0	0.0

For epidemiological sources see Bundy et al. 1996. See explanatory notes for definitions and caveats.

Table 100
Trichuriasis

Cuadro 100
Tricocefalosis

Tableau 100
Tricocéphalose

Massive dysentery syndrome   Síndrome masivo de dysenteria   Syndrome dysentérique massif

Table 100g   LAC - ALC - ALC   Trichuriasis - Massive dysentery syndrome

Age group (years)	Incidence 1990 Number ('000s)	Rate (per 100 000)	Prevalence 1990 Number ('000s)	Rate (per 100 000)	Avg. age at onset (years)	Average duration (years)	Deaths 1990 Number ('000s)	Rate (per 100 000)	Deaths 2000 (Projected) Number ('000s)	Rate (per 100 000)
Males										
0-4	0	0	0	0	-	-	0	0.0	0	0.0
5-14	298	571	298	571	10.0	1.0	0	0.8	0	0.5
15-44	0	0	0	0	-	-	0	0.0	0	0.0
45-59	0	0	0	0	-	-	0	0.0	0	0.0
60+	0	0	0	0	-	-	0	0.0	0	0.0
All ages	298	134	298	134	10.0	1.0	0	0.2	0	0.1
Females										
0-4	0	0	0	0	-	-	0	0.0	0	0.0
5-14	290	571	290	571	10.0	1.0	0	1.0	0	0.5
15-44	0	0	0	0	-	-	0	0.0	0	0.0
45-59	0	0	0	0	-	-	0	0.0	0	0.0
60+	0	0	0	0	-	-	0	0.0	0	0.0
All ages	290	130	290	130	10.0	1.0	0	0.2	0	0.1
Total	587	132	587	132	10.0	1.0	1	0.2	1	0.1

Table 100h   MEC - AOM - CMO   Trichuriasis - Massive dysentery syndrome

Age group (years)	Incidence 1990 Number ('000s)	Rate (per 100 000)	Prevalence 1990 Number ('000s)	Rate (per 100 000)	Avg. age at onset (years)	Average duration (years)	Deaths 1990 Number ('000s)	Rate (per 100 000)	Deaths 2000 (Projected) Number ('000s)	Rate (per 100 000)
Males										
0-4	0	0	0	0	-	-	0	0	0	0
5-14	0	0	0	0	-	-	0	0	0	0
15-44	0	0	0	0	-	-	0	0	0	0
45-59	0	0	0	0	-	-	0	0	0	0
60+	0	0	0	0	-	-	0	0	0	0
All ages	0	0	0	0	-	-	0	0	0	0
Females										
0-4	0	0	0	0	-	-	0	0	0	0
5-14	0	0	0	0	-	-	0	0	0	0
15-44	0	0	0	0	-	-	0	0	0	0
45-59	0	0	0	0	-	-	0	0	0	0
60+	0	0	0	0	-	-	0	0	0	0
All ages	0	0	0	0	-	-	0	0	0	0
Total	0	0	0	0	-	-	0	0	0	0

Table 100i   World - Mundo - Monde   Trichuriasis - Massive dysentery syndrome

Age group (years)	Incidence 1990 Number ('000s)	Rate (per 100 000)	Prevalence 1990 Number ('000s)	Rate (per 100 000)	Avg. age at onset (years)	Average duration (years)	Deaths 1990 Number ('000s)	Rate (per 100 000)	Deaths 2000 (Projected) Number ('000s)	Rate (per 100 000)
Males										
0-4	0	0	0	0	-	-	0	0.0	0	0.0
5-14	1 844	335	1 844	335	10.0	1.0	4	0.7	2	0.3
15-44	0	0	0	0	-	-	0	0.0	0	0.0
45-59	0	0	0	0	-	-	0	0.0	0	0.0
60+	0	0	0	0	-	-	0	0.0	0	0.0
All ages	1 844	69	1 844	69	10.0	1.0	4	0.1	2	0.1
Females										
0-4	0	0	0	0	-	-	0	0.0	0	0.0
5-14	1 752	333	1 752	333	10.0	1.0	3	0.7	2	0.3
15-44	0	0	0	0	-	-	0	0.0	0	0.0
45-59	0	0	0	0	-	-	0	0.0	0	0.0
60+	0	0	0	0	-	-	0	0.0	0	0.0
All ages	1 752	67	1 752	67	10.0	1.0	3	0.1	2	0.1
Total	3 596	68	3 596	68	10.0	1.0	7	0.1	4	0.1

For epidemiological sources see Bundy et al. 1996. See explanatory notes for definitions and caveats.

Table 101
Trichuriasis

Cuadro 101
Tricocefalosis

Tableau 101
Tricocéphalose

Cognitive impairment

Deficiencia cognocitiva

Déficience cognitive

Table 101a — EME - PEMC - EMBE — Trichuriasis - Cognitive impairment

Age group (years)	Incidence 1990 Number ('000s)	Rate (per 100 000)	Prevalence 1990 Number ('000s)	Rate (per 100 000)	Avg. age at onset (years)	Average duration (years)	Deaths 1990 Number ('000s)	Rate (per 100 000)	Deaths 2000 (Projected) Number ('000s)	Rate (per 100 000)
Males										
0-4	0	0	0	0	-	-	0	0	0	0
5-14	0	0	0	0	-	-	0	0	0	0
15-44	0	0	0	0	-	-	0	0	0	0
45-59	0	0	0	0	-	-	0	0	0	0
60+	0	0	0	0	-	-	0	0	0	0
All ages	0	0	0	0	-	-	0	0	0	0
Females										
0-4	0	0	0	0	-	-	0	0	0	0
5-14	0	0	0	0	-	-	0	0	0	0
15-44	0	0	0	0	-	-	0	0	0	0
45-59	0	0	0	0	-	-	0	0	0	0
60+	0	0	0	0	-	-	0	0	0	0
All ages	0	0	0	0	-	-	0	0	0	0
Total	0	0	0	0	-	-	0	0	0	0

Table 101b — FSE - PEAS - AESE — Trichuriasis - Cognitive impairment

Age group (years)	Incidence 1990 Number ('000s)	Rate (per 100 000)	Prevalence 1990 Number ('000s)	Rate (per 100 000)	Avg. age at onset (years)	Average duration (years)	Deaths 1990 Number ('000s)	Rate (per 100 000)	Deaths 2000 (Projected) Number ('000s)	Rate (per 100 000)
Males										
0-4	0	0	0	0	-	-	0	0	0	0
5-14	0	0	0	0	-	-	0	0	0	0
15-44	0	0	0	0	-	-	0	0	0	0
45-59	0	0	0	0	-	-	0	0	0	0
60+	0	0	0	0	-	-	0	0	0	0
All ages	0	0	0	0	-	-	0	0	0	0
Females										
0-4	0	0	0	0	-	-	0	0	0	0
5-14	0	0	0	0	-	-	0	0	0	0
15-44	0	0	0	0	-	-	0	0	0	0
45-59	0	0	0	0	-	-	0	0	0	0
60+	0	0	0	0	-	-	0	0	0	0
All ages	0	0	0	0	-	-	0	0	0	0
Total	0	0	0	0	-	-	0	0	0	0

Table 101c — India - India - Inde — Trichuriasis - Cognitive impairment

Age group (years)	Incidence 1990 Number ('000s)	Rate (per 100 000)	Prevalence 1990 Number ('000s)	Rate (per 100 000)	Avg. age at onset (years)	Average duration (years)	Deaths 1990 Number ('000s)	Rate (per 100 000)	Deaths 2000 (Projected) Number ('000s)	Rate (per 100 000)
Males										
0-4	0	0.3	0	0.7	2.5	59.9	0	0	0	0
5-14	38	37.1	191	187.7	10.0	57.5	0	0	0	0
15-44	0	0.0	748	372.8	-	-	0	0	0	0
45-59	0	0.0	177	372.8	-	-	0	0	0	0
60+	0	0.0	111	372.8	-	-	0	0	0	0
All ages	38	8.6	1 227	279.3	10.0	57.5	0	0	0	0
Females										
0-4	0	0.3	0	0.7	2.5	60.8	0	0	0	0
5-14	35	37.1	179	187.5	10.0	59.1	0	0	0	0
15-44	0	0.0	683	372.8	-	-	0	0	0	0
45-59	0	0.0	172	372.8	-	-	0	0	0	0
60+	0	0.0	108	372.8	-	-	0	0	0	0
All ages	36	8.7	1 142	278.4	10.0	59.1	0	0	0	0
Total	74	8.7	2 369	278.9	10.0	58.2	0	0	0	0

For epidemiological sources see Bundy et al. 1996. See explanatory notes for definitions and caveats.

Table 101 **Cuadro 101** **Tableau 101**
Trichuriasis **Tricocefalosis** **Tricocéphalose**

Cognitive impairment Deficiencia cognocitiva Déficience cognitive

Table 101d China - China - Chine — Trichuriasis - Cognitive impairment

Age group (years)	Incidence 1990 Number ('000s)	Rate (per 100 000)	Prevalence 1990 Number ('000s)	Rate (per 100 000)	Avg. age at onset (years)	Average duration (years)	Deaths 1990 Number ('000s)	Rate (per 100 000)	Deaths 2000 (Projected) Number ('000s)	Rate (per 100 000)
Males										
0-4	0	0.3	0	0.7	2.5	65.5	0	0	0	0
5-14	187	192.4	942	970.7	10.0	59.9	0	0	0	0
15-44	0	0.0	5 897	1 925.3	-	-	0	0	0	0
45-59	0	0.0	1 399	1 925.3	-	-	0	0	0	0
60+	0	0.0	943	1 925.3	-	-	0	0	0	0
All ages	187	31.9	9 182	1 569.0	10.0	59.9	0	0	0	0
Females										
0-4	0	0.3	0	0.7	2.5	68.5	0	0	0	0
5-14	174	192.4	878	970.7	10.0	63.2	0	0	0	0
15-44	0	0.0	5 469	1 925.3	-	-	0	0	0	0
45-59	0	0.0	1 240	1 925.3	-	-	0	0	0	0
60+	0	0.0	995	1 925.3	-	-	0	0	0	0
All ages	174	31.7	8 582	1 564.7	10.0	63.2	0	0	0	0
Total	361	31.8	17 764	1 566.9	10.0	61.5	0	0	0	0

Table 101e OAI - OPAI - APAI — Trichuriasis - Cognitive impairment

Age group (years)	Incidence 1990 Number ('000s)	Rate (per 100 000)	Prevalence 1990 Number ('000s)	Rate (per 100 000)	Avg. age at onset (years)	Average duration (years)	Deaths 1990 Number ('000s)	Rate (per 100 000)	Deaths 2000 (Projected) Number ('000s)	Rate (per 100 000)
Males										
0-4	0	0.6	1	1.5	2.5	59.8	0	0	0	0
5-14	201	238.6	1 012	1 204.0	10.0	56.2	0	0	0	0
15-44	0	0.0	3 842	2 389.2	-	-	0	0	0	0
45-59	0	0.0	816	2 389.2	-	-	0	0	0	0
60+	0	0.0	483	2 389.2	-	-	0	0	0	0
All ages	201	58.5	6 153	1 794.1	10.0	56.2	0	0	0	0
Females										
0-4	0	0.6	1	1.5	2.5	63.2	0	0	0	0
5-14	191	238.6	966	1 204.4	10.0	59.2	0	0	0	0
15-44	0	0.0	3 813	2 389.2	-	-	0	0	0	0
45-59	0	0.0	838	2 389.2	-	-	0	0	0	0
60+	0	0.0	541	2 389.2	-	-	0	0	0	0
All ages	192	56.4	6 160	1 814.1	10.0	59.2	0	0	0	0
Total	392	57.5	12 313	1 804.0	10.0	57.7	0	0	0	0

Table 101f SSA - ASS - ASS — Trichuriasis - Cognitive impairment

Age group (years)	Incidence 1990 Number ('000s)	Rate (per 100 000)	Prevalence 1990 Number ('000s)	Rate (per 100 000)	Avg. age at onset (years)	Average duration (years)	Deaths 1990 Number ('000s)	Rate (per 100 000)	Deaths 2000 (Projected) Number ('000s)	Rate (per 100 000)
Males										
0-4	0	0	0	0	-	-	0	0	0	0
5-14	28	40	140	200	10.0	49.2	0	0	0	0
15-44	0	0	416	401	-	-	0	0	0	0
45-59	0	0	81	401	-	-	0	0	0	0
60+	0	0	42	401	-	-	0	0	0	0
All ages	28	11	680	270	10.0	49.2	0	0	0	0
Females										
0-4	0	0	0	0	-	-	0	0	0	0
5-14	28	40	140	200	10.0	51.9	0	0	0	0
15-44	0	0	426	401	-	-	0	0	0	0
45-59	0	0	89	401	-	-	0	0	0	0
60+	0	0	51	401	-	-	0	0	0	0
All ages	28	11	706	274	10.0	51.9	0	0	0	0
Total	56	11	1 386	272	10.0	50.6	0	0	0	0

For epidemiological sources see Bundy et al. 1996. See explanatory notes for definitions and caveats.

Table 101	Cuadro 101	Tableau 101
Trichuriasis	**Tricocefalosis**	**Tricocéphalose**
Cognitive impairment	Deficiencia cognocitiva	Déficience cognitive

Table 101g LAC - ALC - ALC — Trichuriasis - Cognitive impairment

Age group (years)	Incidence 1990 Number ('000s)	Rate (per 100 000)	Prevalence 1990 Number ('000s)	Rate (per 100 000)	Avg. age at onset (years)	Average duration (years)	Deaths 1990 Number ('000s)	Rate (per 100 000)	Deaths 2000 (Projected) Number ('000s)	Rate (per 100 000)
Males										
0-4	0	0.3	0	0.7	2.5	63.9	0	0	0	0
5-14	90	172.3	453	868.8	10.0	59.3	0	0	0	0
15-44	0	0.0	1 799	1 725.0	-	-	0	0	0	0
45-59	0	0.0	384	1 725.0	-	-	0	0	0	0
60+	0	0.0	245	1 725.0	-	-	0	0	0	0
All ages	90	40.6	2 881	1 300.2	10.0	59.4	0	0	0	0
Females										
0-4	0	0.3	0	0.7	2.5	67.9	0	0	0	0
5-14	87	172.3	441	869.2	10.0	63.0	0	0	0	0
15-44	0	0.0	1 795	1 725.0	-	-	0	0	0	0
45-59	0	0.0	403	1 725.0	-	-	0	0	0	0
60+	0	0.0	290	1 725.0	-	-	0	0	0	0
All ages	88	39.3	2 930	1 315.7	10.0	63.0	0	0	0	0
Total	177	39.9	5 811	1 308.0	10.0	61.2	0	0	0	0

Table 101h MEC - AOM - CMO — Trichuriasis - Cognitive impairment

Age group (years)	Incidence 1990 Number ('000s)	Rate (per 100 000)	Prevalence 1990 Number ('000s)	Rate (per 100 000)	Avg. age at onset (years)	Average duration (years)	Deaths 1990 Number ('000s)	Rate (per 100 000)	Deaths 2000 (Projected) Number ('000s)	Rate (per 100 000)
Males										
0-4	0	0.0	0	0.0	2.5	61.1	0	0	0	0
5-14	1	0.9	4	6.0	10.0	58.1	0	0	0	0
15-44	0	0.0	12	10.5	-	-	0	0	0	0
45-59	0	0.0	2	10.5	-	-	0	0	0	0
60+	0	0.0	1	10.5	-	-	0	0	0	0
All ages	1	0.3	20	7.7	10.0	58.1	0	0	0	0
Females										
0-4	0	0.0	0	0.0	2.5	63.7	0	0	0	0
5-14	1	0.9	4	6.0	10.0	60.9	0	0	0	0
15-44	0	0.0	11	10.5	-	-	0	0	0	0
45-59	0	0.0	2	10.5	-	-	0	0	0	0
60+	0	0.0	2	10.5	-	-	0	0	0	0
All ages	1	0.3	19	7.8	10.0	60.9	0	0	0	0
Total	1	0.3	39	7.7	10.0	59.5	0	0	0	0

Table 101i World - Mundo - Monde — Trichuriasis - Cognitive impairment

Age group (years)	Incidence 1990 Number ('000s)	Rate (per 100 000)	Prevalence 1990 Number ('000s)	Rate (per 100 000)	Avg. age at onset (years)	Average duration (years)	Deaths 1990 Number ('000s)	Rate (per 100 000)	Deaths 2000 (Projected) Number ('000s)	Rate (per 100 000)
Males										
0-4	1	0.2	2	0.5	2.5	61.7	0	0	0	0
5-14	543	98.6	2 741	497.4	10.0	57.7	0	0	0	0
15-44	0	0.0	12 715	1 017.2	-	-	0	0	0	0
45-59	0	0.0	2 860	915.5	-	-	0	0	0	0
60+	0	0.0	1 826	834.3	-	-	0	0	0	0
All ages	544	20.5	20 144	759.1	10.0	57.7	0	0	0	0
Females										
0-4	1	0.2	2	0.5	2.5	64.4	0	0	0	0
5-14	517	98.3	2 607	496.0	10.0	60.8	0	0	0	0
15-44	0	0.0	12 199	1 017.7	-	-	0	0	0	0
45-59	0	0.0	2 744	882.1	-	-	0	0	0	0
60+	0	0.0	1 987	738.0	-	-	0	0	0	0
All ages	517	19.8	19 538	747.5	10.0	60.8	0	0	0	0
Total	1 062	20.2	39 682	753.3	10.0	59.2	0	0	0	0

For epidemiological sources see Bundy et al. 1996. See explanatory notes for definitions and caveats.

Table 102
Ancylostomiasis and
necatoriasis
High intensity infection

Cuadro 102
Anquilostomiasis y
necatoriasis
Infección de alta intensidad

Tableau 102
Ankylostomiase et
nécatoriase
Infection de forte intensité

Table 102a EME - PEMC - EMBE Ancylostomiasis and necatoriasis - High intensity infection

Age group (years)	Incidence 1990 Number ('000s)	Rate (per 100 000)	Prevalence 1990 Number ('000s)	Rate (per 100 000)	Avg. age at onset (years)	Average duration (years)	Deaths 1990 Number ('000s)	Rate (per 100 000)	Deaths 2000 (Projected) Number ('000s)	Rate (per 100 000)
Males										
0-4	-	-	0	0	-	-	0	0	0	0
5-14	-	-	0	0	-	-	0	0	0	0
15-44	-	-	0	0	-	-	0	0	0	0
45-59	-	-	0	0	-	-	0	0	0	0
60+	-	-	0	0	-	-	0	0	0	0
All ages	-	-	0	0	-	-	0	0	0	0
Females										
0-4	-	-	0	0	-	-	0	0	0	0
5-14	-	-	0	0	-	-	0	0	0	0
15-44	-	-	0	0	-	-	0	0	0	0
45-59	-	-	0	0	-	-	0	0	0	0
60+	-	-	0	0	-	-	0	0	0	0
All ages	-	-	0	0	-	-	0	0	0	0
Total	-	-	0	0	-	-	0	0	0	0

Table 102b FSE - PEAS - AESE Ancylostomiasis and necatoriasis - High intensity infection

Age group (years)	Incidence 1990 Number ('000s)	Rate (per 100 000)	Prevalence 1990 Number ('000s)	Rate (per 100 000)	Avg. age at onset (years)	Average duration (years)	Deaths 1990 Number ('000s)	Rate (per 100 000)	Deaths 2000 (Projected) Number ('000s)	Rate (per 100 000)
Males										
0-4	-	-	0	0	-	-	0	0	0	0
5-14	-	-	0	0	-	-	0	0	0	0
15-44	-	-	0	0	-	-	0	0	0	0
45-59	-	-	0	0	-	-	0	0	0	0
60+	-	-	0	0	-	-	0	0	0	0
All ages	-	-	0	0	-	-	0	0	0	0
Females										
0-4	-	-	0	0	-	-	0	0	0	0
5-14	-	-	0	0	-	-	0	0	0	0
15-44	-	-	0	0	-	-	0	0	0	0
45-59	-	-	0	0	-	-	0	0	0	0
60+	-	-	0	0	-	-	0	0	0	0
All ages	-	-	0	0	-	-	0	0	0	0
Total	-	-	0	0	-	-	0	0	0	0

Table 102c India - India - Inde Ancylostomiasis and necatoriasis - High intensity infection

Age group (years)	Incidence 1990 Number ('000s)	Rate (per 100 000)	Prevalence 1990 Number ('000s)	Rate (per 100 000)	Avg. age at onset (years)	Average duration (years)	Deaths 1990 Number ('000s)	Rate (per 100 000)	Deaths 2000 (Projected) Number ('000s)	Rate (per 100 000)
Males										
0-4	-	-	0	0	-	-	0	0.0	0	0.0
5-14	-	-	1 603	1 575	-	-	0	0.0	0	0.0
15-44	-	-	16 343	8 150	-	-	0	0.2	0	0.1
45-59	-	-	3 877	8 150	-	-	0	0.3	0	0.1
60+	-	-	2 426	8 150	-	-	0	0.9	0	0.7
All ages	-	-	24 248	5 518	-	-	1	0.2	0	0.1
Females										
0-4	-	-	0	0	-	-	0	0.0	0	0.0
5-14	-	-	1 500	1 575	-	-	0	0.0	0	0.0
15-44	-	-	14 934	8 150	-	-	0	0.2	0	0.1
45-59	-	-	3 749	8 150	-	-	0	0.3	0	0.1
60+	-	-	2 357	8 150	-	-	0	0.9	0	0.7
All ages	-	-	22 541	5 496	-	-	1	0.2	0	0.1
Total	-	-	46 790	5 508	-	-	1	0.2	1	0.1

For epidemiological sources see Bundy et al. 1996. See explanatory notes for definitions and caveats.

Table 102
Ancylostomiasis and
necatoriasis
High intensity infection

Cuadro 102
Anquilostomiasis y
necatoriasis
Infección de alta intensidad

Tableau 102
Ankylostomiase et
nécatoriase
Infection de forte intensité

Table 102d — China - China - Chine — Ancylostomiasis and necatoriasis - High intensity infection

Age group (years)	Incidence 1990 Number ('000s)	Rate (per 100 000)	Prevalence 1990 Number ('000s)	Rate (per 100 000)	Avg. age at onset (years)	Average duration (years)	Deaths 1990 Number ('000s)	Rate (per 100 000)	Deaths 2000 (Projected) Number ('000s)	Rate (per 100 000)
Males										
0-4	-	-	0	0	-	-	0	0.0	0	0.0
5-14	-	-	524	540	-	-	0	0.0	0	0.0
15-44	-	-	9 986	3 260	-	-	0	0.0	0	0.0
45-59	-	-	2 369	3 260	-	-	0	0.0	0	0.0
60+	-	-	1 597	3 260	-	-	0	0.1	0	0.1
All ages	-	-	14 475	2 474	-	-	0	0.0	0	0.0
Females										
0-4	-	-	0	0	-	-	0	0.0	0	0.0
5-14	-	-	488	540	-	-	0	0.0	0	0.0
15-44	-	-	9 261	3 260	-	-	0	0.0	0	0.0
45-59	-	-	2 100	3 260	-	-	0	0.0	0	0.0
60+	-	-	1 684	3 260	-	-	0	0.1	0	0.1
All ages	-	-	13 533	2 467	-	-	0	0.0	0	0.0
Total	-	-	28 008	2 471	-	-	0	0.0	0	0.0

Table 102e — OAI - OPAI - APAI — Ancylostomiasis and necatoriasis - High intensity infection

Age group (years)	Incidence 1990 Number ('000s)	Rate (per 100 000)	Prevalence 1990 Number ('000s)	Rate (per 100 000)	Avg. age at onset (years)	Average duration (years)	Deaths 1990 Number ('000s)	Rate (per 100 000)	Deaths 2000 (Projected) Number ('000s)	Rate (per 100 000)
Males										
0-4	-	-	0	0	-	-	0	0.0	0	0.0
5-14	-	-	1 298	1 545	-	-	0	0.0	0	0.0
15-44	-	-	12 834	7 980	-	-	0	0.1	0	0.1
45-59	-	-	2 724	7 980	-	-	0	0.3	0	0.2
60+	-	-	1 613	7 980	-	-	0	0.9	0	0.7
All ages	-	-	18 469	5 385	-	-	1	0.2	0	0.1
Females										
0-4	-	-	0	0	-	-	0	0.0	0	0.0
5-14	-	-	1 239	1 545	-	-	0	0.0	0	0.0
15-44	-	-	12 737	7 980	-	-	0	0.1	0	0.0
45-59	-	-	2 800	7 980	-	-	0	0.3	0	0.2
60+	-	-	1 808	7 980	-	-	0	0.8	0	0.7
All ages	-	-	18 585	5 473	-	-	1	0.1	0	0.1
Total	-	-	37 054	5 429	-	-	1	0.2	1	0.1

Table 102f — SSA - ASS - ASS — Ancylostomiasis and necatoriasis - High intensity infection

Age group (years)	Incidence 1990 Number ('000s)	Rate (per 100 000)	Prevalence 1990 Number ('000s)	Rate (per 100 000)	Avg. age at onset (years)	Average duration (years)	Deaths 1990 Number ('000s)	Rate (per 100 000)	Deaths 2000 (Projected) Number ('000s)	Rate (per 100 000)
Males										
0-4	-	-	0	0	-	-	0	0.0	0	0.0
5-14	-	-	885	1 260	-	-	0	0.0	0	0.0
15-44	-	-	5 977	5 760	-	-	0	0.2	0	0.1
45-59	-	-	1 170	5 760	-	-	0	0.4	0	0.2
60+	-	-	605	5 760	-	-	0	1.1	0	0.8
All ages	-	-	8 637	3 423	-	-	0	0.1	0	0.1
Females										
0-4	-	-	0	0	-	-	0	0.0	0	0.0
5-14	-	-	880	1 260	-	-	0	0.0	0	0.0
15-44	-	-	6 120	5 760	-	-	0	0.2	0	0.1
45-59	-	-	1 274	5 760	-	-	0	0.4	0	0.2
60+	-	-	733	5 760	-	-	0	1.2	0	0.8
All ages	-	-	9 007	3 492	-	-	0	0.2	0	0.1
Total	-	-	17 644	3 458	-	-	1	0.2	1	0.1

For epidemiological sources see Bundy et al. 1996. See explanatory notes for definitions and caveats.

Table 102	Cuadro 102	Tableau 102
Ancylostomiasis and necatoriasis	Anquilostomiasis y necatoriasis	Ankylostomiase et nécatoriase
High intensity infection	Infección de alta intensidad	Infection de forte intensité

Table 102g   LAC - ALC - ALC   Ancylostomiasis and necatoriasis - High intensity infection

Age group (years)	Incidence 1990 Number ('000s)	Rate (per 100 000)	Prevalence 1990 Number ('000s)	Rate (per 100 000)	Avg. age at onset (years)	Average duration (years)	Deaths 1990 Number ('000s)	Rate (per 100 000)	Deaths 2000 (Projected) Number ('000s)	Rate (per 100 000)
Males										
0-4	-	-	0	0	-	-	0	0.0	0	0.0
5-14	-	-	493	945	-	-	0	0.0	0	0.0
15-44	-	-	5 246	5 030	-	-	0	0.1	0	0.0
45-59	-	-	1 119	5 030	-	-	0	0.2	0	0.1
60+	-	-	716	5 030	-	-	0	0.5	0	0.4
All ages	-	-	7 573	3 417	-	-	0	0.1	0	0.1
Females										
0-4	-	-	0	0	-	-	0	0.0	0	0.0
5-14	-	-	480	945	-	-	0	0.0	0	0.0
15-44	-	-	5 235	5 030	-	-	0	0.1	0	0.0
45-59	-	-	1 175	5 030	-	-	0	0.2	0	0.1
60+	-	-	846	5 030	-	-	0	0.5	0	0.4
All ages	-	-	7 736	3 474	-	-	0	0.1	0	0.1
Total	-	-	15 309	3 446	-	-	0	0.1	0	0.1

Table 102h   MEC - AOM - CMO   Ancylostomiasis and necatoriasis - High intensity infection

Age group (years)	Incidence 1990 Number ('000s)	Rate (per 100 000)	Prevalence 1990 Number ('000s)	Rate (per 100 000)	Avg. age at onset (years)	Average duration (years)	Deaths 1990 Number ('000s)	Rate (per 100 000)	Deaths 2000 (Projected) Number ('000s)	Rate (per 100 000)
Males										
0-4	-	-	0	0	-	-	0	0.0	0	0.0
5-14	-	-	314	480	-	-	0	0.0	0	0.0
15-44	-	-	2 733	2 400	-	-	0	0.0	0	0.0
45-59	-	-	536	2 400	-	-	0	0.1	0	0.1
60+	-	-	328	2 400	-	-	0	0.3	0	0.2
All ages	-	-	3 911	1 525	-	-	0	0.0	0	0.0
Females										
0-4	-	-	0	0	-	-	0	0.0	0	0.0
5-14	-	-	298	480	-	-	0	0.0	0	0.0
15-44	-	-	2 573	2 400	-	-	0	0.0	0	0.0
45-59	-	-	535	2 400	-	-	0	0.1	0	0.1
60+	-	-	371	2 400	-	-	0	0.3	0	0.2
All ages	-	-	3 776	1 531	-	-	0	0.1	0	0.0
Total	-	-	7 687	1 528	-	-	0	0.0	0	0.0

Table 102i   World - Mundo - Monde   Ancylostomiasis and necatoriasis - High intensity infection

Age group (years)	Incidence 1990 Number ('000s)	Rate (per 100 000)	Prevalence 1990 Number ('000s)	Rate (per 100 000)	Avg. age at onset (years)	Average duration (years)	Deaths 1990 Number ('000s)	Rate (per 100 000)	Deaths 2000 (Projected) Number ('000s)	Rate (per 100 000)
Males										
0-4	-	-	0	0	-	-	0	0.0	0	0.0
5-14	-	-	5 116	928	-	-	0	0.0	0	0.0
15-44	-	-	53 118	4 250	-	-	1	0.1	1	0.0
45-59	-	-	11 795	3 776	-	-	0	0.1	0	0.1
60+	-	-	7 284	3 328	-	-	1	0.3	1	0.3
All ages	-	-	77 313	2 913	-	-	2	0.1	2	0.0
Females										
0-4	-	-	0	0	-	-	0	0.0	0	0.0
5-14	-	-	4 885	929	-	-	0	0.0	0	0.0
15-44	-	-	50 861	4 243	-	-	1	0.1	0	0.0
45-59	-	-	11 633	3 740	-	-	0	0.1	0	0.1
60+	-	-	7 800	2 897	-	-	1	0.3	1	0.2
All ages	-	-	75 179	2 876	-	-	2	0.1	1	0.1
Total	-	-	152 492	2 895	-	-	4	0.1	3	0.1

For epidemiological sources see Bundy et al. 1996. See explanatory notes for definitions and caveats.

Table 103
Ancylostomiasis and necatoriasis
Anaemia

Cuadro 103
Anquilostomiasis y necatoriasis
Anemia

Tableau 103
Ankylostomiase et nécatoriase
Anémie

Table 103a — EME - PEMC - EMBE — Ancylostomiasis and necatoriasis - Anaemia

Age group (years)	Incidence 1990 Number ('000s)	Rate (per 100 000)	Prevalence 1990 Number ('000s)	Rate (per 100 000)	Avg. age at onset (years)	Average duration (years)	Deaths 1990 Number ('000s)	Rate (per 100 000)	Deaths 2000 (Projected) Number ('000s)	Rate (per 100 000)
Males										
0-4	-	-	0	0	-	-	-	-	-	-
5-14	-	-	0	0	-	-	-	-	-	-
15-44	-	-	0	0	-	-	-	-	-	-
45-59	-	-	0	0	-	-	-	-	-	-
60+	-	-	0	0	-	-	-	-	-	-
All ages	-	-	0	0	-	-	-	-	-	-
Females										
0-4	-	-	0	0	-	-	-	-	-	-
5-14	-	-	0	0	-	-	-	-	-	-
15-44	-	-	0	0	-	-	-	-	-	-
45-59	-	-	0	0	-	-	-	-	-	-
60+	-	-	0	0	-	-	-	-	-	-
All ages	-	-	0	0	-	-	-	-	-	-
Total	-	-	0	0	-	-	-	-	-	-

Table 103b — FSE - PEAS - AESE — Ancylostomiasis and necatoriasis - Anaemia

Age group (years)	Incidence 1990 Number ('000s)	Rate (per 100 000)	Prevalence 1990 Number ('000s)	Rate (per 100 000)	Avg. age at onset (years)	Average duration (years)	Deaths 1990 Number ('000s)	Rate (per 100 000)	Deaths 2000 (Projected) Number ('000s)	Rate (per 100 000)
Males										
0-4	-	-	0	0	-	-	-	-	-	-
5-14	-	-	0	0	-	-	-	-	-	-
15-44	-	-	0	0	-	-	-	-	-	-
45-59	-	-	0	0	-	-	-	-	-	-
60+	-	-	0	0	-	-	-	-	-	-
All ages	-	-	0	0	-	-	-	-	-	-
Females										
0-4	-	-	0	0	-	-	-	-	-	-
5-14	-	-	0	0	-	-	-	-	-	-
15-44	-	-	0	0	-	-	-	-	-	-
45-59	-	-	0	0	-	-	-	-	-	-
60+	-	-	0	0	-	-	-	-	-	-
All ages	-	-	0	0	-	-	-	-	-	-
Total	-	-	0	0	-	-	-	-	-	-

Table 103c — India - India - Inde — Ancylostomiasis and necatoriasis - Anaemia

Age group (years)	Incidence 1990 Number ('000s)	Rate (per 100 000)	Prevalence 1990 Number ('000s)	Rate (per 100 000)	Avg. age at onset (years)	Average duration (years)	Deaths 1990 Number ('000s)	Rate (per 100 000)	Deaths 2000 (Projected) Number ('000s)	Rate (per 100 000)
Males										
0-4	-	-	0	0	-	-	-	-	-	-
5-14	-	-	71	70	-	-	-	-	-	-
15-44	-	-	4 151	2 070	-	-	-	-	-	-
45-59	-	-	985	2 070	-	-	-	-	-	-
60+	-	-	616	2 070	-	-	-	-	-	-
All ages	-	-	5 823	1 325	-	-	-	-	-	-
Females										
0-4	-	-	0	0	-	-	-	-	-	-
5-14	-	-	67	70	-	-	-	-	-	-
15-44	-	-	3 793	2 070	-	-	-	-	-	-
45-59	-	-	952	2 070	-	-	-	-	-	-
60+	-	-	599	2 070	-	-	-	-	-	-
All ages	-	-	5 411	1 319	-	-	-	-	-	-
Total	-	-	11 234	1 322	-	-	-	-	-	-

For epidemiological sources see Bundy et al. 1996. See explanatory notes for definitions and caveats.

Table 103
Ancylostomiasis and necatoriasis
Anaemia

Cuadro 103
Anquilostomiasis y necatoriasis
Anemia

Tableau 103
Ankylostomiase et nécatoriase
Anémie

Table 103d China - China - Chine — Ancylostomiasis and necatoriasis - Anaemia

Age group (years)	Incidence 1990 Number ('000s)	Rate (per 100 000)	Prevalence 1990 Number ('000s)	Rate (per 100 000)	Avg. age at onset (years)	Average duration (years)	Deaths 1990 Number ('000s)	Rate (per 100 000)	Deaths 2000 (Projected) Number ('000s)	Rate (per 100 000)
Males										
0-4	-	-	0	0	-	-	-	-	-	-
5-14	-	-	10	10	-	-	-	-	-	-
15-44	-	-	1 011	330	-	-	-	-	-	-
45-59	-	-	240	330	-	-	-	-	-	-
60+	-	-	162	330	-	-	-	-	-	-
All ages	-	-	1 422	243	-	-	-	-	-	-
Females										
0-4	-	-	0	0	-	-	-	-	-	-
5-14	-	-	9	10	-	-	-	-	-	-
15-44	-	-	937	330	-	-	-	-	-	-
45-59	-	-	213	330	-	-	-	-	-	-
60+	-	-	170	330	-	-	-	-	-	-
All ages	-	-	1 330	242	-	-	-	-	-	-
Total	-	-	2 751	243	-	-	-	-	-	-

Table 103e OAI - OPAI - APAI — Ancylostomiasis and necatoriasis - Anaemia

Age group (years)	Incidence 1990 Number ('000s)	Rate (per 100 000)	Prevalence 1990 Number ('000s)	Rate (per 100 000)	Avg. age at onset (years)	Average duration (years)	Deaths 1990 Number ('000s)	Rate (per 100 000)	Deaths 2000 (Projected) Number ('000s)	Rate (per 100 000)
Males										
0-4	-	-	0	0	-	-	-	-	-	-
5-14	-	-	59	70	-	-	-	-	-	-
15-44	-	-	3 313	2 060	-	-	-	-	-	-
45-59	-	-	703	2 060	-	-	-	-	-	-
60+	-	-	416	2 060	-	-	-	-	-	-
All ages	-	-	4 491	1 310	-	-	-	-	-	-
Females										
0-4	-	-	0	0	-	-	-	-	-	-
5-14	-	-	56	70	-	-	-	-	-	-
15-44	-	-	3 288	2 060	-	-	-	-	-	-
45-59	-	-	723	2 060	-	-	-	-	-	-
60+	-	-	467	2 060	-	-	-	-	-	-
All ages	-	-	4 534	1 335	-	-	-	-	-	-
Total	-	-	9 025	1 322	-	-	-	-	-	-

Table 103f SSA - ASS - ASS — Ancylostomiasis and necatoriasis - Anaemia

Age group (years)	Incidence 1990 Number ('000s)	Rate (per 100 000)	Prevalence 1990 Number ('000s)	Rate (per 100 000)	Avg. age at onset (years)	Average duration (years)	Deaths 1990 Number ('000s)	Rate (per 100 000)	Deaths 2000 (Projected) Number ('000s)	Rate (per 100 000)
Males										
0-4	-	-	0	0	-	-	-	-	-	-
5-14	-	-	126	180	-	-	-	-	-	-
15-44	-	-	2 750	2 650	-	-	-	-	-	-
45-59	-	-	538	2 650	-	-	-	-	-	-
60+	-	-	278	2 650	-	-	-	-	-	-
All ages	-	-	3 693	1 464	-	-	-	-	-	-
Females										
0-4	-	-	0	0	-	-	-	-	-	-
5-14	-	-	126	180	-	-	-	-	-	-
15-44	-	-	2 816	2 650	-	-	-	-	-	-
45-59	-	-	586	2 650	-	-	-	-	-	-
60+	-	-	337	2 650	-	-	-	-	-	-
All ages	-	-	3 865	1 498	-	-	-	-	-	-
Total	-	-	7 558	1 481	-	-	-	-	-	-

For epidemiological sources see Bundy et al. 1996. See explanatory notes for definitions and caveats.

Table 103
Ancylostomiasis and
necatoriasis
Anaemia

Cuadro 103
Anquilostomiasis y
necatoriasis
Anemia

Tableau 103
Ankylostomiase et
nécatoriase
Anémie

Table 103g   LAC - ALC - ALC   Ancylostomiasis and necatoriasis - Anaemia

Age group (years)	Incidence 1990 Number ('000s)	Rate (per 100 000)	Prevalence 1990 Number ('000s)	Rate (per 100 000)	Avg. age at onset (years)	Average duration (years)	Deaths 1990 Number ('000s)	Rate (per 100 000)	Deaths 2000 (Projected) Number ('000s)	Rate (per 100 000)
Males										
0-4	-	-	0	0	-	-	-	-	-	-
5-14	-	-	16	30	-	-	-	-	-	-
15-44	-	-	1 137	1 090	-	-	-	-	-	-
45-59	-	-	243	1 090	-	-	-	-	-	-
60+	-	-	155	1 090	-	-	-	-	-	-
All ages	-	-	1 550	699	-	-	-	-	-	-
Females										
0-4	-	-	0	0	-	-	-	-	-	-
5-14	-	-	15	30	-	-	-	-	-	-
15-44	-	-	1 135	1 090	-	-	-	-	-	-
45-59	-	-	255	1 090	-	-	-	-	-	-
60+	-	-	183	1 090	-	-	-	-	-	-
All ages	-	-	1 588	713	-	-	-	-	-	-
Total	-	-	3 138	706	-	-	-	-	-	-

Table 103h   MEC - AOM - CMO   Ancylostomiasis and necatoriasis - Anaemia

Age group (years)	Incidence 1990 Number ('000s)	Rate (per 100 000)	Prevalence 1990 Number ('000s)	Rate (per 100 000)	Avg. age at onset (years)	Average duration (years)	Deaths 1990 Number ('000s)	Rate (per 100 000)	Deaths 2000 (Projected) Number ('000s)	Rate (per 100 000)
Males										
0-4	-	-	0	0	-	-	-	-	-	-
5-14	-	-	20	30	-	-	-	-	-	-
15-44	-	-	877	770	-	-	-	-	-	-
45-59	-	-	172	770	-	-	-	-	-	-
60+	-	-	105	770	-	-	-	-	-	-
All ages	-	-	1 174	458	-	-	-	-	-	-
Females										
0-4	-	-	0	0	-	-	-	-	-	-
5-14	-	-	19	30	-	-	-	-	-	-
15-44	-	-	826	770	-	-	-	-	-	-
45-59	-	-	172	770	-	-	-	-	-	-
60+	-	-	119	770	-	-	-	-	-	-
All ages	-	-	1 135	460	-	-	-	-	-	-
Total	-	-	2 308	459	-	-	-	-	-	-

Table 103i   World - Mundo - Monde   Ancylostomiasis and necatoriasis - Anaemia

Age group (years)	Incidence 1990 Number ('000s)	Rate (per 100 000)	Prevalence 1990 Number ('000s)	Rate (per 100 000)	Avg. age at onset (years)	Average duration (years)	Deaths 1990 Number ('000s)	Rate (per 100 000)	Deaths 2000 (Projected) Number ('000s)	Rate (per 100 000)
Males										
0-4	-	-	0	0	-	-	-	-	-	-
5-14	-	-	301	55	-	-	-	-	-	-
15-44	-	-	13 238	1 059	-	-	-	-	-	-
45-59	-	-	2 880	922	-	-	-	-	-	-
60+	-	-	1 733	792	-	-	-	-	-	-
All ages	-	-	18 153	684	-	-	-	-	-	-
Females										
0-4	-	-	0	0	-	-	-	-	-	-
5-14	-	-	291	55	-	-	-	-	-	-
15-44	-	-	12 794	1 067	-	-	-	-	-	-
45-59	-	-	2 900	932	-	-	-	-	-	-
60+	-	-	1 876	697	-	-	-	-	-	-
All ages	-	-	17 862	683	-	-	-	-	-	-
Total	-	-	36 014	684	-	-	-	-	-	-

For epidemiological sources see Bundy et al. 1996. See explanatory notes for definitions and caveats.

Table 104
Ancylostomiasis and
necatoriasis
Cognitive impairment

Cuadro 104
Anquilostomiasis y
necatoriasis
Deficiencia cognocitiva

Tableau 104
Ankylostomiase et
nécatoriase
Déficience cognitive

Table 104a EME - PEMC - EMBE Ancylostomiasis and necatoriasis - Cognitive impairment

Age group (years)	Incidence 1990 Number ('000s)	Rate (per 100 000)	Prevalence 1990 Number ('000s)	Rate (per 100 000)	Avg. age at onset (years)	Average duration (years)	Deaths 1990 Number ('000s)	Rate (per 100 000)	Deaths 2000 (Projected) Number ('000s)	Rate (per 100 000)
Males										
0-4	0	0	0	0	-	-	0	0	0	0
5-14	0	0	0	0	-	-	0	0	0	0
15-44	0	0	0	0	-	-	0	0	0	0
45-59	0	0	0	0	-	-	0	0	0	0
60+	0	0	0	0	-	-	0	0	0	0
All ages	0	0	0	0	-	-	0	0	0	0
Females										
0-4	0	0	0	0	-	-	0	0	0	0
5-14	0	0	0	0	-	-	0	0	0	0
15-44	0	0	0	0	-	-	0	0	0	0
45-59	0	0	0	0	-	-	0	0	0	0
60+	0	0	0	0	-	-	0	0	0	0
All ages	0	0	0	0	-	-	0	0	0	0
Total	0	0	0	0	-	-	0	0	0	0

Table 104b FSE - PEAS - AESE Ancylostomiasis and necatoriasis - Cognitive impairment

Age group (years)	Incidence 1990 Number ('000s)	Rate (per 100 000)	Prevalence 1990 Number ('000s)	Rate (per 100 000)	Avg. age at onset (years)	Average duration (years)	Deaths 1990 Number ('000s)	Rate (per 100 000)	Deaths 2000 (Projected) Number ('000s)	Rate (per 100 000)
Males										
0-4	0	0	0	0	-	-	0	0	0	0
5-14	0	0	0	0	-	-	0	0	0	0
15-44	0	0	0	0	-	-	0	0	0	0
45-59	0	0	0	0	-	-	0	0	0	0
60+	0	0	0	0	-	-	0	0	0	0
All ages	0	0	0	0	-	-	0	0	0	0
Females										
0-4	0	0	0	0	-	-	0	0	0	0
5-14	0	0	0	0	-	-	0	0	0	0
15-44	0	0	0	0	-	-	0	0	0	0
45-59	0	0	0	0	-	-	0	0	0	0
60+	0	0	0	0	-	-	0	0	0	0
All ages	0	0	0	0	-	-	0	0	0	0
Total	0	0	0	0	-	-	0	0	0	0

Table 104c India - India - Inde Ancylostomiasis and necatoriasis - Cognitive impairment

Age group (years)	Incidence 1990 Number ('000s)	Rate (per 100 000)	Prevalence 1990 Number ('000s)	Rate (per 100 000)	Avg. age at onset (years)	Average duration (years)	Deaths 1990 Number ('000s)	Rate (per 100 000)	Deaths 2000 (Projected) Number ('000s)	Rate (per 100 000)
Males										
0-4	0	0	0	0	-	-	0	0	0	0
5-14	48	47	239	235	10.0	57.5	0	0	0	0
15-44	0	0	940	469	-	-	0	0	0	0
45-59	0	0	223	469	-	-	0	0	0	0
60+	0	0	140	469	-	-	0	0	0	0
All ages	48	11	1 542	351	10.0	57.5	0	0	0	0
Females										
0-4	0	0	0	0	-	-	0	0	0	0
5-14	45	47	224	235	10.0	59.1	0	0	0	0
15-44	0	0	859	469	-	-	0	0	0	0
45-59	0	0	216	469	-	-	0	0	0	0
60+	0	0	136	469	-	-	0	0	0	0
All ages	45	11	1 434	350	10.0	59.1	0	0	0	0
Total	92	11	2 977	350	10.0	58.2	0	0	0	0

For epidemiological sources see Bundy et al. 1996. See explanatory notes for definitions and caveats.

Table 104
Ancylostomiasis and
necatoriasis
Cognitive impairment

Cuadro 104
Anquilostomiasis y
necatoriasis
Deficiencia cognocitiva

Tableau 104
Ankylostomiase et
nécatoriase
Déficience cognitive

Table 104d		China - China - Chine						Ancylostomiasis and necatoriasis - Cognitive impairment			
Age group (years)	Incidence 1990		Prevalence 1990		Avg. age at onset (years)	Average duration (years)	Deaths 1990		Deaths 2000 (Projected)		
	Number ('000s)	Rate (per 100 000)	Number ('000s)	Rate (per 100 000)			Number ('000s)	Rate (per 100 000)	Number ('000s)	Rate (per 100 000)	
Males											
0-4	0	0.0	0	0	-	-	0	0	0	0	
5-14	16	16.0	78	80	10.0	59.9	0	0	0	0	
15-44	0	0.0	490	160	-	-	0	0	0	0	
45-59	0	0.0	116	160	-	-	0	0	0	0	
60+	0	0.0	78	160	-	-	0	0	0	0	
All ages	16	2.6	762	130	10.0	59.9	0	0	0	0	
Females											
0-4	0	0.0	0	0	-	-	0	0	0	0	
5-14	14	16.0	73	80	10.0	63.2	0	0	0	0	
15-44	0	0.0	454	160	-	-	0	0	0	0	
45-59	0	0.0	103	160	-	-	0	0	0	0	
60+	0	0.0	83	160	-	-	0	0	0	0	
All ages	14	2.6	712	130	10.0	63.2	0	0	0	0	
Total	30	2.6	1 474	130	10.0	61.5	0	0	0	0	

Table 104e		OAI - OPAI - APAI						Ancylostomiasis and necatoriasis - Cognitive impairment			
Age group (years)	Incidence 1990		Prevalence 1990		Avg. age at onset (years)	Average duration (years)	Deaths 1990		Deaths 2000 (Projected)		
	Number ('000s)	Rate (per 100 000)	Number ('000s)	Rate (per 100 000)			Number ('000s)	Rate (per 100 000)	Number ('000s)	Rate (per 100 000)	
Males											
0-4	0	0	0	0	-	-	0	0	0	0	
5-14	39	46	193	230	10.0	56.2	0	0	0	0	
15-44	0	0	738	459	-	-	0	0	0	0	
45-59	0	0	157	459	-	-	0	0	0	0	
60+	0	0	93	459	-	-	0	0	0	0	
All ages	39	11	1 181	344	10.0	56.2	0	0	0	0	
Females											
0-4	0	0	0	0	-	-	0	0	0	0	
5-14	37	46	185	230	10.0	59.2	0	0	0	0	
15-44	0	0	733	459	-	-	0	0	0	0	
45-59	0	0	161	459	-	-	0	0	0	0	
60+	0	0	104	459	-	-	0	0	0	0	
All ages	37	11	1 182	348	10.0	59.2	0	0	0	0	
Total	75	11	2 363	346	10.0	57.6	0	0	0	0	

Table 104f		SSA - ASS - ASS						Ancylostomiasis and necatoriasis - Cognitive impairment			
Age group (years)	Incidence 1990		Prevalence 1990		Avg. age at onset (years)	Average duration (years)	Deaths 1990		Deaths 2000 (Projected)		
	Number ('000s)	Rate (per 100 000)	Number ('000s)	Rate (per 100 000)			Number ('000s)	Rate (per 100 000)	Number ('000s)	Rate (per 100 000)	
Males											
0-4	0	0	0	0	-	-	0	0	0	0	
5-14	27	38	133	189	10.0	49.2	0	0	0	0	
15-44	0	0	394	379	-	-	0	0	0	0	
45-59	0	0	77	379	-	-	0	0	0	0	
60+	0	0	40	379	-	-	0	0	0	0	
All ages	27	11	643	255	10.0	49.2	0	0	0	0	
Females											
0-4	0	0	0	0	-	-	0	0	0	0	
5-14	26	38	132	189	10.0	51.9	0	0	0	0	
15-44	0	0	403	379	-	-	0	0	0	0	
45-59	0	0	84	379	-	-	0	0	0	0	
60+	0	0	48	379	-	-	0	0	0	0	
All ages	26	10	667	259	10.0	51.9	0	0	0	0	
Total	53	10	1 311	257	10.0	50.6	0	0	0	0	

For epidemiological sources see Bundy et al. 1996. See explanatory notes for definitions and caveats.

Table 104
Ancylostomiasis and
necatoriasis
Cognitive impairment

Cuadro 104
Anquilostomiasis y
necatoriasis
Deficiencia cognocitiva

Tableau 104
Ankylostomiase et
nécatoriase
Déficience cognitive

Table 104g LAC - ALC - ALC Ancylostomiasis and necatoriasis - Cognitive impairment

Age group (years)	Incidence 1990 Number ('000s)	Rate (per 100 000)	Prevalence 1990 Number ('000s)	Rate (per 100 000)	Avg. age at onset (years)	Average duration (years)	Deaths 1990 Number ('000s)	Rate (per 100 000)	Deaths 2000 (Projected) Number ('000s)	Rate (per 100 000)
Males										
0-4	0	0.0	0	0	-	-	0	0	0	0
5-14	15	28.0	73	140	10.0	59.3	0	0	0	0
15-44	0	0.0	292	280	-	-	0	0	0	0
45-59	0	0.0	62	280	-	-	0	0	0	0
60+	0	0.0	40	280	-	-	0	0	0	0
All ages	15	6.6	467	211	10.0	59.3	0	0	0	0
Females										
0-4	0	0.0	0	0	-	-	0	0	0	0
5-14	14	28.0	71	140	10.0	63.0	0	0	0	0
15-44	0	0.0	291	280	-	-	0	0	0	0
45-59	0	0.0	65	280	-	-	0	0	0	0
60+	0	0.0	47	280	-	-	0	0	0	0
All ages	14	6.4	475	213	10.0	63.0	0	0	0	0
Total	29	6.5	941	212	10.0	61.1	0	0	0	0

Table 104h MEC - AOM - CMO Ancylostomiasis and necatoriasis - Cognitive impairment

Age group (years)	Incidence 1990 Number ('000s)	Rate (per 100 000)	Prevalence 1990 Number ('000s)	Rate (per 100 000)	Avg. age at onset (years)	Average duration (years)	Deaths 1990 Number ('000s)	Rate (per 100 000)	Deaths 2000 (Projected) Number ('000s)	Rate (per 100 000)
Males										
0-4	0	0.0	0	0	-	-	0	0	0	0
5-14	9	14.0	46	70	10.0	58.1	0	0	0	0
15-44	0	0.0	159	140	-	-	0	0	0	0
45-59	0	0.0	31	140	-	-	0	0	0	0
60+	0	0.0	19	140	-	-	0	0	0	0
All ages	9	3.6	256	100	10.0	58.1	0	0	0	0
Females										
0-4	0	0.0	0	0	-	-	0	0	0	0
5-14	9	14.0	44	70	10.0	60.9	0	0	0	0
15-44	0	0.0	150	140	-	-	0	0	0	0
45-59	0	0.0	31	140	-	-	0	0	0	0
60+	0	0.0	22	140	-	-	0	0	0	0
All ages	9	3.5	246	100	10.0	60.9	0	0	0	0
Total	18	3.5	502	100	10.0	59.5	0	0	0	0

Table 104i World - Mundo - Monde Ancylostomiasis and necatoriasis - Cognitive impairment

Age group (years)	Incidence 1990 Number ('000s)	Rate (per 100 000)	Prevalence 1990 Number ('000s)	Rate (per 100 000)	Avg. age at onset (years)	Average duration (years)	Deaths 1990 Number ('000s)	Rate (per 100 000)	Deaths 2000 (Projected) Number ('000s)	Rate (per 100 000)
Males										
0-4	0	0.0	0	0	-	-	0	0	0	0
5-14	152	27.6	762	138	10.0	56.2	0	0	0	0
15-44	0	0.0	3 013	241	-	-	0	0	0	0
45-59	0	0.0	666	213	-	-	0	0	0	0
60+	0	0.0	409	187	-	-	0	0	0	0
All ages	152	5.7	4 851	183	10.0	56.2	0	0	0	0
Females										
0-4	0	0.0	0	0	-	-	0	0	0	0
5-14	145	27.6	728	139	10.0	58.7	0	0	0	0
15-44	0	0.0	2 890	241	-	-	0	0	0	0
45-59	0	0.0	660	212	-	-	0	0	0	0
60+	0	0.0	439	163	-	-	0	0	0	0
All ages	145	5.6	4 717	180	10.0	58.7	0	0	0	0
Total	297	5.6	9 568	182	10.0	57.4	0	0	0	0

For epidemiological sources see Bundy et al. 1996. See explanatory notes for definitions and caveats.

Table 105
Lower respiratory infections

Episodes

Cuadro 105
Infecciones de las vías respiratorias inferiores

Episodios

Tableau 105
Infections des voies respiratoires inférieures

Episodes

Table 105a — EME - PEMC - EMBE — Lower respiratory infections - Episodes

Age group (years)	Incidence 1990 Number ('000s)	Rate (per 100 000)	Prevalence 1990 Number ('000s)	Rate (per 100 000)	Avg. age at onset (years)	Average duration (years)	Deaths 1990 Number ('000s)	Rate (per 100 000)	Deaths 2000 (Projected) Number ('000s)	Rate (per 100 000)
Males										
0-4	950	3 600	18	69	2.5	0.02	2	6.2	1	4.2
5-14	854	1 600	16	31	10.0	0.02	0	0.4	0	0.3
15-44	1 104	600	21	12	29.9	0.02	3	1.5	2	1.0
45-59	397	600	8	12	52.4	0.02	5	8.3	4	5.4
60+	1 150	1 900	22	36	71.1	0.02	119	196.8	137	190.1
All ages	4 455	1 141	85	22	32.9	0.02	129	33.1	145	35.2
Females										
0-4	902	3 600	17	69	2.5	0.02	1	4.5	1	3.1
5-14	811	1 600	16	31	10.0	0.02	0	0.4	0	0.3
15-44	1 075	600	21	12	30.0	0.02	2	0.9	1	0.5
45-59	407	600	8	12	52.4	0.02	3	4.2	2	2.8
60+	1 607	1 900	31	36	72.4	0.02	137	161.4	150	154.1
All ages	4 802	1 179	92	23	37.5	0.02	142	34.9	154	36.1
Total	9 257	1 160	178	22	35.3	0.02	272	34.1	299	35.6

Table 105b — FSE - PEAS - AESE — Lower respiratory infections - Episodes

Age group (years)	Incidence 1990 Number ('000s)	Rate (per 100 000)	Prevalence 1990 Number ('000s)	Rate (per 100 000)	Avg. age at onset (years)	Average duration (years)	Deaths 1990 Number ('000s)	Rate (per 100 000)	Deaths 2000 (Projected) Number ('000s)	Rate (per 100 000)
Males										
0-4	4 678	34 000	90	652	2.5	0.02	10	71.1	7	53.4
5-14	1 641	6 000	31	115	10.0	0.02	0	1.8	0	1.3
15-44	763	1 000	15	19	29.8	0.02	3	3.8	2	2.4
45-59	270	1 000	5	19	52.2	0.02	5	18.0	4	12.3
60+	377	1 800	7	35	70.0	0.02	33	155.9	43	168.1
All ages	7 729	4 675	148	90	11.8	0.02	51	30.7	56	32.5
Females										
0-4	4 466	34 000	86	652	2.5	0.02	7	57.0	5	42.2
5-14	1 585	6 000	30	115	10.0	0.02	0	1.7	0	1.1
15-44	750	1 000	14	19	29.9	0.02	1	1.6	1	0.9
45-59	300	1 000	6	19	52.4	0.02	1	4.7	1	3.2
60+	655	1 800	13	35	71.5	0.02	52	141.9	58	140.1
All ages	7 756	4 287	149	82	14.4	0.02	62	34.4	65	34.7
Total	15 485	4 472	297	86	13.1	0.02	113	32.6	121	33.7

Table 105c — India - India - Inde — Lower respiratory infections - Episodes

Age group (years)	Incidence 1990 Number ('000s)	Rate (per 100 000)	Prevalence 1990 Number ('000s)	Rate (per 100 000)	Avg. age at onset (years)	Average duration (years)	Deaths 1990 Number ('000s)	Rate (per 100 000)	Deaths 2000 (Projected) Number ('000s)	Rate (per 100 000)
Males										
0-4	26 905	45 000	737	1 233	2.5	0.03	363	608	216	380.1
5-14	6 105	6 000	167	164	10.0	0.03	32	31	17	15.4
15-44	2 005	1 000	55	27	29.8	0.03	25	12	14	5.7
45-59	476	1 000	13	27	52.3	0.03	18	38	11	18.6
60+	2 084	7 000	57	192	69.7	0.03	150	505	137	370.0
All ages	37 575	8 551	1 029	234	9.5	0.03	588	134	394	77.0
Females										
0-4	25 506	45 000	699	1 233	2.5	0.03	386	681	220	408.9
5-14	5 716	6 000	157	164	10.0	0.03	57	60	30	28.6
15-44	1 832	1 000	50	27	29.8	0.03	20	11	10	4.5
45-59	460	1 000	13	27	52.4	0.03	18	38	11	19.0
60+	2 025	7 000	55	192	70.1	0.03	126	436	126	323.3
All ages	35 538	8 666	974	237	9.6	0.03	607	148	397	82.1
Total	73 113	8 606	2 003	236	9.6	0.03	1 195	141	791	79.5

For epidemiological sources see Lob-Levyt et al. 1996. For the methods used to estimate and project incidence, prevalence, and deaths see Murray and Lopez 1996a. See explanatory notes for definitions and caveats.

Table 105
Lower respiratory infections
Episodes

Cuadro 105
Infecciones de las vías respiratorias inferiores
Episodios

Tableau 105
Infections des voies respiratoires inférieures
Episodes

Table 105d   China - China - Chine   Lower respiratory infections - Episodes

Age group (years)	Incidence 1990 Number ('000s)	Rate (per 100 000)	Prevalence 1990 Number ('000s)	Rate (per 100 000)	Avg. age at onset (years)	Average duration (years)	Deaths 1990 Number ('000s)	Rate (per 100 000)	Deaths 2000 (Projected) Number ('000s)	Rate (per 100 000)
Males										
0-4	27 109	45 000	743	1 233	2.5	0.03	129	214.7	65	111.1
5-14	5 820	6 000	159	164	10.0	0.03	4	4.3	2	1.7
15-44	3 063	1 000	84	27	29.9	0.03	5	1.6	2	0.6
45-59	727	1 000	20	27	52.3	0.03	5	7.4	3	3.1
60+	980	2 000	27	55	69.8	0.03	82	167.9	84	139.1
All ages	37 699	6 442	1 033	176	8.6	0.03	226	38.6	156	23.8
Females										
0-4	26 076	45 000	714	1 233	2.5	0.03	156	269.6	74	133.5
5-14	5 424	6 000	149	164	10.0	0.03	4	4.7	2	1.9
15-44	2 841	1 000	78	27	29.9	0.03	5	1.7	2	0.6
45-59	644	1 000	18	27	52.4	0.03	3	4.4	2	1.9
60+	1 033	2 000	28	55	70.6	0.03	73	140.6	74	115.4
All ages	36 018	6 567	987	180	8.6	0.03	241	43.9	154	24.7
Total	73 716	6 502	2 020	178	8.6	0.03	467	41.2	311	24.3

Table 105e   OAI - OPAI - APAI   Lower respiratory infections - Episodes

Age group (years)	Incidence 1990 Number ('000s)	Rate (per 100 000)	Prevalence 1990 Number ('000s)	Rate (per 100 000)	Avg. age at onset (years)	Average duration (years)	Deaths 1990 Number ('000s)	Rate (per 100 000)	Deaths 2000 (Projected) Number ('000s)	Rate (per 100 000)
Males										
0-4	19 693	45 000	540	1 233	2.5	0.03	185	423.0	120	272.4
5-14	5 042	6 000	138	164	10.0	0.03	27	32.5	14	17.3
15-44	1 608	1 000	44	27	29.7	0.03	10	6.2	6	3.1
45-59	341	1 000	9	27	52.3	0.03	6	18.0	4	9.7
60+	606	3 000	17	82	69.6	0.03	74	364.3	78	282.5
All ages	27 291	7 957	748	218	7.6	0.03	302	88.1	223	55.2
Females										
0-4	18 895	45 000	518	1 233	2.4	0.03	138	328.4	87	204.6
5-14	4 813	6 000	132	164	10.0	0.03	24	29.7	13	15.6
15-44	1 596	1 000	44	27	29.4	0.03	9	5.5	5	2.5
45-59	351	1 000	10	27	52.2	0.03	6	17.8	5	9.6
60+	680	3 000	19	82	69.2	0.03	64	283.7	75	231.7
All ages	26 334	7 755	721	212	7.8	0.03	241	71.0	184	45.6
Total	53 626	7 857	1 469	215	7.7	0.03	543	79.6	407	50.4

Table 105f   SSA - ASS - ASS   Lower respiratory infections - Episodes

Age group (years)	Incidence 1990 Number ('000s)	Rate (per 100 000)	Prevalence 1990 Number ('000s)	Rate (per 100 000)	Avg. age at onset (years)	Average duration (years)	Deaths 1990 Number ('000s)	Rate (per 100 000)	Deaths 2000 (Projected) Number ('000s)	Rate (per 100 000)
Males										
0-4	21 368	45 000	585	1 233	2.4	0.03	399	841	399	605.3
5-14	4 215	6 000	115	164	10.0	0.03	44	62	34	35.7
15-44	1 038	1 000	28	27	29.4	0.03	12	12	9	6.2
45-59	203	1 000	6	27	52.2	0.03	6	27	4	15.4
60+	736	7 000	20	192	69.2	0.03	75	718	80	553.3
All ages	27 560	10 922	755	299	6.7	0.03	536	212	525	153.1
Females										
0-4	21 164	45 000	580	1 233	2.4	0.03	323	687	303	476.2
5-14	4 189	6 000	115	164	10.0	0.03	37	53	28	29.6
15-44	1 063	1 000	29	27	29.5	0.03	16	15	10	7.0
45-59	221	1 000	6	27	52.2	0.03	6	27	4	15.2
60+	891	7 000	24	192	69.7	0.03	88	693	92	522.3
All ages	27 527	10 672	754	292	7.2	0.03	470	182	437	125.3
Total	55 087	10 796	1 509	296	7.0	0.03	1 006	197	962	139.1

For epidemiological sources see Lob-Levyt et al. 1996. For the methods used to estimate and project incidence, prevalence, and deaths see Murray and Lopez 1996a. See explanatory notes for definitions and caveats.

Table 105	Cuadro 105	Tableau 105
Lower respiratory infections	Infecciones de las vías respiratorias inferiores	Infections des voies respiratoires inférieures
Episodes	Episodios	Episodes

Table 105g LAC - ALC - ALC — Lower respiratory infections - Episodes

Age group (years)	Incidence 1990 Number ('000s)	Rate (per 100 000)	Prevalence 1990 Number ('000s)	Rate (per 100 000)	Avg. age at onset (years)	Average duration (years)	Deaths 1990 Number ('000s)	Rate (per 100 000)	Deaths 2000 (Projected) Number ('000s)	Rate (per 100 000)
Males										
0-4	12 924	45 000	354	1 233	2.5	0.03	58	200.9	41	140.4
5-14	3 127	6 000	86	164	10.0	0.03	4	7.3	3	4.4
15-44	1 043	1 000	29	27	29.8	0.03	5	5.1	4	2.9
45-59	222	1 000	6	27	52.3	0.03	5	23.3	4	13.9
60+	285	2 000	8	55	70.3	0.03	24	167.8	28	142.8
All ages	17 602	7 943	482	218	7.2	0.03	96	43.3	80	30.1
Females										
0-4	12 454	45 000	341	1 233	2.5	0.03	41	148.1	28	100.8
5-14	3 045	6 000	83	164	10.0	0.03	4	8.8	3	5.2
15-44	1 041	1 000	29	27	29.9	0.03	8	7.7	5	3.9
45-59	234	1 000	6	27	52.4	0.03	4	17.5	3	10.4
60+	336	2 000	9	55	71.1	0.03	25	147.5	30	125.9
All ages	17 110	7 683	460	211	7.5	0.03	82	37.0	69	25.9
Total	34 712	7 813	951	214	7.4	0.03	178	40.1	149	28.0

Table 105h MEC - AOM - CMO — Lower respiratory infections - Episodes

Age group (years)	Incidence 1990 Number ('000s)	Rate (per 100 000)	Prevalence 1990 Number ('000s)	Rate (per 100 000)	Avg. age at onset (years)	Average duration (years)	Deaths 1990 Number ('000s)	Rate (per 100 000)	Deaths 2000 (Projected) Number ('000s)	Rate (per 100 000)
Males										
0-4	18 522	45 000	507	1 233	2.5	0.03	193	469.9	173	346.6
5-14	3 921	6 000	107	164	10.0	0.03	18	27.0	14	16.2
15-44	1 139	1 000	31	27	29.8	0.03	4	3.3	3	1.8
45-59	223	1 000	6	27	52.3	0.03	3	11.4	2	6.8
60+	341	2 500	9	68	69.7	0.03	50	368.5	53	281.7
All ages	24 147	9 418	662	258	6.4	0.03	268	104.4	244	73.1
Females										
0-4	17 880	45 000	490	1 233	2.5	0.03	184	462.4	157	330.0
5-14	3 720	6 000	102	164	10.0	0.03	20	31.5	15	18.3
15-44	1 072	1 000	29	27	29.8	0.03	6	5.3	4	2.7
45-59	223	1 000	6	27	52.3	0.03	4	17.4	3	10.1
60+	386	2 500	11	68	70.4	0.03	45	289.1	48	224.3
All ages	23 282	9 438	638	259	6.6	0.03	258	104.4	226	70.3
Total	47 428	9 428	1 299	258	6.5	0.03	525	104.4	470	71.7

Table 105i World - Mundo - Monde — Lower respiratory infections - Episodes

Age group (years)	Incidence 1990 Number ('000s)	Rate (per 100 000)	Prevalence 1990 Number ('000s)	Rate (per 100 000)	Avg. age at onset (years)	Average duration (years)	Deaths 1990 Number ('000s)	Rate (per 100 000)	Deaths 2000 (Projected) Number ('000s)	Rate (per 100 000)
Males										
0-4	132 150	41 130	3 574	1 112	2.5	0.03	1 340	416.9	1 021	295.3
5-14	30 725	5 574	821	149	10.0	0.03	130	23.5	84	13.3
15-44	11 763	941	307	25	29.8	0.03	67	5.3	41	2.8
45-59	2 859	915	73	23	52.3	0.03	53	16.9	37	9.2
60+	6 559	2 997	167	76	69.9	0.03	608	277.6	639	232.1
All ages	184 057	6 936	4 943	186	8.7	0.03	2 196	82.8	1 823	58.9
Females										
0-4	127 342	41 178	3 445	1 114	2.5	0.03	1 237	399.8	875	264.7
5-14	29 303	5 576	783	149	10.0	0.03	147	27.9	90	14.9
15-44	11 270	940	294	25	29.8	0.03	66	5.5	38	2.7
45-59	2 839	913	72	23	52.4	0.03	45	14.5	31	7.8
60+	7 614	2 828	190	71	70.7	0.02	609	226.1	653	193.6
All ages	178 367	6 824	4 784	183	9.1	0.03	2 103	80.5	1 687	55.1
Total	362 424	6 881	9 726	185	8.9	0.03	4 299	81.6	3 510	57.0

For epidemiological sources see Lob-Levyt et al. 1996. For the methods used to estimate and project incidence, prevalence, and deaths see Murray and Lopez 1996a. See explanatory notes for definitions and caveats.

Table 106
Lower respiratory infections

Chronic sequelae

Cuadro 106
Infecciones de las vías respiratorias inferiores

Secuelas crónicas

Tableau 106
Infections des voies respiratoires inférieures

Séquelles chroniques

Table 106a   EME - PEMC - EMBE   Lower respiratory infections - Chronic sequelae

Age group (years)	Incidence 1990 Number ('000s)	Rate (per 100 000)	Prevalence 1990 Number ('000s)	Rate (per 100 000)	Avg. age at onset (years)	Average duration (years)	Deaths 1990 Number ('000s)	Rate (per 100 000)	Deaths 2000 (Projected) Number ('000s)	Rate (per 100 000)
Males										
0-4	0	0	0	0	-	-	0	0	0	0
5-14	0	0	0	0	-	-	0	0	0	0
15-44	0	0	0	0	-	-	0	0	0	0
45-59	0	0	0	0	-	-	0	0	0	0
60+	0	0	0	0	-	-	0	0	0	0
All ages	0	0	0	0	-	-	0	0	0	0
Females										
0-4	0	0	0	0	-	-	0	0	0	0
5-14	0	0	0	0	-	-	0	0	0	0
15-44	0	0	0	0	-	-	0	0	0	0
45-59	0	0	0	0	-	-	0	0	0	0
60+	0	0	0	0	-	-	0	0	0	0
All ages	0	0	0	0	-	-	0	0	0	0
Total	0	0	0	0	-	-	0	0	0	0

Table 106b   FSE - PEAS - AESE   Lower respiratory infections - Chronic sequelae

Age group (years)	Incidence 1990 Number ('000s)	Rate (per 100 000)	Prevalence 1990 Number ('000s)	Rate (per 100 000)	Avg. age at onset (years)	Average duration (years)	Deaths 1990 Number ('000s)	Rate (per 100 000)	Deaths 2000 (Projected) Number ('000s)	Rate (per 100 000)
Males										
0-4	0	0	0	0	-	-	0	0	0	0
5-14	0	0	0	0	-	-	0	0	0	0
15-44	0	0	0	0	-	-	0	0	0	0
45-59	0	0	0	0	-	-	0	0	0	0
60+	0	0	0	0	-	-	0	0	0	0
All ages	0	0	0	0	-	-	0	0	0	0
Females										
0-4	0	0	0	0	-	-	0	0	0	0
5-14	0	0	0	0	-	-	0	0	0	0
15-44	0	0	0	0	-	-	0	0	0	0
45-59	0	0	0	0	-	-	0	0	0	0
60+	0	0	0	0	-	-	0	0	0	0
All ages	0	0	0	0	-	-	0	0	0	0
Total	0	0	0	0	-	-	0	0	0	0

Table 106c   India - India - Inde   Lower respiratory infections - Chronic sequelae

Age group (years)	Incidence 1990 Number ('000s)	Rate (per 100 000)	Prevalence 1990 Number ('000s)	Rate (per 100 000)	Avg. age at onset (years)	Average duration (years)	Deaths 1990 Number ('000s)	Rate (per 100 000)	Deaths 2000 (Projected) Number ('000s)	Rate (per 100 000)
Males										
0-4	94	157	230	385	2.5	59.9	0	0	0	0
5-14	0	0	794	781	-	-	0	0	0	0
15-44	0	0	1 565	781	-	-	0	0	0	0
45-59	0	0	371	781	-	-	0	0	0	0
60+	0	0	232	781	-	-	0	0	0	0
All ages	94	21	3 193	727	2.5	59.9	0	0	0	0
Females										
0-4	89	157	218	384	2.4	60.8	0	0	0	0
5-14	0	0	744	781	-	-	0	0	0	0
15-44	0	0	1 431	781	-	-	0	0	0	0
45-59	0	0	359	781	-	-	0	0	0	0
60+	0	0	226	781	-	-	0	0	0	0
All ages	89	22	2 977	726	2.4	60.8	0	0	0	0
Total	183	22	6 170	726	2.5	60.3	0	0	0	0

For epidemiological sources see Lob-Levyt et al. 1996. For the methods used to estimate and project incidence, prevalence, and deaths see Murray and Lopez 1996a. See explanatory notes for definitions and caveats.

Table 106
Lower respiratory infections

Chronic sequelae

Cuadro 106
Infecciones de las vías respiratorias inferiores

Secuelas crónicas

Tableau 106
Infections des voies respiratoires inférieures

Séquelles chroniques

Table 106d — China - China - Chine — Lower respiratory infections - Chronic sequelae

Age group (years)	Incidence 1990 Number ('000s)	Rate (per 100 000)	Prevalence 1990 Number ('000s)	Rate (per 100 000)	Avg. age at onset (years)	Average duration (years)	Deaths 1990 Number ('000s)	Rate (per 100 000)	Deaths 2000 (Projected) Number ('000s)	Rate (per 100 000)
Males										
0-4	95	157	235	390	2.5	65.5	0	0	0	0
5-14	0	0	757	780	-	-	0	0	0	0
15-44	0	0	2 390	780	-	-	0	0	0	0
45-59	0	0	567	780	-	-	0	0	0	0
60+	0	0	382	780	-	-	0	0	0	0
All ages	95	16	4 331	740	2.5	65.5	0	0	0	0
Females										
0-4	91	157	226	390	2.5	68.5	0	0	0	0
5-14	0	0	705	780	-	-	0	0	0	0
15-44	0	0	2 217	780	-	-	0	0	0	0
45-59	0	0	503	780	-	-	0	0	0	0
60+	0	0	403	780	-	-	0	0	0	0
All ages	91	17	4 054	739	2.5	68.5	0	0	0	0
Total	186	16	8 385	740	2.5	67.0	0	0	0	0

Table 106e — OAI - OPAI - APAI — Lower respiratory infections - Chronic sequelae

Age group (years)	Incidence 1990 Number ('000s)	Rate (per 100 000)	Prevalence 1990 Number ('000s)	Rate (per 100 000)	Avg. age at onset (years)	Average duration (years)	Deaths 1990 Number ('000s)	Rate (per 100 000)	Deaths 2000 (Projected) Number ('000s)	Rate (per 100 000)
Males										
0-4	69	157	169	387	2.5	59.8	0	0	0	0
5-14	0	0	656	781	-	-	0	0	0	0
15-44	0	0	1 255	781	-	-	0	0	0	0
45-59	0	0	266	781	-	-	0	0	0	0
60+	0	0	158	781	-	-	0	0	0	0
All ages	69	20	2 505	730	2.5	59.8	0	0	0	0
Females										
0-4	66	157	163	388	2.5	63.2	0	0	0	0
5-14	0	0	626	780	-	-	0	0	0	0
15-44	0	0	1 246	780	-	-	0	0	0	0
45-59	0	0	274	780	-	-	0	0	0	0
60+	0	0	177	780	-	-	0	0	0	0
All ages	66	19	2 485	732	2.5	63.2	0	0	0	0
Total	135	20	4 990	731	2.5	61.5	0	0	0	0

Table 106f — SSA - ASS - ASS — Lower respiratory infections - Chronic sequelae

Age group (years)	Incidence 1990 Number ('000s)	Rate (per 100 000)	Prevalence 1990 Number ('000s)	Rate (per 100 000)	Avg. age at onset (years)	Average duration (years)	Deaths 1990 Number ('000s)	Rate (per 100 000)	Deaths 2000 (Projected) Number ('000s)	Rate (per 100 000)
Males										
0-4	75	157	180	378	2.4	48.7	0	0	0	0
5-14	0	0	549	781	-	-	0	0	0	0
15-44	0	0	811	781	-	-	0	0	0	0
45-59	0	0	159	781	-	-	0	0	0	0
60+	0	0	82	781	-	-	0	0	0	0
All ages	75	30	1 780	705	2.4	48.7	0	0	0	0
Females										
0-4	74	157	179	380	2.4	51.9	0	0	0	0
5-14	0	0	545	781	-	-	0	0	0	0
15-44	0	0	830	781	-	-	0	0	0	0
45-59	0	0	173	781	-	-	0	0	0	0
60+	0	0	99	781	-	-	0	0	0	0
All ages	74	29	1 826	708	2.4	51.9	0	0	0	0
Total	148	29	3 606	707	2.4	50.3	0	0	0	0

For epidemiological sources see Lob-Levyt et al. 1996. For the methods used to estimate and project incidence, prevalence, and deaths see Murray and Lopez 1996a. See explanatory notes for definitions and caveats.

Table 106
Lower respiratory infections

Chronic sequelae

Cuadro 106
Infecciones de las vías respiratorias inferiores

Secuelas crónicas

Tableau 106
Infections des voies respiratoires inférieures

Séquelles chroniques

Table 106g — LAC - ALC - ALC — Lower respiratory infections - Chronic sequelae

Age group (years)	Incidence 1990 Number ('000s)	Rate (per 100 000)	Prevalence 1990 Number ('000s)	Rate (per 100 000)	Avg. age at onset (years)	Average duration (years)	Deaths 1990 Number ('000s)	Rate (per 100 000)	Deaths 2000 (Projected) Number ('000s)	Rate (per 100 000)
Males										
0-4	45	157	112	389	2.5	63.9	0	0	0	0
5-14	0	0	407	780	-	-	0	0	0	0
15-44	0	0	814	780	-	-	0	0	0	0
45-59	0	0	174	780	-	-	0	0	0	0
60+	0	0	111	780	-	-	0	0	0	0
All ages	45	20	1 617	730	2.5	63.9	0	0	0	0
Females										
0-4	43	157	108	389	2.5	67.9	0	0	0	0
5-14	0	0	396	780	-	-	0	0	0	0
15-44	0	0	812	780	-	-	0	0	0	0
45-59	0	0	182	780	-	-	0	0	0	0
60+	0	0	131	780	-	-	0	0	0	0
All ages	43	20	1 629	732	2.5	67.9	0	0	0	0
Total	89	20	3 246	731	2.5	65.9	0	0	0	0

Table 106h — MEC - AOM - CMO — Lower respiratory infections - Chronic sequelae

Age group (years)	Incidence 1990 Number ('000s)	Rate (per 100 000)	Prevalence 1990 Number ('000s)	Rate (per 100 000)	Avg. age at onset (years)	Average duration (years)	Deaths 1990 Number ('000s)	Rate (per 100 000)	Deaths 2000 (Projected) Number ('000s)	Rate (per 100 000)
Males										
0-4	65	157	159	385	2.5	61.1	0	0	0	0
5-14	0	0	510	781	-	-	0	0	0	0
15-44	0	0	889	781	-	-	0	0	0	0
45-59	0	0	174	781	-	-	0	0	0	0
60+	0	0	107	781	-	-	0	0	0	0
All ages	65	25	1 839	717	2.5	61.1	0	0	0	0
Females										
0-4	62	157	153	386	2.5	63.7	0	0	0	0
5-14	0	0	484	781	-	-	0	0	0	0
15-44	0	0	837	781	-	-	0	0	0	0
45-59	0	0	174	781	-	-	0	0	0	0
60+	0	0	121	781	-	-	0	0	0	0
All ages	62	25	1 769	717	2.5	63.7	0	0	0	0
Total	127	25	3 607	717	2.5	62.4	0	0	0	0

Table 106i — World - Mundo - Monde — Lower respiratory infections - Chronic sequelae

Age group (years)	Incidence 1990 Number ('000s)	Rate (per 100 000)	Prevalence 1990 Number ('000s)	Rate (per 100 000)	Avg. age at onset (years)	Average duration (years)	Deaths 1990 Number ('000s)	Rate (per 100 000)	Deaths 2000 (Projected) Number ('000s)	Rate (per 100 000)
Males										
0-4	441	137	1 084	337	2.5	59.8	0	0	0	0
5-14	0	0	3 673	666	-	-	0	0	0	0
15-44	0	0	7 724	618	-	-	0	0	0	0
45-59	0	0	1 711	548	-	-	0	0	0	0
60+	0	0	1 072	490	-	-	0	0	0	0
All ages	441	17	15 264	575	2.5	59.8	0	0	0	0
Females										
0-4	426	138	1 046	338	2.5	62.4	0	0	0	0
5-14	0	0	3 500	666	-	-	0	0	0	0
15-44	0	0	7 372	615	-	-	0	0	0	0
45-59	0	0	1 665	535	-	-	0	0	0	0
60+	0	0	1 157	430	-	-	0	0	0	0
All ages	426	16	14 740	564	2.5	62.4	0	0	0	0
Total	867	16	30 004	570	2.5	61.1	0	0	0	0

For epidemiological sources see Lob-Levyt et al. 1996. For the methods used to estimate and project incidence, prevalence, and deaths see Murray and Lopez 1996a. See explanatory notes for definitions and caveats.

Table 107	Cuadro 107	Tableau 107
Upper respiratory infections	Infecciones de las vías respiratorias superiores	Infections des voies respiratoires supérieures
Episodes	Episodios	Episodes

Table 107a   EME - PEMC - EMBE   Upper respiratory infections - Episodes

Age group (years)	Incidence 1990 Number ('000s)	Rate (per 100 000)	Prevalence 1990 Number ('000s)	Rate (per 100 000)	Avg. age at onset (years)	Average duration (years)	Deaths 1990 Number ('000s)	Rate (per 100 000)	Deaths 2000 (Projected) Number ('000s)	Rate (per 100 000)
Males										
0-4	105 536	400 000	1 161	4 400	2.5	0.01	0	0.9	0	0.6
5-14	160 044	300 000	1 760	3 300	10.0	0.01	0	0.1	0	0.0
15-44	552 189	300 000	6 074	3 300	29.9	0.01	0	0.0	0	0.0
45-59	198 417	300 000	2 183	3 300	52.4	0.01	0	0.1	0	0.1
60+	242 192	400 000	2 664	4 400	71.1	0.01	1	1.3	1	1.3
All ages	1 258 378	322 263	13 842	3 545	36.5	0.01	1	0.3	1	0.3
Females										
0-4	100 260	400 000	1 103	4 400	2.5	0.01	0	0.5	0	0.3
5-14	152 040	300 000	1 672	3 300	10.0	0.01	0	0.0	0	0.0
15-44	627 197	350 000	6 899	3 850	30.0	0.01	0	0.0	0	0.0
45-59	203 397	300 000	2 237	3 300	52.4	0.01	0	0.1	0	0.1
60+	338 260	400 000	3 721	4 400	72.4	0.01	1	1.6	1	1.5
All ages	1 421 154	348 914	15 633	3 838	39.2	0.01	2	0.4	2	0.4
Total	2 679 532	335 869	29 475	3 695	38.0	0.01	3	0.3	3	0.3

Table 107b   FSE - PEAS - AESE   Upper respiratory infections - Episodes

Age group (years)	Incidence 1990 Number ('000s)	Rate (per 100 000)	Prevalence 1990 Number ('000s)	Rate (per 100 000)	Avg. age at onset (years)	Average duration (years)	Deaths 1990 Number ('000s)	Rate (per 100 000)	Deaths 2000 (Projected) Number ('000s)	Rate (per 100 000)
Males										
0-4	55 036	400 000	605	4 400	2.5	0.01	0	1.0	0	0.7
5-14	82 047	300 000	903	3 300	10.0	0.01	0	0.0	0	0.0
15-44	228 834	300 000	2 517	3 300	29.8	0.01	0	0.0	0	0.0
45-59	80 919	300 000	890	3 300	52.2	0.01	0	0.1	0	0.1
60+	83 852	400 000	922	4 400	70.0	0.01	0	0.7	0	0.7
All ages	530 688	321 003	5 838	3 531	33.7	0.01	0	0.2	0	0.2
Females										
0-4	52 540	400 000	578	4 400	2.5	0.01	0	0.9	0	0.6
5-14	79 263	300 000	872	3 300	10.0	0.01	0	0.0	0	0.0
15-44	262 357	350 000	2 886	3 850	29.9	0.01	0	0.0	0	0.0
45-59	90 018	300 000	990	3 300	52.4	0.01	0	0.1	0	0.0
60+	145 576	400 000	1 601	4 400	71.5	0.01	0	0.6	0	0.6
All ages	629 754	348 094	6 927	3 829	37.9	0.01	0	0.2	0	0.2
Total	1 160 442	335 158	12 765	3 687	36.0	0.01	1	0.2	1	0.2

Table 107c   India - India - Inde   Upper respiratory infections - Episodes

Age group (years)	Incidence 1990 Number ('000s)	Rate (per 100 000)	Prevalence 1990 Number ('000s)	Rate (per 100 000)	Avg. age at onset (years)	Average duration (years)	Deaths 1990 Number ('000s)	Rate (per 100 000)	Deaths 2000 (Projected) Number ('000s)	Rate (per 100 000)
Males										
0-4	418 523	700 000	4 604	7 700	2.5	0.01	4	6.1	2	3.8
5-14	407 008	400 000	4 477	4 400	10.0	0.01	0	0.3	0	0.2
15-44	802 100	400 000	8 823	4 400	29.8	0.01	0	0.1	0	0.1
45-59	142 701	300 000	1 570	3 300	52.3	0.01	0	0.4	0	0.2
60+	119 072	400 000	1 310	4 400	69.7	0.01	2	5.1	1	3.7
All ages	1 889 404	429 995	20 783	4 730	23.7	0.01	6	1.3	4	0.8
Females										
0-4	396 753	700 000	4 364	7 700	2.5	0.01	4	6.8	2	4.1
5-14	381 052	400 000	4 192	4 400	10.0	0.01	1	0.6	0	0.3
15-44	659 671	360 000	7 256	3 960	29.8	0.01	0	0.1	0	0.0
45-59	165 618	360 000	1 822	3 960	52.4	0.01	0	0.4	0	0.2
60+	115 696	400 000	1 273	4 400	70.1	0.01	1	4.4	1	3.3
All ages	1 718 790	419 102	18 907	4 610	24.0	0.01	6	1.5	4	0.8
Total	3 608 194	424 736	39 690	4 672	23.8	0.01	12	1.4	8	0.8

For epidemiological sources see Lob-Levyt et al. 1996. For the methods used to estimate and project incidence, prevalence, and deaths see Murray and Lopez 1996a. See explanatory notes for definitions and caveats.

Table 107
Upper respiratory infections

Episodes

Cuadro 107
Infecciones de las vías respiratorias superiores

Episodios

Tableau 107
Infections des voies respiratoires supérieures

Episodes

Table 107d   China - China - Chine   Upper respiratory infections - Episodes

Age group (years)	Incidence 1990 Number ('000s)	Rate (per 100 000)	Prevalence 1990 Number ('000s)	Rate (per 100 000)	Avg. age at onset (years)	Average duration (years)	Deaths 1990 Number ('000s)	Rate (per 100 000)	Deaths 2000 (Projected) Number ('000s)	Rate (per 100 000)
Males										
0-4	210 851	350 000	2 319	3 850	2.5	0.01	1	2.2	1	1.1
5-14	271 592	280 000	2 988	3 080	10.0	0.01	0	0.0	0	0.0
15-44	765 763	250 000	8 423	2 750	29.9	0.01	0	0.0	0	0.0
45-59	181 685	250 000	1 999	2 750	52.3	0.01	0	0.1	0	0.0
60+	146 940	300 000	1 616	3 300	69.8	0.01	1	1.7	1	1.4
All ages	1 576 830	269 452	17 345	2 964	29.1	0.01	2	0.4	2	0.2
Females										
0-4	202 811	350 000	2 231	3 850	2.5	0.01	2	2.7	1	1.4
5-14	253 123	280 000	2 784	3 080	10.0	0.01	0	0.0	0	0.0
15-44	710 195	250 000	7 812	2 750	29.9	0.01	0	0.0	0	0.0
45-59	161 008	250 000	1 771	2 750	52.4	0.01	0	0.0	0	0.0
60+	154 998	300 000	1 705	3 300	70.6	0.01	1	1.4	1	1.2
All ages	1 482 134	270 219	16 303	2 972	29.5	0.01	2	0.4	2	0.3
Total	3 058 964	269 823	33 649	2 968	29.3	0.01	5	0.4	3	0.2

Table 107e   OAI - OPAI - APAI   Upper respiratory infections - Episodes

Age group (years)	Incidence 1990 Number ('000s)	Rate (per 100 000)	Prevalence 1990 Number ('000s)	Rate (per 100 000)	Avg. age at onset (years)	Average duration (years)	Deaths 1990 Number ('000s)	Rate (per 100 000)	Deaths 2000 (Projected) Number ('000s)	Rate (per 100 000)
Males										
0-4	306 341	700 000	3 370	7 700	2.5	0.01	2	4.3	1	2.8
5-14	336 128	400 000	3 697	4 400	10.0	0.01	0	0.3	0	0.2
15-44	643 300	400 000	7 076	4 400	29.7	0.01	0	0.1	0	0.0
45-59	102 414	300 000	1 127	3 300	52.3	0.01	0	0.2	0	0.1
60+	80 832	400 000	889	4 400	69.6	0.01	1	3.7	1	2.9
All ages	1 469 015	428 327	16 159	4 712	23.3	0.01	3	0.9	2	0.6
Females										
0-4	293 916	700 000	3 233	7 700	2.5	0.01	1	3.3	1	2.1
5-14	320 868	400 000	3 530	4 400	10.0	0.01	0	0.3	0	0.2
15-44	574 600	360 000	6 321	3 960	29.8	0.01	0	0.1	0	0.0
45-59	126 324	360 000	1 390	3 960	52.3	0.01	0	0.2	0	0.1
60+	90 648	400 000	997	4 400	70.3	0.01	1	2.9	1	2.3
All ages	1 406 356	414 160	15 470	4 556	24.2	0.01	2	0.7	2	0.5
Total	2 875 371	421 279	31 629	4 634	23.7	0.01	6	0.8	4	0.5

Table 107f   SSA - ASS - ASS   Upper respiratory infections - Episodes

Age group (years)	Incidence 1990 Number ('000s)	Rate (per 100 000)	Prevalence 1990 Number ('000s)	Rate (per 100 000)	Avg. age at onset (years)	Average duration (years)	Deaths 1990 Number ('000s)	Rate (per 100 000)	Deaths 2000 (Projected) Number ('000s)	Rate (per 100 000)
Males										
0-4	332 388	700 000	3 656	7 700	2.4	0.01	4	8.6	4	6.2
5-14	351 290	500 000	3 864	5 500	10.0	0.01	0	0.6	0	0.4
15-44	311 292	300 000	3 424	3 300	29.4	0.01	0	0.1	0	0.1
45-59	60 924	300 000	670	3 300	52.2	0.01	0	0.3	0	0.2
60+	52 540	500 000	578	5 500	69.2	0.01	1	7.3	1	5.6
All ages	1 108 434	439 293	12 193	4 832	18.3	0.01	5	2.2	5	1.6
Females										
0-4	329 210	700 000	3 621	7 700	2.4	0.01	3	7.0	3	4.8
5-14	349 090	500 000	3 840	5 500	10.0	0.01	0	0.5	0	0.3
15-44	318 771	300 000	3 506	3 300	29.5	0.01	0	0.1	0	0.1
45-59	66 351	300 000	730	3 300	52.2	0.01	0	0.3	0	0.2
60+	63 650	500 000	700	5 500	69.7	0.01	1	7.0	1	5.3
All ages	1 127 072	436 931	12 398	4 806	19.2	0.01	5	1.9	4	1.3
Total	2 235 506	438 099	24 591	4 819	18.7	0.01	10	2.0	10	1.4

For epidemiological sources see Lob-Levyt et al. 1996. For the methods used to estimate and project incidence, prevalence, and deaths see Murray and Lopez 1996a. See explanatory notes for definitions and caveats.

Table 107
Upper respiratory infections

Episodes

Cuadro 107
Infecciones de las vías respiratorias superiores

Episodios

Tableau 107
Infections des voies respiratoires supérieures

Episodes

Table 107g　　LAC - ALC - ALC　　Upper respiratory infections - Episodes

Age group (years)	Incidence 1990 Number ('000s)	Rate (per 100 000)	Prevalence 1990 Number ('000s)	Rate (per 100 000)	Avg. age at onset (years)	Average duration (years)	Deaths 1990 Number ('000s)	Rate (per 100 000)	Deaths 2000 (Projected) Number ('000s)	Rate (per 100 000)
Males										
0-4	129 245	450 000	1 422	4 950	2.5	0.01	1	2.0	0	1.4
5-14	177 222	340 000	1 949	3 740	10.0	0.01	0	0.1	0	0.0
15-44	312 858	300 000	3 441	3 300	29.8	0.01	0	0.1	0	0.0
45-59	66 747	300 000	734	3 300	52.3	0.01	0	0.2	0	0.1
60+	48 385	340 000	532	3 740	70.3	0.01	0	1.7	0	1.4
All ages	734 457	331 417	8 079	3 646	24.9	0.01	1	0.4	1	0.3
Females										
0-4	124 542	450 000	1 370	4 950	2.5	0.01	0	1.5	0	1.0
5-14	172 530	340 000	1 898	3 740	10.0	0.01	0	0.1	0	0.1
15-44	312 255	300 000	3 435	3 300	29.9	0.01	0	0.1	0	0.0
45-59	70 065	300 000	771	3 300	52.4	0.01	0	0.2	0	0.1
60+	57 202	340 000	629	3 740	71.1	0.01	0	1.5	0	1.3
All ages	736 593	330 780	8 103	3 639	25.9	0.01	1	0.4	1	0.3
Total	1 471 050	331 098	16 182	3 642	25.4	0.01	2	0.4	2	0.3

Table 107h　　MEC - AOM - CMO　　Upper respiratory infections - Episodes

Age group (years)	Incidence 1990 Number ('000s)	Rate (per 100 000)	Prevalence 1990 Number ('000s)	Rate (per 100 000)	Avg. age at onset (years)	Average duration (years)	Deaths 1990 Number ('000s)	Rate (per 100 000)	Deaths 2000 (Projected) Number ('000s)	Rate (per 100 000)
Males										
0-4	164 644	400 000	1 811	4 400	2.5	0.01	2	4.8	2	3.5
5-14	196 035	300 000	2 156	3 300	10.0	0.01	0	0.3	0	0.2
15-44	341 685	300 000	3 759	3 300	29.8	0.01	0	0.0	0	0.0
45-59	67 011	300 000	737	3 300	52.3	0.01	0	0.1	0	0.1
60+	54 604	400 000	601	4 400	69.7	0.01	1	3.7	1	2.8
All ages	823 979	321 378	9 064	3 535	22.5	0.01	3	1.1	2	0.7
Females										
0-4	158 936	400 000	1 748	4 400	2.5	0.01	2	4.7	2	3.4
5-14	185 997	300 000	2 046	3 300	10.0	0.01	0	0.3	0	0.2
15-44	375 239	350 000	4 128	3 850	29.8	0.01	0	0.1	0	0.0
45-59	66 876	300 000	736	3 300	52.3	0.01	0	0.2	0	0.1
60+	61 800	400 000	680	4 400	70.4	0.01	0	2.9	0	2.3
All ages	848 848	344 100	9 337	3 785	23.3	0.01	3	1.1	2	0.7
Total	1 672 827	332 520	18 401	3 658	22.9	0.01	5	1.1	5	0.7

Table 107i　　World - Mundo - Monde　　Upper respiratory infections - Episodes

Age group (years)	Incidence 1990 Number ('000s)	Rate (per 100 000)	Prevalence 1990 Number ('000s)	Rate (per 100 000)	Avg. age at onset (years)	Average duration (years)	Deaths 1990 Number ('000s)	Rate (per 100 000)	Deaths 2000 (Projected) Number ('000s)	Rate (per 100 000)
Males										
0-4	1 722 563	536 123	18 948	5 897	2.5	0.01	14	4.3	11	3.0
5-14	1 981 365	359 467	21 795	3 954	10.0	0.01	1	0.2	1	0.1
15-44	3 958 021	316 664	43 538	3 483	29.8	0.01	1	0.1	0	0.0
45-59	900 818	288 381	9 909	3 172	52.3	0.01	1	0.2	0	0.1
60+	828 417	378 520	9 113	4 164	70.2	0.01	6	2.5	6	2.1
All ages	9 391 184	353 899	103 303	3 893	26.4	0.01	22	0.8	18	0.6
Females										
0-4	1 658 968	536 451	18 249	5 901	2.5	0.01	13	4.1	9	2.7
5-14	1 893 962	360 388	20 834	3 964	10.0	0.01	2	0.3	1	0.2
15-44	3 840 283	320 394	42 243	3 524	29.8	0.01	1	0.1	0	0.0
45-59	949 657	305 304	10 446	3 358	52.4	0.01	0	0.2	0	0.1
60+	1 027 830	381 788	11 306	4 200	71.2	0.01	6	2.2	6	1.8
All ages	9 370 700	358 527	103 078	3 944	27.9	0.01	21	0.8	17	0.5
Total	18 761 884	356 195	206 381	3 918	27.2	0.01	43	0.8	35	0.6

For epidemiological sources see Lob-Levyt et al. 1996. For the methods used to estimate and project incidence, prevalence, and deaths see Murray and Lopez 1996a. See explanatory notes for definitions and caveats.

Table 108
Upper respiratory infections

Pharyngitis

Cuadro 108
Infecciones de las vías
respiratorias superiores
Faringuitis

Tableau 108
Infections des voies
respiratoires supérieures
Pharyngite

Table 108a EME - PEMC - EMBE — Upper respiratory infections - Pharyngitis

Age group (years)	Incidence 1990 Number ('000s)	Rate (per 100 000)	Prevalence 1990 Number ('000s)	Rate (per 100 000)	Avg. age at onset (years)	Average duration (years)	Deaths 1990 Number ('000s)	Rate (per 100 000)	Deaths 2000 (Projected) Number ('000s)	Rate (per 100 000)
Males										
0-4	1 055	4 000	14	55	2.5	0.01	-	-	-	-
5-14	1 600	3 000	22	41	10.0	0.01	-	-	-	-
15-44	5 522	3 000	76	41	29.9	0.01	-	-	-	-
45-59	1 984	3 000	27	41	52.4	0.01	-	-	-	-
60+	2 422	4 000	33	55	71.1	0.01	-	-	-	-
All ages	12 584	3 223	172	44	36.5	0.01	-	-	-	-
Females										
0-4	1 003	4 000	14	55	2.5	0.01	-	-	-	-
5-14	1 520	3 000	21	41	10.0	0.01	-	-	-	-
15-44	6 272	3 500	86	48	30.0	0.01	-	-	-	-
45-59	2 034	3 000	28	41	52.4	0.01	-	-	-	-
60+	3 383	4 000	46	55	72.4	0.01	-	-	-	-
All ages	14 212	3 489	195	48	39.2	0.01	-	-	-	-
Total	26 795	3 359	367	46	38.0	0.01	-	-	-	-

Table 108b FSE - PEAS - AESE — Upper respiratory infections - Pharyngitis

Age group (years)	Incidence 1990 Number ('000s)	Rate (per 100 000)	Prevalence 1990 Number ('000s)	Rate (per 100 000)	Avg. age at onset (years)	Average duration (years)	Deaths 1990 Number ('000s)	Rate (per 100 000)	Deaths 2000 (Projected) Number ('000s)	Rate (per 100 000)
Males										
0-4	550	4 000	8	55	2.5	0.01	-	-	-	-
5-14	820	3 000	11	41	10.0	0.01	-	-	-	-
15-44	2 288	3 000	31	41	29.8	0.01	-	-	-	-
45-59	809	3 000	11	41	52.2	0.01	-	-	-	-
60+	839	4 000	11	55	70.0	0.01	-	-	-	-
All ages	5 307	3 210	73	44	33.7	0.01	-	-	-	-
Females										
0-4	525	4 000	7	55	2.5	0.01	-	-	-	-
5-14	793	3 000	11	41	10.0	0.01	-	-	-	-
15-44	2 624	3 500	36	48	29.9	0.01	-	-	-	-
45-59	900	3 000	12	41	52.4	0.01	-	-	-	-
60+	1 456	4 000	20	55	71.5	0.01	-	-	-	-
All ages	6 298	3 481	86	48	37.9	0.01	-	-	-	-
Total	11 604	3 352	159	46	36.0	0.01	-	-	-	-

Table 108c India - India - Inde — Upper respiratory infections - Pharyngitis

Age group (years)	Incidence 1990 Number ('000s)	Rate (per 100 000)	Prevalence 1990 Number ('000s)	Rate (per 100 000)	Avg. age at onset (years)	Average duration (years)	Deaths 1990 Number ('000s)	Rate (per 100 000)	Deaths 2000 (Projected) Number ('000s)	Rate (per 100 000)
Males										
0-4	4 185	7 000	57	96	2.5	0.01	-	-	-	-
5-14	4 070	4 000	56	55	10.0	0.01	-	-	-	-
15-44	8 021	4 000	110	55	29.8	0.01	-	-	-	-
45-59	1 427	3 000	20	41	52.3	0.01	-	-	-	-
60+	1 191	4 000	16	55	69.7	0.01	-	-	-	-
All ages	18 894	4 300	259	59	23.7	0.01	-	-	-	-
Females										
0-4	3 968	7 000	54	96	2.5	0.01	-	-	-	-
5-14	3 811	4 000	52	55	10.0	0.01	-	-	-	-
15-44	6 597	3 600	90	49	29.8	0.01	-	-	-	-
45-59	1 656	3 600	23	49	52.4	0.01	-	-	-	-
60+	1 157	4 000	16	55	70.1	0.01	-	-	-	-
All ages	17 188	4 191	235	57	24.0	0.01	-	-	-	-
Total	36 082	4 247	494	58	23.8	0.01	-	-	-	-

For epidemiological sources see Lob-Levyt et al. 1996. For the methods used to estimate and project incidence, prevalence, and deaths see Murray and Lopez 1996a. See explanatory notes for definitions and caveats.

Table 108
Upper respiratory infections
Pharyngitis

Cuadro 108
Infecciones de las vías respiratorias superiores
Faringuitis

Tableau 108
Infections des voies respiratoires supérieures
Pharyngite

Table 108d　　China - China - Chine　　Upper respiratory infections - Pharyngitis

Age group (years)	Incidence 1990 Number ('000s)	Rate (per 100 000)	Prevalence 1990 Number ('000s)	Rate (per 100 000)	Avg. age at onset (years)	Average duration (years)	Deaths 1990 Number ('000s)	Rate (per 100 000)	Deaths 2000 (Projected) Number ('000s)	Rate (per 100 000)
Males										
0-4	2 109	3 500	29	48	2.5	0.01	-	-	-	-
5-14	2 716	2 800	37	38	10.0	0.01	-	-	-	-
15-44	7 658	2 500	105	34	29.9	0.01	-	-	-	-
45-59	1 817	2 500	25	34	52.3	0.01	-	-	-	-
60+	1 469	3 000	20	41	69.8	0.01	-	-	-	-
All ages	15 768	2 695	216	37	29.1	0.01	-	-	-	-
Females										
0-4	2 028	3 500	28	48	2.5	0.01	-	-	-	-
5-14	2 531	2 800	35	38	10.0	0.01	-	-	-	-
15-44	7 102	2 500	97	34	29.9	0.01	-	-	-	-
45-59	1 610	2 500	22	34	52.4	0.01	-	-	-	-
60+	1 550	3 000	21	41	70.6	0.01	-	-	-	-
All ages	14 821	2 702	203	37	29.5	0.01	-	-	-	-
Total	30 590	2 698	419	37	29.3	0.01	-	-	-	-

Table 108e　　OAI - OPAI - APAI　　Upper respiratory infections - Pharyngitis

Age group (years)	Incidence 1990 Number ('000s)	Rate (per 100 000)	Prevalence 1990 Number ('000s)	Rate (per 100 000)	Avg. age at onset (years)	Average duration (years)	Deaths 1990 Number ('000s)	Rate (per 100 000)	Deaths 2000 (Projected) Number ('000s)	Rate (per 100 000)
Males										
0-4	3 063	7 000	42	96	2.5	0.01	-	-	-	-
5-14	3 361	4 000	46	55	10.0	0.01	-	-	-	-
15-44	6 433	4 000	88	55	29.7	0.01	-	-	-	-
45-59	1 024	3 000	14	41	52.3	0.01	-	-	-	-
60+	808	4 000	11	55	69.6	0.01	-	-	-	-
All ages	14 690	4 283	201	59	23.3	0.01	-	-	-	-
Females										
0-4	2 939	7 000	40	96	2.4	0.01	-	-	-	-
5-14	3 209	4 000	44	55	10.0	0.01	-	-	-	-
15-44	5 746	3 600	79	49	29.4	0.01	-	-	-	-
45-59	1 263	3 600	17	49	52.2	0.01	-	-	-	-
60+	906	4 000	12	55	69.2	0.01	-	-	-	-
All ages	14 064	4 142	193	57	23.9	0.01	-	-	-	-
Total	28 754	4 213	394	58	23.6	0.01	-	-	-	-

Table 108f　　SSA - ASS - ASS　　Upper respiratory infections - Pharyngitis

Age group (years)	Incidence 1990 Number ('000s)	Rate (per 100 000)	Prevalence 1990 Number ('000s)	Rate (per 100 000)	Avg. age at onset (years)	Average duration (years)	Deaths 1990 Number ('000s)	Rate (per 100 000)	Deaths 2000 (Projected) Number ('000s)	Rate (per 100 000)
Males										
0-4	3 324	7 000	46	96	2.4	0.01	-	-	-	-
5-14	3 513	5 000	48	68	10.0	0.01	-	-	-	-
15-44	3 113	3 000	43	41	29.4	0.01	-	-	-	-
45-59	609	3 000	8	41	52.2	0.01	-	-	-	-
60+	525	5 000	7	68	69.2	0.01	-	-	-	-
All ages	11 084	4 393	152	60	18.3	0.01	-	-	-	-
Females										
0-4	3 292	7 000	45	96	2.4	0.01	-	-	-	-
5-14	3 491	5 000	48	68	10.0	0.01	-	-	-	-
15-44	3 188	3 000	44	41	29.5	0.01	-	-	-	-
45-59	664	3 000	9	41	52.2	0.01	-	-	-	-
60+	637	5 000	9	68	69.7	0.01	-	-	-	-
All ages	11 271	4 369	154	60	19.2	0.01	-	-	-	-
Total	22 355	4 381	306	60	18.7	0.01	-	-	-	-

For epidemiological sources see Lob-Levyt et al. 1996. For the methods used to estimate and project incidence, prevalence, and deaths see Murray and Lopez 1996a. See explanatory notes for definitions and caveats.

Table 108
Upper respiratory infections

Pharyngitis

Cuadro 108
Infecciones de las vías
respiratorias superiores
Faringuitis

Tableau 108
Infections des voies
respiratoires supérieures
Pharyngite

Table 108g   LAC - ALC - ALC   Upper respiratory infections - Pharyngitis

Age group (years)	Incidence 1990 Number ('000s)	Rate (per 100 000)	Prevalence 1990 Number ('000s)	Rate (per 100 000)	Avg. age at onset (years)	Average duration (years)	Deaths 1990 Number ('000s)	Rate (per 100 000)	Deaths 2000 (Projected) Number ('000s)	Rate (per 100 000)
Males										
0-4	1 292	4 500	18	62	2.5	0.01	-	-	-	-
5-14	1 772	3 400	24	47	10.0	0.01	-	-	-	-
15-44	3 129	3 000	43	41	29.8	0.01	-	-	-	-
45-59	667	3 000	9	41	52.3	0.01	-	-	-	-
60+	484	3 400	7	47	70.3	0.01	-	-	-	-
All ages	7 345	3 314	101	45	24.9	0.01	-	-	-	-
Females										
0-4	1 245	4 500	17	62	2.5	0.01	-	-	-	-
5-14	1 725	3 400	24	47	10.0	0.01	-	-	-	-
15-44	3 123	3 000	43	41	29.9	0.01	-	-	-	-
45-59	701	3 000	10	41	52.4	0.01	-	-	-	-
60+	572	3 400	8	47	71.1	0.01	-	-	-	-
All ages	7 366	3 308	101	45	25.9	0.01	-	-	-	-
Total	14 710	3 311	202	45	25.4	0.01	-	-	-	-

Table 108h   MEC - AOM - CMO   Upper respiratory infections - Pharyngitis

Age group (years)	Incidence 1990 Number ('000s)	Rate (per 100 000)	Prevalence 1990 Number ('000s)	Rate (per 100 000)	Avg. age at onset (years)	Average duration (years)	Deaths 1990 Number ('000s)	Rate (per 100 000)	Deaths 2000 (Projected) Number ('000s)	Rate (per 100 000)
Males										
0-4	1 646	4 000	23	55	2.5	0.01	-	-	-	-
5-14	1 960	3 000	27	41	10.0	0.01	-	-	-	-
15-44	3 417	3 000	47	41	29.8	0.01	-	-	-	-
45-59	670	3 000	9	41	52.3	0.01	-	-	-	-
60+	546	4 000	7	55	69.7	0.01	-	-	-	-
All ages	8 240	3 214	113	44	22.5	0.01	-	-	-	-
Females										
0-4	1 589	4 000	22	55	2.5	0.01	-	-	-	-
5-14	1 860	3 000	25	41	10.0	0.01	-	-	-	-
15-44	3 752	3 500	51	48	29.8	0.01	-	-	-	-
45-59	669	3 000	9	41	52.3	0.01	-	-	-	-
60+	618	4 000	8	55	70.4	0.01	-	-	-	-
All ages	8 488	3 441	116	47	23.3	0.01	-	-	-	-
Total	16 728	3 325	229	46	22.9	0.01	-	-	-	-

Table 108i   World - Mundo - Monde   Upper respiratory infections - Pharyngitis

Age group (years)	Incidence 1990 Number ('000s)	Rate (per 100 000)	Prevalence 1990 Number ('000s)	Rate (per 100 000)	Avg. age at onset (years)	Average duration (years)	Deaths 1990 Number ('000s)	Rate (per 100 000)	Deaths 2000 (Projected) Number ('000s)	Rate (per 100 000)
Males										
0-4	17 226	5 361	236	73	2.5	0.01	-	-	-	-
5-14	19 814	3 595	271	49	10.0	0.01	-	-	-	-
15-44	39 580	3 167	542	43	29.8	0.01	-	-	-	-
45-59	9 008	2 884	123	40	52.3	0.01	-	-	-	-
60+	8 284	3 785	113	52	70.2	0.01	-	-	-	-
All ages	93 912	3 539	1 286	48	26.4	0.01	-	-	-	-
Females										
0-4	16 590	5 365	227	73	2.5	0.01	-	-	-	-
5-14	18 940	3 604	259	49	10.0	0.01	-	-	-	-
15-44	38 403	3 204	526	44	29.8	0.01	-	-	-	-
45-59	9 497	3 053	130	42	52.4	0.01	-	-	-	-
60+	10 278	3 818	141	52	71.1	0.01	-	-	-	-
All ages	93 707	3 585	1 284	49	27.9	0.01	-	-	-	-
Total	187 619	3 562	2 570	49	27.2	0.01	-	-	-	-

For epidemiological sources see Lob-Levyt et al. 1996. For the methods used to estimate and project incidence, prevalence, and deaths see Murray and Lopez 1996a. See explanatory notes for definitions and caveats.

Table 109
Otitis media

Cuadro 109
Otitis media

Tableau 109
Otite moyenne

Episodes

Episodios

Episodes

Table 109a — EME - PEMC - EMBE — Otitis media - Episodes

Age group (years)	Incidence 1990 Number ('000s)	Rate (per 100 000)	Prevalence 1990 Number ('000s)	Rate (per 100 000)	Avg. age at onset (years)	Average duration (years)	Deaths 1990 Number ('000s)	Rate (per 100 000)	Deaths 2000 (Projected) Number ('000s)	Rate (per 100 000)
Males										
0-4	6 860	26 000	528	2 000	2.5	0.08	0	0.2	0	0.1
5-14	13 870	26 000	1 067	2 000	10.0	0.08	0	0.0	0	0.0
15-44	0	0	0	0	-	-	0	0.0	0	0.0
45-59	0	0	0	0	-	-	0	0.0	0	0.0
60+	0	0	0	0	-	-	0	0.1	0	0.1
All ages	20 730	5 309	1 595	408	7.5	0.08	0	0.0	0	0.0
Females										
0-4	6 517	26 000	501	2 000	2.5	0.08	0	0.1	0	0.1
5-14	13 177	26 000	1 014	2 000	10.0	0.08	0	0.0	0	0.0
15-44	0	0	0	0	-	-	0	0.0	0	0.0
45-59	0	0	0	0	-	-	0	0.0	0	0.0
60+	0	0	0	0	-	-	0	0.1	0	0.1
All ages	19 694	4 835	1 515	372	7.5	0.08	0	0.0	0	0.0
Total	40 424	5 067	3 110	390	7.5	0.08	0	0.0	0	0.0

Table 109b — FSE - PEAS - AESE — Otitis media - Episodes

Age group (years)	Incidence 1990 Number ('000s)	Rate (per 100 000)	Prevalence 1990 Number ('000s)	Rate (per 100 000)	Avg. age at onset (years)	Average duration (years)	Deaths 1990 Number ('000s)	Rate (per 100 000)	Deaths 2000 (Projected) Number ('000s)	Rate (per 100 000)
Males										
0-4	3 577	26 000	275	2 000	2.5	0.08	0	0.8	0	0.6
5-14	7 111	26 000	547	2 000	10.0	0.08	0	0.0	0	0.0
15-44	0	0	0	0	-	-	0	0.0	0	0.0
45-59	0	0	0	0	-	-	0	0.0	0	0.0
60+	0	0	0	0	-	-	0	0.0	0	0.0
All ages	10 688	6 465	822	497	7.5	0.08	0	0.1	0	0.1
Females										
0-4	3 415	26 000	263	2 000	2.5	0.08	0	0.6	0	0.4
5-14	6 869	26 000	528	2 000	10.0	0.08	0	0.0	0	0.0
15-44	0	0	0	0	-	-	0	0.0	0	0.0
45-59	0	0	0	0	-	-	0	0.0	0	0.0
60+	0	0	0	0	-	-	0	0.0	0	0.0
All ages	10 285	5 685	791	437	7.5	0.08	0	0.1	0	0.0
Total	20 973	6 057	1 613	466	7.5	0.08	0	0.1	0	0.1

Table 109c — India - India - Inde — Otitis media - Episodes

Age group (years)	Incidence 1990 Number ('000s)	Rate (per 100 000)	Prevalence 1990 Number ('000s)	Rate (per 100 000)	Avg. age at onset (years)	Average duration (years)	Deaths 1990 Number ('000s)	Rate (per 100 000)	Deaths 2000 (Projected) Number ('000s)	Rate (per 100 000)
Males										
0-4	23 318	39 000	1 794	3 000	2.5	0.08	5	8.2	3	5.1
5-14	39 683	39 000	3 053	3 000	10.0	0.08	0	0.3	0	0.1
15-44	0	0	0	0	-	-	0	0.0	0	0.0
45-59	0	0	0	0	-	-	0	0.0	0	0.0
60+	0	0	0	0	-	-	0	0.0	0	0.0
All ages	63 001	14 338	4 846	1 103	7.2	0.08	5	1.2	3	0.6
Females										
0-4	22 105	39 000	1 700	3 000	2.5	0.08	6	10.3	3	6.2
5-14	37 153	39 000	2 858	3 000	10.0	0.08	0	0.5	0	0.2
15-44	0	0	0	0	-	-	0	0.0	0	0.0
45-59	0	0	0	0	-	-	0	0.0	0	0.0
60+	0	0	0	0	-	-	0	0.0	0	0.0
All ages	59 257	14 449	4 558	1 111	7.2	0.08	6	1.6	4	0.7
Total	122 258	14 392	9 404	1 107	7.2	0.08	12	1.4	7	0.7

For the methods used to estimate and project incidence, prevalence, and deaths see Murray and Lopez 1996a. See explanatory notes for definitions and caveats.

Table 109   **Cuadro 109**   **Tableau 109**
Otitis media   **Otitis media**   **Otite moyenne**

Episodes   Episodios   Episodes

Table 109d   China - China - Chine   Otitis media - Episodes

Age group (years)	Incidence 1990 Number ('000s)	Rate (per 100 000)	Prevalence 1990 Number ('000s)	Rate (per 100 000)	Avg. age at onset (years)	Average duration (years)	Deaths 1990 Number ('000s)	Rate (per 100 000)	Deaths 2000 (Projected) Number ('000s)	Rate (per 100 000)
Males										
0-4	23 495	39 000	1 807	3 000	2.5	0.08	1	1.7	1	0.9
5-14	37 829	39 000	2 910	3 000	10.0	0.08	0	0.0	0	0.0
15-44	0	0	0	0	-	-	0	0.0	0	0.0
45-59	0	0	0	0	-	-	0	0.0	0	0.0
60+	0	0	0	0	-	-	0	0.0	0	0.0
All ages	61 324	10 479	4 717	806	7.1	0.08	1	0.2	1	0.1
Females										
0-4	22 599	39 000	1 738	3 000	2.5	0.08	1	2.2	1	1.1
5-14	35 256	39 000	2 712	3 000	10.0	0.08	0	0.0	0	0.0
15-44	0	0	0	0	-	-	0	0.0	0	0.0
45-59	0	0	0	0	-	-	0	0.0	0	0.0
60+	0	0	0	0	-	-	0	0.0	0	0.0
All ages	57 855	10 548	4 450	811	7.1	0.08	1	0.2	1	0.1
Total	119 179	10 512	9 168	809	7.1	0.08	2	0.2	1	0.1

Table 109e   OAI - OPAI - APAI   Otitis media - Episodes

Age group (years)	Incidence 1990 Number ('000s)	Rate (per 100 000)	Prevalence 1990 Number ('000s)	Rate (per 100 000)	Avg. age at onset (years)	Average duration (years)	Deaths 1990 Number ('000s)	Rate (per 100 000)	Deaths 2000 (Projected) Number ('000s)	Rate (per 100 000)
Males										
0-4	17 068	39 000	1 313	3 000	2.5	0.08	2	3.4	1	2.2
5-14	32 772	39 000	2 521	3 000	10.0	0.08	0	0.3	0	0.1
15-44	0	0	0	0	-	-	0	0.0	0	0.0
45-59	0	0	0	0	-	-	0	0.0	0	0.0
60+	0	0	0	0	-	-	0	0.0	0	0.0
All ages	49 840	14 532	3 834	1 118	7.4	0.08	2	0.5	1	0.3
Females										
0-4	16 375	39 000	1 260	3 000	2.5	0.08	1	2.7	1	1.7
5-14	31 285	39 000	2 407	3 000	10.0	0.08	0	0.2	0	0.1
15-44	0	0	0	0	-	-	0	0.0	0	0.0
45-59	0	0	0	0	-	-	0	0.0	0	0.0
60+	0	0	0	0	-	-	0	0.0	0	0.0
All ages	47 660	14 035	3 666	1 080	7.4	0.08	1	0.4	1	0.2
Total	97 500	14 285	7 500	1 099	7.4	0.08	3	0.5	2	0.2

Table 109f   SSA - ASS - ASS   Otitis media - Episodes

Age group (years)	Incidence 1990 Number ('000s)	Rate (per 100 000)	Prevalence 1990 Number ('000s)	Rate (per 100 000)	Avg. age at onset (years)	Average duration (years)	Deaths 1990 Number ('000s)	Rate (per 100 000)	Deaths 2000 (Projected) Number ('000s)	Rate (per 100 000)
Males										
0-4	18 519	39 000	1 425	3 000	2.4	0.08	3	6.9	3	4.9
5-14	27 401	39 000	2 108	3 000	10.0	0.08	0	0.5	0	0.3
15-44	0	0	0	0	-	-	0	0.1	0	0.0
45-59	0	0	0	0	-	-	0	0.0	0	0.0
60+	0	0	0	0	-	-	0	0.0	0	0.0
All ages	45 919	18 199	3 532	1 400	6.9	0.08	4	1.5	4	1.0
Females										
0-4	18 342	39 000	1 411	3 000	2.4	0.08	3	5.6	2	3.9
5-14	27 229	39 000	2 095	3 000	10.0	0.08	0	0.4	0	0.2
15-44	0	0	0	0	-	-	0	0.1	0	0.0
45-59	0	0	0	0	-	-	0	0.0	0	0.0
60+	0	0	0	0	-	-	0	0.0	0	0.0
All ages	45 571	17 666	3 505	1 359	6.9	0.08	3	1.2	3	0.8
Total	91 490	17 930	7 038	1 379	6.9	0.08	7	1.3	6	0.9

For the methods used to estimate and project incidence, prevalence, and deaths see Murray and Lopez 1996a. See explanatory notes for definitions and caveats.

Table 109
Otitis media

Cuadro 109
Otitis media

Tableau 109
Otite moyenne

Episodes

Episodios

Episodes

Table 109g LAC - ALC - ALC   Otitis media - Episodes

Age group (years)	Incidence 1990 Number ('000s)	Rate (per 100 000)	Prevalence 1990 Number ('000s)	Rate (per 100 000)	Avg. age at onset (years)	Average duration (years)	Deaths 1990 Number ('000s)	Rate (per 100 000)	Deaths 2000 (Projected) Number ('000s)	Rate (per 100 000)
Males										
0-4	11 201	39 000	862	3 000	2.5	0.08	0	0.1	0	0.1
5-14	20 328	39 000	1 564	3 000	10.0	0.08	0	0.0	0	0.0
15-44	0	0	0	0	-	-	0	0.0	0	0.0
45-59	0	0	0	0	-	-	0	0.0	0	0.0
60+	0	0	0	0	-	-	0	0.0	0	0.0
All ages	31 530	14 227	2 425	1 094	7.3	0.08	0	0.0	0	0.0
Females										
0-4	10 794	39 000	830	3 000	2.5	0.08	0	0.2	0	0.1
5-14	19 790	39 000	1 522	3 000	10.0	0.08	0	0.1	0	0.0
15-44	0	0	0	0	-	-	0	0.1	0	0.0
45-59	0	0	0	0	-	-	0	0.0	0	0.0
60+	0	0	0	0	-	-	0	0.1	0	0.0
All ages	30 584	13 734	2 353	1 056	7.4	0.08	0	0.1	0	0.0
Total	62 113	13 980	4 778	1 075	7.3	0.08	0	0.1	0	0.0

Table 109h MEC - AOM - CMO   Otitis media - Episodes

Age group (years)	Incidence 1990 Number ('000s)	Rate (per 100 000)	Prevalence 1990 Number ('000s)	Rate (per 100 000)	Avg. age at onset (years)	Average duration (years)	Deaths 1990 Number ('000s)	Rate (per 100 000)	Deaths 2000 (Projected) Number ('000s)	Rate (per 100 000)
Males										
0-4	16 053	39 000	1 235	3 000	2.5	0.08	2	3.8	1	2.8
5-14	25 485	39 000	1 960	3 000	10.0	0.08	0	0.2	0	0.1
15-44	0	0	0	0	-	-	0	0.0	0	0.0
45-59	0	0	0	0	-	-	0	0.0	0	0.0
60+	0	0	0	0	-	-	0	0.0	0	0.0
All ages	41 537	16 201	3 195	1 246	7.1	0.08	2	0.7	2	0.5
Females										
0-4	15 496	39 000	1 192	3 000	2.5	0.08	1	3.8	1	2.7
5-14	24 180	39 000	1 860	3 000	10.0	0.08	0	0.3	0	0.1
15-44	0	0	0	0	-	-	0	0.0	0	0.0
45-59	0	0	0	0	-	-	0	0.0	0	0.0
60+	0	0	0	0	-	-	0	0.0	0	0.0
All ages	39 676	16 084	3 052	1 237	7.1	0.08	2	0.7	1	0.4
Total	81 213	16 143	6 247	1 242	7.1	0.08	3	0.7	3	0.4

Table 109i World - Mundo - Monde   Otitis media - Episodes

Age group (years)	Incidence 1990 Number ('000s)	Rate (per 100 000)	Prevalence 1990 Number ('000s)	Rate (per 100 000)	Avg. age at onset (years)	Average duration (years)	Deaths 1990 Number ('000s)	Rate (per 100 000)	Deaths 2000 (Projected) Number ('000s)	Rate (per 100 000)
Males										
0-4	120 090	37 376	9 238	2 875	2.5	0.08	12	3.9	9	2.7
5-14	204 479	37 097	15 729	2 854	10.0	0.08	1	0.2	1	0.1
15-44	0	0	0	0	-	-	0	0.0	0	0.0
45-59	0	0	0	0	-	-	0	0.0	0	0.0
60+	0	0	0	0	-	-	0	0.0	0	0.0
All ages	324 569	12 231	24 967	941	7.2	0.08	14	0.5	10	0.3
Females										
0-4	115 643	37 395	8 896	2 877	2.5	0.08	13	4.1	9	2.6
5-14	194 939	37 093	14 995	2 853	10.0	0.08	1	0.2	1	0.1
15-44	0	0	0	0	-	-	0	0.0	0	0.0
45-59	0	0	0	0	-	-	0	0.0	0	0.0
60+	0	0	0	0	-	-	0	0.0	0	0.0
All ages	310 581	11 883	23 891	914	7.2	0.08	14	0.5	10	0.3
Total	635 151	12 058	48 858	928	7.2	0.08	28	0.5	20	0.3

For the methods used to estimate and project incidence, prevalence, and deaths see Murray and Lopez 1996a. See explanatory notes for definitions and caveats.

Table 110
Otitis media

Cuadro 110
Otitis media

Tableau 110
Otite moyenne

Deafness

Sordera

Surdité

Table 110a EME - PEMC - EMBE Otitis media - Deafness

Age group (years)	Incidence 1990 Number ('000s)	Rate (per 100 000)	Prevalence 1990 Number ('000s)	Rate (per 100 000)	Avg. age at onset (years)	Average duration (years)	Deaths 1990 Number ('000s)	Rate (per 100 000)	Deaths 2000 (Projected) Number ('000s)	Rate (per 100 000)
Males										
0-4	0	1.3	1	3.2	2.5	70.2	0	0	0	0
5-14	1	1.3	7	13.0	10.0	63.6	0	0	0	0
15-44	0	0.0	36	19.5	-	-	0	0	0	0
45-59	0	0.0	13	19.5	-	-	0	0	0	0
60+	0	0.0	12	19.5	-	-	0	0	0	0
All ages	1	0.3	68	17.5	7.5	65.8	0	0	0	0
Females										
0-4	0	1.3	1	3.2	2.5	76.1	0	0	0	0
5-14	1	1.3	7	13.0	10.0	69.5	0	0	0	0
15-44	0	0.0	35	19.5	-	-	0	0	0	0
45-59	0	0.0	13	19.5	-	-	0	0	0	0
60+	0	0.0	16	19.5	-	-	0	0	0	0
All ages	1	0.2	72	17.7	7.5	71.7	0	0	0	0
Total	2	0.3	140	17.6	7.5	68.7	0	0	0	0

Table 110b FSE - PEAS - AESE Otitis media - Deafness

Age group (years)	Incidence 1990 Number ('000s)	Rate (per 100 000)	Prevalence 1990 Number ('000s)	Rate (per 100 000)	Avg. age at onset (years)	Average duration (years)	Deaths 1990 Number ('000s)	Rate (per 100 000)	Deaths 2000 (Projected) Number ('000s)	Rate (per 100 000)
Males										
0-4	0	1.3	0	3.2	2.5	63.5	0	0	0	0
5-14	0	1.3	4	13.0	10.0	57.3	0	0	0	0
15-44	0	0.0	15	19.5	-	-	0	0	0	0
45-59	0	0.0	5	19.5	-	-	0	0	0	0
60+	0	0.0	4	19.5	-	-	0	0	0	0
All ages	1	0.3	28	17.0	7.5	59.4	0	0	0	0
Females										
0-4	0	1.3	0	3.2	2.5	72.4	0	0	0	0
5-14	0	1.3	3	13.0	10.0	66.0	0	0	0	0
15-44	0	0.0	15	19.5	-	-	0	0	0	0
45-59	0	0.0	6	19.5	-	-	0	0	0	0
60+	0	0.0	7	19.5	-	-	0	0	0	0
All ages	1	0.3	31	17.3	7.5	68.1	0	0	0	0
Total	1	0.3	60	17.2	7.5	63.7	0	0	0	0

Table 110c India - India - Inde Otitis media - Deafness

Age group (years)	Incidence 1990 Number ('000s)	Rate (per 100 000)	Prevalence 1990 Number ('000s)	Rate (per 100 000)	Avg. age at onset (years)	Average duration (years)	Deaths 1990 Number ('000s)	Rate (per 100 000)	Deaths 2000 (Projected) Number ('000s)	Rate (per 100 000)
Males										
0-4	1	2.0	3	4.9	2.5	59.9	0	0	0	0
5-14	2	2.0	20	20.0	10.0	57.4	0	0	0	0
15-44	0	0.0	60	29.9	-	-	0	0	0	0
45-59	0	0.0	14	29.9	-	-	0	0	0	0
60+	0	0.0	9	29.9	-	-	0	0	0	0
All ages	3	0.7	106	24.2	7.2	58.3	0	0	0	0
Females										
0-4	1	2.0	3	4.9	2.5	60.8	0	0	0	0
5-14	2	2.0	19	20.0	10.0	59.1	0	0	0	0
15-44	0	0.0	55	29.9	-	-	0	0	0	0
45-59	0	0.0	14	29.9	-	-	0	0	0	0
60+	0	0.0	9	29.9	-	-	0	0	0	0
All ages	3	0.7	99	24.2	7.2	59.7	0	0	0	0
Total	6	0.7	206	24.2	7.2	59.0	0	0	0	0

For the methods used to estimate and project incidence, prevalence, and deaths see Murray and Lopez 1996a. See explanatory notes for definitions and caveats.

Table 110
Otitis media

Cuadro 110
Otitis media

Tableau 110
Otite moyenne

Deafness   Sordera   Surdité

Table 110d   China - China - Chine   Otitis media - Deafness

Age group (years)	Incidence 1990 Number ('000s)	Rate (per 100 000)	Prevalence 1990 Number ('000s)	Rate (per 100 000)	Avg. age at onset (years)	Average duration (years)	Deaths 1990 Number ('000s)	Rate (per 100 000)	Deaths 2000 (Projected) Number ('000s)	Rate (per 100 000)
Males										
0-4	1	2.0	3	5.0	2.5	65.5	0	0	0	0
5-14	2	2.0	19	20.0	10.0	59.9	0	0	0	0
15-44	0	0.0	92	29.9	-	-	0	0	0	0
45-59	0	0.0	22	29.9	-	-	0	0	0	0
60+	0	0.0	15	29.9	-	-	0	0	0	0
All ages	3	0.5	151	25.7	7.1	62.1	0	0	0	0
Females										
0-4	1	2.0	3	5.0	2.5	68.5	0	0	0	0
5-14	2	2.0	18	20.0	10.0	63.2	0	0	0	0
15-44	0	0.0	85	29.9	-	-	0	0	0	0
45-59	0	0.0	19	29.9	-	-	0	0	0	0
60+	0	0.0	15	29.9	-	-	0	0	0	0
All ages	3	0.5	141	25.7	7.1	65.3	0	0	0	0
Total	6	0.5	291	25.7	7.1	63.6	0	0	0	0

Table 110e   OAI - OPAI - APAI   Otitis media - Deafness

Age group (years)	Incidence 1990 Number ('000s)	Rate (per 100 000)	Prevalence 1990 Number ('000s)	Rate (per 100 000)	Avg. age at onset (years)	Average duration (years)	Deaths 1990 Number ('000s)	Rate (per 100 000)	Deaths 2000 (Projected) Number ('000s)	Rate (per 100 000)
Males										
0-4	1	2.0	2	4.9	2.5	59.8	0	0	0	0
5-14	2	2.0	17	20.0	10.0	56.2	0	0	0	0
15-44	0	0.0	48	29.9	-	-	0	0	0	0
45-59	0	0.0	10	29.9	-	-	0	0	0	0
60+	0	0.0	6	29.9	-	-	0	0	0	0
All ages	3	0.7	83	24.3	7.4	57.4	0	0	0	0
Females										
0-4	1	2.0	2	4.9	2.5	63.2	0	0	0	0
5-14	2	2.0	16	20.0	10.0	59.2	0	0	0	0
15-44	0	0.0	48	29.9	-	-	0	0	0	0
45-59	0	0.0	11	29.9	-	-	0	0	0	0
60+	0	0.0	7	29.9	-	-	0	0	0	0
All ages	2	0.7	83	24.5	7.4	60.5	0	0	0	0
Total	5	0.7	167	24.4	7.4	59.0	0	0	0	0

Table 110f   SSA - ASS - ASS   Otitis media - Deafness

Age group (years)	Incidence 1990 Number ('000s)	Rate (per 100 000)	Prevalence 1990 Number ('000s)	Rate (per 100 000)	Avg. age at onset (years)	Average duration (years)	Deaths 1990 Number ('000s)	Rate (per 100 000)	Deaths 2000 (Projected) Number ('000s)	Rate (per 100 000)
Males										
0-4	1	2.0	2	4.8	2.4	48.7	0	0	0	0
5-14	1	2.0	14	19.9	10.0	49.2	0	0	0	0
15-44	0	0.0	31	30.0	-	-	0	0	0	0
45-59	0	0.0	6	30.0	-	-	0	0	0	0
60+	0	0.0	3	30.0	-	-	0	0	0	0
All ages	2	0.9	57	22.4	6.9	49.0	0	0	0	0
Females										
0-4	1	2.0	2	4.8	2.4	51.9	0	0	0	0
5-14	1	2.0	14	19.9	10.0	51.9	0	0	0	0
15-44	0	0.0	32	30.0	-	-	0	0	0	0
45-59	0	0.0	7	30.0	-	-	0	0	0	0
60+	0	0.0	4	30.0	-	-	0	0	0	0
All ages	2	0.9	58	22.7	6.9	51.9	0	0	0	0
Total	5	0.9	115	22.5	6.9	50.5	0	0	0	0

For the methods used to estimate and project incidence, prevalence, and deaths see Murray and Lopez 1996a. See explanatory notes for definitions and caveats.

Table 110　　　　　　　　**Cuadro 110**　　　　　　　　**Tableau 110**
Otitis media　　　　　　　**Otitis media**　　　　　　　**Otite moyenne**

Deafness　　　　　　　　　　Sordera　　　　　　　　　　Surdité

Table 110g   LAC - ALC - ALC   Otitis media - Deafness

Age group (years)	Incidence 1990 Number ('000s)	Rate (per 100 000)	Prevalence 1990 Number ('000s)	Rate (per 100 000)	Avg. age at onset (years)	Average duration (years)	Deaths 1990 Number ('000s)	Rate (per 100 000)	Deaths 2000 (Projected) Number ('000s)	Rate (per 100 000)
Males										
0-4	1	2.0	1	4.9	2.5	63.9	0	0	0	0
5-14	1	2.0	10	20.0	10.0	59.3	0	0	0	0
15-44	0	0.0	31	29.9	-	-	0	0	0	0
45-59	0	0.0	7	29.9	-	-	0	0	0	0
60+	0	0.0	4	29.9	-	-	0	0	0	0
All ages	2	0.7	54	24.4	7.3	60.9	0	0	0	0
Females										
0-4	1	2.0	1	5.0	2.5	67.9	0	0	0	0
5-14	1	2.0	10	20.0	10.0	63.0	0	0	0	0
15-44	0	0.0	31	29.9	-	-	0	0	0	0
45-59	0	0.0	7	29.9	-	-	0	0	0	0
60+	0	0.0	5	29.9	-	-	0	0	0	0
All ages	2	0.7	55	24.6	7.4	64.7	0	0	0	0
Total	3	0.7	109	24.5	7.3	62.8	0	0	0	0

Table 110h   MEC - AOM - CMO   Otitis media - Deafness

Age group (years)	Incidence 1990 Number ('000s)	Rate (per 100 000)	Prevalence 1990 Number ('000s)	Rate (per 100 000)	Avg. age at onset (years)	Average duration (years)	Deaths 1990 Number ('000s)	Rate (per 100 000)	Deaths 2000 (Projected) Number ('000s)	Rate (per 100 000)
Males										
0-4	1	2.0	2	4.9	2.5	61.1	0	0	0	0
5-14	1	2.0	13	20.0	10.0	58.1	0	0	0	0
15-44	0	0.0	34	29.9	-	-	0	0	0	0
45-59	0	0.0	7	29.9	-	-	0	0	0	0
60+	0	0.0	4	29.9	-	-	0	0	0	0
All ages	2	0.8	60	23.4	7.1	59.3	0	0	0	0
Females										
0-4	1	2.0	2	4.9	2.5	63.7	0	0	0	0
5-14	1	2.0	12	20.0	10.0	60.9	0	0	0	0
15-44	0	0.0	32	29.9	-	-	0	0	0	0
45-59	0	0.0	7	29.9	-	-	0	0	0	0
60+	0	0.0	5	29.9	-	-	0	0	0	0
All ages	2	0.8	58	23.4	7.1	62.0	0	0	0	0
Total	4	0.8	118	23.4	7.1	60.6	0	0	0	0

Table 110i   World - Mundo - Monde   Otitis media - Deafness

Age group (years)	Incidence 1990 Number ('000s)	Rate (per 100 000)	Prevalence 1990 Number ('000s)	Rate (per 100 000)	Avg. age at onset (years)	Average duration (years)	Deaths 1990 Number ('000s)	Rate (per 100 000)	Deaths 2000 (Projected) Number ('000s)	Rate (per 100 000)
Males										
0-4	6	1.9	15	4.7	2.5	60.5	0	0	0	0
5-14	10	1.9	104	18.9	10.0	57.3	0	0	0	0
15-44	0	0.0	347	27.8	-	-	0	0	0	0
45-59	0	0.0	84	26.8	-	-	0	0	0	0
60+	0	0.0	57	26.0	-	-	0	0	0	0
All ages	17	0.6	607	22.9	7.2	58.5	0	0	0	0
Females										
0-4	6	1.9	15	4.7	2.5	63.5	0	0	0	0
5-14	10	1.9	100	18.9	10.0	60.4	0	0	0	0
15-44	0	0.0	332	27.7	-	-	0	0	0	0
45-59	0	0.0	83	26.7	-	-	0	0	0	0
60+	0	0.0	68	25.2	-	-	0	0	0	0
All ages	16	0.6	597	22.9	7.2	61.5	0	0	0	0
Total	33	0.6	1 205	22.9	7.2	60.0	0	0	0	0

For the methods used to estimate and project incidence, prevalence, and deaths see Murray and Lopez 1996a. See explanatory notes for definitions and caveats.

Table 111
Maternal haemorrhage

Cuadro 111
Hemorragia materna

Tableau 111
Hémorragie maternelle

Episodes

Episodios

Episodes

Table 111a EME - PEMC - EMBE — Maternal haemorrhage - Episodes

Age group (years)	Incidence 1990 Number ('000s)	Rate (per 100 000)	Prevalence 1990 Number ('000s)	Rate (per 100 000)	Avg. age at onset (years)	Average duration (years)	Deaths 1990 Number ('000s)	Rate (per 100 000)	Deaths 2000 (Projected) Number ('000s)	Rate (per 100 000)
Males										
0-4	0	0	-	-	-	-	0	0	0	0
5-14	0	0	-	-	-	-	0	0	0	0
15-44	0	0	-	-	-	-	0	0	0	0
45-59	0	0	-	-	-	-	0	0	0	0
60+	0	0	-	-	-	-	0	0	0	0
All ages	0	0	-	-	-	-	0	0	0	0
Females										
0-4	0	0	-	-	-	-	0	0.0	0	0
5-14	0	0	-	-	-	-	0	0.0	0	0
15-44	1 040	580	-	-	30.0	-	0	0.1	0	0
45-59	0	0	-	-	-	-	0	0.0	0	0
60+	0	0	-	-	-	-	0	0.0	0	0
All ages	1 040	255	-	-	30.0	-	0	0.0	0	0
Total	1 040	130	-	-	30.0	-	0	0.0	0	0

Table 111b FSE - PEAS - AESE — Maternal haemorrhage - Episodes

Age group (years)	Incidence 1990 Number ('000s)	Rate (per 100 000)	Prevalence 1990 Number ('000s)	Rate (per 100 000)	Avg. age at onset (years)	Average duration (years)	Deaths 1990 Number ('000s)	Rate (per 100 000)	Deaths 2000 (Projected) Number ('000s)	Rate (per 100 000)
Males										
0-4	0	0	-	-	-	-	0	0	0	0
5-14	0	0	-	-	-	-	0	0	0	0
15-44	0	0	-	-	-	-	0	0	0	0
45-59	0	0	-	-	-	-	0	0	0	0
60+	0	0	-	-	-	-	0	0	0	0
All ages	0	0	-	-	-	-	0	0	0	0
Females										
0-4	0	0	-	-	-	-	0	0.0	0	0.0
5-14	0	0	-	-	-	-	0	0.0	0	0.0
15-44	529	706	-	-	29.9	-	0	0.3	0	0.2
45-59	5	17	-	-	52.4	-	0	0.0	0	0.0
60+	0	0	-	-	-	-	0	0.0	0	0.0
All ages	534	295	-	-	30.1	-	0	0.1	0	0.1
Total	534	154	-	-	30.1	-	0	0.1	0	0.0

Table 111c India - India - Inde — Maternal haemorrhage - Episodes

Age group (years)	Incidence 1990 Number ('000s)	Rate (per 100 000)	Prevalence 1990 Number ('000s)	Rate (per 100 000)	Avg. age at onset (years)	Average duration (years)	Deaths 1990 Number ('000s)	Rate (per 100 000)	Deaths 2000 (Projected) Number ('000s)	Rate (per 100 000)
Males										
0-4	0	0	-	-	-	-	0	0	0	0
5-14	0	0	-	-	-	-	0	0	0	0
15-44	0	0	-	-	-	-	0	0	0	0
45-59	0	0	-	-	-	-	0	0	0	0
60+	0	0	-	-	-	-	0	0	0	0
All ages	0	0	-	-	-	-	0	0	0	0
Females										
0-4	0	0	-	-	-	-	0	0.0	0	0.0
5-14	0	0	-	-	-	-	0	0.0	0	0.0
15-44	2 581	1 409	-	-	29.8	-	27	14.5	12	5.3
45-59	84	183	-	-	52.4	-	1	1.9	0	0.9
60+	0	0	-	-	-	-	0	0.0	0	0.0
All ages	2 665	650	-	-	30.5	-	28	6.7	13	2.6
Total	2 665	314	-	-	30.5	-	28	3.2	13	1.3

For epidemiological sources see Abou-Zahr 1996. For the methods used to estimate and project incidence, prevalence, and deaths see Murray and Lopez 1996a. See explanatory notes for definitions and caveats.

Table 111
Maternal haemorrhage

Cuadro 111
Hemorragia materna

Tableau 111
Hémorragie maternelle

Episodes

Episodios

Episodes

Table 111d   China - China - Chine

Maternal haemorrhage - Episodes

Age group (years)	Incidence 1990 Number ('000s)	Rate (per 100 000)	Prevalence 1990 Number ('000s)	Rate (per 100 000)	Avg. age at onset (years)	Average duration (years)	Deaths 1990 Number ('000s)	Rate (per 100 000)	Deaths 2000 (Projected) Number ('000s)	Rate (per 100 000)
Males										
0-4	0	0	-	-	-	-	0	0	0	0
5-14	0	0	-	-	-	-	0	0	0	0
15-44	0	0	-	-	-	-	0	0	0	0
45-59	0	0	-	-	-	-	0	0	0	0
60+	0	0	-	-	-	-	0	0	0	0
All ages	0	0	-	-	-	-	0	0	0	0
Females										
0-4	0	0	-	-	-	-	0	0.0	0	0.0
5-14	0	0	-	-	-	-	0	0.0	0	0.0
15-44	2 513	885	-	-	29.9	-	11	3.9	3	1.1
45-59	159	246	-	-	52.4	-	1	1.1	0	0.4
60+	0	0	-	-	-	-	0	0.0	0	0.0
All ages	2 672	487	-	-	31.2	-	12	2.2	4	0.6
Total	2 672	236	-	-	31.2	-	12	1.0	4	0.3

Table 111e   OAI - OPAI - APAI

Maternal haemorrhage - Episodes

Age group (years)	Incidence 1990 Number ('000s)	Rate (per 100 000)	Prevalence 1990 Number ('000s)	Rate (per 100 000)	Avg. age at onset (years)	Average duration (years)	Deaths 1990 Number ('000s)	Rate (per 100 000)	Deaths 2000 (Projected) Number ('000s)	Rate (per 100 000)
Males										
0-4	0	0	-	-	-	-	0	0	0	0
5-14	0	0	-	-	-	-	0	0	0	0
15-44	0	0	-	-	-	-	0	0	0	0
45-59	0	0	-	-	-	-	0	0	0	0
60+	0	0	-	-	-	-	0	0	0	0
All ages	0	0	-	-	-	-	0	0	0	0
Females										
0-4	0	0	-	-	-	-	0	0.0	0	0.0
5-14	0	0	-	-	-	-	0	0.0	0	0.0
15-44	1 887	1 182	-	-	29.4	-	12	7.5	6	3.1
45-59	79	224	-	-	52.2	-	1	1.4	0	0.7
60+	0	0	-	-	-	-	0	0.0	0	0.0
All ages	1 966	579	-	-	30.3	-	13	3.7	7	1.6
Total	1 966	288	-	-	30.3	-	13	1.8	7	0.8

Table 111f   SSA - ASS - ASS

Maternal haemorrhage - Episodes

Age group (years)	Incidence 1990 Number ('000s)	Rate (per 100 000)	Prevalence 1990 Number ('000s)	Rate (per 100 000)	Avg. age at onset (years)	Average duration (years)	Deaths 1990 Number ('000s)	Rate (per 100 000)	Deaths 2000 (Projected) Number ('000s)	Rate (per 100 000)
Males										
0-4	0	0	-	-	-	-	0	0	0	0
5-14	0	0	-	-	-	-	0	0	0	0
15-44	0	0	-	-	-	-	0	0	0	0
45-59	0	0	-	-	-	-	0	0	0	0
60+	0	0	-	-	-	-	0	0	0	0
All ages	0	0	-	-	-	-	0	0	0	0
Females										
0-4	0	0	-	-	-	-	0	0.0	0	0.0
5-14	142	204	-	-	10.0	-	2	3.4	2	1.8
15-44	2 518	2 370	-	-	29.5	-	42	39.8	25	17.3
45-59	5	25	-	-	52.2	-	0	0.4	0	0.2
60+	0	0	-	-	-	-	0	0.0	0	0.0
All ages	2 666	1 033	-	-	28.5	-	45	17.3	27	7.7
Total	2 666	522	-	-	28.5	-	45	8.8	27	3.9

For epidemiological sources see Abou-Zahr 1996. For the methods used to estimate and project incidence, prevalence, and deaths see Murray and Lopez 1996a. See explanatory notes for definitions and caveats.

Table 111
Maternal haemorrhage

Cuadro 111
Hemorragia materna

Tableau 111
Hémorragie maternelle

Episodes

Episodios

Episodes

Table 111g LAC - ALC - ALC Maternal haemorrhage - Episodes

Age group (years)	Incidence 1990 Number ('000s)	Rate (per 100 000)	Prevalence 1990 Number ('000s)	Rate (per 100 000)	Avg. age at onset (years)	Average duration (years)	Deaths 1990 Number ('000s)	Rate (per 100 000)	Deaths 2000 (Projected) Number ('000s)	Rate (per 100 000)
Males										
0-4	0	0	-	-	-	-	0	0	0	0
5-14	0	0	-	-	-	-	0	0	0	0
15-44	0	0	-	-	-	-	0	0	0	0
45-59	0	0	-	-	-	-	0	0	0	0
60+	0	0	-	-	-	-	0	0	0	0
All ages	0	0	-	-	-	-	0	0	0	0
Females										
0-4	0	0	-	-	-	-	0	0.0	0	0.0
5-14	9	18	-	-	10.0	-	0	0.1	0	0.0
15-44	1 246	1 197	-	-	29.9	-	5	4.4	3	2.1
45-59	8	35	-	-	52.4	-	0	0.1	0	0.1
60+	0	0	-	-	-	-	0	0.0	0	0.0
All ages	1 263	567	-	-	29.9	-	5	2.1	3	1.0
Total	1 263	284	-	-	29.9	-	5	1.0	3	0.5

Table 111h MEC - AOM - CMO Maternal haemorrhage - Episodes

Age group (years)	Incidence 1990 Number ('000s)	Rate (per 100 000)	Prevalence 1990 Number ('000s)	Rate (per 100 000)	Avg. age at onset (years)	Average duration (years)	Deaths 1990 Number ('000s)	Rate (per 100 000)	Deaths 2000 (Projected) Number ('000s)	Rate (per 100 000)
Males										
0-4	0	0	-	-	-	-	0	0	0	0
5-14	0	0	-	-	-	-	0	0	0	0
15-44	0	0	-	-	-	-	0	0	0	0
45-59	0	0	-	-	-	-	0	0	0	0
60+	0	0	-	-	-	-	0	0	0	0
All ages	0	0	-	-	-	-	0	0	0	0
Females										
0-4	0	0	-	-	-	-	0	0.0	0	0.0
5-14	2	4	-	-	10.0	-	0	0.0	0	0.0
15-44	1 958	1 826	-	-	29.8	-	11	10.4	7	4.8
45-59	125	562	-	-	52.3	-	1	3.2	1	1.7
60+	0	0	-	-	-	-	0	0.0	0	0.0
All ages	2 086	846	-	-	31.1	-	12	4.8	7	2.3
Total	2 086	415	-	-	31.1	-	12	2.4	7	1.1

Table 111i World - Mundo - Monde Maternal haemorrhage - Episodes

Age group (years)	Incidence 1990 Number ('000s)	Rate (per 100 000)	Prevalence 1990 Number ('000s)	Rate (per 100 000)	Avg. age at onset (years)	Average duration (years)	Deaths 1990 Number ('000s)	Rate (per 100 000)	Deaths 2000 (Projected) Number ('000s)	Rate (per 100 000)
Males										
0-4	0	0	-	-	-	-	0	0	0	0
5-14	0	0	-	-	-	-	0	0	0	0
15-44	0	0	-	-	-	-	0	0	0	0
45-59	0	0	-	-	-	-	0	0	0	0
60+	0	0	-	-	-	-	0	0	0	0
All ages	0	0	-	-	-	-	0	0	0	0
Females										
0-4	0	0	-	-	-	-	0	0.0	0	0.0
5-14	154	29	-	-	10.0	-	2	0.5	2	0.3
15-44	14 272	1 191	-	-	29.8	-	108	9.0	56	4.1
45-59	466	150	-	-	52.4	-	3	0.9	2	0.5
60+	0	0	-	-	-	-	0	0.0	0	0.0
All ages	14 892	570	-	-	30.3	-	114	4.3	60	2.0
Total	14 892	283	-	-	30.3	-	114	2.2	60	1.0

For epidemiological sources see Abou-Zahr 1996. For the methods used to estimate and project incidence, prevalence, and deaths see Murray and Lopez 1996a. See explanatory notes for definitions and caveats.

Table 112 | **Cuadro 112** | **Tableau 112**
Maternal haemorrhage | **Hemorragia materna** | **Hémorragie maternelle**

Sheehan syndrome | Sindrome de Sheehan | Syndrome de Sheehan

Table 112a   EME - PEMC - EMBE   Maternal haemorrhage - Sheehan syndrome

Age group (years)	Incidence 1990 Number ('000s)	Rate (per 100 000)	Prevalence 1990 Number ('000s)	Rate (per 100 000)	Avg. age at onset (years)	Average duration (years)	Deaths 1990 Number ('000s)	Rate (per 100 000)	Deaths 2000 (Projected) Number ('000s)	Rate (per 100 000)
Males										
0-4	0	0	0	0	-	-	-	-	-	-
5-14	0	0	0	0	-	-	-	-	-	-
15-44	0	0	0	0	-	-	-	-	-	-
45-59	0	0	0	0	-	-	-	-	-	-
60+	0	0	0	0	-	-	-	-	-	-
All ages	0	0	0	0	-	-	-	-	-	-
Females										
0-4	0	0.0	0	0	-	-	-	-	-	-
5-14	0	0.0	0	0	-	-	-	-	-	-
15-44	8	4.5	120	67	30.0	50.0	-	-	-	-
45-59	0	0.0	91	134	-	-	-	-	-	-
60+	0	0.0	113	134	-	-	-	-	-	-
All ages	8	2.0	324	79	30.0	50.0	-	-	-	-
Total	8	1.0	324	41	30.0	50.0	-	-	-	-

Table 112b   FSE - PEAS - AESE   Maternal haemorrhage - Sheehan syndrome

Age group (years)	Incidence 1990 Number ('000s)	Rate (per 100 000)	Prevalence 1990 Number ('000s)	Rate (per 100 000)	Avg. age at onset (years)	Average duration (years)	Deaths 1990 Number ('000s)	Rate (per 100 000)	Deaths 2000 (Projected) Number ('000s)	Rate (per 100 000)
Males										
0-4	0	0	0	0	-	-	-	-	-	-
5-14	0	0	0	0	-	-	-	-	-	-
15-44	0	0	0	0	-	-	-	-	-	-
45-59	0	0	0	0	-	-	-	-	-	-
60+	0	0	0	0	-	-	-	-	-	-
All ages	0	0	0	0	-	-	-	-	-	-
Females										
0-4	0	0.0	0	0	-	-	-	-	-	-
5-14	0	0.0	0	0	-	-	-	-	-	-
15-44	4	5.3	60	80	29.9	46.8	-	-	-	-
45-59	0	0.0	48	160	-	-	-	-	-	-
60+	0	0.0	58	160	-	-	-	-	-	-
All ages	4	2.2	166	92	29.9	46.8	-	-	-	-
Total	4	1.2	166	48	29.9	46.8	-	-	-	-

Table 112c   India - India - Inde   Maternal haemorrhage - Sheehan syndrome

Age group (years)	Incidence 1990 Number ('000s)	Rate (per 100 000)	Prevalence 1990 Number ('000s)	Rate (per 100 000)	Avg. age at onset (years)	Average duration (years)	Deaths 1990 Number ('000s)	Rate (per 100 000)	Deaths 2000 (Projected) Number ('000s)	Rate (per 100 000)
Males										
0-4	0	0	0	0	-	-	-	-	-	-
5-14	0	0	0	0	-	-	-	-	-	-
15-44	0	0	0	0	-	-	-	-	-	-
45-59	0	0	0	0	-	-	-	-	-	-
60+	0	0	0	0	-	-	-	-	-	-
All ages	0	0	0	0	-	-	-	-	-	-
Females										
0-4	0	0.0	0	0	-	-	-	-	-	-
5-14	0	0.0	0	0	-	-	-	-	-	-
15-44	21	11.4	310	169	29.8	41.7	-	-	-	-
45-59	0	0.0	158	343	-	-	-	-	-	-
60+	0	0.0	99	343	-	-	-	-	-	-
All ages	21	5.1	567	138	29.8	41.7	-	-	-	-
Total	21	2.5	567	67	29.8	41.7	-	-	-	-

For epidemiological sources see Abou-Zahr 1996. For the methods used to estimate and project incidence, prevalence, and deaths see Murray and Lopez 1996a. See explanatory notes for definitions and caveats.

Table 112
Maternal haemorrhage

Cuadro 112
Hemorragia materna

Tableau 112
Hémorragie maternelle

Sheehan syndrome

Sindrome de Sheehan

Syndrome de Sheehan

Table 112d   China - China - Chine   Maternal haemorrhage - Sheehan syndrome

Age group (years)	Incidence 1990 Number ('000s)	Rate (per 100 000)	Prevalence 1990 Number ('000s)	Rate (per 100 000)	Avg. age at onset (years)	Average duration (years)	Deaths 1990 Number ('000s)	Rate (per 100 000)	Deaths 2000 (Projected) Number ('000s)	Rate (per 100 000)
Males										
0-4	0	0	0	0	-	-	-	-	-	-
5-14	0	0	0	0	-	-	-	-	-	-
15-44	0	0	0	0	-	-	-	-	-	-
45-59	0	0	0	0	-	-	-	-	-	-
60+	0	0	0	0	-	-	-	-	-	-
All ages	0	0	0	0	-	-	-	-	-	-
Females										
0-4	0	0.0	0	0	-	-	-	-	-	-
5-14	0	0.0	0	0	-	-	-	-	-	-
15-44	20	7.0	298	105	29.9	44.2	-	-	-	-
45-59	0	0.0	136	211	-	-	-	-	-	-
60+	0	0.0	109	211	-	-	-	-	-	-
All ages	20	3.6	543	99	29.9	44.2	-	-	-	-
Total	20	1.8	543	48	29.9	44.2	-	-	-	-

Table 112e   OAI - OPAI - APAI   Maternal haemorrhage - Sheehan syndrome

Age group (years)	Incidence 1990 Number ('000s)	Rate (per 100 000)	Prevalence 1990 Number ('000s)	Rate (per 100 000)	Avg. age at onset (years)	Average duration (years)	Deaths 1990 Number ('000s)	Rate (per 100 000)	Deaths 2000 (Projected) Number ('000s)	Rate (per 100 000)
Males										
0-4	0	0	0	0	-	-	-	-	-	-
5-14	0	0	0	0	-	-	-	-	-	-
15-44	0	0	0	0	-	-	-	-	-	-
45-59	0	0	0	0	-	-	-	-	-	-
60+	0	0	0	0	-	-	-	-	-	-
All ages	0	0	0	0	-	-	-	-	-	-
Females										
0-4	0	0.0	0	0	-	-	-	-	-	-
5-14	0	0.0	0	0	-	-	-	-	-	-
15-44	15	9.4	222	139	29.4	41.5	-	-	-	-
45-59	0	0.0	99	282	-	-	-	-	-	-
60+	0	0.0	64	282	-	-	-	-	-	-
All ages	15	4.4	384	113	29.4	41.5	-	-	-	-
Total	15	2.2	384	56	29.4	41.5	-	-	-	-

Table 112f   SSA - ASS - ASS   Maternal haemorrhage - Sheehan syndrome

Age group (years)	Incidence 1990 Number ('000s)	Rate (per 100 000)	Prevalence 1990 Number ('000s)	Rate (per 100 000)	Avg. age at onset (years)	Average duration (years)	Deaths 1990 Number ('000s)	Rate (per 100 000)	Deaths 2000 (Projected) Number ('000s)	Rate (per 100 000)
Males										
0-4	0	0	0	0	-	-	-	-	-	-
5-14	0	0	0	0	-	-	-	-	-	-
15-44	0	0	0	0	-	-	-	-	-	-
45-59	0	0	0	0	-	-	-	-	-	-
60+	0	0	0	0	-	-	-	-	-	-
All ages	0	0	0	0	-	-	-	-	-	-
Females										
0-4	0	0.0	0	0	-	-	-	-	-	-
5-14	0	0.0	0	0	-	-	-	-	-	-
15-44	20	19.0	289	272	29.5	37.2	-	-	-	-
45-59	0	0.0	125	563	-	-	-	-	-	-
60+	0	0.0	72	563	-	-	-	-	-	-
All ages	20	7.8	486	188	29.5	37.2	-	-	-	-
Total	20	4.0	486	95	29.5	37.2	-	-	-	-

For epidemiological sources see Abou-Zahr 1996. For the methods used to estimate and project incidence, prevalence, and deaths see Murray and Lopez 1996a. See explanatory notes for definitions and caveats.

Table 112   **Cuadro 112**   **Tableau 112**
Maternal haemorrhage   **Hemorragia materna**   **Hémorragie maternelle**

Sheehan syndrome   Sindrome de Sheehan   Syndrome de Sheehan

Table 112g   LAC - ALC - ALC   Maternal haemorrhage - Sheehan syndrome

Age group (years)	Incidence 1990 Number ('000s)	Rate (per 100 000)	Prevalence 1990 Number ('000s)	Rate (per 100 000)	Avg. age at onset (years)	Average duration (years)	Deaths 1990 Number ('000s)	Rate (per 100 000)	Deaths 2000 (Projected) Number ('000s)	Rate (per 100 000)
Males										
0-4	0	0	0	0	-	-	-	-	-	-
5-14	0	0	0	0	-	-	-	-	-	-
15-44	0	0	0	0	-	-	-	-	-	-
45-59	0	0	0	0	-	-	-	-	-	-
60+	0	0	0	0	-	-	-	-	-	-
All ages	0	0	0	0	-	-	-	-	-	-
Females										
0-4	0	0.0	0	0	-	-	-	-	-	-
5-14	0	0.0	0	0	-	-	-	-	-	-
15-44	10	9.6	149	143	29.9	44.6	-	-	-	-
45-59	0	0.0	67	288	-	-	-	-	-	-
60+	0	0.0	48	288	-	-	-	-	-	-
All ages	10	4.5	265	119	29.9	44.6	-	-	-	-
Total	10	2.2	265	60	29.9	44.6	-	-	-	-

Table 112h   MEC - AOM - CMO   Maternal haemorrhage - Sheehan syndrome

Age group (years)	Incidence 1990 Number ('000s)	Rate (per 100 000)	Prevalence 1990 Number ('000s)	Rate (per 100 000)	Avg. age at onset (years)	Average duration (years)	Deaths 1990 Number ('000s)	Rate (per 100 000)	Deaths 2000 (Projected) Number ('000s)	Rate (per 100 000)
Males										
0-4	0	0	0	0	-	-	-	-	-	-
5-14	0	0	0	0	-	-	-	-	-	-
15-44	0	0	0	0	-	-	-	-	-	-
45-59	0	0	0	0	-	-	-	-	-	-
60+	0	0	0	0	-	-	-	-	-	-
All ages	0	0	0	0	-	-	-	-	-	-
Females										
0-4	0	0.0	0	0	-	-	-	-	-	-
5-14	0	0.0	0	0	-	-	-	-	-	-
15-44	16	14.9	237	221	29.8	42.6	-	-	-	-
45-59	0	0.0	100	447	-	-	-	-	-	-
60+	0	0.0	69	447	-	-	-	-	-	-
All ages	16	6.5	406	165	29.8	42.6	-	-	-	-
Total	16	3.2	406	81	29.8	42.6	-	-	-	-

Table 112i   World - Mundo - Monde   Maternal haemorrhage - Sheehan syndrome

Age group (years)	Incidence 1990 Number ('000s)	Rate (per 100 000)	Prevalence 1990 Number ('000s)	Rate (per 100 000)	Avg. age at onset (years)	Average duration (years)	Deaths 1990 Number ('000s)	Rate (per 100 000)	Deaths 2000 (Projected) Number ('000s)	Rate (per 100 000)
Males										
0-4	0	0	0	0	-	-	-	-	-	-
5-14	0	0	0	0	-	-	-	-	-	-
15-44	0	0	0	0	-	-	-	-	-	-
45-59	0	0	0	0	-	-	-	-	-	-
60+	0	0	0	0	-	-	-	-	-	-
All ages	0	0	0	0	-	-	-	-	-	-
Females										
0-4	0	0.0	0	0	-	-	-	-	-	-
5-14	0	0.0	0	0	-	-	-	-	-	-
15-44	114	9.5	1 685	141	29.7	42.4	-	-	-	-
45-59	0	0.0	823	265	-	-	-	-	-	-
60+	0	0.0	633	235	-	-	-	-	-	-
All ages	114	4.4	3 141	120	29.7	42.4	-	-	-	-
Total	114	2.2	3 141	60	29.7	42.4	-	-	-	-

For epidemiological sources see Abou-Zahr 1996. For the methods used to estimate and project incidence, prevalence, and deaths see Murray and Lopez 1996a. See explanatory notes for definitions and caveats.

Table 113
Maternal haemorrhage

Cuadro 113
Hemorragia materna

Tableau 113
Hémorragie maternelle

Severe anaemia

Anemia severa

Anémie grave

Table 113a   EME - PEMC - EMBE   Maternal haemorrhage - Severe anaemia

Age group (years)	Incidence 1990 Number ('000s)	Rate (per 100 000)	Prevalence 1990 Number ('000s)	Rate (per 100 000)	Avg. age at onset (years)	Average duration (years)	Deaths 1990 Number ('000s)	Rate (per 100 000)	Deaths 2000 (Projected) Number ('000s)	Rate (per 100 000)
Males										
0-4	0	0	0	0	-	-	-	-	-	-
5-14	0	0	0	0	-	-	-	-	-	-
15-44	0	0	0	0	-	-	-	-	-	-
45-59	0	0	0	0	-	-	-	-	-	-
60+	0	0	0	0	-	-	-	-	-	-
All ages	0	0	0	0	-	-	-	-	-	-
Females										
0-4	0	0.0	0	0.0	-	-	-	-	-	-
5-14	0	0.0	0	0.0	-	-	-	-	-	-
15-44	10	5.6	5	2.8	30.0	0.50	-	-	-	-
45-59	0	0.0	0	0.0	-	-	-	-	-	-
60+	0	0.0	0	0.0	-	-	-	-	-	-
All ages	10	2.5	5	1.2	30.0	0.50	-	-	-	-
Total	10	1.3	5	0.6	30.0	0.50	-	-	-	-

Table 113b   FSE - PEAS - AESE   Maternal haemorrhage - Severe anaemia

Age group (years)	Incidence 1990 Number ('000s)	Rate (per 100 000)	Prevalence 1990 Number ('000s)	Rate (per 100 000)	Avg. age at onset (years)	Average duration (years)	Deaths 1990 Number ('000s)	Rate (per 100 000)	Deaths 2000 (Projected) Number ('000s)	Rate (per 100 000)
Males										
0-4	0	0	0	0	-	-	-	-	-	-
5-14	0	0	0	0	-	-	-	-	-	-
15-44	0	0	0	0	-	-	-	-	-	-
45-59	0	0	0	0	-	-	-	-	-	-
60+	0	0	0	0	-	-	-	-	-	-
All ages	0	0	0	0	-	-	-	-	-	-
Females										
0-4	0	0.0	0	0.0	-	-	-	-	-	-
5-14	0	0.0	0	0.0	-	-	-	-	-	-
15-44	5	6.7	2	3.3	29.9	0.50	-	-	-	-
45-59	0	0.0	0	0.0	-	-	-	-	-	-
60+	0	0.0	0	0.0	-	-	-	-	-	-
All ages	5	2.8	2	1.4	29.9	0.50	-	-	-	-
Total	5	1.4	2	0.7	29.9	0.50	-	-	-	-

Table 113c   India - India - Inde   Maternal haemorrhage - Severe anaemia

Age group (years)	Incidence 1990 Number ('000s)	Rate (per 100 000)	Prevalence 1990 Number ('000s)	Rate (per 100 000)	Avg. age at onset (years)	Average duration (years)	Deaths 1990 Number ('000s)	Rate (per 100 000)	Deaths 2000 (Projected) Number ('000s)	Rate (per 100 000)
Males										
0-4	0	0	0	0	-	-	-	-	-	-
5-14	0	0	0	0	-	-	-	-	-	-
15-44	0	0	0	0	-	-	-	-	-	-
45-59	0	0	0	0	-	-	-	-	-	-
60+	0	0	0	0	-	-	-	-	-	-
All ages	0	0	0	0	-	-	-	-	-	-
Females										
0-4	0	0.0	0	0.0	-	-	-	-	-	-
5-14	0	0.0	0	0.0	-	-	-	-	-	-
15-44	26	14.2	65	35.5	29.8	2.5	-	-	-	-
45-59	0	0.0	0	0.0	-	-	-	-	-	-
60+	0	0.0	0	0.0	-	-	-	-	-	-
All ages	26	6.3	65	15.8	29.8	2.5	-	-	-	-
Total	26	3.1	65	7.7	29.8	2.5	-	-	-	-

For epidemiological sources see Abou-Zahr 1996. For the methods used to estimate and project incidence, prevalence, and deaths see Murray and Lopez 1996a. See explanatory notes for definitions and caveats.

Table 113
Maternal haemorrhage

Cuadro 113
Hemorragia materna

Tableau 113
Hémorragie maternelle

Severe anaemia

Anemia severa

Anémie grave

| Table 113d | China - China - Chine | | | | | | Maternal haemorrhage - Severe anaemia | | | |

Age group (years)	Incidence 1990		Prevalence 1990		Avg. age at onset (years)	Average duration (years)	Deaths 1990		Deaths 2000 (Projected)	
	Number ('000s)	Rate (per 100 000)	Number ('000s)	Rate (per 100 000)			Number ('000s)	Rate (per 100 000)	Number ('000s)	Rate (per 100 000)
Males										
0-4	0	0	0	0	-	-	-	-	-	-
5-14	0	0	0	0	-	-	-	-	-	-
15-44	0	0	0	0	-	-	-	-	-	-
45-59	0	0	0	0	-	-	-	-	-	-
60+	0	0	0	0	-	-	-	-	-	-
All ages	0	0	0	0	-	-	-	-	-	-
Females										
0-4	0	0.0	0	0.0	-	-	-	-	-	-
5-14	0	0.0	0	0.0	-	-	-	-	-	-
15-44	25	8.8	13	4.4	29.9	0.50	-	-	-	-
45-59	0	0.0	0	0.0	-	-	-	-	-	-
60+	0	0.0	0	0.0	-	-	-	-	-	-
All ages	25	4.6	13	2.3	29.9	0.50	-	-	-	-
Total	25	2.2	13	1.1	29.9	0.50	-	-	-	-

| Table 113e | OAI - OPAI - APAI | | | | | | Maternal haemorrhage - Severe anaemia | | | |

Age group (years)	Incidence 1990		Prevalence 1990		Avg. age at onset (years)	Average duration (years)	Deaths 1990		Deaths 2000 (Projected)	
	Number ('000s)	Rate (per 100 000)	Number ('000s)	Rate (per 100 000)			Number ('000s)	Rate (per 100 000)	Number ('000s)	Rate (per 100 000)
Males										
0-4	0	0	0	0	-	-	-	-	-	-
5-14	0	0	0	0	-	-	-	-	-	-
15-44	0	0	0	0	-	-	-	-	-	-
45-59	0	0	0	0	-	-	-	-	-	-
60+	0	0	0	0	-	-	-	-	-	-
All ages	0	0	0	0	-	-	-	-	-	-
Females										
0-4	0	0.0	0	0.0	-	-	-	-	-	-
5-14	0	0.0	0	0.0	-	-	-	-	-	-
15-44	19	11.9	14	8.9	29.4	0.75	-	-	-	-
45-59	0	0.0	0	0.0	-	-	-	-	-	-
60+	0	0.0	0	0.0	-	-	-	-	-	-
All ages	19	5.6	14	4.2	29.4	0.75	-	-	-	-
Total	19	2.8	14	2.1	29.4	0.75	-	-	-	-

| Table 113f | SSA - ASS - ASS | | | | | | Maternal haemorrhage - Severe anaemia | | | |

Age group (years)	Incidence 1990		Prevalence 1990		Avg. age at onset (years)	Average duration (years)	Deaths 1990		Deaths 2000 (Projected)	
	Number ('000s)	Rate (per 100 000)	Number ('000s)	Rate (per 100 000)			Number ('000s)	Rate (per 100 000)	Number ('000s)	Rate (per 100 000)
Males										
0-4	0	0	0	0	-	-	-	-	-	-
5-14	0	0	0	0	-	-	-	-	-	-
15-44	0	0	0	0	-	-	-	-	-	-
45-59	0	0	0	0	-	-	-	-	-	-
60+	0	0	0	0	-	-	-	-	-	-
All ages	0	0	0	0	-	-	-	-	-	-
Females										
0-4	0	0.0	0	0	-	-	-	-	-	-
5-14	0	0.0	0	0	-	-	-	-	-	-
15-44	25	23.5	63	59	29.5	2.5	-	-	-	-
45-59	0	0.0	0	0	-	-	-	-	-	-
60+	0	0.0	0	0	-	-	-	-	-	-
All ages	25	9.7	63	24	29.5	2.5	-	-	-	-
Total	25	4.9	63	12	29.5	2.5	-	-	-	-

For epidemiological sources see Abou-Zahr 1996. For the methods used to estimate and project incidence, prevalence, and deaths see Murray and Lopez 1996a. See explanatory notes for definitions and caveats.

Table 113 — **Cuadro 113** — **Tableau 113**
Maternal haemorrhage — **Hemorragia materna** — **Hémorragie maternelle**

Severe anaemia — Anemia severa — Anémie grave

Table 113g — LAC - ALC - ALC — Maternal haemorrhage - Severe anaemia

Age group (years)	Incidence 1990 Number ('000s)	Rate (per 100 000)	Prevalence 1990 Number ('000s)	Rate (per 100 000)	Avg. age at onset (years)	Average duration (years)	Deaths 1990 Number ('000s)	Rate (per 100 000)	Deaths 2000 (Projected) Number ('000s)	Rate (per 100 000)
Males										
0-4	0	0	0	0	-	-	-	-	-	-
5-14	0	0	0	0	-	-	-	-	-	-
15-44	0	0	0	0	-	-	-	-	-	-
45-59	0	0	0	0	-	-	-	-	-	-
60+	0	0	0	0	-	-	-	-	-	-
All ages	0	0	0	0	-	-	-	-	-	-
Females										
0-4	0	0.0	0	0.0	-	-	-	-	-	-
5-14	0	0.0	0	0.0	-	-	-	-	-	-
15-44	12	11.5	9	8.6	29.9	0.75	-	-	-	-
45-59	0	0.0	0	0.0	-	-	-	-	-	-
60+	0	0.0	0	0.0	-	-	-	-	-	-
All ages	12	5.4	9	4.0	29.9	0.75	-	-	-	-
Total	12	2.7	9	2.0	29.9	0.75	-	-	-	-

Table 113h — MEC - AOM - CMO — Maternal haemorrhage - Severe anaemia

Age group (years)	Incidence 1990 Number ('000s)	Rate (per 100 000)	Prevalence 1990 Number ('000s)	Rate (per 100 000)	Avg. age at onset (years)	Average duration (years)	Deaths 1990 Number ('000s)	Rate (per 100 000)	Deaths 2000 (Projected) Number ('000s)	Rate (per 100 000)
Males										
0-4	0	0	0	0	-	-	-	-	-	-
5-14	0	0	0	0	-	-	-	-	-	-
15-44	0	0	0	0	-	-	-	-	-	-
45-59	0	0	0	0	-	-	-	-	-	-
60+	0	0	0	0	-	-	-	-	-	-
All ages	0	0	0	0	-	-	-	-	-	-
Females										
0-4	0	0.0	0	0.0	-	-	-	-	-	-
5-14	0	0.0	0	0.0	-	-	-	-	-	-
15-44	20	18.7	15	14.0	29.8	0.75	-	-	-	-
45-59	0	0.0	0	0.0	-	-	-	-	-	-
60+	0	0.0	0	0.0	-	-	-	-	-	-
All ages	20	8.1	15	6.1	29.8	0.75	-	-	-	-
Total	20	4.0	15	3.0	29.8	0.75	-	-	-	-

Table 113i — World - Mundo - Monde — Maternal haemorrhage - Severe anaemia

Age group (years)	Incidence 1990 Number ('000s)	Rate (per 100 000)	Prevalence 1990 Number ('000s)	Rate (per 100 000)	Avg. age at onset (years)	Average duration (years)	Deaths 1990 Number ('000s)	Rate (per 100 000)	Deaths 2000 (Projected) Number ('000s)	Rate (per 100 000)
Males										
0-4	0	0	0	0	-	-	-	-	-	-
5-14	0	0	0	0	-	-	-	-	-	-
15-44	0	0	0	0	-	-	-	-	-	-
45-59	0	0	0	0	-	-	-	-	-	-
60+	0	0	0	0	-	-	-	-	-	-
All ages	0	0	0	0	-	-	-	-	-	-
Females										
0-4	0	0	0	0.0	-	-	-	-	-	-
5-14	0	0	0	0.0	-	-	-	-	-	-
15-44	142	0	142	11.8	29.7	1.3	-	-	-	-
45-59	0	0	0	0.0	-	-	-	-	-	-
60+	0	0	0	0.0	-	-	-	-	-	-
All ages	142	0	142	5.4	29.7	1.3	-	-	-	-
Total	142	0	142	2.7	29.7	1.3	-	-	-	-

For epidemiological sources see Abou-Zahr 1996. For the methods used to estimate and project incidence, prevalence, and deaths see Murray and Lopez 1996a. See explanatory notes for definitions and caveats.

Table 114
Maternal sepsis

Cuadro 114
Sepsis puerperal

Tableau 114
Septicémie maternelle

Episodes

Episodios

Episodes

Table 114a   EME - PEMC - EMBE   Maternal sepsis - Episodes

Age group (years)	Incidence 1990 Number ('000s)	Rate (per 100 000)	Prevalence 1990 Number ('000s)	Rate (per 100 000)	Avg. age at onset (years)	Average duration (years)	Deaths 1990 Number ('000s)	Rate (per 100 000)	Deaths 2000 (Projected) Number ('000s)	Rate (per 100 000)
Males										
0-4	0	0	-	-	-	-	0	0	0	0
5-14	0	0	-	-	-	-	0	0	0	0
15-44	0	0	-	-	-	-	0	0	0	0
45-59	0	0	-	-	-	-	0	0	0	0
60+	0	0	-	-	-	-	0	0	0	0
All ages	0	0	-	-	-	-	0	0	0	0
Females										
0-4	0	0	-	-	-	-	0	0	0	0
5-14	0	0	-	-	-	-	0	0	0	0
15-44	520	290	-	-	25.0	-	0	0	0	0
45-59	0	0	-	-	-	-	0	0	0	0
60+	0	0	-	-	-	-	0	0	0	0
All ages	520	128	-	-	25.0	-	0	0	0	0
Total	520	65	-	-	25.0	-	0	0	0	0

Table 114b   FSE - PEAS - AESE   Maternal sepsis - Episodes

Age group (years)	Incidence 1990 Number ('000s)	Rate (per 100 000)	Prevalence 1990 Number ('000s)	Rate (per 100 000)	Avg. age at onset (years)	Average duration (years)	Deaths 1990 Number ('000s)	Rate (per 100 000)	Deaths 2000 (Projected) Number ('000s)	Rate (per 100 000)
Males										
0-4	0	0	-	-	-	-	0	0	0	0
5-14	0	0	-	-	-	-	0	0	0	0
15-44	0	0	-	-	-	-	0	0	0	0
45-59	0	0	-	-	-	-	0	0	0	0
60+	0	0	-	-	-	-	0	0	0	0
All ages	0	0	-	-	-	-	0	0	0	0
Females										
0-4	0	0	-	-	-	-	0	0.0	0	0.0
5-14	0	0	-	-	-	-	0	0.0	0	0.0
15-44	370	494	-	-	25.0	-	0	0.2	0	0.1
45-59	0	0	-	-	-	-	0	0.0	0	0.0
60+	0	0	-	-	-	-	0	0.0	0	0.0
All ages	370	205	-	-	25.0	-	0	0.1	0	0.0
Total	370	107	-	-	25.0	-	0	0.0	0	0.0

Table 114c   India - India - Inde   Maternal sepsis - Episodes

Age group (years)	Incidence 1990 Number ('000s)	Rate (per 100 000)	Prevalence 1990 Number ('000s)	Rate (per 100 000)	Avg. age at onset (years)	Average duration (years)	Deaths 1990 Number ('000s)	Rate (per 100 000)	Deaths 2000 (Projected) Number ('000s)	Rate (per 100 000)
Males										
0-4	0	0	-	-	-	-	0	0	0	0
5-14	0	0	-	-	-	-	0	0	0	0
15-44	0	0	-	-	-	-	0	0	0	0
45-59	0	0	-	-	-	-	0	0	0	0
60+	0	0	-	-	-	-	0	0	0	0
All ages	0	0	-	-	-	-	0	0	0	0
Females										
0-4	0	0	-	-	-	-	0	0.0	0	0.0
5-14	0	0	-	-	-	-	0	0.0	0	0.0
15-44	2 581	1 409	-	-	25.0	-	18	9.7	8	3.5
45-59	84	183	-	-	52.4	-	1	1.3	0	0.6
60+	0	0	-	-	-	-	0	0.0	0	0.0
All ages	2 665	650	-	-	25.9	-	18	4.5	8	1.7
Total	2 665	314	-	-	25.9	-	18	2.2	8	0.8

For epidemiological sources see Abou-Zahr and Guidotti 1996. For the methods used to estimate and project incidence, prevalence, and deaths see Murray and Lopez 1996a. See explanatory notes for definitions and caveats.

Table 114
Maternal sepsis

Cuadro 114
Sepsis puerperal

Tableau 114
Septicémie maternelle

Episodes

Episodios

Episodes

Table 114d   China - China - Chine   Maternal sepsis - Episodes

Age group (years)	Incidence 1990 Number ('000s)	Rate (per 100 000)	Prevalence 1990 Number ('000s)	Rate (per 100 000)	Avg. age at onset (years)	Average duration (years)	Deaths 1990 Number ('000s)	Rate (per 100 000)	Deaths 2000 (Projected) Number ('000s)	Rate (per 100 000)
Males										
0-4	0	0	-	-	-	-	0	0	0	0
5-14	0	0	-	-	-	-	0	0	0	0
15-44	0	0	-	-	-	-	0	0	0	0
45-59	0	0	-	-	-	-	0	0	0	0
60+	0	0	-	-	-	-	0	0	0	0
All ages	0	0	-	-	-	-	0	0	0	0
Females										
0-4	0	0	-	-	-	-	0	0.0	0	0.0
5-14	0	0	-	-	-	-	0	0.0	0	0.0
15-44	1 509	531	-	-	25.0	-	1	0.5	0	0.1
45-59	95	148	-	-	52.4	-	0	0.1	0	0.1
60+	0	0	-	-	-	-	0	0.0	0	0.0
All ages	1 604	292	-	-	26.6	-	1	0.3	0	0.1
Total	1 604	141	-	-	26.6	-	1	0.1	0	0.0

Table 114e   OAI - OPAI - APAI   Maternal sepsis - Episodes

Age group (years)	Incidence 1990 Number ('000s)	Rate (per 100 000)	Prevalence 1990 Number ('000s)	Rate (per 100 000)	Avg. age at onset (years)	Average duration (years)	Deaths 1990 Number ('000s)	Rate (per 100 000)	Deaths 2000 (Projected) Number ('000s)	Rate (per 100 000)
Males										
0-4	0	0	-	-	-	-	0	0	0	0
5-14	0	0	-	-	-	-	0	0	0	0
15-44	0	0	-	-	-	-	0	0	0	0
45-59	0	0	-	-	-	-	0	0	0	0
60+	0	0	-	-	-	-	0	0	0	0
All ages	0	0	-	-	-	-	0	0	0	0
Females										
0-4	0	0	-	-	-	-	0	0.0	0	0.0
5-14	0	0	-	-	-	-	0	0.0	0	0.0
15-44	1 672	1 048	-	-	25.0	-	8	5.0	4	2.1
45-59	70	199	-	-	52.2	-	0	1.0	0	0.5
60+	0	0	-	-	-	-	0	0.0	0	0.0
All ages	1 742	513	-	-	26.1	-	8	2.5	4	1.1
Total	1 742	255	-	-	26.1	-	8	1.2	4	0.5

Table 114f   SSA - ASS - ASS   Maternal sepsis - Episodes

Age group (years)	Incidence 1990 Number ('000s)	Rate (per 100 000)	Prevalence 1990 Number ('000s)	Rate (per 100 000)	Avg. age at onset (years)	Average duration (years)	Deaths 1990 Number ('000s)	Rate (per 100 000)	Deaths 2000 (Projected) Number ('000s)	Rate (per 100 000)
Males										
0-4	0	0	-	-	-	-	0	0	0	0
5-14	0	0	-	-	-	-	0	0	0	0
15-44	0	0	-	-	-	-	0	0	0	0
45-59	0	0	-	-	-	-	0	0	0	0
60+	0	0	-	-	-	-	0	0	0	0
All ages	0	0	-	-	-	-	0	0	0	0
Females										
0-4	0	0	-	-	-	-	0	0.0	0	0.0
5-14	142	204	-	-	10.0	-	2	2.3	1	1.2
15-44	2 518	2 370	-	-	25.0	-	28	26.5	17	11.5
45-59	5	25	-	-	52.2	-	0	0.3	0	0.1
60+	0	0	-	-	-	-	0	0.0	0	0.0
All ages	2 666	1 033	-	-	24.3	-	30	11.5	18	5.1
Total	2 666	522	-	-	24.3	-	30	5.8	18	2.6

For epidemiological sources see Abou-Zahr and Guidotti 1996. For the methods used to estimate and project incidence, prevalence, and deaths see Murray and Lopez 1996a. See explanatory notes for definitions and caveats.

Table 114
Maternal sepsis

Cuadro 114
Sepsis puerperal

Tableau 114
Septicémie maternelle

Episodes

Episodios

Episodes

Table 114g   LAC - ALC - ALC   Maternal sepsis - Episodes

Age group (years)	Incidence 1990 Number ('000s)	Rate (per 100 000)	Prevalence 1990 Number ('000s)	Rate (per 100 000)	Avg. age at onset (years)	Average duration (years)	Deaths 1990 Number ('000s)	Rate (per 100 000)	Deaths 2000 (Projected) Number ('000s)	Rate (per 100 000)
Males										
0-4	0	0	-	-	-	-	0	0	0	0
5-14	0	0	-	-	-	-	0	0	0	0
15-44	0	0	-	-	-	-	0	0	0	0
45-59	0	0	-	-	-	-	0	0	0	0
60+	0	0	-	-	-	-	0	0	0	0
All ages	0	0	-	-	-	-	0	0	0	0
Females										
0-4	0	0	-	-	-	-	0	0.0	0	0.0
5-14	6	12	-	-	10.0	-	0	0.0	0	0.0
15-44	872	838	-	-	25.0	-	2	1.5	1	0.7
45-59	6	24	-	-	52.4	-	0	0.0	0	0.0
60+	0	0	-	-	-	-	0	0.0	0	0.0
All ages	884	397	-	-	25.1	-	2	0.7	1	0.3
Total	884	199	-	-	25.1	-	2	0.4	1	0.2

Table 114h   MEC - AOM - CMO   Maternal sepsis - Episodes

Age group (years)	Incidence 1990 Number ('000s)	Rate (per 100 000)	Prevalence 1990 Number ('000s)	Rate (per 100 000)	Avg. age at onset (years)	Average duration (years)	Deaths 1990 Number ('000s)	Rate (per 100 000)	Deaths 2000 (Projected) Number ('000s)	Rate (per 100 000)
Males										
0-4	0	0	-	-	-	-	0	0	0	0
5-14	0	0	-	-	-	-	0	0	0	0
15-44	0	0	-	-	-	-	0	0	0	0
45-59	0	0	-	-	-	-	0	0	0	0
60+	0	0	-	-	-	-	0	0	0	0
All ages	0	0	-	-	-	-	0	0	0	0
Females										
0-4	0	0	-	-	-	-	0	0.0	0	0.0
5-14	2	4	-	-	10.0	-	0	0.0	0	0.0
15-44	1 958	1 826	-	-	25.0	-	8	7.0	5	3.2
45-59	125	562	-	-	52.3	-	0	2.2	0	1.2
60+	0	0	-	-	-	-	0	0.0	0	0.0
All ages	2 086	846	-	-	26.6	-	8	3.2	5	1.5
Total	2 086	415	-	-	26.6	-	8	1.6	5	0.8

Table 114i   World - Mundo - Monde   Maternal sepsis - Episodes

Age group (years)	Incidence 1990 Number ('000s)	Rate (per 100 000)	Prevalence 1990 Number ('000s)	Rate (per 100 000)	Avg. age at onset (years)	Average duration (years)	Deaths 1990 Number ('000s)	Rate (per 100 000)	Deaths 2000 (Projected) Number ('000s)	Rate (per 100 000)
Males										
0-4	0	0	-	-	-	-	0	0	0	0
5-14	0	0	-	-	-	-	0	0	0	0
15-44	0	0	-	-	-	-	0	0	0	0
45-59	0	0	-	-	-	-	0	0	0	0
60+	0	0	-	-	-	-	0	0	0	0
All ages	0	0	-	-	-	-	0	0	0	0
Females										
0-4	0	0	-	-	-	-	0	0.0	0	0.0
5-14	151	29	-	-	10.0	-	2	0.3	1	0.2
15-44	12 000	1 001	-	-	25.0	-	64	5.4	35	2.5
45-59	386	124	-	-	52.4	-	2	0.5	1	0.3
60+	0	0	-	-	-	-	0	0.0	0	0.0
All ages	12 537	480	-	-	25.7	-	68	2.6	37	1.2
Total	12 537	238	-	-	25.7	-	68	1.3	37	0.6

For epidemiological sources see Abou-Zahr and Guidotti 1996. For the methods used to estimate and project incidence, prevalence, and deaths see Murray and Lopez 1996a. See explanatory notes for definitions and caveats.

Table 115	Cuadro 115	Tableau 115
Maternal sepsis	**Sepsis puerperal**	**Septicémie maternelle**
Infertility	Infertilidad	Stérilité

Table 115a　　EME - PEMC - EMBE　　　Maternal sepsis - Infertility

Age group (years)	Incidence 1990 Number ('000s)	Rate (per 100 000)	Prevalence 1990 Number ('000s)	Rate (per 100 000)	Avg. age at onset (years)	Average duration (years)	Deaths 1990 Number ('000s)	Rate (per 100 000)	Deaths 2000 (Projected) Number ('000s)	Rate (per 100 000)
Males										
0-4	0	0	0	0	-	-	0	0	0	0
5-14	0	0	0	0	-	-	0	0	0	0
15-44	0	0	0	0	-	-	0	0	0	0
45-59	0	0	0	0	-	-	0	0	0	0
60+	0	0	0	0	-	-	0	0	0	0
All ages	0	0	0	0	-	-	0	0	0	0
Females										
0-4	0	0.0	0	0	-	-	0	0	0	0
5-14	0	0.0	0	0	-	-	0	0	0	0
15-44	10	5.6	150	84	25.0	15.0	0	0	0	0
45-59	0	0.0	0	0	-	-	0	0	0	0
60+	0	0.0	0	0	-	-	0	0	0	0
All ages	10	2.5	150	37	25.0	15.0	0	0	0	0
Total	10	1.3	150	19	25.0	15.0	0	0	0	0

Table 115b　　FSE - PEAS - AESE　　　Maternal sepsis - Infertility

Age group (years)	Incidence 1990 Number ('000s)	Rate (per 100 000)	Prevalence 1990 Number ('000s)	Rate (per 100 000)	Avg. age at onset (years)	Average duration (years)	Deaths 1990 Number ('000s)	Rate (per 100 000)	Deaths 2000 (Projected) Number ('000s)	Rate (per 100 000)
Males										
0-4	0	0	0	0	-	-	0	0	0	0
5-14	0	0	0	0	-	-	0	0	0	0
15-44	0	0	0	0	-	-	0	0	0	0
45-59	0	0	0	0	-	-	0	0	0	0
60+	0	0	0	0	-	-	0	0	0	0
All ages	0	0	0	0	-	-	0	0	0	0
Females										
0-4	0	0.0	0	0	-	-	0	0	0	0
5-14	0	0.0	0	0	-	-	0	0	0	0
15-44	33	43.7	491	655	25.0	15.0	0	0	0	0
45-59	0	0.0	0	0	-	-	0	0	0	0
60+	0	0.0	0	0	-	-	0	0	0	0
All ages	33	18.1	491	272	25.0	15.0	0	0	0	0
Total	33	9.5	491	142	25.0	15.0	0	0	0	0

Table 115c　　India - India - Inde　　　Maternal sepsis - Infertility

Age group (years)	Incidence 1990 Number ('000s)	Rate (per 100 000)	Prevalence 1990 Number ('000s)	Rate (per 100 000)	Avg. age at onset (years)	Average duration (years)	Deaths 1990 Number ('000s)	Rate (per 100 000)	Deaths 2000 (Projected) Number ('000s)	Rate (per 100 000)
Males										
0-4	0	0	0	0	-	-	0	0	0	0
5-14	0	0	0	0	-	-	0	0	0	0
15-44	0	0	0	0	-	-	0	0	0	0
45-59	0	0	0	0	-	-	0	0	0	0
60+	0	0	0	0	-	-	0	0	0	0
All ages	0	0	0	0	-	-	0	0	0	0
Females										
0-4	0	0	0	0	-	-	0	0	0	0
5-14	0	0	0	0	-	-	0	0	0	0
15-44	228	124	3 387	1 849	25.0	15.0	0	0	0	0
45-59	0	0	0	0	-	-	0	0	0	0
60+	0	0	0	0	-	-	0	0	0	0
All ages	228	56	3 387	826	25.0	15.0	0	0	0	0
Total	228	27	3 387	399	25.0	15.0	0	0	0	0

For epidemiological sources see Abou-Zahr and Guidotti 1996. For the methods used to estimate and project incidence, prevalence, and deaths see Murray and Lopez 1996a. See explanatory notes for definitions and caveats.

Table 115
Maternal sepsis

Cuadro 115
Sepsis puerperal

Tableau 115
Septicémie maternelle

Infertility

Infertilidad

Stérilité

Table 115d China - China - Chine — Maternal sepsis - Infertility

Age group (years)	Incidence 1990 Number ('000s)	Rate (per 100 000)	Prevalence 1990 Number ('000s)	Rate (per 100 000)	Avg. age at onset (years)	Average duration (years)	Deaths 1990 Number ('000s)	Rate (per 100 000)	Deaths 2000 (Projected) Number ('000s)	Rate (per 100 000)
Males										
0-4	0	0	0	0	-	-	0	0	0	0
5-14	0	0	0	0	-	-	0	0	0	0
15-44	0	0	0	0	-	-	0	0	0	0
45-59	0	0	0	0	-	-	0	0	0	0
60+	0	0	0	0	-	-	0	0	0	0
All ages	0	0	0	0	-	-	0	0	0	0
Females										
0-4	0	0	0	0	-	-	0	0	0	0
5-14	0	0	0	0	-	-	0	0	0	0
15-44	135	48	2 020	711	25.0	15.0	0	0	0	0
45-59	0	0	0	0	-	-	0	0	0	0
60+	0	0	0	0	-	-	0	0	0	0
All ages	135	25	2 020	368	25.0	15.0	0	0	0	0
Total	135	12	2 020	178	25.0	15.0	0	0	0	0

Table 115e OAI - OPAI - APAI — Maternal sepsis - Infertility

Age group (years)	Incidence 1990 Number ('000s)	Rate (per 100 000)	Prevalence 1990 Number ('000s)	Rate (per 100 000)	Avg. age at onset (years)	Average duration (years)	Deaths 1990 Number ('000s)	Rate (per 100 000)	Deaths 2000 (Projected) Number ('000s)	Rate (per 100 000)
Males										
0-4	0	0	0	0	-	-	0	0	0	0
5-14	0	0	0	0	-	-	0	0	0	0
15-44	0	0	0	0	-	-	0	0	0	0
45-59	0	0	0	0	-	-	0	0	0	0
60+	0	0	0	0	-	-	0	0	0	0
All ages	0	0	0	0	-	-	0	0	0	0
Females										
0-4	0	0	0	0	-	-	0	0	0	0
5-14	0	0	0	0	-	-	0	0	0	0
15-44	148	93	2 199	1 377	25.0	15.0	0	0	0	0
45-59	0	0	0	0	-	-	0	0	0	0
60+	0	0	0	0	-	-	0	0	0	0
All ages	148	44	2 199	647	25.0	15.0	0	0	0	0
Total	148	22	2 199	322	25.0	15.0	0	0	0	0

Table 115f SSA - ASS - ASS — Maternal sepsis - Infertility

Age group (years)	Incidence 1990 Number ('000s)	Rate (per 100 000)	Prevalence 1990 Number ('000s)	Rate (per 100 000)	Avg. age at onset (years)	Average duration (years)	Deaths 1990 Number ('000s)	Rate (per 100 000)	Deaths 2000 (Projected) Number ('000s)	Rate (per 100 000)
Males										
0-4	0	0	0	0	-	-	0	0	0	0
5-14	0	0	0	0	-	-	0	0	0	0
15-44	0	0	0	0	-	-	0	0	0	0
45-59	0	0	0	0	-	-	0	0	0	0
60+	0	0	0	0	-	-	0	0	0	0
All ages	0	0	0	0	-	-	0	0	0	0
Females										
0-4	0	0	0	0	-	-	0	0	0	0
5-14	0	0	0	0	-	-	0	0	0	0
15-44	290	273	4 260	4 009	25.0	15.0	0	0	0	0
45-59	0	0	0	0	-	-	0	0	0	0
60+	0	0	0	0	-	-	0	0	0	0
All ages	290	112	4 260	1 651	25.0	15.0	0	0	0	0
Total	290	57	4 260	835	25.0	15.0	0	0	0	0

For epidemiological sources see Abou-Zahr and Guidotti 1996. For the methods used to estimate and project incidence, prevalence, and deaths see Murray and Lopez 1996a. See explanatory notes for definitions and caveats.

Table 115 — **Cuadro 115** — **Tableau 115**
Maternal sepsis — **Sepsis puerperal** — **Septicémie maternelle**

Infertility — Infertilidad — Stérilité

Table 115g LAC - ALC - ALC — Maternal sepsis - Infertility

Age group (years)	Incidence 1990 Number ('000s)	Rate (per 100 000)	Prevalence 1990 Number ('000s)	Rate (per 100 000)	Avg. age at onset (years)	Average duration (years)	Deaths 1990 Number ('000s)	Rate (per 100 000)	Deaths 2000 (Projected) Number ('000s)	Rate (per 100 000)
Males										
0-4	0	0	0	0	-	-	0	0	0	0
5-14	0	0	0	0	-	-	0	0	0	0
15-44	0	0	0	0	-	-	0	0	0	0
45-59	0	0	0	0	-	-	0	0	0	0
60+	0	0	0	0	-	-	0	0	0	0
All ages	0	0	0	0	-	-	0	0	0	0
Females										
0-4	0	0	0	0	-	-	0	0	0	0
5-14	0	0	0	0	-	-	0	0	0	0
15-44	77	74	1 151	1 106	25.0	15.0	0	0	0	0
45-59	0	0	0	0	-	-	0	0	0	0
60+	0	0	0	0	-	-	0	0	0	0
All ages	77	35	1 151	517	25.0	15.0	0	0	0	0
Total	77	17	1 151	259	25.0	15.0	0	0	0	0

Table 115h MEC - AOM - CMO — Maternal sepsis - Infertility

Age group (years)	Incidence 1990 Number ('000s)	Rate (per 100 000)	Prevalence 1990 Number ('000s)	Rate (per 100 000)	Avg. age at onset (years)	Average duration (years)	Deaths 1990 Number ('000s)	Rate (per 100 000)	Deaths 2000 (Projected) Number ('000s)	Rate (per 100 000)
Males										
0-4	0	0	0	0	-	-	0	0	0	0
5-14	0	0	0	0	-	-	0	0	0	0
15-44	0	0	0	0	-	-	0	0	0	0
45-59	0	0	0	0	-	-	0	0	0	0
60+	0	0	0	0	-	-	0	0	0	0
All ages	0	0	0	0	-	-	0	0	0	0
Females										
0-4	0	0	0	0	-	-	0	0	0	0
5-14	0	0	0	0	-	-	0	0	0	0
15-44	172	160	2 573	2 400	25.0	15.0	0	0	0	0
45-59	0	0	0	0	-	-	0	0	0	0
60+	0	0	0	0	-	-	0	0	0	0
All ages	172	70	2 573	1 043	25.0	15.0	0	0	0	0
Total	172	34	2 573	512	25.0	15.0	0	0	0	0

Table 115i World - Mundo - Monde — Maternal sepsis - Infertility

Age group (years)	Incidence 1990 Number ('000s)	Rate (per 100 000)	Prevalence 1990 Number ('000s)	Rate (per 100 000)	Avg. age at onset (years)	Average duration (years)	Deaths 1990 Number ('000s)	Rate (per 100 000)	Deaths 2000 (Projected) Number ('000s)	Rate (per 100 000)
Males										
0-4	0	0	0	0	-	-	0	0	0	0
5-14	0	0	0	0	-	-	0	0	0	0
15-44	0	0	0	0	-	-	0	0	0	0
45-59	0	0	0	0	-	-	0	0	0	0
60+	0	0	0	0	-	-	0	0	0	0
All ages	0	0	0	0	-	-	0	0	0	0
Females										
0-4	0	0	0	0	-	-	0	0	0	0
5-14	0	0	0	0	-	-	0	0	0	0
15-44	1 092	91	16 231	1 354	25.0	15.0	0	0	0	0
45-59	0	0	0	0	-	-	0	0	0	0
60+	0	0	0	0	-	-	0	0	0	0
All ages	1 092	42	16 231	621	25.0	15.0	0	0	0	0
Total	1 092	21	16 231	308	25.0	15.0	0	0	0	0

For epidemiological sources see Abou-Zahr and Guidotti 1996. For the methods used to estimate and project incidence, prevalence, and deaths see Murray and Lopez 1996a. See explanatory notes for definitions and caveats.

Table 116
Hypertensive disorders of pregnancy
Episodes

Cuadro 116
Trastornos hipertensivos del embarazo
Episodios

Tableau 116
Troubles hypertensifs de la grossesse
Episodes

Table 116a EME - PEMC - EMBE Hypertensive disorders of pregnancy - Episodes

Age group (years)	Incidence 1990 Number ('000s)	Rate (per 100 000)	Prevalence 1990 Number ('000s)	Rate (per 100 000)	Avg. age at onset (years)	Average duration (years)	Deaths 1990 Number ('000s)	Rate (per 100 000)	Deaths 2000 (Projected) Number ('000s)	Rate (per 100 000)
Males										
0-4	0	0	-	-	-	-	0	0	0	0
5-14	0	0	-	-	-	-	0	0	0	0
15-44	0	0	-	-	-	-	0	0	0	0
45-59	0	0	-	-	-	-	0	0	0	0
60+	0	0	-	-	-	-	0	0	0	0
All ages	0	0	-	-	-	-	0	0	0	0
Females										
0-4	0	0	-	-	-	-	0	0.0	0	0.0
5-14	0	0	-	-	-	-	0	0.0	0	0.0
15-44	447	249	-	-	30.0	-	0	0.2	0	0.1
45-59	0	0	-	-	-	-	0	0.0	0	0.0
60+	0	0	-	-	-	-	0	0.0	0	0.0
All ages	447	110	-	-	30.0	-	0	0.1	0	0.0
Total	447	56	-	-	30.0	-	0	0.0	0	0.0

Table 116b FSE - PEAS - AESE Hypertensive disorders of pregnancy - Episodes

Age group (years)	Incidence 1990 Number ('000s)	Rate (per 100 000)	Prevalence 1990 Number ('000s)	Rate (per 100 000)	Avg. age at onset (years)	Average duration (years)	Deaths 1990 Number ('000s)	Rate (per 100 000)	Deaths 2000 (Projected) Number ('000s)	Rate (per 100 000)
Males										
0-4	0	0	-	-	-	-	0	0	0	0
5-14	0	0	-	-	-	-	0	0	0	0
15-44	0	0	-	-	-	-	0	0	0	0
45-59	0	0	-	-	-	-	0	0	0	0
60+	0	0	-	-	-	-	0	0	0	0
All ages	0	0	-	-	-	-	0	0	0	0
Females										
0-4	0	0	-	-	-	-	0	0.0	0	0.0
5-14	0	0	-	-	-	-	0	0.0	0	0.0
15-44	264	352	-	-	29.9	-	0	0.4	0	0.2
45-59	0	0	-	-	-	-	0	0.0	0	0.0
60+	0	0	-	-	-	-	0	0.0	0	0.0
All ages	264	146	-	-	29.9	-	0	0.2	0	0.1
Total	264	76	-	-	29.9	-	0	0.1	0	0.0

Table 116c India - India - Inde Hypertensive disorders of pregnancy - Episodes

Age group (years)	Incidence 1990 Number ('000s)	Rate (per 100 000)	Prevalence 1990 Number ('000s)	Rate (per 100 000)	Avg. age at onset (years)	Average duration (years)	Deaths 1990 Number ('000s)	Rate (per 100 000)	Deaths 2000 (Projected) Number ('000s)	Rate (per 100 000)
Males										
0-4	0	0	-	-	-	-	0	0	0	0
5-14	0	0	-	-	-	-	0	0	0	0
15-44	0	0	-	-	-	-	0	0	0	0
45-59	0	0	-	-	-	-	0	0	0	0
60+	0	0	-	-	-	-	0	0	0	0
All ages	0	0	-	-	-	-	0	0	0	0
Females										
0-4	0	0	-	-	-	-	0	0.0	0	0.0
5-14	0	0	-	-	-	-	0	0.0	0	0.0
15-44	1 290	704	-	-	29.8	-	13	5.8	6	2.6
45-59	42	92	-	-	52.4	-	0	0.8	0	0.4
60+	0	0	-	-	-	-	0	0.0	0	0.0
All ages	1 332	325	-	-	30.5	-	14	2.8	6	1.3
Total	1 332	157	-	-	30.5	-	14	1.4	6	0.6

For epidemiological sources see Abou-Zahr and Guidotti 1996. For the methods used to estimate and project incidence, prevalence, and deaths see Murray and Lopez 1996a. See explanatory notes for definitions and caveats.

Table 116
Hypertensive disorders of pregnancy
Episodes

Cuadro 116
Trastornos hipertensivos del embarazo
Episodios

Tableau 116
Troubles hypertensifs de la grossesse
Episodes

Table 116d   China - China - Chine   Hypertensive disorders of pregnancy - Episodes

Age group (years)	Incidence 1990 Number ('000s)	Rate (per 100 000)	Prevalence 1990 Number ('000s)	Rate (per 100 000)	Avg. age at onset (years)	Average duration (years)	Deaths 1990 Number ('000s)	Rate (per 100 000)	Deaths 2000 (Projected) Number ('000s)	Rate (per 100 000)
Males										
0-4	0	0	-	-	-	-	0	0	0	0
5-14	0	0	-	-	-	-	0	0	0	0
15-44	0	0	-	-	-	-	0	0	0	0
45-59	0	0	-	-	-	-	0	0	0	0
60+	0	0	-	-	-	-	0	0	0	0
All ages	0	0	-	-	-	-	0	0	0	0
Females										
0-4	0	0	-	-	-	-	0	0.0	0	0.0
5-14	0	0	-	-	-	-	0	0.0	0	0.0
15-44	1 257	442	-	-	29.9	-	2	0.8	1	0.2
45-59	79	123	-	-	52.4	-	0	0.2	0	0.1
60+	0	0	-	-	-	-	0	0.0	0	0.0
All ages	1 336	244	-	-	31.2	-	2	0.4	1	0.1
Total	1 336	118	-	-	31.2	-	2	0.2	1	0.1

Table 116e   OAI - OPAI - APAI   Hypertensive disorders of pregnancy - Episodes

Age group (years)	Incidence 1990 Number ('000s)	Rate (per 100 000)	Prevalence 1990 Number ('000s)	Rate (per 100 000)	Avg. age at onset (years)	Average duration (years)	Deaths 1990 Number ('000s)	Rate (per 100 000)	Deaths 2000 (Projected) Number ('000s)	Rate (per 100 000)
Males										
0-4	0	0	-	-	-	-	0	0	0	0
5-14	0	0	-	-	-	-	0	0	0	0
15-44	0	0	-	-	-	-	0	0	0	0
45-59	0	0	-	-	-	-	0	0	0	0
60+	0	0	-	-	-	-	0	0	0	0
All ages	0	0	-	-	-	-	0	0	0	0
Females										
0-4	0	0	-	-	-	-	0	0.0	0	0.0
5-14	0	0	-	-	-	-	0	0.0	0	0.0
15-44	943	591	-	-	29.8	-	6	3.0	3	1.6
45-59	39	112	-	-	52.2	-	0	0.5	0	0.4
60+	0	0	-	-	-	-	0	0.0	0	0.0
All ages	982	289	-	-	30.7	-	6	1.6	3	0.8
Total	982	144	-	-	30.7	-	6	0.8	3	0.4

Table 116f   SSA - ASS - ASS   Hypertensive disorders of pregnancy - Episodes

Age group (years)	Incidence 1990 Number ('000s)	Rate (per 100 000)	Prevalence 1990 Number ('000s)	Rate (per 100 000)	Avg. age at onset (years)	Average duration (years)	Deaths 1990 Number ('000s)	Rate (per 100 000)	Deaths 2000 (Projected) Number ('000s)	Rate (per 100 000)
Males										
0-4	0	0	-	-	-	-	0	0	0	0
5-14	0	0	-	-	-	-	0	0	0	0
15-44	0	0	-	-	-	-	0	0	0	0
45-59	0	0	-	-	-	-	0	0	0	0
60+	0	0	-	-	-	-	0	0	0	0
All ages	0	0	-	-	-	-	0	0	0	0
Females										
0-4	0	0	-	-	-	-	0	0.0	0	0.0
5-14	71	102	-	-	10.0	-	1	1.3	1	0.9
15-44	1 259	1 185	-	-	29.5	-	21	14.6	13	8.7
45-59	3	12	-	-	52.2	-	0	0.2	0	0.1
60+	0	0	-	-	-	-	0	0.0	0	0.0
All ages	1 333	517	-	-	28.5	-	22	6.4	13	3.8
Total	1 333	261	-	-	28.5	-	22	3.2	13	1.9

For epidemiological sources see Abou-Zahr and Guidotti 1996. For the methods used to estimate and project incidence, prevalence, and deaths see Murray and Lopez 1996a. See explanatory notes for definitions and caveats.

Table 116
Hypertensive disorders of pregnancy
Episodes

Cuadro 116
Trastornos hipertensivos del embarazo
Episodios

Tableau 116
Troubles hypertensifs de la grossesse
Episodes

Table 116g   LAC - ALC - ALC   Hypertensive disorders of pregnancy - Episodes

Age group (years)	Incidence 1990 Number ('000s)	Rate (per 100 000)	Prevalence 1990 Number ('000s)	Rate (per 100 000)	Avg. age at onset (years)	Average duration (years)	Deaths 1990 Number ('000s)	Rate (per 100 000)	Deaths 2000 (Projected) Number ('000s)	Rate (per 100 000)
Males										
0-4	0	0	-	-	-	-	0	0	0	0
5-14	0	0	-	-	-	-	0	0	0	0
15-44	0	0	-	-	-	-	0	0	0	0
45-59	0	0	-	-	-	-	0	0	0	0
60+	0	0	-	-	-	-	0	0	0	0
All ages	0	0	-	-	-	-	0	0	0	0
Females										
0-4	0	0	-	-	-	-	0	0.0	0	0.0
5-14	4	9	-	-	10.0	-	0	0.0	0	0.0
15-44	623	599	-	-	29.8	-	3	2.4	2	1.4
45-59	4	17	-	-	52.4	-	0	0.1	0	0.0
60+	0	-	-	-	-	-	0	0.0	0	0.0
All ages	632	284	-	-	29.8	-	3	1.1	2	0.7
Total	632	142	-	-	29.8	-	3	0.6	2	0.3

Table 116h   MEC - AOM - CMO   Hypertensive disorders of pregnancy - Episodes

Age group (years)	Incidence 1990 Number ('000s)	Rate (per 100 000)	Prevalence 1990 Number ('000s)	Rate (per 100 000)	Avg. age at onset (years)	Average duration (years)	Deaths 1990 Number ('000s)	Rate (per 100 000)	Deaths 2000 (Projected) Number ('000s)	Rate (per 100 000)
Males										
0-4	0	0	-	-	-	-	0	0	0	0
5-14	0	0	-	-	-	-	0	0	0	0
15-44	0	0	-	-	-	-	0	0	0	0
45-59	0	0	-	-	-	-	0	0	0	0
60+	0	0	-	-	-	-	0	0	0	0
All ages	0	0	-	-	-	-	0	0	0	0
Females										
0-4	0	0	-	-	-	-	0	0.0	0	0.0
5-14	1	2	-	-	10.0	-	0	0.0	0	0.0
15-44	979	913	-	-	29.8	-	8	5.3	5	3.2
45-59	63	281	-	-	52.3	-	0	1.5	0	1.2
60+	0	0	-	-	-	-	0	0.0	0	0.0
All ages	1 043	423	-	-	31.1	-	8	2.5	5	1.5
Total	1 043	207	-	-	31.1	-	8	1.2	5	0.8

Table 116i   World - Mundo - Monde   Hypertensive disorders of pregnancy - Episodes

Age group (years)	Incidence 1990 Number ('000s)	Rate (per 100 000)	Prevalence 1990 Number ('000s)	Rate (per 100 000)	Avg. age at onset (years)	Average duration (years)	Deaths 1990 Number ('000s)	Rate (per 100 000)	Deaths 2000 (Projected) Number ('000s)	Rate (per 100 000)
Males										
0-4	0	0	-	-	-	-	0	0	0	0
5-14	0	0	-	-	-	-	0	0	0	0
15-44	0	0	-	-	-	-	0	0	0	0
45-59	0	0	-	-	-	-	0	0	0	0
60+	0	0	-	-	-	-	0	0	0	0
All ages	0	0	-	-	-	-	0	0	0	0
Females										
0-4	0	0	-	-	-	-	0	0.0	0	0.0
5-14	77	15	-	-	10.0	-	1	0.2	1	0.1
15-44	7 062	589	-	-	29.8	-	54	3.9	29	2.1
45-59	230	74	-	-	52.4	-	1	0.3	1	0.2
60+	0	0	-	-	-	-	0	0.0	0	0.0
All ages	7 369	282	-	-	30.4	-	57	1.8	31	1.0
Total	7 369	140	-	-	30.4	-	57	0.9	31	0.5

For epidemiological sources see Abou-Zahr and Guidotti 1996. For the methods used to estimate and project incidence, prevalence, and deaths see Murray and Lopez 1996a. See explanatory notes for definitions and caveats.

Table 117
Hypertensive disorders of pregnancy
Neurological sequelae

Cuadro 117
Trastornos hipertensivos del embarazo
Secuelas neurológicas

Tableau 117
Troubles hypertensifs de la grossesse
Séquelles neurologiques

Table 117a   EME - PEMC - EMBE   Hypertensive disorders of pregnancy - Neurological sequelae

Age group (years)	Incidence 1990 Number ('000s)	Rate (per 100 000)	Prevalence 1990 Number ('000s)	Rate (per 100 000)	Avg. age at onset (years)	Average duration (years)	Deaths 1990 Number ('000s)	Rate (per 100 000)	Deaths 2000 (Projected) Number ('000s)	Rate (per 100 000)
Males										
0-4	0	0	0	0	-	-	0	0	0	0
5-14	0	0	0	0	-	-	0	0	0	0
15-44	0	0	0	0	-	-	0	0	0	0
45-59	0	0	0	0	-	-	0	0	0	0
60+	0	0	0	0	-	-	0	0	0	0
All ages	0	0	0	0	-	-	0	0	0	0
Females										
0-4	0	0.0	0	0.0	-	-	0	0	0	0
5-14	0	0.0	0	0.0	-	-	0	0	0	0
15-44	0	0.1	4	2.1	30.0	50.0	0	0	0	0
45-59	0	0.0	3	4.2	-	-	0	0	0	0
60+	0	0.0	4	4.2	-	-	0	0	0	0
All ages	0	0.1	10	2.5	30.0	50.0	0	0	0	0
Total	0	0.0	10	1.3	30.0	50.0	0	0	0	0

Table 117b   FSE - PEAS - AESE   Hypertensive disorders of pregnancy - Neurological sequelae

Age group (years)	Incidence 1990 Number ('000s)	Rate (per 100 000)	Prevalence 1990 Number ('000s)	Rate (per 100 000)	Avg. age at onset (years)	Average duration (years)	Deaths 1990 Number ('000s)	Rate (per 100 000)	Deaths 2000 (Projected) Number ('000s)	Rate (per 100 000)
Males										
0-4	0	0	0	0	-	-	0	0	0	0
5-14	0	0	0	0	-	-	0	0	0	0
15-44	0	0	0	0	-	-	0	0	0	0
45-59	0	0	0	0	-	-	0	0	0	0
60+	0	0	0	0	-	-	0	0	0	0
All ages	0	0	0	0	-	-	0	0	0	0
Females										
0-4	0	0.0	0	0.0	-	-	0	0	0	0
5-14	0	0.0	0	0.0	-	-	0	0	0	0
15-44	0	0.2	2	3.0	29.9	46.8	0	0	0	0
45-59	0	0.0	2	6.0	-	-	0	0	0	0
60+	0	0.0	2	6.0	-	-	0	0	0	0
All ages	0	0.1	6	3.4	29.9	46.8	0	0	0	0
Total	0	0.0	6	1.8	29.9	46.8	0	0	0	0

Table 117c   India - India - Inde   Hypertensive disorders of pregnancy - Neurological sequelae

Age group (years)	Incidence 1990 Number ('000s)	Rate (per 100 000)	Prevalence 1990 Number ('000s)	Rate (per 100 000)	Avg. age at onset (years)	Average duration (years)	Deaths 1990 Number ('000s)	Rate (per 100 000)	Deaths 2000 (Projected) Number ('000s)	Rate (per 100 000)
Males										
0-4	0	0	0	0	-	-	0	0	0	0
5-14	0	0	0	0	-	-	0	0	0	0
15-44	0	0	0	0	-	-	0	0	0	0
45-59	0	0	0	0	-	-	0	0	0	0
60+	0	0	0	0	-	-	0	0	0	0
All ages	0	0	0	0	-	-	0	0	0	0
Females										
0-4	0	0.0	0	0.0	-	-	0	0	0	0
5-14	0	0.0	0	0.0	-	-	0	0	0	0
15-44	1	0.7	19	10.5	29.8	41.7	0	0	0	0
45-59	0	0.0	10	21.3	-	-	0	0	0	0
60+	0	0.0	6	21.3	-	-	0	0	0	0
All ages	1	0.3	35	8.6	29.8	41.7	0	0	0	0
Total	1	0.2	35	4.1	29.8	41.7	0	0	0	0

For epidemiological sources see Abou-Zahr and Guidotti 1996. For the methods used to estimate and project incidence, prevalence, and deaths see Murray and Lopez 1996a. See explanatory notes for definitions and caveats.

Table 117
Hypertensive disorders of pregnancy
Neurological sequelae

Cuadro 117
Trastornos hipertensivos del embarazo
Secuelas neurológicas

Tableau 117
Troubles hypertensifs de la grossesse
Séquelles neurologiques

Table 117d   China - China - Chine   Hypertensive disorders of pregnancy - Neurological sequelae

Age group (years)	Incidence 1990 Number ('000s)	Rate (per 100 000)	Prevalence 1990 Number ('000s)	Rate (per 100 000)	Avg. age at onset (years)	Average duration (years)	Deaths 1990 Number ('000s)	Rate (per 100 000)	Deaths 2000 (Projected) Number ('000s)	Rate (per 100 000)
Males										
0-4	0	0	0	0	-	-	0	0	0	0
5-14	0	0	0	0	-	-	0	0	0	0
15-44	0	0	0	0	-	-	0	0	0	0
45-59	0	0	0	0	-	-	0	0	0	0
60+	0	0	0	0	-	-	0	0	0	0
All ages	0	0	0	0	-	-	0	0	0	0
Females										
0-4	0	0.0	0	0.0	-	-	0	0	0	0
5-14	0	0.0	0	0.0	-	-	0	0	0	0
15-44	1	0.5	19	6.8	29.9	44.2	0	0	0	0
45-59	0	0.0	9	13.7	-	-	0	0	0	0
60+	0	0.0	7	13.7	-	-	0	0	0	0
All ages	1	0.2	35	6.4	29.9	44.2	0	0	0	0
Total	1	0.1	35	3.1	29.9	44.2	0	0	0	0

Table 117e   OAI - OPAI - APAI   Hypertensive disorders of pregnancy - Neurological sequelae

Age group (years)	Incidence 1990 Number ('000s)	Rate (per 100 000)	Prevalence 1990 Number ('000s)	Rate (per 100 000)	Avg. age at onset (years)	Average duration (years)	Deaths 1990 Number ('000s)	Rate (per 100 000)	Deaths 2000 (Projected) Number ('000s)	Rate (per 100 000)
Males										
0-4	0	0	0	0	-	-	0	0	0	0
5-14	0	0	0	0	-	-	0	0	0	0
15-44	0	0	0	0	-	-	0	0	0	0
45-59	0	0	0	0	-	-	0	0	0	0
60+	0	0	0	0	-	-	0	0	0	0
All ages	0	0	0	0	-	-	0	0	0	0
Females										
0-4	0	0.0	0	0.0	-	-	0	0	0	0
5-14	0	0.0	0	0.0	-	-	0	0	0	0
15-44	1	0.6	13	8.3	29.8	41.4	0	0	0	0
45-59	0	0.0	6	16.9	-	-	0	0	0	0
60+	0	0.0	4	16.9	-	-	0	0	0	0
All ages	1	0.3	23	6.8	29.8	41.4	0	0	0	0
Total	1	0.1	23	3.4	29.8	41.4	0	0	0	0

Table 117f   SSA - ASS - ASS   Hypertensive disorders of pregnancy - Neurological sequelae

Age group (years)	Incidence 1990 Number ('000s)	Rate (per 100 000)	Prevalence 1990 Number ('000s)	Rate (per 100 000)	Avg. age at onset (years)	Average duration (years)	Deaths 1990 Number ('000s)	Rate (per 100 000)	Deaths 2000 (Projected) Number ('000s)	Rate (per 100 000)
Males										
0-4	0	0	0	0	-	-	0	0	0	0
5-14	0	0	0	0	-	-	0	0	0	0
15-44	0	0	0	0	-	-	0	0	0	0
45-59	0	0	0	0	-	-	0	0	0	0
60+	0	0	0	0	-	-	0	0	0	0
All ages	0	0	0	0	-	-	0	0	0	0
Females										
0-4	0	0.0	0	0.0	-	-	0	0	0	0
5-14	0	0.0	0	0.0	-	-	0	0	0	0
15-44	1	1.2	19	17.7	29.5	37.2	0	0	0	0
45-59	0	0.0	8	36.7	-	-	0	0	0	0
60+	0	0.0	5	36.7	-	-	0	0	0	0
All ages	1	0.5	32	12.3	29.5	37.2	0	0	0	0
Total	1	0.3	32	6.2	29.5	37.2	0	0	0	0

For epidemiological sources see Abou-Zahr and Guidotti 1996. For the methods used to estimate and project incidence, prevalence, and deaths see Murray and Lopez 1996a. See explanatory notes for definitions and caveats.

Table 117
Hypertensive disorders of pregnancy
Neurological sequelae

Cuadro 117
Trastornos hipertensivos del embarazo
Secuelas neurológicas

Tableau 117
Troubles hypertensifs de la grossesse
Séquelles neurologiques

Table 117g   LAC - ALC - ALC   Hypertensive disorders of pregnancy - Neurological sequelae

Age group (years)	Incidence 1990 Number ('000s)	Rate (per 100 000)	Prevalence 1990 Number ('000s)	Rate (per 100 000)	Avg. age at onset (years)	Average duration (years)	Deaths 1990 Number ('000s)	Rate (per 100 000)	Deaths 2000 (Projected) Number ('000s)	Rate (per 100 000)
Males										
0-4	0	0	0	0	-	-	0	0	0	0
5-14	0	0	0	0	-	-	0	0	0	0
15-44	0	0	0	0	-	-	0	0	0	0
45-59	0	0	0	0	-	-	0	0	0	0
60+	0	0	0	0	-	-	0	0	0	0
All ages	0	0	0	0	-	-	0	0	0	0
Females										
0-4	0	0.0	0	0.0	-	-	0	0	0	0
5-14	0	0.0	0	0.0	-	-	0	0	0	0
15-44	1	0.6	9	8.6	29.8	44.6	0	0	0	0
45-59	0	0.0	4	17.3	-	-	0	0	0	0
60+	0	0.0	3	17.3	-	-	0	0	0	0
All ages	1	0.3	16	7.1	29.8	44.6	0	0	0	0
Total	1	0.1	16	3.6	29.8	44.6	0	0	0	0

Table 117h   MEC - AOM - CMO   Hypertensive disorders of pregnancy - Neurological sequelae

Age group (years)	Incidence 1990 Number ('000s)	Rate (per 100 000)	Prevalence 1990 Number ('000s)	Rate (per 100 000)	Avg. age at onset (years)	Average duration (years)	Deaths 1990 Number ('000s)	Rate (per 100 000)	Deaths 2000 (Projected) Number ('000s)	Rate (per 100 000)
Males										
0-4	0	0	0	0	-	-	0	0	0	0
5-14	0	0	0	0	-	-	0	0	0	0
15-44	0	0	0	0	-	-	0	0	0	0
45-59	0	0	0	0	-	-	0	0	0	0
60+	0	0	0	0	-	-	0	0	0	0
All ages	0	0	0	0	-	-	0	0	0	0
Females										
0-4	0	0.0	0	0.0	-	-	0	0	0	0
5-14	0	0.0	0	0.0	-	-	0	0	0	0
15-44	1	0.9	15	13.9	29.8	42.6	0	0	0	0
45-59	0	0.0	6	28.0	-	-	0	0	0	0
60+	0	0.0	4	28.0	-	-	0	0	0	0
All ages	1	0.4	25	10.3	29.8	42.6	0	0	0	0
Total	1	0.2	25	5.1	29.8	42.6	0	0	0	0

Table 117i   World - Mundo - Monde   Hypertensive disorders of pregnancy - Neurological sequelae

Age group (years)	Incidence 1990 Number ('000s)	Rate (per 100 000)	Prevalence 1990 Number ('000s)	Rate (per 100 000)	Avg. age at onset (years)	Average duration (years)	Deaths 1990 Number ('000s)	Rate (per 100 000)	Deaths 2000 (Projected) Number ('000s)	Rate (per 100 000)
Males										
0-4	0	0	0	0	-	-	0	0	0	0
5-14	0	0	0	0	-	-	0	0	0	0
15-44	0	0	0	0	-	-	0	0	0	0
45-59	0	0	0	0	-	-	0	0	0	0
60+	0	0	0	0	-	-	0	0	0	0
All ages	0	0	0	0	-	-	0	0	0	0
Females										
0-4	0	0.0	0	0.0	-	-	0	0	0	0
5-14	0	0.0	0	0.0	-	-	0	0	0	0
15-44	7	0.6	101	8.4	29.8	42.1	0	0	0	0
45-59	0	0.0	48	15.3	-	-	0	0	0	0
60+	0	0.0	35	12.9	-	-	0	0	0	0
All ages	7	0.3	183	7.0	29.8	42.1	0	0	0	0
Total	7	0.1	183	3.5	29.8	42.1	0	0	0	0

For epidemiological sources see Abou-Zahr and Guidotti 1996. For the methods used to estimate and project incidence, prevalence, and deaths see Murray and Lopez 1996a. See explanatory notes for definitions and caveats.

Table 118
Obstructed labour

Cuadro 118
Parto obstruido

Tableau 118
Dystocie d'obstacle

Episodes

Episodios

Episodes

Table 118a EME - PEMC - EMBE — Obstructed labour - Episodes

Age group (years)	Incidence 1990 Number ('000s)	Rate (per 100 000)	Prevalence 1990 Number ('000s)	Rate (per 100 000)	Avg. age at onset (years)	Average duration (years)	Deaths 1990 Number ('000s)	Rate (per 100 000)	Deaths 2000 (Projected) Number ('000s)	Rate (per 100 000)
Males										
0-4	0	0	-	-	-	-	0	0	0	0
5-14	0	0	-	-	-	-	0	0	0	0
15-44	0	0	-	-	-	-	0	0	0	0
45-59	0	0	-	-	-	-	0	0	0	0
60+	0	0	-	-	-	-	0	0	0	0
All ages	0	0	-	-	-	-	0	0	0	0
Females										
0-4	0	0	-	-	-	-	0	0	0	0
5-14	0	0	-	-	-	-	0	0	0	0
15-44	312	174	-	-	19.0	-	0	0	0	0
45-59	0	0	-	-	-	-	0	0	0	0
60+	0	0	-	-	-	-	0	0	0	0
All ages	312	77	-	-	19.0	-	0	0	0	0
Total	312	39	-	-	19.0	-	0	0	0	0

Table 118b FSE - PEAS - AESE — Obstructed labour - Episodes

Age group (years)	Incidence 1990 Number ('000s)	Rate (per 100 000)	Prevalence 1990 Number ('000s)	Rate (per 100 000)	Avg. age at onset (years)	Average duration (years)	Deaths 1990 Number ('000s)	Rate (per 100 000)	Deaths 2000 (Projected) Number ('000s)	Rate (per 100 000)
Males										
0-4	0	0	-	-	-	-	0	0	0	0
5-14	0	0	-	-	-	-	0	0	0	0
15-44	0	0	-	-	-	-	0	0	0	0
45-59	0	0	-	-	-	-	0	0	0	0
60+	0	0	-	-	-	-	0	0	0	0
All ages	0	0	-	-	-	-	0	0	0	0
Females										
0-4	0	0	-	-	-	-	0	0	0	0
5-14	0	0	-	-	-	-	0	0	0	0
15-44	212	283	-	-	19.0	-	0	0	0	0
45-59	0	0	-	-	-	-	0	0	0	0
60+	0	0	-	-	-	-	0	0	0	0
All ages	212	117	-	-	19.0	-	0	0	0	0
Total	212	61	-	-	19.0	-	0	0	0	0

Table 118c India - India - Inde — Obstructed labour - Episodes

Age group (years)	Incidence 1990 Number ('000s)	Rate (per 100 000)	Prevalence 1990 Number ('000s)	Rate (per 100 000)	Avg. age at onset (years)	Average duration (years)	Deaths 1990 Number ('000s)	Rate (per 100 000)	Deaths 2000 (Projected) Number ('000s)	Rate (per 100 000)
Males										
0-4	0	0	-	-	-	-	0	0	0	0
5-14	0	0	-	-	-	-	0	0	0	0
15-44	0	0	-	-	-	-	0	0	0	0
45-59	0	0	-	-	-	-	0	0	0	0
60+	0	0	-	-	-	-	0	0	0	0
All ages	0	0	-	-	-	-	0	0	0	0
Females										
0-4	0	0	-	-	-	-	0	0.0	0	0.0
5-14	0	0	-	-	-	-	0	0.0	0	0.0
15-44	1 549	845	-	-	19.0	-	9	4.9	4	1.8
45-59	51	110	-	-	52.4	-	0	0.6	0	0.3
60+	0	0	-	-	-	-	0	0.0	0	0.0
All ages	1 600	390	-	-	20.1	-	9	2.2	4	0.9
Total	1 600	188	-	-	20.1	-	9	1.1	4	0.4

For epidemiological sources see Abou-Zahr 1996. For the methods used to estimate and project incidence, prevalence, and deaths see Murray and Lopez 1996a. See explanatory notes for definitions and caveats.

Table 118
Obstructed labour

Cuadro 118
Parto obstruido

Tableau 118
Dystocie d'obstacle

Episodes

Episodios

Episodes

Table 118d **China - China - Chine**   Obstructed labour - Episodes

Age group (years)	Incidence 1990 Number ('000s)	Rate (per 100 000)	Prevalence 1990 Number ('000s)	Rate (per 100 000)	Avg. age at onset (years)	Average duration (years)	Deaths 1990 Number ('000s)	Rate (per 100 000)	Deaths 2000 (Projected) Number ('000s)	Rate (per 100 000)
Males										
0-4	0	0	-	-	-	-	0	0	0	0
5-14	0	0	-	-	-	-	0	0	0	0
15-44	0	0	-	-	-	-	0	0	0	0
45-59	0	0	-	-	-	-	0	0	0	0
60+	0	0	-	-	-	-	0	0	0	0
All ages	0	0	-	-	-	-	0	0	0	0
Females										
0-4	0	0	-	-	-	-	0	0.0	0	0
5-14	0	0	-	-	-	-	0	0.0	0	0
15-44	1 005	354	-	-	19.0	-	0	0.1	0	0
45-59	63	98	-	-	52.4	-	0	0.0	0	0
60+	0	0	-	-	-	-	0	0.0	0	0
All ages	1 068	195	-	-	21.0	-	0	0.1	0	0
Total	1 068	94	-	-	21.0	-	0	0.0	0	0

Table 118e **OAI - OPAI - APAI**   Obstructed labour - Episodes

Age group (years)	Incidence 1990 Number ('000s)	Rate (per 100 000)	Prevalence 1990 Number ('000s)	Rate (per 100 000)	Avg. age at onset (years)	Average duration (years)	Deaths 1990 Number ('000s)	Rate (per 100 000)	Deaths 2000 (Projected) Number ('000s)	Rate (per 100 000)
Males										
0-4	0	0	-	-	-	-	0	0	0	0
5-14	0	0	-	-	-	-	0	0	0	0
15-44	0	0	-	-	-	-	0	0	0	0
45-59	0	0	-	-	-	-	0	0	0	0
60+	0	0	-	-	-	-	0	0	0	0
All ages	0	0	-	-	-	-	0	0	0	0
Females										
0-4	0	0	-	-	-	-	0	0.0	0	0.0
5-14	0	0	-	-	-	-	0	0.0	0	0.0
15-44	1 046	655	-	-	19.0	-	4	2.5	2	1.0
45-59	44	124	-	-	52.2	-	0	0.5	0	0.2
60+	0	0	-	-	-	-	0	0.0	0	0.0
All ages	1 090	321	-	-	20.3	-	4	1.2	2	0.5
Total	1 090	160	-	-	20.3	-	4	0.6	2	0.3

Table 118f **SSA - ASS - ASS**   Obstructed labour - Episodes

Age group (years)	Incidence 1990 Number ('000s)	Rate (per 100 000)	Prevalence 1990 Number ('000s)	Rate (per 100 000)	Avg. age at onset (years)	Average duration (years)	Deaths 1990 Number ('000s)	Rate (per 100 000)	Deaths 2000 (Projected) Number ('000s)	Rate (per 100 000)
Males										
0-4	0	0	-	-	-	-	0	0	0	0
5-14	0	0	-	-	-	-	0	0	0	0
15-44	0	0	-	-	-	-	0	0	0	0
45-59	0	0	-	-	-	-	0	0	0	0
60+	0	0	-	-	-	-	0	0	0	0
All ages	0	0	-	-	-	-	0	0	0	0
Females										
0-4	0	0	-	-	-	-	0	0.0	0	0.0
5-14	85	122	-	-	10.0	-	1	1.1	1	0.6
15-44	1 511	1 422	-	-	19.0	-	14	13.3	8	5.8
45-59	3	15	-	-	52.2	-	0	0.1	0	0.1
60+	0	0	-	-	-	-	0	0.0	0	0.0
All ages	1 600	620	-	-	18.6	-	15	5.8	9	2.6
Total	1 600	314	-	-	18.6	-	15	2.9	9	1.3

For epidemiological sources see Abou-Zahr 1996. For the methods used to estimate and project incidence, prevalence, and deaths see Murray and Lopez 1996a. See explanatory notes for definitions and caveats.

Table 118 Obstructed labour

Cuadro 118 Parto obstruido

Tableau 118 Dystocie d'obstacle

Episodes

Episodios

Episodes

Table 118g   LAC - ALC - ALC   Obstructed labour - Episodes

Age group (years)	Incidence 1990 Number ('000s)	Rate (per 100 000)	Prevalence 1990 Number ('000s)	Rate (per 100 000)	Avg. age at onset (years)	Average duration (years)	Deaths 1990 Number ('000s)	Rate (per 100 000)	Deaths 2000 (Projected) Number ('000s)	Rate (per 100 000)
Males										
0-4	0	0	-	-	-	-	0	0	0	0
5-14	0	0	-	-	-	-	0	0	0	0
15-44	0	0	-	-	-	-	0	0	0	0
45-59	0	0	-	-	-	-	0	0	0	0
60+	0	0	-	-	-	-	0	0	0	0
All ages	0	0	-	-	-	-	0	0	0	0
Females										
0-4	0	0	-	-	-	-	0	0.0	0	0.0
5-14	4	7	-	-	10.0	-	0	0.0	0	0.0
15-44	498	478	-	-	19.0	-	2	1.5	1	0.7
45-59	3	14	-	-	52.4	-	0	0.0	0	0.0
60+	0	0	-	-	-	-	0	0.0	0	0.0
All ages	505	227	-	-	19.2	-	2	0.7	1	0.3
Total	505	114	-	-	19.2	-	2	0.4	1	0.2

Table 118h   MEC - AOM - CMO   Obstructed labour - Episodes

Age group (years)	Incidence 1990 Number ('000s)	Rate (per 100 000)	Prevalence 1990 Number ('000s)	Rate (per 100 000)	Avg. age at onset (years)	Average duration (years)	Deaths 1990 Number ('000s)	Rate (per 100 000)	Deaths 2000 (Projected) Number ('000s)	Rate (per 100 000)
Males										
0-4	0	0	-	-	-	-	0	0	0	0
5-14	0	0	-	-	-	-	0	0	0	0
15-44	0	0	-	-	-	-	0	0	0	0
45-59	0	0	-	-	-	-	0	0	0	0
60+	0	0	-	-	-	-	0	0	0	0
All ages	0	0	-	-	-	-	0	0	0	0
Females										
0-4	0	0	-	-	-	-	0	0.0	0	0.0
5-14	1	2	-	-	10.0	-	0	0.0	0	0.0
15-44	1 175	1 096	-	-	19.0	-	4	3.5	2	1.6
45-59	75	337	-	-	52.3	-	0	1.1	0	0.6
60+	0	0	-	-	-	-	0	0.0	0	0.0
All ages	1 252	507	-	-	21.0	-	4	1.6	2	0.8
Total	1 252	249	-	-	21.0	-	4	0.8	2	0.4

Table 118i   World - Mundo - Monde   Obstructed labour - Episodes

Age group (years)	Incidence 1990 Number ('000s)	Rate (per 100 000)	Prevalence 1990 Number ('000s)	Rate (per 100 000)	Avg. age at onset (years)	Average duration (years)	Deaths 1990 Number ('000s)	Rate (per 100 000)	Deaths 2000 (Projected) Number ('000s)	Rate (per 100 000)
Males										
0-4	0	0	-	-	-	-	0	0	0	0
5-14	0	0	-	-	-	-	0	0	0	0
15-44	0	0	-	-	-	-	0	0	0	0
45-59	0	0	-	-	-	-	0	0	0	0
60+	0	0	-	-	-	-	0	0	0	0
All ages	0	0	-	-	-	-	0	0	0	0
Females										
0-4	0	0	-	-	-	-	0	0.0	0	0.0
5-14	90	17	-	-	10.0	-	1	0.2	1	0.1
15-44	7 308	610	-	-	19.0	-	33	2.7	18	1.3
45-59	239	77	-	-	52.4	-	1	0.2	1	0.1
60+	0	0	-	-	-	-	0	0.0	0	0.0
All ages	7 638	292	-	-	19.9	-	34	1.3	19	0.6
Total	7 638	145	-	-	19.9	-	34	0.7	19	0.3

For epidemiological sources see Abou-Zahr 1996. For the methods used to estimate and project incidence, prevalence, and deaths see Murray and Lopez 1996a. See explanatory notes for definitions and caveats.

Table 119
Obstructed labour

Cuadro 119
Parto obstruido

Tableau 119
Dystocie d'obstacle

Stress incontinence

Incontinencia por stress

Incontinence urinaire de stress

Table 119a   **EME - PEMC - EMBE**   Obstructed labour - Stress incontinence

Age group (years)	Incidence 1990 Number ('000s)	Rate (per 100 000)	Prevalence 1990 Number ('000s)	Rate (per 100 000)	Avg. age at onset (years)	Average duration (years)	Deaths 1990 Number ('000s)	Rate (per 100 000)	Deaths 2000 (Projected) Number ('000s)	Rate (per 100 000)
Males										
0-4	0	0	0	0	-	-	0	0	0	0
5-14	0	0	0	0	-	-	0	0	0	0
15-44	0	0	0	0	-	-	0	0	0	0
45-59	0	0	0	0	-	-	0	0	0	0
60+	0	0	0	0	-	-	0	0	0	0
All ages	0	0	0	0	-	-	0	0	0	0
Females										
0-4	0	0	0	0	-	-	0	0	0	0
5-14	0	0	0	0	-	-	0	0	0	0
15-44	312	174	4 715	2 631	29.8	50.1	0	0	0	0
45-59	0	0	3 541	5 223	-	-	0	0	0	0
60+	0	0	4 417	5 223	-	-	0	0	0	0
All ages	312	77	12 673	3 111	29.8	50.1	0	0	0	0
Total	312	39	12 673	1 589	29.8	50.1	0	0	0	0

Table 119b   **FSE - PEAS - AESE**   Obstructed labour - Stress incontinence

Age group (years)	Incidence 1990 Number ('000s)	Rate (per 100 000)	Prevalence 1990 Number ('000s)	Rate (per 100 000)	Avg. age at onset (years)	Average duration (years)	Deaths 1990 Number ('000s)	Rate (per 100 000)	Deaths 2000 (Projected) Number ('000s)	Rate (per 100 000)
Males										
0-4	0	0	0	0	-	-	0	0	0	0
5-14	0	0	0	0	-	-	0	0	0	0
15-44	0	0	0	0	-	-	0	0	0	0
45-59	0	0	0	0	-	-	0	0	0	0
60+	0	0	0	0	-	-	0	0	0	0
All ages	0	0	0	0	-	-	0	0	0	0
Females										
0-4	0	0	0	0	-	-	0	0	0	0
5-14	0	0	0	0	-	-	0	0	0	0
15-44	212	283	3 217	4 292	29.7	47.0	0	0	0	0
45-59	0	0	2 546	8 484	-	-	0	0	0	0
60+	0	0	3 088	8 484	-	-	0	0	0	0
All ages	212	117	8 850	4 892	29.7	47.0	0	0	0	0
Total	212	61	8 850	2 556	29.7	47.0	0	0	0	0

Table 119c   **India - India - Inde**   Obstructed labour - Stress incontinence

Age group (years)	Incidence 1990 Number ('000s)	Rate (per 100 000)	Prevalence 1990 Number ('000s)	Rate (per 100 000)	Avg. age at onset (years)	Average duration (years)	Deaths 1990 Number ('000s)	Rate (per 100 000)	Deaths 2000 (Projected) Number ('000s)	Rate (per 100 000)
Males										
0-4	0	0	0	0	-	-	0	0	0	0
5-14	0	0	0	0	-	-	0	0	0	0
15-44	0	0	0	0	-	-	0	0	0	0
45-59	0	0	0	0	-	-	0	0	0	0
60+	0	0	0	0	-	-	0	0	0	0
All ages	0	0	0	0	-	-	0	0	0	0
Females										
0-4	0	0	0	0	-	-	0	0	0	0
5-14	0	0	0	0	-	-	0	0	0	0
15-44	1 528	834	23 639	12 901	29.1	42.4	0	0	0	0
45-59	0	0	11 485	24 966	-	-	0	0	0	0
60+	0	0	7 221	24 966	-	-	0	0	0	0
All ages	1 528	373	42 346	10 325	29.1	42.4	0	0	0	0
Total	1 528	180	42 346	4 985	29.1	42.4	0	0	0	0

For epidemiological sources see Abou-Zahr 1996. For the methods used to estimate and project incidence, prevalence, and deaths see Murray and Lopez 1996a. See explanatory notes for definitions and caveats.

Table 119
Obstructed labour

Cuadro 119
Parto obstruido

Tableau 119
Dystocie d'obstacle

Stress incontinence

Incontinencia por stress

Incontinence urinaire de stress

Table 119d China - China - Chine   Obstructed labour - Stress incontinence

Age group (years)	Incidence 1990 Number ('000s)	Rate (per 100 000)	Prevalence 1990 Number ('000s)	Rate (per 100 000)	Avg. age at onset (years)	Average duration (years)	Deaths 1990 Number ('000s)	Rate (per 100 000)	Deaths 2000 (Projected) Number ('000s)	Rate (per 100 000)
Males										
0-4	0	0	0	0	-	-	0	0	0	0
5-14	0	0	0	0	-	-	0	0	0	0
15-44	0	0	0	0	-	-	0	0	0	0
45-59	0	0	0	0	-	-	0	0	0	0
60+	0	0	0	0	-	-	0	0	0	0
All ages	0	0	0	0	-	-	0	0	0	0
Females										
0-4	0	0	0	0	-	-	0	0	0	0
5-14	0	0	0	0	-	-	0	0	0	0
15-44	746	263	11 284	3 972	29.7	44.4	0	0	0	0
45-59	0	0	5 073	7 877	-	-	0	0	0	0
60+	0	0	4 070	7 877	-	-	0	0	0	0
All ages	746	136	20 427	3 724	29.7	44.4	0	0	0	0
Total	746	66	20 427	1 802	29.7	44.4	0	0	0	0

Table 119e OAI - OPAI - APAI   Obstructed labour - Stress incontinence

Age group (years)	Incidence 1990 Number ('000s)	Rate (per 100 000)	Prevalence 1990 Number ('000s)	Rate (per 100 000)	Avg. age at onset (years)	Average duration (years)	Deaths 1990 Number ('000s)	Rate (per 100 000)	Deaths 2000 (Projected) Number ('000s)	Rate (per 100 000)
Males										
0-4	0	0	0	0	-	-	0	0	0	0
5-14	0	0	0	0	-	-	0	0	0	0
15-44	0	0	0	0	-	-	0	0	0	0
45-59	0	0	0	0	-	-	0	0	0	0
60+	0	0	0	0	-	-	0	0	0	0
All ages	0	0	0	0	-	-	0	0	0	0
Females										
0-4	0	0	0	0	-	-	0	0	0	0
5-14	0	0	0	0	-	-	0	0	0	0
15-44	1 026	643	15 705	9 839	29.3	41.9	0	0	0	0
45-59	0	0	6 757	19 257	-	-	0	0	0	0
60+	0	0	4 364	19 257	-	-	0	0	0	0
All ages	1 026	302	26 826	7 900	29.3	41.9	0	0	0	0
Total	1 026	150	26 826	3 930	29.3	41.9	0	0	0	0

Table 119f SSA - ASS - ASS   Obstructed labour - Stress incontinence

Age group (years)	Incidence 1990 Number ('000s)	Rate (per 100 000)	Prevalence 1990 Number ('000s)	Rate (per 100 000)	Avg. age at onset (years)	Average duration (years)	Deaths 1990 Number ('000s)	Rate (per 100 000)	Deaths 2000 (Projected) Number ('000s)	Rate (per 100 000)
Males										
0-4	0	0	0	0	-	-	0	0	0	0
5-14	0	0	0	0	-	-	0	0	0	0
15-44	0	0	0	0	-	-	0	0	0	0
45-59	0	0	0	0	-	-	0	0	0	0
60+	0	0	0	0	-	-	0	0	0	0
All ages	0	0	0	0	-	-	0	0	0	0
Females										
0-4	0	0	0	0	-	-	0	0	0	0
5-14	0	0	0	0	-	-	0	0	0	0
15-44	1 491	1 403	23 422	22 043	28.4	38.2	0	0	0	0
45-59	0	0	9 229	41 727	-	-	0	0	0	0
60+	0	0	5 312	41 727	-	-	0	0	0	0
All ages	1 491	578	37 963	14 717	28.4	38.2	0	0	0	0
Total	1 491	292	37 963	7 440	28.4	38.2	0	0	0	0

For epidemiological sources see Abou-Zahr 1996. For the methods used to estimate and project incidence, prevalence, and deaths see Murray and Lopez 1996a. See explanatory notes for definitions and caveats.

Table 119
Obstructed labour

Cuadro 119
Parto obstruido

Tableau 119
Dystocie d'obstacle

Stress incontinence

Incontinencia por stress

Incontinence urinaire de stress

Table 119g LAC - ALC - ALC — Obstructed labour - Stress incontinence

Age group (years)	Incidence 1990 Number ('000s)	Rate (per 100 000)	Prevalence 1990 Number ('000s)	Rate (per 100 000)	Avg. age at onset (years)	Average duration (years)	Deaths 1990 Number ('000s)	Rate (per 100 000)	Deaths 2000 (Projected) Number ('000s)	Rate (per 100 000)
Males										
0-4	0	0	0	0	-	-	0	0	0	0
5-14	0	0	0	0	-	-	0	0	0	0
15-44	0	0	0	0	-	-	0	0	0	0
45-59	0	0	0	0	-	-	0	0	0	0
60+	0	0	0	0	-	-	0	0	0	0
All ages	0	0	0	0	-	-	0	0	0	0
Females										
0-4	0	0	0	0	-	-	0	0	0	0
5-14	0	0	0	0	-	-	0	0	0	0
15-44	486	467	7 403	7 113	29.5	45.0	0	0	0	0
45-59	0	0	3 269	13 999	-	-	0	0	0	0
60+	0	0	2 355	13 999	-	-	0	0	0	0
All ages	486	218	13 028	5 850	29.5	45.0	0	0	0	0
Total	486	109	13 028	2 932	29.5	45.0	0	0	0	0

Table 119h MEC - AOM - CMO — Obstructed labour - Stress incontinence

Age group (years)	Incidence 1990 Number ('000s)	Rate (per 100 000)	Prevalence 1990 Number ('000s)	Rate (per 100 000)	Avg. age at onset (years)	Average duration (years)	Deaths 1990 Number ('000s)	Rate (per 100 000)	Deaths 2000 (Projected) Number ('000s)	Rate (per 100 000)
Males										
0-4	0	0	0	0	-	-	0	0	0	0
5-14	0	0	0	0	-	-	0	0	0	0
15-44	0	0	0	0	-	-	0	0	0	0
45-59	0	0	0	0	-	-	0	0	0	0
60+	0	0	0	0	-	-	0	0	0	0
All ages	0	0	0	0	-	-	0	0	0	0
Females										
0-4	0	0	0	0	-	-	0	0	0	0
5-14	0	0	0	0	-	-	0	0	0	0
15-44	1 159	1 081	18 324	17 092	29.0	43.5	0	0	0	0
45-59	0	0	7 217	32 374	-	-	0	0	0	0
60+	0	0	5 002	32 374	-	-	0	0	0	0
All ages	1 159	470	30 543	12 381	29.0	43.5	0	0	0	0
Total	1 159	230	30 543	6 071	29.0	43.5	0	0	0	0

Table 119i World - Mundo - Monde — Obstructed labour - Stress incontinence

Age group (years)	Incidence 1990 Number ('000s)	Rate (per 100 000)	Prevalence 1990 Number ('000s)	Rate (per 100 000)	Avg. age at onset (years)	Average duration (years)	Deaths 1990 Number ('000s)	Rate (per 100 000)	Deaths 2000 (Projected) Number ('000s)	Rate (per 100 000)
Males										
0-4	0	0	0	0	-	-	0	0	0	0
5-14	0	0	0	0	-	-	0	0	0	0
15-44	0	0	0	0	-	-	0	0	0	0
45-59	0	0	0	0	-	-	0	0	0	0
60+	0	0	0	0	-	-	0	0	0	0
All ages	0	0	0	0	-	-	0	0	0	0
Females										
0-4	0	0	0	0	-	-	0	0	0	0
5-14	0	0	0	0	-	-	0	0	0	0
15-44	6 960	581	107 710	8 986	29.1	42.5	0	0	0	0
45-59	0	0	49 118	15 791	-	-	0	0	0	0
60+	0	0	35 828	13 308	-	-	0	0	0	0
All ages	6 960	266	192 656	7 371	29.1	42.5	0	0	0	0
Total	6 960	132	192 656	3 658	29.1	42.5	0	0	0	0

For epidemiological sources see Abou-Zahr 1996. For the methods used to estimate and project incidence, prevalence, and deaths see Murray and Lopez 1996a. See explanatory notes for definitions and caveats.

Table 120
Obstructed labour

Cuadro 120
Parto obstruido

Tableau 120
Dystocie d'obstacle

Rectovaginal fistula

Fístula rectovaginal

Fistule recto-vaginale

Table 120a **EME - PEMC - EMBE** Obstructed labour - Rectovaginal fistula

Age group (years)	Incidence 1990 Number ('000s)	Rate (per 100 000)	Prevalence 1990 Number ('000s)	Rate (per 100 000)	Avg. age at onset (years)	Average duration (years)	Deaths 1990 Number ('000s)	Rate (per 100 000)	Deaths 2000 (Projected) Number ('000s)	Rate (per 100 000)
Males										
0-4	0	0	0	0	-	-	-	-	-	-
5-14	0	0	0	0	-	-	-	-	-	-
15-44	0	0	0	0	-	-	-	-	-	-
45-59	0	0	0	0	-	-	-	-	-	-
60+	0	0	0	0	-	-	-	-	-	-
All ages	0	0	0	0	-	-	-	-	-	-
Females										
0-4	0	0	0	0	-	-	-	-	-	-
5-14	0	0	0	0	-	-	-	-	-	-
15-44	0	0	0	0	-	-	-	-	-	-
45-59	0	0	0	0	-	-	-	-	-	-
60+	0	0	0	0	-	-	-	-	-	-
All ages	0	0	0	0	-	-	-	-	-	-
Total	0	0	0	0	-	-	-	-	-	-

Table 120b **FSE - PEAS - AESE** Obstructed labour - Rectovaginal fistula

Age group (years)	Incidence 1990 Number ('000s)	Rate (per 100 000)	Prevalence 1990 Number ('000s)	Rate (per 100 000)	Avg. age at onset (years)	Average duration (years)	Deaths 1990 Number ('000s)	Rate (per 100 000)	Deaths 2000 (Projected) Number ('000s)	Rate (per 100 000)
Males										
0-4	0	0	0	0	-	-	-	-	-	-
5-14	0	0	0	0	-	-	-	-	-	-
15-44	0	0	0	0	-	-	-	-	-	-
45-59	0	0	0	0	-	-	-	-	-	-
60+	0	0	0	0	-	-	-	-	-	-
All ages	0	0	0	0	-	-	-	-	-	-
Females										
0-4	0	0	0	0	-	-	-	-	-	-
5-14	0	0	0	0	-	-	-	-	-	-
15-44	0	0	0	0	-	-	-	-	-	-
45-59	0	0	0	0	-	-	-	-	-	-
60+	0	0	0	0	-	-	-	-	-	-
All ages	0	0	0	0	-	-	-	-	-	-
Total	0	0	0	0	-	-	-	-	-	-

Table 120c **India - India - Inde** Obstructed labour - Rectovaginal fistula

Age group (years)	Incidence 1990 Number ('000s)	Rate (per 100 000)	Prevalence 1990 Number ('000s)	Rate (per 100 000)	Avg. age at onset (years)	Average duration (years)	Deaths 1990 Number ('000s)	Rate (per 100 000)	Deaths 2000 (Projected) Number ('000s)	Rate (per 100 000)
Males										
0-4	0	0	0	0	-	-	-	-	-	-
5-14	0	0	0	0	-	-	-	-	-	-
15-44	0	0	0	0	-	-	-	-	-	-
45-59	0	0	0	0	-	-	-	-	-	-
60+	0	0	0	0	-	-	-	-	-	-
All ages	0	0	0	0	-	-	-	-	-	-
Females										
0-4	0	0.0	0	0	-	-	-	-	-	-
5-14	0	0.0	0	0	-	-	-	-	-	-
15-44	21	11.5	139	76	19.0	12.4	-	-	-	-
45-59	0	0.0	34	74	-	-	-	-	-	-
60+	0	0.0	21	74	-	-	-	-	-	-
All ages	21	5.1	194	47	19.0	12.4	-	-	-	-
Total	21	2.5	194	23	19.0	12.4	-	-	-	-

For epidemiological sources see Abou-Zahr 1996. For the methods used to estimate and project incidence, prevalence, and deaths see Murray and Lopez 1996a. See explanatory notes for definitions and caveats.

Table 120	Cuadro 120	Tableau 120
Obstructed labour	Parto obstruido	Dystocie d'obstacle

Rectovaginal fistula   Fístula rectovaginal   Fistule recto-vaginale

Table 120d   China - China - Chine   Obstructed labour - Rectovaginal fistula

Age group (years)	Incidence 1990 Number ('000s)	Rate (per 100 000)	Prevalence 1990 Number ('000s)	Rate (per 100 000)	Avg. age at onset (years)	Average duration (years)	Deaths 1990 Number ('000s)	Rate (per 100 000)	Deaths 2000 (Projected) Number ('000s)	Rate (per 100 000)
Males										
0-4	0	0	0	0	-	-	-	-	-	-
5-14	0	0	0	0	-	-	-	-	-	-
15-44	0	0	0	0	-	-	-	-	-	-
45-59	0	0	0	0	-	-	-	-	-	-
60+	0	0	0	0	-	-	-	-	-	-
All ages	0	0	0	0	-	-	-	-	-	-
Females										
0-4	0	0.0	0	0.0	-	-	-	-	-	-
5-14	0	0.0	0	0.0	-	-	-	-	-	-
15-44	8	2.8	27	9.4	19.0	6.2	-	-	-	-
45-59	0	0.0	5	8.2	-	-	-	-	-	-
60+	0	0.0	4	8.2	-	-	-	-	-	-
All ages	8	1.5	36	6.6	19.0	6.2	-	-	-	-
Total	8	0.7	36	3.2	19.0	6.2	-	-	-	-

Table 120e   OAI - OPAI - APAI   Obstructed labour - Rectovaginal fistula

Age group (years)	Incidence 1990 Number ('000s)	Rate (per 100 000)	Prevalence 1990 Number ('000s)	Rate (per 100 000)	Avg. age at onset (years)	Average duration (years)	Deaths 1990 Number ('000s)	Rate (per 100 000)	Deaths 2000 (Projected) Number ('000s)	Rate (per 100 000)
Males										
0-4	0	0	0	0	-	-	-	-	-	-
5-14	0	0	0	0	-	-	-	-	-	-
15-44	0	0	0	0	-	-	-	-	-	-
45-59	0	0	0	0	-	-	-	-	-	-
60+	0	0	0	0	-	-	-	-	-	-
All ages	0	0	0	0	-	-	-	-	-	-
Females										
0-4	0	0.0	0	0	-	-	-	-	-	-
5-14	0	0.0	0	0	-	-	-	-	-	-
15-44	13	8.0	58	36	19.0	8.0	-	-	-	-
45-59	0	0.0	12	33	-	-	-	-	-	-
60+	0	0.0	7	33	-	-	-	-	-	-
All ages	13	3.8	77	23	19.0	8.0	-	-	-	-
Total	13	1.9	77	11	19.0	8.0	-	-	-	-

Table 120f   SSA - ASS - ASS   Obstructed labour - Rectovaginal fistula

Age group (years)	Incidence 1990 Number ('000s)	Rate (per 100 000)	Prevalence 1990 Number ('000s)	Rate (per 100 000)	Avg. age at onset (years)	Average duration (years)	Deaths 1990 Number ('000s)	Rate (per 100 000)	Deaths 2000 (Projected) Number ('000s)	Rate (per 100 000)
Males										
0-4	0	0	0	0	-	-	-	-	-	-
5-14	0	0	0	0	-	-	-	-	-	-
15-44	0	0	0	0	-	-	-	-	-	-
45-59	0	0	0	0	-	-	-	-	-	-
60+	0	0	0	0	-	-	-	-	-	-
All ages	0	0	0	0	-	-	-	-	-	-
Females										
0-4	0	0.0	0	0	-	-	-	-	-	-
5-14	0	0.0	0	0	-	-	-	-	-	-
15-44	20	18.8	196	184	19.0	17.4	-	-	-	-
45-59	0	0.0	42	190	-	-	-	-	-	-
60+	0	0.0	24	190	-	-	-	-	-	-
All ages	20	7.7	262	102	19.0	17.4	-	-	-	-
Total	20	3.9	262	51	19.0	17.4	-	-	-	-

For epidemiological sources see Abou-Zahr 1996. For the methods used to estimate and project incidence, prevalence, and deaths see Murray and Lopez 1996a. See explanatory notes for definitions and caveats.

Table 120	Cuadro 120	Tableau 120
Obstructed labour	**Parto obstruido**	**Dystocie d'obstacle**
Rectovaginal fistula	Fístula rectovaginal	Fistule recto-vaginale

Table 120g   LAC - ALC - ALC   Obstructed labour - Rectovaginal fistula

Age group (years)	Incidence 1990 Number ('000s)	Rate (per 100 000)	Prevalence 1990 Number ('000s)	Rate (per 100 000)	Avg. age at onset (years)	Average duration (years)	Deaths 1990 Number ('000s)	Rate (per 100 000)	Deaths 2000 (Projected) Number ('000s)	Rate (per 100 000)
Males										
0-4	0	0	0	0	-	-	-	-	-	-
5-14	0	0	0	0	-	-	-	-	-	-
15-44	0	0	0	0	-	-	-	-	-	-
45-59	0	0	0	0	-	-	-	-	-	-
60+	0	0	0	0	-	-	-	-	-	-
All ages	0	0	0	0	-	-	-	-	-	-
Females										
0-4	0	0.0	0	0.0	-	-	-	-	-	-
5-14	0	0.0	0	0.0	-	-	-	-	-	-
15-44	4	3.8	13	12.7	19.0	6.1	-	-	-	-
45-59	0	0.0	3	11.0	-	-	-	-	-	-
60+	0	0.0	2	11.0	-	-	-	-	-	-
All ages	4	1.8	18	7.9	19.0	6.1	-	-	-	-
Total	4	0.9	18	4.0	19.0	6.1	-	-	-	-

Table 120h   MEC - AOM - CMO   Obstructed labour - Rectovaginal fistula

Age group (years)	Incidence 1990 Number ('000s)	Rate (per 100 000)	Prevalence 1990 Number ('000s)	Rate (per 100 000)	Avg. age at onset (years)	Average duration (years)	Deaths 1990 Number ('000s)	Rate (per 100 000)	Deaths 2000 (Projected) Number ('000s)	Rate (per 100 000)
Males										
0-4	0	0	0	0	-	-	-	-	-	-
5-14	0	0	0	0	-	-	-	-	-	-
15-44	0	0	0	0	-	-	-	-	-	-
45-59	0	0	0	0	-	-	-	-	-	-
60+	0	0	0	0	-	-	-	-	-	-
All ages	0	0	0	0	-	-	-	-	-	-
Females										
0-4	0	0.0	0	0	-	-	-	-	-	-
5-14	0	0.0	0	0	-	-	-	-	-	-
15-44	16	14.9	52	48	19.0	5.8	-	-	-	-
45-59	0	0.0	9	41	-	-	-	-	-	-
60+	0	0.0	6	41	-	-	-	-	-	-
All ages	16	6.5	67	27	19.0	5.8	-	-	-	-
Total	16	3.2	67	13	19.0	5.8	-	-	-	-

Table 120i   World - Mundo - Monde   Obstructed labour - Rectovaginal fistula

Age group (years)	Incidence 1990 Number ('000s)	Rate (per 100 000)	Prevalence 1990 Number ('000s)	Rate (per 100 000)	Avg. age at onset (years)	Average duration (years)	Deaths 1990 Number ('000s)	Rate (per 100 000)	Deaths 2000 (Projected) Number ('000s)	Rate (per 100 000)
Males										
0-4	0	0	0	0	-	-	-	-	-	-
5-14	0	0	0	0	-	-	-	-	-	-
15-44	0	0	0	0	-	-	-	-	-	-
45-59	0	0	0	0	-	-	-	-	-	-
60+	0	0	0	0	-	-	-	-	-	-
All ages	0	0	0	0	-	-	-	-	-	-
Females										
0-4	0	0.0	0	0	-	-	-	-	-	-
5-14	0	0.0	0	0	-	-	-	-	-	-
15-44	82	6.8	484	40	19.0	10.7	-	-	-	-
45-59	0	0.0	105	34	-	-	-	-	-	-
60+	0	0.0	65	24	-	-	-	-	-	-
All ages	82	3.1	654	25	19.0	10.7	-	-	-	-
Total	82	1.6	654	12	19.0	10.7	-	-	-	-

For epidemiological sources see Abou-Zahr 1996. For the methods used to estimate and project incidence, prevalence, and deaths see Murray and Lopez 1996a. See explanatory notes for definitions and caveats.

Table 121	Cuadro 121	Tableau 121
Abortion	Aborto	Avortement

Episodes	Episodios	Episodes

Table 121a EME - PEMC - EMBE — Abortion - Episodes

Age group (years)	Incidence 1990 Number ('000s)	Rate (per 100 000)	Prevalence 1990 Number ('000s)	Rate (per 100 000)	Avg. age at onset (years)	Average duration (years)	Deaths 1990 Number ('000s)	Rate (per 100 000)	Deaths 2000 (Projected) Number ('000s)	Rate (per 100 000)
Males										
0-4	0	0	-	-	-	-	0	0	0	0
5-14	0	0	-	-	-	-	0	0	0	0
15-44	0	0	-	-	-	-	0	0	0	0
45-59	0	0	-	-	-	-	0	0	0	0
60+	0	0	-	-	-	-	0	0	0	0
All ages	0	0	-	-	-	-	0	0	0	0
Females										
0-4	0	0	-	-	-	-	0	0.0	0	0
5-14	0	0	-	-	-	-	0	0.0	0	0
15-44	123	69	-	-	30.0	-	0	0.1	0	0
45-59	3	4	-	-	52.4	-	0	0.0	0	0
60+	0	0	-	-	-	-	0	0.0	0	0
All ages	126	31	-	-	30.4	-	0	0.0	0	0
Total	126	16	-	-	30.4	-	0	0.0	0	0

Table 121b FSE - PEAS - AESE — Abortion - Episodes

Age group (years)	Incidence 1990 Number ('000s)	Rate (per 100 000)	Prevalence 1990 Number ('000s)	Rate (per 100 000)	Avg. age at onset (years)	Average duration (years)	Deaths 1990 Number ('000s)	Rate (per 100 000)	Deaths 2000 (Projected) Number ('000s)	Rate (per 100 000)
Males										
0-4	0	0	-	-	-	-	0	0	0	0
5-14	0	0	-	-	-	-	0	0	0	0
15-44	0	0	-	-	-	-	0	0	0	0
45-59	0	0	-	-	-	-	0	0	0	0
60+	0	0	-	-	-	-	0	0	0	0
All ages	0	0	-	-	-	-	0	0	0	0
Females										
0-4	0	0	-	-	-	-	0	0.0	0	0.0
5-14	0	0	-	-	-	-	0	0.0	0	0.0
15-44	1 948	2 599	-	-	29.9	-	1	1.4	1	0.8
45-59	10	33	-	-	52.4	-	0	0.0	0	0.0
60+	0	0	-	-	-	-	0	0.0	0	0.0
All ages	1 958	1 082	-	-	30.0	-	1	0.6	1	0.3
Total	1 958	565	-	-	30.0	-	1	0.3	1	0.2

Table 121c India - India - Inde — Abortion - Episodes

Age group (years)	Incidence 1990 Number ('000s)	Rate (per 100 000)	Prevalence 1990 Number ('000s)	Rate (per 100 000)	Avg. age at onset (years)	Average duration (years)	Deaths 1990 Number ('000s)	Rate (per 100 000)	Deaths 2000 (Projected) Number ('000s)	Rate (per 100 000)
Males										
0-4	0	0	-	-	-	-	0	0	0	0
5-14	0	0	-	-	-	-	0	0	0	0
15-44	0	0	-	-	-	-	0	0	0	0
45-59	0	0	-	-	-	-	0	0	0	0
60+	0	0	-	-	-	-	0	0	0	0
All ages	0	0	-	-	-	-	0	0	0	0
Females										
0-4	0	0	-	-	-	-	0	0.0	0	0.0
5-14	0	0	-	-	-	-	0	0.0	0	0.0
15-44	4 156	2 268	-	-	29.6	-	16	9.0	8	3.3
45-59	136	295	-	-	52.4	-	1	1.2	0	0.5
60+	0	0	-	-	-	-	0	0.0	0	0.0
All ages	4 292	1 047	-	-	30.3	-	17	4.2	8	1.6
Total	4 292	505	-	-	30.3	-	17	2.0	8	0.8

For epidemiological sources see Abou-Zahr and Ahman 1996. For the methods used to estimate and project incidence, prevalence, and deaths see Murray and Lopez 1996a. See explanatory notes for definitions and caveats.

Table 121	Cuadro 121	Tableau 121
Abortion	Aborto	Avortement

Episodes · Episodios · Episodes

Table 121d China - China - Chine — Abortion - Episodes

Age group (years)	Incidence 1990 Number ('000s)	Rate (per 100 000)	Prevalence 1990 Number ('000s)	Rate (per 100 000)	Avg. age at onset (years)	Average duration (years)	Deaths 1990 Number ('000s)	Rate (per 100 000)	Deaths 2000 (Projected) Number ('000s)	Rate (per 100 000)
Males										
0-4	0	0	-	-	-	-	0	0	0	0
5-14	0	0	-	-	-	-	0	0	0	0
15-44	0	0	-	-	-	-	0	0	0	0
45-59	0	0	-	-	-	-	0	0	0	0
60+	0	0	-	-	-	-	0	0	0	0
All ages	0	0	-	-	-	-	0	0	0	0
Females										
0-4	0	0	-	-	-	-	0	0.0	0	0.0
5-14	0	0	-	-	-	-	0	0.0	0	0.0
15-44	0	0	-	-	-	-	2	0.8	1	0.2
45-59	0	0	-	-	-	-	0	0.2	0	0.1
60+	0	0	-	-	-	-	0	0.0	0	0.0
All ages	0	0	-	-	-	-	3	0.5	1	0.1
Total	0	0	-	-	-	-	3	0.2	1	0.1

Table 121e OAI - OPAI - APAI — Abortion - Episodes

Age group (years)	Incidence 1990 Number ('000s)	Rate (per 100 000)	Prevalence 1990 Number ('000s)	Rate (per 100 000)	Avg. age at onset (years)	Average duration (years)	Deaths 1990 Number ('000s)	Rate (per 100 000)	Deaths 2000 (Projected) Number ('000s)	Rate (per 100 000)
Males										
0-4	0	0	-	-	-	-	0	0	0	0
5-14	0	0	-	-	-	-	0	0	0	0
15-44	0	0	-	-	-	-	0	0	0	0
45-59	0	0	-	-	-	-	0	0	0	0
60+	0	0	-	-	-	-	0	0	0	0
All ages	0	0	-	-	-	-	0	0	0	0
Females										
0-4	0	0	-	-	-	-	0	0.0	0	0.0
5-14	0	0	-	-	-	-	0	0.0	0	0.0
15-44	3 402	2 131	-	-	29.7	-	7	4.2	3	1.7
45-59	142	404	-	-	52.2	-	0	0.8	0	0.4
60+	0	0	-	-	-	-	0	0.0	0	0.0
All ages	3 544	1 044	-	-	30.6	-	7	2.0	4	0.9
Total	3 544	519	-	-	30.6	-	7	1.0	4	0.5

Table 121f SSA - ASS - ASS — Abortion - Episodes

Age group (years)	Incidence 1990 Number ('000s)	Rate (per 100 000)	Prevalence 1990 Number ('000s)	Rate (per 100 000)	Avg. age at onset (years)	Average duration (years)	Deaths 1990 Number ('000s)	Rate (per 100 000)	Deaths 2000 (Projected) Number ('000s)	Rate (per 100 000)
Males										
0-4	0	0	-	-	-	-	0	0	0	0
5-14	0	0	-	-	-	-	0	0	0	0
15-44	0	0	-	-	-	-	0	0	0	0
45-59	0	0	-	-	-	-	0	0	0	0
60+	0	0	-	-	-	-	0	0	0	0
All ages	0	0	-	-	-	-	0	0	0	0
Females										
0-4	0	0	-	-	-	-	0	0.0	0	0.0
5-14	194	277	-	-	10.0	-	1	1.9	1	1.0
15-44	3 424	3 222	-	-	29.2	-	24	22.4	14	9.7
45-59	7	34	-	-	52.2	-	0	0.2	0	0.1
60+	0	0	-	-	-	-	0	0.0	0	0.0
All ages	3 625	1 405	-	-	28.2	-	25	9.8	15	4.3
Total	3 625	710	-	-	28.2	-	25	4.9	15	2.2

For epidemiological sources see Abou-Zahr and Ahman 1996. For the methods used to estimate and project incidence, prevalence, and deaths see Murray and Lopez 1996a. See explanatory notes for definitions and caveats.

Table 121
Abortion

Cuadro 121
Aborto

Tableau 121
Avortement

Episodes

Episodios

Episodes

Table 121g   LAC - ALC - ALC   Abortion - Episodes

Age group (years)	Incidence 1990 Number ('000s)	Incidence 1990 Rate (per 100 000)	Prevalence 1990 Number ('000s)	Prevalence 1990 Rate (per 100 000)	Avg. age at onset (years)	Average duration (years)	Deaths 1990 Number ('000s)	Deaths 1990 Rate (per 100 000)	Deaths 2000 (Projected) Number ('000s)	Deaths 2000 (Projected) Rate (per 100 000)
Males										
0-4	0	0	-	-	-	-	0	0	0	0
5-14	0	0	-	-	-	-	0	0	0	0
15-44	0	0	-	-	-	-	0	0	0	0
45-59	0	0	-	-	-	-	0	0	0	0
60+	0	0	-	-	-	-	0	0	0	0
All ages	0	0	-	-	-	-	0	0	0	0
Females										
0-4	0	0	-	-	-	-	0	0.0	0	0.0
5-14	33	66	-	-	10.0	-	0	0.1	0	0.0
15-44	4 655	4 472	-	-	29.7	-	4	4.1	2	1.9
45-59	30	131	-	-	52.4	-	0	0.1	0	0.1
60+	0	0	-	-	-	-	0	0.0	0	0.0
All ages	4 719	2 119	-	-	29.7	-	4	2.0	3	0.9
Total	4 719	1 062	-	-	29.7	-	4	1.0	3	0.5

Table 121h   MEC - AOM - CMO   Abortion - Episodes

Age group (years)	Incidence 1990 Number ('000s)	Incidence 1990 Rate (per 100 000)	Prevalence 1990 Number ('000s)	Prevalence 1990 Rate (per 100 000)	Avg. age at onset (years)	Average duration (years)	Deaths 1990 Number ('000s)	Deaths 1990 Rate (per 100 000)	Deaths 2000 (Projected) Number ('000s)	Deaths 2000 (Projected) Rate (per 100 000)
Males										
0-4	0	0	-	-	-	-	0	0	0	0
5-14	0	0	-	-	-	-	0	0	0	0
15-44	0	0	-	-	-	-	0	0	0	0
45-59	0	0	-	-	-	-	0	0	0	0
60+	0	0	-	-	-	-	0	0	0	0
All ages	0	0	-	-	-	-	0	0	0	0
Females										
0-4	0	0	-	-	-	-	0	0.0	0	0.0
5-14	3	4	-	-	10.0	-	0	0.0	0	0.0
15-44	2 190	2 043	-	-	29.8	-	4	3.5	2	1.6
45-59	140	629	-	-	52.3	-	0	1.1	0	0.6
60+	0	0	-	-	-	-	0	0.0	0	0.0
All ages	2 333	946	-	-	31.1	-	4	1.6	2	0.8
Total	2 333	464	-	-	31.1	-	4	0.8	2	0.4

Table 121i   World - Mundo - Monde   Abortion - Episodes

Age group (years)	Incidence 1990 Number ('000s)	Incidence 1990 Rate (per 100 000)	Prevalence 1990 Number ('000s)	Prevalence 1990 Rate (per 100 000)	Avg. age at onset (years)	Average duration (years)	Deaths 1990 Number ('000s)	Deaths 1990 Rate (per 100 000)	Deaths 2000 (Projected) Number ('000s)	Deaths 2000 (Projected) Rate (per 100 000)
Males										
0-4	0	0	-	-	-	-	0	0	0	0
5-14	0	0	-	-	-	-	0	0	0	0
15-44	0	0	-	-	-	-	0	0	0	0
45-59	0	0	-	-	-	-	0	0	0	0
60+	0	0	-	-	-	-	0	0	0	0
All ages	0	0	-	-	-	-	0	0	0	0
Females										
0-4	0	0	-	-	-	-	0	0.0	0	0.0
5-14	230	44	-	-	10.0	-	1	0.3	1	0.2
15-44	19 898	1 660	-	-	29.8	-	59	4.9	31	2.2
45-59	468	151	-	-	52.4	-	1	0.4	1	0.2
60+	0	0	-	-	-	-	0	0.0	0	0.0
All ages	20 596	788	-	-	30.0	-	61	2.3	33	1.1
Total	20 596	391	-	-	30.0	-	61	1.2	33	0.5

For epidemiological sources see Abou-Zahr and Ahman 1996. For the methods used to estimate and project incidence, prevalence, and deaths see Murray and Lopez 1996a. See explanatory notes for definitions and caveats.

Table 122   **Cuadro 122**   **Tableau 122**
Abortion   **Aborto**   **Avortement**

Infertility   Infertilidad   Stérilité

Table 122a   EME - PEMC - EMBE   Abortion - Infertility

Age group (years)	Incidence 1990 Number ('000s)	Rate (per 100 000)	Prevalence 1990 Number ('000s)	Rate (per 100 000)	Avg. age at onset (years)	Average duration (years)	Deaths 1990 Number ('000s)	Rate (per 100 000)	Deaths 2000 (Projected) Number ('000s)	Rate (per 100 000)
Males										
0-4	0	0	0	0	-	-	0	0	0	0
5-14	0	0	0	0	-	-	0	0	0	0
15-44	0	0	0	0	-	-	0	0	0	0
45-59	0	0	0	0	-	-	0	0	0	0
60+	0	0	0	0	-	-	0	0	0	0
All ages	0	0	0	0	-	-	0	0	0	0
Females										
0-4	0	0.0	0	0.0	-	-	0	0	0	0
5-14	0	0.0	0	0.0	-	-	0	0	0	0
15-44	4	2.2	60	33.5	25.0	15.0	0	0	0	0
45-59	0	0.0	0	0.0	-	-	0	0	0	0
60+	0	0.0	0	0.0	-	-	0	0	0	0
All ages	4	1.0	60	14.7	25.0	15.0	0	0	0	0
Total	4	0.5	60	7.5	25.0	15.0	0	0	0	0

Table 122b   FSE - PEAS - AESE   Abortion - Infertility

Age group (years)	Incidence 1990 Number ('000s)	Rate (per 100 000)	Prevalence 1990 Number ('000s)	Rate (per 100 000)	Avg. age at onset (years)	Average duration (years)	Deaths 1990 Number ('000s)	Rate (per 100 000)	Deaths 2000 (Projected) Number ('000s)	Rate (per 100 000)
Males										
0-4	0	0	0	0	-	-	0	0	0	0
5-14	0	0	0	0	-	-	0	0	0	0
15-44	0	0	0	0	-	-	0	0	0	0
45-59	0	0	0	0	-	-	0	0	0	0
60+	0	0	0	0	-	-	0	0	0	0
All ages	0	0	0	0	-	-	0	0	0	0
Females										
0-4	0	0	0	0	-	-	0	0	0	0
5-14	0	0	0	0	-	-	0	0	0	0
15-44	57	76	860	1 147	25.0	15.0	0	0	0	0
45-59	0	0	0	0	-	-	0	0	0	0
60+	0	0	0	0	-	-	0	0	0	0
All ages	57	32	860	475	25.0	15.0	0	0	0	0
Total	57	17	860	248	25.0	15.0	0	0	0	0

Table 122c   India - India - Inde   Abortion - Infertility

Age group (years)	Incidence 1990 Number ('000s)	Rate (per 100 000)	Prevalence 1990 Number ('000s)	Rate (per 100 000)	Avg. age at onset (years)	Average duration (years)	Deaths 1990 Number ('000s)	Rate (per 100 000)	Deaths 2000 (Projected) Number ('000s)	Rate (per 100 000)
Males										
0-4	0	0	0	0	-	-	0	0	0	0
5-14	0	0	0	0	-	-	0	0	0	0
15-44	0	0	0	0	-	-	0	0	0	0
45-59	0	0	0	0	-	-	0	0	0	0
60+	0	0	0	0	-	-	0	0	0	0
All ages	0	0	0	0	-	-	0	0	0	0
Females										
0-4	0	0	0	0	-	-	0	0	0	0
5-14	0	0	0	0	-	-	0	0	0	0
15-44	479	262	7 192	3 925	25.0	15.0	0	0	0	0
45-59	0	0	0	0	-	-	0	0	0	0
60+	0	0	0	0	-	-	0	0	0	0
All ages	479	117	7 192	1 754	25.0	15.0	0	0	0	0
Total	479	56	7 192	847	25.0	15.0	0	0	0	0

For epidemiological sources see Abou-Zahr and Ahman 1996. For the methods used to estimate and project incidence, prevalence, and deaths see Murray and Lopez 1996a. See explanatory notes for definitions and caveats.

Table 122	Cuadro 122	Tableau 122
Abortion	**Aborto**	**Avortement**
Infertility	Infertilidad	Stérilité

Table 122d — China - China - Chine — Abortion - Infertility

Age group (years)	Incidence 1990 Number ('000s)	Rate (per 100 000)	Prevalence 1990 Number ('000s)	Rate (per 100 000)	Avg. age at onset (years)	Average duration (years)	Deaths 1990 Number ('000s)	Rate (per 100 000)	Deaths 2000 (Projected) Number ('000s)	Rate (per 100 000)
Males										
0-4	0	0	0	0	-	-	0	0	0	0
5-14	0	0	0	0	-	-	0	0	0	0
15-44	0	0	0	0	-	-	0	0	0	0
45-59	0	0	0	0	-	-	0	0	0	0
60+	0	0	0	0	-	-	0	0	0	0
All ages	0	0	0	0	-	-	0	0	0	0
Females										
0-4	0	0	0	0	-	-	0	0	0	0
5-14	0	0	0	0	-	-	0	0	0	0
15-44	0	0	0	0	-	-	0	0	0	0
45-59	0	0	0	0	-	-	0	0	0	0
60+	0	0	0	0	-	-	0	0	0	0
All ages	0	0	0	0	-	*	0	0	0	0
Total	0	0	0	0	-	-	0	0	0	0

Table 122e — OAI - OPAI - APAI — Abortion - Infertility

Age group (years)	Incidence 1990 Number ('000s)	Rate (per 100 000)	Prevalence 1990 Number ('000s)	Rate (per 100 000)	Avg. age at onset (years)	Average duration (years)	Deaths 1990 Number ('000s)	Rate (per 100 000)	Deaths 2000 (Projected) Number ('000s)	Rate (per 100 000)
Males										
0-4	0	0	0	0	-	-	0	0	0	0
5-14	0	0	0	0	-	-	0	0	0	0
15-44	0	0	0	0	-	-	0	0	0	0
45-59	0	0	0	0	-	-	0	0	0	0
60+	0	0	0	0	-	-	0	0	0	0
All ages	0	0	0	0	-	-	0	0	0	0
Females										
0-4	0	0	0	0	-	-	0	0	0	0
5-14	0	0	0	0	-	-	0	0	0	0
15-44	252	158	3 779	2 368	25.0	15.0	0	0	0	0
45-59	0	0	0	0	-	-	0	0	0	0
60+	0	0	0	0	-	-	0	0	0	0
All ages	252	74	3 779	1 113	25.0	15.0	0	0	0	0
Total	252	37	3 779	554	25.0	15.0	0	0	0	0

Table 122f — SSA - ASS - ASS — Abortion - Infertility

Age group (years)	Incidence 1990 Number ('000s)	Rate (per 100 000)	Prevalence 1990 Number ('000s)	Rate (per 100 000)	Avg. age at onset (years)	Average duration (years)	Deaths 1990 Number ('000s)	Rate (per 100 000)	Deaths 2000 (Projected) Number ('000s)	Rate (per 100 000)
Males										
0-4	0	0	0	0	-	-	0	0	0	0
5-14	0	0	0	0	-	-	0	0	0	0
15-44	0	0	0	0	-	-	0	0	0	0
45-59	0	0	0	0	-	-	0	0	0	0
60+	0	0	0	0	-	-	0	0	0	0
All ages	0	0	0	0	-	-	0	0	0	0
Females										
0-4	0	0	0	0	-	-	0	0	0	0
5-14	0	0	0	0	-	-	0	0	0	0
15-44	389	366	5 833	5 489	25.0	15.0	0	0	0	0
45-59	0	0	0	0	-	-	0	0	0	0
60+	0	0	0	0	-	-	0	0	0	0
All ages	389	151	5 833	2 261	25.0	15.0	0	0	0	0
Total	389	76	5 833	1 143	25.0	15.0	0	0	0	0

For epidemiological sources see Abou-Zahr and Ahman 1996. For the methods used to estimate and project incidence, prevalence, and deaths see Murray and Lopez 1996a. See explanatory notes for definitions and caveats.

Table 122	Cuadro 122	Tableau 122
Abortion	Aborto	Avortement

Infertility | Infertilidad | Stérilité

Table 122g   LAC - ALC - ALC   Abortion - Infertility

Age group (years)	Incidence 1990 Number ('000s)	Rate (per 100 000)	Prevalence 1990 Number ('000s)	Rate (per 100 000)	Avg. age at onset (years)	Average duration (years)	Deaths 1990 Number ('000s)	Rate (per 100 000)	Deaths 2000 (Projected) Number ('000s)	Rate (per 100 000)
Males										
0-4	0	0	0	0	-	-	0	0	0	0
5-14	0	0	0	0	-	-	0	0	0	0
15-44	0	0	0	0	-	-	0	0	0	0
45-59	0	0	0	0	-	-	0	0	0	0
60+	0	0	0	0	-	-	0	0	0	0
All ages	0	0	0	0	-	-	0	0	0	0
Females										
0-4	0	0	0	0	-	-	0	0	0	0
5-14	0	0	0	0	-	-	0	0	0	0
15-44	137	132	2 059	1 978	25.0	15.0	0	0	0	0
45-59	0	0	0	0	-	-	0	0	0	0
60+	0	0	0	0	-	-	0	0	0	0
All ages	137	62	2 059	924	25.0	15.0	0	0	0	0
Total	137	31	2 059	463	25.0	15.0	0	0	0	0

Table 122h   MEC - AOM - CMO   Abortion - Infertility

Age group (years)	Incidence 1990 Number ('000s)	Rate (per 100 000)	Prevalence 1990 Number ('000s)	Rate (per 100 000)	Avg. age at onset (years)	Average duration (years)	Deaths 1990 Number ('000s)	Rate (per 100 000)	Deaths 2000 (Projected) Number ('000s)	Rate (per 100 000)
Males										
0-4	0	0	0	0	-	-	0	0	0	0
5-14	0	0	0	0	-	-	0	0	0	0
15-44	0	0	0	0	-	-	0	0	0	0
45-59	0	0	0	0	-	-	0	0	0	0
60+	0	0	0	0	-	-	0	0	0	0
All ages	0	0	0	0	-	-	0	0	0	0
Females										
0-4	0	0	0	0	-	-	0	0	0	0
5-14	0	0	0	0	-	-	0	0	0	0
15-44	107	100	1 611	1 502	25.0	15.0	0	0	0	0
45-59	0	0	0	0	-	-	0	0	0	0
60+	0	0	0	0	-	-	0	0	0	0
All ages	107	44	1 611	653	25.0	15.0	0	0	0	0
Total	107	21	1 611	320	25.0	15.0	0	0	0	0

Table 122i   World - Mundo - Monde   Abortion - Infertility

Age group (years)	Incidence 1990 Number ('000s)	Rate (per 100 000)	Prevalence 1990 Number ('000s)	Rate (per 100 000)	Avg. age at onset (years)	Average duration (years)	Deaths 1990 Number ('000s)	Rate (per 100 000)	Deaths 2000 (Projected) Number ('000s)	Rate (per 100 000)
Males										
0-4	0	0	0	0	-	-	0	0	0	0
5-14	0	0	0	0	-	-	0	0	0	0
15-44	0	0	0	0	-	-	0	0	0	0
45-59	0	0	0	0	-	-	0	0	0	0
60+	0	0	0	0	-	-	0	0	0	0
All ages	0	0	0	0	-	-	0	0	0	0
Females										
0-4	0	0	0	0	-	-	0	0	0	0
5-14	0	0	0	0	-	-	0	0	0	0
15-44	1 426	119	21 394	1 785	25.0	15.0	0	0	0	0
45-59	0	0	0	0	-	-	0	0	0	0
60+	0	0	0	0	-	-	0	0	0	0
All ages	1 426	55	21 394	819	25.0	15.0	0	0	0	0
Total	1 426	27	21 394	406	25.0	15.0	0	0	0	0

For epidemiological sources see Abou-Zahr and Ahman 1996. For the methods used to estimate and project incidence, prevalence, and deaths see Murray and Lopez 1996a. See explanatory notes for definitions and caveats.

Table 123
Low birth weight

All sequelae

Cuadro 123
Bajo peso al nacer

Todas las secuelas

Tableau 123
Poids insuffisant à la naissance

Toutes les séquelles

Table 123a EME - PEMC - EMBE — Low birth weight - All sequelae

Age group (years)	Incidence 1990 Number ('000s)	Rate (per 100 000)	Prevalence 1990 Number ('000s)	Rate (per 100 000)	Avg. age at onset (years)	Average duration (years)	Deaths 1990 Number ('000s)	Rate (per 100 000)	Deaths 2000 (Projected) Number ('000s)	Rate (per 100 000)
Males										
0-4	2	7.0	9	35	0.0	68.1	6	20.5	4	15.5
5-14	0	0.0	19	35	-	-	0	0.0	0	0.0
15-44	0	0.0	64	35	-	-	0	0.0	0	0.0
45-59	0	0.0	23	35	-	-	0	0.0	0	0.0
60+	0	0.0	21	35	-	-	0	0.0	0	0.0
All ages	2	0.5	136	35	0.0	68.1	6	1.4	4	1.1
Females										
0-4	2	7.0	9	35	0.0	73.8	5	16.6	3	12.5
5-14	0	0.0	18	35	-	-	0	0.0	0	0.0
15-44	0	0.0	62	35	-	-	0	0.0	0	0.0
45-59	0	0.0	24	35	-	-	0	0.0	0	0.0
60+	0	0.0	29	35	-	-	0	0.0	0	0.0
All ages	2	0.4	142	35	0.0	73.8	5	1.1	3	0.8
Total	4	0.5	278	35	0.0	70.9	10	1.2	8	0.9

Table 123b FSE - PEAS - AESE — Low birth weight - All sequelae

Age group (years)	Incidence 1990 Number ('000s)	Rate (per 100 000)	Prevalence 1990 Number ('000s)	Rate (per 100 000)	Avg. age at onset (years)	Average duration (years)	Deaths 1990 Number ('000s)	Rate (per 100 000)	Deaths 2000 (Projected) Number ('000s)	Rate (per 100 000)
Males										
0-4	2	11.3	8	56	0.0	62.8	3	24.1	2	17.0
5-14	0	0.0	15	56	-	-	0	0.0	0	0.0
15-44	0	0.0	43	56	-	-	0	0.0	0	0.0
45-59	0	0.0	15	56	-	-	0	0.0	0	0.0
60+	0	0.0	12	56	-	-	0	0.0	0	0.0
All ages	2	0.9	93	56	0.0	62.8	3	1.8	2	1.3
Females										
0-4	1	11.3	7	56	0.0	70.7	2	18.9	2	13.2
5-14	0	0.0	15	56	-	-	0	0.0	0	0.0
15-44	0	0.0	42	56	-	-	0	0.0	0	0.0
45-59	0	0.0	17	56	-	-	0	0.0	0	0.0
60+	0	0.0	20	56	-	-	0	0.0	0	0.0
All ages	1	0.8	102	56	0.0	70.7	2	1.2	2	0.9
Total	3	0.9	195	56	0.0	66.7	5	1.5	4	1.1

Table 123c India - India - Inde — Low birth weight - All sequelae

Age group (years)	Incidence 1990 Number ('000s)	Rate (per 100 000)	Prevalence 1990 Number ('000s)	Rate (per 100 000)	Avg. age at onset (years)	Average duration (years)	Deaths 1990 Number ('000s)	Rate (per 100 000)	Deaths 2000 (Projected) Number ('000s)	Rate (per 100 000)
Males										
0-4	77	128	382	639	0.0	58.8	164	289	100	175
5-14	0	0	650	639	-	-	0	0	0	0
15-44	0	0	1 281	639	-	-	0	0	0	0
45-59	0	0	304	639	-	-	0	0	0	0
60+	0	0	190	639	-	-	0	0	0	0
All ages	77	17	2 807	639	0.0	58.8	164	32	100	19
Females										
0-4	73	128	362	639	0.0	59.7	169	313	99	184
5-14	0	0	609	639	-	-	0	0	0	0
15-44	0	0	1 171	639	-	-	0	0	0	0
45-59	0	0	294	639	-	-	0	0	0	0
60+	0	0	185	639	-	-	0	0	0	0
All ages	73	18	2 620	639	0.0	59.7	169	35	99	20
Total	150	18	5 427	639	0.0	59.2	333	33	199	20

For epidemiological sources see Shibuya and Murray 1996c. For the methods used to estimate and project incidence, prevalence, and deaths see Murray and Lopez 1996a. See explanatory notes for definitions and caveats.

Table 123	Cuadro 123	Tableau 123
Low birth weight	Bajo peso al nacer	Poids insuffisant à la naissance
All sequelae	Todas las secuelas	Toutes les séquelles

Table 123d   China - China - Chine   Low birth weight - All sequelae

Age group (years)	Incidence 1990 Number ('000s)	Rate (per 100 000)	Prevalence 1990 Number ('000s)	Rate (per 100 000)	Avg. age at onset (years)	Average duration (years)	Deaths 1990 Number ('000s)	Rate (per 100 000)	Deaths 2000 (Projected) Number ('000s)	Rate (per 100 000)
Males										
0-4	5	8.4	25	42	0.0	64.1	24	41.5	13	21.6
5-14	0	0.0	41	42	-	-	0	0.0	0	0.0
15-44	0	0.0	128	42	-	-	0	0.0	0	0.0
45-59	0	0.0	30	42	-	-	0	0.0	0	0.0
60+	0	0.0	20	42	-	-	0	0.0	0	0.0
All ages	5	0.9	244	42	0.0	64.1	24	3.7	13	1.9
Females										
0-4	5	8.4	24	42	0.0	66.9	22	39.2	11	19.4
5-14	0	0.0	38	42	-	-	0	0.0	0	0.0
15-44	0	0.0	119	42	-	-	0	0.0	0	0.0
45-59	0	0.0	27	42	-	-	0	0.0	0	0.0
60+	0	0.0	22	42	-	-	0	0.0	0	0.0
All ages	5	0.9	229	42	0.0	66.9	22	3.5	11	1.7
Total	10	0.9	474	42	0.0	65.5	46	3.6	23	1.8

Table 123e   OAI - OPAI - APAI   Low birth weight - All sequelae

Age group (years)	Incidence 1990 Number ('000s)	Rate (per 100 000)	Prevalence 1990 Number ('000s)	Rate (per 100 000)	Avg. age at onset (years)	Average duration (years)	Deaths 1990 Number ('000s)	Rate (per 100 000)	Deaths 2000 (Projected) Number ('000s)	Rate (per 100 000)
Males										
0-4	12	27.5	60	137	0.0	60.6	91	206	60	136
5-14	0	0.0	115	137	-	-	0	0	0	0
15-44	0	0.0	220	137	-	-	0	0	0	0
45-59	0	0.0	47	137	-	-	0	0	0	0
60+	0	0.0	28	137	-	-	0	0	0	0
All ages	12	3.5	469	137	0.0	60.6	91	22	60	15
Females										
0-4	12	27.5	57	137	0.0	64.5	73	173	47	111
5-14	0	0.0	110	137	-	-	0	0	0	0
15-44	0	0.0	218	137	-	-	0	0	0	0
45-59	0	0.0	48	137	-	-	0	0	0	0
60+	0	0.0	31	137	-	-	0	0	0	0
All ages	12	3.4	464	137	0.0	64.5	73	18	47	12
Total	24	3.5	933	137	0.0	62.5	164	20	107	13

Table 123f   SSA - ASS - ASS   Low birth weight - All sequelae

Age group (years)	Incidence 1990 Number ('000s)	Rate (per 100 000)	Prevalence 1990 Number ('000s)	Rate (per 100 000)	Avg. age at onset (years)	Average duration (years)	Deaths 1990 Number ('000s)	Rate (per 100 000)	Deaths 2000 (Projected) Number ('000s)	Rate (per 100 000)
Males										
0-4	28	59	139	293	0.0	51.1	127	193	129	196
5-14	0	0	206	293	-	-	0	0	0	0
15-44	0	0	304	293	-	-	0	0	0	0
45-59	0	0	60	293	-	-	0	0	0	0
60+	0	0	31	293	-	-	0	0	0	0
All ages	28	11	740	293	0.0	51.1	127	37	129	38
Females										
0-4	28	59	138	293	0.0	54.1	122	191	117	183
5-14	0	0	205	293	-	-	0	0	0	0
15-44	0	0	312	293	-	-	0	0	0	0
45-59	0	0	65	293	-	-	0	0	0	0
60+	0	0	37	293	-	-	0	0	0	0
All ages	28	11	756	293	0.0	54.1	122	35	117	33
Total	56	11	1 497	293	0.0	52.6	249	36	246	36

For epidemiological sources see Shibuya and Murray 1996c. For the methods used to estimate and project incidence, prevalence, and deaths see Murray and Lopez 1996a. See explanatory notes for definitions and caveats.

Table 123 / **Cuadro 123** / **Tableau 123**
Low birth weight / Bajo peso al nacer / Poids insuffisant à la naissance

All sequelae / Todas las secuelas / Toutes les séquelles

Table 123g   LAC - ALC - ALC   Low birth weight - All sequelae

Age group (years)	Incidence 1990 Number ('000s)	Rate (per 100 000)	Prevalence 1990 Number ('000s)	Rate (per 100 000)	Avg. age at onset (years)	Average duration (years)	Deaths 1990 Number ('000s)	Rate (per 100 000)	Deaths 2000 (Projected) Number ('000s)	Rate (per 100 000)
Males										
0-4	10	35.8	51	178	0.0	63.4	16	56	12	40
5-14	0	0.0	93	178	-	-	0	0	0	0
15-44	0	0.0	186	178	-	-	0	0	0	0
45-59	0	0.0	40	178	-	-	0	0	0	0
60+	0	0.0	25	178	-	-	0	0	0	0
All ages	10	4.6	394	178	0.0	63.4	16	6	12	4
Females										
0-4	10	35.8	49	178	0.0	67.3	12	44	9	31
5-14	0	0.0	90	178	-	-	0	0	0	0
15-44	0	0.0	185	178	-	-	0	0	0	0
45-59	0	0.0	42	178	-	-	0	0	0	0
60+	0	0.0	30	178	-	-	0	0	0	0
All ages	10	4.4	396	178	0.0	67.3	12	5	9	3
Total	20	4.5	791	178	0.0	65.3	29	5	21	4

Table 123h   MEC - AOM - CMO   Low birth weight - All sequelae

Age group (years)	Incidence 1990 Number ('000s)	Rate (per 100 000)	Prevalence 1990 Number ('000s)	Rate (per 100 000)	Avg. age at onset (years)	Average duration (years)	Deaths 1990 Number ('000s)	Rate (per 100 000)	Deaths 2000 (Projected) Number ('000s)	Rate (per 100 000)
Males										
0-4	18	44.2	90	220	0.0	61.5	101	204	92	184
5-14	0	0.0	144	220	-	-	0	0	0	0
15-44	0	0.0	250	220	-	-	0	0	0	0
45-59	0	0.0	49	220	-	-	0	0	0	0
60+	0	0.0	30	220	-	-	0	0	0	0
All ages	18	7.1	563	220	0.0	61.5	101	30	92	28
Females										
0-4	18	44.2	87	220	0.0	64.1	98	206	85	179
5-14	0	0.0	136	220	-	-	0	0	0	0
15-44	0	0.0	236	220	-	-	0	0	0	0
45-59	0	0.0	49	220	-	-	0	0	0	0
60+	0	0.0	34	220	-	-	0	0	0	0
All ages	18	7.1	542	220	0.0	64.1	98	30	85	26
Total	36	7.1	1 106	220	0.0	62.8	199	30	177	27

Table 123i   World - Mundo - Monde   Low birth weight - All sequelae

Age group (years)	Incidence 1990 Number ('000s)	Rate (per 100 000)	Prevalence 1990 Number ('000s)	Rate (per 100 000)	Avg. age at onset (years)	Average duration (years)	Deaths 1990 Number ('000s)	Rate (per 100 000)	Deaths 2000 (Projected) Number ('000s)	Rate (per 100 000)
Males										
0-4	154	47.8	765	238	0.0	60.6	533	154	412	119
5-14	0	0.0	1 282	233	-	-	0	0	0	0
15-44	0	0.0	2 476	198	-	-	0	0	0	0
45-59	0	0.0	567	182	-	-	0	0	0	0
60+	0	0.0	357	163	-	-	0	0	0	0
All ages	154	5.8	5 447	205	0.0	61.7	533	17	412	13
Females										
0-4	148	47.7	734	237	0.0	63.7	503	152	373	113
5-14	0	0.0	1 220	232	-	-	0	0	0	0
15-44	0	0.0	2 345	196	-	-	0	0	0	0
45-59	0	0.0	565	182	-	-	0	0	0	0
60+	0	0.0	388	144	-	-	0	0	0	0
All ages	148	5.6	5 252	201	0.0	65.3	503	16	373	12
Total	301	5.7	10 699	203	0.0	63.5	1 036	17	784	13

For epidemiological sources see Shibuya and Murray 1996c. For the methods used to estimate and project incidence, prevalence, and deaths see Murray and Lopez 1996a. See explanatory notes for definitions and caveats.

Table 124
Birth asphyxia and birth trauma
All sequelae

Cuadro 124
Asfixia y trauma al nacer
Todas las secuelas

Tableau 124
Asphyxie néonatale et traumatismes de l'accouchement
Toutes les séquelles

Table 124a   EME - PEMC - EMBE   Birth asphyxia and birth trauma - All sequelae

Age group (years)	Incidence 1990 Number ('000s)	Rate (per 100 000)	Prevalence 1990 Number ('000s)	Rate (per 100 000)	Avg. age at onset (years)	Average duration (years)	Deaths 1990 Number ('000s)	Rate (per 100 000)	Deaths 2000 (Projected) Number ('000s)	Rate (per 100 000)
Males										
0-4	9	35.6	47	177	0.0	68.1	12	41.2	9	31.1
5-14	0	0.0	94	177	-	-	0	0.0	0	0.0
15-44	0	0.0	326	177	-	-	0	0.0	0	0.0
45-59	0	0.0	117	177	-	-	0	0.0	0	0.0
60+	0	0.0	107	177	-	-	0	0.0	0	0.0
All ages	9	2.4	691	177	0.0	68.1	12	2.9	9	2.2
Females										
0-4	9	35.6	44	177	0.0	73.8	8	29.4	6	22.0
5-14	0	0.0	90	177	-	-	0	0.0	0	0.0
15-44	0	0.0	317	177	-	-	0	0.0	0	0.0
45-59	0	0.0	120	177	-	-	0	0.0	0	0.0
60+	0	0.0	150	177	-	-	0	0.0	0	0.0
All ages	9	2.2	721	177	0.0	73.8	8	1.9	6	1.4
Total	18	2.3	1 413	177	0.0	70.9	20	2.4	15	1.8

Table 124b   FSE - PEAS - AESE   Birth asphyxia and birth trauma - All sequelae

Age group (years)	Incidence 1990 Number ('000s)	Rate (per 100 000)	Prevalence 1990 Number ('000s)	Rate (per 100 000)	Avg. age at onset (years)	Average duration (years)	Deaths 1990 Number ('000s)	Rate (per 100 000)	Deaths 2000 (Projected) Number ('000s)	Rate (per 100 000)
Males										
0-4	5	35.6	24	177	0.0	62.8	5	41.0	4	28.9
5-14	0	0.0	48	177	-	-	0	0.0	0	0.0
15-44	0	0.0	135	177	-	-	0	0.0	0	0.0
45-59	0	0.0	48	177	-	-	0	0.0	0	0.0
60+	0	0.0	37	177	-	-	0	0.0	0	0.0
All ages	5	3.0	293	177	0.0	62.8	5	3.1	4	2.2
Females										
0-4	5	35.6	23	177	0.0	70.7	3	28.2	2	19.7
5-14	0	0.0	47	177	-	-	0	0.0	0	0.0
15-44	0	0.0	133	177	-	-	0	0.0	0	0.0
45-59	0	0.0	53	177	-	-	0	0.0	0	0.0
60+	0	0.0	64	177	-	-	0	0.0	0	0.0
All ages	5	2.6	320	177	0.0	70.7	3	1.8	2	1.3
Total	10	2.8	613	177	0.0	66.7	9	2.4	6	1.7

Table 124c   India - India - Inde   Birth asphyxia and birth trauma - All sequelae

Age group (years)	Incidence 1990 Number ('000s)	Rate (per 100 000)	Prevalence 1990 Number ('000s)	Rate (per 100 000)	Avg. age at onset (years)	Average duration (years)	Deaths 1990 Number ('000s)	Rate (per 100 000)	Deaths 2000 (Projected) Number ('000s)	Rate (per 100 000)
Males										
0-4	78	131	390	651	0.0	58.8	87	153	53	92.6
5-14	0	0	663	651	-	-	0	0	0	0.0
15-44	0	0	1 306	651	-	-	0	0	0	0.0
45-59	0	0	310	651	-	-	0	0	0	0.0
60+	0	0	194	651	-	-	0	0	0	0.0
All ages	78	18	2 863	651	0.0	58.8	87	17	53	10.3
Females										
0-4	74	131	369	652	0.0	59.7	82	153	48	89.6
5-14	0	0	621	652	-	-	0	0	0	0.0
15-44	0	0	1 194	652	-	-	0	0	0	0.0
45-59	0	0	300	652	-	-	0	0	0	0.0
60+	0	0	188	652	-	-	0	0	0	0.0
All ages	74	18	2 672	652	0.0	59.7	82	17	48	10.0
Total	153	18	5 535	652	0.0	59.2	169	17	101	10.1

For epidemiological sources see Shibuya and Murray 1996b. For the methods used to estimate and project incidence, prevalence, and deaths see Murray and Lopez 1996a. See explanatory notes for definitions and caveats.

Table 124
Birth asphyxia and birth trauma
All sequelae

Cuadro 124
Asfixia y trauma al nacer
Todas las secuelas

Tableau 124
Asphyxie néonatale et traumatismes de l'accouchement
Toutes les séquelles

Table 124d China - China - Chine — Birth asphyxia and birth trauma - All sequelae

Age group (years)	Incidence 1990 Number ('000s)	Rate (per 100 000)	Prevalence 1990 Number ('000s)	Rate (per 100 000)	Avg. age at onset (years)	Average duration (years)	Deaths 1990 Number ('000s)	Rate (per 100 000)	Deaths 2000 (Projected) Number ('000s)	Rate (per 100 000)
Males										
0-4	38	63.7	189	313	0.0	64.1	67	114	35	59.2
5-14	0	0.0	304	313	-	-	0	0	0	0.0
15-44	0	0.0	959	313	-	-	0	0	0	0.0
45-59	0	0.0	227	313	-	-	0	0	0	0.0
60+	0	0.0	153	313	-	-	0	0	0	0.0
All ages	38	6.6	1 831	313	0.0	64.1	67	10	35	5.3
Females										
0-4	36	62.9	181	313	0.0	66.9	80	143	40	71.1
5-14	0	0.0	283	313	-	-	0	0	0	0.0
15-44	0	0.0	889	313	-	-	0	0	0	0.0
45-59	0	0.0	202	313	-	-	0	0	0	0.0
60+	0	0.0	162	313	-	-	0	0	0	0.0
All ages	36	6.6	1 717	313	0.0	66.9	80	13	40	6.4
Total	75	6.6	3 548	313	0.0	65.5	147	11	74	5.8

Table 124e OAI - OPAI - APAI — Birth asphyxia and birth trauma - All sequelae

Age group (years)	Incidence 1990 Number ('000s)	Rate (per 100 000)	Prevalence 1990 Number ('000s)	Rate (per 100 000)	Avg. age at onset (years)	Average duration (years)	Deaths 1990 Number ('000s)	Rate (per 100 000)	Deaths 2000 (Projected) Number ('000s)	Rate (per 100 000)
Males										
0-4	37	84	183	417	0.0	60.6	43	97	28	64.2
5-14	0	0	351	417	-	-	0	0	0	0.0
15-44	0	0	671	417	-	-	0	0	0	0.0
45-59	0	0	142	417	-	-	0	0	0	0.0
60+	0	0	84	417	-	-	0	0	0	0.0
All ages	37	11	1 431	417	0.0	60.6	43	11	28	7.0
Females										
0-4	35	84	175	417	0.0	64.5	34	81	22	52.4
5-14	0	0	335	417	-	-	0	0	0	0.0
15-44	0	0	666	417	-	-	0	0	0	0.0
45-59	0	0	146	417	-	-	0	0	0	0.0
60+	0	0	95	417	-	-	0	0	0	0.0
All ages	35	10	1 417	417	0.0	64.5	34	9	22	5.5
Total	72	11	2 848	417	0.0	62.5	77	10	50	6.2

Table 124f SSA - ASS - ASS — Birth asphyxia and birth trauma - All sequelae

Age group (years)	Incidence 1990 Number ('000s)	Rate (per 100 000)	Prevalence 1990 Number ('000s)	Rate (per 100 000)	Avg. age at onset (years)	Average duration (years)	Deaths 1990 Number ('000s)	Rate (per 100 000)	Deaths 2000 (Projected) Number ('000s)	Rate (per 100 000)
Males										
0-4	75	158	372	784	0.0	51.1	82	124	83	126
5-14	0	0	551	784	-	-	0	0	0	0
15-44	0	0	813	784	-	-	0	0	0	0
45-59	0	0	159	784	-	-	0	0	0	0
60+	0	0	82	784	-	-	0	0	0	0
All ages	75	30	1 977	784	0.0	51.1	82	24	83	24
Females										
0-4	74	158	368	783	0.0	54.1	82	129	78	123
5-14	0	0	547	783	-	-	0	0	0	0
15-44	0	0	832	783	-	-	0	0	0	0
45-59	0	0	173	783	-	-	0	0	0	0
60+	0	0	100	783	-	-	0	0	0	0
All ages	74	29	2 021	783	0.0	54.1	82	23	78	23
Total	149	29	3 998	784	0.0	52.6	164	24	161	23

For epidemiological sources see Shibuya and Murray 1996b. For the methods used to estimate and project incidence, prevalence, and deaths see Murray and Lopez 1996a. See explanatory notes for definitions and caveats.

Table 124
Birth asphyxia and birth trauma
All sequelae

Cuadro 124
Asfixia y trauma al nacer
Todas las secuelas

Tableau 124
Asphyxie néonatale et trauma-tismes de l'accouchement
Toutes les séquelles

Table 124g — LAC - ALC - ALC — Birth asphyxia and birth trauma - All sequelae

Age group (years)	Incidence 1990 Number ('000s)	Rate (per 100 000)	Prevalence 1990 Number ('000s)	Rate (per 100 000)	Avg. age at onset (years)	Average duration (years)	Deaths 1990 Number ('000s)	Rate (per 100 000)	Deaths 2000 (Projected) Number ('000s)	Rate (per 100 000)
Males										
0-4	21	73.4	105	365	0.0	63.4	54	183.9	39	133.3
5-14	0	0.0	190	365	-	-	0	0.0	0	0.0
15-44	0	0.0	381	365	-	-	0	0.0	0	0.0
45-59	0	0.0	81	365	-	-	0	0.0	0	0.0
60+	0	0.0	52	365	-	-	0	0.0	0	0.0
All ages	21	9.5	809	365	0.0	63.4	54	20.3	39	14.7
Females										
0-4	20	73.4	101	365	0.0	67.3	37	131.9	26	93.1
5-14	0	0.0	185	365	-	-	0	0.0	0	0.0
15-44	0	0.0	380	365	-	-	0	0.0	0	0.0
45-59	0	0.0	85	365	-	-	0	0.0	0	0.0
60+	0	0.0	61	365	-	-	0	0.0	0	0.0
All ages	20	9.1	813	365	0.0	67.3	37	13.9	26	9.8
Total	41	9.3	1 622	365	0.0	65.3	91	17.1	65	12.2

Table 124h — MEC - AOM - CMO — Birth asphyxia and birth trauma - All sequelae

Age group (years)	Incidence 1990 Number ('000s)	Rate (per 100 000)	Prevalence 1990 Number ('000s)	Rate (per 100 000)	Avg. age at onset (years)	Average duration (years)	Deaths 1990 Number ('000s)	Rate (per 100 000)	Deaths 2000 (Projected) Number ('000s)	Rate (per 100 000)
Males										
0-4	43	105	215	521	0.0	61.5	48	96	43	87
5-14	0	0	341	521	-	-	0	0	0	0
15-44	0	0	594	521	-	-	0	0	0	0
45-59	0	0	116	521	-	-	0	0	0	0
60+	0	0	71	521	-	-	0	0	0	0
All ages	43	17	1 337	521	0.0	61.5	48	14	43	13
Females										
0-4	42	105	207	521	0.0	64.1	46	97	40	84
5-14	0	0	323	521	-	-	0	0	0	0
15-44	0	0	559	521	-	-	0	0	0	0
45-59	0	0	116	521	-	-	0	0	0	0
60+	0	0	81	521	-	-	0	0	0	0
All ages	42	17	1 286	521	0.0	64.1	46	14	40	12
Total	85	17	2 623	521	0.0	62.8	94	14	83	13

Table 124i — World - Mundo - Monde — Birth asphyxia and birth trauma - All sequelae

Age group (years)	Incidence 1990 Number ('000s)	Rate (per 100 000)	Prevalence 1990 Number ('000s)	Rate (per 100 000)	Avg. age at onset (years)	Average duration (years)	Deaths 1990 Number ('000s)	Rate (per 100 000)	Deaths 2000 (Projected) Number ('000s)	Rate (per 100 000)
Males										
0-4	307	95	1 523	474	0.0	60.6	397	115	293	84.8
5-14	0	0	2 542	461	-	-	0	0	0	0.0
15-44	0	0	5 185	415	-	-	0	0	0	0.0
45-59	0	0	1 201	385	-	-	0	0	0	0.0
60+	0	0	781	357	-	-	0	0	0	0.0
All ages	307	12	11 232	423	0.0	61.7	397	13	293	9.5
Females										
0-4	296	96	1 470	475	0.0	63.7	373	113	263	79.6
5-14	0	0	2 430	462	-	-	0	0	0	0.0
15-44	0	0	4 970	415	-	-	0	0	0	0.0
45-59	0	0	1 196	384	-	-	0	0	0	0.0
60+	0	0	901	335	-	-	0	0	0	0.0
All ages	296	11	10 967	420	0.0	65.3	373	12	263	8.6
Total	602	11	22 200	421	0.0	63.5	770	13	557	9.0

For epidemiological sources see Shibuya and Murray 1996b. For the methods used to estimate and project incidence, prevalence, and deaths see Murray and Lopez 1996a. See explanatory notes for definitions and caveats.

Table 125
Protein-energy malnutrition
Wasting

Cuadro 125
Desnutrición proteínico-calórica
Emaciación

Tableau 125
Malnutrition protéino-calorique
Insuffisance pondérale

Table 125a EME - PEMC - EMBE Protein-energy malnutrition - Wasting

Age group (years)	Incidence 1990 Number ('000s)	Rate (per 100 000)	Prevalence 1990 Number ('000s)	Rate (per 100 000)	Avg. age at onset (years)	Average duration (years)	Deaths 1990 Number ('000s)	Rate (per 100 000)	Deaths 2000 (Projected) Number ('000s)	Rate (per 100 000)
Males										
0-4	-	-	607	2 300	-	-	0	0.1	0	0.0
5-14	-	-	0	0	-	-	0	0.0	0	0.0
15-44	-	-	0	0	-	-	0	0.0	0	0.0
45-59	-	-	0	0	-	-	0	0.2	0	0.1
60+	-	-	0	0	-	-	2	3.2	2	3.0
All ages	-	-	607	155	-	-	2	0.5	2	0.6
Females										
0-4	-	-	576	2 300	-	-	0	0.0	0	0.0
5-14	-	-	0	0	-	-	0	0.0	0	0.0
15-44	-	-	0	0	-	-	0	0.0	0	0.0
45-59	-	-	0	0	-	-	0	0.1	0	0.1
60+	-	-	0	0	-	-	4	4.3	4	4.1
All ages	-	-	576	142	-	-	4	0.9	4	1.0
Total	-	-	1 183	148	-	-	6	0.7	6	0.8

Table 125b FSE - PEAS - AESE Protein-energy malnutrition - Wasting

Age group (years)	Incidence 1990 Number ('000s)	Rate (per 100 000)	Prevalence 1990 Number ('000s)	Rate (per 100 000)	Avg. age at onset (years)	Average duration (years)	Deaths 1990 Number ('000s)	Rate (per 100 000)	Deaths 2000 (Projected) Number ('000s)	Rate (per 100 000)
Males										
0-4	-	-	482	3 500	-	-	0	0.2	0	0.1
5-14	-	-	0	0	-	-	0	0.0	0	0.0
15-44	-	-	0	0	-	-	0	0.0	0	0.0
45-59	-	-	0	0	-	-	0	0.2	0	0.1
60+	-	-	0	0	-	-	1	2.5	1	2.7
All ages	-	-	482	291	-	-	1	0.4	1	0.4
Females										
0-4	-	-	460	3 500	-	-	0	0.2	0	0.1
5-14	-	-	0	0	-	-	0	0.0	0	0.0
15-44	-	-	0	0	-	-	0	0.0	0	0.0
45-59	-	-	0	0	-	-	0	0.1	0	0.1
60+	-	-	0	0	-	-	1	3.8	2	3.7
All ages	-	-	460	254	-	-	1	0.8	2	0.8
Total	-	-	941	272	-	-	2	0.6	2	0.7

Table 125c India - India - Inde Protein-energy malnutrition - Wasting

Age group (years)	Incidence 1990 Number ('000s)	Rate (per 100 000)	Prevalence 1990 Number ('000s)	Rate (per 100 000)	Avg. age at onset (years)	Average duration (years)	Deaths 1990 Number ('000s)	Rate (per 100 000)	Deaths 2000 (Projected) Number ('000s)	Rate (per 100 000)
Males										
0-4	-	-	11 479	19 200	-	-	23	38.1	14	23.8
5-14	-	-	0	0	-	-	1	1.0	1	0.5
15-44	-	-	0	0	-	-	2	0.8	1	0.3
45-59	-	-	0	0	-	-	1	1.5	0	0.7
60+	-	-	0	0	-	-	4	13.1	3	9.4
All ages	-	-	11 479	2 613	-	-	30	6.8	19	3.7
Females										
0-4	-	-	10 882	19 200	-	-	30	53.2	17	31.9
5-14	-	-	0	0	-	-	3	3.0	1	1.3
15-44	-	-	0	0	-	-	1	0.5	0	0.2
45-59	-	-	0	0	-	-	1	1.2	0	0.6
60+	-	-	0	0	-	-	4	14.0	4	10.3
All ages	-	-	10 882	2 654	-	-	39	9.4	23	4.8
Total	-	-	22 362	2 632	-	-	69	8.1	42	4.2

For epidemiological sources see Bailey et al. 1996. For the methods used to estimate and project incidence, prevalence, and deaths see Murray and Lopez 1996a. See explanatory notes for definitions and caveats.

Table 125
Protein-energy malnutrition

Wasting

Cuadro 125
Desnutrición proteínico-calórica

Emaciación

Tableau 125
Malnutrition protéino-calorique

Insuffisance pondérale

Table 125d   China - China - Chine   Protein-energy malnutrition - Wasting

Age group (years)	Incidence 1990 Number ('000s)	Rate (per 100 000)	Prevalence 1990 Number ('000s)	Rate (per 100 000)	Avg. age at onset (years)	Average duration (years)	Deaths 1990 Number ('000s)	Rate (per 100 000)	Deaths 2000 (Projected) Number ('000s)	Rate (per 100 000)
Males										
0-4	-	-	2 169	3 600	-	-	8	14.1	4	7.3
5-14	-	-	0	0	-	-	0	0.1	0	0.0
15-44	-	-	0	0	-	-	0	0.1	0	0.0
45-59	-	-	0	0	-	-	0	0.5	0	0.2
60+	-	-	0	0	-	-	5	9.8	5	7.8
All ages	-	-	2 169	371	-	-	14	2.4	9	1.4
Females										
0-4	-	-	2 086	3 600	-	-	19	33.4	9	16.6
5-14	-	-	0	0	-	-	0	0.1	0	0.0
15-44	-	-	0	0	-	-	0	0.1	0	0.0
45-59	-	-	0	0	-	-	0	0.3	0	0.1
60+	-	-	0	0	-	-	4	7.5	4	6.0
All ages	-	-	2 086	380	-	-	24	4.4	13	2.1
Total	-	-	4 255	375	-	-	38	3.3	23	1.8

Table 125e   OAI - OPAI - APAI   Protein-energy malnutrition - Wasting

Age group (years)	Incidence 1990 Number ('000s)	Rate (per 100 000)	Prevalence 1990 Number ('000s)	Rate (per 100 000)	Avg. age at onset (years)	Average duration (years)	Deaths 1990 Number ('000s)	Rate (per 100 000)	Deaths 2000 (Projected) Number ('000s)	Rate (per 100 000)
Males										
0-4	-	-	4 726	10 800	-	-	19	44.4	13	28.6
5-14	-	-	0	0	-	-	0	0.4	0	0.2
15-44	-	-	0	0	-	-	0	0.1	0	0.1
45-59	-	-	0	0	-	-	0	1.0	0	0.5
60+	-	-	0	0	-	-	1	5.4	1	4.1
All ages	-	-	4 726	1 378	-	-	21	6.3	14	3.5
Females										
0-4	-	-	4 535	10 800	-	-	17	41.6	11	25.9
5-14	-	-	0	0	-	-	0	0.4	0	0.2
15-44	-	-	0	0	-	-	0	0.2	0	0.1
45-59	-	-	0	0	-	-	0	0.8	0	0.4
60+	-	-	0	0	-	-	1	3.8	1	3.0
All ages	-	-	4 535	1 335	-	-	19	5.6	12	3.1
Total	-	-	9 261	1 357	-	-	41	6.0	27	3.3

Table 125f   SSA - ASS - ASS   Protein-energy malnutrition - Wasting

Age group (years)	Incidence 1990 Number ('000s)	Rate (per 100 000)	Prevalence 1990 Number ('000s)	Rate (per 100 000)	Avg. age at onset (years)	Average duration (years)	Deaths 1990 Number ('000s)	Rate (per 100 000)	Deaths 2000 (Projected) Number ('000s)	Rate (per 100 000)
Males										
0-4	-	-	3 656	7 700	-	-	47	98.4	47	70.8
5-14	-	-	0	0	-	-	1	1.4	1	0.8
15-44	-	-	0	0	-	-	1	0.7	1	0.4
45-59	-	-	0	0	-	-	1	3.1	0	1.6
60+	-	-	0	0	-	-	3	26.7	3	20.5
All ages	-	-	3 656	1 449	-	-	52	20.6	51	14.9
Females										
0-4	-	-	3 621	7 700	-	-	44	92.9	41	64.4
5-14	-	-	0	0	-	-	1	1.6	1	0.8
15-44	-	-	0	0	-	-	2	1.6	1	0.7
45-59	-	-	0	0	-	-	1	2.5	0	1.3
60+	-	-	0	0	-	-	3	21.9	3	16.4
All ages	-	-	3 621	1 404	-	-	50	19.3	46	13.2
Total	-	-	7 278	1 426	-	-	102	19.9	97	14.1

For epidemiological sources see Bailey et al. 1996. For the methods used to estimate and project incidence, prevalence, and deaths see Murray and Lopez 1996a. See explanatory notes for definitions and caveats.

Table 125	Cuadro 125	Tableau 125
Protein-energy malnutrition	**Desnutrición proteínico-calórica**	**Malnutrition protéino-calorique**
Wasting	Emaciación	Insuffisance pondérale

Table 125g   LAC - ALC - ALC   Protein-energy malnutrition - Wasting

Age group (years)	Incidence 1990 Number ('000s)	Rate (per 100 000)	Prevalence 1990 Number ('000s)	Rate (per 100 000)	Avg. age at onset (years)	Average duration (years)	Deaths 1990 Number ('000s)	Rate (per 100 000)	Deaths 2000 (Projected) Number ('000s)	Rate (per 100 000)
Males										
0-4	-	-	1 005	3 500	-	-	18	62.6	13	43.8
5-14	-	-	0	0	-	-	1	2.0	1	1.1
15-44	-	-	0	0	-	-	1	1.0	1	0.5
45-59	-	-	0	0	-	-	1	5.1	1	2.9
60+	-	-	0	0	-	-	6	42.3	7	36.0
All ages	-	-	1 005	454	-	-	27	12.3	22	8.3
Females										
0-4	-	-	969	3 500	-	-	13	48.2	9	32.8
5-14	-	-	0	0	-	-	1	2.7	1	1.5
15-44	-	-	0	0	-	-	2	1.6	1	0.7
45-59	-	-	0	0	-	-	1	4.2	1	2.3
60+	-	-	0	0	-	-	7	43.0	9	36.8
All ages	-	-	969	435	-	-	25	11.0	20	7.6
Total	-	-	1 974	444	-	-	52	11.7	43	8.0

Table 125h   MEC - AOM - CMO   Protein-energy malnutrition - Wasting

Age group (years)	Incidence 1990 Number ('000s)	Rate (per 100 000)	Prevalence 1990 Number ('000s)	Rate (per 100 000)	Avg. age at onset (years)	Average duration (years)	Deaths 1990 Number ('000s)	Rate (per 100 000)	Deaths 2000 (Projected) Number ('000s)	Rate (per 100 000)
Males										
0-4	-	-	2 182	5 300	-	-	30	73.1	27	53.9
5-14	-	-	0	0	-	-	0	0.3	0	0.2
15-44	-	-	0	0	-	-	0	0.2	0	0.1
45-59	-	-	0	0	-	-	0	0.8	0	0.5
60+	-	-	0	0	-	-	1	9.4	1	7.2
All ages	-	-	2 182	851	-	-	32	12.5	29	8.6
Females										
0-4	-	-	2 106	5 300	-	-	29	73.1	25	52.2
5-14	-	-	0	0	-	-	0	0.3	0	0.2
15-44	-	-	0	0	-	-	0	0.4	0	0.2
45-59	-	-	0	0	-	-	0	0.7	0	0.4
60+	-	-	0	0	-	-	1	7.3	1	5.7
All ages	-	-	2 106	854	-	-	31	12.5	27	8.2
Total	-	-	4 287	852	-	-	63	12.5	55	8.4

Table 125i   World - Mundo - Monde   Protein-energy malnutrition - Wasting

Age group (years)	Incidence 1990 Number ('000s)	Rate (per 100 000)	Prevalence 1990 Number ('000s)	Rate (per 100 000)	Avg. age at onset (years)	Average duration (years)	Deaths 1990 Number ('000s)	Rate (per 100 000)	Deaths 2000 (Projected) Number ('000s)	Rate (per 100 000)
Males										
0-4	-	-	26 306	8 187	-	-	146	45.3	117	33.8
5-14	-	-	0	0	-	-	4	0.7	2	0.4
15-44	-	-	0	0	-	-	4	0.3	2	0.2
45-59	-	-	0	0	-	-	4	1.1	2	0.6
60+	-	-	0	0	-	-	22	10.2	24	8.6
All ages	-	-	26 306	991	-	-	179	6.8	147	4.8
Females										
0-4	-	-	25 235	8 160	-	-	153	49.5	112	34.0
5-14	-	-	0	0	-	-	6	1.1	3	0.5
15-44	-	-	0	0	-	-	5	0.5	3	0.2
45-59	-	-	0	0	-	-	3	0.9	2	0.5
60+	-	-	0	0	-	-	25	9.3	27	8.1
All ages	-	-	25 235	966	-	-	192	7.4	148	4.8
Total	-	-	51 541	979	-	-	372	7.1	295	4.8

For epidemiological sources see Bailey et al. 1996. For the methods used to estimate and project incidence, prevalence, and deaths see Murray and Lopez 1996a. See explanatory notes for definitions and caveats.

Table 126
Protein-energy malnutrition

Stunting

Cuadro 126
Desnutrición proteínico-calórica
Retraso de crecimiento

Tableau 126
Malnutrition protéino-calorique
Insuffisance staturale

Table 126a   EME - PEMC - EMBE Protein-energy malnutrition - Stunting

Age group (years)	Incidence 1990 Number ('000s)	Rate (per 100 000)	Prevalence 1990 Number ('000s)	Rate (per 100 000)	Avg. age at onset (years)	Average duration (years)	Deaths 1990 Number ('000s)	Rate (per 100 000)	Deaths 2000 (Projected) Number ('000s)	Rate (per 100 000)
Males										
0-4	-	-	607	2 300	-	-	-	-	-	-
5-14	-	-	0	0	-	-	-	-	-	-
15-44	-	-	0	0	-	-	-	-	-	-
45-59	-	-	0	0	-	-	-	-	-	-
60+	-	-	0	0	-	-	-	-	-	-
All ages	-	-	607	155	-	-	-	-	-	-
Females										
0-4	-	-	576	2 300	-	-	-	-	-	-
5-14	-	-	0	0	-	-	-	-	-	-
15-44	-	-	0	0	-	-	-	-	-	-
45-59	-	-	0	0	-	-	-	-	-	-
60+	-	-	0	0	-	-	-	-	-	-
All ages	-	-	576	142	-	-	-	-	-	-
Total	-	-	1 183	148	-	-	-	-	-	-

Table 126b   FSE - PEAS - AESE Protein-energy malnutrition - Stunting

Age group (years)	Incidence 1990 Number ('000s)	Rate (per 100 000)	Prevalence 1990 Number ('000s)	Rate (per 100 000)	Avg. age at onset (years)	Average duration (years)	Deaths 1990 Number ('000s)	Rate (per 100 000)	Deaths 2000 (Projected) Number ('000s)	Rate (per 100 000)
Males										
0-4	-	-	2 078	15 100	-	-	-	-	-	-
5-14	-	-	0	0	-	-	-	-	-	-
15-44	-	-	0	0	-	-	-	-	-	-
45-59	-	-	0	0	-	-	-	-	-	-
60+	-	-	0	0	-	-	-	-	-	-
All ages	-	-	2 078	1 257	-	-	-	-	-	-
Females										
0-4	-	-	1 983	15 100	-	-	-	-	-	-
5-14	-	-	0	0	-	-	-	-	-	-
15-44	-	-	0	0	-	-	-	-	-	-
45-59	-	-	0	0	-	-	-	-	-	-
60+	-	-	0	0	-	-	-	-	-	-
All ages	-	-	1 983	1 096	-	-	-	-	-	-
Total	-	-	4 061	1 173	-	-	-	-	-	-

Table 126c   India - India - Inde Protein-energy malnutrition - Stunting

Age group (years)	Incidence 1990 Number ('000s)	Rate (per 100 000)	Prevalence 1990 Number ('000s)	Rate (per 100 000)	Avg. age at onset (years)	Average duration (years)	Deaths 1990 Number ('000s)	Rate (per 100 000)	Deaths 2000 (Projected) Number ('000s)	Rate (per 100 000)
Males										
0-4	-	-	37 129	62 100	-	-	-	-	-	-
5-14	-	-	0	0	-	-	-	-	-	-
15-44	-	-	0	0	-	-	-	-	-	-
45-59	-	-	0	0	-	-	-	-	-	-
60+	-	-	0	0	-	-	-	-	-	-
All ages	-	-	37 129	8 450	-	-	-	-	-	-
Females										
0-4	-	-	35 198	62 100	-	-	-	-	-	-
5-14	-	-	0	0	-	-	-	-	-	-
15-44	-	-	0	0	-	-	-	-	-	-
45-59	-	-	0	0	-	-	-	-	-	-
60+	-	-	0	0	-	-	-	-	-	-
All ages	-	-	35 198	8 582	-	-	-	-	-	-
Total	-	-	72 327	8 514	-	-	-	-	-	-

For epidemiological sources see Bailey et al. 1996. For the methods used to estimate and project incidence, prevalence, and deaths see Murray and Lopez 1996a. See explanatory notes for definitions and caveats.

Table 126
Protein-energy malnutrition

Stunting

Cuadro 126
Desnutrición proteínico-calórica

Retraso de crecimiento

Tableau 126
Malnutrition protéino-calorique

Insuffisance staturale

Table 126d   China - China - Chine

Protein-energy malnutrition - Stunting

Age group (years)	Incidence 1990 Number ('000s)	Rate (per 100 000)	Prevalence 1990 Number ('000s)	Rate (per 100 000)	Avg. age at onset (years)	Average duration (years)	Deaths 1990 Number ('000s)	Rate (per 100 000)	Deaths 2000 (Projected) Number ('000s)	Rate (per 100 000)
Males										
0-4	-	-	19 338	32 100	-	-	-	-	-	-
5-14	-	-	0	0	-	-	-	-	-	-
15-44	-	-	0	0	-	-	-	-	-	-
45-59	-	-	0	0	-	-	-	-	-	-
60+	-	-	0	0	-	-	-	-	-	-
All ages	-	-	19 338	3 305	-	-	-	-	-	-
Females										
0-4	-	-	18 601	32 100	-	-	-	-	-	-
5-14	-	-	0	0	-	-	-	-	-	-
15-44	-	-	0	0	-	-	-	-	-	-
45-59	-	-	0	0	-	-	-	-	-	-
60+	-	-	0	0	-	-	-	-	-	-
All ages	-	-	18 601	3 391	-	-	-	-	-	-
Total	-	-	37 939	3 346	-	-	-	-	-	-

Table 126e   OAI - OPAI - APAI

Protein-energy malnutrition - Stunting

Age group (years)	Incidence 1990 Number ('000s)	Rate (per 100 000)	Prevalence 1990 Number ('000s)	Rate (per 100 000)	Avg. age at onset (years)	Average duration (years)	Deaths 1990 Number ('000s)	Rate (per 100 000)	Deaths 2000 (Projected) Number ('000s)	Rate (per 100 000)
Males										
0-4	-	-	20 831	47 600	-	-	-	-	-	-
5-14	-	-	0	0	-	-	-	-	-	-
15-44	-	-	0	0	-	-	-	-	-	-
45-59	-	-	0	0	-	-	-	-	-	-
60+	-	-	0	0	-	-	-	-	-	-
All ages	-	-	20 831	6 074	-	-	-	-	-	-
Females										
0-4	-	-	19 986	47 600	-	-	-	-	-	-
5-14	-	-	0	0	-	-	-	-	-	-
15-44	-	-	0	0	-	-	-	-	-	-
45-59	-	-	0	0	-	-	-	-	-	-
60+	-	-	0	0	-	-	-	-	-	-
All ages	-	-	19 986	5 886	-	-	-	-	-	-
Total	-	-	40 817	5 980	-	-	-	-	-	-

Table 126f   SSA - ASS - ASS

Protein-energy malnutrition - Stunting

Age group (years)	Incidence 1990 Number ('000s)	Rate (per 100 000)	Prevalence 1990 Number ('000s)	Rate (per 100 000)	Avg. age at onset (years)	Average duration (years)	Deaths 1990 Number ('000s)	Rate (per 100 000)	Deaths 2000 (Projected) Number ('000s)	Rate (per 100 000)
Males										
0-4	-	-	19 706	41 500	-	-	-	-	-	-
5-14	-	-	0	0	-	-	-	-	-	-
15-44	-	-	0	0	-	-	-	-	-	-
45-59	-	-	0	0	-	-	-	-	-	-
60+	-	-	0	0	-	-	-	-	-	-
All ages	-	-	19 706	7 810	-	-	-	-	-	-
Females										
0-4	-	-	19 517	41 500	-	-	-	-	-	-
5-14	-	-	0	0	-	-	-	-	-	-
15-44	-	-	0	0	-	-	-	-	-	-
45-59	-	-	0	0	-	-	-	-	-	-
60+	-	-	0	0	-	-	-	-	-	-
All ages	-	-	19 517	7 566	-	-	-	-	-	-
Total	-	-	39 223	7 687	-	-	-	-	-	-

For epidemiological sources see Bailey et al. 1996. For the methods used to estimate and project incidence, prevalence, and deaths see Murray and Lopez 1996a. See explanatory notes for definitions and caveats.

Table 126	Cuadro 126	Tableau 126
Protein-energy malnutrition	**Desnutrición proteínico-calórica**	**Malnutrition protéino-calorique**
Stunting	Retraso de crecimiento	Insuffisance staturale

Table 126g   LAC - ALC - ALC   Protein-energy malnutrition - Stunting

Age group (years)	Incidence 1990 Number ('000s)	Rate (per 100 000)	Prevalence 1990 Number ('000s)	Rate (per 100 000)	Avg. age at onset (years)	Average duration (years)	Deaths 1990 Number ('000s)	Rate (per 100 000)	Deaths 2000 (Projected) Number ('000s)	Rate (per 100 000)
Males										
0-4	-	-	7 611	26 500	-	-	-	-	-	-
5-14	-	-	0	0	-	-	-	-	-	-
15-44	-	-	0	0	-	-	-	-	-	-
45-59	-	-	0	0	-	-	-	-	-	-
60+	-	-	0	0	-	-	-	-	-	-
All ages	-	-	7 611	3 434	-	-	-	-	-	-
Females										
0-4	-	-	7 334	26 500	-	-	-	-	-	-
5-14	-	-	0	0	-	-	-	-	-	-
15-44	-	-	0	0	-	-	-	-	-	-
45-59	-	-	0	0	-	-	-	-	-	-
60+	-	-	0	0	-	-	-	-	-	-
All ages	-	-	7 334	3 294	-	-	-	-	-	-
Total	-	-	14 945	3 364	-	-	-	-	-	-

Table 126h   MEC - AOM - CMO   Protein-energy malnutrition - Stunting

Age group (years)	Incidence 1990 Number ('000s)	Rate (per 100 000)	Prevalence 1990 Number ('000s)	Rate (per 100 000)	Avg. age at onset (years)	Average duration (years)	Deaths 1990 Number ('000s)	Rate (per 100 000)	Deaths 2000 (Projected) Number ('000s)	Rate (per 100 000)
Males										
0-4	-	-	14 612	35 500	-	-	-	-	-	-
5-14	-	-	0	0	-	-	-	-	-	-
15-44	-	-	0	0	-	-	-	-	-	-
45-59	-	-	0	0	-	-	-	-	-	-
60+	-	-	0	0	-	-	-	-	-	-
All ages	-	-	14 612	5 699	-	-	-	-	-	-
Females										
0-4	-	-	14 106	35 500	-	-	-	-	-	-
5-14	-	-	0	0	-	-	-	-	-	-
15-44	-	-	0	0	-	-	-	-	-	-
45-59	-	-	0	0	-	-	-	-	-	-
60+	-	-	0	0	-	-	-	-	-	-
All ages	-	-	14 106	5 718	-	-	-	-	-	-
Total	-	-	28 718	5 708	-	-	-	-	-	-

Table 126i   World - Mundo - Monde   Protein-energy malnutrition - Stunting

Age group (years)	Incidence 1990 Number ('000s)	Rate (per 100 000)	Prevalence 1990 Number ('000s)	Rate (per 100 000)	Avg. age at onset (years)	Average duration (years)	Deaths 1990 Number ('000s)	Rate (per 100 000)	Deaths 2000 (Projected) Number ('000s)	Rate (per 100 000)
Males										
0-4	-	-	121 912	37 943	-	-	-	-	-	-
5-14	-	-	0	0	-	-	-	-	-	-
15-44	-	-	0	0	-	-	-	-	-	-
45-59	-	-	0	0	-	-	-	-	-	-
60+	-	-	0	0	-	-	-	-	-	-
All ages	-	-	121 912	4 594	-	-	-	-	-	-
Females										
0-4	-	-	117 302	37 931	-	-	-	-	-	-
5-14	-	-	0	0	-	-	-	-	-	-
15-44	-	-	0	0	-	-	-	-	-	-
45-59	-	-	0	0	-	-	-	-	-	-
60+	-	-	0	0	-	-	-	-	-	-
All ages	-	-	117 302	4 488	-	-	-	-	-	-
Total	-	-	239 213	4 541	-	-	-	-	-	-

For epidemiological sources see Bailey et al. 1996. For the methods used to estimate and project incidence, prevalence, and deaths see Murray and Lopez 1996a. See explanatory notes for definitions and caveats.

Table 127
Protein-energy malnutrition

Developmental disability

Cuadro 127
Desnutrición proteínico-calórica

Discapacidad en el desarrollo

Tableau 127
Malnutrition protéino-calorique

Déficit du developpement

Table 127a EME - PEMC - EMBE Protein-energy malnutrition - Developmental disability

Age group (years)	Incidence 1990 Number ('000s)	Rate (per 100 000)	Prevalence 1990 Number ('000s)	Rate (per 100 000)	Avg. age at onset (years)	Average duration (years)	Deaths 1990 Number ('000s)	Rate (per 100 000)	Deaths 2000 (Projected) Number ('000s)	Rate (per 100 000)
Males										
0-4	23	86.5	79	300	1.5	70.8	0	0	0	0
5-14	0	0.0	228	427	-	-	0	0	0	0
15-44	0	0.0	787	427	-	-	0	0	0	0
45-59	0	0.0	283	427	-	-	0	0	0	0
60+	0	0.0	259	427	-	-	0	0	0	0
All ages	23	5.8	1 635	419	1.5	70.8	0	0	0	0
Females										
0-4	22	86.4	75	300	1.5	76.7	0	0	0	0
5-14	0	0.0	217	427	-	-	0	0	0	0
15-44	0	0.0	766	427	-	-	0	0	0	0
45-59	0	0.0	290	427	-	-	0	0	0	0
60+	0	0.0	361	427	-	-	0	0	0	0
All ages	22	5.3	1 708	419	1.5	76.7	0	0	0	0
Total	44	5.6	3 343	419	1.5	73.7	0	0	0	0

Table 127b FSE - PEAS - AESE Protein-energy malnutrition - Developmental disability

Age group (years)	Incidence 1990 Number ('000s)	Rate (per 100 000)	Prevalence 1990 Number ('000s)	Rate (per 100 000)	Avg. age at onset (years)	Average duration (years)	Deaths 1990 Number ('000s)	Rate (per 100 000)	Deaths 2000 (Projected) Number ('000s)	Rate (per 100 000)
Males										
0-4	48	347	165	1 200	1.5	64.0	0	0	0	0
5-14	0	0	468	1 710	-	-	0	0	0	0
15-44	0	0	1 304	1 710	-	-	0	0	0	0
45-59	0	0	461	1 710	-	-	0	0	0	0
60+	0	0	358	1 710	-	-	0	0	0	0
All ages	48	29	2 757	1 668	1.5	64.0	0	0	0	0
Females										
0-4	45	346	158	1 200	1.5	72.8	0	0	0	0
5-14	0	0	452	1 709	-	-	0	0	0	0
15-44	0	0	1 281	1 709	-	-	0	0	0	0
45-59	0	0	513	1 709	-	-	0	0	0	0
60+	0	0	622	1 709	-	-	0	0	0	0
All ages	45	25	3 025	1 672	1.5	72.8	0	0	0	0
Total	93	27	5 782	1 670	1.5	68.3	0	0	0	0

Table 127c India - India - Inde Protein-energy malnutrition - Developmental disability

Age group (years)	Incidence 1990 Number ('000s)	Rate (per 100 000)	Prevalence 1990 Number ('000s)	Rate (per 100 000)	Avg. age at onset (years)	Average duration (years)	Deaths 1990 Number ('000s)	Rate (per 100 000)	Deaths 2000 (Projected) Number ('000s)	Rate (per 100 000)
Males										
0-4	1 596	2 669	5 381	9 000	1.5	59.1	0	0	0	0
5-14	0	0	13 107	12 881	-	-	0	0	0	0
15-44	0	0	25 830	12 881	-	-	0	0	0	0
45-59	0	0	6 127	12 881	-	-	0	0	0	0
60+	0	0	3 834	12 881	-	-	0	0	0	0
All ages	1 596	363	54 279	12 353	1.5	59.1	0	0	0	0
Females										
0-4	1 519	2 679	5 101	9 000	1.5	59.9	0	0	0	0
5-14	0	0	12 289	12 900	-	-	0	0	0	0
15-44	0	0	23 638	12 900	-	-	0	0	0	0
45-59	0	0	5 935	12 900	-	-	0	0	0	0
60+	0	0	3 731	12 900	-	-	0	0	0	0
All ages	1 519	370	50 694	12 361	1.5	59.9	0	0	0	0
Total	3 114	367	104 973	12 357	1.5	59.5	0	0	0	0

For epidemiological sources see Bailey et al. 1996. For the methods used to estimate and project incidence, prevalence, and deaths see Murray and Lopez 1996a. See explanatory notes for definitions and caveats.

Table 127
Protein-energy malnutrition

Developmental disability

Cuadro 127
Desnutrición proteínico-calórica

Discapacidad en el desarrollo

Tableau 127
Malnutrition protéino-calorique

Déficit du developpement

Table 127d   China - China - Chine   Protein-energy malnutrition - Developmental disability

Age group (years)	Incidence 1990 Number ('000s)	Rate (per 100 000)	Prevalence 1990 Number ('000s)	Rate (per 100 000)	Avg. age at onset (years)	Average duration (years)	Deaths 1990 Number ('000s)	Rate (per 100 000)	Deaths 2000 (Projected) Number ('000s)	Rate (per 100 000)
Males										
0-4	559	928	1 928	3 200	1.5	65.8	0	0	0	0
5-14	0	0	4 423	4 560	-	-	0	0	0	0
15-44	0	0	13 966	4 560	-	-	0	0	0	0
45-59	0	0	3 314	4 560	-	-	0	0	0	0
60+	0	0	2 233	4 560	-	-	0	0	0	0
All ages	559	95	25 864	4 420	1.5	65.8	0	0	0	0
Females										
0-4	538	929	1 854	3 200	1.5	68.6	0	0	0	0
5-14	0	0	4 125	4 562	-	-	0	0	0	0
15-44	0	0	12 961	4 562	-	-	0	0	0	0
45-59	0	0	2 938	4 562	-	-	0	0	0	0
60+	0	0	2 357	4 562	-	-	0	0	0	0
All ages	538	98	24 235	4 419	1.5	68.6	0	0	0	0
Total	1 097	97	50 099	4 419	1.5	67.2	0	0	0	0

Table 127e   OAI - OPAI - APAI   Protein-energy malnutrition - Developmental disability

Age group (years)	Incidence 1990 Number ('000s)	Rate (per 100 000)	Prevalence 1990 Number ('000s)	Rate (per 100 000)	Avg. age at onset (years)	Average duration (years)	Deaths 1990 Number ('000s)	Rate (per 100 000)	Deaths 2000 (Projected) Number ('000s)	Rate (per 100 000)
Males										
0-4	901	2 058	3 063	7 000	1.5	59.5	0	0	0	0
5-14	0	0	8 404	10 001	-	-	0	0	0	0
15-44	0	0	16 084	10 001	-	-	0	0	0	0
45-59	0	0	3 414	10 001	-	-	0	0	0	0
60+	0	0	2 021	10 001	-	-	0	0	0	0
All ages	901	263	32 987	9 618	1.5	59.5	0	0	0	0
Females										
0-4	860	2 047	2 939	7 000	1.5	63.0	0	0	0	0
5-14	0	0	8 007	9 981	-	-	0	0	0	0
15-44	0	0	15 931	9 981	-	-	0	0	0	0
45-59	0	0	3 502	9 981	-	-	0	0	0	0
60+	0	0	2 262	9 981	-	-	0	0	0	0
All ages	860	253	32 641	9 613	1.5	63.0	0	0	0	0
Total	1 760	258	65 628	9 615	1.5	61.2	0	0	0	0

Table 127f   SSA - ASS - ASS   Protein-energy malnutrition - Developmental disability

Age group (years)	Incidence 1990 Number ('000s)	Rate (per 100 000)	Prevalence 1990 Number ('000s)	Rate (per 100 000)	Avg. age at onset (years)	Average duration (years)	Deaths 1990 Number ('000s)	Rate (per 100 000)	Deaths 2000 (Projected) Number ('000s)	Rate (per 100 000)
Males										
0-4	1 340	2 821	4 369	9 200	1.4	47.2	0	0	0	0
5-14	0	0	9 370	13 337	-	-	0	0	0	0
15-44	0	0	13 839	13 337	-	-	0	0	0	0
45-59	0	0	2 708	13 337	-	-	0	0	0	0
60+	0	0	1 401	13 337	-	-	0	0	0	0
All ages	1 340	531	31 687	12 558	1.4	47.2	0	0	0	0
Females										
0-4	1 313	2 793	4 327	9 200	1.4	50.6	0	0	0	0
5-14	0	0	9 274	13 284	-	-	0	0	0	0
15-44	0	0	14 115	13 284	-	-	0	0	0	0
45-59	0	0	2 938	13 284	-	-	0	0	0	0
60+	0	0	1 691	13 284	-	-	0	0	0	0
All ages	1 313	509	32 345	12 539	1.4	50.6	0	0	0	0
Total	2 653	520	64 032	12 549	1.4	48.9	0	0	0	0

For epidemiological sources see Bailey et al. 1996. For the methods used to estimate and project incidence, prevalence, and deaths see Murray and Lopez 1996a. See explanatory notes for definitions and caveats.

Table 127
Protein-energy malnutrition

Developmental disability

Cuadro 127
Desnutrición proteínico-calórica

Discapacidad en el desarrollo

Tableau 127
Malnutrition protéino-calorique

Déficit du developpement

Table 127g LAC - ALC - ALC — Protein-energy malnutrition - Developmental disability

Age group (years)	Incidence 1990 Number ('000s)	Rate (per 100 000)	Prevalence 1990 Number ('000s)	Rate (per 100 000)	Avg. age at onset (years)	Average duration (years)	Deaths 1990 Number ('000s)	Rate (per 100 000)	Deaths 2000 (Projected) Number ('000s)	Rate (per 100 000)
Males										
0-4	193	674	661	2 300	1.5	63.7	0	0	0	0
5-14	0	0	1 716	3 292	-	-	0	0	0	0
15-44	0	0	3 434	3 292	-	-	0	0	0	0
45-59	0	0	733	3 292	-	-	0	0	0	0
60+	0	0	469	3 292	-	-	0	0	0	0
All ages	193	87	7 011	3 164	1.5	63.7	0	0	0	0
Females										
0-4	186	671	637	2 300	1.5	67.9	0	0	0	0
5-14	0	0	1 668	3 286	-	-	0	0	0	0
15-44	0	0	3 421	3 286	-	-	0	0	0	0
45-59	0	0	768	3 286	-	-	0	0	0	0
60+	0	0	553	3 286	-	-	0	0	0	0
All ages	186	83	7 045	3 164	1.5	67.9	0	0	0	0
Total	379	85	14 057	3 164	1.5	65.8	0	0	0	0

Table 127h MEC - AOM - CMO — Protein-energy malnutrition - Developmental disability

Age group (years)	Incidence 1990 Number ('000s)	Rate (per 100 000)	Prevalence 1990 Number ('000s)	Rate (per 100 000)	Avg. age at onset (years)	Average duration (years)	Deaths 1990 Number ('000s)	Rate (per 100 000)	Deaths 2000 (Projected) Number ('000s)	Rate (per 100 000)
Males										
0-4	925	2 248	3 128	7 600	1.5	60.4	0	0	0	0
5-14	0	0	7 109	10 879	-	-	0	0	0	0
15-44	0	0	12 391	10 879	-	-	0	0	0	0
45-59	0	0	2 430	10 879	-	-	0	0	0	0
60+	0	0	1 485	10 879	-	-	0	0	0	0
All ages	925	361	26 544	10 353	1.5	60.4	0	0	0	0
Females										
0-4	893	2 248	3 020	7 600	1.5	63.0	0	0	0	0
5-14	0	0	6 744	10 878	-	-	0	0	0	0
15-44	0	0	11 662	10 878	-	-	0	0	0	0
45-59	0	0	2 425	10 878	-	-	0	0	0	0
60+	0	0	1 681	10 878	-	-	0	0	0	0
All ages	893	362	25 532	10 350	1.5	63.0	0	0	0	0
Total	1 819	361	52 075	10 351	1.5	61.7	0	0	0	0

Table 127i World - Mundo - Monde — Protein-energy malnutrition - Developmental disability

Age group (years)	Incidence 1990 Number ('000s)	Rate (per 100 000)	Prevalence 1990 Number ('000s)	Rate (per 100 000)	Avg. age at onset (years)	Average duration (years)	Deaths 1990 Number ('000s)	Rate (per 100 000)	Deaths 2000 (Projected) Number ('000s)	Rate (per 100 000)
Males										
0-4	5 584	1 738	18 774	5 843	1.5	57.4	0	0	0	0
5-14	0	0	44 825	8 132	-	-	0	0	0	0
15-44	0	0	87 635	7 011	-	-	0	0	0	0
45-59	0	0	19 470	6 233	-	-	0	0	0	0
60+	0	0	12 061	5 511	-	-	0	0	0	0
All ages	5 584	210	182 764	6 887	1.5	57.4	0	0	0	0
Females										
0-4	5 376	1 738	18 110	5 856	1.5	60.0	0	0	0	0
5-14	0	0	42 774	8 139	-	-	0	0	0	0
15-44	0	0	83 775	6 989	-	-	0	0	0	0
45-59	0	0	19 308	6 207	-	-	0	0	0	0
60+	0	0	13 258	4 925	-	-	0	0	0	0
All ages	5 376	206	177 226	6 781	1.5	60.0	0	0	0	0
Total	10 960	208	359 990	6 834	1.5	58.7	0	0	0	0

For epidemiological sources see Bailey et al. 1996. For the methods used to estimate and project incidence, prevalence, and deaths see Murray and Lopez 1996a. See explanatory notes for definitions and caveats.

Table 128
Iodine deficiency

Cuadro 128
Deficiencia de yodo

Tableau 128
Déficience en iode

Goitre - grade 0   Bocio - grado 0   Goitre - grade 0

Table 128a   **EME - PEMC - EMBE**   Iodine deficiency - Goitre - grade 0

Age group (years)	Incidence 1990 Number ('000s)	Rate (per 100 000)	Prevalence 1990 Number ('000s)	Rate (per 100 000)	Avg. age at onset (years)	Average duration (years)	Deaths 1990 Number ('000s)	Rate (per 100 000)	Deaths 2000 (Projected) Number ('000s)	Rate (per 100 000)
Males										
0-4	-	-	1 225	4 643	-	-	0	0	0	0
5-14	-	-	2 112	3 959	-	-	0	0	0	0
15-44	-	-	3 481	1 891	-	-	0	0	0	0
45-59	-	-	1 251	1 891	-	-	0	0	0	0
60+	-	-	1 025	1 693	-	-	0	0	0	0
All ages	-	-	9 094	2 329	-	-	0	0	0	0
Females										
0-4	-	-	1 164	4 643	-	-	0	0	0	0
5-14	-	-	2 698	5 324	-	-	0	0	0	0
15-44	-	-	6 919	3 861	-	-	0	0	0	0
45-59	-	-	2 618	3 861	-	-	0	0	0	0
60+	-	-	2 934	3 469	-	-	0	0	0	0
All ages	-	-	16 332	4 010	-	-	0	0	0	0
Total	-	-	25 427	3 187	-	-	0	0	0	0

Table 128b   **FSE - PEAS - AESE**   Iodine deficiency - Goitre - grade 0

Age group (years)	Incidence 1990 Number ('000s)	Rate (per 100 000)	Prevalence 1990 Number ('000s)	Rate (per 100 000)	Avg. age at onset (years)	Average duration (years)	Deaths 1990 Number ('000s)	Rate (per 100 000)	Deaths 2000 (Projected) Number ('000s)	Rate (per 100 000)
Males										
0-4	-	-	1 286	9 347	-	-	0	0	0	0
5-14	-	-	2 219	8 113	-	-	0	0	0	0
15-44	-	-	3 616	4 740	-	-	0	0	0	0
45-59	-	-	1 279	4 740	-	-	0	0	0	0
60+	-	-	891	4 252	-	-	0	0	0	0
All ages	-	-	9 291	5 620	-	-	0	0	0	0
Females										
0-4	-	-	1 228	9 347	-	-	0	0	0	0
5-14	-	-	2 495	9 442	-	-	0	0	0	0
15-44	-	-	7 077	9 442	-	-	0	0	0	0
45-59	-	-	2 833	9 442	-	-	0	0	0	0
60+	-	-	3 091	8 494	-	-	0	0	0	0
All ages	-	-	16 724	9 244	-	-	0	0	0	0
Total	-	-	26 015	7 514	-	-	0	0	0	0

Table 128c   **India - India - Inde**   Iodine deficiency - Goitre - grade 0

Age group (years)	Incidence 1990 Number ('000s)	Rate (per 100 000)	Prevalence 1990 Number ('000s)	Rate (per 100 000)	Avg. age at onset (years)	Average duration (years)	Deaths 1990 Number ('000s)	Rate (per 100 000)	Deaths 2000 (Projected) Number ('000s)	Rate (per 100 000)
Males										
0-4	-	-	5 249	8 779	-	-	0	0	0	0
5-14	-	-	7 672	7 540	-	-	0	0	0	0
15-44	-	-	8 919	4 448	-	-	0	0	0	0
45-59	-	-	2 116	4 448	-	-	0	0	0	0
60+	-	-	1 179	3 959	-	-	0	0	0	0
All ages	-	-	25 134	5 720	-	-	0	0	0	0
Females										
0-4	-	-	4 976	8 779	-	-	0	0	0	0
5-14	-	-	9 533	10 007	-	-	0	0	0	0
15-44	-	-	15 913	8 684	-	-	0	0	0	0
45-59	-	-	3 995	8 684	-	-	0	0	0	0
60+	-	-	2 264	7 827	-	-	0	0	0	0
All ages	-	-	36 681	8 944	-	-	0	0	0	0
Total	-	-	61 816	7 277	-	-	0	0	0	0

For epidemiological sources see Bailey 1996. For the methods used to estimate and project incidence, prevalence, and deaths see Murray and Lopez 1996a. See explanatory notes for definitions and caveats.

Table 128 Iodine deficiency	Cuadro 128 Deficiencia de yodo	Tableau 128 Déficience en iode
Goitre - grade 0	Bocio - grado 0	Goitre - grade 0

Table 128d   China - China - Chine   Iodine deficiency - Goitre - grade 0

Age group (years)	Incidence 1990 Number ('000s)	Rate (per 100 000)	Prevalence 1990 Number ('000s)	Rate (per 100 000)	Avg. age at onset (years)	Average duration (years)	Deaths 1990 Number ('000s)	Rate (per 100 000)	Deaths 2000 (Projected) Number ('000s)	Rate (per 100 000)
Males										
0-4	-	-	5 403	8 969	-	-	0	0	0	0
5-14	-	-	7 499	7 732	-	-	0	0	0	0
15-44	-	-	13 922	4 545	-	-	0	0	0	0
45-59	-	-	3 303	4 545	-	-	0	0	0	0
60+	-	-	1 987	4 057	-	-	0	0	0	0
All ages	-	-	32 115	5 488	-	-	0	0	0	0
Females										
0-4	-	-	5 197	8 969	-	-	0	0	0	0
5-14	-	-	9 217	10 196	-	-	0	0	0	0
15-44	-	-	25 478	8 969	-	-	0	0	0	0
45-59	-	-	5 776	8 969	-	-	0	0	0	0
60+	-	-	4 192	8 113	-	-	0	0	0	0
All ages	-	-	49 860	9 090	-	-	0	0	0	0
Total	-	-	81 975	7 231	-	-	0	0	0	0

Table 128e   OAI - OPAI - APAI   Iodine deficiency - Goitre - grade 0

Age group (years)	Incidence 1990 Number ('000s)	Rate (per 100 000)	Prevalence 1990 Number ('000s)	Rate (per 100 000)	Avg. age at onset (years)	Average duration (years)	Deaths 1990 Number ('000s)	Rate (per 100 000)	Deaths 2000 (Projected) Number ('000s)	Rate (per 100 000)
Males										
0-4	-	-	3 925	8 969	-	-	0	0	0	0
5-14	-	-	6 497	7 732	-	-	0	0	0	0
15-44	-	-	7 310	4 545	-	-	0	0	0	0
45-59	-	-	1 552	4 545	-	-	0	0	0	0
60+	-	-	820	4 057	-	-	0	0	0	0
All ages	-	-	20 103	5 862	-	-	0	0	0	0
Females										
0-4	-	-	3 766	8 969	-	-	0	0	0	0
5-14	-	-	8 179	10 196	-	-	0	0	0	0
15-44	-	-	14 315	8 969	-	-	0	0	0	0
45-59	-	-	3 147	8 969	-	-	0	0	0	0
60+	-	-	1 839	8 113	-	-	0	0	0	0
All ages	-	-	31 245	9 201	-	-	0	0	0	0
Total	-	-	51 348	7 523	-	-	0	0	0	0

Table 128f   SSA - ASS - ASS   Iodine deficiency - Goitre - grade 0

Age group (years)	Incidence 1990 Number ('000s)	Rate (per 100 000)	Prevalence 1990 Number ('000s)	Rate (per 100 000)	Avg. age at onset (years)	Average duration (years)	Deaths 1990 Number ('000s)	Rate (per 100 000)	Deaths 2000 (Projected) Number ('000s)	Rate (per 100 000)
Males										
0-4	-	-	6 298	13 262	-	-	0	0	0	0
5-14	-	-	9 318	13 262	-	-	0	0	0	0
15-44	-	-	8 715	8 399	-	-	0	0	0	0
45-59	-	-	1 706	8 399	-	-	0	0	0	0
60+	-	-	792	7 540	-	-	0	0	0	0
All ages	-	-	26 829	10 633	-	-	0	0	0	0
Females										
0-4	-	-	8 110	17 244	-	-	0	0	0	0
5-14	-	-	12 039	17 244	-	-	0	0	0	0
15-44	-	-	17 373	16 350	-	-	0	0	0	0
45-59	-	-	3 616	16 350	-	-	0	0	0	0
60+	-	-	1 886	14 815	-	-	0	0	0	0
All ages	-	-	43 025	16 679	-	-	0	0	0	0
Total	-	-	69 853	13 689	-	-	0	0	0	0

For epidemiological sources see Bailey 1996. For the methods used to estimate and project incidence, prevalence, and deaths see Murray and Lopez 1996a. See explanatory notes for definitions and caveats.

Table 128
Iodine deficiency

Cuadro 128
Deficiencia de yodo

Tableau 128
Déficience en iode

Goitre - grade 0

Bocio - grado 0

Goitre - grade 0

Table 128g   LAC - ALC - ALC   Iodine deficiency - Goitre - grade 0

Age group (years)	Incidence 1990 Number ('000s)	Rate (per 100 000)	Prevalence 1990 Number ('000s)	Rate (per 100 000)	Avg. age at onset (years)	Average duration (years)	Deaths 1990 Number ('000s)	Rate (per 100 000)	Deaths 2000 (Projected) Number ('000s)	Rate (per 100 000)
Males										
0-4	-	-	3 809	13 262	-	-	0	0	0	0
5-14	-	-	5 900	11 319	-	-	0	0	0	0
15-44	-	-	7 564	7 253	-	-	0	0	0	0
45-59	-	-	1 614	7 253	-	-	0	0	0	0
60+	-	-	936	6 580	-	-	0	0	0	0
All ages	-	-	19 823	8 945	-	-	0	0	0	0
Females										
0-4	-	-	3 671	13 262	-	-	0	0	0	0
5-14	-	-	7 610	14 997	-	-	0	0	0	0
15-44	-	-	14 662	14 087	-	-	0	0	0	0
45-59	-	-	3 290	14 087	-	-	0	0	0	0
60+	-	-	2 138	12 710	-	-	0	0	0	0
All ages	-	-	31 371	14 088	-	-	0	0	0	0
Total	-	-	51 194	11 523	-	-	0	0	0	0

Table 128h   MEC - AOM - CMO   Iodine deficiency - Goitre - grade 0

Age group (years)	Incidence 1990 Number ('000s)	Rate (per 100 000)	Prevalence 1990 Number ('000s)	Rate (per 100 000)	Avg. age at onset (years)	Average duration (years)	Deaths 1990 Number ('000s)	Rate (per 100 000)	Deaths 2000 (Projected) Number ('000s)	Rate (per 100 000)
Males										
0-4	-	-	8 791	21 358	-	-	0	0	0	0
5-14	-	-	12 136	18 573	-	-	0	0	0	0
15-44	-	-	13 950	12 248	-	-	0	0	0	0
45-59	-	-	2 736	12 248	-	-	0	0	0	0
60+	-	-	1 095	8 018	-	-	0	0	0	0
All ages	-	-	38 708	15 097	-	-	0	0	0	0
Females										
0-4	-	-	8 487	21 358	-	-	0	0	0	0
5-14	-	-	14 927	24 077	-	-	0	0	0	0
15-44	-	-	25 272	23 572	-	-	0	0	0	0
45-59	-	-	5 255	23 572	-	-	0	0	0	0
60+	-	-	3 300	21 358	-	-	0	0	0	0
All ages	-	-	57 240	23 204	-	-	0	0	0	0
Total	-	-	95 948	19 072	-	-	0	0	0	0

Table 128i   World - Mundo - Monde   Iodine deficiency - Goitre - grade 0

Age group (years)	Incidence 1990 Number ('000s)	Rate (per 100 000)	Prevalence 1990 Number ('000s)	Rate (per 100 000)	Avg. age at onset (years)	Average duration (years)	Deaths 1990 Number ('000s)	Rate (per 100 000)	Deaths 2000 (Projected) Number ('000s)	Rate (per 100 000)
Males										
0-4	-	-	35 986	11 200	-	-	0	0	0	0
5-14	-	-	53 354	9 680	-	-	0	0	0	0
15-44	-	-	67 477	5 399	-	-	0	0	0	0
45-59	-	-	15 555	4 980	-	-	0	0	0	0
60+	-	-	8 725	3 987	-	-	0	0	0	0
All ages	-	-	181 097	6 824	-	-	0	0	0	0
Females										
0-4	-	-	36 597	11 834	-	-	0	0	0	0
5-14	-	-	66 698	12 691	-	-	0	0	0	0
15-44	-	-	127 010	10 596	-	-	0	0	0	0
45-59	-	-	30 530	9 815	-	-	0	0	0	0
60+	-	-	21 643	8 039	-	-	0	0	0	0
All ages	-	-	282 479	10 808	-	-	0	0	0	0
Total	-	-	463 576	8 801	-	-	0	0	0	0

For epidemiological sources see Bailey 1996. For the methods used to estimate and project incidence, prevalence, and deaths see Murray and Lopez 1996a. See explanatory notes for definitions and caveats.

Table 129
Iodine deficiency

Cuadro 129
Deficiencia de yodo

Tableau 129
Déficience en iode

Goitre - grade 1

Bocio - grado 1

Goitre - grade 1

Table 129a   EME - PEMC - EMBE   Iodine deficiency - Goitre - grade 1

Age group (years)	Incidence 1990 Number ('000s)	Rate (per 100 000)	Prevalence 1990 Number ('000s)	Rate (per 100 000)	Avg. age at onset (years)	Average duration (years)	Deaths 1990 Number ('000s)	Rate (per 100 000)	Deaths 2000 (Projected) Number ('000s)	Rate (per 100 000)
Males										
0-4	-	-	14	51.5	-	-	0	0	0	0
5-14	-	-	20	36.8	-	-	0	0	0	0
15-44	-	-	14	7.8	-	-	0	0	0	0
45-59	-	-	5	7.8	-	-	0	0	0	0
60+	-	-	4	6.2	-	-	0	0	0	0
All ages	-	-	57	14.5	-	-	0	0	0	0
Females										
0-4	-	-	13	51.5	-	-	0	0	0	0
5-14	-	-	35	68.7	-	-	0	0	0	0
15-44	-	-	63	34.9	-	-	0	0	0	0
45-59	-	-	24	34.9	-	-	0	0	0	0
60ı	-	-	24	27.9	-	-	0	0	0	0
All ages	-	-	158	38./	-	-	0	0	0	0
Total	-	-	214	26.8	-	-	0	0	0	0

Table 129b   FSE - PEAS - AESE   Iodine deficiency - Goitre - grade 1

Age group (years)	Incidence 1990 Number ('000s)	Rate (per 100 000)	Prevalence 1990 Number ('000s)	Rate (per 100 000)	Avg. age at onset (years)	Average duration (years)	Deaths 1990 Number ('000s)	Rate (per 100 000)	Deaths 2000 (Projected) Number ('000s)	Rate (per 100 000)
Males										
0-4	-	-	31	227	-	-	0	0	0	0
5-14	-	-	46	168	-	-	0	0	0	0
15-44	-	-	41	54	-	-	0	0	0	0
45-59	-	-	15	54	-	-	0	0	0	0
60+	-	-	9	43	-	-	0	0	0	0
All ages	-	-	142	86	-	-	0	0	0	0
Females										
0-4	-	-	30	227	-	-	0	0	0	0
5-14	-	-	61	232	-	-	0	0	0	0
15-44	-	-	174	232	-	-	0	0	0	0
45-59	-	-	70	232	-	-	0	0	0	0
60+	-	-	67	185	-	-	0	0	0	0
All ages	-	-	403	223	-	-	0	0	0	0
Total	-	-	544	157	-	-	0	0	0	0

Table 129c   India - India - Inde   Iodine deficiency - Goitre - grade 1

Age group (years)	Incidence 1990 Number ('000s)	Rate (per 100 000)	Prevalence 1990 Number ('000s)	Rate (per 100 000)	Avg. age at onset (years)	Average duration (years)	Deaths 1990 Number ('000s)	Rate (per 100 000)	Deaths 2000 (Projected) Number ('000s)	Rate (per 100 000)
Males										
0-4	-	-	119	199	-	-	0	0	0	0
5-14	-	-	146	144	-	-	0	0	0	0
15-44	-	-	94	47	-	-	0	0	0	0
45-59	-	-	22	47	-	-	0	0	0	0
60+	-	-	11	37	-	-	0	0	0	0
All ages	-	-	393	89	-	-	0	0	0	0
Females										
0-4	-	-	113	199	-	-	0	0	0	0
5-14	-	-	251	263	-	-	0	0	0	0
15-44	-	-	356	194	-	-	0	0	0	0
45-59	-	-	89	194	-	-	0	0	0	0
60+	-	-	45	156	-	-	0	0	0	0
All ages	-	-	854	208	-	-	0	0	0	0
Total	-	-	1 247	147	-	-	0	0	0	0

For epidemiological sources see Bailey 1996. For the methods used to estimate and project incidence, prevalence, and deaths see Murray and Lopez 1996a. See explanatory notes for definitions and caveats.

Table 129
Iodine deficiency

Cuadro 129
Deficiencia de yodo

Tableau 129
Déficience en iode

Goitre - grade 1

Bocio - grado 1

Goitre - grade 1

Table 129d   China - China - Chine   Iodine deficiency - Goitre - grade 1

Age group (years)	Incidence 1990 Number ('000s)	Rate (per 100 000)	Prevalence 1990 Number ('000s)	Rate (per 100 000)	Avg. age at onset (years)	Average duration (years)	Deaths 1990 Number ('000s)	Rate (per 100 000)	Deaths 2000 (Projected) Number ('000s)	Rate (per 100 000)
Males										
0-4	-	-	125	208	-	-	0	0	0	0
5-14	-	-	147	152	-	-	0	0	0	0
15-44	-	-	151	49	-	-	0	0	0	0
45-59	-	-	36	49	-	-	0	0	0	0
60+	-	-	19	39	-	-	0	0	0	0
All ages	-	-	478	82	-	-	0	0	0	0
Females										
0-4	-	-	121	208	-	-	0	0	0	0
5-14	-	-	248	274	-	-	0	0	0	0
15-44	-	-	591	208	-	-	0	0	0	0
45-59	-	-	134	208	-	-	0	0	0	0
60+	-	-	87	168	-	-	0	0	0	0
All ages	-	-	1 181	215	-	-	0	0	0	0
Total	-	-	1 659	146	-	-	0	0	0	0

Table 129e   OAI - OPAI - APAI   Iodine deficiency - Goitre - grade 1

Age group (years)	Incidence 1990 Number ('000s)	Rate (per 100 000)	Prevalence 1990 Number ('000s)	Rate (per 100 000)	Avg. age at onset (years)	Average duration (years)	Deaths 1990 Number ('000s)	Rate (per 100 000)	Deaths 2000 (Projected) Number ('000s)	Rate (per 100 000)
Males										
0-4	-	-	91	208	-	-	0	0	0	0
5-14	-	-	127	152	-	-	0	0	0	0
15-44	-	-	79	49	-	-	0	0	0	0
45-59	-	-	17	49	-	-	0	0	0	0
60+	-	-	8	39	-	-	0	0	0	0
All ages	-	-	322	94	-	-	0	0	0	0
Females										
0-4	-	-	87	208	-	-	0	0	0	0
5-14	-	-	220	274	-	-	0	0	0	0
15-44	-	-	332	208	-	-	0	0	0	0
45-59	-	-	73	208	-	-	0	0	0	0
60+	-	-	38	168	-	-	0	0	0	0
All ages	-	-	751	221	-	-	0	0	0	0
Total	-	-	1 073	157	-	-	0	0	0	0

Table 129f   SSA - ASS - ASS   Iodine deficiency - Goitre - grade 1

Age group (years)	Incidence 1990 Number ('000s)	Rate (per 100 000)	Prevalence 1990 Number ('000s)	Rate (per 100 000)	Avg. age at onset (years)	Average duration (years)	Deaths 1990 Number ('000s)	Rate (per 100 000)	Deaths 2000 (Projected) Number ('000s)	Rate (per 100 000)
Males										
0-4	-	-	230	484	-	-	0	0	0	0
5-14	-	-	340	484	-	-	0	0	0	0
15-44	-	-	188	181	-	-	0	0	0	0
45-59	-	-	37	181	-	-	0	0	0	0
60+	-	-	15	144	-	-	0	0	0	0
All ages	-	-	809	321	-	-	0	0	0	0
Females										
0-4	-	-	405	860	-	-	0	0	0	0
5-14	-	-	601	860	-	-	0	0	0	0
15-44	-	-	813	765	-	-	0	0	0	0
45-59	-	-	169	765	-	-	0	0	0	0
60+	-	-	78	616	-	-	0	0	0	0
All ages	-	-	2 066	801	-	-	0	0	0	0
Total	-	-	2 875	563	-	-	0	0	0	0

For epidemiological sources see Bailey 1996. For the methods used to estimate and project incidence, prevalence, and deaths see Murray and Lopez 1996a. See explanatory notes for definitions and caveats.

Table 129
Iodine deficiency

Cuadro 129
Deficiencia de yodo

Tableau 129
Déficience en iode

Goitre - grade 1

Bocio - grado 1

Goitre - grade 1

Table 129g LAC - ALC - ALC Iodine deficiency - Goitre - grade 1

Age group (years)	Incidence 1990 Number ('000s)	Rate (per 100 000)	Prevalence 1990 Number ('000s)	Rate (per 100 000)	Avg. age at onset (years)	Average duration (years)	Deaths 1990 Number ('000s)	Rate (per 100 000)	Deaths 2000 (Projected) Number ('000s)	Rate (per 100 000)
Males										
0-4	-	-	139	484	-	-	0	0	0	0
5-14	-	-	179	343	-	-	0	0	0	0
15-44	-	-	138	132	-	-	0	0	0	0
45-59	-	-	29	132	-	-	0	0	0	0
60+	-	-	15	108	-	-	0	0	0	0
All ages	-	-	501	226	-	-	0	0	0	0
Females										
0-4	-	-	134	484	-	-	0	0	0	0
5-14	-	-	321	633	-	-	0	0	0	0
15-44	-	-	574	552	-	-	0	0	0	0
45-59	-	-	129	552	-	-	0	0	0	0
60+	-	-	74	441	-	-	0	0	0	0
All ages	-	-	1 232	553	-	-	0	0	0	0
Total	-	-	1 733	390	-	-	0	0	0	0

Table 129h MEC - AOM - CMO Iodine deficiency - Goitre - grade 1

Age group (years)	Incidence 1990 Number ('000s)	Rate (per 100 000)	Prevalence 1990 Number ('000s)	Rate (per 100 000)	Avg. age at onset (years)	Average duration (years)	Deaths 1990 Number ('000s)	Rate (per 100 000)	Deaths 2000 (Projected) Number ('000s)	Rate (per 100 000)
Males										
0-4	-	-	571	1 387	-	-	0	0	0	0
5-14	-	-	663	1 014	-	-	0	0	0	0
15-44	-	-	464	407	-	-	0	0	0	0
45-59	-	-	91	407	-	-	0	0	0	0
60+	-	-	22	164	-	-	0	0	0	0
All ages	-	-	1 811	706	-	-	0	0	0	0
Females										
0-4	-	-	551	1 387	-	-	0	0	0	0
5-14	-	-	1 129	1 821	-	-	0	0	0	0
15-44	-	-	1 860	1 735	-	-	0	0	0	0
45-59	-	-	387	1 735	-	-	0	0	0	0
60+	-	-	214	1 387	-	-	0	0	0	0
All ages	-	-	4 142	1 679	-	-	0	0	0	0
Total	-	-	5 953	1 183	-	-	0	0	0	0

Table 129i World - Mundo - Monde Iodine deficiency - Goitre - grade 1

Age group (years)	Incidence 1990 Number ('000s)	Rate (per 100 000)	Prevalence 1990 Number ('000s)	Rate (per 100 000)	Avg. age at onset (years)	Average duration (years)	Deaths 1990 Number ('000s)	Rate (per 100 000)	Deaths 2000 (Projected) Number ('000s)	Rate (per 100 000)
Males										
0-4	-	-	1 320	411	-	-	0	0	0	0
5-14	-	-	1 668	303	-	-	0	0	0	0
15-44	-	-	1 169	94	-	-	0	0	0	0
45-59	-	-	252	81	-	-	0	0	0	0
60+	-	-	103	47	-	-	0	0	0	0
All ages	-	-	4 512	170	-	-	0	0	0	0
Females										
0-4	-	-	1 453	470	-	-	0	0	0	0
5-14	-	-	2 865	545	-	-	0	0	0	0
15-44	-	-	4 764	397	-	-	0	0	0	0
45-59	-	-	1 075	346	-	-	0	0	0	0
60+	-	-	628	233	-	-	0	0	0	0
All ages	-	-	10 785	413	-	-	0	0	0	0
Total	-	-	15 297	290	-	-	0	0	0	0

For epidemiological sources see Bailey 1996. For the methods used to estimate and project incidence, prevalence, and deaths see Murray and Lopez 1996a. See explanatory notes for definitions and caveats.

Table 130	Cuadro 130	Tableau 130
Iodine deficiency	**Deficiencia de yodo**	**Déficience en iode**
Goitre - grade 2	Bocio - grado 2	Goitre - grade 2

Table 130a   EME - PEMC - EMBE   Iodine deficiency - Goitre - grade 2

Age group (years)	Incidence 1990 Number ('000s)	Rate (per 100 000)	Prevalence 1990 Number ('000s)	Rate (per 100 000)	Avg. age at onset (years)	Average duration (years)	Deaths 1990 Number ('000s)	Rate (per 100 000)	Deaths 2000 (Projected) Number ('000s)	Rate (per 100 000)
Males										
0-4	-	-	2	5.7	-	-	-	-	-	-
5-14	-	-	2	4.1	-	-	-	-	-	-
15-44	-	-	2	0.9	-	-	-	-	-	-
45-59	-	-	1	0.9	-	-	-	-	-	-
60+	-	-	0	0.7	-	-	-	-	-	-
All ages	-	-	6	1.6	-	-	-	-	-	-
Females										
0-4	-	-	1	5.7	-	-	-	-	-	-
5-14	-	-	4	7.6	-	-	-	-	-	-
15-44	-	-	7	3.9	-	-	-	-	-	-
45-59	-	-	3	3.9	-	-	-	-	-	-
60+	-	-	3	3.1	-	-	-	-	-	-
All ages	-	-	18	4.3	-	-	-	-	-	-
Total	-	-	24	3.0	-	-	-	-	-	-

Table 130b   FSE - PEAS - AESE   Iodine deficiency - Goitre - grade 2

Age group (years)	Incidence 1990 Number ('000s)	Rate (per 100 000)	Prevalence 1990 Number ('000s)	Rate (per 100 000)	Avg. age at onset (years)	Average duration (years)	Deaths 1990 Number ('000s)	Rate (per 100 000)	Deaths 2000 (Projected) Number ('000s)	Rate (per 100 000)
Males										
0-4	-	-	3	25.3	-	-	-	-	-	-
5-14	-	-	0	18.7	-	-	-	-	-	-
15-44	-	-	5	6.0	-	-	-	-	-	-
45-59	-	-	2	6.0	-	-	-	-	-	-
60+	-	-	1	4.8	-	-	-	-	-	-
All ages	-	-	11	7.7	-	-	-	-	-	-
Females										
0-4	-	-	3	25.3	-	-	-	-	-	-
5-14	-	-	7	25.8	-	-	-	-	-	-
15-44	-	-	19	25.8	-	-	-	-	-	-
45-59	-	-	8	25.8	-	-	-	-	-	-
60+	-	-	7	20.6	-	-	-	-	-	-
All ages	-	-	45	24.7	-	-	-	-	-	-
Total	-	-	55	17.4	-	-	-	-	-	-

Table 130c   India - India - Inde   Iodine deficiency - Goitre - grade 2

Age group (years)	Incidence 1990 Number ('000s)	Rate (per 100 000)	Prevalence 1990 Number ('000s)	Rate (per 100 000)	Avg. age at onset (years)	Average duration (years)	Deaths 1990 Number ('000s)	Rate (per 100 000)	Deaths 2000 (Projected) Number ('000s)	Rate (per 100 000)
Males										
0-4	-	-	13	22.1	-	-	-	-	-	-
5-14	-	-	16	16.0	-	-	-	-	-	-
15-44	-	-	10	5.2	-	-	-	-	-	-
45-59	-	-	2	5.2	-	-	-	-	-	-
60+	-	-	1	4.1	-	-	-	-	-	-
All ages	-	-	44	9.9	-	-	-	-	-	-
Females										
0-4	-	-	13	22.1	-	-	-	-	-	-
5-14	-	-	28	29.3	-	-	-	-	-	-
15-44	-	-	40	21.6	-	-	-	-	-	-
45-59	-	-	10	21.6	-	-	-	-	-	-
60+	-	-	5	17.3	-	-	-	-	-	-
All ages	-	-	95	23.1	-	-	-	-	-	-
Total	-	-	139	16.3	-	-	-	-	-	-

For epidemiological sources see Bailey 1996. For the methods used to estimate and project incidence, prevalence, and deaths see Murray and Lopez 1996a. See explanatory notes for definitions and caveats.

Table 130
Iodine deficiency

Cuadro 130
Deficiencia de yodo

Tableau 130
Déficience en iode

Goitre - grade 2

Bocio - grado 2

Goitre - grade 2

Table 130d China - China - Chine — Iodine deficiency - Goitre - grade 2

Age group (years)	Incidence 1990 Number ('000s)	Rate (per 100 000)	Prevalence 1990 Number ('000s)	Rate (per 100 000)	Avg. age at onset (years)	Average duration (years)	Deaths 1990 Number ('000s)	Rate (per 100 000)	Deaths 2000 (Projected) Number ('000s)	Rate (per 100 000)
Males										
0-4	-	-	14	23.1	-	-	-	-	-	-
5-14	-	-	16	16.8	-	-	-	-	-	-
15-44	-	-	17	5.5	-	-	-	-	-	-
45-59	-	-	4	5.5	-	-	-	-	-	-
60+	-	-	2	4.3	-	-	-	-	-	-
All ages	-	-	53	9.1	-	-	-	-	-	-
Females										
0-4	-	-	13	23.1	-	-	-	-	-	-
5-14	-	-	28	30.4	-	-	-	-	-	-
15-44	-	-	66	23.1	-	-	-	-	-	-
45-59	-	-	15	23.1	-	-	-	-	-	-
60+	-	-	10	18.7	-	-	-	-	-	-
All ages	-	-	131	23.9	-	-	-	-	-	-
Total	-	-	184	16.3	-	-	-	-	-	-

Table 130e OAI - OPAI - APAI — Iodine deficiency - Goitre - grade 2

Age group (years)	Incidence 1990 Number ('000s)	Rate (per 100 000)	Prevalence 1990 Number ('000s)	Rate (per 100 000)	Avg. age at onset (years)	Average duration (years)	Deaths 1990 Number ('000s)	Rate (per 100 000)	Deaths 2000 (Projected) Number ('000s)	Rate (per 100 000)
Males										
0-4	-	-	10	23.1	-	-	-	-	-	-
5-14	-	-	14	16.8	-	-	-	-	-	-
15-44	-	-	9	5.5	-	-	-	-	-	-
45-59	-	-	2	5.5	-	-	-	-	-	-
60+	-	-	1	4.3	-	-	-	-	-	-
All ages	-	-	36	10.4	-	-	-	-	-	-
Females										
0-4	-	-	10	23.1	-	-	-	-	-	-
5-14	-	-	24	30.4	-	-	-	-	-	-
15-44	-	-	37	23.1	-	-	-	-	-	-
45-59	-	-	8	23.1	-	-	-	-	-	-
60+	-	-	4	18.7	-	-	-	-	-	-
All ages	-	-	83	24.6	-	-	-	-	-	-
Total	-	-	119	17.5	-	-	-	-	-	-

Table 130f SSA - ASS - ASS — Iodine deficiency - Goitre - grade 2

Age group (years)	Incidence 1990 Number ('000s)	Rate (per 100 000)	Prevalence 1990 Number ('000s)	Rate (per 100 000)	Avg. age at onset (years)	Average duration (years)	Deaths 1990 Number ('000s)	Rate (per 100 000)	Deaths 2000 (Projected) Number ('000s)	Rate (per 100 000)
Males										
0-4	-	-	26	54	-	-	-	-	-	-
5-14	-	-	38	54	-	-	-	-	-	-
15-44	-	-	21	20	-	-	-	-	-	-
45-59	-	-	4	20	-	-	-	-	-	-
60+	-	-	2	16	-	-	-	-	-	-
All ages	-	-	90	36	-	-	-	-	-	-
Females										
0-4	-	-	45	96	-	-	-	-	-	-
5-14	-	-	67	96	-	-	-	-	-	-
15-44	-	-	90	85	-	-	-	-	-	-
45-59	-	-	19	85	-	-	-	-	-	-
60+	-	-	9	68	-	-	-	-	-	-
All ages	-	-	230	89	-	-	-	-	-	-
Total	-	-	319	63	-	-	-	-	-	-

For epidemiological sources see Bailey 1996. For the methods used to estimate and project incidence, prevalence, and deaths see Murray and Lopez 1996a. See explanatory notes for definitions and caveats.

Table 130 | **Cuadro 130** | **Tableau 130**
Iodine deficiency | Deficiencia de yodo | Déficience en iode

Goitre - grade 2 | Bocio - grado 2 | Goitre - grade 2

Table 130g — LAC - ALC - ALC — Iodine deficiency - Goitre - grade 2

Age group (years)	Incidence 1990 Number ('000s)	Rate (per 100 000)	Prevalence 1990 Number ('000s)	Rate (per 100 000)	Avg. age at onset (years)	Average duration (years)	Deaths 1990 Number ('000s)	Rate (per 100 000)	Deaths 2000 (Projected) Number ('000s)	Rate (per 100 000)
Males										
0-4	-	-	15	54	-	-	-	-	-	-
5-14	-	-	20	38	-	-	-	-	-	-
15-44	-	-	15	15	-	-	-	-	-	-
45-59	-	-	3	15	-	-	-	-	-	-
60+	-	-	2	12	-	-	-	-	-	-
All ages	-	-	56	25	-	-	-	-	-	-
Females										
0-4	-	-	15	54	-	-	-	-	-	-
5-14	-	-	36	70	-	-	-	-	-	-
15-44	-	-	64	61	-	-	-	-	-	-
45-59	-	-	14	61	-	-	-	-	-	-
60+	-	-	8	49	-	-	-	-	-	-
All ages	-	-	137	61	-	-	-	-	-	-
Total	-	-	193	43	-	-	-	-	-	-

Table 130h — MEC - AOM - CMO — Iodine deficiency - Goitre - grade 2

Age group (years)	Incidence 1990 Number ('000s)	Rate (per 100 000)	Prevalence 1990 Number ('000s)	Rate (per 100 000)	Avg. age at onset (years)	Average duration (years)	Deaths 1990 Number ('000s)	Rate (per 100 000)	Deaths 2000 (Projected) Number ('000s)	Rate (per 100 000)
Males										
0-4	-	-	63	154	-	-	-	-	-	-
5-14	-	-	74	113	-	-	-	-	-	-
15-44	-	-	52	45	-	-	-	-	-	-
45-59	-	-	10	45	-	-	-	-	-	-
60+	-	-	2	18	-	-	-	-	-	-
All ages	-	-	201	78	-	-	-	-	-	-
Females										
0-4	-	-	61	154	-	-	-	-	-	-
5-14	-	-	125	202	-	-	-	-	-	-
15-44	-	-	207	193	-	-	-	-	-	-
45-59	-	-	43	193	-	-	-	-	-	-
60+	-	-	24	154	-	-	-	-	-	-
All ages	-	-	460	187	-	-	-	-	-	-
Total	-	-	661	131	-	-	-	-	-	-

Table 130i — World - Mundo - Monde — Iodine deficiency - Goitre - grade 2

Age group (years)	Incidence 1990 Number ('000s)	Rate (per 100 000)	Prevalence 1990 Number ('000s)	Rate (per 100 000)	Avg. age at onset (years)	Average duration (years)	Deaths 1990 Number ('000s)	Rate (per 100 000)	Deaths 2000 (Projected) Number ('000s)	Rate (per 100 000)
Males										
0-4	-	-	147	45.6	-	-	-	-	-	-
5-14	-	-	180	32.7	-	-	-	-	-	-
15-44	-	-	130	10.4	-	-	-	-	-	-
45-59	-	-	28	9.0	-	-	-	-	-	-
60+	-	-	11	5.2	-	-	-	-	-	-
All ages	-	-	496	18.7	-	-	-	-	-	-
Females										
0-4	-	-	161	52.2	-	-	-	-	-	-
5-14	-	-	318	60.6	-	-	-	-	-	-
15-44	-	-	529	44.2	-	-	-	-	-	-
45-59	-	-	119	38.4	-	-	-	-	-	-
60+	-	-	70	25.9	-	-	-	-	-	-
All ages	-	-	1 198	45.8	-	-	-	-	-	-
Total	-	-	1 695	32.2	-	-	-	-	-	-

For epidemiological sources see Bailey 1996. For the methods used to estimate and project incidence, prevalence, and deaths see Murray and Lopez 1996a. See explanatory notes for definitions and caveats.

Table 131
Iodine deficiency

Cuadro 131
Deficiencia de yodo

Tableau 131
Déficience en iode

Mild developmental disability | Discapacidad leve en el desarrollo | Déficit léger du développement

Table 131a EME - PEMC - EMBE   Iodine deficiency - Mild developmental disability

Age group (years)	Incidence 1990 Number ('000s)	Rate (per 100 000)	Prevalence 1990 Number ('000s)	Rate (per 100 000)	Avg. age at onset (years)	Average duration (years)	Deaths 1990 Number ('000s)	Rate (per 100 000)	Deaths 2000 (Projected) Number ('000s)	Rate (per 100 000)
Males										
0-4	0	1.6	1	3.9	2.5	70.2	0	0	0	0
5-14	0	0.0	4	7.8	-	-	0	0	0	0
15-44	0	0.0	14	7.8	-	-	0	0	0	0
45-59	0	0.0	5	7.8	-	-	0	0	0	0
60+	0	0.0	5	7.8	-	-	0	0	0	0
All ages	0	0.1	29	7.5	2.5	70.2	0	0	0	0
Females										
0-4	0	1.6	1	3.9	2.5	76.1	0	0	0	0
5-14	0	0.0	4	7.8	-	-	0	0	0	0
15-44	0	0.0	14	7.8	-	-	0	0	0	0
45-59	0	0.0	5	7.8	-	-	0	0	0	0
60+	0	0.0	7	7.8	-	-	0	0	0	0
All ages	0	0.1	31	7.5	2.5	76.1	0	0	0	0
Total	1	0.1	60	7.5	2.5	73.1	0	0	0	0

Table 131b FSE - PEAS - AESE   Iodine deficiency - Mild developmental disability

Age group (years)	Incidence 1990 Number ('000s)	Rate (per 100 000)	Prevalence 1990 Number ('000s)	Rate (per 100 000)	Avg. age at onset (years)	Average duration (years)	Deaths 1990 Number ('000s)	Rate (per 100 000)	Deaths 2000 (Projected) Number ('000s)	Rate (per 100 000)
Males										
0-4	0	3.2	1	7.8	2.5	63.5	0	0	0	0
5-14	0	0.0	4	15.7	-	-	0	0	0	0
15-44	0	0.0	12	15.7	-	-	0	0	0	0
45-59	0	0.0	4	15.7	-	-	0	0	0	0
60+	0	0.0	3	15.7	-	-	0	0	0	0
All ages	0	0.3	25	15.0	2.5	63.5	0	0	0	0
Females										
0-4	0	3.2	1	7.9	2.5	72.4	0	0	0	0
5-14	0	0.0	4	15.7	-	-	0	0	0	0
15-44	0	0.0	12	15.7	-	-	0	0	0	0
45-59	0	0.0	5	15.7	-	-	0	0	0	0
60+	0	0.0	6	15.7	-	-	0	0	0	0
All ages	0	0.2	27	15.1	2.5	72.4	0	0	0	0
Total	1	0.2	52	15.1	2.5	67.8	0	0	0	0

Table 131c India - India - Inde   Iodine deficiency - Mild developmental disability

Age group (years)	Incidence 1990 Number ('000s)	Rate (per 100 000)	Prevalence 1990 Number ('000s)	Rate (per 100 000)	Avg. age at onset (years)	Average duration (years)	Deaths 1990 Number ('000s)	Rate (per 100 000)	Deaths 2000 (Projected) Number ('000s)	Rate (per 100 000)
Males										
0-4	6	9.7	14	24	2.5	59.9	0	0	0	0
5-14	0	0.0	49	48	-	-	0	0	0	0
15-44	0	0.0	97	48	-	-	0	0	0	0
45-59	0	0.0	23	48	-	-	0	0	0	0
60+	0	0.0	14	48	-	-	0	0	0	0
All ages	6	1.3	198	45	2.5	59.9	0	0	0	0
Females										
0-4	6	9.7	13	24	2.5	60.8	0	0	0	0
5-14	0	0.0	46	48	-	-	0	0	0	0
15-44	0	0.0	89	48	-	-	0	0	0	0
45-59	0	0.0	22	48	-	-	0	0	0	0
60+	0	0.0	14	48	-	-	0	0	0	0
All ages	6	1.3	184	45	2.5	60.8	0	0	0	0
Total	11	1.3	382	45	2.5	60.3	0	0	0	0

For epidemiological sources see Bailey 1996. For the methods used to estimate and project incidence, prevalence, and deaths see Murray and Lopez 1996a. See explanatory notes for definitions and caveats.

Table 131
Iodine deficiency

Cuadro 131
Deficiencia de yodo

Tableau 131
Déficience en iode

Mild developmental disability   Discapacidad leve en el desarrollo   Déficit léger du développement

Table 131d   China - China - Chine   Iodine deficiency - Mild developmental disability

Age group (years)	Incidence 1990 Number ('000s)	Rate (per 100 000)	Prevalence 1990 Number ('000s)	Rate (per 100 000)	Avg. age at onset (years)	Average duration (years)	Deaths 1990 Number ('000s)	Rate (per 100 000)	Deaths 2000 (Projected) Number ('000s)	Rate (per 100 000)
Males										
0-4	6	9.6	14	24	2.5	65.5	0	0	0	0
5-14	0	0.0	46	48	-	-	0	0	0	0
15-44	0	0.0	146	48	-	-	0	0	0	0
45-59	0	0.0	35	48	-	-	0	0	0	0
60+	0	0.0	23	48	-	-	0	0	0	0
All ages	6	1.0	264	45	2.5	65.5	0	0	0	0
Females										
0-4	6	9.6	14	24	2.5	68.5	0	0	0	0
5-14	0	0.0	43	48	-	-	0	0	0	0
15-44	0	0.0	135	48	-	-	0	0	0	0
45-59	0	0.0	31	48	-	-	0	0	0	0
60+	0	0.0	25	48	-	-	0	0	0	0
All ages	6	1.0	247	45	2.5	68.5	0	0	0	0
Total	11	1.0	510	45	2.5	67.0	0	0	0	0

Table 131e   OAI - OPAI - APAI   Iodine deficiency - Mild developmental disability

Age group (years)	Incidence 1990 Number ('000s)	Rate (per 100 000)	Prevalence 1990 Number ('000s)	Rate (per 100 000)	Avg. age at onset (years)	Average duration (years)	Deaths 1990 Number ('000s)	Rate (per 100 000)	Deaths 2000 (Projected) Number ('000s)	Rate (per 100 000)
Males										
0-4	3	5.8	6	14	2.5	59.8	0	0	0	0
5-14	0	0.0	24	29	-	-	0	0	0	0
15-44	0	0.0	46	29	-	-	0	0	0	0
45-59	0	0.0	10	29	-	-	0	0	0	0
60+	0	0.0	6	29	-	-	0	0	0	0
All ages	3	0.7	93	27	2.5	59.8	0	0	0	0
Females										
0-4	2	5.8	6	14	2.5	63.2	0	0	0	0
5-14	0	0.0	23	29	-	-	0	0	0	0
15-44	0	0.0	46	29	-	-	0	0	0	0
45-59	0	0.0	10	29	-	-	0	0	0	0
60+	0	0.0	7	29	-	-	0	0	0	0
All ages	2	0.7	92	27	2.5	63.2	0	0	0	0
Total	5	0.7	184	27	2.5	61.5	0	0	0	0

Table 131f   SSA - ASS - ASS   Iodine deficiency - Mild developmental disability

Age group (years)	Incidence 1990 Number ('000s)	Rate (per 100 000)	Prevalence 1990 Number ('000s)	Rate (per 100 000)	Avg. age at onset (years)	Average duration (years)	Deaths 1990 Number ('000s)	Rate (per 100 000)	Deaths 2000 (Projected) Number ('000s)	Rate (per 100 000)
Males										
0-4	3	5.3	6	13	2.5	48.7	0	0	0	0
5-14	0	0.0	19	27	-	-	0	0	0	0
15-44	0	0.0	28	27	-	-	0	0	0	0
45-59	0	0.0	5	27	-	-	0	0	0	0
60+	0	0.0	3	27	-	-	0	0	0	0
All ages	3	1.0	61	24	2.5	48.7	0	0	0	0
Females										
0-4	3	5.3	6	13	2.5	51.9	0	0	0	0
5-14	0	0.0	19	27	-	-	0	0	0	0
15-44	0	0.0	28	27	-	-	0	0	0	0
45-59	0	0.0	6	27	-	-	0	0	0	0
60+	0	0.0	3	27	-	-	0	0	0	0
All ages	3	1.0	62	24	2.5	51.9	0	0	0	0
Total	5	1.0	123	24	2.5	50.3	0	0	0	0

For epidemiological sources see Bailey 1996. For the methods used to estimate and project incidence, prevalence, and deaths see Murray and Lopez 1996a. See explanatory notes for definitions and caveats.

Table 131
Iodine deficiency

Cuadro 131
Deficiencia de yodo

Tableau 131
Déficience en iode

Mild developmental disability   Discapacidad leve en el desarrollo   Déficit léger du développement

Table 131g   LAC - ALC - ALC   Iodine deficiency - Mild developmental disability

Age group (years)	Incidence 1990 Number ('000s)	Rate (per 100 000)	Prevalence 1990 Number ('000s)	Rate (per 100 000)	Avg. age at onset (years)	Average duration (years)	Deaths 1990 Number ('000s)	Rate (per 100 000)	Deaths 2000 (Projected) Number ('000s)	Rate (per 100 000)
Males										
0-4	1	4.5	3	11	2.5	63.9	0	0	0	0
5-14	0	0.0	12	22	-	-	0	0	0	0
15-44	0	0.0	23	22	-	-	0	0	0	0
45-59	0	0.0	5	22	-	-	0	0	0	0
60+	0	0.0	3	22	-	-	0	0	0	0
All ages	1	0.6	47	21	2.5	63.9	0	0	0	0
Females										
0-4	1	4.5	3	11	2.5	67.9	0	0	0	0
5-14	0	0.0	11	22	-	-	0	0	0	0
15-44	0	0.0	23	22	-	-	0	0	0	0
45-59	0	0.0	5	22	-	-	0	0	0	0
60+	0	0.0	4	22	-	-	0	0	0	0
All ages	1	0.6	47	21	2.5	67.9	0	0	0	0
Total	3	0.6	93	21	2.5	65.9	0	0	0	0

Table 131h   MEC - AOM - CMO   Iodine deficiency - Mild developmental disability

Age group (years)	Incidence 1990 Number ('000s)	Rate (per 100 000)	Prevalence 1990 Number ('000s)	Rate (per 100 000)	Avg. age at onset (years)	Average duration (years)	Deaths 1990 Number ('000s)	Rate (per 100 000)	Deaths 2000 (Projected) Number ('000s)	Rate (per 100 000)
Males										
0-4	4	9.9	10	24	2.5	61.1	0	0	0	0
5-14	0	0.0	32	49	-	-	0	0	0	0
15-44	0	0.0	56	49	-	-	0	0	0	0
45-59	0	0.0	11	49	-	-	0	0	0	0
60+	0	0.0	7	49	-	-	0	0	0	0
All ages	4	1.6	116	45	2.5	61.1	0	0	0	0
Females										
0-4	4	9.9	10	24	2.5	63.7	0	0	0	0
5-14	0	0.0	30	49	-	-	0	0	0	0
15-44	0	0.0	53	49	-	-	0	0	0	0
45-59	0	0.0	11	49	-	-	0	0	0	0
60+	0	0.0	8	49	-	-	0	0	0	0
All ages	4	1.6	111	45	2.5	63.7	0	0	0	0
Total	8	1.6	227	45	2.5	62.4	0	0	0	0

Table 131i   World - Mundo - Monde   Iodine deficiency - Mild developmental disability

Age group (years)	Incidence 1990 Number ('000s)	Rate (per 100 000)	Prevalence 1990 Number ('000s)	Rate (per 100 000)	Avg. age at onset (years)	Average duration (years)	Deaths 1990 Number ('000s)	Rate (per 100 000)	Deaths 2000 (Projected) Number ('000s)	Rate (per 100 000)
Males										
0-4	23	7.1	56	17	2.5	60.7	0	0	0	0
5-14	0	0.0	190	35	-	-	0	0	0	0
15-44	0	0.0	422	34	-	-	0	0	0	0
45-59	0	0.0	98	31	-	-	0	0	0	0
60+	0	0.0	64	29	-	-	0	0	0	0
All ages	23	0.9	831	31	2.5	60.7	0	0	0	0
Females										
0-4	22	7.1	54	17	2.5	63.4	0	0	0	0
5-14	0	0.0	180	34	-	-	0	0	0	0
15-44	0	0.0	399	33	-	-	0	0	0	0
45-59	0	0.0	95	31	-	-	0	0	0	0
60+	0	0.0	72	27	-	-	0	0	0	0
All ages	22	0.8	801	31	2.5	63.4	0	0	0	0
Total	45	0.9	1 631	31	2.5	62.1	0	0	0	0

For epidemiological sources see Bailey 1996. For the methods used to estimate and project incidence, prevalence, and deaths see Murray and Lopez 1996a. See explanatory notes for definitions and caveats.

Table 132 | **Cuadro 132** | **Tableau 132**
Iodine deficiency | **Deficiencia de yodo** | **Déficience en iode**

Cretinoidism | Cretinoidismo | Crétinoidisme

Table 132a EME - PEMC - EMBE Iodine deficiency - Cretinoidism

Age group (years)	Incidence 1990 Number ('000s)	Rate (per 100 000)	Prevalence 1990 Number ('000s)	Rate (per 100 000)	Avg. age at onset (years)	Average duration (years)	Deaths 1990 Number ('000s)	Rate (per 100 000)	Deaths 2000 (Projected) Number ('000s)	Rate (per 100 000)
Males										
0-4	0	0.5	0	1.3	2.5	70.2	-	-	-	-
5-14	0	0.0	1	2.6	-	-	-	-	-	-
15-44	0	0.0	5	2.6	-	-	-	-	-	-
45-59	0	0.0	2	2.6	-	-	-	-	-	-
60+	0	0.0	2	2.6	-	-	-	-	-	-
All ages	0	0.0	10	2.5	2.5	70.2	-	-	-	-
Females										
0-4	0	0.5	0	1.3	2.5	76.1	-	-	-	-
5-14	0	0.0	1	2.6	-	-	-	-	-	-
15-44	0	0.0	5	2.6	-	-	-	-	-	-
45-59	0	0.0	2	2.6	-	-	-	-	-	-
60+	0	0.0	2	2.6	-	-	-	-	-	-
All ages	0	0.0	10	2.5	2.5	76.1	-	-	-	-
Total	0	0.0	20	2.5	2.5	73.1	-	-	-	-

Table 132b FSE - PEAS - AESE Iodine deficiency - Cretinoidism

Age group (years)	Incidence 1990 Number ('000s)	Rate (per 100 000)	Prevalence 1990 Number ('000s)	Rate (per 100 000)	Avg. age at onset (years)	Average duration (years)	Deaths 1990 Number ('000s)	Rate (per 100 000)	Deaths 2000 (Projected) Number ('000s)	Rate (per 100 000)
Males										
0-4	0	1.1	0	2.6	2.5	63.5	-	-	-	-
5-14	0	0.0	1	5.2	-	-	-	-	-	-
15-44	0	0.0	4	5.2	-	-	-	-	-	-
45-59	0	0.0	1	5.2	-	-	-	-	-	-
60+	0	0.0	1	5.2	-	-	-	-	-	-
All ages	0	0.1	8	5.0	2.5	63.5	-	-	-	-
Females										
0-4	0	1.1	0	2.6	2.5	72.4	-	-	-	-
5-14	0	0.0	1	5.2	-	-	-	-	-	-
15-44	0	0.0	4	5.2	-	-	-	-	-	-
45-59	0	0.0	2	5.2	-	-	-	-	-	-
60+	0	0.0	2	5.2	-	-	-	-	-	-
All ages	0	0.1	9	5.0	2.5	72.4	-	-	-	-
Total	0	0.1	17	5.0	2.5	67.8	-	-	-	-

Table 132c India - India - Inde Iodine deficiency - Cretinoidism

Age group (years)	Incidence 1990 Number ('000s)	Rate (per 100 000)	Prevalence 1990 Number ('000s)	Rate (per 100 000)	Avg. age at onset (years)	Average duration (years)	Deaths 1990 Number ('000s)	Rate (per 100 000)	Deaths 2000 (Projected) Number ('000s)	Rate (per 100 000)
Males										
0-4	2	3.2	5	7.9	2.5	59.9	-	-	-	-
5-14	0	0.0	16	16.1	-	-	-	-	-	-
15-44	0	0.0	32	16.1	-	-	-	-	-	-
45-59	0	0.0	8	16.1	-	-	-	-	-	-
60+	0	0.0	5	16.1	-	-	-	-	-	-
All ages	2	0.4	66	15.0	2.5	59.9	-	-	-	-
Females										
0-4	2	3.2	4	7.9	2.5	60.8	-	-	-	-
5-14	0	0.0	15	16.1	-	-	-	-	-	-
15-44	0	0.0	30	16.1	-	-	-	-	-	-
45-59	0	0.0	7	16.1	-	-	-	-	-	-
60+	0	0.0	5	16.1	-	-	-	-	-	-
All ages	2	0.4	61	15.0	2.5	60.8	-	-	-	-
Total	4	0.4	127	15.0	2.5	60.3	-	-	-	-

For epidemiological sources see Bailey 1996. For the methods used to estimate and project incidence, prevalence, and deaths see Murray and Lopez 1996a. See explanatory notes for definitions and caveats.

Table 132
Iodine deficiency

Cuadro 132
Deficiencia de yodo

Tableau 132
Déficience en iode

Cretinoidism — Cretinoidismo — Crétinoidisme

Table 132d   China - China - Chine — Iodine deficiency - Cretinoidism

Age group (years)	Incidence 1990 Number ('000s)	Rate (per 100 000)	Prevalence 1990 Number ('000s)	Rate (per 100 000)	Avg. age at onset (years)	Average duration (years)	Deaths 1990 Number ('000s)	Rate (per 100 000)	Deaths 2000 (Projected) Number ('000s)	Rate (per 100 000)
Males										
0-4	2	3.2	5	7.9	2.5	65.5	-	-	-	-
5-14	0	0.0	15	15.8	-	-	-	-	-	-
15-44	0	0.0	49	15.8	-	-	-	-	-	-
45-59	0	0.0	12	15.8	-	-	-	-	-	-
60+	0	0.0	8	15.8	-	-	-	-	-	-
All ages	2	0.3	88	15.0	2.5	65.5	-	-	-	-
Females										
0-4	2	3.2	5	7.9	2.5	68.5	-	-	-	-
5-14	0	0.0	14	15.8	-	-	-	-	-	-
15-44	0	0.0	45	15.8	-	-	-	-	-	-
45-59	0	0.0	10	15.8	-	-	-	-	-	-
60+	0	0.0	8	15.8	-	-	-	-	-	-
All ages	2	0.3	82	15.0	2.5	68.5	-	-	-	-
Total	4	0.3	170	15.0	2.5	67.0	-	-	-	-

Table 132e   OAI - OPAI - APAI — Iodine deficiency - Cretinoidism

Age group (years)	Incidence 1990 Number ('000s)	Rate (per 100 000)	Prevalence 1990 Number ('000s)	Rate (per 100 000)	Avg. age at onset (years)	Average duration (years)	Deaths 1990 Number ('000s)	Rate (per 100 000)	Deaths 2000 (Projected) Number ('000s)	Rate (per 100 000)
Males										
0-4	1	1.9	2	4.8	2.5	59.8	-	-	-	-
5-14	0	0.0	8	9.6	-	-	-	-	-	-
15-44	0	0.0	15	9.6	-	-	-	-	-	-
45-59	0	0.0	3	9.6	-	-	-	-	-	-
60+	0	0.0	2	9.6	-	-	-	-	-	-
All ages	1	0.2	31	9.0	2.5	59.8	-	-	-	-
Females										
0-4	1	1.9	2	4.8	2.5	63.2	-	-	-	-
5-14	0	0.0	8	9.6	-	-	-	-	-	-
15-44	0	0.0	15	9.6	-	-	-	-	-	-
45-59	0	0.0	3	9.6	-	-	-	-	-	-
60+	0	0.0	2	9.6	-	-	-	-	-	-
All ages	1	0.2	31	9.0	2.5	63.2	-	-	-	-
Total	2	0.2	61	9.0	2.5	61.5	-	-	-	-

Table 132f   SSA - ASS - ASS — Iodine deficiency - Cretinoidism

Age group (years)	Incidence 1990 Number ('000s)	Rate (per 100 000)	Prevalence 1990 Number ('000s)	Rate (per 100 000)	Avg. age at onset (years)	Average duration (years)	Deaths 1990 Number ('000s)	Rate (per 100 000)	Deaths 2000 (Projected) Number ('000s)	Rate (per 100 000)
Males										
0-4	1	1.8	2	4.3	2.5	48.7	-	-	-	-
5-14	0	0.0	6	8.9	-	-	-	-	-	-
15-44	0	0.0	9	8.9	-	-	-	-	-	-
45-59	0	0.0	2	8.9	-	-	-	-	-	-
60+	0	0.0	1	8.9	-	-	-	-	-	-
All ages	1	0.3	20	8.0	2.5	48.7	-	-	-	-
Females										
0-4	1	1.8	2	4.3	2.5	51.9	-	-	-	-
5-14	0	0.0	6	8.8	-	-	-	-	-	-
15-44	0	0.0	9	8.8	-	-	-	-	-	-
45-59	0	0.0	2	8.8	-	-	-	-	-	-
60+	0	0.0	1	8.8	-	-	-	-	-	-
All ages	1	0.3	21	8.0	2.5	51.9	-	-	-	-
Total	2	0.3	41	8.0	2.5	50.3	-	-	-	-

For epidemiological sources see Bailey 1996. For the methods used to estimate and project incidence, prevalence, and deaths see Murray and Lopez 1996a. See explanatory notes for definitions and caveats.

Table 132
Iodine deficiency

Cuadro 132
Deficiencia de yodo

Tableau 132
Déficience en iode

Cretinoidism

Cretinoidismo

Crétinoidisme

Table 132g		LAC - ALC - ALC								Iodine deficiency - Cretinoidism	
Age group (years)	Incidence 1990		Prevalence 1990		Avg. age at onset (years)	Average duration (years)	Deaths 1990		Deaths 2000 (Projected)		
	Number ('000s)	Rate (per 100 000)	Number ('000s)	Rate (per 100 000)			Number ('000s)	Rate (per 100 000)	Number ('000s)	Rate (per 100 000)	
Males											
0-4	0	1.5	1	3.7	2.5	63.9	-	-	-	-	
5-14	0	0.0	4	7.5	-	-	-	-	-	-	
15-44	0	0.0	8	7.5	-	-	-	-	-	-	
45-59	0	0.0	2	7.5	-	-	-	-	-	-	
60+	0	0.0	1	7.5	-	-	-	-	-	-	
All ages	0	0.2	16	7.0	2.5	63.9	-	-	-	-	
Females											
0-4	0	1.5	1	3.7	2.5	67.9	-	-	-	-	
5-14	0	0.0	4	7.5	-	-	-	-	-	-	
15-44	0	0.0	8	7.5	-	-	-	-	-	-	
45-59	0	0.0	2	7.5	-	-	-	-	-	-	
60+	0	0.0	1	7.5	-	-	-	-	-	-	
All ages	0	0.2	16	7.0	2.5	67.9	-	-	-	-	
Total	1	0.2	31	7.0	2.5	65.9	-	-	-	-	

Table 132h		MEC - AOM - CMO								Iodine deficiency - Cretinoidism	
Age group (years)	Incidence 1990		Prevalence 1990		Avg. age at onset (years)	Average duration (years)	Deaths 1990		Deaths 2000 (Projected)		
	Number ('000s)	Rate (per 100 000)	Number ('000s)	Rate (per 100 000)			Number ('000s)	Rate (per 100 000)	Number ('000s)	Rate (per 100 000)	
Males											
0-4	1	3.3	3	8.1	2.5	61.1	-	-	-	-	
5-14	0	0.0	11	16.4	-	-	-	-	-	-	
15-44	0	0.0	19	16.4	-	-	-	-	-	-	
45-59	0	0.0	4	16.4	-	-	-	-	-	-	
60+	0	0.0	2	16.4	-	-	-	-	-	-	
All ages	1	0.5	39	15.0	2.5	61.1	-	-	-	-	
Females											
0-4	1	3.3	3	8.1	2.5	63.7	-	-	-	-	
5-14	0	0.0	10	16.4	-	-	-	-	-	-	
15-44	0	0.0	18	16.4	-	-	-	-	-	-	
45-59	0	0.0	4	16.4	-	-	-	-	-	-	
60+	0	0.0	3	16.4	-	-	-	-	-	-	
All ages	1	0.5	37	15.0	2.5	63.7	-	-	-	-	
Total	3	0.5	76	15.0	2.5	62.4	-	-	-	-	

Table 132i		World - Mundo - Monde								Iodine deficiency - Cretinoidism	
Age group (years)	Incidence 1990		Prevalence 1990		Avg. age at onset (years)	Average duration (years)	Deaths 1990		Deaths 2000 (Projected)		
	Number ('000s)	Rate (per 100 000)	Number ('000s)	Rate (per 100 000)			Number ('000s)	Rate (per 100 000)	Number ('000s)	Rate (per 100 000)	
Males											
0-4	8	2.4	19	5.8	2.5	60.7	-	-	-	-	
5-14	0	0.0	63	11.5	-	-	-	-	-	-	
15-44	0	0.0	141	11.3	-	-	-	-	-	-	
45-59	0	0.0	33	10.5	-	-	-	-	-	-	
60+	0	0.0	21	9.8	-	-	-	-	-	-	
All ages	8	0.3	277	10.4	2.5	60.7	-	-	-	-	
Females											
0-4	7	2.4	18	5.8	2.5	63.4	-	-	-	-	
5-14	0	0.0	60	11.4	-	-	-	-	-	-	
15-44	0	0.0	133	11.1	-	-	-	-	-	-	
45-59	0	0.0	32	10.2	-	-	-	-	-	-	
60+	0	0.0	24	8.9	-	-	-	-	-	-	
All ages	7	0.3	267	10.2	2.5	63.4	-	-	-	-	
Total	15	0.3	544	10.3	2.5	62.1	-	-	-	-	

For epidemiological sources see Bailey 1996. For the methods used to estimate and project incidence, prevalence, and deaths see Murray and Lopez 1996a. See explanatory notes for definitions and caveats.

Table 133
Iodine deficiency

Cuadro 133
Deficiencia de yodo

Tableau 133
Déficience en iode

Cretinism

Cretinismo

Crétinisme

Table 133a   EME - PEMC - EMBE

Iodine deficiency - Cretinism

Age group (years)	Incidence 1990 Number ('000s)	Rate (per 100 000)	Prevalence 1990 Number ('000s)	Rate (per 100 000)	Avg. age at onset (years)	Average duration (years)	Deaths 1990 Number ('000s)	Rate (per 100 000)	Deaths 2000 (Projected) Number ('000s)	Rate (per 100 000)
Males										
0-4	2	7.0	7	25.0	0.5	10.0	0	0	0	0
5-14	0	0.0	13	25.0	-	-	0	0	0	0
15-44	0	0.0	26	14.3	-	-	0	0	0	0
45-59	0	0.0	2	2.8	-	-	0	0	0	0
60+	0	0.0	0	0.3	-	-	0	0	0	0
All ages	2	0.5	48	12.3	0.5	10.0	0	0	0	0
Females										
0-4	2	7.6	7	27.1	0.5	10.0	0	0	0	0
5-14	0	0.0	8	15.5	-	-	0	0	0	0
15-44	0	0.0	5	3.1	-	-	0	0	0	0
45-59	0	0.0	0	0.3	-	-	0	0	0	0
60+	0	0.0	0	0.1	-	-	0	0	0	0
All ages	2	0.5	20	5.0	0.5	10.0	0	0	0	0
Total	4	0.5	69	8.6	0.5	10.0	0	0	0	0

Table 133b   FSE - PEAS - AESE

Iodine deficiency - Cretinism

Age group (years)	Incidence 1990 Number ('000s)	Rate (per 100 000)	Prevalence 1990 Number ('000s)	Rate (per 100 000)	Avg. age at onset (years)	Average duration (years)	Deaths 1990 Number ('000s)	Rate (per 100 000)	Deaths 2000 (Projected) Number ('000s)	Rate (per 100 000)
Males										
0-4	2	12.1	6	42.9	0.5	10.0	0	0	0	0
5-14	0	0.0	7	24.5	-	-	0	0	0	0
15-44	0	0.0	4	4.9	-	-	0	0	0	0
45-59	0	0.0	0	0.5	-	-	0	0	0	0
60+	0	0.0	0	0.1	-	-	0	0	0	0
All ages	2	1.0	17	10.0	0.5	10.0	0	0	0	0
Females										
0-4	2	14.0	7	50.0	0.5	10.0	0	0	0	0
5-14	0	0.0	8	28.6	-	-	0	0	0	0
15-44	0	0.0	4	5.7	-	-	0	0	0	0
45-59	0	0.0	0	0.5	-	-	0	0	0	0
60+	0	0.0	0	0.1	-	-	0	0	0	0
All ages	2	1.0	19	10.3	0.5	10.0	0	0	0	0
Total	4	1.0	35	10.1	0.5	10.0	0	0	0	0

Table 133c   India - India - Inde

Iodine deficiency - Cretinism

Age group (years)	Incidence 1990 Number ('000s)	Rate (per 100 000)	Prevalence 1990 Number ('000s)	Rate (per 100 000)	Avg. age at onset (years)	Average duration (years)	Deaths 1990 Number ('000s)	Rate (per 100 000)	Deaths 2000 (Projected) Number ('000s)	Rate (per 100 000)
Males										
0-4	15	25.3	52	87.2	0.5	10.0	2	3.8	1	2.3
5-14	0	0.0	54	53.2	-	-	1	0.5	0	0.2
15-44	0	0.0	24	12.2	-	-	0	0.1	0	0.0
45-59	0	0.0	1	1.5	-	-	0	0.0	0	0.0
60+	0	0.0	0	0.4	-	-	0	0.0	0	0.0
All ages	15	3.4	132	29.9	0.5	10.0	3	0.7	2	0.3
Females										
0-4	14	25.2	49	86.6	0.5	10.0	2	3.8	1	2.3
5-14	0	0.0	50	53.0	-	-	1	0.6	0	0.2
15-44	0	0.0	22	12.2	-	-	0	0.1	0	0.0
45-59	0	0.0	1	1.5	-	-	0	0.0	0	0.0
60+	0	0.0	0	0.4	-	-	0	0.0	0	0.0
All ages	14	3.5	123	29.9	0.5	10.0	3	0.7	2	0.3
Total	29	3.5	254	29.9	0.5	10.0	6	0.7	3	0.3

For epidemiological sources see Bailey 1996. For the methods used to estimate and project incidence, prevalence, and deaths see Murray and Lopez 1996a. See explanatory notes for definitions and caveats.

Table 133
Iodine deficiency

Cuadro 133
Deficiencia de yodo

Tableau 133
Déficience en iode

Cretinism   Cretinismo   Crétinisme

Table 133d   China - China - Chine   Iodine deficiency - Cretinism

Age group (years)	Incidence 1990 Number ('000s)	Rate (per 100 000)	Prevalence 1990 Number ('000s)	Rate (per 100 000)	Avg. age at onset (years)	Average duration (years)	Deaths 1990 Number ('000s)	Rate (per 100 000)	Deaths 2000 (Projected) Number ('000s)	Rate (per 100 000)
Males										
0-4	20	32.5	69	114.6	0.5	10.0	3	5.2	2	2.7
5-14	0	0.0	64	66.3	-	-	1	0.6	0	0.2
15-44	0	0.0	42	13.6	-	-	0	0.1	0	0.0
45-59	0	0.0	1	1.3	-	-	0	0.0	0	0.0
60+	0	0.0	0	0.3	-	-	0	0.0	0	0.0
All ages	20	3.3	176	30.1	0.5	10.0	4	0.7	2	0.3
Females										
0-4	19	32.2	66	113.3	0.5	10.0	3	5.1	1	2.5
5-14	0	0.0	59	65.8	-	-	1	0.6	0	0.2
15-44	0	0.0	38	13.5	-	-	0	0.1	0	0.0
45-59	0	0.0	1	1.3	-	-	0	0.0	0	0.0
60+	0	0.0	0	0.3	-	-	0	0.0	0	0.0
All ages	19	3.4	164	30.0	0.5	10.0	4	0.7	2	0.3
Total	38	3.4	340	30.0	0.5	10.0	8	0.7	4	0.3

Table 133e   OAI - OPAI - APAI   Iodine deficiency - Cretinism

Age group (years)	Incidence 1990 Number ('000s)	Rate (per 100 000)	Prevalence 1990 Number ('000s)	Rate (per 100 000)	Avg. age at onset (years)	Average duration (years)	Deaths 1990 Number ('000s)	Rate (per 100 000)	Deaths 2000 (Projected) Number ('000s)	Rate (per 100 000)
Males										
0-4	7	15.4	23	53.5	0.5	10.0	1	2.4	1	1.5
5-14	0	0.0	27	32.0	-	-	0	0.3	0	0.2
15-44	0	0.0	11	7.1	-	-	0	0.1	0	0.0
45-59	0	0.0	0	0.8	-	-	0	0.0	0	0.0
60+	0	0.0	0	0.2	-	-	0	0.0	0	0.0
All ages	7	2.0	62	18.1	0.5	10.0	1	0.4	1	0.2
Females										
0-4	7	15.9	23	55.6	0.5	10.0	1	2.3	1	1.4
5-14	0	0.0	26	32.9	-	-	0	0.3	0	0.1
15-44	0	0.0	11	7.1	-	-	0	0.1	0	0.0
45-59	0	0.0	0	0.8	-	-	0	0.0	0	0.0
60+	0	0.0	0	0.2	-	-	0	0.0	0	0.0
All ages	7	2.0	61	18.1	0.5	10.0	1	0.4	1	0.2
Total	13	2.0	123	18.1	0.5	10.0	3	0.4	2	0.2

Table 133f   SSA - ASS - ASS   Iodine deficiency - Cretinism

Age group (years)	Incidence 1990 Number ('000s)	Rate (per 100 000)	Prevalence 1990 Number ('000s)	Rate (per 100 000)	Avg. age at onset (years)	Average duration (years)	Deaths 1990 Number ('000s)	Rate (per 100 000)	Deaths 2000 (Projected) Number ('000s)	Rate (per 100 000)
Males										
0-4	5	10.7	17	35.9	0.5	10.0	1	1.3	1	0.9
5-14	0	0.0	16	23.5	-	-	0	0.2	0	0.1
15-44	0	0.0	7	6.4	-	-	0	0.0	0	0.0
45-59	0	0.0	0	1.0	-	-	0	0.0	0	0.0
60+	0	0.0	0	0.3	-	-	0	0.0	0	0.0
All ages	5	2.0	40	16.0	0.5	10.0	1	0.3	1	0.2
Females										
0-4	5	11.1	18	37.6	0.5	10.0	1	1.3	1	0.9
5-14	0	0.0	17	24.1	-	-	0	0.2	0	0.1
15-44	0	0.0	7	6.3	-	-	0	0.1	0	0.0
45-59	0	0.0	0	0.9	-	-	0	0.0	0	0.0
60+	0	0.0	0	0.2	-	-	0	0.0	0	0.0
All ages	5	2.0	41	16.0	0.5	10.0	1	0.3	1	0.2
Total	10	2.0	82	16.0	0.5	10.0	2	0.3	1	0.2

For epidemiological sources see Bailey 1996. For the methods used to estimate and project incidence, prevalence, and deaths see Murray and Lopez 1996a. See explanatory notes for definitions and caveats.

Table 133
Iodine deficiency

Cuadro 133
Deficiencia de yodo

Tableau 133
Déficience en iode

Cretinism

Cretinismo

Crétinisme

Table 133g LAC - ALC - ALC   Iodine deficiency - Cretinism

Age group (years)	Incidence 1990 Number ('000s)	Rate (per 100 000)	Prevalence 1990 Number ('000s)	Rate (per 100 000)	Avg. age at onset (years)	Average duration (years)	Deaths 1990 Number ('000s)	Rate (per 100 000)	Deaths 2000 (Projected) Number ('000s)	Rate (per 100 000)
Males										
0-4	3	12.1	12	42.5	0.5	10.0	1	1.9	0	1.3
5-14	0	0.0	13	25.0	-	-	0	0.2	0	0.1
15-44	0	0.0	6	5.3	-	-	0	0.0	0	0.0
45-59	0	0.0	0	0.6	-	-	0	0.0	0	0.0
60+	0	0.0	0	0.1	-	-	0	0.0	0	0.0
All ages	3	1.6	31	14.0	0.5	10.0	1	0.3	0	0.2
Females										
0-4	4	12.7	12	44.5	0.5	10.0	1	1.9	0	1.3
5-14	0	0.0	13	25.9	-	-	0	0.2	0	0.1
15-44	0	0.0	6	5.4	-	-	0	0.1	0	0.0
45-59	0	0.0	0	0.5	-	-	0	0.0	0	0.0
60+	0	0.0	0	0.1	-	-	0	0.0	0	0.0
All ages	4	1.6	31	14.0	0.5	10.0	1	0.3	0	0.2
Total	7	1.6	62	14.0	0.5	10.0	1	0.3	1	0.2

Table 133h MEC - AOM - CMO   Iodine deficiency - Cretinism

Age group (years)	Incidence 1990 Number ('000s)	Rate (per 100 000)	Prevalence 1990 Number ('000s)	Rate (per 100 000)	Avg. age at onset (years)	Average duration (years)	Deaths 1990 Number ('000s)	Rate (per 100 000)	Deaths 2000 (Projected) Number ('000s)	Rate (per 100 000)
Males										
0-4	9	23.1	33	79.7	0.5	10.0	1	3.5	1	2.6
5-14	0	0.0	31	48.1	-	-	0	0.4	0	0.2
15-44	0	0.0	12	10.8	-	-	0	0.1	0	0.0
45-59	0	0.0	0	1.2	-	-	0	0.0	0	0.0
60+	0	0.0	0	0.3	-	-	0	0.0	0	0.0
All ages	9	3.7	77	30.0	0.5	10.0	2	0.7	2	0.5
Females										
0-4	9	23.3	32	80.4	0.5	10.0	1	3.5	1	2.5
5-14	0	0.0	30	48.3	-	-	0	0.5	0	0.2
15-44	0	0.0	11	10.7	-	-	0	0.1	0	0.0
45-59	0	0.0	0	1.2	-	-	0	0.0	0	0.0
60+	0	0.0	0	0.3	-	-	0	0.0	0	0.0
All ages	9	3.7	74	29.9	0.5	10.0	2	0.7	1	0.4
Total	19	3.7	151	29.9	0.5	10.0	4	0.7	3	0.5

Table 133i World - Mundo - Monde   Iodine deficiency - Cretinism

Age group (years)	Incidence 1990 Number ('000s)	Rate (per 100 000)	Prevalence 1990 Number ('000s)	Rate (per 100 000)	Avg. age at onset (years)	Average duration (years)	Deaths 1990 Number ('000s)	Rate (per 100 000)	Deaths 2000 (Projected) Number ('000s)	Rate (per 100 000)
Males										
0-4	63	19.6	219	68.2	0.5	10.0	9	2.8	6	1.7
5-14	0	0.0	226	41.1	-	-	2	0.3	1	0.2
15-44	0	0.0	132	10.5	-	-	1	0.1	0	0.0
45-59	0	0.0	4	1.4	-	-	0	0.0	0	0.0
60+	0	0.0	1	0.2	-	-	0	0.0	0	0.0
All ages	63	2.4	582	21.9	0.5	10.0	12	0.4	7	0.2
Females										
0-4	61	19.8	213	69.0	0.5	10.0	9	2.8	5	1.6
5-14	0	0.0	212	40.3	-	-	2	0.4	1	0.2
15-44	0	0.0	106	8.8	-	-	1	0.1	0	0.0
45-59	0	0.0	3	0.9	-	-	0	0.0	0	0.0
60+	0	0.0	0	0.2	-	-	0	0.0	0	0.0
All ages	61	2.3	534	20.4	0.5	10.0	11	0.4	7	0.2
Total	124	2.4	1 116	21.2	0.5	10.0	23	0.4	14	0.2

For epidemiological sources see Bailey 1996. For the methods used to estimate and project incidence, prevalence, and deaths see Murray and Lopez 1996a. See explanatory notes for definitions and caveats.

Table 134
Vitamin A deficiency

Cuadro 134
Deficiencia de vitamina A

Tableau 134
Avitaminose A

Xerophthalmia

Xeroftalmia

Xérophtalmie

Table 134a   EME - PEMC - EMBE — Vitamin A deficiency - Xerophthalmia

Age group (years)	Incidence 1990 Number ('000s)	Rate (per 100 000)	Prevalence 1990 Number ('000s)	Rate (per 100 000)	Avg. age at onset (years)	Average duration (years)	Deaths 1990 Number ('000s)	Rate (per 100 000)	Deaths 2000 (Projected) Number ('000s)	Rate (per 100 000)
Males										
0-4	0	0	0	0	-	-	-	-	-	-
5-14	0	0	0	0	-	-	-	-	-	-
15-44	0	0	0	0	-	-	-	-	-	-
45-59	0	0	0	0	-	-	-	-	-	-
60+	0	0	0	0	-	-	-	-	-	-
All ages	0	0	0	0	-	-	-	-	-	-
Females										
0-4	0	0	0	0	-	-	-	-	-	-
5-14	0	0	0	0	-	-	-	-	-	-
15-44	0	0	0	0	-	-	-	-	-	-
45-59	0	0	0	0	-	-	-	-	-	-
60+	0	0	0	0	-	-	-	-	-	-
All ages	0	0	0	0	-	-	-	-	-	-
Total	0	0	0	0	-	-	-	-	-	-

Table 134b   FSE - PEAS - AESE — Vitamin A deficiency - Xerophthalmia

Age group (years)	Incidence 1990 Number ('000s)	Rate (per 100 000)	Prevalence 1990 Number ('000s)	Rate (per 100 000)	Avg. age at onset (years)	Average duration (years)	Deaths 1990 Number ('000s)	Rate (per 100 000)	Deaths 2000 (Projected) Number ('000s)	Rate (per 100 000)
Males										
0-4	0	0	0	0	-	-	-	-	-	-
5-14	0	0	0	0	-	-	-	-	-	-
15-44	0	0	0	0	-	-	-	-	-	-
45-59	0	0	0	0	-	-	-	-	-	-
60+	0	0	0	0	-	-	-	-	-	-
All ages	0	0	0	0	-	-	-	-	-	-
Females										
0-4	0	0	0	0	-	-	-	-	-	-
5-14	0	0	0	0	-	-	-	-	-	-
15-44	0	0	0	0	-	-	-	-	-	-
45-59	0	0	0	0	-	-	-	-	-	-
60+	0	0	0	0	-	-	-	-	-	-
All ages	0	0	0	0	-	-	-	-	-	-
Total	0	0	0	0	-	-	-	-	-	-

Table 134c   India - India - Inde — Vitamin A deficiency - Xerophthalmia

Age group (years)	Incidence 1990 Number ('000s)	Rate (per 100 000)	Prevalence 1990 Number ('000s)	Rate (per 100 000)	Avg. age at onset (years)	Average duration (years)	Deaths 1990 Number ('000s)	Rate (per 100 000)	Deaths 2000 (Projected) Number ('000s)	Rate (per 100 000)
Males										
0-4	102	170	298	498	2.0	59.9	-	-	-	-
5-14	0	0	857	842	-	-	-	-	-	-
15-44	0	0	1 688	842	-	-	-	-	-	-
45-59	0	0	400	842	-	-	-	-	-	-
60+	0	0	251	842	-	-	-	-	-	-
All ages	102	23	3 493	795	2.0	59.9	-	-	-	-
Females										
0-4	97	171	282	498	2.0	60.8	-	-	-	-
5-14	0	0	804	844	-	-	-	-	-	-
15-44	0	0	1 546	844	-	-	-	-	-	-
45-59	0	0	388	844	-	-	-	-	-	-
60+	0	0	244	844	-	-	-	-	-	-
All ages	97	24	3 264	796	2.0	60.8	-	-	-	-
Total	199	23	6 758	795	2.0	60.4	-	-	-	-

For epidemiological sources see Underwood 1996. For the methods used to estimate and project incidence, prevalence, and deaths see Murray and Lopez 1996a. See explanatory notes for definitions and caveats.

Table 134
Vitamin A deficiency

Cuadro 134
Deficiencia de vitamina A

Tableau 134
Avitaminose A

Xerophthalmia

Xeroftalmia

Xérophtalmie

Table 134d — China - China - Chine — Vitamin A deficiency - Xerophthalmia

Age group (years)	Incidence 1990 Number ('000s)	Rate (per 100 000)	Prevalence 1990 Number ('000s)	Rate (per 100 000)	Avg. age at onset (years)	Average duration (years)	Deaths 1990 Number ('000s)	Rate (per 100 000)	Deaths 2000 (Projected) Number ('000s)	Rate (per 100 000)
Males										
0-4	50	83.6	151	250	2.0	66.1	-	-	-	-
5-14	0	0.0	404	416	-	-	-	-	-	-
15-44	0	0.0	1 275	416	-	-	-	-	-	-
45-59	0	0.0	302	416	-	-	-	-	-	-
60+	0	0.0	204	416	-	-	-	-	-	-
All ages	50	8.6	2 336	399	2.0	66.1	-	-	-	-
Females										
0-4	48	83.7	145	250	2.0	69.1	-	-	-	-
5-14	0	0.0	377	417	-	-	-	-	-	-
15-44	0	0.0	1 183	417	-	-	-	-	-	-
45-59	0	0.0	268	417	-	-	-	-	-	-
60+	0	0.0	215	417	-	-	-	-	-	-
All ages	48	8.8	2 189	399	2.0	69.1	-	-	-	-
Total	99	8.7	4 525	399	2.0	67.6	-	-	-	-

Table 134e — OAI - OPAI - APAI — Vitamin A deficiency - Xerophthalmia

Age group (years)	Incidence 1990 Number ('000s)	Rate (per 100 000)	Prevalence 1990 Number ('000s)	Rate (per 100 000)	Avg. age at onset (years)	Average duration (years)	Deaths 1990 Number ('000s)	Rate (per 100 000)	Deaths 2000 (Projected) Number ('000s)	Rate (per 100 000)
Males										
0-4	89	203	261	597	2.0	60.1	-	-	-	-
5-14	0	0	844	1 004	-	-	-	-	-	-
15-44	0	0	1 614	1 004	-	-	-	-	-	-
45-59	0	0	343	1 004	-	-	-	-	-	-
60+	0	0	203	1 004	-	-	-	-	-	-
All ages	89	26	3 265	952	2.0	60.1	-	-	-	-
Females										
0-4	85	202	251	597	2.0	63.6	-	-	-	-
5-14	0	0	803	1 001	-	-	-	-	-	-
15-44	0	0	1 597	1 001	-	-	-	-	-	-
45-59	0	0	351	1 001	-	-	-	-	-	-
60+	0	0	227	1 001	-	-	-	-	-	-
All ages	85	25	3 229	951	2.0	63.6	-	-	-	-
Total	173	25	6 494	951	2.0	61.8	-	-	-	-

Table 134f — SSA - ASS - ASS — Vitamin A deficiency - Xerophthalmia

Age group (years)	Incidence 1990 Number ('000s)	Rate (per 100 000)	Prevalence 1990 Number ('000s)	Rate (per 100 000)	Avg. age at onset (years)	Average duration (years)	Deaths 1990 Number ('000s)	Rate (per 100 000)	Deaths 2000 (Projected) Number ('000s)	Rate (per 100 000)
Males										
0-4	185	389	524	1 104	2.0	48.4	-	-	-	-
5-14	0	0	1 337	1 903	-	-	-	-	-	-
15-44	0	0	1 975	1 903	-	-	-	-	-	-
45-59	0	0	386	1 903	-	-	-	-	-	-
60+	0	0	200	1 903	-	-	-	-	-	-
All ages	185	73	4 423	1 753	2.0	48.4	-	-	-	-
Females										
0-4	181	385	519	1 104	2.0	51.7	-	-	-	-
5-14	0	0	1 321	1 892	-	-	-	-	-	-
15-44	0	0	2 010	1 892	-	-	-	-	-	-
45-59	0	0	418	1 892	-	-	-	-	-	-
60+	0	0	241	1 892	-	-	-	-	-	-
All ages	181	70	4 509	1 748	2.0	51.7	-	-	-	-
Total	366	72	8 931	1 750	2.0	50.0	-	-	-	-

For epidemiological sources see Underwood 1996. For the methods used to estimate and project incidence, prevalence, and deaths see Murray and Lopez 1996a. See explanatory notes for definitions and caveats.

Table 134	Cuadro 134	Tableau 134
Vitamin A deficiency	**Deficiencia de vitamina A**	**Avitaminose A**
Xerophthalmia	Xeroftalmia	Xérophtalmie

Table 134g   LAC - ALC - ALC   Vitamin A deficiency - Xerophthalmia

Age group (years)	Incidence 1990 Number ('000s)	Rate (per 100 000)	Prevalence 1990 Number ('000s)	Rate (per 100 000)	Avg. age at onset (years)	Average duration (years)	Deaths 1990 Number ('000s)	Rate (per 100 000)	Deaths 2000 (Projected) Number ('000s)	Rate (per 100 000)
Males										
0-4	28	98	84	293	2.0	64.3	-	-	-	-
5-14	0	0	255	489	-	-	-	-	-	-
15-44	0	0	510	489	-	-	-	-	-	-
45-59	0	0	109	489	-	-	-	-	-	-
60+	0	0	70	489	-	-	-	-	-	-
All ages	28	13	1 028	464	2.0	64.3	-	-	-	-
Females										
0-4	27	98	81	293	2.0	68.5	-	-	-	-
5-14	0	0	248	488	-	-	-	-	-	-
15-44	0	0	508	488	-	-	-	-	-	-
45-59	0	0	114	488	-	-	-	-	-	-
60+	0	0	82	488	-	-	-	-	-	-
All ages	27	12	1 032	464	2.0	68.5	-	-	-	-
Total	55	12	2 060	464	2.0	66.3	-	-	-	-

Table 134h   MEC - AOM - CMO   Vitamin A deficiency - Xerophthalmia

Age group (years)	Incidence 1990 Number ('000s)	Rate (per 100 000)	Prevalence 1990 Number ('000s)	Rate (per 100 000)	Avg. age at onset (years)	Average duration (years)	Deaths 1990 Number ('000s)	Rate (per 100 000)	Deaths 2000 (Projected) Number ('000s)	Rate (per 100 000)
Males										
0-4	109	265	320	777	2.0	61.2	-	-	-	-
5-14	0	0	857	1 311	-	-	-	-	-	-
15-44	0	0	1 493	1 311	-	-	-	-	-	-
45-59	0	0	293	1 311	-	-	-	-	-	-
60+	0	0	179	1 311	-	-	-	-	-	-
All ages	109	43	3 142	1 226	2.0	61.2	-	-	-	-
Females										
0-4	105	265	309	777	2.0	63.8	-	-	-	-
5-14	0	0	813	1 311	-	-	-	-	-	-
15-44	0	0	1 406	1 311	-	-	-	-	-	-
45-59	0	0	292	1 311	-	-	-	-	-	-
60+	0	0	203	1 311	-	-	-	-	-	-
All ages	105	43	3 022	1 225	2.0	63.8	-	-	-	-
Total	214	43	6 164	1 225	2.0	62.5	-	-	-	-

Table 134i   World - Mundo - Monde   Vitamin A deficiency - Xerophthalmia

Age group (years)	Incidence 1990 Number ('000s)	Rate (per 100 000)	Prevalence 1990 Number ('000s)	Rate (per 100 000)	Avg. age at onset (years)	Average duration (years)	Deaths 1990 Number ('000s)	Rate (per 100 000)	Deaths 2000 (Projected) Number ('000s)	Rate (per 100 000)
Males										
0-4	563	175	1 638	510	2.0	57.2	-	-	-	-
5-14	0	0	4 553	826	-	-	-	-	-	-
15-44	0	0	8 556	685	-	-	-	-	-	-
45-59	0	0	1 834	587	-	-	-	-	-	-
60+	0	0	1 106	505	-	-	-	-	-	-
All ages	563	21	17 686	666	2.0	57.2	-	-	-	-
Females										
0-4	544	176	1 587	513	2.0	59.9	-	-	-	-
5-14	0	0	4 364	830	-	-	-	-	-	-
15-44	0	0	8 250	688	-	-	-	-	-	-
45-59	0	0	1 832	589	-	-	-	-	-	-
60+	0	0	1 211	450	-	-	-	-	-	-
All ages	544	21	17 245	660	2.0	59.9	-	-	-	-
Total	1 107	21	34 931	663	2.0	58.5	-	-	-	-

For epidemiological sources see Underwood 1996. For the methods used to estimate and project incidence, prevalence, and deaths see Murray and Lopez 1996a. See explanatory notes for definitions and caveats.

Table 135
Vitamin A deficiency

Cuadro 135
Deficiencia de vitamina A

Tableau 135
Avitaminose A

Corneal scar

Cicatriz de la córnea

Cicatrice de la cornée

Table 135a   EME - PEMC - EMBE   Vitamin A deficiency - Corneal scar

Age group (years)	Incidence 1990 Number ('000s)	Rate (per 100 000)	Prevalence 1990 Number ('000s)	Rate (per 100 000)	Avg. age at onset (years)	Average duration (years)	Deaths 1990 Number ('000s)	Rate (per 100 000)	Deaths 2000 (Projected) Number ('000s)	Rate (per 100 000)
Males										
0-4	0	0	0	0	-	-	0	0	0	0
5-14	0	0	0	0	-	-	0	0	0	0
15-44	0	0	0	0	-	-	0	0	0	0
45-59	0	0	0	0	-	-	0	0	0	0
60+	0	0	0	0	-	-	0	0	0	0
All ages	0	0	0	0	-	-	0	0	0	0
Females										
0-4	0	0	0	0	-	-	0	0	0	0
5-14	0	0	0	0	-	-	0	0	0	0
15-44	0	0	0	0	-	-	0	0	0	0
45-59	0	0	0	0	-	-	0	0	0	0
60+	0	0	0	0	-	-	0	0	0	0
All ages	0	0	0	0	-	-	0	0	0	0
Total	0	0	0	0	-	-	0	0	0	0

Table 135b   FSE - PEAS - AESE   Vitamin A deficiency - Corneal scar

Age group (years)	Incidence 1990 Number ('000s)	Rate (per 100 000)	Prevalence 1990 Number ('000s)	Rate (per 100 000)	Avg. age at onset (years)	Average duration (years)	Deaths 1990 Number ('000s)	Rate (per 100 000)	Deaths 2000 (Projected) Number ('000s)	Rate (per 100 000)
Males										
0-4	0	0	0	0	-	-	0	0	0	0
5-14	0	0	0	0	-	-	0	0	0	0
15-44	0	0	0	0	-	-	0	0	0	0
45-59	0	0	0	0	-	-	0	0	0	0
60+	0	0	0	0	-	-	0	0	0	0
All ages	0	0	0	0	-	-	0	0	0	0
Females										
0-4	0	0	0	0	-	-	0	0	0	0
5-14	0	0	0	0	-	-	0	0	0	0
15-44	0	0	0	0	-	-	0	0	0	0
45-59	0	0	0	0	-	-	0	0	0	0
60+	0	0	0	0	-	-	0	0	0	0
All ages	0	0	0	0	-	-	0	0	0	0
Total	0	0	0	0	-	-	0	0	0	0

Table 135c   India - India - Inde   Vitamin A deficiency - Corneal scar

Age group (years)	Incidence 1990 Number ('000s)	Rate (per 100 000)	Prevalence 1990 Number ('000s)	Rate (per 100 000)	Avg. age at onset (years)	Average duration (years)	Deaths 1990 Number ('000s)	Rate (per 100 000)	Deaths 2000 (Projected) Number ('000s)	Rate (per 100 000)
Males										
0-4	15	25.2	33	55.3	2.0	4.7	7	11.0	4	6.9
5-14	0	0.0	30	29.8	-	-	4	3.5	2	1.6
15-44	0	0.0	3	1.6	-	-	0	0.2	0	0.1
45-59	0	0.0	0	0.0	-	-	0	0.0	0	0.0
60+	0	0.0	0	0.0	-	-	0	0.0	0	0.0
All ages	15	3.4	67	15.2	2.0	4.7	10	2.4	6	1.1
Females										
0-4	14	25.3	31	55.3	2.0	4.7	6	11.3	4	6.8
5-14	0	0.0	29	29.9	-	-	4	3.8	2	1.6
15-44	0	0.0	3	1.6	-	-	0	0.1	0	0.0
45-59	0	0.0	0	0.0	-	-	0	0.0	0	0.0
60+	0	0.0	0	0.0	-	-	0	0.0	0	0.0
All ages	14	3.5	63	15.3	2.0	4.7	10	2.5	5	1.1
Total	29	3.5	129	15.2	2.0	4.7	21	2.4	11	1.1

For epidemiological sources see Underwood 1996. For the methods used to estimate and project incidence, prevalence, and deaths see Murray and Lopez 1996a. See explanatory notes for definitions and caveats.

Table 135 | **Cuadro 135** | **Tableau 135**
Vitamin A deficiency | **Deficiencia de vitamina A** | **Avitaminose A**

Corneal scar | Cicatriz de la córnea | Cicatrice de la cornée

Table 135d   China - China - Chine   Vitamin A deficiency - Corneal scar

Age group (years)	Incidence 1990 Number ('000s)	Rate (per 100 000)	Prevalence 1990 Number ('000s)	Rate (per 100 000)	Avg. age at onset (years)	Average duration (years)	Deaths 1990 Number ('000s)	Rate (per 100 000)	Deaths 2000 (Projected) Number ('000s)	Rate (per 100 000)
Males										
0-4	7	12.4	17	27.8	2.0	4.9	3	5.4	2	2.8
5-14	0	0.0	14	14.6	-	-	1	1.4	1	0.5
15-44	0	0.0	2	0.8	-	-	0	0.1	0	0.0
45-59	0	0.0	0	0.0	-	-	0	0.0	0	0.0
60+	0	0.0	0	0.0	-	-	0	0.0	0	0.0
All ages	7	1.3	33	5.7	2.0	4.9	5	0.8	2	0.4
Females										
0-4	7	12.4	16	27.8	2.0	4.9	3	5.4	1	2.7
5-14	0	0.0	13	14.7	-	-	1	1.4	1	0.5
15-44	0	0.0	2	0.8	-	-	0	0.1	0	0.0
45-59	0	0.0	0	0.0	-	-	0	0.0	0	0.0
60+	0	0.0	0	0.0	-	-	0	0.0	0	0.0
All ages	7	1.3	32	5.8	2.0	4.9	5	0.8	2	0.3
Total	15	1.3	65	5.7	2.0	4.9	9	0.8	4	0.3

Table 135e   OAI - OPAI - APAI   Vitamin A deficiency - Corneal scar

Age group (years)	Incidence 1990 Number ('000s)	Rate (per 100 000)	Prevalence 1990 Number ('000s)	Rate (per 100 000)	Avg. age at onset (years)	Average duration (years)	Deaths 1990 Number ('000s)	Rate (per 100 000)	Deaths 2000 (Projected) Number ('000s)	Rate (per 100 000)
Males										
0-4	13	30.1	29	66.4	2.0	4.8	6	13.1	4	8.4
5-14	0	0.0	30	35.4	-	-	3	4.0	2	1.9
15-44	0	0.0	3	1.9	-	-	0	0.2	0	0.1
45-59	0	0.0	0	0.0	-	-	0	0.0	0	0.0
60+	0	0.0	0	0.0	-	-	0	0.0	0	0.0
All ages	13	3.8	62	18.0	2.0	4.8	9	2.7	5	1.4
Females										
0-4	13	29.9	28	66.4	2.0	4.8	5	12.3	3	7.7
5-14	0	0.0	28	35.3	-	-	3	3.6	1	1.7
15-44	0	0.0	3	1.9	-	-	0	0.1	0	0.0
45-59	0	0.0	0	0.0	-	-	0	0.0	0	0.0
60+	0	0.0	0	0.0	-	-	0	0.0	0	0.0
All ages	13	3.7	59	17.4	2.0	4.8	8	2.4	5	1.2
Total	26	3.8	121	17.7	2.0	4.8	18	2.6	10	1.3

Table 135f   SSA - ASS - ASS   Vitamin A deficiency - Corneal scar

Age group (years)	Incidence 1990 Number ('000s)	Rate (per 100 000)	Prevalence 1990 Number ('000s)	Rate (per 100 000)	Avg. age at onset (years)	Average duration (years)	Deaths 1990 Number ('000s)	Rate (per 100 000)	Deaths 2000 (Projected) Number ('000s)	Rate (per 100 000)
Males										
0-4	27	57	58	122.6	2.0	4.4	11	22.9	11	16.5
5-14	0	0	48	67.7	-	-	6	7.9	4	4.3
15-44	0	0	4	3.8	-	-	0	0.3	0	0.1
45-59	0	0	0	0.0	-	-	0	0.0	0	0.0
60+	0	0	0	0.0	-	-	0	0.0	0	0.0
All ages	27	11	110	43.5	2.0	4.4	17	6.6	15	4.4
Females										
0-4	27	57	58	122.6	2.0	4.5	10	21.6	10	15.0
5-14	0	0	47	67.5	-	-	6	8.1	4	4.2
15-44	0	0	4	3.8	-	-	0	0.3	0	0.1
45-59	0	0	0	0.0	-	-	0	0.0	0	0.0
60+	0	0	0	0.0	-	-	0	0.0	0	0.0
All ages	27	10	109	42.2	2.0	4.5	16	6.3	14	3.9
Total	54	11	219	42.8	2.0	4.5	33	6.4	29	4.1

For epidemiological sources see Underwood 1996. For the methods used to estimate and project incidence, prevalence, and deaths see Murray and Lopez 1996a. See explanatory notes for definitions and caveats.

Table 135	Cuadro 135	Tableau 135
Vitamin A deficiency	**Deficiencia de vitamina A**	**Avitaminose A**
Corneal scar	Cicatriz de la córnea	Cicatrice de la cornée

Table 135g   LAC - ALC - ALC — Vitamin A deficiency - Corneal scar

Age group (years)	Incidence 1990 Number ('000s)	Rate (per 100 000)	Prevalence 1990 Number ('000s)	Rate (per 100 000)	Avg. age at onset (years)	Average duration (years)	Deaths 1990 Number ('000s)	Rate (per 100 000)	Deaths 2000 (Projected) Number ('000s)	Rate (per 100 000)
Males										
0-4	4	14.6	2	6.4	2.0	4.8	2	6.4	1	4.5
5-14	0	0.0	2	3.5	-	-	1	1.3	0	0.7
15-44	0	0.0	0	0.2	-	-	0	0.1	0	0.0
45-59	0	0.0	0	0.0	-	-	0	0.0	0	0.0
60+	0	0.0	0	0.0	-	-	0	0.0	0	0.0
All ages	4	1.9	4	1.7	2.0	4.8	3	1.2	2	0.7
Females										
0-4	4	14.6	2	6.4	2.0	4.8	2	6.0	1	4.1
5-14	0	0.0	2	3.5	-	-	1	1.5	0	0.8
15-44	0	0.0	0	0.2	-	-	0	0.1	0	0.0
45-59	0	0.0	0	0.0	-	-	0	0.0	0	0.0
60+	0	0.0	0	0.0	-	-	0	0.0	0	0.0
All ages	4	1.8	4	1.7	2.0	4.8	3	1.1	2	0.6
Total	8	1.9	8	1.7	2.0	4.8	5	1.1	3	0.6

Table 135h   MEC - AOM - CMO — Vitamin A deficiency - Corneal scar

Age group (years)	Incidence 1990 Number ('000s)	Rate (per 100 000)	Prevalence 1990 Number ('000s)	Rate (per 100 000)	Avg. age at onset (years)	Average duration (years)	Deaths 1990 Number ('000s)	Rate (per 100 000)	Deaths 2000 (Projected) Number ('000s)	Rate (per 100 000)
Males										
0-4	16	39.3	36	86.4	2.0	4.8	7	16.4	6	12.1
5-14	0	0.0	30	46.5	-	-	3	4.6	2	2.6
15-44	0	0.0	3	2.5	-	-	0	0.1	0	0.1
45-59	0	0.0	0	0.0	-	-	0	0.0	0	0.0
60+	0	0.0	0	0.0	-	-	0	0.0	0	0.0
All ages	16	6.3	69	26.8	2.0	4.8	10	3.9	8	2.5
Females										
0-4	16	39.3	34	86.4	2.0	4.7	7	17.6	6	12.5
5-14	0	0.0	29	46.4	-	-	3	5.3	2	2.8
15-44	0	0.0	3	2.5	-	-	0	0.2	0	0.1
45-59	0	0.0	0	0.0	-	-	0	0.0	0	0.0
60+	0	0.0	0	0.0	-	-	0	0.0	0	0.0
All ages	16	6.3	66	26.7	2.0	4.7	10	4.2	8	2.6
Total	32	6.3	135	26.8	2.0	4.7	20	4.1	17	2.5

Table 135i   World - Mundo - Monde — Vitamin A deficiency - Corneal scar

Age group (years)	Incidence 1990 Number ('000s)	Rate (per 100 000)	Prevalence 1990 Number ('000s)	Rate (per 100 000)	Avg. age at onset (years)	Average duration (years)	Deaths 1990 Number ('000s)	Rate (per 100 000)	Deaths 2000 (Projected) Number ('000s)	Rate (per 100 000)
Males										
0-4	83	25.9	175	54.3	2.0	4.7	35	10.9	27	7.9
5-14	0	0.0	154	28.0	-	-	18	3.2	11	1.7
15-44	0	0.0	16	1.2	-	-	1	0.1	1	0.0
45-59	0	0.0	0	0.0	-	-	0	0.0	0	0.0
60+	0	0.0	0	0.0	-	-	0	0.0	0	0.0
All ages	83	3.1	344	13.0	2.0	4.7	54	2.0	39	1.3
Females										
0-4	81	26.0	169	54.7	2.0	4.7	33	10.8	25	7.6
5-14	0	0.0	148	28.1	-	-	17	3.3	10	1.7
15-44	0	0.0	15	1.2	-	-	1	0.1	1	0.0
45-59	0	0.0	0	0.0	-	-	0	0.0	0	0.0
60+	0	0.0	0	0.0	-	-	0	0.0	0	0.0
All ages	81	3.1	332	12.7	2.0	4.7	52	2.0	36	1.2
Total	164	3.1	676	12.8	2.0	4.7	106	2.0	75	1.2

For epidemiological sources see Underwood 1996. For the methods used to estimate and project incidence, prevalence, and deaths see Murray and Lopez 1996a. See explanatory notes for definitions and caveats.

Table 136
Iron-deficiency anaemia

All forms

Cuadro 136
Anemia por deficiencia de hierro

Todas las formas

Tableau 136
Anémie ferriprive

Toutes les formes

Table 136a — EME - PEMC - EMBE — Iron-deficiency anaemia - All forms

Age group (years)	Incidence 1990 Number ('000s)	Rate (per 100 000)	Prevalence 1990 Number ('000s)	Rate (per 100 000)	Avg. age at onset (years)	Average duration (years)	Deaths 1990 Number ('000s)	Rate (per 100 000)	Deaths 2000 (Projected) Number ('000s)	Rate (per 100 000)
Males										
0-4	-	-	2 520	9 550	-	-	0	0.4	0	0.3
5-14	-	-	4 268	8 000	-	-	0	0.2	0	0.1
15-44	-	-	3 681	2 000	-	-	1	0.3	0	0.2
45-59	-	-	1 323	2 000	-	-	0	0.6	0	0.4
60+	-	-	6 055	10 000	-	-	5	7.8	5	7.4
All ages	-	-	17 846	4 570	-	-	6	1.5	6	1.5
Females										
0-4	-	-	2 258	9 010	-	-	0	0.4	0	0.2
5-14	-	-	4 054	8 000	-	-	0	0.2	0	0.1
15-44	-	-	16 146	9 010	-	-	0	0.2	0	0.1
45-59	-	-	6 780	10 000	-	-	0	0.5	0	0.3
60+	-	-	8 457	10 000	-	-	7	8.5	8	8.0
All ages	-	-	37 695	9 255	-	-	8	2.0	8	2.0
Total	-	-	55 541	6 962	-	-	14	1.8	14	1.7

Table 136b — FSE - PEAS - AESE — Iron-deficiency anaemia - All forms

Age group (years)	Incidence 1990 Number ('000s)	Rate (per 100 000)	Prevalence 1990 Number ('000s)	Rate (per 100 000)	Avg. age at onset (years)	Average duration (years)	Deaths 1990 Number ('000s)	Rate (per 100 000)	Deaths 2000 (Projected) Number ('000s)	Rate (per 100 000)
Males										
0-4	-	-	2 752	20 000	-	-	0	0.5	0	0.4
5-14	-	-	4 923	18 000	-	-	0	0.2	0	0.1
15-44	-	-	1 526	2 000	-	-	0	0.2	0	0.1
45-59	-	-	539	2 000	-	-	0	0.7	0	0.4
60+	-	-	2 096	10 000	-	-	1	5.2	1	5.4
All ages	-	-	11 836	7 159	-	-	2	0.9	2	1.0
Females										
0-4	-	-	2 627	20 000	-	-	0	0.3	0	0.3
5-14	-	-	4 756	18 000	-	-	0	0.2	0	0.1
15-44	-	-	6 754	9 010	-	-	0	0.2	0	0.1
45-59	-	-	3 001	10 000	-	-	0	0.6	0	0.4
60+	-	-	3 639	10 000	-	-	3	7.1	3	6.8
All ages	-	-	20 777	11 484	-	-	3	1.7	3	1.6
Total	-	-	32 613	9 419	-	-	5	1.3	5	1.3

Table 136c — India - India - Inde — Iron-deficiency anaemia - All forms

Age group (years)	Incidence 1990 Number ('000s)	Rate (per 100 000)	Prevalence 1990 Number ('000s)	Rate (per 100 000)	Avg. age at onset (years)	Average duration (years)	Deaths 1990 Number ('000s)	Rate (per 100 000)	Deaths 2000 (Projected) Number ('000s)	Rate (per 100 000)
Males										
0-4	-	-	31 090	52 000	-	-	3	4.3	2	2.7
5-14	-	-	57 999	57 000	-	-	2	1.5	1	0.7
15-44	-	-	64 168	32 000	-	-	3	1.6	2	0.6
45-59	-	-	15 221	32 000	-	-	1	2.9	1	1.3
60+	-	-	18 158	61 000	-	-	5	15.2	4	11.5
All ages	-	-	186 637	42 475	-	-	13	3.0	9	1.7
Females										
0-4	-	-	29 473	52 000	-	-	3	4.5	1	2.7
5-14	-	-	54 300	57 000	-	-	2	1.6	1	0.7
15-44	-	-	111 778	61 000	-	-	5	2.8	2	0.9
45-59	-	-	28 063	61 000	-	-	3	5.5	1	2.5
60+	-	-	17 644	61 000	-	-	4	15.3	4	11.5
All ages	-	-	241 257	58 827	-	-	16	3.9	10	2.1
Total	-	-	427 894	50 369	-	-	29	3.4	19	1.9

For epidemiological sources see Bailey and Abou-Zahr 1996. For the methods used to estimate and project incidence, prevalence, and deaths see Murray and Lopez 1996a. See explanatory notes for definitions and caveats.

Table 136
Iron-deficiency anaemia

All forms

Cuadro 136
Anemia por deficiencia de hierro

Todas las formas

Tableau 136
Anémie ferriprive

Toutes les formes

Table 136d China - China - Chine — Iron-deficiency anaemia - All forms

Age group (years)	Incidence 1990 Number ('000s)	Rate (per 100 000)	Prevalence 1990 Number ('000s)	Rate (per 100 000)	Avg. age at onset (years)	Average duration (years)	Deaths 1990 Number ('000s)	Rate (per 100 000)	Deaths 2000 (Projected) Number ('000s)	Rate (per 100 000)
Males										
0-4	-	-	21 687	36 000	-	-	2	2.7	1	1.4
5-14	-	-	50 438	52 000	-	-	1	0.6	0	0.2
15-44	-	-	134 774	44 000	-	-	2	0.7	1	0.2
45-59	-	-	31 977	44 000	-	-	1	0.7	0	0.3
60+	-	-	25 964	53 010	-	-	3	6.2	3	4.3
All ages	-	-	264 841	45 257	-	-	8	1.3	5	0.7
Females										
0-4	-	-	20 861	36 000	-	-	5	8.8	2	4.3
5-14	-	-	47 009	52 000	-	-	2	2.0	1	0.7
15-44	-	-	90 905	32 000	-	-	4	1.3	1	0.4
45-59	-	-	34 140	53 010	-	-	1	1.1	0	0.4
60+	-	-	27 388	53 010	-	-	5	10.4	5	7.1
All ages	-	-	220 302	40 165	-	-	17	3.1	9	1.5
Total	-	-	485 143	42 793	-	-	25	2.2	14	1.1

Table 136e OAI - OPAI - APAI — Iron-deficiency anaemia - All forms

Age group (years)	Incidence 1990 Number ('000s)	Rate (per 100 000)	Prevalence 1990 Number ('000s)	Rate (per 100 000)	Avg. age at onset (years)	Average duration (years)	Deaths 1990 Number ('000s)	Rate (per 100 000)	Deaths 2000 (Projected) Number ('000s)	Rate (per 100 000)
Males										
0-4	-	-	21 448	49 010	-	-	2	4.0	1	2.6
5-14	-	-	27 739	33 010	-	-	1	0.8	0	0.4
15-44	-	-	51 464	32 000	-	-	2	1.3	1	0.6
45-59	-	-	10 924	32 000	-	-	1	2.9	1	1.5
60+	-	-	9 700	48 000	-	-	2	12.3	3	9.8
All ages	-	-	121 275	35 361	-	-	8	2.4	6	1.5
Females										
0-4	-	-	17 370	41 370	-	-	2	3.8	1	2.4
5-14	-	-	26 480	33 010	-	-	1	0.7	0	0.4
15-44	-	-	94 186	59 010	-	-	4	2.2	2	0.8
45-59	-	-	16 843	48 000	-	-	2	4.4	1	2.2
60+	-	-	10 878	48 000	-	-	3	11.8	3	9.5
All ages	-	-	165 757	48 814	-	-	10	2.9	7	1.8
Total	-	-	287 033	42 054	-	-	18	2.6	13	1.6

Table 136f SSA - ASS - ASS — Iron-deficiency anaemia - All forms

Age group (years)	Incidence 1990 Number ('000s)	Rate (per 100 000)	Prevalence 1990 Number ('000s)	Rate (per 100 000)	Avg. age at onset (years)	Average duration (years)	Deaths 1990 Number ('000s)	Rate (per 100 000)	Deaths 2000 (Projected) Number ('000s)	Rate (per 100 000)
Males										
0-4	-	-	21 843	46 000	-	-	2	3.6	2	2.6
5-14	-	-	30 914	44 000	-	-	1	1.1	1	0.6
15-44	-	-	24 903	24 000	-	-	1	0.9	1	0.4
45-59	-	-	4 874	24 000	-	-	0	2.2	0	1.2
60+	-	-	4 519	43 010	-	-	1	10.5	1	7.9
All ages	-	-	87 053	34 501	-	-	5	2.0	4	1.3
Females										
0-4	-	-	21 634	46 000	-	-	2	3.4	2	2.4
5-14	-	-	30 720	44 000	-	-	1	1.2	1	0.6
15-44	-	-	36 669	34 510	-	-	2	2.2	1	0.9
45-59	-	-	7 150	32 330	-	-	1	4.0	1	2.1
60+	-	-	5 475	43 010	-	-	1	11.2	1	8.3
All ages	-	-	101 649	39 406	-	-	7	2.7	5	1.6
Total	-	-	188 702	36 980	-	-	12	2.4	10	1.4

For epidemiological sources see Bailey and Abou-Zahr 1996. For the methods used to estimate and project incidence, prevalence, and deaths see Murray and Lopez 1996a. See explanatory notes for definitions and caveats.

Table 136	Cuadro 136	Tableau 136
Iron-deficiency anaemia	Anemia por deficiencia de hierro	Anémie ferriprive
All forms	Todas las formas	Toutes les formes

Table 136g LAC - ALC - ALC Iron-deficiency anaemia - All forms

Age group (years)	Incidence 1990 Number ('000s)	Rate (per 100 000)	Prevalence 1990 Number ('000s)	Rate (per 100 000)	Avg. age at onset (years)	Average duration (years)	Deaths 1990 Number ('000s)	Rate (per 100 000)	Deaths 2000 (Projected) Number ('000s)	Rate (per 100 000)
Males										
0-4	-	-	11 776	41 000	-	-	2	6.5	1	4.5
5-14	-	-	10 946	21 000	-	-	1	1.9	1	1.1
15-44	-	-	8 343	8 000	-	-	1	0.9	1	0.5
45-59	-	-	1 780	8 000	-	-	1	3.2	1	1.8
60+	-	-	2 136	15 010	-	-	3	18.1	3	15.0
All ages	-	-	34 981	15 785	-	-	7	3.2	6	2.3
Females										
0-4	-	-	11 347	41 000	-	-	1	5.3	1	3.6
5-14	-	-	10 656	21 000	-	-	1	2.3	1	1.3
15-44	-	-	37 471	36 000	-	-	3	2.6	1	1.2
45-59	-	-	3 506	15 010	-	-	1	4.4	1	2.4
60+	-	-	2 525	15 010	-	-	3	20.2	4	16.5
All ages	-	-	65 505	29 416	-	-	10	4.4	8	2.9
Total	-	-	100 485	22 617	-	-	17	3.8	14	2.6

Table 136h MEC - AOM - CMO Iron-deficiency anaemia - All forms

Age group (years)	Incidence 1990 Number ('000s)	Rate (per 100 000)	Prevalence 1990 Number ('000s)	Rate (per 100 000)	Avg. age at onset (years)	Average duration (years)	Deaths 1990 Number ('000s)	Rate (per 100 000)	Deaths 2000 (Projected) Number ('000s)	Rate (per 100 000)
Males										
0-4	-	-	21 819	53 010	-	-	2	4.4	2	3.2
5-14	-	-	21 570	33 010	-	-	0	0.8	0	0.4
15-44	-	-	15 945	14 000	-	-	1	0.5	0	0.3
45-59	-	-	3 127	14 000	-	-	0	1.3	0	0.7
60+	-	-	3 003	22 000	-	-	1	5.2	1	4.1
All ages	-	-	65 466	25 534	-	-	4	1.5	3	1.0
Females										
0-4	-	-	21 063	53 010	-	-	2	4.4	1	3.1
5-14	-	-	20 466	33 010	-	-	0	0.8	0	0.4
15-44	-	-	56 833	53 010	-	-	2	1.9	1	0.8
45-59	-	-	4 904	22 000	-	-	0	2.0	0	1.1
60+	-	-	3 399	22 000	-	-	1	5.3	1	4.2
All ages	-	-	106 665	43 239	-	-	6	2.2	4	1.3
Total	-	-	172 130	34 216	-	-	9	1.9	8	1.2

Table 136i World - Mundo - Monde Iron-deficiency anaemia - All forms

Age group (years)	Incidence 1990 Number ('000s)	Rate (per 100 000)	Prevalence 1990 Number ('000s)	Rate (per 100 000)	Avg. age at onset (years)	Average duration (years)	Deaths 1990 Number ('000s)	Rate (per 100 000)	Deaths 2000 (Projected) Number ('000s)	Rate (per 100 000)
Males										
0-4	-	-	134 935	41 997	-	-	12	3.6	8	2.4
5-14	-	-	208 797	37 881	-	-	5	0.9	3	0.5
15-44	-	-	304 805	24 386	-	-	11	0.8	5	0.4
45-59	-	-	69 765	22 334	-	-	5	1.6	3	0.8
60+	-	-	71 633	32 730	-	-	20	9.3	21	7.7
All ages	-	-	789 934	29 768	-	-	52	2.0	41	1.3
Females										
0-4	-	-	126 633	40 949	-	-	14	4.6	9	2.7
5-14	-	-	198 440	37 760	-	-	7	1.2	4	0.6
15-44	-	-	450 741	37 605	-	-	20	1.7	9	0.7
45-59	-	-	104 387	33 559	-	-	8	2.5	5	1.2
60+	-	-	79 405	29 495	-	-	28	10.3	29	8.6
All ages	-	-	959 607	36 715	-	-	76	2.9	56	1.8
Total	-	-	1 749 541	33 215	-	-	129	2.4	97	1.6

For epidemiological sources see Bailey and Abou-Zahr 1996. For the methods used to estimate and project incidence, prevalence, and deaths see Murray and Lopez 1996a. See explanatory notes for definitions and caveats.

Table 137
Iron-deficiency anaemia

Mild

Cuadro 137
Anemia por deficiencia de hierro

Leve

Tableau 137
Anémie ferriprive

Légère

Table 137a EME - PEMC - EMBE Iron-deficiency anaemia - Mild

Age group (years)	Incidence 1990 Number ('000s)	Rate (per 100 000)	Prevalence 1990 Number ('000s)	Rate (per 100 000)	Avg. age at onset (years)	Average duration (years)	Deaths 1990 Number ('000s)	Rate (per 100 000)	Deaths 2000 (Projected) Number ('000s)	Rate (per 100 000)
Males										
0-4	-	-	950	3 600	-	-	-	-	-	-
5-14	-	-	1 707	3 200	-	-	-	-	-	-
15-44	-	-	1 473	800	-	-	-	-	-	-
45-59	-	-	529	800	-	-	-	-	-	-
60+	-	-	2 422	4 000	-	-	-	-	-	-
All ages	-	-	7 080	1 813	-	-	-	-	-	-
Females										
0-4	-	-	902	3 600	-	-	-	-	-	-
5-14	-	-	1 622	3 200	-	-	-	-	-	-
15-44	-	-	6 451	3 600	-	-	-	-	-	-
45-59	-	-	2 712	4 000	-	-	-	-	-	-
60+	-	-	3 383	4 000	-	-	-	-	-	-
All ages	-	-	15 070	3 700	-	-	-	-	-	-
Total	-	-	22 150	2 776	-	-	-	-	-	-

Table 137b FSE - PEAS - AESE Iron-deficiency anaemia - Mild

Age group (years)	Incidence 1990 Number ('000s)	Rate (per 100 000)	Prevalence 1990 Number ('000s)	Rate (per 100 000)	Avg. age at onset (years)	Average duration (years)	Deaths 1990 Number ('000s)	Rate (per 100 000)	Deaths 2000 (Projected) Number ('000s)	Rate (per 100 000)
Males										
0-4	-	-	1 101	8 000	-	-	-	-	-	-
5-14	-	-	1 969	7 200	-	-	-	-	-	-
15-44	-	-	610	800	-	-	-	-	-	-
45-59	-	-	216	800	-	-	-	-	-	-
60+	-	-	839	4 000	-	-	-	-	-	-
All ages	-	-	4 734	2 864	-	-	-	-	-	-
Females										
0-4	-	-	1 051	8 000	-	-	-	-	-	-
5-14	-	-	1 902	7 200	-	-	-	-	-	-
15-44	-	-	2 699	3 600	-	-	-	-	-	-
45-59	-	-	1 200	4 000	-	-	-	-	-	-
60+	-	-	1 456	4 000	-	-	-	-	-	-
All ages	-	-	8 308	4 592	-	-	-	-	-	-
Total	-	-	13 042	3 767	-	-	-	-	-	-

Table 137c India - India - Inde Iron-deficiency anaemia - Mild

Age group (years)	Incidence 1990 Number ('000s)	Rate (per 100 000)	Prevalence 1990 Number ('000s)	Rate (per 100 000)	Avg. age at onset (years)	Average duration (years)	Deaths 1990 Number ('000s)	Rate (per 100 000)	Deaths 2000 (Projected) Number ('000s)	Rate (per 100 000)
Males										
0-4	-	-	12 436	20 800	-	-	-	-	-	-
5-14	-	-	23 199	22 800	-	-	-	-	-	-
15-44	-	-	25 667	12 800	-	-	-	-	-	-
45-59	-	-	6 089	12 800	-	-	-	-	-	-
60+	-	-	7 263	24 400	-	-	-	-	-	-
All ages	-	-	74 655	16 990	-	-	-	-	-	-
Females										
0-4	-	-	11 789	20 800	-	-	-	-	-	-
5-14	-	-	21 720	22 800	-	-	-	-	-	-
15-44	-	-	44 711	24 400	-	-	-	-	-	-
45-59	-	-	11 225	24 400	-	-	-	-	-	-
60+	-	-	7 057	24 400	-	-	-	-	-	-
All ages	-	-	96 503	23 531	-	-	-	-	-	-
Total	-	-	171 158	20 148	-	-	-	-	-	-

For epidemiological sources see Bailey and Abou-Zahr 1996. For the methods used to estimate and project incidence, prevalence, and deaths see Murray and Lopez 1996a. See explanatory notes for definitions and caveats.

Table 137
Iron-deficiency anaemia

Mild

Cuadro 137
Anemia por deficiencia de hierro

Leve

Tableau 137
Anémie ferriprive

Légère

Table 137d — China - China - Chine — Iron-deficiency anaemia - Mild

Age group (years)	Incidence 1990 Number ('000s)	Rate (per 100 000)	Prevalence 1990 Number ('000s)	Rate (per 100 000)	Avg. age at onset (years)	Average duration (years)	Deaths 1990 Number ('000s)	Rate (per 100 000)	Deaths 2000 (Projected) Number ('000s)	Rate (per 100 000)
Males										
0-4	-	-	8 675	14 400	-	-	-	-	-	-
5-14	-	-	20 175	20 800	-	-	-	-	-	-
15-44	-	-	53 910	17 600	-	-	-	-	-	-
45-59	-	-	12 791	17 600	-	-	-	-	-	-
60+	-	-	10 384	21 200	-	-	-	-	-	-
All ages	-	-	105 934	18 102	-	-	-	-	-	-
Females										
0-4	-	-	8 344	14 400	-	-	-	-	-	-
5-14	-	-	18 803	20 800	-	-	-	-	-	-
15-44	-	-	36 362	12 800	-	-	-	-	-	-
45-59	-	-	13 653	21 200	-	-	-	-	-	-
60+	-	-	10 953	21 200	-	-	-	-	-	-
All ages	-	-	88 116	16 065	-	-	-	-	-	-
Total	-	-	194 051	17 117	-	-	-	-	-	-

Table 137e — OAI - OPAI - APAI — Iron-deficiency anaemia - Mild

Age group (years)	Incidence 1990 Number ('000s)	Rate (per 100 000)	Prevalence 1990 Number ('000s)	Rate (per 100 000)	Avg. age at onset (years)	Average duration (years)	Deaths 1990 Number ('000s)	Rate (per 100 000)	Deaths 2000 (Projected) Number ('000s)	Rate (per 100 000)
Males										
0-4	-	-	8 578	19 600	-	-	-	-	-	-
5-14	-	-	11 092	13 200	-	-	-	-	-	-
15-44	-	-	20 586	12 800	-	-	-	-	-	-
45-59	-	-	4 370	12 800	-	-	-	-	-	-
60+	-	-	3 880	19 200	-	-	-	-	-	-
All ages	-	-	48 505	14 143	-	-	-	-	-	-
Females										
0-4	-	-	5 022	11 960	-	-	-	-	-	-
5-14	-	-	10 589	13 200	-	-	-	-	-	-
15-44	-	-	37 668	23 600	-	-	-	-	-	-
45-59	-	-	6 737	19 200	-	-	-	-	-	-
60+	-	-	4 351	19 200	-	-	-	-	-	-
All ages	-	-	64 367	18 956	-	-	-	-	-	-
Total	-	-	112 872	16 537	-	-	-	-	-	-

Table 137f — SSA - ASS - ASS — Iron-deficiency anaemia - Mild

Age group (years)	Incidence 1990 Number ('000s)	Rate (per 100 000)	Prevalence 1990 Number ('000s)	Rate (per 100 000)	Avg. age at onset (years)	Average duration (years)	Deaths 1990 Number ('000s)	Rate (per 100 000)	Deaths 2000 (Projected) Number ('000s)	Rate (per 100 000)
Males										
0-4	-	-	8 737	18 400	-	-	-	-	-	-
5-14	-	-	12 365	17 600	-	-	-	-	-	-
15-44	-	-	9 961	9 600	-	-	-	-	-	-
45-59	-	-	1 950	9 600	-	-	-	-	-	-
60+	-	-	1 807	17 200	-	-	-	-	-	-
All ages	-	-	34 821	13 800	-	-	-	-	-	-
Females										
0-4	-	-	8 654	18 400	-	-	-	-	-	-
5-14	-	-	12 288	17 600	-	-	-	-	-	-
15-44	-	-	20 401	19 200	-	-	-	-	-	-
45-59	-	-	3 804	17 200	-	-	-	-	-	-
60+	-	-	2 190	17 200	-	-	-	-	-	-
All ages	-	-	47 337	18 351	-	-	-	-	-	-
Total	-	-	82 157	16 101	-	-	-	-	-	-

For epidemiological sources see Bailey and Abou-Zahr 1996. For the methods used to estimate and project incidence, prevalence, and deaths see Murray and Lopez 1996a. See explanatory notes for definitions and caveats.

Table 137 Iron-deficiency anaemia	Cuadro 137 Anemia por deficiencia de hierro	Tableau 137 Anémie ferriprive
Mild	Leve	Légère

Table 137g   LAC - ALC - ALC   Iron-deficiency anaemia - Mild

Age group (years)	Incidence 1990 Number ('000s)	Rate (per 100 000)	Prevalence 1990 Number ('000s)	Rate (per 100 000)	Avg. age at onset (years)	Average duration (years)	Deaths 1990 Number ('000s)	Rate (per 100 000)	Deaths 2000 (Projected) Number ('000s)	Rate (per 100 000)
Males										
0-4	-	-	4 710	16 400	-	-	-	-	-	-
5-14	-	-	4 378	8 400	-	-	-	-	-	-
15-44	-	-	3 337	3 200	-	-	-	-	-	-
45-59	-	-	712	3 200	-	-	-	-	-	-
60+	-	-	854	6 000	-	-	-	-	-	-
All ages	-	-	13 992	6 314	-	-	-	-	-	-
Females										
0-4	-	-	4 539	16 400	-	-	-	-	-	-
5-14	-	-	4 262	8 400	-	-	-	-	-	-
15-44	-	-	14 988	14 400	-	-	-	-	-	-
45-59	-	-	1 401	6 000	-	-	-	-	-	-
60+	-	-	1 009	6 000	-	-	-	-	-	-
All ages	-	-	26 200	11 766	-	-	-	-	-	-
Total	-	-	40 192	9 046	-	-	-	-	-	-

Table 137h   MEC - AOM - CMO   Iron-deficiency anaemia - Mild

Age group (years)	Incidence 1990 Number ('000s)	Rate (per 100 000)	Prevalence 1990 Number ('000s)	Rate (per 100 000)	Avg. age at onset (years)	Average duration (years)	Deaths 1990 Number ('000s)	Rate (per 100 000)	Deaths 2000 (Projected) Number ('000s)	Rate (per 100 000)
Males										
0-4	-	-	8 726	21 200	-	-	-	-	-	-
5-14	-	-	8 626	13 200	-	-	-	-	-	-
15-44	-	-	6 378	5 600	-	-	-	-	-	-
45-59	-	-	1 251	5 600	-	-	-	-	-	-
60+	-	-	1 201	8 800	-	-	-	-	-	-
All ages	-	-	26 182	10 212	-	-	-	-	-	-
Females										
0-4	-	-	8 424	21 200	-	-	-	-	-	-
5-14	-	-	8 184	13 200	-	-	-	-	-	-
15-44	-	-	22 729	21 200	-	-	-	-	-	-
45-59	-	-	1 962	8 800	-	-	-	-	-	-
60+	-	-	1 360	8 800	-	-	-	-	-	-
All ages	-	-	42 658	17 292	-	-	-	-	-	-
Total	-	-	68 839	13 684	-	-	-	-	-	-

Table 137i   World - Mundo - Monde   Iron-deficiency anaemia - Mild

Age group (years)	Incidence 1990 Number ('000s)	Rate (per 100 000)	Prevalence 1990 Number ('000s)	Rate (per 100 000)	Avg. age at onset (years)	Average duration (years)	Deaths 1990 Number ('000s)	Rate (per 100 000)	Deaths 2000 (Projected) Number ('000s)	Rate (per 100 000)
Males										
0-4	-	-	53 913	16 780	-	-	-	-	-	-
5-14	-	-	83 513	15 151	-	-	-	-	-	-
15-44	-	-	121 922	9 754	-	-	-	-	-	-
45-59	-	-	27 906	8 934	-	-	-	-	-	-
60+	-	-	28 650	13 091	-	-	-	-	-	-
All ages	-	-	315 903	11 905	-	-	-	-	-	-
Females										
0-4	-	-	48 724	15 756	-	-	-	-	-	-
5-14	-	-	79 370	15 103	-	-	-	-	-	-
15-44	-	-	186 009	15 519	-	-	-	-	-	-
45-59	-	-	42 695	13 726	-	-	-	-	-	-
60+	-	-	31 759	11 797	-	-	-	-	-	-
All ages	-	-	388 558	14 866	-	-	-	-	-	-
Total	-	-	704 461	13 374	-	-	-	-	-	-

For epidemiological sources see Bailey and Abou-Zahr 1996. For the methods used to estimate and project incidence, prevalence, and deaths see Murray and Lopez 1996a. See explanatory notes for definitions and caveats.

Table 138
Iron-deficiency anaemia

Moderate

Cuadro 138
Anemia por deficiencia de hierro

Moderada

Tableau 138
Anémie ferriprive

Modérée

Table 138a EME - PEMC - EMBE — Iron-deficiency anaemia - Moderate

Age group (years)	Incidence 1990 Number ('000s)	Rate (per 100 000)	Prevalence 1990 Number ('000s)	Rate (per 100 000)	Avg. age at onset (years)	Average duration (years)	Deaths 1990 Number ('000s)	Rate (per 100 000)	Deaths 2000 (Projected) Number ('000s)	Rate (per 100 000)
Males										
0-4	-	-	1 478	5 600	-	-	-	-	-	-
5-14	-	-	2 401	4 500	-	-	-	-	-	-
15-44	-	-	2 062	1 120	-	-	-	-	-	-
45-59	-	-	741	1 120	-	-	-	-	-	-
60+	-	-	3 403	5 620	-	-	-	-	-	-
All ages	-	-	10 083	2 582	-	-	-	-	-	-
Females										
0-4	-	-	1 268	5 060	-	-	-	-	-	-
5-14	-	-	2 281	4 500	-	-	-	-	-	-
15-44	-	-	9 067	5 060	-	-	-	-	-	-
45-59	-	-	3 810	5 620	-	-	-	-	-	-
60+	-	-	4 753	5 620	-	-	-	-	-	-
All ages	-	-	21 179	5 200	-	-	-	-	-	-
Total	-	-	31 262	3 919	-	-	-	-	-	-

Table 138b FSE - PEAS - AESE — Iron-deficiency anaemia - Moderate

Age group (years)	Incidence 1990 Number ('000s)	Rate (per 100 000)	Prevalence 1990 Number ('000s)	Rate (per 100 000)	Avg. age at onset (years)	Average duration (years)	Deaths 1990 Number ('000s)	Rate (per 100 000)	Deaths 2000 (Projected) Number ('000s)	Rate (per 100 000)
Males										
0-4	-	-	1 547	11 240	-	-	-	-	-	-
5-14	-	-	2 768	10 120	-	-	-	-	-	-
15-44	-	-	854	1 120	-	-	-	-	-	-
45-59	-	-	302	1 120	-	-	-	-	-	-
60+	-	-	1 178	5 620	-	-	-	-	-	-
All ages	-	-	6 649	4 022	-	-	-	-	-	-
Females										
0-4	-	-	1 476	11 240	-	-	-	-	-	-
5-14	-	-	2 674	10 120	-	-	-	-	-	-
15-44	-	-	3 793	5 060	-	-	-	-	-	-
45-59	-	-	1 686	5 620	-	-	-	-	-	-
60+	-	-	2 045	5 620	-	-	-	-	-	-
All ages	-	-	11 675	6 453	-	-	-	-	-	-
Total	-	-	18 324	5 292	-	-	-	-	-	-

Table 138c India - India - Inde — Iron-deficiency anaemia - Moderate

Age group (years)	Incidence 1990 Number ('000s)	Rate (per 100 000)	Prevalence 1990 Number ('000s)	Rate (per 100 000)	Avg. age at onset (years)	Average duration (years)	Deaths 1990 Number ('000s)	Rate (per 100 000)	Deaths 2000 (Projected) Number ('000s)	Rate (per 100 000)
Males										
0-4	-	-	17 470	29 220	-	-	-	-	-	-
5-14	-	-	32 591	32 030	-	-	-	-	-	-
15-44	-	-	36 054	17 980	-	-	-	-	-	-
45-59	-	-	8 553	17 980	-	-	-	-	-	-
60+	-	-	10 204	34 280	-	-	-	-	-	-
All ages	-	-	104 873	23 867	-	-	-	-	-	-
Females										
0-4	-	-	16 562	29 220	-	-	-	-	-	-
5-14	-	-	30 513	32 030	-	-	-	-	-	-
15-44	-	-	62 815	34 280	-	-	-	-	-	-
45-59	-	-	15 771	34 280	-	-	-	-	-	-
60+	-	-	9 915	34 280	-	-	-	-	-	-
All ages	-	-	135 575	33 058	-	-	-	-	-	-
Total	-	-	240 448	28 304	-	-	-	-	-	-

For epidemiological sources see Bailey and Abou-Zahr 1996. For the methods used to estimate and project incidence, prevalence, and deaths see Murray and Lopez 1996a. See explanatory notes for definitions and caveats.

Table 138
Iron-deficiency anaemia

Moderate

Cuadro 138
Anemia por deficiencia de hierro

Moderada

Tableau 138
Anémie ferriprive

Modérée

Table 138d   China - China - Chine   Iron-deficiency anaemia - Moderate

Age group (years)	Incidence 1990 Number ('000s)	Rate (per 100 000)	Prevalence 1990 Number ('000s)	Rate (per 100 000)	Avg. age at onset (years)	Average duration (years)	Deaths 1990 Number ('000s)	Rate (per 100 000)	Deaths 2000 (Projected) Number ('000s)	Rate (per 100 000)
Males										
0-4	-	-	12 187	20 230	-	-	-	-	-	-
5-14	-	-	28 343	29 220	-	-	-	-	-	-
15-44	-	-	75 749	24 730	-	-	-	-	-	-
45-59	-	-	17 972	24 730	-	-	-	-	-	-
60+	-	-	14 591	29 790	-	-	-	-	-	-
All ages	-	-	148 842	25 434	-	-	-	-	-	-
Females										
0-4	-	-	11 722	20 230	-	-	-	-	-	-
5-14	-	-	26 415	29 220	-	-	-	-	-	-
15-44	-	-	51 077	17 980	-	-	-	-	-	-
45-59	-	-	19 186	29 790	-	-	-	-	-	-
60+	-	-	15 391	29 790	-	-	-	-	-	-
All ages	-	-	123 792	22 569	-	-	-	-	-	-
Total	-	-	272 634	24 048	-	-	-	-	-	-

Table 138e   OAI - OPAI - APAI   Iron-deficiency anaemia - Moderate

Age group (years)	Incidence 1990 Number ('000s)	Rate (per 100 000)	Prevalence 1990 Number ('000s)	Rate (per 100 000)	Avg. age at onset (years)	Average duration (years)	Deaths 1990 Number ('000s)	Rate (per 100 000)	Deaths 2000 (Projected) Number ('000s)	Rate (per 100 000)
Males										
0-4	-	-	12 052	27 540	-	-	-	-	-	-
5-14	-	-	15 588	18 550	-	-	-	-	-	-
15-44	-	-	28 916	17 980	-	-	-	-	-	-
45-59	-	-	6 138	17 980	-	-	-	-	-	-
60+	-	-	5 452	26 980	-	-	-	-	-	-
All ages	-	-	68 147	19 870	-	-	-	-	-	-
Females										
0-4	-	-	11 563	27 540	-	-	-	-	-	-
5-14	-	-	14 880	18 550	-	-	-	-	-	-
15-44	-	-	52 927	33 160	-	-	-	-	-	-
45-59	-	-	9 467	26 980	-	-	-	-	-	-
60+	-	-	6 114	26 980	-	-	-	-	-	-
All ages	-	-	94 952	27 963	-	-	-	-	-	-
Total	-	-	163 099	23 896	-	-	-	-	-	-

Table 138f   SSA - ASS - ASS   Iron-deficiency anaemia - Moderate

Age group (years)	Incidence 1990 Number ('000s)	Rate (per 100 000)	Prevalence 1990 Number ('000s)	Rate (per 100 000)	Avg. age at onset (years)	Average duration (years)	Deaths 1990 Number ('000s)	Rate (per 100 000)	Deaths 2000 (Projected) Number ('000s)	Rate (per 100 000)
Males										
0-4	-	-	12 275	25 850	-	-	-	-	-	-
5-14	-	-	17 375	24 730	-	-	-	-	-	-
15-44	-	-	13 998	13 490	-	-	-	-	-	-
45-59	-	-	2 740	13 490	-	-	-	-	-	-
60+	-	-	2 540	24 170	-	-	-	-	-	-
All ages	-	-	48 927	19 391	-	-	-	-	-	-
Females										
0-4	-	-	12 157	25 850	-	-	-	-	-	-
5-14	-	-	17 266	24 730	-	-	-	-	-	-
15-44	-	-	14 334	13 490	-	-	-	-	-	-
45-59	-	-	2 984	13 490	-	-	-	-	-	-
60+	-	-	3 077	24 170	-	-	-	-	-	-
All ages	-	-	49 818	19 313	-	-	-	-	-	-
Total	-	-	98 744	19 351	-	-	-	-	-	-

For epidemiological sources see Bailey and Abou-Zahr 1996. For the methods used to estimate and project incidence, prevalence, and deaths see Murray and Lopez 1996a. See explanatory notes for definitions and caveats.

Table 138	Cuadro 138	Tableau 138
Iron-deficiency anaemia	Anemia por deficiencia de hierro	Anémie ferriprive
Moderate	Moderada	Modérée

Table 138g LAC - ALC - ALC Iron-deficiency anaemia - Moderate

Age group (years)	Incidence 1990 Number ('000s)	Rate (per 100 000)	Prevalence 1990 Number ('000s)	Rate (per 100 000)	Avg. age at onset (years)	Average duration (years)	Deaths 1990 Number ('000s)	Rate (per 100 000)	Deaths 2000 (Projected) Number ('000s)	Rate (per 100 000)
Males										
0-4	-	-	6 617	23 040	-	-	-	-	-	-
5-14	-	-	6 151	11 800	-	-	-	-	-	-
15-44	-	-	4 693	4 500	-	-	-	-	-	-
45-59	-	-	1 001	4 500	-	-	-	-	-	-
60+	-	-	1 200	8 430	-	-	-	-	-	-
All ages	-	-	19 662	8 872	-	-	-	-	-	-
Females										
0-4	-	-	6 377	23 040	-	-	-	-	-	-
5-14	-	-	5 988	11 800	-	-	-	-	-	-
15-44	-	-	21 056	20 230	-	-	-	-	-	-
45-59	-	-	1 969	8 430	-	-	-	-	-	-
60+	-	-	1 418	8 430	-	-	-	-	-	-
All ages	-	-	36 808	16 529	-	-	-	-	-	-
Total	-	-	56 470	12 710	-	-	-	-	-	-

Table 138h MEC - AOM - CMO Iron-deficiency anaemia - Moderate

Age group (years)	Incidence 1990 Number ('000s)	Rate (per 100 000)	Prevalence 1990 Number ('000s)	Rate (per 100 000)	Avg. age at onset (years)	Average duration (years)	Deaths 1990 Number ('000s)	Rate (per 100 000)	Deaths 2000 (Projected) Number ('000s)	Rate (per 100 000)
Males										
0-4	-	-	12 262	29 790	-	-	-	-	-	-
5-14	-	-	12 121	18 550	-	-	-	-	-	-
15-44	-	-	8 964	7 870	-	-	-	-	-	-
45-59	-	-	1 758	7 870	-	-	-	-	-	-
60+	-	-	1 687	12 360	-	-	-	-	-	-
All ages	-	-	36 792	14 350	-	-	-	-	-	-
Females										
0-4	-	-	11 837	29 790	-	-	-	-	-	-
5-14	-	-	11 501	18 550	-	-	-	-	-	-
15-44	-	-	31 938	29 790	-	-	-	-	-	-
45-59	-	-	2 755	12 360	-	-	-	-	-	-
60+	-	-	1 910	12 360	-	-	-	-	-	-
All ages	-	-	59 941	24 298	-	-	-	-	-	-
Total	-	-	96 733	19 228	-	-	-	-	-	-

Table 138i World - Mundo - Monde Iron-deficiency anaemia - Moderate

Age group (years)	Incidence 1990 Number ('000s)	Rate (per 100 000)	Prevalence 1990 Number ('000s)	Rate (per 100 000)	Avg. age at onset (years)	Average duration (years)	Deaths 1990 Number ('000s)	Rate (per 100 000)	Deaths 2000 (Projected) Number ('000s)	Rate (per 100 000)
Males										
0-4	-	-	75 888	23 619	-	-	-	-	-	-
5-14	-	-	117 337	21 288	-	-	-	-	-	-
15-44	-	-	171 290	13 704	-	-	-	-	-	-
45-59	-	-	39 204	12 551	-	-	-	-	-	-
60+	-	-	40 255	18 393	-	-	-	-	-	-
All ages	-	-	443 974	16 731	-	-	-	-	-	-
Females										
0-4	-	-	72 963	23 594	-	-	-	-	-	-
5-14	-	-	111 517	21 220	-	-	-	-	-	-
15-44	-	-	247 009	20 608	-	-	-	-	-	-
45-59	-	-	57 628	18 527	-	-	-	-	-	-
60+	-	-	44 623	16 575	-	-	-	-	-	-
All ages	-	-	533 740	20 421	-	-	-	-	-	-
Total	-	-	977 714	18 562	-	-	-	-	-	-

For epidemiological sources see Bailey and Abou-Zahr 1996. For the methods used to estimate and project incidence, prevalence, and deaths see Murray and Lopez 1996a. See explanatory notes for definitions and caveats.

Table 139
Iron-deficiency anaemia

Severe

Cuadro 139
Anemia por deficiencia de hierro

Severa

Tableau 139
Anémie ferriprive

Grave

Table 139a   EME - PEMC - EMBE

Iron deficiency anaemia - Severe

Age group (years)	Incidence 1990 Number ('000s)	Rate (per 100 000)	Prevalence 1990 Number ('000s)	Rate (per 100 000)	Avg. age at onset (years)	Average duration (years)	Deaths 1990 Number ('000s)	Rate (per 100 000)	Deaths 2000 (Projected) Number ('000s)	Rate (per 100 000)
Males										
0-4	-	-	84	320	-	-	-	-	-	-
5-14	-	-	149	280	-	-	-	-	-	-
15-44	-	-	129	70	-	-	-	-	-	-
45-59	-	-	46	70	-	-	-	-	-	-
60+	-	-	212	350	-	-	-	-	-	-
All ages	-	-	621	159	-	-	-	-	-	-
Females										
0-4	-	-	80	320	-	-	-	-	-	-
5-14	-	-	142	280	-	-	-	-	-	-
15-44	-	-	573	320	-	-	-	-	-	-
45-59	-	-	237	350	-	-	-	-	-	-
60+	-	-	296	350	-	-	-	-	-	-
All ages	-	-	1 329	326	-	-	-	-	-	-
Total	-	-	1 950	244	-	-	-	-	-	-

Table 139b   FSE - PEAS - AESE

Iron deficiency anaemia - Severe

Age group (years)	Incidence 1990 Number ('000s)	Rate (per 100 000)	Prevalence 1990 Number ('000s)	Rate (per 100 000)	Avg. age at onset (years)	Average duration (years)	Deaths 1990 Number ('000s)	Rate (per 100 000)	Deaths 2000 (Projected) Number ('000s)	Rate (per 100 000)
Males										
0-4	-	-	96	700	-	-	-	-	-	-
5-14	-	-	172	630	-	-	-	-	-	-
15-44	-	-	53	70	-	-	-	-	-	-
45-59	-	-	19	70	-	-	-	-	-	-
60+	-	-	73	350	-	-	-	-	-	-
All ages	-	-	414	251	-	-	-	-	-	-
Females										
0-4	-	-	92	700	-	-	-	-	-	-
5-14	-	-	166	630	-	-	-	-	-	-
15-44	-	-	240	320	-	-	-	-	-	-
45-59	-	-	105	350	-	-	-	-	-	-
60+	-	-	127	350	-	-	-	-	-	-
All ages	-	-	731	404	-	-	-	-	-	-
Total	-	-	1 145	331	-	-	-	-	-	-

Table 139c   India - India - Inde

Iron deficiency anaemia - Severe

Age group (years)	Incidence 1990 Number ('000s)	Rate (per 100 000)	Prevalence 1990 Number ('000s)	Rate (per 100 000)	Avg. age at onset (years)	Average duration (years)	Deaths 1990 Number ('000s)	Rate (per 100 000)	Deaths 2000 (Projected) Number ('000s)	Rate (per 100 000)
Males										
0-4	-	-	1 088	1 820	-	-	-	-	-	-
5-14	-	-	2 035	2 000	-	-	-	-	-	-
15-44	-	-	2 246	1 120	-	-	-	-	-	-
45-59	-	-	533	1 120	-	-	-	-	-	-
60+	-	-	637	2 140	-	-	-	-	-	-
All ages	-	-	6 539	1 488	-	-	-	-	-	-
Females										
0-4	-	-	1 032	1 820	-	-	-	-	-	-
5-14	-	-	1 905	2 000	-	-	-	-	-	-
15-44	-	-	3 921	2 140	-	-	-	-	-	-
45-59	-	-	985	2 140	-	-	-	-	-	-
60+	-	-	619	2 140	-	-	-	-	-	-
All ages	-	-	8 462	2 063	-	-	-	-	-	-
Total	-	-	15 001	1 766	-	-	-	-	-	-

For epidemiological sources see Bailey and Abou-Zahr 1996. For the methods used to estimate and project incidence, prevalence, and deaths see Murray and Lopez 1996a. See explanatory notes for definitions and caveats.

Table 139
Iron-deficiency anaemia

Severe

Cuadro 139
Anemia por deficiencia de hierro

Severa

Tableau 139
Anémie ferriprive

Grave

Table 139d China - China - Chine   Iron-deficiency anaemia - Severe

Age group (years)	Incidence 1990 Number ('000s)	Rate (per 100 000)	Prevalence 1990 Number ('000s)	Rate (per 100 000)	Avg. age at onset (years)	Average duration (years)	Deaths 1990 Number ('000s)	Rate (per 100 000)	Deaths 2000 (Projected) Number ('000s)	Rate (per 100 000)
Males										
0-4	-	-	759	1 260	-	-	-	-	-	-
5-14	-	-	1 765	1 820	-	-	-	-	-	-
15-44	-	-	4 717	1 540	-	-	-	-	-	-
45-59	-	-	1 119	1 540	-	-	-	-	-	-
60+	-	-	911	1 860	-	-	-	-	-	-
All ages	-	-	9 272	1 584	-	-	-	-	-	-
Females										
0-4	-	-	730	1 260	-	-	-	-	-	-
5-14	-	-	1 645	1 820	-	-	-	-	-	-
15-44	-	-	3 182	1 120	-	-	-	-	-	-
45-59	-	-	1 198	1 860	-	-	-	-	-	-
60+	-	-	961	1 860	-	-	-	-	-	-
All ages	-	-	7 716	1 407	-	-	-	-	-	-
Total	-	-	16 988	1 498	-	-	-	-	-	-

Table 139e OAI - OPAI - APAI   Iron-deficiency anaemia - Severe

Age group (years)	Incidence 1990 Number ('000s)	Rate (per 100 000)	Prevalence 1990 Number ('000s)	Rate (per 100 000)	Avg. age at onset (years)	Average duration (years)	Deaths 1990 Number ('000s)	Rate (per 100 000)	Deaths 2000 (Projected) Number ('000s)	Rate (per 100 000)
Males										
0-4	-	-	753	1 720	-	-	-	-	-	-
5-14	-	-	975	1 160	-	-	-	-	-	-
15-44	-	-	1 801	1 120	-	-	-	-	-	-
45-59	-	-	382	1 120	-	-	-	-	-	-
60+	-	-	339	1 680	-	-	-	-	-	-
All ages	-	-	4 251	1 239	-	-	-	-	-	-
Females										
0-4	-	-	722	1 720	-	-	-	-	-	-
5-14	-	-	931	1 160	-	-	-	-	-	-
15-44	-	-	3 304	2 070	-	-	-	-	-	-
45-59	-	-	590	1 680	-	-	-	-	-	-
60+	-	-	381	1 680	-	-	-	-	-	-
All ages	-	-	5 927	1 745	-	-	-	-	-	-
Total	-	-	10 177	1 491	-	-	-	-	-	-

Table 139f SSA - ASS - ASS   Iron-deficiency anaemia - Severe

Age group (years)	Incidence 1990 Number ('000s)	Rate (per 100 000)	Prevalence 1990 Number ('000s)	Rate (per 100 000)	Avg. age at onset (years)	Average duration (years)	Deaths 1990 Number ('000s)	Rate (per 100 000)	Deaths 2000 (Projected) Number ('000s)	Rate (per 100 000)
Males										
0-4	-	-	764	1 610	-	-	-	-	-	-
5-14	-	-	1 082	1 540	-	-	-	-	-	-
15-44	-	-	872	840	-	-	-	-	-	-
45-59	-	-	171	840	-	-	-	-	-	-
60+	-	-	159	1 510	-	-	-	-	-	-
All ages	-	-	3 047	1 208	-	-	-	-	-	-
Females										
0-4	-	-	757	1 610	-	-	-	-	-	-
5-14	-	-	1 075	1 540	-	-	-	-	-	-
15-44	-	-	1 785	1 680	-	-	-	-	-	-
45-59	-	-	334	1 510	-	-	-	-	-	-
60+	-	-	192	1 510	-	-	-	-	-	-
All ages	-	-	4 144	1 606	-	-	-	-	-	-
Total	-	-	7 191	1 409	-	-	-	-	-	-

For epidemiological sources see Bailey and Abou-Zahr 1996. For the methods used to estimate and project incidence, prevalence, and deaths see Murray and Lopez 1996a. See explanatory notes for definitions and caveats.

Table 139
Iron-deficiency anaemia
Severe

Cuadro 139
Anemia por deficiencia de hierro
Severa

Tableau 139
Anémie ferriprive
Grave

Table 139g — LAC - ALC - ALC — Iron-deficiency anaemia - Severe

Age group (years)	Incidence 1990 Number ('000s)	Incidence 1990 Rate (per 100 000)	Prevalence 1990 Number ('000s)	Prevalence 1990 Rate (per 100 000)	Avg. age at onset (years)	Average duration (years)	Deaths 1990 Number ('000s)	Deaths 1990 Rate (per 100 000)	Deaths 2000 (Projected) Number ('000s)	Deaths 2000 (Projected) Rate (per 100 000)
Males										
0-4	-	-	414	1 440	-	-	-	-	-	-
5-14	-	-	386	740	-	-	-	-	-	-
15-44	-	-	292	280	-	-	-	-	-	-
45-59	-	-	62	280	-	-	-	-	-	-
60+	-	-	75	530	-	-	-	-	-	-
All ages	-	-	1 229	555	-	-	-	-	-	-
Females										
0-4	-	-	399	1 440	-	-	-	-	-	-
5-14	-	-	376	740	-	-	-	-	-	-
15-44	-	-	1 311	1 260	-	-	-	-	-	-
45-59	-	-	124	530	-	-	-	-	-	-
60+	-	-	89	530	-	-	-	-	-	-
All ages	-	-	2 298	1 032	-	-	-	-	-	-
Total	-	-	3 527	794	-	-	-	-	-	-

Table 139h — MEC - AOM - CMO — Iron-deficiency anaemia - Severe

Age group (years)	Incidence 1990 Number ('000s)	Incidence 1990 Rate (per 100 000)	Prevalence 1990 Number ('000s)	Prevalence 1990 Rate (per 100 000)	Avg. age at onset (years)	Average duration (years)	Deaths 1990 Number ('000s)	Deaths 1990 Rate (per 100 000)	Deaths 2000 (Projected) Number ('000s)	Deaths 2000 (Projected) Rate (per 100 000)
Males										
0-4	-	-	766	1 860	-	-	-	-	-	-
5-14	-	-	758	1 160	-	-	-	-	-	-
15-44	-	-	558	490	-	-	-	-	-	-
45-59	-	-	109	490	-	-	-	-	-	-
60+	-	-	105	770	-	-	-	-	-	-
All ages	-	-	2 296	896	-	-	-	-	-	-
Females										
0-4	-	-	739	1 860	-	-	-	-	-	-
5-14	-	-	719	1 160	-	-	-	-	-	-
15-44	-	-	1 994	1 860	-	-	-	-	-	-
45-59	-	-	172	770	-	-	-	-	-	-
60+	-	-	119	770	-	-	-	-	-	-
All ages	-	-	3 743	1 517	-	-	-	-	-	-
Total	-	-	6 039	1 200	-	-	-	-	-	-

Table 139i — World - Mundo - Monde — Iron-deficiency anaemia - Severe

Age group (years)	Incidence 1990 Number ('000s)	Incidence 1990 Rate (per 100 000)	Prevalence 1990 Number ('000s)	Prevalence 1990 Rate (per 100 000)	Avg. age at onset (years)	Average duration (years)	Deaths 1990 Number ('000s)	Deaths 1990 Rate (per 100 000)	Deaths 2000 (Projected) Number ('000s)	Deaths 2000 (Projected) Rate (per 100 000)
Males										
0-4	-	-	4 724	1 470	-	-	-	-	-	-
5-14	-	-	7 323	1 328	-	-	-	-	-	-
15-44	-	-	10 668	854	-	-	-	-	-	-
45-59	-	-	2 442	782	-	-	-	-	-	-
60+	-	-	2 512	1 148	-	-	-	-	-	-
All ages	-	-	27 669	1 043	-	-	-	-	-	-
Females										
0-4	-	-	4 551	1 472	-	-	-	-	-	-
5-14	-	-	6 959	1 324	-	-	-	-	-	-
15-44	-	-	16 311	1 361	-	-	-	-	-	-
45-59	-	-	3 744	1 204	-	-	-	-	-	-
60+	-	-	2 784	1 034	-	-	-	-	-	-
All ages	-	-	34 349	1 314	-	-	-	-	-	-
Total	-	-	62 018	1 177	-	-	-	-	-	-

For epidemiological sources see Bailey and Abou-Zahr 1996. For the methods used to estimate and project incidence, prevalence, and deaths see Murray and Lopez 1996a. See explanatory notes for definitions and caveats.

Table 140
Iron-deficiency anaemia

Very severe

Cuadro 140
Anemia por deficiencia de hierro

Muy severa

Tableau 140
Anémie ferriprive

Très grave

Table 140a EME - PEMC - EMBE

Iron-deficiency anaemia - Very severe

Age group (years)	Incidence 1990 Number ('000s)	Rate (per 100 000)	Prevalence 1990 Number ('000s)	Rate (per 100 000)	Avg. age at onset (years)	Average duration (years)	Deaths 1990 Number ('000s)	Rate (per 100 000)	Deaths 2000 (Projected) Number ('000s)	Rate (per 100 000)
Males										
0-4	-	-	8	30	-	-	-	-	-	-
5-14	-	-	11	20	-	-	-	-	-	-
15-44	-	-	18	10	-	-	-	-	-	-
45-59	-	-	7	10	-	-	-	-	-	-
60+	-	-	18	30	-	-	-	-	-	-
All ages	-	-	62	16	-	-	-	-	-	-
Females										
0-4	-	-	8	30	-	-	-	-	-	-
5-14	-	-	10	20	-	-	-	-	-	-
15-44	-	-	54	30	-	-	-	-	-	-
45-59	-	-	20	30	-	-	-	-	-	-
60+	-	-	25	30	-	-	-	-	-	-
All ages	-	-	117	29	-	-	-	-	-	-
Total	-	-	179	22	-	-	-	-	-	-

Table 140b FSE - PEAS - AESE

Iron-deficiency anaemia - Very severe

Age group (years)	Incidence 1990 Number ('000s)	Rate (per 100 000)	Prevalence 1990 Number ('000s)	Rate (per 100 000)	Avg. age at onset (years)	Average duration (years)	Deaths 1990 Number ('000s)	Rate (per 100 000)	Deaths 2000 (Projected) Number ('000s)	Rate (per 100 000)
Males										
0-4	-	-	8	60	-	-	-	-	-	-
5-14	-	-	14	50	-	-	-	-	-	-
15-44	-	-	8	10	-	-	-	-	-	-
45-59	-	-	3	10	-	-	-	-	-	-
60+	-	-	6	30	-	-	-	-	-	-
All ages	-	-	39	23	-	-	-	-	-	-
Females										
0-4	-	-	8	60	-	-	-	-	-	-
5-14	-	-	13	50	-	-	-	-	-	-
15-44	-	-	22	30	-	-	-	-	-	-
45-59	-	-	9	30	-	-	-	-	-	-
60+	-	-	11	30	-	-	-	-	-	-
All ages	-	-	63	35	-	-	-	-	-	-
Total	-	-	102	29	-	-	-	-	-	-

Table 140c India - India - Inde

Iron-deficiency anaemia - Very severe

Age group (years)	Incidence 1990 Number ('000s)	Rate (per 100 000)	Prevalence 1990 Number ('000s)	Rate (per 100 000)	Avg. age at onset (years)	Average duration (years)	Deaths 1990 Number ('000s)	Rate (per 100 000)	Deaths 2000 (Projected) Number ('000s)	Rate (per 100 000)
Males										
0-4	-	-	96	160	-	-	-	-	-	-
5-14	-	-	173	170	-	-	-	-	-	-
15-44	-	-	201	100	-	-	-	-	-	-
45-59	-	-	48	100	-	-	-	-	-	-
60+	-	-	54	180	-	-	-	-	-	-
All ages	-	-	570	130	-	-	-	-	-	-
Females										
0-4	-	-	91	160	-	-	-	-	-	-
5-14	-	-	162	170	-	-	-	-	-	-
15-44	-	-	330	180	-	-	-	-	-	-
45-59	-	-	83	180	-	-	-	-	-	-
60+	-	-	52	180	-	-	-	-	-	-
All ages	-	-	717	175	-	-	-	-	-	-
Total	-	-	1 288	152	-	-	-	-	-	-

For epidemiological sources see Bailey and Abou-Zahr 1996. For the methods used to estimate and project incidence, prevalence, and deaths see Murray and Lopez 1996a. See explanatory notes for definitions and caveats.

Table 140
Iron-deficiency anaemia

Very severe

Cuadro 140
Anemia por deficiencia de hierro

Muy severa

Tableau 140
Anémie ferriprive

Très grave

Table 140d   China - China - Chine   Iron-deficiency anaemia - Very severe

Age group (years)	Incidence 1990 Number ('000s)	Rate (per 100 000)	Prevalence 1990 Number ('000s)	Rate (per 100 000)	Avg. age at onset (years)	Average duration (years)	Deaths 1990 Number ('000s)	Rate (per 100 000)	Deaths 2000 (Projected) Number ('000s)	Rate (per 100 000)
Males										
0-4	-	-	66	110	-	-	-	-	-	-
5-14	-	-	155	160	-	-	-	-	-	-
15-44	-	-	398	130	-	-	-	-	-	-
45-59	-	-	94	130	-	-	-	-	-	-
60+	-	-	78	160	-	-	-	-	-	-
All ages	-	-	793	135	-	-	-	-	-	-
Females										
0-4	-	-	64	110	-	-	-	-	-	-
5-14	-	-	145	160	-	-	-	-	-	-
15-44	-	-	284	100	-	-	-	-	-	-
45-59	-	-	103	160	-	-	-	-	-	-
60+	-	-	83	160	-	-	-	-	-	-
All ages	-	-	678	124	-	-	-	-	-	-
Total	-	-	1 471	130	-	-	-	-	-	-

Table 140e   OAI - OPAI - APAI   Iron-deficiency anaemia - Very severe

Age group (years)	Incidence 1990 Number ('000s)	Rate (per 100 000)	Prevalence 1990 Number ('000s)	Rate (per 100 000)	Avg. age at onset (years)	Average duration (years)	Deaths 1990 Number ('000s)	Rate (per 100 000)	Deaths 2000 (Projected) Number ('000s)	Rate (per 100 000)
Males										
0-4	-	-	66	150	-	-	-	-	-	-
5-14	-	-	84	100	-	-	-	-	-	-
15-44	-	-	161	100	-	-	-	-	-	-
45-59	-	-	34	100	-	-	-	-	-	-
60+	-	-	28	140	-	-	-	-	-	-
All ages	-	-	373	109	-	-	-	-	-	-
Females										
0-4	-	-	63	150	-	-	-	-	-	-
5-14	-	-	80	100	-	-	-	-	-	-
15-44	-	-	287	180	-	-	-	-	-	-
45-59	-	-	49	140	-	-	-	-	-	-
60+	-	-	32	140	-	-	-	-	-	-
All ages	-	-	511	151	-	-	-	-	-	-
Total	-	-	884	130	-	-	-	-	-	-

Table 140f   SSA - ASS - ASS   Iron-deficiency anaemia - Very severe

Age group (years)	Incidence 1990 Number ('000s)	Rate (per 100 000)	Prevalence 1990 Number ('000s)	Rate (per 100 000)	Avg. age at onset (years)	Average duration (years)	Deaths 1990 Number ('000s)	Rate (per 100 000)	Deaths 2000 (Projected) Number ('000s)	Rate (per 100 000)
Males										
0-4	-	-	66	140	-	-	-	-	-	-
5-14	-	-	91	130	-	-	-	-	-	-
15-44	-	-	73	70	-	-	-	-	-	-
45-59	-	-	14	70	-	-	-	-	-	-
60+	-	-	14	130	-	-	-	-	-	-
All ages	-	-	258	102	-	-	-	-	-	-
Females										
0-4	-	-	66	140	-	-	-	-	-	-
5-14	-	-	91	130	-	-	-	-	-	-
15-44	-	-	149	140	-	-	-	-	-	-
45-59	-	-	29	130	-	-	-	-	-	-
60+	-	-	17	130	-	-	-	-	-	-
All ages	-	-	351	136	-	-	-	-	-	-
Total	-	-	609	119	-	-	-	-	-	-

For epidemiological sources see Bailey and Abou-Zahr 1996. For the methods used to estimate and project incidence, prevalence, and deaths see Murray and Lopez 1996a. See explanatory notes for definitions and caveats.

Table 140
Iron-deficiency anaemia

Very severe

Cuadro 140
Anemia por deficiencia de hierro

Muy severa

Tableau 140
Anémie ferriprive

Très grave

Table 140g — LAC - ALC - ALC — Iron-deficiency anaemia - Very severe

Age group (years)	Incidence 1990 Number ('000s)	Rate (per 100 000)	Prevalence 1990 Number ('000s)	Rate (per 100 000)	Avg. age at onset (years)	Average duration (years)	Deaths 1990 Number ('000s)	Rate (per 100 000)	Deaths 2000 (Projected) Number ('000s)	Rate (per 100 000)
Males										
0-4	-	-	34	120	-	-	-	-	-	-
5-14	-	-	31	60	-	-	-	-	-	-
15-44	-	-	21	20	-	-	-	-	-	-
45-59	-	-	4	20	-	-	-	-	-	-
60+	-	-	7	50	-	-	-	-	-	-
All ages	-	-	98	44	-	-	-	-	-	-
Females										
0-4	-	-	33	120	-	-	-	-	-	-
5-14	-	-	30	60	-	-	-	-	-	-
15-44	-	-	114	110	-	-	-	-	-	-
45-59	-	-	12	50	-	-	-	-	-	-
60+	-	-	8	50	-	-	-	-	-	-
All ages	-	-	198	89	-	-	-	-	-	-
Total	-	-	296	67	-	-	-	-	-	-

Table 140h — MEC - AOM - CMO — Iron-deficiency anaemia - Very severe

Age group (years)	Incidence 1990 Number ('000s)	Rate (per 100 000)	Prevalence 1990 Number ('000s)	Rate (per 100 000)	Avg. age at onset (years)	Average duration (years)	Deaths 1990 Number ('000s)	Rate (per 100 000)	Deaths 2000 (Projected) Number ('000s)	Rate (per 100 000)
Males										
0-4	-	-	66	160	-	-	-	-	-	-
5-14	-	-	65	100	-	-	-	-	-	-
15-44	-	-	46	40	-	-	-	-	-	-
45-59	-	-	9	40	-	-	-	-	-	-
60+	-	-	10	70	-	-	-	-	-	-
All ages	-	-	195	76	-	-	-	-	-	-
Females										
0-4	-	-	64	160	-	-	-	-	-	-
5-14	-	-	62	100	-	-	-	-	-	-
15-44	-	-	172	160	-	-	-	-	-	-
45-59	-	-	16	70	-	-	-	-	-	-
60+	-	-	11	70	-	-	-	-	-	-
All ages	-	-	324	131	-	-	-	-	-	-
Total	-	-	519	103	-	-	-	-	-	-

Table 140i — World - Mundo - Monde — Iron-deficiency anaemia - Very severe

Age group (years)	Incidence 1990 Number ('000s)	Rate (per 100 000)	Prevalence 1990 Number ('000s)	Rate (per 100 000)	Avg. age at onset (years)	Average duration (years)	Deaths 1990 Number ('000s)	Rate (per 100 000)	Deaths 2000 (Projected) Number ('000s)	Rate (per 100 000)
Males										
0-4	-	-	411	128	-	-	-	-	-	-
5-14	-	-	625	113	-	-	-	-	-	-
15-44	-	-	925	74	-	-	-	-	-	-
45-59	-	-	213	68	-	-	-	-	-	-
60+	-	-	215	98	-	-	-	-	-	-
All ages	-	-	2 388	90	-	-	-	-	-	-
Females										
0-4	-	-	395	128	-	-	-	-	-	-
5-14	-	-	593	113	-	-	-	-	-	-
15-44	-	-	1 412	118	-	-	-	-	-	-
45-59	-	-	320	103	-	-	-	-	-	-
60+	-	-	239	89	-	-	-	-	-	-
All ages	-	-	2 960	113	-	-	-	-	-	-
Total	-	-	5 348	102	-	-	-	-	-	-

For epidemiological sources see Bailey and Abou-Zahr 1996. For the methods used to estimate and project incidence, prevalence, and deaths see Murray and Lopez 1996a. See explanatory notes for definitions and caveats.

Table 141
Iron-deficiency anaemia

Cognitive impairment

Cuadro 141
Anemia por deficiencia de hierro

Deficiencia cognocitivo

Tableau 141
Anémie ferriprive

Déficience cognitive

Table 141a EME - PEMC - EMBE — Iron-deficiency anaemia - Cognitive impairment

Age group (years)	Incidence 1990 Number ('000s)	Rate (per 100 000)	Prevalence 1990 Number ('000s)	Rate (per 100 000)	Avg. age at onset (years)	Average duration (years)	Deaths 1990 Number ('000s)	Rate (per 100 000)	Deaths 2000 (Projected) Number ('000s)	Rate (per 100 000)
Males										
0-4	18	68.3	45	171	2.5	70.2	0	0	0	0
5-14	0	0.0	181	340	-	-	0	0	0	0
15-44	0	0.0	625	340	-	-	0	0	0	0
45-59	0	0.0	225	340	-	-	0	0	0	0
60+	0	0.0	206	340	-	-	0	0	0	0
All ages	18	4.6	1 281	328	2.5	70.2	0	0	0	0
Females										
0-4	17	68.3	43	171	2.5	76.1	0	0	0	0
5-14	0	3.2	172	340	-	-	0	0	0	0
15-44	0	3.6	608	340	-	-	0	0	0	0
45-59	0	4.0	230	340	-	-	0	0	0	0
60+	0	4.0	287	340	-	-	0	0	0	0
All ages	17	4.2	1 341	329	2.5	76.1	0	0	0	0
Total	35	4.4	2 622	329	2.5	73.1	0	0	0	0

Table 141b FSE - PEAS - AESE — Iron-deficiency anaemia - Cognitive impairment

Age group (years)	Incidence 1990 Number ('000s)	Rate (per 100 000)	Prevalence 1990 Number ('000s)	Rate (per 100 000)	Avg. age at onset (years)	Average duration (years)	Deaths 1990 Number ('000s)	Rate (per 100 000)	Deaths 2000 (Projected) Number ('000s)	Rate (per 100 000)
Males										
0-4	21	151	52	378	2.5	63.5	0	0	0	0
5-14	0	0	206	753	-	-	0	0	0	0
15-44	0	0	574	753	-	-	0	0	0	0
45-59	0	0	203	753	-	-	0	0	0	0
60+	0	0	158	753	-	-	0	0	0	0
All ages	21	13	1 193	722	2.5	63.5	0	0	0	0
Females										
0-4	20	151	50	378	2.5	72.4	0	0	0	0
5-14	0	0	199	753	-	-	0	0	0	0
15-44	0	0	564	753	-	-	0	0	0	0
45-59	0	0	226	753	-	-	0	0	0	0
60+	0	0	274	753	-	-	0	0	0	0
All ages	20	11	1 313	726	2.5	72.4	0	0	0	0
Total	41	12	2 506	724	2.5	67.9	0	0	0	0

Table 141c India - India - Inde — Iron-deficiency anaemia - Cognitive impairment

Age group (years)	Incidence 1990 Number ('000s)	Rate (per 100 000)	Prevalence 1990 Number ('000s)	Rate (per 100 000)	Avg. age at onset (years)	Average duration (years)	Deaths 1990 Number ('000s)	Rate (per 100 000)	Deaths 2000 (Projected) Number ('000s)	Rate (per 100 000)
Males										
0-4	234	392	575	962	2.4	59.9	0	0	0	0
5-14	0	0	1 981	1 947	-	-	0	0	0	0
15-44	0	0	3 905	1 947	-	-	0	0	0	0
45-59	0	0	926	1 947	-	-	0	0	0	0
60+	0	0	580	1 947	-	-	0	0	0	0
All ages	234	53	7 967	1 813	2.4	59.9	0	0	0	0
Females										
0-4	222	392	544	960	2.4	60.8	0	0	0	0
5-14	0	0	1 855	1 947	-	-	0	0	0	0
15-44	0	0	3 569	1 947	-	-	0	0	0	0
45-59	0	0	896	1 947	-	-	0	0	0	0
60+	0	0	563	1 947	-	-	0	0	0	0
All ages	222	54	7 427	1 811	2.4	60.8	0	0	0	0
Total	456	54	15 394	1 812	2.4	60.3	0	0	0	0

For epidemiological sources see Bailey and Abou-Zahr 1996. For the methods used to estimate and project incidence, prevalence, and deaths see Murray and Lopez 1996a. See explanatory notes for definitions and caveats.

Table 141
Iron-deficiency anaemia

Cognitive impairment

Cuadro 141
Anemia por deficiencia de hierro

Deficiencia cognocitivo

Tableau 141
Anémie ferriprive

Déficience cognitive

Table 141d — China - China - Chine — Iron-deficiency anaemia - Cognitive impairment

Age group (years)	Incidence 1990 Number ('000s)	Rate (per 100 000)	Prevalence 1990 Number ('000s)	Rate (per 100 000)	Avg. age at onset (years)	Average duration (years)	Deaths 1990 Number ('000s)	Rate (per 100 000)	Deaths 2000 (Projected) Number ('000s)	Rate (per 100 000)
Males										
0-4	164	272	408	677	2.5	65.5	0	0	0	0
5-14	0	0	1 311	1 352	-	-	0	0	0	0
15-44	0	0	4 140	1 352	-	-	0	0	0	0
45-59	0	0	982	1 352	-	-	0	0	0	0
60+	0	0	662	1 352	-	-	0	0	0	0
All ages	164	28	7 503	1 282	2.5	65.5	0	0	0	0
Females										
0-4	157	272	392	676	2.5	68.5	0	0	0	0
5-14	0	0	1 222	1 352	-	-	0	0	0	0
15-44	0	0	3 840	1 352	-	-	0	0	0	0
45-59	0	0	870	1 352	-	-	0	0	0	0
60+	0	0	698	1 352	-	-	0	0	0	0
All ages	157	29	7 022	1 280	2.5	68.5	0	0	0	0
Total	321	28	14 525	1 281	2.5	67.0	0	0	0	0

Table 141e — OAI - OPAI - APAI — Iron-deficiency anaemia - Cognitive impairment

Age group (years)	Incidence 1990 Number ('000s)	Rate (per 100 000)	Prevalence 1990 Number ('000s)	Rate (per 100 000)	Avg. age at onset (years)	Average duration (years)	Deaths 1990 Number ('000s)	Rate (per 100 000)	Deaths 2000 (Projected) Number ('000s)	Rate (per 100 000)
Males										
0-4	162	369	399	911	2.5	59.8	0	0	0	0
5-14	0	0	1 543	1 836	-	-	0	0	0	0
15-44	0	0	2 952	1 836	-	-	0	0	0	0
45-59	0	0	627	1 836	-	-	0	0	0	0
60+	0	0	371	1 836	-	-	0	0	0	0
All ages	162	47	5 891	1 718	2.5	59.8	0	0	0	0
Females										
0-4	155	369	384	914	2.5	63.2	0	0	0	0
5-14	0	0	1 472	1 836	-	-	0	0	0	0
15-44	0	0	2 930	1 836	-	-	0	0	0	0
45-59	0	0	644	1 836	-	-	0	0	0	0
60+	0	0	416	1 836	-	-	0	0	0	0
All ages	155	46	5 846	1 722	2.5	63.2	0	0	0	0
Total	317	46	11 737	1 720	2.5	61.5	0	0	0	0

Table 141f — SSA - ASS - ASS — Iron-deficiency anaemia - Cognitive impairment

Age group (years)	Incidence 1990 Number ('000s)	Rate (per 100 000)	Prevalence 1990 Number ('000s)	Rate (per 100 000)	Avg. age at onset (years)	Average duration (years)	Deaths 1990 Number ('000s)	Rate (per 100 000)	Deaths 2000 (Projected) Number ('000s)	Rate (per 100 000)
Males										
0-4	165	347	397	837	2.4	48.7	0	0	0	0
5-14	0	0	1 212	1 726	-	-	0	0	0	0
15-44	0	0	1 791	1 726	-	-	0	0	0	0
45-59	0	0	350	1 726	-	-	0	0	0	0
60+	0	0	181	1 726	-	-	0	0	0	0
All ages	165	65	3 932	1 558	2.4	48.7	0	0	0	0
Females										
0-4	163	347	396	841	2.4	51.9	0	0	0	0
5-14	0	0	1 205	1 725	-	-	0	0	0	0
15-44	0	0	1 833	1 725	-	-	0	0	0	0
45-59	0	0	382	1 725	-	-	0	0	0	0
60+	0	0	220	1 725	-	-	0	0	0	0
All ages	163	63	4 035	1 564	2.4	51.9	0	0	0	0
Total	328	64	7 967	1 561	2.4	50.3	0	0	0	0

For epidemiological sources see Bailey and Abou-Zahr 1996. For the methods used to estimate and project incidence, prevalence, and deaths see Murray and Lopez 1996a. See explanatory notes for definitions and caveats.

Table 141 Iron-deficiency anaemia Cognitive impairment	Cuadro 141 Anemia por deficiencia de hierro Deficiencia cognocitivo	Tableau 141 Anémie ferriprive Déficience cognitive

Table 141g LAC - ALC - ALC — Iron-deficiency anaemia - Cognitive impairment

Age group (years)	Incidence 1990 Number ('000s)	Rate (per 100 000)	Prevalence 1990 Number ('000s)	Rate (per 100 000)	Avg. age at onset (years)	Average duration (years)	Deaths 1990 Number ('000s)	Rate (per 100 000)	Deaths 2000 (Projected) Number ('000s)	Rate (per 100 000)
Males										
0-4	89	309	220	767	2.5	63.9	0	0	0	0
5-14	0	0	802	1 538	-	-	0	0	0	0
15-44	0	0	1 604	1 538	-	-	0	0	0	0
45-59	0	0	342	1 538	-	-	0	0	0	0
60+	0	0	219	1 538	-	-	0	0	0	0
All ages	89	40	3 187	1 438	2.5	63.9	0	0	0	0
Females										
0-4	86	309	213	769	2.5	67.9	0	0	0	0
5-14	0	0	780	1 538	-	-	0	0	0	0
15-44	0	0	1 601	1 538	-	-	0	0	0	0
45-59	0	0	359	1 538	-	-	0	0	0	0
60+	0	0	259	1 538	-	-	0	0	0	0
All ages	86	38	3 212	1 442	2.5	67.9	0	0	0	0
Total	174	39	6 399	1 440	2.5	65.9	0	0	0	0

Table 141h MEC - AOM - CMO — Iron-deficiency anaemia - Cognitive impairment

Age group (years)	Incidence 1990 Number ('000s)	Rate (per 100 000)	Prevalence 1990 Number ('000s)	Rate (per 100 000)	Avg. age at onset (years)	Average duration (years)	Deaths 1990 Number ('000s)	Rate (per 100 000)	Deaths 2000 (Projected) Number ('000s)	Rate (per 100 000)
Males										
0-4	164	399	404	982	2.5	61.1	0	0	0	0
5-14	0	0	1 297	1 984	-	-	0	0	0	0
15-44	0	0	2 260	1 984	-	-	0	0	0	0
45-59	0	0	443	1 984	-	-	0	0	0	0
60+	0	0	271	1 984	-	-	0	0	0	0
All ages	164	64	4 675	1 823	2.5	61.1	0	0	0	0
Females										
0-4	159	399	390	982	2.5	63.7	0	0	0	0
5-14	0	0	1 230	1 984	-	-	0	0	0	0
15-44	0	0	2 127	1 984	-	-	0	0	0	0
45-59	0	0	442	1 984	-	-	0	0	0	0
60+	0	0	307	1 984	-	-	0	0	0	0
All ages	159	64	4 497	1 823	2.5	63.7	0	0	0	0
Total	323	64	9 172	1 823	2.5	62.4	0	0	0	0

Table 141i World - Mundo - Monde — Iron-deficiency anaemia - Cognitive impairment

Age group (years)	Incidence 1990 Number ('000s)	Rate (per 100 000)	Prevalence 1990 Number ('000s)	Rate (per 100 000)	Avg. age at onset (years)	Average duration (years)	Deaths 1990 Number ('000s)	Rate (per 100 000)	Deaths 2000 (Projected) Number ('000s)	Rate (per 100 000)
Males										
0-4	1 016	316	2 500	778	2.5	59.8	0	0	0	0
5-14	0	0	8 533	1 548	-	-	0	0	0	0
15-44	0	0	17 851	1 428	-	-	0	0	0	0
45-59	0	0	4 099	1 312	-	-	0	0	0	0
60+	0	0	2 647	1 210	-	-	0	0	0	0
All ages	1 016	38	35 630	1 343	2.5	59.8	0	0	0	0
Females										
0-4	979	316	2 410	779	2.5	62.5	0	0	0	0
5-14	0	0	8 136	1 548	-	-	0	0	0	0
15-44	0	0	17 072	1 424	-	-	0	0	0	0
45-59	0	0	4 050	1 302	-	-	0	0	0	0
60+	0	0	3 024	1 123	-	-	0	0	0	0
All ages	979	37	34 692	1 327	2.5	62.5	0	0	0	0
Total	1 995	38	70 322	1 335	2.5	61.1	0	0	0	0

For epidemiological sources see Bailey and Abou-Zahr 1996. For the methods used to estimate and project incidence, prevalence, and deaths see Murray and Lopez 1996a. See explanatory notes for definitions and caveats.

Table 142
Mouth and oropharynx cancers
Cases

Cuadro 142
Cánceres de boca y orofaringue
Casos

Tableau 142
Cancers de la bouche et de l'oropharynx
Cas

Table 142a   EME - PEMC - EMBE   Mouth and oropharynx cancers - Cases

Age group (years)	Incidence 1990 Number ('000s)	Rate (per 100 000)	Prevalence 1990 Number ('000s)	Rate (per 100 000)	Avg. age at onset (years)	Average duration (years)	Deaths 1990 Number ('000s)	Rate (per 100 000)	Deaths 2000 (Projected) Number ('000s)	Rate (per 100 000)
Males										
0-4	0	0.2	0	0.4	2.5	4.7	0	0.0	0	0.0
5-14	0	0.2	0	0.7	10.0	4.7	0	0.0	0	0.0
15-44	13	7.2	62	33.5	29.9	4.7	2	0.9	2	0.9
45-59	32	48.2	138	207.9	52.4	4.3	8	12.6	10	12.4
60+	48	78.8	199	328.1	71.1	4.2	15	24.8	17	23.0
All ages	93	23.8	398	102.0	58.8	4.3	25	6.4	28	6.8
Females										
0-4	0	0.2	0	0.4	2.5	4.7	0	0.0	0	0.0
5-14	0	0.2	0	0.7	10.0	4.7	0	0.0	0	0.0
15-44	4	2.2	18	10.2	30.0	4.7	0	0.2	0	0.2
45-59	7	9.9	30	43.6	52.4	4.4	1	2.2	2	1.9
60+	17	20.5	70	83.0	72.4	4.0	6	7.3	7	6.8
All ages	28	6.9	119	29.1	61.6	4.2	8	2.0	9	2.0
Total	121	15.2	517	64.8	59.4	4.3	33	4.1	37	4.4

Table 142b   FSE - PEAS - AESE   Mouth and oropharynx cancers - Cases

Age group (years)	Incidence 1990 Number ('000s)	Rate (per 100 000)	Prevalence 1990 Number ('000s)	Rate (per 100 000)	Avg. age at onset (years)	Average duration (years)	Deaths 1990 Number ('000s)	Rate (per 100 000)	Deaths 2000 (Projected) Number ('000s)	Rate (per 100 000)
Males										
0-4	0	0.5	0	1.0	2.5	4.7	0	0.1	0	0.1
5-14	0	0.4	1	2.0	10.0	4.7	0	0.1	0	0.1
15-44	11	14.0	50	65.3	29.8	4.7	1	1.7	1	1.8
45-59	25	93.8	109	403.1	52.2	4.3	7	24.5	9	30.3
60+	20	96.6	84	401.0	70.0	4.1	6	30.4	8	32.0
All ages	56	34.1	243	147.1	54.3	4.3	14	8.7	19	11.1
Females										
0-4	0	0.4	0	0.7	2.5	4.7	0	0.0	0	0.0
5-14	0	0.2	0	1.2	10.0	4.7	0	0.0	0	0.0
15-44	2	2.9	10	13.8	29.9	4.7	0	0.3	0	0.3
45-59	3	9.3	12	41.1	52.4	4.4	1	2.1	1	1.9
60+	6	16.3	24	65.9	71.5	4.0	2	5.8	2	5.8
All ages	11	6.1	47	26.0	58.0	4.3	3	1.6	3	1.8
Total	67	19.5	290	83.8	54.9	4.3	17	5.0	22	6.2

Table 142c   India - India - Inde   Mouth and oropharynx cancers - Cases

Age group (years)	Incidence 1990 Number ('000s)	Rate (per 100 000)	Prevalence 1990 Number ('000s)	Rate (per 100 000)	Avg. age at onset (years)	Average duration (years)	Deaths 1990 Number ('000s)	Rate (per 100 000)	Deaths 2000 (Projected) Number ('000s)	Rate (per 100 000)
Males										
0-4	1	0.9	1	1.7	2.5	4.6	0	0.1	0	0.1
5-14	1	0.8	4	3.7	10.0	4.6	0	0.1	0	0.1
15-44	33	16.4	152	75.8	29.8	4.6	4	2.2	6	2.3
45-59	62	129.7	262	551.7	52.3	4.3	16	34.7	22	37.1
60+	84	282.8	346	1 162.3	69.7	4.1	27	90.4	35	95.7
All ages	180	41.0	765	174.2	56.1	4.3	48	10.9	63	12.4
Females										
0-4	1	0.9	1	1.8	2.5	4.7	0	0.1	0	0.1
5-14	1	1.0	4	4.6	10.0	4.7	0	0.1	0	0.1
15-44	34	18.6	159	86.8	29.8	4.7	4	2.1	5	2.0
45-59	57	124.2	249	542.2	52.4	4.4	13	28.2	16	27.5
60+	42	144.0	166	575.4	70.1	4.0	15	51.8	20	52.5
All ages	134	32.8	580	141.5	51.8	4.3	32	7.8	41	8.5
Total	315	37.0	1 346	158.4	54.3	4.3	80	9.4	104	10.5

For epidemiological sources see Murray et al. 1996. For the methods used to estimate and project incidence, prevalence, and deaths see Murray and Lopez 1996a. See explanatory notes for definitions and caveats.

Table 142
Mouth and oropharynx cancers
Cases

Cuadro 142
Cánceres de boca y orofaringue
Casos

Tableau 142
Cancers de la bouche et de l'oropharynx
Cas

Table 142d   China - China - Chine   Mouth and oropharynx cancers - Cases

Age group (years)	Incidence 1990 Number ('000s)	Rate (per 100 000)	Prevalence 1990 Number ('000s)	Rate (per 100 000)	Avg. age at onset (years)	Average duration (years)	Deaths 1990 Number ('000s)	Rate (per 100 000)	Deaths 2000 (Projected) Number ('000s)	Rate (per 100 000)
Males										
0-4	1	2.4	3	4.4	2.5	4.6	0	0.4	0	0.4
5-14	1	1.4	7	6.7	10.0	4.6	0	0.2	0	0.2
15-44	42	13.8	196	63.9	29.9	4.6	6	2.1	9	2.8
45-59	24	32.4	101	138.3	52.3	4.3	7	9.1	11	10.9
60+	35	70.8	143	292.5	69.8	4.1	12	23.6	17	27.5
All ages	103	17.6	449	76.7	48.4	4.4	25	4.3	37	5.6
Females										
0-4	0	0.0	0	0.0	-	-	0	0.0	0	0.0
5-14	2	1.7	7	8.1	10.0	4.7	0	0.0	0	0.0
15-44	20	7.2	96	33.7	29.9	4.7	3	0.9	3	1.1
45-59	14	21.5	61	94.1	52.4	4.4	3	5.2	5	5.4
60+	14	27.8	58	111.5	70.6	4.0	5	10.4	7	11.4
All ages	50	9.2	221	40.4	47.1	4.4	11	2.1	16	2.5
Total	153	13.5	670	59.1	48.0	4.4	36	3.2	52	4.1

Table 142e   OAI - OPAI - APAI   Mouth and oropharynx cancers - Cases

Age group (years)	Incidence 1990 Number ('000s)	Rate (per 100 000)	Prevalence 1990 Number ('000s)	Rate (per 100 000)	Avg. age at onset (years)	Average duration (years)	Deaths 1990 Number ('000s)	Rate (per 100 000)	Deaths 2000 (Projected) Number ('000s)	Rate (per 100 000)
Males										
0-4	1	3.2	3	6	2.5	4.6	0	0.5	0	0.4
5-14	3	4.0	15	18	10.0	4.6	0	0.6	0	0.5
15-44	31	19.0	141	88	29.7	4.6	4	2.7	6	3.0
45-59	23	67.1	98	286	52.3	4.3	6	18.5	9	19.4
60+	93	459.2	382	1 893	69.6	4.1	30	150.3	44	159.5
All ages	151	44.0	640	186.5	57.5	4.3	42	12.1	60	14.8
Females										
0-4	2	4.7	4	9	2.5	4.7	0	0.6	0	0.6
5-14	3	3.9	15	18	10.0	4.7	0	0.5	0	0.4
15-44	24	15.1	113	71	29.8	4.7	3	1.9	4	1.9
45-59	13	37.4	57	164	52.3	4.4	3	8.8	4	8.4
60+	53	235.2	214	943	70.3	4.0	20	86.3	28	86.3
All ages	96	28.2	402	118.5	55.3	4.3	26	7.7	36	9.0
Total	247	36.1	1 042	152.7	56.6	4.3	68	9.9	96	11.9

Table 142f   SSA - ASS - ASS   Mouth and oropharynx cancers - Cases

Age group (years)	Incidence 1990 Number ('000s)	Rate (per 100 000)	Prevalence 1990 Number ('000s)	Rate (per 100 000)	Avg. age at onset (years)	Average duration (years)	Deaths 1990 Number ('000s)	Rate (per 100 000)	Deaths 2000 (Projected) Number ('000s)	Rate (per 100 000)
Males										
0-4	0	0.4	0	0.7	2.4	4.6	0	0.1	0	0.1
5-14	1	0.9	3	4.0	10.0	4.6	0	0.1	0	0.1
15-44	10	10.1	48	46.5	29.4	4.6	2	1.4	2	1.5
45-59	8	40.6	35	172.4	52.2	4.2	2	11.3	3	11.0
60+	30	289.5	125	1 187.9	69.2	4.1	10	95.4	14	98.3
All ages	50	19.8	211	83.7	57.3	4.2	14	5.5	19	5.6
Females										
0-4	1	2.4	2	4.4	2.4	4.7	0	0.3	0	0.3
5-14	3	4.7	15	21.8	10.0	4.7	0	0.6	0	0.5
15-44	9	8.5	42	39.6	29.5	4.7	1	0.7	1	0.6
45-59	5	22.1	21	96.1	52.2	4.4	1	5.3	1	4.9
60+	18	143.4	73	572.2	69.7	4.0	7	52.9	9	50.5
All ages	37	14.2	153	59.5	51.5	4.3	9	3.5	12	3.4
Total	86	16.9	365	71.5	54.9	4.3	23	4.5	31	4.5

For epidemiological sources see Murray et al. 1996. For the methods used to estimate and project incidence, prevalence, and deaths see Murray and Lopez 1996a. See explanatory notes for definitions and caveats.

Table 142	Cuadro 142	Tableau 142
Mouth and oropharynx cancers	Cánceres de boca y orofaringue	Cancers de la bouche et de l'oropharynx
Cases	Casos	Cas

Table 142g LAC - ALC - ALC   Mouth and oropharynx cancers - Cases

Age group (years)	Incidence 1990 Number ('000s)	Rate (per 100 000)	Prevalence 1990 Number ('000s)	Rate (per 100 000)	Avg. age at onset (years)	Average duration (years)	Deaths 1990 Number ('000s)	Rate (per 100 000)	Deaths 2000 (Projected) Number ('000s)	Rate (per 100 000)
Males										
0-4	0	0.4	0	0.7	2.5	4.6	0	0.1	0	0.1
5-14	0	0.5	1	2.5	10.0	4.6	0	0.1	0	0.1
15-44	6	5.9	29	27.6	29.8	4.6	1	0.9	1	0.9
45-59	11	49.8	47	213.2	52.3	4.3	3	14.2	4	14.0
60+	14	95.1	56	393.2	70.3	4.1	5	31.9	7	33.2
All ages	31	14.1	134	60.3	55.3	4.3	9	3.9	12	4.6
Females										
0-4	0	0.3	0	0.6	2.5	4.7	0	0.0	0	0.0
5-14	0	0.5	1	2.4	10.0	4.7	0	0.1	0	0.1
15-44	2	2.1	10	9.8	29.9	4.7	0	0.3	0	0.3
45-59	3	13.9	14	60.9	52.4	4.4	1	3.4	1	3.3
60+	7	38.6	26	155.3	71.1	4.0	2	14.5	3	14.5
All ages	12	5.5	52	23.3	57.5	4.3	4	1.6	5	1.8
Total	43	9.8	186	41.8	55.9	4.3	12	2.8	17	3.2

Table 142h MEC - AOM - CMO   Mouth and oropharynx cancers - Cases

Age group (years)	Incidence 1990 Number ('000s)	Rate (per 100 000)	Prevalence 1990 Number ('000s)	Rate (per 100 000)	Avg. age at onset (years)	Average duration (years)	Deaths 1990 Number ('000s)	Rate (per 100 000)	Deaths 2000 (Projected) Number ('000s)	Rate (per 100 000)
Males										
0-4	0	0.6	0	1.1	2.5	4.6	0	0.1	0	0.1
5-14	1	1.4	4	6.5	10.0	4.6	0	0.2	0	0.2
15-44	13	11.2	59	51.8	29.8	4.6	2	1.5	2	1.6
45-59	7	33.5	32	143.1	52.3	4.3	2	9.2	3	9.1
60+	19	142.4	80	587.1	69.7	4.1	6	46.3	8	45.3
All ages	41	15.9	176	68.6	52.6	4.3	10	4.0	14	4.2
Females										
0-4	0	0.8	1	1.5	2.5	4.7	0	0.1	0	0.1
5-14	1	1.9	5	8.7	10.0	4.7	0	0.2	0	0.2
15-44	8	7.3	36	33.9	29.8	4.7	1	0.9	1	0.8
45-59	4	19.6	19	85.9	52.3	4.4	1	4.6	1	4.1
60+	10	66.6	41	267.0	70.4	4.0	4	24.3	5	21.9
All ages	24	9.7	103	41.7	50.7	4.3	6	2.4	7	2.3
Total	65	12.9	279	55.4	51.9	4.3	16	3.2	21	3.2

Table 142i World - Mundo - Monde   Mouth and oropharynx cancers - Cases

Age group (years)	Incidence 1990 Number ('000s)	Rate (per 100 000)	Prevalence 1990 Number ('000s)	Rate (per 100 000)	Avg. age at onset (years)	Average duration (years)	Deaths 1990 Number ('000s)	Rate (per 100 000)	Deaths 2000 (Projected) Number ('000s)	Rate (per 100 000)
Males										
0-4	4	1.3	7	2.3	2.5	4.6	1	0.2	1	0.2
5-14	8	1.4	35	6.4	10.0	4.6	1	0.2	1	0.2
15-44	159	12.7	737	58.9	29.8	4.6	22	1.8	29	2.0
45-59	192	61.5	821	262.9	52.3	4.3	52	16.6	71	17.6
60+	343	156.7	1 415	646.7	69.9	4.1	111	50.8	150	54.5
All ages	706	26.6	3 016	113.7	55.0	4.3	187	7.0	252	8.1
Females										
0-4	4	1.3	8	2.5	2.5	4.7	1	0.2	1	0.2
5-14	10	2.0	49	9.3	10.0	4.7	1	0.2	1	0.2
15-44	104	8.7	485	40.5	29.8	4.7	12	1.0	15	1.1
45-59	106	34.1	464	149.2	52.4	4.4	24	7.9	31	7.6
60+	168	62.3	672	249.6	70.5	4.0	61	22.7	82	24.3
All ages	392	15.0	1 678	64.2	52.5	4.3	99	3.8	129	4.2
Total	1 098	20.8	4 694	89.1	54.1	4.3	286	5.4	381	6.2

For epidemiological sources see Murray et al. 1996. For the methods used to estimate and project incidence, prevalence, and deaths see Murray and Lopez 1996a. See explanatory notes for definitions and caveats.

Table 143   **Cuadro 143**   **Tableau 143**
Oesophagus cancer   **Cáncer de esófago**   **Cancer de l'oesophage**

Cases   Casos   Cas

Table 143a   EME - PEMC - EMBE   Oesophagus cancer - Cases

Age group (years)	Incidence 1990 Number ('000s)	Rate (per 100 000)	Prevalence 1990 Number ('000s)	Rate (per 100 000)	Avg. age at onset (years)	Average duration (years)	Deaths 1990 Number ('000s)	Rate (per 100 000)	Deaths 2000 (Projected) Number ('000s)	Rate (per 100 000)
Males										
0-4	0	0.0	0	0.0	2.5	2.1	0	0.0	0	0.0
5-14	0	0.0	0	0.0	10.0	2.1	0	0.0	0	0.0
15-44	1	0.6	2	1.2	29.9	2.1	1	0.5	1	0.5
45-59	8	12.8	15	22.0	52.4	1.7	8	11.9	9	11.7
60+	24	40.5	42	68.9	71.1	1.7	23	37.9	26	35.7
All ages	34	8.7	58	15.0	65.2	1.7	32	8.1	36	8.8
Females										
0-4	0	0.0	0	0.0	-	-	0	0.0	0	0.0
5-14	0	0.0	0	0.0	10.0	2.9	0	0.0	0	0.0
15-44	0	0.1	0	0.3	30.0	2.9	0	0.1	0	0.1
45-59	2	2.5	5	7.4	52.4	2.9	1	1.8	1	1.6
60+	10	12.1	21	25.0	72.4	2.1	9	10.6	10	10.1
All ages	12	3.0	27	6.6	69.0	2.2	10	2.5	11	2.6
Total	46	5.8	85	10.7	66.2	1.8	42	5.3	47	5.6

Table 143b   FSE - PEAS - AESE   Oesophagus cancer - Cases

Age group (years)	Incidence 1990 Number ('000s)	Rate (per 100 000)	Prevalence 1990 Number ('000s)	Rate (per 100 000)	Avg. age at onset (years)	Average duration (years)	Deaths 1990 Number ('000s)	Rate (per 100 000)	Deaths 2000 (Projected) Number ('000s)	Rate (per 100 000)
Males										
0-4	0	0.0	0	0.0	2.5	2.0	0	0.0	0	0.0
5-14	0	0.0	0	0.0	-	-	0	0.0	0	0.0
15-44	1	0.7	1	1.4	29.8	2.0	0	0.6	0	0.6
45-59	4	13.9	6	22.7	52.2	1.6	4	13.1	5	16.1
60+	5	22.0	7	35.7	70.0	1.6	4	20.8	6	22.2
All ages	9	5.4	15	8.9	60.1	1.7	8	5.1	11	6.5
Females										
0-4	0	0.0	0	0.0	-	-	0	0.0	0	0.0
5-14	0	0.0	0	0.0	10.0	2.7	0	0.0	0	0.0
15-44	0	0.1	0	0.3	29.9	2.7	0	0.1	0	0.1
45-59	0	1.6	1	4.4	52.4	2.7	0	1.2	0	1.1
60+	2	4.4	3	8.6	71.5	2.0	1	4.0	2	4.0
All ages	2	1.2	5	2.6	65.7	2.2	2	1.0	2	1.1
Total	11	3.2	19	5.6	61.2	1.8	10	3.0	13	3.7

Table 143c   India - India - Inde   Oesophagus cancer - Cases

Age group (years)	Incidence 1990 Number ('000s)	Rate (per 100 000)	Prevalence 1990 Number ('000s)	Rate (per 100 000)	Avg. age at onset (years)	Average duration (years)	Deaths 1990 Number ('000s)	Rate (per 100 000)	Deaths 2000 (Projected) Number ('000s)	Rate (per 100 000)
Males										
0-4	0	0.0	0	0.0	-	-	0	0.0	0	0.0
5-14	0	0.0	0	0.0	-	-	0	0.0	0	0.0
15-44	2	0.9	3	1.6	29.8	1.6	2	0.9	2	0.9
45-59	9	18.9	12	26.0	52.3	1.4	9	18.4	12	19.7
60+	16	54.2	22	73.9	69.7	1.4	16	52.7	21	56.2
All ages	27	6.2	38	8.5	61.1	1.4	26	6.0	35	6.8
Females										
0-4	0	0.0	0	0.0	-	-	0	0.0	0	0.0
5-14	0	0.0	0	0.0	-	-	0	0.0	0	0.0
15-44	2	1.2	5	2.5	29.8	2.2	2	1.1	3	1.1
45-59	10	21.5	21	46.6	52.4	2.2	9	18.6	10	18.1
60+	15	50.8	24	81.8	70.1	1.6	14	48.1	19	49.3
All ages	27	6.5	50	12.1	60.4	1.9	25	6.0	32	6.6
Total	54	6.3	87	10.3	60.7	1.6	51	6.0	67	6.7

For epidemiological sources see Murray et al. 1996. For the methods used to estimate and project incidence, prevalence, and deaths see Murray and Lopez 1996a. See explanatory notes for definitions and caveats.

Table 143
Oesophagus cancer

Cuadro 143
Cáncer de esófago

Tableau 143
Cancer de l'oesophage

Cases   Casos   Cas

Table 143d   China - China - Chine   Oesophagus cancer - Cases

Age group (years)	Incidence 1990 Number ('000s)	Rate (per 100 000)	Prevalence 1990 Number ('000s)	Rate (per 100 000)	Avg. age at onset (years)	Average duration (years)	Deaths 1990 Number ('000s)	Rate (per 100 000)	Deaths 2000 (Projected) Number ('000s)	Rate (per 100 000)
Males										
0-4	0	0.0	0	0.0	-	-	0	0.0	0	0.0
5-14	0	0.0	0	0.0	-	-	0	0.0	0	0.0
15-44	8	2.5	14	4.5	29.9	1.8	7	2.3	11	3.3
45-59	33	44.8	49	67.6	52.3	1.5	31	43.0	50	51.3
60+	94	192.1	141	287.0	69.8	1.5	90	184.4	130	215.7
All ages	134	23.0	204	34.8	63.3	1.5	129	22.0	191	29.1
Females										
0-4	0	0.0	0	0.0	-	-	0	0.0	0	0.0
5-14	0	0.0	0	0.0	-	-	0	0.0	0	0.0
15-44	1	0.5	4	1.3	29.9	2.5	1	0.5	2	0.6
45-59	14	22.5	36	55.2	52.4	2.5	12	18.1	17	18.8
60+	51	98.7	91	176.2	70.6	1.8	47	91.3	65	101.2
All ages	67	12.2	130	23.7	65.8	1.9	60	11.0	84	13.5
Total	201	17.8	334	29.4	64.1	1.7	189	16.7	275	21.5

Table 143e   OAI - OPAI - APAI   Oesophagus cancer - Cases

Age group (years)	Incidence 1990 Number ('000s)	Rate (per 100 000)	Prevalence 1990 Number ('000s)	Rate (per 100 000)	Avg. age at onset (years)	Average duration (years)	Deaths 1990 Number ('000s)	Rate (per 100 000)	Deaths 2000 (Projected) Number ('000s)	Rate (per 100 000)
Males										
0-4	0	0.0	0	0.0	-	-	0	0.0	0	0.0
5-14	0	0.0	0	0.0	-	-	0	0.0	0	0.0
15-44	1	0.5	1	0.8	29.7	1.8	1	0.4	1	0.5
45-59	5	14.6	7	21.4	52.3	1.5	5	14.0	7	14.8
60+	10	50.5	15	73.4	69.6	1.5	10	48.7	14	51.7
All ages	16	4.7	23	6.9	62.3	1.5	15	4.5	22	5.5
Females										
0-4	0	0.0	0	0.0	-	-	0	0.0	0	0.0
5-14	0	0.0	0	0.0	-	-	0	0.0	0	0.0
15-44	0	0.3	1	0.6	29.8	2.4	0	0.3	1	0.3
45-59	2	6.5	5	15.3	52.3	2.4	2	5.3	2	5.1
60+	5	22.8	9	39.4	70.3	1.7	5	21.2	7	21.2
All ages	8	2.3	15	4.5	62.9	1.9	7	2.1	10	2.4
Total	24	3.5	39	5.7	62.5	1.6	22	3.3	32	4.0

Table 143f   SSA - ASS - ASS   Oesophagus cancer - Cases

Age group (years)	Incidence 1990 Number ('000s)	Rate (per 100 000)	Prevalence 1990 Number ('000s)	Rate (per 100 000)	Avg. age at onset (years)	Average duration (years)	Deaths 1990 Number ('000s)	Rate (per 100 000)	Deaths 2000 (Projected) Number ('000s)	Rate (per 100 000)
Males										
0-4	0	0.0	0	0.0	-	-	0	0.0	0	0.0
5-14	0	0.0	0	0.0	-	-	0	0.0	0	0.0
15-44	2	1.6	3	2.5	29.4	1.6	2	1.5	2	1.6
45-59	7	36.1	10	47.8	52.2	1.3	7	35.2	9	34.2
60+	9	81.9	11	107.6	69.2	1.3	8	79.9	12	82.4
All ages	18	7.0	24	9.4	58.3	1.3	17	6.8	23	6.8
Females										
0-4	0	0.0	0	0.0	-	-	0	0.0	0	0.0
5-14	0	0.0	0	0.0	-	-	0	0.0	0	0.0
15-44	0	0.3	1	0.7	29.5	2.1	0	0.3	0	0.3
45-59	2	9.2	4	19.1	52.2	2.1	2	8.2	2	7.6
60+	4	34.0	7	52.5	69.7	1.5	4	32.5	5	31.0
All ages	7	2.6	12	4.5	62.2	1.7	6	2.4	8	2.3
Total	24	4.8	35	6.9	59.4	1.4	23	4.6	31	4.5

For epidemiological sources see Murray et al. 1996. For the methods used to estimate and project incidence, prevalence, and deaths see Murray and Lopez 1996a. See explanatory notes for definitions and caveats.

Table 143	Cuadro 143	Tableau 143
Oesophagus cancer	Cáncer de esófago	Cancer de l'oesophage

Cases	Casos	Cas

Table 143g   LAC - ALC - ALC   Oesophagus cancer - Cases

Age group (years)	Incidence 1990 Number ('000s)	Rate (per 100 000)	Prevalence 1990 Number ('000s)	Rate (per 100 000)	Avg. age at onset (years)	Average duration (years)	Deaths 1990 Number ('000s)	Rate (per 100 000)	Deaths 2000 (Projected) Number ('000s)	Rate (per 100 000)
Males										
0-4	0	0.0	0	0.0	-	-	0	0.0	0	0.0
5-14	0	0.0	0	0.0	-	-	0	0.0	0	0.0
15-44	0	0.3	1	0.6	29.8	1.9	0	0.3	0	0.3
45-59	2	10.5	4	16.2	52.3	1.5	2	10.0	3	9.9
60+	5	32.3	7	49.6	70.3	1.5	4	30.9	6	32.0
All ages	7	3.3	11	5.1	62.7	1.6	7	3.1	10	3.7
Females										
0-4	0	0.0	0	0.0	-	-	0	0.0	0	0.0
5-14	0	0.0	0	0.0	-	-	0	0.0	0	0.0
15-44	0	0.1	0	0.2	29.9	2.5	0	0.1	0	0.1
45-59	1	3.0	2	7.7	52.4	2.5	1	2.4	1	2.3
60+	3	17.6	5	32.4	71.1	1.8	3	16.2	4	16.5
All ages	4	1.7	7	3.4	66.6	2.0	3	1.5	5	1.8
Total	11	2.5	19	4.2	64.0	1.7	10	2.3	14	2.7

Table 143h   MEC - AOM - CMO   Oesophagus cancer - Cases

Age group (years)	Incidence 1990 Number ('000s)	Rate (per 100 000)	Prevalence 1990 Number ('000s)	Rate (per 100 000)	Avg. age at onset (years)	Average duration (years)	Deaths 1990 Number ('000s)	Rate (per 100 000)	Deaths 2000 (Projected) Number ('000s)	Rate (per 100 000)
Males										
0-4	0	0.0	0	0.0	2.5	1.8	0	0.0	0	0.0
5-14	0	0.0	0	0.1	10.0	1.8	0	0.0	0	0.0
15-44	1	0.5	1	0.9	29.8	1.8	1	0.5	1	0.5
45-59	2	10.4	3	15.3	52.3	1.5	2	10.0	3	9.9
60+	3	22.5	4	32.7	69.7	1.5	3	21.7	4	21.2
All ages	6	2.3	9	3.5	58.8	1.5	6	2.3	8	2.4
Females										
0-4	0	0.0	0	0.0	2.5	2.4	0	0.0	0	0.0
5-14	0	0.1	0	0.2	10.0	2.4	0	0.1	0	0.1
15-44	0	0.4	1	0.9	29.8	2.4	0	0.4	1	0.4
45-59	2	6.9	4	16.3	52.3	2.4	1	5.7	2	5.1
60+	2	16.2	4	28.0	70.4	1.7	2	15.1	3	13.6
All ages	5	1.8	9	3.7	59.7	2.0	4	1.6	5	1.6
Total	11	2.1	18	3.6	59.2	1.7	10	2.0	13	2.0

Table 143i   World - Mundo - Monde   Oesophagus cancer - Cases

Age group (years)	Incidence 1990 Number ('000s)	Rate (per 100 000)	Prevalence 1990 Number ('000s)	Rate (per 100 000)	Avg. age at onset (years)	Average duration (years)	Deaths 1990 Number ('000s)	Rate (per 100 000)	Deaths 2000 (Projected) Number ('000s)	Rate (per 100 000)
Males										
0-4	0	0.0	0	0.0	2.5	1.8	0	0.0	0	0.0
5-14	0	0.0	0	0.0	10.0	1.8	0	0.0	0	0.0
15-44	14	1.2	26	2.1	29.8	1.8	13	1.1	19	1.3
45-59	71	22.7	106	34.0	52.3	1.5	68	21.7	98	24.4
60+	166	75.8	249	114.0	70.1	1.5	159	72.6	219	79.4
All ages	251	9.5	382	14.4	61.9	1.5	240	9.0	336	10.8
Females										
0-4	0	0.0	0	0.0	2.5	2.4	0	0.0	0	0.0
5-14	0	0.0	0	0.0	10.0	2.4	0	0.0	0	0.0
15-44	5	0.4	12	1.0	29.8	2.5	5	0.4	6	0.4
45-59	33	10.6	78	25.2	52.4	2.5	27	8.8	36	8.9
60+	92	34.4	164	61.1	71.2	1.9	86	31.8	115	34.1
All ages	131	5.0	255	9.7	64.2	2.0	118	4.5	157	5.1
Total	382	7.2	636	12.1	62.7	1.7	358	6.8	493	8.0

For epidemiological sources see Murray et al. 1996. For the methods used to estimate and project incidence, prevalence, and deaths see Murray and Lopez 1996a. See explanatory notes for definitions and caveats.

Table 144
Stomach cancer

Cuadro 144
Cáncer de estómago

Tableau 144
Cancer de l'estomac

Cases

Casos

Cas

Table 144a   EME - PEMC - EMBE   Stomach cancer - Cases

Age group (years)	Incidence 1990 Number ('000s)	Rate (per 100 000)	Prevalence 1990 Number ('000s)	Rate (per 100 000)	Avg. age at onset (years)	Average duration (years)	Deaths 1990 Number ('000s)	Rate (per 100 000)	Deaths 2000 (Projected) Number ('000s)	Rate (per 100 000)
Males										
0-4	0	0.0	0	0.0	2.5	3.5	0	0.0	0	0.0
5-14	0	0.0	0	0.0	10.0	3.5	0	0.0	0	0.0
15-44	5	2.8	18	9.9	29.9	3.5	3	1.5	3	1.5
45-59	22	33.6	72	108.8	52.4	3.2	14	20.5	16	20.1
60+	111	183.7	363	599.6	71.1	3.3	67	110.7	77	106.9
All ages	139	35.5	453	116.1	66.6	3.3	83	21.3	96	23.3
Females										
0-4	0	0.0	0	0.0	2.5	3.5	0	0.0	0	0.0
5-14	0	0.0	0	0.0	10.0	3.5	0	0.0	0	0.0
15-44	5	2.5	16	8.8	30.0	3.5	2	1.4	2	1.4
45-59	11	16.6	39	57.0	52.4	3.4	6	9.2	7	8.2
60+	56	66.2	122	143.9	72.4	2.2	48	57.1	54	54.9
All ages	72	17.6	176	43.3	66.6	2.5	57	14.0	63	14.6
Total	210	26.4	629	78.9	66.6	3.0	140	17.6	158	18.9

Table 144b   FSE - PEAS - AESE   Stomach cancer - Cases

Age group (years)	Incidence 1990 Number ('000s)	Rate (per 100 000)	Prevalence 1990 Number ('000s)	Rate (per 100 000)	Avg. age at onset (years)	Average duration (years)	Deaths 1990 Number ('000s)	Rate (per 100 000)	Deaths 2000 (Projected) Number ('000s)	Rate (per 100 000)
Males										
0-4	0	0.1	0	0.1	2.5	3.4	0	0.0	0	0.0
5-14	0	0.0	0	0.0	10.0	3.4	0	0.0	0	0.0
15-44	6	7.8	20	26.7	29.8	3.4	3	4.4	3	4.5
45-59	29	105.9	89	331.0	52.2	3.1	18	67.9	26	83.8
60+	59	279.7	185	882.1	70.0	3.2	37	177.3	50	197.2
All ages	93	56.4	295	178.2	62.0	3.2	59	35.6	80	46.6
Females										
0-4	0	0.0	0	0.0	2.5	3.3	0	0.0	0	0.0
5-14	0	0.0	0	0.1	10.0	3.3	0	0.0	0	0.0
15-44	4	4.9	12	16.4	29.9	3.3	2	2.9	2	2.6
45-59	13	42.5	42	140.8	52.4	3.3	8	25.0	8	23.5
60+	37	102.4	79	216.5	71.5	2.1	33	89.4	37	89.2
All ages	54	29.7	133	73.7	64.1	2.5	42	23.3	47	25.0
Total	147	42.4	428	123.6	62.7	2.9	101	29.2	126	35.3

Table 144c   India - India - Inde   Stomach cancer - Cases

Age group (years)	Incidence 1990 Number ('000s)	Rate (per 100 000)	Prevalence 1990 Number ('000s)	Rate (per 100 000)	Avg. age at onset (years)	Average duration (years)	Deaths 1990 Number ('000s)	Rate (per 100 000)	Deaths 2000 (Projected) Number ('000s)	Rate (per 100 000)
Males										
0-4	0	0.0	0	0.0	2.5	3.1	0	0.0	0	0.0
5-14	0	0.0	0	0.1	10.0	3.1	0	0.0	0	0.0
15-44	4	2.0	13	6.3	29.8	3.1	3	1.3	4	1.4
45-59	14	29.0	39	81.9	52.3	2.8	10	20.9	13	22.4
60+	21	71.8	61	204.4	69.7	2.8	15	51.3	20	54.8
All ages	39	8.9	112	25.6	59.4	2.9	28	6.4	37	7.2
Females										
0-4	0	0.0	0	0.0	-	-	0	0.0	0	0.0
5-14	0	0.0	0	0.0	-	-	0	0.0	0	0.0
15-44	3	1.7	9	5.1	29.8	3.0	2	1.1	3	1.1
45-59	8	17.6	24	52.5	52.4	3.0	6	12.0	7	11.7
60+	9	32.3	18	62.9	70.1	1.9	8	29.1	12	29.7
All ages	21	5.0	52	12.6	57.0	2.5	16	3.9	21	4.3
Total	60	7.0	164	19.3	58.6	2.7	44	5.2	58	5.8

For epidemiological sources see Murray et al. 1996. For the methods used to estimate and project incidence, prevalence, and deaths see Murray and Lopez 1996a. See explanatory notes for definitions and caveats.

Table 144
Stomach cancer

Cuadro 144
Cáncer de estómago

Tableau 144
Cancer de l'estomac

Cases

Casos

Cas

Table 144d China - China - Chine — Stomach cancer - Cases

Age group (years)	Incidence 1990 Number ('000s)	Rate (per 100 000)	Prevalence 1990 Number ('000s)	Rate (per 100 000)	Avg. age at onset (years)	Average duration (years)	Deaths 1990 Number ('000s)	Rate (per 100 000)	Deaths 2000 (Projected) Number ('000s)	Rate (per 100 000)
Males										
0-4	0	0.0	0	0.0	-	-	0	0.0	0	0.0
5-14	0	0.3	1	1.1	10.0	3.2	0	0.2	0	0.2
15-44	17	5.5	55	17.9	29.9	3.2	10	3.4	15	4.8
45-59	80	110.7	239	328.5	52.3	3.0	55	75.7	88	90.4
60+	212	433.2	635	1 296.4	69.8	3.0	144	293.5	206	342.0
All ages	310	53.0	930	158.9	63.0	3.0	209	35.8	310	47.3
Females										
0-4	0	0.0	0	0.0	-	-	0	0.0	0	0.0
5-14	0	0.4	1	1.1	10.0	3.2	0	0.2	0	0.2
15-44	18	6.4	57	20.1	29.9	3.2	11	4.0	15	4.9
45-59	34	53.5	108	167.9	52.4	3.1	22	34.1	32	35.4
60+	86	166.2	174	336.8	70.6	2.0	76	147.7	106	165.0
All ages	139	25.3	340	62.0	60.6	2.5	110	20.0	153	24.6
Total	449	39.6	1 270	112.0	62.3	2.8	319	28.2	464	36.2

Table 144e OAI - OPAI - APAI — Stomach cancer - Cases

Age group (years)	Incidence 1990 Number ('000s)	Rate (per 100 000)	Prevalence 1990 Number ('000s)	Rate (per 100 000)	Avg. age at onset (years)	Average duration (years)	Deaths 1990 Number ('000s)	Rate (per 100 000)	Deaths 2000 (Projected) Number ('000s)	Rate (per 100 000)
Males										
0-4	0	0.1	0	0.1	2.5	3.2	0	0.0	0	0.0
5-14	0	0.1	0	0.3	10.0	3.2	0	0.1	0	0.1
15-44	5	3.2	16	10.0	29.7	3.2	3	2.0	4	2.2
45-59	17	50.3	50	146.9	52.3	2.9	12	35.0	17	36.8
60+	31	153.2	91	451.3	69.6	2.9	21	105.8	31	112.4
All ages	53	15.5	158	46.0	60.1	3.0	37	10.7	53	13.0
Females										
0-4	0	0.0	0	0.1	2.5	3.1	0	0.0	0	0.0
5-14	0	0.0	0	0.1	10.0	3.1	0	0.0	0	0.0
15-44	3	1.9	10	6.0	29.8	3.1	2	1.3	3	1.3
45-59	8	22.8	25	70.2	52.3	3.1	5	14.8	7	14.1
60+	15	64.6	29	129.2	70.3	2.0	13	57.7	19	57.7
All ages	26	7.6	64	18.7	59.7	2.5	20	6.0	28	6.9
Total	79	11.6	221	32.4	60.0	2.8	57	8.3	81	10.0

Table 144f SSA - ASS - ASS — Stomach cancer - Cases

Age group (years)	Incidence 1990 Number ('000s)	Rate (per 100 000)	Prevalence 1990 Number ('000s)	Rate (per 100 000)	Avg. age at onset (years)	Average duration (years)	Deaths 1990 Number ('000s)	Rate (per 100 000)	Deaths 2000 (Projected) Number ('000s)	Rate (per 100 000)
Males										
0-4	0	0.0	0	0.0	2.4	3.0	0	0.0	0	0.0
5-14	0	0.1	0	0.2	10.0	3.0	0	0.1	0	0.1
15-44	3	2.5	8	7.5	29.4	3.0	2	1.7	2	1.7
45-59	9	45.3	26	125.8	52.2	2.8	7	33.2	9	32.3
60+	14	132.0	39	369.2	69.2	2.8	10	96.0	14	99.0
All ages	26	10.2	72	28.7	59.0	2.8	19	7.4	25	7.4
Females										
0-4	0	0.0	0	0.0	-	-	0	0.0	0	0.0
5-14	0	0.0	0	0.0	-	-	0	0.0	0	0.0
15-44	2	2.1	6	6.1	29.5	3.0	1	0.9	1	0.8
45-59	7	32.9	21	96.3	52.2	2.9	5	22.8	6	21.2
60+	8	61.6	15	118.2	69.7	1.9	7	55.8	9	53.4
All ages	17	6.7	43	16.6	57.3	2.5	13	5.1	17	4.8
Total	43	8.4	115	22.6	58.3	2.7	32	6.2	42	6.1

For epidemiological sources see Murray et al. 1996. For the methods used to estimate and project incidence, prevalence, and deaths see Murray and Lopez 1996a. See explanatory notes for definitions and caveats.

Table 144   **Cuadro 144**   **Tableau 144**
Stomach cancer   Cáncer de estómago   Cancer de l'estomac

Cases   Casos   Cas

Table 144g   LAC - ALC - ALC   Stomach cancer - Cases

Age group (years)	Incidence 1990 Number ('000s)	Rate (per 100 000)	Prevalence 1990 Number ('000s)	Rate (per 100 000)	Avg. age at onset (years)	Average duration (years)	Deaths 1990 Number ('000s)	Rate (per 100 000)	Deaths 2000 (Projected) Number ('000s)	Rate (per 100 000)
Males										
0-4	0	0.0	0	0.0	2.5	3.3	0	0.0	0	0.0
5-14	0	0.0	0	0.1	10.0	3.3	0	0.0	0	0.0
15-44	2	2.3	8	7.7	29.8	3.3	1	1.4	2	1.5
45-59	8	35.7	24	107.5	52.3	3.0	5	24.0	7	23.7
60+	23	164.3	71	499.4	70.3	3.0	16	109.3	23	114.1
All ages	34	15.2	103	46.5	63.1	3.1	22	10.1	32	11.9
Females										
0-4	0	0.0	0	0.0	2.5	3.2	0	0.0	0	0.0
5-14	0	0.0	0	0.0	10.0	3.2	0	0.0	0	0.0
15-44	2	1.6	5	5.1	29.9	3.2	1	1.0	1	1.0
45-59	4	18.9	14	60.2	52.4	3.2	3	11.8	4	11.4
60+	13	77.6	27	159.1	71.1	2.1	12	68.6	16	69.5
All ages	19	8.6	46	20.7	63.2	2.4	15	6.9	21	8.0
Total	53	11.9	149	33.6	63.1	2.8	38	8.5	53	9.9

Table 144h   MEC - AOM - CMO   Stomach cancer - Cases

Age group (years)	Incidence 1990 Number ('000s)	Rate (per 100 000)	Prevalence 1990 Number ('000s)	Rate (per 100 000)	Avg. age at onset (years)	Average duration (years)	Deaths 1990 Number ('000s)	Rate (per 100 000)	Deaths 2000 (Projected) Number ('000s)	Rate (per 100 000)
Males										
0-4	0	0.1	0	0.1	2.5	3.2	0	0.0	0	0.0
5-14	0	0.1	0	0.4	10.0	3.2	0	0.1	0	0.1
15-44	2	2.1	8	6.7	29.8	3.2	2	1.3	2	1.3
45-59	7	29.5	19	86.0	52.3	2.9	5	20.5	6	20.3
60+	9	66.5	27	195.9	69.7	2.9	6	45.9	8	44.9
All ages	18	7.1	54	21.0	57.8	3.0	12	4.8	17	5.1
Females										
0-4	0	0.0	0	0.0	2.5	3.1	0	0.0	0	0.0
5-14	0	0.1	0	0.2	10.0	3.1	0	0.0	0	0.0
15-44	1	1.4	5	4.2	29.8	3.1	1	0.9	1	0.8
45-59	3	15.3	11	47.2	52.3	3.1	2	10.0	3	8.9
60+	6	39.7	12	79.3	70.4	2.0	5	35.4	7	32.0
All ages	11	4.5	27	11.1	59.1	2.5	9	3.5	11	3.4
Total	29	5.8	81	16.2	58.3	2.8	21	4.2	28	4.2

Table 144i   World - Mundo - Monde   Stomach cancer - Cases

Age group (years)	Incidence 1990 Number ('000s)	Rate (per 100 000)	Prevalence 1990 Number ('000s)	Rate (per 100 000)	Avg. age at onset (years)	Average duration (years)	Deaths 1990 Number ('000s)	Rate (per 100 000)	Deaths 2000 (Projected) Number ('000s)	Rate (per 100 000)
Males										
0-4	0	0.0	0	0.0	2.5	3.2	0	0.0	0	0.0
5-14	1	0.1	2	0.4	10.0	3.2	0	0.1	0	0.1
15-44	45	3.6	146	11.7	29.8	3.3	27	2.2	36	2.5
45-59	186	59.5	558	178.5	52.3	3.0	125	40.2	183	45.5
60+	481	219.6	1 472	672.4	70.1	3.1	317	144.6	430	156.2
All ages	712	26.8	2 177	82.0	62.9	3.1	469	17.7	649	21.0
Females										
0-4	0	0.0	0	0.0	2.5	3.2	0	0.0	0	0.0
5-14	0	0.1	1	0.2	10.0	3.2	0	0.0	0	0.1
15-44	38	3.2	120	10.1	29.9	3.2	23	1.9	27	2.0
45-59	90	28.8	284	91.2	52.4	3.2	56	18.2	73	18.1
60+	230	85.5	476	176.8	71.1	2.1	203	75.3	259	77.0
All ages	358	13.7	882	33.7	62.0	2.5	282	10.8	360	11.8
Total	1 070	20.3	3 059	58.1	62.6	2.9	752	14.3	1 010	16.4

For epidemiological sources see Murray et al. 1996. For the methods used to estimate and project incidence, prevalence, and deaths see Murray and Lopez 1996a. See explanatory notes for definitions and caveats.

Table 145
Colon and rectum cancers

Cuadro 145
Cánceres de colon y recto

Tableau 145
Cancers du côlon et du rectum

Cases

Casos

Cas

Table 145a   EME - PEMC - EMBE   Colon and rectum cancers - Cases

Age group (years)	Incidence 1990 Number ('000s)	Rate (per 100 000)	Prevalence 1990 Number ('000s)	Rate (per 100 000)	Avg. age at onset (years)	Average duration (years)	Deaths 1990 Number ('000s)	Rate (per 100 000)	Deaths 2000 (Projected) Number ('000s)	Rate (per 100 000)
Males										
0-4	0	0.0	0	0.1	2.5	4.0	0	0.0	0	0.0
5-14	0	0.0	0	0.2	10.0	4.0	0	0.0	0	0.0
15-44	8	4.2	31	17.0	29.9	4.0	3	1.5	3	1.6
45-59	43	65.3	175	265.2	52.4	4.1	15	22.9	18	22.4
60+	208	343.8	809	1 336.6	71.1	3.9	85	140.7	98	136.0
All ages	259	66.4	1 016	260.2	66.7	3.9	103	26.4	119	28.9
Females										
0-4	0	0.0	0	0.0	2.5	4.1	0	0.0	0	0.0
5-14	0	0.0	0	0.0	-	-	0	0.0	0	0.0
15-44	7	4.1	30	17.0	30.0	4.1	2	1.4	2	1.4
45-59	33	48.4	134	197.2	52.4	4.1	11	16.7	12	14.9
60+	200	236.0	746	882.2	72.4	3.7	92	108.2	101	103.8
All ages	240	58.9	910	223.4	68.4	3.8	105	25.8	116	27.0
Total	499	62.5	1 926	241.5	67.5	3.9	208	26.1	234	27.9

Table 145b   FSE - PEAS - AESE   Colon and rectum cancers - Cases

Age group (years)	Incidence 1990 Number ('000s)	Rate (per 100 000)	Prevalence 1990 Number ('000s)	Rate (per 100 000)	Avg. age at onset (years)	Average duration (years)	Deaths 1990 Number ('000s)	Rate (per 100 000)	Deaths 2000 (Projected) Number ('000s)	Rate (per 100 000)
Males										
0-4	0	0.2	0	0.2	2.5	3.8	0	0.1	0	0.1
5-14	0	0.1	0	0.3	10.0	3.8	0	0.0	0	0.0
15-44	4	5.0	14	19.0	29.8	3.8	2	2.1	2	2.2
45-59	18	65.2	68	252.3	52.2	3.9	7	27.0	10	33.4
60+	49	234.4	182	869.3	70.0	3.7	23	109.7	32	126.1
All ages	71	42.7	265	160.2	63.4	3.8	32	19.3	44	25.8
Females										
0-4	0	0.1	0	0.2	2.5	3.9	0	0.0	0	0.0
5-14	0	0.0	0	0.2	10.0	3.9	0	0.0	0	0.0
15-44	4	4.9	14	19.1	29.9	3.9	1	1.9	1	1.8
45-59	16	52.0	61	202.2	52.4	3.9	6	21.3	7	20.0
60+	57	156.1	203	556.8	71.5	3.6	29	80.0	33	79.9
All ages	76	42.1	278	153.5	65.6	3.6	37	20.4	41	22.0
Total	147	42.4	543	156.7	64.5	3.7	69	19.9	85	23.8

Table 145c   India - India - Inde   Colon and rectum cancers - Cases

Age group (years)	Incidence 1990 Number ('000s)	Rate (per 100 000)	Prevalence 1990 Number ('000s)	Rate (per 100 000)	Avg. age at onset (years)	Average duration (years)	Deaths 1990 Number ('000s)	Rate (per 100 000)	Deaths 2000 (Projected) Number ('000s)	Rate (per 100 000)
Males										
0-4	0	0.0	0	0.0	2.5	3.3	0	0.0	0	0.0
5-14	0	0.0	0	0.0	10.0	3.3	0	0.0	0	0.0
15-44	3	1.4	10	4.8	29.8	3.3	2	0.9	2	0.9
45-59	5	10.3	16	34.2	52.3	3.3	3	6.0	4	6.4
60+	10	33.8	32	108.2	69.7	3.2	6	21.0	8	22.5
All ages	18	4.1	58	13.2	58.4	3.3	11	2.5	14	2.8
Females										
0-4	0	0.0	0	0.0	2.5	3.4	0	0.0	0	0.0
5-14	0	0.0	0	0.1	10.0	3.4	0	0.0	0	0.0
15-44	2	1.0	6	3.3	29.8	3.4	1	0.6	1	0.5
45-59	5	11.4	17	38.0	52.4	3.3	3	6.6	4	6.4
60+	9	30.8	27	95.0	70.1	3.1	6	20.1	8	20.5
All ages	16	3.9	51	12.5	59.7	3.2	10	2.4	13	2.7
Total	34	4.0	109	12.8	59.0	3.2	21	2.4	27	2.7

For epidemiological sources see Murray et al. 1996. For the methods used to estimate and project incidence, prevalence, and deaths see Murray and Lopez 1996a. See explanatory notes for definitions and caveats.

Table 145
Colon and rectum cancers

Cuadro 145
Cánceres de colon y recto

Tableau 145
Cancers du côlon et du rectum

Cases   Casos   Cas

Table 145d   China - China - Chine   Colon and rectum cancers - Cases

Age group (years)	Incidence 1990 Number ('000s)	Rate (per 100 000)	Prevalence 1990 Number ('000s)	Rate (per 100 000)	Avg. age at onset (years)	Average duration (years)	Deaths 1990 Number ('000s)	Rate (per 100 000)	Deaths 2000 (Projected) Number ('000s)	Rate (per 100 000)
Males										
0-4	0	0.0	0	0.0	-	-	0	0.0	0	0.0
5-14	0	0.4	1	1.5	10.0	3.6	0	0.2	0	0.2
15-44	13	4.2	46	15.1	29.9	3.6	7	2.2	9	2.8
45-59	21	28.8	75	103.4	52.3	3.6	11	14.6	17	17.4
60+	53	107.3	181	369.5	69.8	3.4	29	59.0	42	69.7
All ages	87	14.9	304	51.9	59.3	3.5	46	7.9	68	10.4
Females										
0-4	0	0.0	0	0.0	-	-	0	0.0	0	0.0
5-14	0	0.5	2	1.9	10.0	3.6	0	0.3	0	0.3
15-44	9	3.1	32	11.2	29.9	3.6	4	1.5	5	1.8
45-59	18	27.4	64	98.9	52.4	3.6	9	13.7	13	14.3
60+	40	77.6	133	257.4	70.6	3.3	24	45.6	33	50.8
All ages	67	12.2	230	42.0	60.0	3.4	37	6.7	52	8.3
Total	154	13.6	534	47.1	59.6	3.5	83	7.3	120	9.3

Table 145e   OAI - OPAI - APAI   Colon and rectum cancers - Cases

Age group (years)	Incidence 1990 Number ('000s)	Rate (per 100 000)	Prevalence 1990 Number ('000s)	Rate (per 100 000)	Avg. age at onset (years)	Average duration (years)	Deaths 1990 Number ('000s)	Rate (per 100 000)	Deaths 2000 (Projected) Number ('000s)	Rate (per 100 000)
Males										
0-4	0	0.3	0	0.4	2.5	3.5	0	0.2	0	0.2
5-14	0	0.4	1	1.3	10.0	3.5	0	0.2	0	0.2
15-44	4	2.7	15	9.2	29.7	3.5	2	1.4	3	1.6
45-59	6	16.7	20	58.6	52.3	3.5	3	8.9	4	9.3
60+	26	131.1	89	441.2	69.6	3.4	15	75.2	22	80.0
All ages	37	10.8	125	36.5	61.6	3.4	21	6.1	30	7.4
Females										
0-4	0	0.4	0	0.5	2.5	3.6	0	0.2	0	0.2
5-14	0	0.3	1	1.1	10.0	3.6	0	0.2	0	0.1
15-44	4	2.3	13	8.2	29.8	3.6	2	1.2	2	1.2
45-59	5	15.4	19	54.1	52.3	3.5	3	8.1	4	7.7
60+	24	105.2	77	341.1	70.3	3.2	15	64.1	21	64.1
All ages	33	9.8	110	32.5	62.1	3.3	19	5.7	27	6.7
Total	70	10.3	236	34.5	61.8	3.4	40	5.9	57	7.1

Table 145f   SSA - ASS - ASS   Colon and rectum cancers - Cases

Age group (years)	Incidence 1990 Number ('000s)	Rate (per 100 000)	Prevalence 1990 Number ('000s)	Rate (per 100 000)	Avg. age at onset (years)	Average duration (years)	Deaths 1990 Number ('000s)	Rate (per 100 000)	Deaths 2000 (Projected) Number ('000s)	Rate (per 100 000)
Males										
0-4	0	0.0	0	0.1	2.4	3.2	0	0.0	0	0.0
5-14	0	0.1	0	0.3	10.0	3.2	0	0.1	0	0.1
15-44	2	1.6	5	5.2	29.4	3.2	1	1.0	1	1.0
45-59	2	11.2	7	36.3	52.2	3.2	1	6.8	2	6.6
60+	8	78.2	26	244.0	69.2	3.1	5	50.4	7	51.9
All ages	12	4.9	39	15.3	60.2	3.2	8	3.1	11	3.1
Females										
0-4	0	0.0	0	0.0	2.4	3.3	0	0.0	0	0.0
5-14	0	0.1	0	0.2	10.0	3.3	0	0.0	0	0.0
15-44	1	1.4	5	4.5	29.5	3.3	1	0.5	1	0.5
45-59	2	8.0	6	26.0	52.2	3.3	1	4.8	1	4.5
60+	8	64.7	25	194.6	69.7	3.0	6	43.6	7	41.7
All ages	12	4.5	35	13.7	61.7	3.1	7	2.8	9	2.7
Total	24	4.7	74	14.5	60.9	3.1	15	2.9	20	2.9

For epidemiological sources see Murray et al. 1996. For the methods used to estimate and project incidence, prevalence, and deaths see Murray and Lopez 1996a. See explanatory notes for definitions and caveats.

Table 145
Colon and rectum cancers

Cuadro 145
Cánceres de colon y recto

Tableau 145
Cancers du côlon et du rectum

Cases

Casos

Cas

Table 145g   LAC - ALC - ALC   Colon and rectum cancers - Cases

Age group (years)	Incidence 1990 Number ('000s)	Rate (per 100 000)	Prevalence 1990 Number ('000s)	Rate (per 100 000)	Avg. age at onset (years)	Average duration (years)	Deaths 1990 Number ('000s)	Rate (per 100 000)	Deaths 2000 (Projected) Number ('000s)	Rate (per 100 000)
Males										
0-4	0	0.0	0	0.0	2.5	3.6	0	0.0	0	0.0
5-14	0	0.1	0	0.2	10.0	3.6	0	0.0	0	0.0
15-44	2	1.9	7	6.9	29.8	3.6	1	0.9	1	1.0
45-59	5	21.7	18	79.6	52.3	3.7	2	10.4	3	10.3
60+	13	92.5	46	325.7	70.3	3.5	7	48.7	10	51.3
All ages	20	9.0	71	32.2	61.8	3.6	10	4.6	15	5.5
Females										
0-4	0	0.0	0	0.0	2.5	3.7	0	0.0	0	0.0
5-14	0	0.0	0	0.1	10.0	3.7	0	0.0	0	0.0
15-44	2	1.7	7	6.4	29.9	3.7	1	0.8	1	0.8
45-59	5	21.0	18	77.3	52.4	3.7	2	10.0	3	9.6
60+	17	99.0	56	335.7	71.1	3.4	9	56.0	13	56.4
All ages	23	10.5	81	36.5	64.0	3.5	13	5.7	17	6.5
Total	43	9.8	153	34.3	63.0	3.5	23	5.1	32	6.0

Table 145h   MEC - AOM - CMO   Colon and rectum cancers - Cases

Age group (years)	Incidence 1990 Number ('000s)	Rate (per 100 000)	Prevalence 1990 Number ('000s)	Rate (per 100 000)	Avg. age at onset (years)	Average duration (years)	Deaths 1990 Number ('000s)	Rate (per 100 000)	Deaths 2000 (Projected) Number ('000s)	Rate (per 100 000)
Males										
0-4	0	0.0	0	0.1	2.5	3.5	0	0.0	0	0.0
5-14	0	0.1	0	0.4	10.0	3.5	0	0.1	0	0.1
15-44	2	1.7	7	5.9	29.8	3.5	1	0.9	1	0.9
45-59	2	10.2	8	35.8	52.3	3.5	1	5.4	2	5.4
60+	7	51.3	24	172.6	69.7	3.4	4	29.4	5	28.8
All ages	11	4.4	39	15.0	58.9	3.4	6	2.5	9	2.6
Females										
0-4	0	0.1	0	0.2	2.5	3.6	0	0.1	0	0.1
5-14	0	0.3	1	0.9	10.0	3.6	0	0.1	0	0.1
15-44	1	1.4	5	4.9	29.8	3.6	1	0.7	1	0.7
45-59	2	7.7	6	27.2	52.3	3.5	1	4.1	1	3.6
60+	8	52.2	26	169.3	70.4	3.2	5	31.8	6	28.8
All ages	11	4.6	38	15.4	61.3	3.3	7	2.7	8	2.6
Total	23	4.5	77	15.2	60.1	3.4	13	2.6	17	2.6

Table 145i   World - Mundo - Monde   Colon and rectum cancers - Cases

Age group (years)	Incidence 1990 Number ('000s)	Rate (per 100 000)	Prevalence 1990 Number ('000s)	Rate (per 100 000)	Avg. age at onset (years)	Average duration (years)	Deaths 1990 Number ('000s)	Rate (per 100 000)	Deaths 2000 (Projected) Number ('000s)	Rate (per 100 000)
Males										
0-4	0	0.1	0	0.1	2.5	3.5	0	0.0	0	0.0
5-14	1	0.2	3	0.6	10.0	3.5	0	0.1	1	0.1
15-44	37	3.0	136	10.9	29.8	3.6	18	1.5	23	1.6
45-59	102	32.5	388	124.2	52.3	3.8	44	14.0	60	14.9
60+	375	171.3	1 389	634.8	70.5	3.7	175	79.8	226	82.0
All ages	515	19.4	1 917	72.2	63.8	3.7	237	8.9	309	10.0
Females										
0-4	0	0.1	0	0.1	2.5	3.6	0	0.0	0	0.0
5-14	1	0.2	4	0.7	10.0	3.6	0	0.1	1	0.1
15-44	30	2.5	112	9.4	29.9	3.8	13	1.1	15	1.1
45-59	85	27.4	324	104.3	52.4	3.8	37	11.8	45	11.1
60+	362	134.5	1 294	480.6	71.7	3.6	184	68.5	222	66.0
All ages	478	18.3	1 734	66.4	65.5	3.6	235	9.0	283	9.2
Total	993	18.9	3 651	69.3	64.6	3.7	472	9.0	592	9.6

For epidemiological sources see Murray et al. 1996. For the methods used to estimate and project incidence, prevalence, and deaths see Murray and Lopez 1996a. See explanatory notes for definitions and caveats.

Table 146	Cuadro 146	Tableau 146
Liver cancer	Cáncer de higado	Cancer du foie

Cases   Casos   Cas

Table 146a   EME - PEMC - EMBE   Liver cancer - Cases

Age group (years)	Incidence 1990 Number ('000s)	Rate (per 100 000)	Prevalence 1990 Number ('000s)	Rate (per 100 000)	Avg. age at onset (years)	Average duration (years)	Deaths 1990 Number ('000s)	Rate (per 100 000)	Deaths 2000 (Projected) Number ('000s)	Rate (per 100 000)
Males										
0-4	0	0.5	0	0.8	2.5	4.11	0	0.2	0	0.1
5-14	0	0.1	0	0.4	10.0	4.11	0	0.0	0	0.0
15-44	1	0.7	4	2.0	29.9	2.92	1	0.5	1	0.5
45-59	10	14.8	28	42.8	52.4	2.88	7	10.5	8	10.3
60+	20	33.1	31	51.8	71.1	1.56	19	31.6	21	29.1
All ages	31	8.0	64	16.4	63.2	2.05	27	6.9	30	7.3
Females										
0-4	0	0.4	0	0.7	2.5	4.48	0	0.1	0	0.1
5-14	0	0.2	0	0.7	10.0	4.48	0	0.0	0	0.0
15-44	0	0.2	0	0.2	30.0	1.45	0	0.2	0	0.1
45-59	1	2.0	3	3.9	52.4	1.91	1	1.9	1	1.7
60+	9	10.5	6	7.6	72.4	0.72	9	10.5	10	9.8
All ages	11	2.6	10	2.5	67.6	0.96	10	2.6	11	2.6
Total	42	5.3	74	9.3	64.3	1.77	37	4.7	41	4.9

Table 146b   FSE - PEAS - AESE   Liver cancer - Cases

Age group (years)	Incidence 1990 Number ('000s)	Rate (per 100 000)	Prevalence 1990 Number ('000s)	Rate (per 100 000)	Avg. age at onset (years)	Average duration (years)	Deaths 1990 Number ('000s)	Rate (per 100 000)	Deaths 2000 (Projected) Number ('000s)	Rate (per 100 000)
Males										
0-4	0	0.5	0	0.7	2.5	3.69	0	0.2	0	0.2
5-14	0	0.2	0	0.6	10.0	3.69	0	0.1	0	0.1
15-44	1	0.9	2	2.5	29.8	2.66	1	0.7	1	0.7
45-59	4	14.5	10	38.0	52.2	2.63	3	11.1	4	13.7
60+	8	36.5	11	53.5	70.0	1.47	7	35.1	10	38.5
All ages	12	7.5	24	14.3	61.5	1.92	11	6.6	15	8.6
Females										
0-4	0	0.5	0	0.7	2.5	4.00	0	0.2	0	0.2
5-14	0	0.2	0	0.6	10.0	4.00	0	0.1	0	0.1
15-44	0	0.4	0	0.6	29.9	1.36	0	0.4	0	0.4
45-59	2	5.5	3	9.8	52.4	1.78	2	5.1	2	4.8
60+	8	21.3	6	15.4	71.5	0.72	8	21.3	9	21.0
All ages	10	5.4	9	5.1	66.3	0.95	10	5.3	11	5.7
Total	22	6.4	33	9.5	63.6	1.49	21	5.9	25	7.1

Table 146c   India - India - Inde   Liver cancer - Cases

Age group (years)	Incidence 1990 Number ('000s)	Rate (per 100 000)	Prevalence 1990 Number ('000s)	Rate (per 100 000)	Avg. age at onset (years)	Average duration (years)	Deaths 1990 Number ('000s)	Rate (per 100 000)	Deaths 2000 (Projected) Number ('000s)	Rate (per 100 000)
Males										
0-4	0	0.1	0	0.1	2.5	2.28	0	0.1	0	0.1
5-14	0	0.1	0	0.2	10.0	2.28	0	0.1	0	0.1
15-44	1	0.5	2	0.8	29.8	1.76	1	0.4	1	0.5
45-59	3	6.7	6	11.6	52.3	1.74	3	6.2	4	6.6
60+	5	16.0	5	17.6	69.7	1.10	5	15.8	6	17.3
All ages	9	2.1	13	2.9	58.5	1.41	9	2.0	12	2.3
Females										
0-4	0	0.0	0	0.0	2.5	2.43	0	0.0	0	0.0
5-14	0	0.0	0	0.1	10.0	2.43	0	0.0	0	0.0
15-44	0	0.2	0	0.2	29.8	1.04	0	0.2	1	0.2
45-59	1	2.6	2	3.4	52.4	1.28	1	2.6	1	2.5
60+	2	8.0	2	5.8	70.1	0.72	2	8.0	3	8.4
All ages	4	1.0	4	0.9	59.4	0.95	4	1.0	5	1.1
Total	13	1.5	17	1.9	58.8	1.27	13	1.5	17	1.7

For epidemiological sources see Murray et al. 1996. For the methods used to estimate and project incidence, prevalence, and deaths see Murray and Lopez 1996a. See explanatory notes for definitions and caveats.

Table 146 / **Cuadro 146** / **Tableau 146**
Liver cancer / Cáncer de higado / Cancer du foie

Cases / Casos / Cas

Table 146d — China - China - Chine — Liver cancer - Cases

Age group (years)	Incidence 1990 Number ('000s)	Rate (per 100 000)	Prevalence 1990 Number ('000s)	Rate (per 100 000)	Avg. age at onset (years)	Average duration (years)	Deaths 1990 Number ('000s)	Rate (per 100 000)	Deaths 2000 (Projected) Number ('000s)	Rate (per 100 000)
Males										
0-4	0	0.5	0	0.6	2.5	3.01	0	0.4	0	0.4
5-14	1	1.0	3	2.9	10.0	3.01	1	0.6	1	0.7
15-44	54	17.7	121	39.6	29.9	2.24	46	15.1	68	21.2
45-59	89	123.0	198	271.9	52.3	2.21	77	105.3	123	125.7
60+	91	186.3	119	242.1	69.8	1.30	89	182.0	128	211.6
All ages	236	40.3	441	75.3	53.7	1.87	213	36.3	319	48.7
Females										
0-4	0	0.6	0	0.8	2.5	3.25	0	0.4	0	0.4
5-14	1	1.1	3	3.7	10.0	3.25	1	0.7	1	0.6
15-44	11	4.0	14	4.9	29.9	1.22	11	3.9	15	4.9
45-59	24	37.0	37	57.3	52.4	1.55	23	35.3	33	36.7
60+	45	87.9	33	63.6	70.6	0.72	45	87.8	63	98.1
All ages	82	15.0	87	15.9	58.6	1.07	80	14.6	112	18.0
Total	318	28.1	528	46.6	55.0	1.66	293	25.8	432	33.7

Table 146e — OAI - OPAI - APAI — Liver cancer - Cases

Age group (years)	Incidence 1990 Number ('000s)	Rate (per 100 000)	Prevalence 1990 Number ('000s)	Rate (per 100 000)	Avg. age at onset (years)	Average duration (years)	Deaths 1990 Number ('000s)	Rate (per 100 000)	Deaths 2000 (Projected) Number ('000s)	Rate (per 100 000)
Males										
0-4	0	0.8	0	0.9	2.5	2.79	0	0.6	0	0.6
5-14	1	1.0	2	2.9	10.0	2.79	1	0.8	1	0.7
15-44	8	4.7	16	9.8	29.7	2.10	7	4.1	9	4.5
45-59	23	66.5	47	137.8	52.3	2.07	20	58.6	28	61.6
60+	22	107.8	27	133.9	69.6	1.24	21	105.7	31	112.7
All ages	53	15.5	93	27.0	55.2	1.75	49	14.2	70	17.2
Females										
0-4	0	0.7	0	0.9	2.5	3.00	0	0.5	0	0.5
5-14	0	0.6	1	1.8	10.0	3.00	0	0.4	0	0.4
15-44	2	1.1	2	1.3	29.8	1.17	2	1.1	2	1.1
45-59	5	14.0	7	20.5	52.3	1.47	5	13.4	6	12.8
60+	11	47.9	8	34.6	70.3	0.72	11	47.8	16	47.8
All ages	18	5.4	19	5.6	58.9	1.07	18	5.2	24	6.0
Total	72	10.5	112	16.3	56.1	1.58	67	9.8	94	11.6

Table 146f — SSA - ASS - ASS — Liver cancer - Cases

Age group (years)	Incidence 1990 Number ('000s)	Rate (per 100 000)	Prevalence 1990 Number ('000s)	Rate (per 100 000)	Avg. age at onset (years)	Average duration (years)	Deaths 1990 Number ('000s)	Rate (per 100 000)	Deaths 2000 (Projected) Number ('000s)	Rate (per 100 000)
Males										
0-4	0	0.2	0	0.2	2.4	1.96	0	0.2	0	0.2
5-14	0	0.4	1	0.9	10.0	1.96	0	0.4	0	0.4
15-44	12	11.6	19	18.0	29.4	1.55	11	11.1	16	11.2
45-59	17	82.3	26	126.4	52.2	1.54	16	78.7	20	76.5
60+	13	126.6	13	127.4	69.2	1.01	13	125.7	19	129.7
All ages	42	16.8	58	23.1	50.6	1.38	41	16.3	55	16.1
Females										
0-4	0	0.3	0	0.2	2.4	2.08	0	0.2	0	0.2
5-14	0	0.5	1	1.0	10.0	2.08	0	0.4	0	0.4
15-44	3	3.2	3	3.1	29.5	0.95	2	2.0	3	1.8
45-59	5	22.1	6	25.5	52.2	1.16	5	21.8	6	20.2
60+	8	62.1	6	44.9	69.7	0.72	8	62.1	10	59.2
All ages	17	6.5	15	6.0	54.6	0.94	15	5.9	19	5.6
Total	59	11.6	74	14.5	51.8	1.25	56	11.0	75	10.8

For epidemiological sources see Murray et al. 1996. For the methods used to estimate and project incidence, prevalence, and deaths see Murray and Lopez 1996a. See explanatory notes for definitions and caveats.

Table 146	Cuadro 146	Tableau 146
Liver cancer	Cáncer de higado	Cancer du foie
Cases	Casos	Cas

Table 146g   LAC - ALC - ALC — Liver cancer - Cases

Age group (years)	Incidence 1990 Number ('000s)	Rate (per 100 000)	Prevalence 1990 Number ('000s)	Rate (per 100 000)	Avg. age at onset (years)	Average duration (years)	Deaths 1990 Number ('000s)	Rate (per 100 000)	Deaths 2000 (Projected) Number ('000s)	Rate (per 100 000)
Males										
0-4	0	0.1	0	0.1	2.5	3.22	0	0.1	0	0.1
5-14	0	0.1	0	0.5	10.0	3.22	0	0.1	0	0.1
15-44	0	0.3	1	0.7	29.8	2.37	0	0.2	0	0.3
45-59	1	3.5	2	8.2	52.3	2.34	1	2.9	1	2.9
60+	2	12.2	2	16.4	70.3	1.35	2	11.8	2	12.4
All ages	3	1.3	5	2.3	59.0	1.79	3	1.2	4	1.4
Females										
0-4	0	0.1	0	0.1	2.5	3.48	0	0.0	0	0.0
5-14	0	0.1	0	0.4	10.0	3.48	0	0.1	0	0.1
15-44	0	0.2	0	0.2	29.9	1.26	0	0.2	0	0.2
45-59	1	2.4	1	3.9	52.4	1.62	1	2.3	1	2.2
60+	2	12.8	2	9.2	71.1	0.72	2	12.8	3	12.8
All ages	3	1.3	3	1.3	63.5	1.00	3	1.3	4	1.5
Total	6	1.3	8	1.8	61.2	1.39	6	1.2	8	1.4

Table 146h   MEC - AOM - CMO — Liver cancer - Cases

Age group (years)	Incidence 1990 Number ('000s)	Rate (per 100 000)	Prevalence 1990 Number ('000s)	Rate (per 100 000)	Avg. age at onset (years)	Average duration (years)	Deaths 1990 Number ('000s)	Rate (per 100 000)	Deaths 2000 (Projected) Number ('000s)	Rate (per 100 000)
Males										
0-4	0	0.1	0	0.1	2.5	2.79	0	0.1	0	0.1
5-14	0	0.2	0	0.6	10.0	2.79	0	0.2	0	0.2
15-44	1	0.6	2	1.3	29.8	2.10	1	0.6	1	0.6
45-59	2	9.9	5	20.6	52.3	2.07	2	8.7	3	8.7
60+	3	19.3	3	23.9	69.7	1.24	3	18.9	3	18.6
All ages	6	2.3	10	3.8	55.9	1.72	5	2.1	7	2.2
Females										
0-4	0	0.1	0	0.1	2.5	3.00	0	0.1	0	0.1
5-14	0	0.2	0	0.7	10.0	3.00	0	0.2	0	0.1
15-44	0	0.3	0	0.4	29.8	1.17	0	0.3	0	0.3
45-59	1	4.5	1	6.6	52.3	1.47	1	4.3	1	3.9
60+	2	12.7	1	9.2	70.4	0.72	2	12.7	2	11.5
All ages	4	1.4	4	1.5	57.9	1.10	3	1.4	4	1.3
Total	9	1.8	14	2.7	56.7	1.49	9	1.7	11	1.7

Table 146i   World - Mundo - Monde — Liver cancer - Cases

Age group (years)	Incidence 1990 Number ('000s)	Rate (per 100 000)	Prevalence 1990 Number ('000s)	Rate (per 100 000)	Avg. age at onset (years)	Average duration (years)	Deaths 1990 Number ('000s)	Rate (per 100 000)	Deaths 2000 (Projected) Number ('000s)	Rate (per 100 000)
Males										
0-4	1	0.3	1	0.4	2.5	2.98	1	0.2	1	0.2
5-14	3	0.5	7	1.3	10.0	2.81	2	0.3	2	0.3
15-44	78	6.2	165	13.2	29.8	2.12	67	5.4	97	6.7
45-59	149	47.6	321	102.7	52.3	2.16	128	41.0	191	47.5
60+	163	74.6	212	97.1	69.9	1.30	159	72.7	221	80.1
All ages	393	14.8	707	26.6	54.7	1.80	357	13.5	512	16.5
Females										
0-4	1	0.3	1	0.4	2.5	3.18	1	0.2	1	0.2
5-14	2	0.4	7	1.3	10.0	3.05	1	0.3	2	0.3
15-44	18	1.5	21	1.8	29.8	1.16	16	1.4	21	1.5
45-59	39	12.7	59	19.1	52.4	1.50	38	12.1	52	12.8
60+	87	32.4	63	23.4	70.7	0.72	87	32.4	116	34.4
All ages	148	5.7	152	5.8	59.5	1.04	143	5.5	191	6.2
Total	541	10.3	858	16.3	56.0	1.59	501	9.5	703	11.4

For epidemiological sources see Murray et al. 1996. For the methods used to estimate and project incidence, prevalence, and deaths see Murray and Lopez 1996a. See explanatory notes for definitions and caveats.

Table 147
Pancreas cancer

Cuadro 147
Cáncer de páncreas

Tableau 147
Cancer du pancréas

Cases

Casos

Cas

Table 147a   EME - PEMC - EMBE   Pancreas cancer - Cases

Age group (years)	Incidence 1990 Number ('000s)	Rate (per 100 000)	Prevalence 1990 Number ('000s)	Rate (per 100 000)	Avg. age at onset (years)	Average duration (years)	Deaths 1990 Number ('000s)	Rate (per 100 000)	Deaths 2000 (Projected) Number ('000s)	Rate (per 100 000)
Males										
0-4	0	0.0	0	0.0	2.5	2.36	0	0.0	0	0.0
5-14	0	0.0	0	0.0	10.0	2.36	0	0.0	0	0.0
15-44	1	0.8	3	1.9	29.9	2.36	1	0.7	1	0.7
45-59	8	12.0	12	17.6	52.4	1.47	8	11.5	9	11.3
60+	36	59.1	53	86.8	71.1	1.47	34	56.9	39	54.0
All ages	45	11.6	68	17.3	66.5	1.50	43	11.1	49	12.0
Females										
0-4	0	0.0	0	0.0	2.5	2.99	0	0.0	0	0.0
5-14	0	0.0	0	0.0	10.0	2.99	0	0.0	0	0.0
15-44	1	0.5	3	1.6	29.9	2.99	1	0.4	1	0.4
45-59	5	7.7	13	18.6	52.4	2.40	4	6.3	5	5.7
60+	37	44.0	27	31.8	72.4	0.72	37	44.0	41	41.6
All ages	43	10.7	42	10.4	69.0	0.98	42	10.3	46	10.7
Total	89	11.1	110	13.8	67.7	1.24	85	10.7	95	11.3

Table 147b   FSE - PEAS - AESE   Pancreas cancer - Cases

Age group (years)	Incidence 1990 Number ('000s)	Rate (per 100 000)	Prevalence 1990 Number ('000s)	Rate (per 100 000)	Avg. age at onset (years)	Average duration (years)	Deaths 1990 Number ('000s)	Rate (per 100 000)	Deaths 2000 (Projected) Number ('000s)	Rate (per 100 000)
Males										
0-4	0	0.0	0	0.0	-	-	0	0.0	0	0.0
5-14	0	0.0	0	0.0	-	-	0	0.0	0	0.0
15-44	1	1.4	2	3.1	29.8	2.21	1	1.2	1	1.2
45-59	5	18.9	7	26.4	52.2	1.40	5	18.3	7	22.5
60+	10	49.2	14	68.9	70.0	1.40	10	47.7	13	52.6
All ages	16	10.0	24	14.5	61.9	1.45	16	9.6	21	12.5
Females										
0-4	0	0.0	0	0.0	2.5	2.78	0	0.0	0	0.0
5-14	0	0.0	0	0.1	10.0	2.78	0	0.0	0	0.0
15-44	1	0.7	1	1.9	29.9	2.78	0	0.5	0	0.5
45-59	3	8.4	6	18.8	52.4	2.25	2	7.1	2	6.7
60+	11	29.2	8	21.1	71.5	0.72	11	29.2	12	28.7
All ages	14	7.6	15	8.2	66.3	1.08	13	7.3	14	7.7
Total	30	8.7	39	11.2	63.9	1.28	29	8.4	36	10.0

Table 147c   India - India - Inde   Pancreas cancer - Cases

Age group (years)	Incidence 1990 Number ('000s)	Rate (per 100 000)	Prevalence 1990 Number ('000s)	Rate (per 100 000)	Avg. age at onset (years)	Average duration (years)	Deaths 1990 Number ('000s)	Rate (per 100 000)	Deaths 2000 (Projected) Number ('000s)	Rate (per 100 000)
Males										
0-4	0	0.0	0	0.0	-	-	0	0.0	0	0.0
5-14	0	0.0	0	0.0	-	-	0	0.0	0	0.0
15-44	0	0.2	1	0.4	29.8	1.74	0	0.2	1	0.2
45-59	2	3.3	2	3.8	52.3	1.17	2	3.2	2	3.4
60+	3	8.4	3	9.9	69.7	1.17	2	8.3	3	8.9
All ages	4	1.0	6	1.3	59.8	1.23	4	1.0	6	1.1
Females										
0-4	0	0.0	0	0.0	2.5	2.13	0	0.0	0	0.0
5-14	0	0.0	0	0.0	10.0	2.13	0	0.0	0	0.0
15-44	0	0.2	1	0.4	29.8	2.13	0	0.2	0	0.2
45-59	1	2.0	2	3.6	52.4	1.77	1	1.9	1	1.8
60+	2	6.6	1	4.8	70.1	0.72	2	6.6	3	6.9
All ages	3	0.8	4	0.9	60.0	1.20	3	0.8	4	0.9
Total	8	0.9	9	1.1	59.9	1.21	8	0.9	10	1.0

For epidemiological sources see Murray et al. 1996. For the methods used to estimate and project incidence, prevalence, and deaths see Murray and Lopez 1996a. See explanatory notes for definitions and caveats.

Table 147	Cuadro 147	Tableau 147
Pancreas cancer	Cáncer de páncreas	Cancer du pancréas
Cases	Casos	Cas

Table 147d   China - China - Chine   Pancreas cancer - Cases

Age group (years)	Incidence 1990 Number ('000s)	Rate (per 100 000)	Prevalence 1990 Number ('000s)	Rate (per 100 000)	Avg. age at onset (years)	Average duration (years)	Deaths 1990 Number ('000s)	Rate (per 100 000)	Deaths 2000 (Projected) Number ('000s)	Rate (per 100 000)
Males										
0-4	0	0.0	0	0.0	-	-	0	0.0	0	0.0
5-14	0	0.0	0	0.0	-	-	0	0.0	0	0.0
15-44	2	0.5	3	1.1	29.9	1.98	1	0.5	2	0.6
45-59	4	5.8	5	7.4	52.3	1.29	4	5.6	7	6.7
60+	14	29.4	19	38.0	69.8	1.29	14	28.8	21	34.1
All ages	20	3.5	27	4.7	63.0	1.34	20	3.4	29	4.4
Females										
0-4	0	0.0	0	0.0	2.5	2.46	0	0.0	0	0.0
5-14	0	0.0	0	0.0	10.0	2.46	0	0.0	0	0.0
15-44	1	0.2	1	0.4	29.9	2.46	0	0.1	0	0.2
45-59	2	3.2	4	6.4	52.4	2.01	2	2.8	3	3.0
60+	10	19.8	7	14.3	70.6	0.72	10	19.8	14	22.2
All ages	13	2.3	13	2.3	65.9	1.00	13	2.3	18	2.8
Total	33	2.9	40	3.5	64.1	1.21	32	2.8	47	3.6

Table 147e   OAI - OPAI - APAI   Pancreas cancer - Cases

Age group (years)	Incidence 1990 Number ('000s)	Rate (per 100 000)	Prevalence 1990 Number ('000s)	Rate (per 100 000)	Avg. age at onset (years)	Average duration (years)	Deaths 1990 Number ('000s)	Rate (per 100 000)	Deaths 2000 (Projected) Number ('000s)	Rate (per 100 000)
Males										
0-4	0	0.0	0	0.0	-	-	0	0.0	0	0.0
5-14	0	0.0	0	0.0	-	-	0	0.0	0	0.0
15-44	1	0.4	1	0.7	29.7	1.91	1	0.3	1	0.4
45-59	2	4.9	2	6.1	52.3	1.25	2	4.8	2	5.0
60+	4	19.0	5	23.8	69.6	1.25	4	18.6	5	19.8
All ages	6	1.8	8	2.3	61.1	1.32	6	1.7	9	2.1
Females										
0-4	0	0.1	0	0.1	2.5	2.35	0	0.1	0	0.1
5-14	0	0.1	0	0.1	10.0	2.35	0	0.0	0	0.0
15-44	0	0.1	0	0.3	29.8	2.35	0	0.1	0	0.1
45-59	1	2.8	2	5.3	52.3	1.93	1	2.5	1	2.4
60+	3	11.7	2	8.5	70.3	0.72	3	11.7	4	11.7
All ages	4	1.1	4	1.3	62.7	1.14	4	1.1	5	1.3
Total	10	1.5	12	1.8	61.7	1.25	10	1.4	14	1.7

Table 147f   SSA - ASS - ASS   Pancreas cancer - Cases

Age group (years)	Incidence 1990 Number ('000s)	Rate (per 100 000)	Prevalence 1990 Number ('000s)	Rate (per 100 000)	Avg. age at onset (years)	Average duration (years)	Deaths 1990 Number ('000s)	Rate (per 100 000)	Deaths 2000 (Projected) Number ('000s)	Rate (per 100 000)
Males										
0-4	0	0.0	0	0.0	-	-	0	0.0	0	0.0
5-14	0	0.0	0	0.0	-	-	0	0.0	0	0.0
15-44	0	0.4	1	0.7	29.4	1.65	0	0.4	1	0.4
45-59	2	7.7	2	8.7	52.2	1.13	2	7.6	2	7.4
60+	2	18.6	2	21.0	69.2	1.13	2	18.4	3	19.0
All ages	4	1.6	5	1.9	57.9	1.19	4	1.6	5	1.5
Females										
0-4	0	0.0	0	0.0	-	-	0	0.0	0	0.0
5-14	0	0.0	0	0.0	-	-	0	0.0	0	0.0
15-44	0	0.4	1	0.9	29.5	2.00	0	0.2	0	0.2
45-59	1	5.4	2	9.1	52.2	1.67	1	5.1	1	4.7
60+	2	12.0	1	8.7	69.7	0.72	2	12.0	2	11.5
All ages	3	1.2	4	1.6	57.3	1.27	3	1.1	4	1.1
Total	7	1.4	9	1.7	57.6	1.22	7	1.3	9	1.3

For epidemiological sources see Murray et al. 1996. For the methods used to estimate and project incidence, prevalence, and deaths see Murray and Lopez 1996a. See explanatory notes for definitions and caveats.

Table 147   **Cuadro 147**   **Tableau 147**
Pancreas cancer   **Cáncer de páncreas**   **Cancer du pancréas**

Cases   Casos   Cas

Table 147g   LAC - ALC - ALC   Pancreas cancer - Cases

Age group (years)	Incidence 1990 Number ('000s)	Rate (per 100 000)	Prevalence 1990 Number ('000s)	Rate (per 100 000)	Avg. age at onset (years)	Average duration (years)	Deaths 1990 Number ('000s)	Rate (per 100 000)	Deaths 2000 (Projected) Number ('000s)	Rate (per 100 000)
Males										
0-4	0	0.0	0	0.0	2.5	2.05	0	0.0	0	0.0
5-14	0	0.0	0	0.0	10.0	2.05	0	0.0	0	0.0
15-44	0	0.2	1	0.5	29.8	2.05	0	0.2	0	0.2
45-59	1	4.6	1	6.1	52.3	1.32	1	4.5	1	4.4
60+	3	19.3	4	25.5	70.3	1.32	3	18.8	4	19.5
All ages	4	1.8	6	2.5	63.0	1.37	4	1.8	6	2.1
Females										
0-4	0	0.0	0	0.0	2.5	2.55	0	0.0	0	0.0
5-14	0	0.0	0	0.0	10.0	2.55	0	0.0	0	0.0
15-44	0	0.2	0	0.4	29.9	2.55	0	0.1	0	0.1
45-59	1	3.6	2	7.4	52.4	2.08	1	3.1	1	3.0
60+	3	19.9	2	14.4	71.1	0.72	3	19.9	5	20.2
All ages	4	2.0	5	2.1	65.8	1.06	4	1.9	6	2.2
Total	8	1.9	10	2.3	64.4	1.21	8	1.8	11	2.1

Table 147h   MEC - AOM - CMO   Pancreas cancer - Cases

Age group (years)	Incidence 1990 Number ('000s)	Rate (per 100 000)	Prevalence 1990 Number ('000s)	Rate (per 100 000)	Avg. age at onset (years)	Average duration (years)	Deaths 1990 Number ('000s)	Rate (per 100 000)	Deaths 2000 (Projected) Number ('000s)	Rate (per 100 000)
Males										
0-4	0	0.0	0	0.0	-	-	0	0.0	0	0.0
5-14	0	0.0	0	0.0	-	-	0	0.0	0	0.0
15-44	0	0.3	1	0.6	29.8	1.91	0	0.3	0	0.3
45-59	1	4.9	1	6.1	52.3	1.25	1	4.8	1	4.7
60+	1	10.2	2	12.8	69.7	1.25	1	10.0	2	9.9
All ages	3	1.1	4	1.5	57.7	1.34	3	1.1	4	1.1
Females										
0-4	0	0.0	0	0.0	-	-	0	0.0	0	0.0
5-14	0	0.0	0	0.0	-	-	0	0.0	0	0.0
15-44	0	0.2	0	0.4	29.8	2.35	0	0.1	0	0.1
45-59	1	2.9	1	5.6	52.3	1.93	1	2.6	1	2.3
60+	1	8.3	1	6.0	70.4	0.72	1	8.2	2	7.4
All ages	2	0.8	3	1.0	61.6	1.22	2	0.8	2	0.8
Total	5	1.0	6	1.3	59.4	1.29	5	0.9	6	1.0

Table 147i   World - Mundo - Monde   Pancreas cancer - Cases

Age group (years)	Incidence 1990 Number ('000s)	Rate (per 100 000)	Prevalence 1990 Number ('000s)	Rate (per 100 000)	Avg. age at onset (years)	Average duration (years)	Deaths 1990 Number ('000s)	Rate (per 100 000)	Deaths 2000 (Projected) Number ('000s)	Rate (per 100 000)
Males										
0-4	0	0.0	0	0.0	2.5	2.20	0	0.0	0	0.0
5-14	0	0.0	0	0.0	10.0	2.11	0	0.0	0	0.0
15-44	6	0.5	13	1.0	29.8	2.06	6	0.4	7	0.5
45-59	24	7.7	32	10.4	52.3	1.35	23	7.5	32	7.9
60+	73	33.4	101	46.1	70.5	1.38	71	32.3	90	32.7
All ages	103	3.9	146	5.5	63.7	1.42	100	3.8	129	4.2
Females										
0-4	0	0.0	0	0.0	2.5	2.44	0	0.0	0	0.0
5-14	0	0.0	0	0.0	10.0	2.42	0	0.0	0	0.0
15-44	3	0.3	9	0.7	29.9	2.56	2	0.2	3	0.2
45-59	14	4.6	31	9.9	52.4	2.14	12	4.0	15	3.7
60+	69	25.6	50	18.5	71.7	0.72	69	25.5	82	24.2
All ages	87	3.3	90	3.4	66.7	1.03	84	3.2	99	3.2
Total	190	3.6	236	4.5	65.1	1.24	183	3.5	228	3.7

For epidemiological sources see Murray et al. 1996. For the methods used to estimate and project incidence, prevalence, and deaths see Murray and Lopez 1996a. See explanatory notes for definitions and caveats.

Table 148
Trachea, bronchus and
lung cancers
Cases

Cuadro 148
Cánceres de traquea,
bronquios y pulmones
Casos

Tableau 148
Cancers de la trachée, des
bronches et du poumon
Cas

Table 148a   EME - PEMC - EMBE   Trachea, bronchus and lung cancers - Cases

Age group (years)	Incidence 1990 Number ('000s)	Rate (per 100 000)	Prevalence 1990 Number ('000s)	Rate (per 100 000)	Avg. age at onset (years)	Average duration (years)	Deaths 1990 Number ('000s)	Rate (per 100 000)	Deaths 2000 (Projected) Number ('000s)	Rate (per 100 000)
Males										
0-4	0	0.1	0	0.1	2.5	2.7	0	0.1	0	0.1
5-14	0	0.0	0	0.1	10.0	2.7	0	0.0	0	0.0
15-44	8	4.2	21	11.5	29.9	2.7	6	3.1	8	4.4
45-59	57	86.5	121	182.4	52.4	2.1	50	75.6	68	86.3
60+	241	397.7	426	702.9	71.1	1.8	223	368.8	238	330.2
All ages	306	78.3	567	145.3	66.5	1.9	279	71.5	315	76.6
Females										
0-4	0	0.0	0	0.0	2.5	3.1	0	0.0	0	0.0
5-14	0	0.0	0	0.1	10.0	3.1	0	0.0	0	0.0
15-44	4	2.3	13	7.1	30.0	3.1	3	1.5	3	1.7
45-59	24	34.7	68	100.4	52.4	2.9	17	24.4	22	26.9
60+	97	114.8	226	266.9	72.4	2.3	81	95.7	100	102.6
All ages	125	30.6	307	75.3	67.2	2.5	100	24.6	125	29.1
Total	430	54.0	874	109.6	66.7	2.0	379	47.5	439	52.4

Table 148b   FSE - PEAS - AESE   Trachea, bronchus and lung cancers - Cases

Age group (years)	Incidence 1990 Number ('000s)	Rate (per 100 000)	Prevalence 1990 Number ('000s)	Rate (per 100 000)	Avg. age at onset (years)	Average duration (years)	Deaths 1990 Number ('000s)	Rate (per 100 000)	Deaths 2000 (Projected) Number ('000s)	Rate (per 100 000)
Males										
0-4	0	0.3	0	0.3	2.5	2.6	0	0.2	0	0.2
5-14	0	0.1	0	0.4	10.0	2.6	0	0.1	0	0.1
15-44	6	8.4	17	21.7	29.8	2.6	5	6.6	6	7.6
45-59	51	189.4	102	379.8	52.2	2.0	46	168.9	62	198.5
60+	74	352.2	125	595.0	70.0	1.7	69	330.2	99	389.3
All ages	131	79.5	244	147.5	61.1	1.9	120	72.5	167	97.6
Females										
0-4	0	0.0	0	0.0	2.5	2.9	0	0.0	0	0.0
5-14	0	0.1	0	0.3	10.0	2.9	0	0.1	0	0.1
15-44	2	2.5	5	7.3	29.9	2.9	1	1.7	1	1.5
45-59	8	25.8	21	70.3	52.4	2.7	6	19.2	7	19.4
60+	20	53.8	43	118.6	71.5	2.2	17	46.1	23	56.2
All ages	29	16.2	70	38.6	63.7	2.4	24	13.2	31	16.6
Total	161	46.4	314	90.6	61.6	2.0	144	41.5	198	55.3

Table 148c   India - India - Inde   Trachea, bronchus and lung cancers - Cases

Age group (years)	Incidence 1990 Number ('000s)	Rate (per 100 000)	Prevalence 1990 Number ('000s)	Rate (per 100 000)	Avg. age at onset (years)	Average duration (years)	Deaths 1990 Number ('000s)	Rate (per 100 000)	Deaths 2000 (Projected) Number ('000s)	Rate (per 100 000)
Males										
0-4	0	0.0	0	0.0	2.5	2.1	0	0.0	0	0.0
5-14	0	0.0	0	0.0	10.0	2.1	0	0.0	0	0.0
15-44	2	1.1	5	2.4	29.8	2.1	2	1.0	6	2.6
45-59	11	22.5	18	38.0	52.3	1.7	10	21.1	30	50.0
60+	17	58.5	25	84.7	69.7	1.4	17	56.4	38	103.2
All ages	30	6.9	48	10.9	60.6	1.6	29	6.6	74	14.5
Females										
0-4	0	0.0	0	0.0	2.5	2.4	0	0.0	0	0.0
5-14	0	0.0	0	0.0	10.0	2.4	0	0.0	0	0.0
15-44	1	0.3	1	0.8	29.8	2.4	1	0.3	2	0.8
45-59	2	4.4	5	9.8	52.4	2.2	2	3.8	5	9.5
60+	4	14.2	8	26.2	70.1	1.8	4	13.1	10	26.5
All ages	7	1.7	14	3.3	60.9	2.0	6	1.5	18	3.7
Total	37	4.4	62	7.3	60.6	1.7	35	4.1	92	9.2

For epidemiological sources see Murray et al. 1996. For the methods used to estimate and project incidence, prevalence, and deaths see Murray and Lopez 1996a. See explanatory notes for definitions and caveats.

Table 148 Trachea, bronchus and lung cancers Cases	Cuadro 148 Cánceres de traquea, bronquios y pulmones Casos	Tableau 148 Cancers de la trachée, des bronches et du poumon Cas

Table 148d   China - China - Chine   Trachea, bronchus and lung cancers - Cases

Age group (years)	Incidence 1990 Number ('000s)	Rate (per 100 000)	Prevalence 1990 Number ('000s)	Rate (per 100 000)	Avg. age at onset (years)	Average duration (years)	Deaths 1990 Number ('000s)	Rate (per 100 000)	Deaths 2000 (Projected) Number ('000s)	Rate (per 100 000)
Males										
0-4	0	0.4	0	0.4	2.5	2.3	0	0.3	0	0.4
5-14	0	0.5	1	1.1	10.0	2.3	0	0.4	0	0.4
15-44	6	2.0	15	4.8	29.9	2.3	5	1.7	11	3.6
45-59	38	52.5	70	96.9	52.3	1.8	35	48.1	73	74.7
60+	117	239.0	184	374.9	69.8	1.6	111	227.5	150	249.1
All ages	162	27.7	270	46.1	63.9	1.7	152	26.0	235	35.9
Females										
0-4	0	0.0	0	0.0	-	-	0	0.0	0	0.0
5-14	0	0.0	0	0.0	-	-	0	0.0	0	0.0
15-44	4	1.2	9	3.3	29.9	2.6	3	0.9	3	1.1
45-59	19	29.8	47	73.6	52.4	2.5	15	24.0	24	26.0
60+	54	103.9	108	209.8	70.6	2.0	48	92.4	63	97.2
All ages	76	13.9	165	30.1	64.2	2.2	66	12.0	90	14.3
Total	239	21.0	435	38.4	64.0	1.8	218	19.2	325	25.4

Table 148e   OAI - OPAI - APAI   Trachea, bronchus and lung cancers - Cases

Age group (years)	Incidence 1990 Number ('000s)	Rate (per 100 000)	Prevalence 1990 Number ('000s)	Rate (per 100 000)	Avg. age at onset (years)	Average duration (years)	Deaths 1990 Number ('000s)	Rate (per 100 000)	Deaths 2000 (Projected) Number ('000s)	Rate (per 100 000)
Males										
0-4	0	0.2	0	0.2	2.5	2.3	0	0.2	0	0.2
5-14	0	0.3	1	0.7	10.0	2.3	0	0.3	0	0.2
15-44	4	2.3	8	5.2	29.7	2.3	3	2.0	6	3.0
45-59	21	60.6	37	108.8	52.3	1.8	19	56.0	32	69.9
60+	43	214.9	66	328.9	69.6	1.5	42	205.4	60	218.0
All ages	68	19.9	113	32.9	61.9	1.7	64	18.7	99	24.5
Females										
0-4	0	0.2	0	0.3	2.5	2.6	0	0.2	0	0.2
5-14	0	0.2	0	0.5	10.0	2.6	0	0.2	0	0.1
15-44	1	0.9	4	2.4	29.8	2.6	1	0.7	1	0.7
45-59	6	17.3	15	41.4	52.3	2.4	5	14.2	8	16.2
60+	17	73.6	33	144.2	70.3	2.0	15	66.1	23	70.8
All ages	24	7.2	52	15.2	62.7	2.1	21	6.3	32	8.0
Total	93	13.6	164	24.1	62.1	1.8	85	12.5	131	16.3

Table 148f   SSA - ASS - ASS   Trachea, bronchus and lung cancers - Cases

Age group (years)	Incidence 1990 Number ('000s)	Rate (per 100 000)	Prevalence 1990 Number ('000s)	Rate (per 100 000)	Avg. age at onset (years)	Average duration (years)	Deaths 1990 Number ('000s)	Rate (per 100 000)	Deaths 2000 (Projected) Number ('000s)	Rate (per 100 000)
Males										
0-4	0	0.0	0	0.0	2.4	2.0	0	0.0	0	0.0
5-14	0	0.0	0	0.0	10.0	2.0	0	0.0	0	0.0
15-44	1	1.2	3	2.4	29.4	2.0	1	1.1	2	1.4
45-59	6	29.0	10	47.3	52.2	1.6	6	27.4	7	25.9
60+	8	80.8	12	113.4	69.2	1.4	8	78.3	11	79.5
All ages	16	6.2	24	9.5	59.6	1.5	15	5.9	20	5.9
Females										
0-4	0	0.0	0	0.0	-	-	0	0.0	0	0.0
5-14	0	0.0	0	0.0	-	-	0	0.0	0	0.0
15-44	1	0.5	1	1.1	29.5	2.3	0	0.3	1	0.7
45-59	2	8.9	4	18.9	52.2	2.1	2	7.7	3	9.7
60+	3	23.3	5	41.3	69.7	1.8	3	21.6	5	25.8
All ages	5	2.1	11	4.1	59.6	1.9	5	1.8	8	2.4
Total	21	4.1	35	6.8	59.6	1.6	20	3.8	29	4.1

For epidemiological sources see Murray et al. 1996. For the methods used to estimate and project incidence, prevalence, and deaths see Murray and Lopez 1996a. See explanatory notes for definitions and caveats.

Table 148	Cuadro 148	Tableau 148
Trachea, bronchus and lung cancers	Cánceres de traquea, bronquios y pulmones	Cancers de la trachée, des bronches et du poumon
Cases	Casos	Cas

Table 148g   LAC - ALC - ALC   Trachea, bronchus and lung cancers - Cases

Age group (years)	Incidence 1990 Number ('000s)	Rate (per 100 000)	Prevalence 1990 Number ('000s)	Rate (per 100 000)	Avg. age at onset (years)	Average duration (years)	Deaths 1990 Number ('000s)	Rate (per 100 000)	Deaths 2000 (Projected) Number ('000s)	Rate (per 100 000)
Males										
0-4	0	0.0	0	0.0	2.5	2.4	0	0.0	0	0.0
5-14	0	0.1	0	0.1	10.0	2.4	0	0.0	0	0.0
15-44	2	1.6	4	3.8	29.8	2.4	1	1.3	3	2.0
45-59	7	33.3	14	63.1	52.3	1.9	7	30.3	11	36.1
60+	18	124.4	28	199.6	70.3	1.6	17	117.9	23	118.5
All ages	27	12.1	46	21.0	62.8	1.7	25	11.2	37	14.0
Females										
0-4	0	0.0	0	0.0	2.5	2.7	0	0.0	0	0.0
5-14	0	0.0	0	0.1	10.0	2.7	0	0.0	0	0.0
15-44	1	0.8	2	2.1	29.9	2.7	1	0.6	1	0.9
45-59	3	11.0	7	28.0	52.4	2.5	2	8.6	5	14.3
60+	7	43.9	15	91.0	71.1	2.1	6	38.6	10	41.4
All ages	11	4.8	24	10.8	63.5	2.2	9	4.1	15	5.8
Total	38	8.5	71	15.9	63.0	1.9	34	7.7	53	9.9

Table 148h   MEC - AOM - CMO   Trachea, bronchus and lung cancers - Cases

Age group (years)	Incidence 1990 Number ('000s)	Rate (per 100 000)	Prevalence 1990 Number ('000s)	Rate (per 100 000)	Avg. age at onset (years)	Average duration (years)	Deaths 1990 Number ('000s)	Rate (per 100 000)	Deaths 2000 (Projected) Number ('000s)	Rate (per 100 000)
Males										
0-4	0	0.1	0	0.1	2.5	2.3	0	0.1	0	0.1
5-14	0	0.2	0	0.6	10.0	2.3	0	0.2	0	0.2
15-44	2	2.0	5	4.6	29.8	2.3	2	1.7	4	2.8
45-59	10	46.5	19	83.4	52.3	1.8	10	42.9	19	61.2
60+	13	94.2	20	144.2	69.7	1.5	12	90.1	26	139.5
All ages	26	10.1	44	17.2	58.6	1.7	24	9.4	50	14.9
Females										
0-4	0	0.1	0	0.1	2.5	2.6	0	0.1	0	0.1
5-14	0	0.3	0	0.7	10.0	2.6	0	0.2	0	0.2
15-44	1	0.6	2	1.6	29.8	2.6	1	0.5	1	0.8
45-59	2	9.1	5	21.8	52.3	2.4	2	7.5	4	12.4
60+	4	26.7	8	52.3	70.4	2.0	4	24.0	9	40.5
All ages	7	2.8	15	6.1	59.5	2.2	6	2.5	14	4.3
Total	33	6.5	59	11.7	58.8	1.8	30	6.0	64	9.7

Table 148i   World - Mundo - Monde   Trachea, bronchus and lung cancers - Cases

Age group (years)	Incidence 1990 Number ('000s)	Rate (per 100 000)	Prevalence 1990 Number ('000s)	Rate (per 100 000)	Avg. age at onset (years)	Average duration (years)	Deaths 1990 Number ('000s)	Rate (per 100 000)	Deaths 2000 (Projected) Number ('000s)	Rate (per 100 000)
Males										
0-4	0	0.1	0	0.1	2.5	2.3	0	0.1	0	0.1
5-14	1	0.2	2	0.4	10.0	2.3	1	0.2	1	0.2
15-44	32	2.5	77	6.2	29.8	2.3	25	2.0	46	3.2
45-59	202	64.5	391	125.2	52.3	1.9	182	58.1	303	75.2
60+	532	242.9	886	404.7	70.1	1.6	500	228.3	647	235.0
All ages	766	28.9	1 357	51.1	62.3	1.7	708	26.7	997	32.2
Females										
0-4	0	0.1	0	0.1	2.5	2.6	0	0.0	0	0.0
5-14	0	0.1	1	0.2	10.0	2.6	0	0.1	0	0.1
15-44	14	1.1	38	3.2	29.8	2.6	10	0.8	14	1.0
45-59	65	20.9	171	55.0	52.4	2.5	50	16.0	76	19.0
60+	206	76.4	446	165.7	71.2	2.1	177	65.8	242	71.8
All ages	285	10.9	656	25.1	63.0	2.2	237	9.1	333	10.9
Total	1 051	20.0	2 013	38.2	62.5	1.8	945	17.9	1 331	21.6

For epidemiological sources see Murray et al. 1996. For the methods used to estimate and project incidence, prevalence, and deaths see Murray and Lopez 1996a. See explanatory notes for definitions and caveats.

Table 149
Melanoma and other skin cancers
Cases

Cuadro 149
Melanoma y otros tumores de la piel
Casos

Tableau 149
Mélanome et autres tumeurs cutanées
Cas

Table 149a   EME - PEMC - EMBE   Melanoma and other skin cancers - Cases

Age group (years)	Incidence 1990 Number ('000s)	Rate (per 100 000)	Prevalence 1990 Number ('000s)	Rate (per 100 000)	Avg. age at onset (years)	Average duration (years)	Deaths 1990 Number ('000s)	Rate (per 100 000)	Deaths 2000 (Projected) Number ('000s)	Rate (per 100 000)
Males										
0-4	0	0.1	0	0.1	2.5	4.6	0	0.0	0	0.0
5-14	0	0.0	0	0.2	10.0	4.6	0	0.0	0	0.0
15-44	13	6.9	59	32.1	29.9	4.6	2	1.0	2	1.0
45-59	13	20.2	59	90.0	52.4	4.4	3	4.3	3	4.3
60+	28	46.0	118	194.7	71.1	4.2	8	13.3	9	12.6
All ages	54	13.8	237	60.6	56.7	4.4	13	3.3	14	3.5
Females										
0-4	0	0.0	0	0.0	-	-	0	0.0	0	0.0
5-14	0	0.1	0	0.6	10.0	4.8	0	0.0	0	0.0
15-44	16	9.1	79	44.0	30.0	4.8	1	0.7	1	0.7
45-59	11	16.0	50	73.5	52.4	4.6	2	2.5	2	2.2
60+	22	26.6	95	112.3	72.4	4.2	7	7.8	7	7.4
All ages	50	12.2	224	55.0	54.0	4.5	10	2.3	10	2.4
Total	104	13.0	460	57.7	55.4	4.4	22	2.8	24	2.9

Table 149b   FSE - PEAS - AESE   Melanoma and other skin cancers - Cases

Age group (years)	Incidence 1990 Number ('000s)	Rate (per 100 000)	Prevalence 1990 Number ('000s)	Rate (per 100 000)	Avg. age at onset (years)	Average duration (years)	Deaths 1990 Number ('000s)	Rate (per 100 000)	Deaths 2000 (Projected) Number ('000s)	Rate (per 100 000)
Males										
0-4	0	0.1	0	0.2	2.5	4.4	0	0.0	0	0.0
5-14	0	0.1	0	0.3	10.0	4.4	0	0.0	0	0.0
15-44	3	3.7	12	16.3	29.8	4.4	1	0.9	1	0.9
45-59	4	13.3	15	56.2	52.2	4.2	1	4.0	2	4.9
60+	6	29.3	25	117.6	70.0	4.0	2	10.7	3	12.6
All ages	13	7.6	52	31.7	55.7	4.2	4	2.4	5	3.2
Females										
0-4	0	0.4	0	0.7	2.5	4.6	0	0.1	0	0.1
5-14	0	0.1	0	0.5	10.0	4.6	0	0.0	0	0.0
15-44	4	4.9	17	22.4	29.9	4.6	1	0.9	1	0.8
45-59	3	10.5	14	45.9	52.4	4.4	1	2.6	1	2.4
60+	8	22.9	33	91.7	71.5	4.0	3	8.4	4	8.7
All ages	15	8.4	64	35.5	57.1	4.2	5	2.5	5	2.7
Total	28	8.0	117	33.7	56.5	4.2	8	2.5	10	2.9

Table 149c   India - India - Inde   Melanoma and other skin cancers - Cases

Age group (years)	Incidence 1990 Number ('000s)	Rate (per 100 000)	Prevalence 1990 Number ('000s)	Rate (per 100 000)	Avg. age at onset (years)	Average duration (years)	Deaths 1990 Number ('000s)	Rate (per 100 000)	Deaths 2000 (Projected) Number ('000s)	Rate (per 100 000)
Males										
0-4	0	0.0	0	0.0	2.5	3.7	0	0.0	0	0.0
5-14	0	0.0	0	0.1	10.0	3.7	0	0.0	0	0.0
15-44	0	0.1	1	0.3	29.8	3.7	0	0.0	0	0.0
45-59	0	0.9	2	3.2	52.3	3.6	0	0.5	0	0.5
60+	0	1.2	1	4.0	69.7	3.4	0	0.7	0	0.7
All ages	1	0.2	3	0.8	53.4	3.5	1	0.1	1	0.1
Females										
0-4	0	0.0	0	0.0	2.5	3.8	0	0.0	0	0.0
5-14	0	0.0	0	0.1	10.0	3.8	0	0.0	0	0.0
15-44	0	0.1	1	0.4	29.8	3.8	0	0.0	0	0.0
45-59	0	1.0	2	3.6	52.4	3.7	0	0.5	0	0.5
60+	0	1.5	2	5.2	70.1	3.4	0	0.9	0	0.9
All ages	1	0.3	4	1.0	54.5	3.6	1	0.1	1	0.2
Total	2	0.2	7	0.9	54.0	3.6	1	0.1	1	0.1

For epidemiological sources see Murray et al. 1996. For the methods used to estimate and project incidence, prevalence, and deaths see Murray and Lopez 1996a. See explanatory notes for definitions and caveats.

Table 149
Melanoma and other skin cancers
Cases

Cuadro 149
Melanoma y otros tumores de la piel
Casos

Tableau 149
Mélanome et autres tumeurs cutanées
Cas

Table 149d   China - China - Chine   Melanoma and other skin cancers - Cases

Age group (years)	Incidence 1990 Number ('000s)	Rate (per 100 000)	Prevalence 1990 Number ('000s)	Rate (per 100 000)	Avg. age at onset (years)	Average duration (years)	Deaths 1990 Number ('000s)	Rate (per 100 000)	Deaths 2000 (Projected) Number ('000s)	Rate (per 100 000)
Males										
0-4	0	0.0	0	0.0	2.5	4.0	0	0.0	0	0.0
5-14	0	0.0	0	0.1	10.0	4.0	0	0.0	0	0.0
15-44	0	0.1	1	0.4	29.9	4.0	0	0.0	0	0.0
45-59	0	0.5	1	1.9	52.3	3.9	0	0.2	0	0.2
60+	1	1.8	3	6.7	69.8	3.7	0	0.9	1	1.0
All ages	2	0.3	6	1.0	57.0	3.8	1	0.1	1	0.2
Females										
0-4	0	0.0	0	0.0	-	-	0	0.0	0	0.0
5-14	0	0.0	0	0.0	-	-	0	0.0	0	0.0
15-44	0	0.1	1	0.3	29.9	4.2	0	0.0	0	0.0
45-59	0	0.4	1	1.7	52.4	4.0	0	0.2	0	0.2
60+	1	1.3	2	4.6	70.6	3.7	0	0.6	0	0.7
All ages	1	0.2	4	0.8	58.6	3.9	0	0.1	1	0.1
Total	3	0.2	10	0.9	57.7	3.8	1	0.1	2	0.1

Table 149e   OAI - OPAI - APAI   Melanoma and other skin cancers - Cases

Age group (years)	Incidence 1990 Number ('000s)	Rate (per 100 000)	Prevalence 1990 Number ('000s)	Rate (per 100 000)	Avg. age at onset (years)	Average duration (years)	Deaths 1990 Number ('000s)	Rate (per 100 000)	Deaths 2000 (Projected) Number ('000s)	Rate (per 100 000)
Males										
0-4	0	0.1	0	0.1	2.5	3.9	0	0.0	0	0.0
5-14	0	0.1	0	0.3	10.0	3.9	0	0.0	0	0.0
15-44	0	0.2	2	1.0	29.7	3.9	0	0.1	0	0.1
45-59	1	1.9	3	7.3	52.3	3.8	0	0.9	0	0.9
60+	1	4.2	3	15.1	69.6	3.6	0	2.1	1	2.2
All ages	2	0.6	7	2.1	53.3	3.7	1	0.3	1	0.3
Females										
0-4	0	0.0	0	0.0	-	-	0	0.0	0	0.0
5-14	0	0.0	0	0.0	-	-	0	0.0	0	0.0
15-44	0	0.3	2	1.2	29.8	4.1	0	0.1	0	0.1
45-59	1	2.2	3	8.5	52.3	3.9	0	0.9	0	0.8
60+	2	7.8	6	28.2	70.3	3.6	1	4.0	1	4.0
All ages	3	0.9	11	3.3	59.3	3.7	1	0.4	2	0.5
Total	5	0.7	19	2.7	56.9	3.7	2	0.3	3	0.4

Table 149f   SSA - ASS - ASS   Melanoma and other skin cancers - Cases

Age group (years)	Incidence 1990 Number ('000s)	Rate (per 100 000)	Prevalence 1990 Number ('000s)	Rate (per 100 000)	Avg. age at onset (years)	Average duration (years)	Deaths 1990 Number ('000s)	Rate (per 100 000)	Deaths 2000 (Projected) Number ('000s)	Rate (per 100 000)
Males										
0-4	0	0.0	0	0.0	2.4	3.6	0	0.0	0	0.0
5-14	0	0.0	0	0.1	10.0	3.6	0	0.0	0	0.0
15-44	1	0.5	2	1.9	29.4	3.6	0	0.3	0	0.3
45-59	2	11.5	8	39.6	52.2	3.4	1	6.3	2	6.1
60+	3	27.7	10	91.5	69.2	3.3	2	16.4	2	16.9
All ages	6	2.3	20	7.8	58.3	3.4	3	1.3	4	1.3
Females										
0-4	0	0.0	0	0.0	2.4	3.7	0	0.0	0	0.0
5-14	0	0.1	0	0.2	10.0	3.7	0	0.0	0	0.0
15-44	1	0.7	3	2.4	29.5	3.7	0	0.2	0	0.2
45-59	3	11.9	9	42.3	52.2	3.6	1	6.1	2	5.7
60+	6	45.1	19	148.7	69.7	3.3	3	26.8	4	25.6
All ages	9	3.5	31	12.0	61.2	3.4	5	1.9	6	1.8
Total	15	2.9	51	10.0	60.0	3.4	8	1.6	11	1.6

For epidemiological sources see Murray et al. 1996. For the methods used to estimate and project incidence, prevalence, and deaths see Murray and Lopez 1996a. See explanatory notes for definitions and caveats.

Table 149
Melanoma and other skin cancers
Cases

Cuadro 149
Melanoma y otros tumores de la piel
Casos

Tableau 149
Mélanome et autres tumeurs cutanées
Cas

Table 149g   LAC - ALC - ALC   Melanoma and other skin cancers - Cases

Age group (years)	Incidence 1990 Number ('000s)	Rate (per 100 000)	Prevalence 1990 Number ('000s)	Rate (per 100 000)	Avg. age at onset (years)	Average duration (years)	Deaths 1990 Number ('000s)	Rate (per 100 000)	Deaths 2000 (Projected) Number ('000s)	Rate (per 100 000)
Males										
0-4	0	0.0	0	0.1	2.5	4.1	0	0.0	0	0.0
5-14	0	0.1	0	0.3	10.0	4.1	0	0.0	0	0.0
15-44	1	0.9	4	3.8	29.8	4.1	0	0.3	0	0.3
45-59	1	4.9	4	19.5	52.3	4.0	0	1.9	1	1.9
60+	1	10.5	6	39.9	70.3	3.8	1	4.6	1	4.8
All ages	4	1.6	14	6.4	53.0	3.9	1	0.6	2	0.7
Females										
0-4	0	0.1	0	0.2	2.5	4.3	0	0.0	0	0.0
5-14	0	0.2	0	0.6	10.0	4.3	0	0.0	0	0.0
15-44	1	1.1	5	4.8	29.9	4.3	0	0.3	0	0.3
45-59	1	5.4	5	22.0	52.4	4.1	0	1.8	1	1.7
60+	2	11.9	8	44.9	71.1	3.8	1	5.3	1	5.3
All ages	5	2.0	18	8.1	53.9	4.0	2	0.7	2	0.8
Total	8	1.8	32	7.3	53.5	4.0	3	0.7	4	0.8

Table 149h   MEC - AOM - CMO   Melanoma and other skin cancers - Cases

Age group (years)	Incidence 1990 Number ('000s)	Rate (per 100 000)	Prevalence 1990 Number ('000s)	Rate (per 100 000)	Avg. age at onset (years)	Average duration (years)	Deaths 1990 Number ('000s)	Rate (per 100 000)	Deaths 2000 (Projected) Number ('000s)	Rate (per 100 000)
Males										
0-4	0	0.0	0	0.0	2.5	3.9	0	0.0	0	0.0
5-14	0	0.0	0	0.1	10.0	3.9	0	0.0	0	0.0
15-44	0	0.3	1	1.3	29.8	3.9	0	0.1	0	0.1
45-59	1	3.1	3	11.7	52.3	3.8	0	1.4	0	1.4
60+	0	3.5	2	12.6	69.7	3.6	0	1.8	0	1.7
All ages	2	0.6	6	2.3	51.5	3.8	1	0.3	1	0.3
Females										
0-4	0	0.0	0	0.0	-	-	0	0.0	0	0.0
5-14	0	0.0	0	0.0	-	-	0	0.0	0	0.0
15-44	0	0.3	1	1.4	29.8	4.1	0	0.1	0	0.1
45-59	0	1.5	1	5.9	52.3	3.9	0	0.6	0	0.6
60+	0	2.6	1	9.2	70.4	3.6	0	1.3	0	1.2
All ages	1	0.4	4	1.7	51.3	3.8	0	0.2	1	0.2
Total	3	0.5	10	2.0	51.4	3.8	1	0.2	2	0.2

Table 149i   World - Mundo - Monde   Melanoma and other skin cancers - Cases

Age group (years)	Incidence 1990 Number ('000s)	Rate (per 100 000)	Prevalence 1990 Number ('000s)	Rate (per 100 000)	Avg. age at onset (years)	Average duration (years)	Deaths 1990 Number ('000s)	Rate (per 100 000)	Deaths 2000 (Projected) Number ('000s)	Rate (per 100 000)
Males										
0-4	0	0.0	0	0.1	2.5	4.1	0	0.0	0	0.0
5-14	0	0.0	1	0.2	10.0	4.0	0	0.0	0	0.0
15-44	18	1.5	82	6.6	29.9	4.5	4	0.3	4	0.3
45-59	23	7.2	95	30.4	52.3	4.2	7	2.1	8	2.1
60+	41	18.7	167	76.3	70.7	4.1	14	6.4	18	6.4
All ages	82	3.1	346	13.0	56.3	4.2	24	0.9	30	1.0
Females										
0-4	0	0.0	0	0.1	2.5	4.3	0	0.0	0	0.0
5-14	0	0.0	1	0.2	10.0	4.3	0	0.0	0	0.0
15-44	23	1.9	108	9.0	30.0	4.7	3	0.2	3	0.2
45-59	20	6.3	85	27.4	52.4	4.3	5	1.6	6	1.4
60+	42	15.5	167	61.9	71.6	4.0	16	5.8	19	5.6
All ages	85	3.3	361	13.8	55.6	4.2	24	0.9	28	0.9
Total	167	3.2	707	13.4	55.9	4.2	48	0.9	58	0.9

For epidemiological sources see Murray et al. 1996. For the methods used to estimate and project incidence, prevalence, and deaths see Murray and Lopez 1996a. See explanatory notes for definitions and caveats.

Table 150
Breast cancer

Cuadro 150
Cáncer de mama

Tableau 150
Cancer du sein

Cases

Casos

Cas

Table 150a — EME - PEMC - EMBE — Breast cancer - Cases

Age group (years)	Incidence 1990 Number ('000s)	Incidence 1990 Rate (per 100 000)	Prevalence 1990 Number ('000s)	Prevalence 1990 Rate (per 100 000)	Avg. age at onset (years)	Average duration (years)	Deaths 1990 Number ('000s)	Deaths 1990 Rate (per 100 000)	Deaths 2000 (Projected) Number ('000s)	Deaths 2000 (Projected) Rate (per 100 000)
Males										
0-4	0	0	0	0	-	-	0	0	0	0
5-14	0	0	0	0	-	-	0	0	0	0
15-44	0	0	0	0	-	-	0	0	0	0
45-59	0	0	0	0	-	-	0	0	0	0
60+	0	0	0	0	-	-	0	0	0	0
All ages	0	0	0	0	-	-	0	0	0	0
Females										
0-4	0	0	0	0.1	2.5	4.6	0	0.0	0	0.0
5-14	0	0	0	0.1	10.0	4.6	0	0.0	0	0.0
15-44	83	46	386	215.5	30.0	4.6	11	6.4	11	6.4
45-59	140	207	618	910.8	52.4	4.4	32	47.9	35	42.8
60+	299	354	1 259	1 488.3	72.4	4.2	90	106.5	96	98.7
All ages	523	128	2 262	555.5	60.3	4.3	134	32.9	142	33.1
Total	523	66	2 262	283.6	60.3	4.3	134	16.8	142	16.9

Table 150b — FSE - PEAS - AESE — Breast cancer - Cases

Age group (years)	Incidence 1990 Number ('000s)	Incidence 1990 Rate (per 100 000)	Prevalence 1990 Number ('000s)	Prevalence 1990 Rate (per 100 000)	Avg. age at onset (years)	Average duration (years)	Deaths 1990 Number ('000s)	Deaths 1990 Rate (per 100 000)	Deaths 2000 (Projected) Number ('000s)	Deaths 2000 (Projected) Rate (per 100 000)
Males										
0-4	0	0	0	0	-	-	0	0	0	0
5-14	0	0	0	0	-	-	0	0	0	0
15-44	0	0	0	0	-	-	0	0	0	0
45-59	0	0	0	0	-	-	0	0	0	0
60+	0	0	0	0	-	-	0	0	0	0
All ages	0	0	0	0	-	-	0	0	0	0
Females										
0-4	0	0	0	0.1	2.5	4.5	0	0.0	0	0.0
5-14	0	0	0	0.1	10.0	4.5	0	0.0	0	0.0
15-44	24	32	107	143.3	29.9	4.5	5	6.2	4	5.6
45-59	48	159	203	674.9	52.4	4.3	13	44.7	14	42.0
60+	62	171	254	698.0	71.5	4.1	22	59.5	23	56.4
All ages	134	74	564	311.7	57.3	4.2	40	22.0	42	22.4
Total	134	39	564	162.9	57.3	4.2	40	11.5	42	11.7

Table 150c — India - India - Inde — Breast cancer - Cases

Age group (years)	Incidence 1990 Number ('000s)	Incidence 1990 Rate (per 100 000)	Prevalence 1990 Number ('000s)	Prevalence 1990 Rate (per 100 000)	Avg. age at onset (years)	Average duration (years)	Deaths 1990 Number ('000s)	Deaths 1990 Rate (per 100 000)	Deaths 2000 (Projected) Number ('000s)	Deaths 2000 (Projected) Rate (per 100 000)
Males										
0-4	0	0	0	0	-	-	0	0	0	0
5-14	0	0	0	0	-	-	0	0	0	0
15-44	0	0	0	0	-	-	0	0	0	0
45-59	0	0	0	0	-	-	0	0	0	0
60+	0	0	0	0	-	-	0	0	0	0
All ages	0	0	0	0	-	-	0	0	0	0
Females										
0-4	0	0	0	0.0	2.5	4.1	0	0.0	0	0.0
5-14	0	0	0	0.1	10.0	4.1	0	0.0	0	0.0
15-44	21	12	87	47.6	29.8	4.1	7	4.0	9	3.8
45-59	34	75	133	289.9	52.4	3.9	14	31.0	17	30.2
60+	28	96	103	356.1	70.1	3.7	13	44.9	18	45.3
All ages	84	20	324	78.9	52.5	3.9	35	8.4	44	9.1
Total	84	10	324	38.1	52.5	3.9	35	4.1	44	4.4

For epidemiological sources see Murray et al. 1996. For the methods used to estimate and project incidence, prevalence, and deaths see Murray and Lopez 1996a. See explanatory notes for definitions and caveats.

Table 150
Breast cancer

Cuadro 150
Cáncer de mama

Tableau 150
Cancer du sein

Cases

Casos

Cas

Table 150d   China - China - Chine

Breast cancer - Cases

Age group (years)	Incidence 1990 Number ('000s)	Rate (per 100 000)	Prevalence 1990 Number ('000s)	Rate (per 100 000)	Avg. age at onset (years)	Average duration (years)	Deaths 1990 Number ('000s)	Rate (per 100 000)	Deaths 2000 (Projected) Number ('000s)	Rate (per 100 000)
Males										
0-4	0	0	0	0	-	-	0	0	0	0
5-14	0	0	0	0	-	-	0	0	0	0
15-44	0	0	0	0	-	-	0	0	0	0
45-59	0	0	0	0	-	-	0	0	0	0
60+	0	0	0	0	-	-	0	0	0	0
All ages	0	0	0	0	-	-	0	0	0	0
Females										
0-4	0	0.0	0	0.1	2.5	4.3	0	0.0	0	0.0
5-14	0	0.0	0	0.1	10.0	4.3	0	0.0	0	0.0
15-44	24	8.4	102	35.8	29.9	4.3	7	2.3	9	3.0
45-59	23	36.3	95	147.0	52.4	4.1	8	12.8	12	13.3
60+	27	52.8	106	204.7	70.6	3.9	11	21.7	16	24.2
All ages	74	13.0	302	55.1	51.9	4.1	26	4.7	37	5.9
Total	74	6.6	302	26.6	51.9	4.1	26	2.3	37	2.9

Table 150e   OAI - OPAI - APAI

Breast cancer - Cases

Age group (years)	Incidence 1990 Number ('000s)	Rate (per 100 000)	Prevalence 1990 Number ('000s)	Rate (per 100 000)	Avg. age at onset (years)	Average duration (years)	Deaths 1990 Number ('000s)	Rate (per 100 000)	Deaths 2000 (Projected) Number ('000s)	Rate (per 100 000)
Males										
0-4	0	0	0	0	-	-	0	0	0	0
5-14	0	0	0	0	-	-	0	0	0	0
15-44	0	0	0	0	-	-	0	0	0	0
45-59	0	0	0	0	-	-	0	0	0	0
60+	0	0	0	0	-	-	0	0	0	0
All ages	0	0	0	0	-	-	0	0	0	0
Females										
0-4	0	0	0	0.1	2.5	4.2	0	0.1	0	0.1
5-14	0	0	0	0.1	10.0	4.2	0	0.1	0	0.1
15-44	20	13	85	53.2	29.8	4.2	6	3.8	8	3.8
45-59	29	82	114	325.9	52.3	4.0	11	30.5	14	29.1
60+	26	113	98	433.1	70.3	3.8	11	48.7	16	48.8
All ages	74	22	297	87.6	52.4	4.0	28	8.2	37	9.3
Total	74	11	297	43.6	52.4	4.0	28	4.1	37	4.6

Table 150f   SSA - ASS - ASS

Breast cancer - Cases

Age group (years)	Incidence 1990 Number ('000s)	Rate (per 100 000)	Prevalence 1990 Number ('000s)	Rate (per 100 000)	Avg. age at onset (years)	Average duration (years)	Deaths 1990 Number ('000s)	Rate (per 100 000)	Deaths 2000 (Projected) Number ('000s)	Rate (per 100 000)
Males										
0-4	0	0	0	0	-	-	0	0	0	0
5-14	0	0	0	0	-	-	0	0	0	0
15-44	0	0	0	0	-	-	0	0	0	0
45-59	0	0	0	0	-	-	0	0	0	0
60+	0	0	0	0	-	-	0	0	0	0
All ages	0	0	0	0	-	-	0	0	0	0
Females										
0-4	0	0.0	0	0.0	2.4	4.0	0	0.0	0	0.0
5-14	0	0.0	0	0.1	10.0	4.0	0	0.1	0	0.1
15-44	9	8.9	38	35.7	29.5	4.0	2	2.0	3	1.8
45-59	15	68.3	58	260.4	52.2	3.8	7	29.7	8	27.6
60+	17	133.8	62	488.5	69.7	3.7	8	65.0	11	62.2
All ages	42	16.1	158	61.2	54.2	3.8	17	6.6	22	6.2
Total	42	8.2	158	30.9	54.2	3.8	17	3.3	22	3.1

For epidemiological sources see Murray et al. 1996. For the methods used to estimate and project incidence, prevalence, and deaths see Murray and Lopez 1996a. See explanatory notes for definitions and caveats.

Table 150   **Cuadro 150**   **Tableau 150**
Breast cancer   **Cáncer de mama**   **Cancer du sein**

Cases   Casos   Cas

Table 150g   LAC - ALC - ALC   Breast cancer - Cases

Age group (years)	Incidence 1990 Number ('000s)	Rate (per 100 000)	Prevalence 1990 Number ('000s)	Rate (per 100 000)	Avg. age at onset (years)	Average duration (years)	Deaths 1990 Number ('000s)	Rate (per 100 000)	Deaths 2000 (Projected) Number ('000s)	Rate (per 100 000)
Males										
0-4	0	0	0	0	-	-	0	0	0	0
5-14	0	0	0	0	-	-	0	0	0	0
15-44	0	0	0	0	-	-	0	0	0	0
45-59	0	0	0	0	-	-	0	0	0	0
60+	0	0	0	0	-	-	0	0	0	0
All ages	0	0	0	0	-	-	0	0	0	0
Females										
0-4	0	0	0	0.1	2.5	4.3	0	0.0	0	0.0
5-14	0	0	0	0.1	10.0	4.3	0	0.0	0	0.0
15-44	21	20	91	87.8	29.9	4.3	5	5.1	7	5.1
45-59	31	135	129	553.6	52.4	4.1	10	44.8	14	43.3
60+	36	216	143	849.6	71.1	3.9	14	84.9	20	84.4
All ages	89	40	364	163.3	54.7	4.1	30	13.5	40	15.1
Total	89	20	364	81.8	54.7	4.1	30	6.8	40	7.6

Table 150h   MEC - AOM - CMO   Breast cancer - Cases

Age group (years)	Incidence 1990 Number ('000s)	Rate (per 100 000)	Prevalence 1990 Number ('000s)	Rate (per 100 000)	Avg. age at onset (years)	Average duration (years)	Deaths 1990 Number ('000s)	Rate (per 100 000)	Deaths 2000 (Projected) Number ('000s)	Rate (per 100 000)
Males										
0-4	0	0	0	0	-	-	0	0	0	0
5-14	0	0	0	0	-	-	0	0	0	0
15-44	0	0	0	0	-	-	0	0	0	0
45-59	0	0	0	0	-	-	0	0	0	0
60+	0	0	0	0	-	-	0	0	0	0
All ages	0	0	0	0	-	-	0	0	0	0
Females										
0-4	0	0.0	0	0.1	2.5	4.2	0	0.0	0	0.0
5-14	0	0.0	0	0.1	10.0	4.2	0	0.1	0	0.1
15-44	11	10.0	45	42.3	29.8	4.2	3	3.0	4	2.8
45-59	13	59.0	53	235.5	52.3	4.0	5	22.0	6	19.7
60+	11	72.4	43	276.7	70.4	3.8	5	31.1	6	28.2
All ages	35	14.2	141	57.0	51.1	4.0	13	5.3	16	5.0
Total	35	7.0	141	28.0	51.1	4.0	13	2.6	16	2.5

Table 150i   World - Mundo - Monde   Breast cancer - Cases

Age group (years)	Incidence 1990 Number ('000s)	Rate (per 100 000)	Prevalence 1990 Number ('000s)	Rate (per 100 000)	Avg. age at onset (years)	Average duration (years)	Deaths 1990 Number ('000s)	Rate (per 100 000)	Deaths 2000 (Projected) Number ('000s)	Rate (per 100 000)
Males										
0-4	0	0	0	0	-	-	0	0	0	0
5-14	0	0	0	0	-	-	0	0	0	0
15-44	0	0	0	0	-	-	0	0	0	0
45-59	0	0	0	0	-	-	0	0	0	0
60+	0	0	0	0	-	-	0	0	0	0
All ages	0	0	0	0	-	-	0	0	0	0
Females										
0-4	0	0	0	0.1	2.5	4.2	0	0.0	0	0.0
5-14	0	0	0	0.1	10.0	4.2	0	0.0	0	0.0
15-44	214	18	942	78.6	29.9	4.4	47	3.9	54	3.9
45-59	334	107	1 402	450.7	52.4	4.2	101	32.5	120	29.8
60+	507	188	2 067	767.9	71.7	4.1	174	64.7	205	61.0
All ages	1 055	40	4 412	168.8	57.1	4.2	322	12.3	380	12.4
Total	1 055	20	4 412	83.8	57.1	4.2	322	6.1	380	6.2

For epidemiological sources see Murray et al. 1996. For the methods used to estimate and project incidence, prevalence, and deaths see Murray and Lopez 1996a. See explanatory notes for definitions and caveats.

Table 151
Cervix uteri cancer

Cuadro 151
Cáncer cervicouterino

Tableau 151
Cancer du col de l'utérus

Cases

Casos

Cas

Table 151a — EME - PEMC - EMBE — Cervix uteri cancer - Cases

Age group (years)	Incidence 1990 Number ('000s)	Rate (per 100 000)	Prevalence 1990 Number ('000s)	Rate (per 100 000)	Avg. age at onset (years)	Average duration (years)	Deaths 1990 Number ('000s)	Rate (per 100 000)	Deaths 2000 (Projected) Number ('000s)	Rate (per 100 000)
Males										
0-4	0	0	0	0	-	-	0	0	0	0
5-14	0	0	0	0	-	-	0	0	0	0
15-44	0	0	0	0	-	-	0	0	0	0
45-59	0	0	0	0	-	-	0	0	0	0
60+	0	0	0	0	-	-	0	0	0	0
All ages	0	0	0	0	-	-	0	0	0	0
Females										
0-4	0	0.0	0	0.0	-	-	0	0.0	0	0.0
5-14	0	0.0	0	0.1	10.0	4.5	0	0.0	0	0.0
15-44	15	8.5	69	38.6	30.0	4.5	3	1.6	3	1.6
45-59	10	14.8	40	58.9	52.4	4.0	4	5.5	4	4.9
60+	16	18.9	54	64.2	72.4	3.4	9	10.7	10	9.8
All ages	41	10.1	164	40.1	51.0	4.0	16	3.8	16	3.8
Total	41	5.2	164	20.5	51.8	4.0	16	2.0	16	1.9

Table 151b — FSE - PEAS - AESE — Cervix uteri cancer - Cases

Age group (years)	Incidence 1990 Number ('000s)	Rate (per 100 000)	Prevalence 1990 Number ('000s)	Rate (per 100 000)	Avg. age at onset (years)	Average duration (years)	Deaths 1990 Number ('000s)	Rate (per 100 000)	Deaths 2000 (Projected) Number ('000s)	Rate (per 100 000)
Males										
0-4	0	0	0	0	-	-	0	0	0	0
5-14	0	0	0	0	-	-	0	0	0	0
15-44	0	0	0	0	-	-	0	0	0	0
45-59	0	0	0	0	-	-	0	0	0	0
60+	0	0	0	0	-	-	0	0	0	0
All ages	0	0	0	0	-	-	0	0	0	0
Females										
0-4	0	0.1	0	0.1	2.5	4.4	0	0.0	0	0.0
5-14	0	0.0	0	0.1	10.0	4.4	0	0.0	0	0.0
15-44	10	13.5	45	60.1	29.9	4.4	2	2.9	2	2.7
45-59	10	33.2	39	130.2	52.4	3.9	4	13.2	4	12.4
60+	16	43.3	53	144.3	71.5	3.3	9	25.3	10	24.1
All ages	36	19.8	137	75.5	54.4	3.8	15	8.5	16	8.7
Total	36	10.4	137	39.5	54.4	3.8	15	4.4	16	4.5

Table 151c — India - India - Inde — Cervix uteri cancer - Cases

Age group (years)	Incidence 1990 Number ('000s)	Rate (per 100 000)	Prevalence 1990 Number ('000s)	Rate (per 100 000)	Avg. age at onset (years)	Average duration (years)	Deaths 1990 Number ('000s)	Rate (per 100 000)	Deaths 2000 (Projected) Number ('000s)	Rate (per 100 000)
Males										
0-4	0	0	0	0	-	-	0	0	0	0
5-14	0	0	0	0	-	-	0	0	0	0
15-44	0	0	0	0	-	-	0	0	0	0
45-59	0	0	0	0	-	-	0	0	0	0
60+	0	0	0	0	-	-	0	0	0	0
All ages	0	0	0	0	-	-	0	0	0	0
Females										
0-4	0	0	0	0	-	-	0	0.0	0	0.0
5-14	0	0	0	0	-	-	0	0.0	0	0.0
15-44	24	13	103	56	29.8	4.2	7	4.0	9	3.8
45-59	54	116	200	434	52.4	3.7	25	53.8	30	52.5
60+	26	91	84	290	70.1	3.2	17	57.1	22	57.3
All ages	104	25	386	94	51.6	3.7	49	11.9	61	12.6
Total	104	12	386	45	51.6	3.7	49	5.7	61	6.1

For epidemiological sources see Murray et al. 1996. For the methods used to estimate and project incidence, prevalence, and deaths see Murray and Lopez 1996a. See explanatory notes for definitions and caveats.

Table 151
Cervix uteri cancer

Cuadro 151
Cáncer cervicouterino

Tableau 151
Cancer du col de l'utérus

Cases

Casos

Cas

Table 151d — China - China - Chine — Cervix uteri cancer - Cases

Age group (years)	Incidence 1990 Number ('000s)	Rate (per 100 000)	Prevalence 1990 Number ('000s)	Rate (per 100 000)	Avg. age at onset (years)	Average duration (years)	Deaths 1990 Number ('000s)	Rate (per 100 000)	Deaths 2000 (Projected) Number ('000s)	Rate (per 100 000)
Males										
0-4	0	0	0	0	-	-	0	0	0	0
5-14	0	0	0	0	-	-	0	0	0	0
15-44	0	0	0	0	-	-	0	0	0	0
45-59	0	0	0	0	-	-	0	0	0	0
60+	0	0	0	0	-	-	0	0	0	0
All ages	0	0	0	0	-	-	0	0	0	0
Females										
0-4	0	0.0	0	0	-	-	0	0.0	0	0.0
5-14	0	0.0	0	0	-	-	0	0.0	0	0.0
15-44	11	4.0	49	17	29.9	4.3	3	1.0	4	1.3
45-59	15	23.7	58	90	52.4	3.8	7	10.2	10	10.6
60+	19	36.9	62	120	70.6	3.3	12	22.4	16	24.7
All ages	46	8.3	169	31	54.5	3.7	21	3.8	29	4.7
Total	46	4.0	169	15	54.5	3.7	21	1.9	29	2.3

Table 151e — OAI - OPAI - APAI — Cervix uteri cancer - Cases

Age group (years)	Incidence 1990 Number ('000s)	Rate (per 100 000)	Prevalence 1990 Number ('000s)	Rate (per 100 000)	Avg. age at onset (years)	Average duration (years)	Deaths 1990 Number ('000s)	Rate (per 100 000)	Deaths 2000 (Projected) Number ('000s)	Rate (per 100 000)
Males										
0-4	0	0	0	0	-	-	0	0	0	0
5-14	0	0	0	0	-	-	0	0	0	0
15-44	0	0	0	0	-	-	0	0	0	0
45-59	0	0	0	0	-	-	0	0	0	0
60+	0	0	0	0	-	-	0	0	0	0
All ages	0	0	0	0	-	-	0	0	0	0
Females										
0-4	0	0.1	0	0.2	2.5	4.3	0	0.0	0	0.0
5-14	0	0.1	0	0.4	10.0	4.3	0	0.0	0	0.0
15-44	21	13.2	90	56.5	29.8	4.3	6	3.6	7	3.7
45-59	32	92.6	123	350.5	52.3	3.8	14	41.0	18	39.0
60+	21	94.1	69	303.7	70.3	3.2	13	57.7	19	57.7
All ages	75	22.1	282	83.1	51.0	3.8	33	9.8	45	11.0
Total	75	11.0	282	41.4	51.0	3.8	33	4.9	45	5.5

Table 151f — SSA - ASS - ASS — Cervix uteri cancer - Cases

Age group (years)	Incidence 1990 Number ('000s)	Rate (per 100 000)	Prevalence 1990 Number ('000s)	Rate (per 100 000)	Avg. age at onset (years)	Average duration (years)	Deaths 1990 Number ('000s)	Rate (per 100 000)	Deaths 2000 (Projected) Number ('000s)	Rate (per 100 000)
Males										
0-4	0	0	0	0	-	-	0	0	0	0
5-14	0	0	0	0	-	-	0	0	0	0
15-44	0	0	0	0	-	-	0	0	0	0
45-59	0	0	0	0	-	-	0	0	0	0
60+	0	0	0	0	-	-	0	0	0	0
All ages	0	0	0	0	-	-	0	0	0	0
Females										
0-4	0	0.1	0	0.1	2.4	4.2	0	0.0	0	0.0
5-14	0	0.1	0	0.4	10.0	4.2	0	0.0	0	0.0
15-44	17	15.9	71	66.4	29.5	4.2	3	3.1	4	2.8
45-59	27	121.4	99	448.5	52.2	3.7	13	57.3	16	53.2
60+	27	212.7	85	670.8	69.7	3.2	17	134.8	23	128.6
All ages	71	27.5	256	99.1	53.4	3.6	33	12.8	42	12.1
Total	71	13.9	256	50.1	53.4	3.6	33	6.5	42	6.1

For epidemiological sources see Murray et al. 1996. For the methods used to estimate and project incidence, prevalence, and deaths see Murray and Lopez 1996a. See explanatory notes for definitions and caveats.

Table 151
Cervix uteri cancer

Cuadro 151
Cáncer cervicouterino

Tableau 151
Cancer du col de l'utérus

Cases

Casos

Cas

Table 151g LAC - ALC - ALC — Cervix uteri cancer - Cases

Age group (years)	Incidence 1990 Number ('000s)	Rate (per 100 000)	Prevalence 1990 Number ('000s)	Rate (per 100 000)	Avg. age at onset (years)	Average duration (years)	Deaths 1990 Number ('000s)	Rate (per 100 000)	Deaths 2000 (Projected) Number ('000s)	Rate (per 100 000)
Males										
0-4	0	0	0	0	-	-	0	0	0	0
5-14	0	0	0	0	-	-	0	0	0	0
15-44	0	0	0	0	-	-	0	0	0	0
45-59	0	0	0	0	-	-	0	0	0	0
60+	0	0	0	0	-	-	0	0	0	0
All ages	0	0	0	0	-	-	0	0	0	0
Females										
0-4	0	0	0	0.0	2.5	4.3	0	0.0	0	0.0
5-14	0	0	0	0.1	10.0	4.3	0	0.0	0	0.0
15-44	23	22	100	96.0	29.9	4.3	6	5.5	7	5.5
45-59	21	89	80	343.4	52.4	3.8	9	37.8	12	36.5
60+	17	100	55	328.4	71.1	3.3	10	60.2	14	59.7
All ages	61	27	235	105.7	49.1	3.9	25	11.1	33	12.3
Total	61	14	235	53.0	49.1	3.9	25	5.5	33	6.2

Table 151h MEC - AOM - CMO — Cervix uteri cancer - Cases

Age group (years)	Incidence 1990 Number ('000s)	Rate (per 100 000)	Prevalence 1990 Number ('000s)	Rate (per 100 000)	Avg. age at onset (years)	Average duration (years)	Deaths 1990 Number ('000s)	Rate (per 100 000)	Deaths 2000 (Projected) Number ('000s)	Rate (per 100 000)
Males										
0-4	0	0	0	0	-	-	0	0	0	0
5-14	0	0	0	0	-	-	0	0	0	0
15-44	0	0	0	0	-	-	0	0	0	0
45-59	0	0	0	0	-	-	0	0	0	0
60+	0	0	0	0	-	-	0	0	0	0
All ages	0	0	0	0	-	-	0	0	0	0
Females										
0-4	0	0.0	0	0.1	2.5	4.3	0	0.0	0	0.0
5-14	0	0.1	0	0.4	10.0	4.3	0	0.0	0	0.0
15-44	6	5.6	26	23.9	29.8	4.3	2	1.5	2	1.4
45-59	8	34.4	29	130.3	52.3	3.8	3	15.2	4	13.6
60+	5	34.8	17	112.3	70.4	3.2	3	21.4	4	19.3
All ages	19	7.7	72	29.3	50.2	3.8	8	3.4	10	3.2
Total	19	3.8	72	14.4	50.2	3.8	8	1.7	10	1.6

Table 151i World - Mundo - Monde — Cervix uteri cancer - Cases

Age group (years)	Incidence 1990 Number ('000s)	Rate (per 100 000)	Prevalence 1990 Number ('000s)	Rate (per 100 000)	Avg. age at onset (years)	Average duration (years)	Deaths 1990 Number ('000s)	Rate (per 100 000)	Deaths 2000 (Projected) Number ('000s)	Rate (per 100 000)
Males										
0-4	0	0	0	0	-	-	0	0	0	0
5-14	0	0	0	0	-	-	0	0	0	0
15-44	0	0	0	0	-	-	0	0	0	0
45-59	0	0	0	0	-	-	0	0	0	0
60+	0	0	0	0	-	-	0	0	0	0
All ages	0	0	0	0	-	-	0	0	0	0
Females										
0-4	0	0.0	0	0.1	2.5	4.3	0	0.0	0	0.0
5-14	0	0.0	1	0.2	10.0	4.3	0	0.0	0	0.0
15-44	128	10.7	552	46.1	29.8	4.3	32	2.6	38	2.7
45-59	177	56.8	668	214.9	52.3	3.8	78	25.2	98	24.3
60+	148	54.9	479	178.0	70.6	3.2	90	33.4	117	34.8
All ages	453	17.3	1 701	65.1	51.9	3.8	200	7.7	253	8.3
Total	453	8.6	1 701	32.3	51.9	3.8	200	3.8	253	4.1

For epidemiological sources see Murray et al. 1996. For the methods used to estimate and project incidence, prevalence, and deaths see Murray and Lopez 1996a. See explanatory notes for definitions and caveats.

Table 152
Corpus uteri cancer

Cuadro 152
Cáncer de cuerpo de utero

Tableau 152
Cancer du corps de l'utérus

Cases   Casos   Cas

Table 152a   EME - PEMC - EMBE   Corpus uteri cancer - Cases

Age group (years)	Incidence 1990 Number ('000s)	Rate (per 100 000)	Prevalence 1990 Number ('000s)	Rate (per 100 000)	Avg. age at onset (years)	Average duration (years)	Deaths 1990 Number ('000s)	Rate (per 100 000)	Deaths 2000 (Projected) Number ('000s)	Rate (per 100 000)
Males										
0-4	0	0	0	0	-	-	0	0	0	0
5-14	0	0	0	0	-	-	0	0	0	0
15-44	0	0	0	0	-	-	0	0	0	0
45-59	0	0	0	0	-	-	0	0	0	0
60+	0	0	0	0	-	-	0	0	0	0
All ages	0	0	0	0	-	-	0	0	0	0
Females										
0-4	0	0.1	0	0.1	2.5	4.8	0	0.0	0	0.0
5-14	0	0.0	0	0.1	10.0	4.8	0	0.0	0	0.0
15-44	10	5.6	48	27.0	30.0	4.8	1	0.4	1	0.4
45-59	36	53.6	173	255.7	52.4	4.8	3	4.8	3	4.3
60+	86	101.8	377	446.2	72.4	4.4	20	24.1	22	22.5
All ages	133	32.5	599	147.1	63.7	4.5	24	6.0	26	6.1
Total	133	16.6	599	75.1	63.7	4.5	24	3.1	26	3.1

Table 152b   FSE - PEAS - AESE   Corpus uteri cancer - Cases

Age group (years)	Incidence 1990 Number ('000s)	Rate (per 100 000)	Prevalence 1990 Number ('000s)	Rate (per 100 000)	Avg. age at onset (years)	Average duration (years)	Deaths 1990 Number ('000s)	Rate (per 100 000)	Deaths 2000 (Projected) Number ('000s)	Rate (per 100 000)
Males										
0-4	0	0	0	0	-	-	0	0	0	0
5-14	0	0	0	0	-	-	0	0	0	0
15-44	0	0	0	0	-	-	0	0	0	0
45-59	0	0	0	0	-	-	0	0	0	0
60+	0	0	0	0	-	-	0	0	0	0
All ages	0	0	0	0	-	-	0	0	0	0
Females										
0-4	0	0.1	0	0.3	2.5	4.7	0	0.0	0	0.0
5-14	0	0.1	0	0.3	10.0	4.7	0	0.0	0	0.0
15-44	6	8.4	30	39.8	29.9	4.7	1	0.9	1	0.9
45-59	24	80.7	113	377.8	52.4	4.7	3	10.0	3	9.4
60+	35	97.0	152	417.6	71.5	4.3	9	25.8	10	24.8
All ages	66	36.4	295	163.2	60.5	4.5	13	7.2	14	7.5
Total	66	19.0	295	85.3	60.5	4.5	13	3.8	14	3.9

Table 152c   India - India - Inde   Corpus uteri cancer - Cases

Age group (years)	Incidence 1990 Number ('000s)	Rate (per 100 000)	Prevalence 1990 Number ('000s)	Rate (per 100 000)	Avg. age at onset (years)	Average duration (years)	Deaths 1990 Number ('000s)	Rate (per 100 000)	Deaths 2000 (Projected) Number ('000s)	Rate (per 100 000)
Males										
0-4	0	0	0	0	-	-	0	0	0	0
5-14	0	0	0	0	-	-	0	0	0	0
15-44	0	0	0	0	-	-	0	0	0	0
45-59	0	0	0	0	-	-	0	0	0	0
60+	0	0	0	0	-	-	0	0	0	0
All ages	0	0	0	0	-	-	0	0	0	0
Females										
0-4	0	0.0	0	0.0	-	-	0	0.0	0	0.0
5-14	0	0.0	0	0.0	-	-	0	0.0	0	0.0
15-44	1	0.5	4	2.0	29.8	4.5	0	0.1	0	0.1
45-59	5	11.0	22	48.7	52.4	4.4	1	2.3	1	2.3
60+	6	21.5	25	87.8	70.1	4.1	2	7.3	3	7.5
All ages	12	2.9	52	12.6	59.9	4.3	3	0.8	4	0.9
Total	12	1.4	52	6.1	59.9	4.3	3	0.4	4	0.4

For epidemiological sources see Murray et al. 1996. For the methods used to estimate and project incidence, prevalence, and deaths see Murray and Lopez 1996a. See explanatory notes for definitions and caveats.

Table 152
Corpus uteri cancer

Cuadro 152
Cáncer de cuerpo de utero

Tableau 152
Cancer du corps de l'utérus

Cases

Casos

Cas

Table 152d   China - China - Chine — Corpus uteri cancer - Cases

Age group (years)	Incidence 1990 Number ('000s)	Rate (per 100 000)	Prevalence 1990 Number ('000s)	Rate (per 100 000)	Avg. age at onset (years)	Average duration (years)	Deaths 1990 Number ('000s)	Rate (per 100 000)	Deaths 2000 (Projected) Number ('000s)	Rate (per 100 000)
Males										
0-4	0	0	0	0	-	-	0	0	0	0
5-14	0	0	0	0	-	-	0	0	0	0
15-44	0	0	0	0	-	-	0	0	0	0
45-59	0	0	0	0	-	-	0	0	0	0
60+	0	0	0	0	-	-	0	0	0	0
All ages	0	0	0	0	-	-	0	0	0	0
Females										
0-4	0	0.0	0	0.0	-	-	0	0.0	0	0.0
5-14	0	0.0	0	0.0	-	-	0	0.0	0	0.0
15-44	4	1.5	20	7.1	29.9	4.6	1	0.2	1	0.3
45-59	17	26.5	78	120.6	52.4	4.6	3	4.6	4	4.7
60+	9	16.7	36	70.0	70.6	4.2	3	5.1	4	5.7
All ages	30	5.5	134	24.4	54.3	4.5	6	1.1	9	1.4
Total	30	2.7	134	11.8	54.3	4.5	6	0.6	9	0.7

Table 152e   OAI - OPAI - APAI — Corpus uteri cancer - Cases

Age group (years)	Incidence 1990 Number ('000s)	Rate (per 100 000)	Prevalence 1990 Number ('000s)	Rate (per 100 000)	Avg. age at onset (years)	Average duration (years)	Deaths 1990 Number ('000s)	Rate (per 100 000)	Deaths 2000 (Projected) Number ('000s)	Rate (per 100 000)
Males										
0-4	0	0	0	0	-	-	0	0	0	0
5-14	0	0	0	0	-	-	0	0	0	0
15-44	0	0	0	0	-	-	0	0	0	0
45-59	0	0	0	0	-	-	0	0	0	0
60+	0	0	0	0	-	-	0	0	0	0
All ages	0	0	0	0	-	-	0	0	0	0
Females										
0-4	0	0.5	0	0.9	2.5	4.6	0	0.1	0	0.1
5-14	0	0.4	1	1.8	10.0	4.6	0	0.1	0	0.1
15-44	2	1.1	8	4.9	29.8	4.6	0	0.2	0	0.2
45-59	6	18.2	29	82.4	52.3	4.5	1	3.4	2	3.2
60+	8	34.3	32	142.5	70.3	4.2	2	10.9	4	10.9
All ages	16	4.8	71	20.9	57.0	4.4	4	1.2	6	1.4
Total	16	2.4	71	10.4	57.0	4.4	4	0.6	6	0.7

Table 152f   SSA - ASS - ASS — Corpus uteri cancer - Cases

Age group (years)	Incidence 1990 Number ('000s)	Rate (per 100 000)	Prevalence 1990 Number ('000s)	Rate (per 100 000)	Avg. age at onset (years)	Average duration (years)	Deaths 1990 Number ('000s)	Rate (per 100 000)	Deaths 2000 (Projected) Number ('000s)	Rate (per 100 000)
Males										
0-4	0	0	0	0	-	-	0	0	0	0
5-14	0	0	0	0	-	-	0	0	0	0
15-44	0	0	0	0	-	-	0	0	0	0
45-59	0	0	0	0	-	-	0	0	0	0
60+	0	0	0	0	-	-	0	0	0	0
All ages	0	0	0	0	-	-	0	0	0	0
Females										
0-4	0	0.1	0	0.1	2.4	4.4	0	0.0	0	0.0
5-14	0	0.1	0	0.6	10.0	4.4	0	0.0	0	0.0
15-44	1	1.1	5	4.8	29.5	4.4	0	0.1	0	0.1
45-59	4	19.7	19	86.7	52.2	4.4	1	4.5	1	4.2
60+	7	53.8	28	218.1	69.7	4.1	2	18.9	3	18.1
All ages	12	4.8	53	20.4	59.2	4.2	4	1.4	5	1.3
Total	12	2.4	53	10.3	59.2	4.2	4	0.7	5	0.7

For epidemiological sources see Murray et al. 1996. For the methods used to estimate and project incidence, prevalence, and deaths see Murray and Lopez 1996a. See explanatory notes for definitions and caveats.

Table 152 — **Cuadro 152** — **Tableau 152**

Corpus uteri cancer — **Cáncer de cuerpo de utero** — **Cancer du corps de l'utérus**

Cases — Casos — Cas

Table 152g   LAC - ALC - ALC — Corpus uteri cancer - Cases

Age group (years)	Incidence 1990 Number ('000s)	Rate (per 100 000)	Prevalence 1990 Number ('000s)	Rate (per 100 000)	Avg. age at onset (years)	Average duration (years)	Deaths 1990 Number ('000s)	Rate (per 100 000)	Deaths 2000 (Projected) Number ('000s)	Rate (per 100 000)
Males										
0-4	0	0	0	0	-	-	0	0	0	0
5-14	0	0	0	0	-	-	0	0	0	0
15-44	0	0	0	0	-	-	0	0	0	0
45-59	0	0	0	0	-	-	0	0	0	0
60+	0	0	0	0	-	-	0	0	0	0
All ages	0	0	0	0	-	-	0	0	0	0
Females										
0-4	0	0.0	0	0.1	2.5	4.6	0	0.0	0	0.0
5-14	0	0.1	0	0.2	10.0	4.6	0	0.0	0	0.0
15-44	4	3.4	17	15.9	29.9	4.6	1	0.5	1	0.5
45-59	13	56.2	60	258.0	52.4	4.6	2	8.9	3	8.6
60+	14	82.3	58	347.5	71.1	4.2	4	24.2	6	24.1
All ages	31	13.7	135	60.8	58.2	4.4	7	3.0	9	3.4
Total	31	6.9	135	30.5	58.2	4.4	7	1.5	9	1.7

Table 152h   MEC - AOM - CMO — Corpus uteri cancer - Cases

Age group (years)	Incidence 1990 Number ('000s)	Rate (per 100 000)	Prevalence 1990 Number ('000s)	Rate (per 100 000)	Avg. age at onset (years)	Average duration (years)	Deaths 1990 Number ('000s)	Rate (per 100 000)	Deaths 2000 (Projected) Number ('000s)	Rate (per 100 000)
Males										
0-4	0	0	0	0	-	-	0	0	0	0
5-14	0	0	0	0	-	-	0	0	0	0
15-44	0	0	0	0	-	-	0	0	0	0
45-59	0	0	0	0	-	-	0	0	0	0
60+	0	0	0	0	-	-	0	0	0	0
All ages	0	0	0	0	-	-	0	0	0	0
Females										
0-4	0	0.1	0	0.1	2.5	4.6	0	0.0	0	0.0
5-14	0	0.1	0	0.6	10.0	4.6	0	0.0	0	0.0
15-44	1	1.0	5	4.7	29.8	4.6	0	0.2	0	0.2
45-59	4	15.8	16	71.6	52.3	4.5	1	3.0	1	2.6
60+	4	27.3	18	113.5	70.4	4.2	1	8.7	2	7.8
All ages	9	3.6	39	15.8	57.5	4.4	2	0.9	3	0.9
Total	9	1.8	39	7.7	57.5	4.4	2	0.4	3	0.4

Table 152i   World - Mundo - Monde — Corpus uteri cancer - Cases

Age group (years)	Incidence 1990 Number ('000s)	Rate (per 100 000)	Prevalence 1990 Number ('000s)	Rate (per 100 000)	Avg. age at onset (years)	Average duration (years)	Deaths 1990 Number ('000s)	Rate (per 100 000)	Deaths 2000 (Projected) Number ('000s)	Rate (per 100 000)
Males										
0-4	0	0	0	0	-	-	0	0	0	0
5-14	0	0	0	0	-	-	0	0	0	0
15-44	0	0	0	0	-	-	0	0	0	0
45-59	0	0	0	0	-	-	0	0	0	0
60+	0	0	0	0	-	-	0	0	0	0
All ages	0	0	0	0	-	-	0	0	0	0
Females										
0-4	0	0.1	1	0.2	2.5	4.6	0	0.0	0	0.0
5-14	1	0.1	3	0.5	10.0	4.5	0	0.0	0	0.0
15-44	29	2.4	137	11.4	29.9	4.7	3	0.3	4	0.3
45-59	110	35.4	511	164.3	52.4	4.6	15	4.9	19	4.6
60+	169	62.8	727	270.0	71.7	4.3	45	16.6	53	15.7
All ages	309	11.8	1 378	52.7	60.7	4.5	64	2.4	76	2.5
Total	309	5.9	1 378	26.2	60.7	4.5	64	1.2	76	1.2

For epidemiological sources see Murray et al. 1996. For the methods used to estimate and project incidence, prevalence, and deaths see Murray and Lopez 1996a. See explanatory notes for definitions and caveats.

Table 153	Cuadro 153	Tableau 153
Ovary cancer	Cáncer de ovario	Cancer de l'ovaire
Cases	Casos	Cas

Table 153a — EME - PEMC - EMBE — Ovary cancer - Cases

Age group (years)	Incidence 1990 Number ('000s)	Rate (per 100 000)	Prevalence 1990 Number ('000s)	Rate (per 100 000)	Avg. age at onset (years)	Average duration (years)	Deaths 1990 Number ('000s)	Rate (per 100 000)	Deaths 2000 (Projected) Number ('000s)	Rate (per 100 000)
Males										
0-4	0	0	0	0	-	-	0	0	0	0
5-14	0	0	0	0	-	-	0	0	0	0
15-44	0	0	0	0	-	-	0	0	0	0
45-59	0	0	0	0	-	-	0	0	0	0
60+	0	0	0	0	-	-	0	0	0	0
All ages	0	0	0	0	-	-	0	0	0	0
Females										
0-4	0	0.1	0	0.1	2.5	4.6	0	0.0	0	0.0
5-14	0	0.2	0	0.8	10.0	4.6	0	0.0	0	0.0
15-44	14	7.6	63	34.9	30.0	4.6	2	1.2	2	1.2
45-59	20	29.8	77	113.2	52.4	3.8	9	13.1	9	11.7
60+	40	47.2	107	126.5	72.4	2.7	30	35.7	32	32.7
All ages	74	18.1	247	60.6	59.0	3.3	41	10.1	43	10.1
Total	74	9.3	247	30.9	59.0	3.3	41	5.2	43	5.2

Table 153b — FSE - PEAS - AESE — Ovary cancer - Cases

Age group (years)	Incidence 1990 Number ('000s)	Rate (per 100 000)	Prevalence 1990 Number ('000s)	Rate (per 100 000)	Avg. age at onset (years)	Average duration (years)	Deaths 1990 Number ('000s)	Rate (per 100 000)	Deaths 2000 (Projected) Number ('000s)	Rate (per 100 000)
Males										
0-4	0	0	0	0	-	-	0	0	0	0
5-14	0	0	0	0	-	-	0	0	0	0
15-44	0	0	0	0	-	-	0	0	0	0
45-59	0	0	0	0	-	-	0	0	0	0
60+	0	0	0	0	-	-	0	0	0	0
All ages	0	0	0	0	-	-	0	0	0	0
Females										
0-4	0	0.1	0	0.2	2.5	4.4	0	0.0	0	0.0
5-14	0	0.3	0	1.4	10.0	4.4	0	0.1	0	0.1
15-44	7	9.2	31	40.9	29.9	4.4	1	2.0	1	1.8
45-59	11	35.8	39	131.5	52.4	3.7	5	17.1	5	16.1
60+	12	31.7	30	82.7	71.5	2.6	9	24.5	9	22.7
All ages	29	16.2	101	55.6	54.5	3.4	16	8.6	16	8.7
Total	29	8.5	101	29.0	54.5	3.4	16	4.5	16	4.5

Table 153c — India - India - Inde — Ovary cancer - Cases

Age group (years)	Incidence 1990 Number ('000s)	Rate (per 100 000)	Prevalence 1990 Number ('000s)	Rate (per 100 000)	Avg. age at onset (years)	Average duration (years)	Deaths 1990 Number ('000s)	Rate (per 100 000)	Deaths 2000 (Projected) Number ('000s)	Rate (per 100 000)
Males										
0-4	0	0	0	0	-	-	0	0	0	0
5-14	0	0	0	0	-	-	0	0	0	0
15-44	0	0	0	0	-	-	0	0	0	0
45-59	0	0	0	0	-	-	0	0	0	0
60+	0	0	0	0	-	-	0	0	0	0
All ages	0	0	0	0	-	-	0	0	0	0
Females										
0-4	0	0.1	0	0.2	2.5	4.0	0	0.0	0	0.0
5-14	0	0.1	0	0.4	10.0	4.0	0	0.0	0	0.0
15-44	8	4.1	30	16.5	29.8	4.0	3	1.5	3	1.5
45-59	6	12.6	19	42.0	52.4	3.3	3	7.3	4	7.1
60+	7	23.3	16	56.0	70.1	2.4	6	19.0	7	19.2
All ages	20	4.9	66	16.1	49.5	3.3	12	2.9	15	3.1
Total	20	2.4	66	7.8	49.5	3.3	12	1.4	15	1.5

For epidemiological sources see Murray et al. 1996. For the methods used to estimate and project incidence, prevalence, and deaths see Murray and Lopez 1996a. See explanatory notes for definitions and caveats.

Table 153	Cuadro 153	Tableau 153
Ovary cancer	Cáncer de ovario	Cancer de l'ovaire
Cases	Casos	Cas

Table 153d   China - China - Chine   Ovary cancer - Cases

Age group (years)	Incidence 1990 Number ('000s)	Rate (per 100 000)	Prevalence 1990 Number ('000s)	Rate (per 100 000)	Avg. age at onset (years)	Average duration (years)	Deaths 1990 Number ('000s)	Rate (per 100 000)	Deaths 2000 (Projected) Number ('000s)	Rate (per 100 000)
Males										
0-4	0	0	0	0	-	-	0	0	0	0
5-14	0	0	0	0	-	-	0	0	0	0
15-44	0	0	0	0	-	-	0	0	0	0
45-59	0	0	0	0	-	-	0	0	0	0
60+	0	0	0	0	-	-	0	0	0	0
All ages	0	0	0	0	-	-	0	0	0	0
Females										
0-4	0	0.8	1	1.3	2.5	4.2	0	0.2	0	0.3
5-14	1	0.7	3	3.0	10.0	4.2	0	0.2	0	0.2
15-44	10	3.4	41	14.5	29.9	4.2	3	1.0	3	1.2
45-59	6	9.0	20	31.6	52.4	3.5	3	4.8	5	5.0
60+	5	10.1	13	25.3	70.6	2.5	4	8.1	6	9.0
All ages	22	4.0	78	14.2	44.5	3.6	10	1.9	14	2.3
Total	22	1.9	78	6.9	44.5	3.6	10	0.9	14	1.1

Table 153e   OAI - OPAI - APAI   Ovary cancer - Cases

Age group (years)	Incidence 1990 Number ('000s)	Rate (per 100 000)	Prevalence 1990 Number ('000s)	Rate (per 100 000)	Avg. age at onset (years)	Average duration (years)	Deaths 1990 Number ('000s)	Rate (per 100 000)	Deaths 2000 (Projected) Number ('000s)	Rate (per 100 000)
Males										
0-4	0	0	0	0	-	-	0	0	0	0
5-14	0	0	0	0	-	-	0	0	0	0
15-44	0	0	0	0	-	-	0	0	0	0
45-59	0	0	0	0	-	-	0	0	0	0
60+	0	0	0	0	-	-	0	0	0	0
All ages	0	0	0	0	-	-	0	0	0	0
Females										
0-4	1	2.1	1	3.4	2.5	4.1	0	0.7	0	0.7
5-14	1	1.7	6	7.1	10.0	4.1	0	0.6	0	0.5
15-44	10	6.6	43	27.2	29.8	4.1	3	2.1	4	2.1
45-59	5	14.8	18	50.9	52.3	3.4	3	8.1	4	7.7
60+	5	20.8	12	51.5	70.3	2.5	4	16.8	5	16.7
All ages	23	6.7	80	23.6	41.2	3.6	11	3.2	14	3.5
Total	23	3.3	80	11.7	41.2	3.6	11	1.6	14	1.7

Table 153f   SSA - ASS - ASS   Ovary cancer - Cases

Age group (years)	Incidence 1990 Number ('000s)	Rate (per 100 000)	Prevalence 1990 Number ('000s)	Rate (per 100 000)	Avg. age at onset (years)	Average duration (years)	Deaths 1990 Number ('000s)	Rate (per 100 000)	Deaths 2000 (Projected) Number ('000s)	Rate (per 100 000)
Males										
0-4	0	0	0	0	-	-	0	0	0	0
5-14	0	0	0	0	-	-	0	0	0	0
15-44	0	0	0	0	-	-	0	0	0	0
45-59	0	0	0	0	-	-	0	0	0	0
60+	0	0	0	0	-	-	0	0	0	0
All ages	0	0	0	0	-	-	0	0	0	0
Females										
0-4	0	0.6	0	1.0	2.4	3.9	0	0.3	0	0.3
5-14	1	1.3	3	5.0	10.0	3.9	0	0.5	0	0.4
15-44	4	4.0	17	15.8	29.5	3.9	1	1.0	1	0.9
45-59	4	20.1	15	66.2	52.2	3.3	3	12.0	3	11.2
60+	4	32.2	10	76.5	69.7	2.4	3	26.6	4	25.3
All ages	14	5.4	45	17.5	46.7	3.3	8	2.9	10	2.7
Total	14	2.7	45	8.8	46.7	3.3	8	1.5	10	1.4

For epidemiological sources see Murray et al. 1996. For the methods used to estimate and project incidence, prevalence, and deaths see Murray and Lopez 1996a. See explanatory notes for definitions and caveats.

Table 153
Ovary cancer

Cuadro 153
Cáncer de ovario

Tableau 153
Cancer de l'ovaire

Cases

Casos

Cas

Table 153g LAC - ALC - ALC — Ovary cancer - Cases

Age group (years)	Incidence 1990 Number ('000s)	Rate (per 100 000)	Prevalence 1990 Number ('000s)	Rate (per 100 000)	Avg. age at onset (years)	Average duration (years)	Deaths 1990 Number ('000s)	Rate (per 100 000)	Deaths 2000 (Projected) Number ('000s)	Rate (per 100 000)
Males										
0-4	0	0	0	0	-	-	0	0	0	0
5-14	0	0	0	0	-	-	0	0	0	0
15-44	0	0	0	0	-	-	0	0	0	0
45-59	0	0	0	0	-	-	0	0	0	0
60+	0	0	0	0	-	-	0	0	0	0
All ages	0	0	0	0	-	-	0	0	0	0
Females										
0-4	0	0.7	0	1.1	2.5	4.3	0	0.2	0	0.2
5-14	0	1.0	2	4.2	10.0	4.3	0	0.3	0	0.2
15-44	5	4.6	21	19.9	29.9	4.3	1	1.3	2	1.3
45-59	3	12.7	10	44.9	52.4	3.6	2	6.6	2	6.3
60+	4	21.5	9	54.3	71.1	2.5	3	17.0	4	16.7
All ages	12	5.4	43	19.2	46.5	3.6	6	2.6	8	2.9
Total	12	2.7	43	9.6	46.5	3.6	6	1.3	8	1.5

Table 153h MEC - AOM - CMO — Ovary cancer - Cases

Age group (years)	Incidence 1990 Number ('000s)	Rate (per 100 000)	Prevalence 1990 Number ('000s)	Rate (per 100 000)	Avg. age at onset (years)	Average duration (years)	Deaths 1990 Number ('000s)	Rate (per 100 000)	Deaths 2000 (Projected) Number ('000s)	Rate (per 100 000)
Males										
0-4	0	0	0	0	-	-	0	0	0	0
5-14	0	0	0	0	-	-	0	0	0	0
15-44	0	0	0	0	-	-	0	0	0	0
45-59	0	0	0	0	-	-	0	0	0	0
60+	0	0	0	0	-	-	0	0	0	0
All ages	0	0	0	0	-	-	0	0	0	0
Females										
0-4	0	0.3	0	0.6	2.5	4.1	0	0.1	0	0.1
5-14	0	0.8	2	3.2	10.0	4.1	0	0.2	0	0.2
15-44	4	3.4	15	14.1	29.8	4.1	1	1.1	1	1.0
45-59	2	10.2	8	35.2	52.3	3.4	1	5.6	2	5.0
60+	2	10.1	4	25.0	70.4	2.5	1	8.1	2	7.3
All ages	8	3.3	29	11.8	42.3	3.6	4	1.6	5	1.5
Total	8	1.6	29	5.8	42.3	3.6	4	0.8	5	0.7

Table 153i World - Mundo - Monde — Ovary cancer - Cases

Age group (years)	Incidence 1990 Number ('000s)	Rate (per 100 000)	Prevalence 1990 Number ('000s)	Rate (per 100 000)	Avg. age at onset (years)	Average duration (years)	Deaths 1990 Number ('000s)	Rate (per 100 000)	Deaths 2000 (Projected) Number ('000s)	Rate (per 100 000)
Males										
0-4	0	0	0	0	-	-	0	0	0	0
5-14	0	0	0	0	-	-	0	0	0	0
15-44	0	0	0	0	-	-	0	0	0	0
45-59	0	0	0	0	-	-	0	0	0	0
60+	0	0	0	0	-	-	0	0	0	0
All ages	0	0	0	0	-	-	0	0	0	0
Females										
0-4	2	0.7	3	1.1	2.5	4.1	1	0.2	1	0.2
5-14	4	0.8	17	3.3	10.0	4.1	1	0.3	1	0.2
15-44	61	5.1	261	21.7	29.9	4.3	16	1.4	19	1.4
45-59	57	18.5	207	66.4	52.4	3.6	29	9.2	34	8.4
60+	77	28.8	201	74.5	71.6	2.6	60	22.3	70	20.8
All ages	202	7.7	688	26.3	51.6	3.4	107	4.1	125	4.1
Total	202	3.8	688	13.1	51.6	3.4	107	2.0	125	2.0

For epidemiological sources see Murray et al. 1996. For the methods used to estimate and project incidence, prevalence, and deaths see Murray and Lopez 1996a. See explanatory notes for definitions and caveats.

Table 154 · **Prostate cancer** — **Cuadro 154** · **Cáncer de próstata** — **Tableau 154** · **Cancer de la prostate**

Cases · Casos · Cas

Table 154a — EME - PEMC - EMBE — Prostate cancer - Cases

Age group (years)	Incidence 1990 Number ('000s)	Rate (per 100 000)	Prevalence 1990 Number ('000s)	Rate (per 100 000)	Avg. age at onset (years)	Average duration (years)	Deaths 1990 Number ('000s)	Rate (per 100 000)	Deaths 2000 (Projected) Number ('000s)	Rate (per 100 000)
Males										
0-4	0	0.1	0	0.2	2.5	4.8	0	0.0	0	0.0
5-14	0	0.0	0	0.1	10.0	4.8	0	0.0	0	0.0
15-44	1	0.7	6	3.4	29.9	4.8	0	0.1	0	0.1
45-59	29	43.7	137	206.9	52.4	4.7	3	4.5	3	4.4
60+	422	696.7	1 877	3 100.3	71.1	4.4	89	147.4	106	146.6
All ages	452	115.8	2 020	517.4	69.8	4.5	92	23.7	109	26.7
Females										
0-4	0	0	0	0	-	-	0	0	0	0
5-14	0	0	0	0	-	-	0	0	0	0
15-44	0	0	0	0	-	-	0	0	0	0
45-59	0	0	0	0	-	-	0	0	0	0
60+	0	0	0	0	-	-	0	0	0	0
All ages	0	0	0	0	-	-	0	0	0	0
Total	452	56.7	2 020	253.2	69.8	4.5	92	11.6	109	13.0

Table 154b — FSE - PEAS - AESE — Prostate cancer - Cases

Age group (years)	Incidence 1990 Number ('000s)	Rate (per 100 000)	Prevalence 1990 Number ('000s)	Rate (per 100 000)	Avg. age at onset (years)	Average duration (years)	Deaths 1990 Number ('000s)	Rate (per 100 000)	Deaths 2000 (Projected) Number ('000s)	Rate (per 100 000)
Males										
0-4	0	0.1	0	0.1	2.5	4.5	0	0.0	0	0.0
5-14	0	0.0	0	0.1	10.0	4.5	0	0.0	0	0.0
15-44	1	0.7	2	3.2	29.8	4.5	0	0.1	0	0.1
45-59	6	23.0	28	102.7	52.2	4.5	1	4.8	2	5.9
60+	44	207.9	183	871.8	70.0	4.2	13	63.3	20	77.9
All ages	50	30.5	213	128.8	67.3	4.2	15	8.9	22	12.7
Females										
0-4	0	0	0	0	-	-	0	0	0	0
5-14	0	0	0	0	-	-	0	0	0	0
15-44	0	0	0	0	-	-	0	0	0	0
45-59	0	0	0	0	-	-	0	0	0	0
60+	0	0	0	0	-	-	0	0	0	0
All ages	0	0	0	0	-	-	0	0	0	0
Total	50	14.5	213	61.5	67.3	4.2	15	4.2	22	6.1

Table 154c — India - India - Inde — Prostate cancer - Cases

Age group (years)	Incidence 1990 Number ('000s)	Rate (per 100 000)	Prevalence 1990 Number ('000s)	Rate (per 100 000)	Avg. age at onset (years)	Average duration (years)	Deaths 1990 Number ('000s)	Rate (per 100 000)	Deaths 2000 (Projected) Number ('000s)	Rate (per 100 000)
Males										
0-4	0	0.0	0	0.0	-	-	0	0.0	0	0.0
5-14	0	0.0	0	0.0	-	-	0	0.0	0	0.0
15-44	0	0.1	1	0.3	29.8	3.7	0	0.0	0	0.0
45-59	2	4.3	7	15.7	52.3	3.7	1	2.1	1	2.2
60+	19	64.9	67	224.4	69.7	3.5	11	35.4	15	39.9
All ages	22	4.9	75	17.0	67.7	3.5	12	2.6	16	3.2
Females										
0-4	0	0	0	0	-	-	0	0	0	0
5-14	0	0	0	0	-	-	0	0	0	0
15-44	0	0	0	0	-	-	0	0	0	0
45-59	0	0	0	0	-	-	0	0	0	0
60+	0	0	0	0	-	-	0	0	0	0
All ages	0	0	0	0	-	-	0	0	0	0
Total	22	2.5	75	8.8	67.7	3.5	12	1.4	16	1.6

For epidemiological sources see Murray et al. 1996. For the methods used to estimate and project incidence, prevalence, and deaths see Murray and Lopez 1996a. See explanatory notes for definitions and caveats.

Table 154	Cuadro 154	Tableau 154
Prostate cancer	Cáncer de próstata	Cancer de la prostate
Cases	Casos	Cas

Table 154d — China - China - Chine — Prostate cancer - Cases

Age group (years)	Incidence 1990 Number ('000s)	Rate (per 100 000)	Prevalence 1990 Number ('000s)	Rate (per 100 000)	Avg. age at onset (years)	Average duration (years)	Deaths 1990 Number ('000s)	Rate (per 100 000)	Deaths 2000 (Projected) Number ('000s)	Rate (per 100 000)
Males										
0-4	0	0.0	0	0.0	-	-	0	0.0	0	0.0
5-14	0	0.0	0	0.0	-	-	0	0.0	0	0.0
15-44	0	0.1	1	0.4	29.9	4.1	0	0.0	0	0.0
45-59	1	1.1	3	4.4	52.3	4.0	0	0.4	0	0.5
60+	10	20.7	39	79.1	69.8	3.8	4	9.0	6	10.6
All ages	11	1.9	43	7.4	67.5	3.8	5	0.8	7	1.1
Females										
0-4	0	0	0	0	-	-	0	0	0	0
5-14	0	0	0	0	-	-	0	0	0	0
15-44	0	0	0	0	-	-	0	0	0	0
45-59	0	0	0	0	-	-	0	0	0	0
60+	0	0	0	0	-	-	0	0	0	0
All ages	0	0	0	0	-	-	0	0	0	0
Total	11	1.0	43	3.8	67.5	3.8	5	0.4	7	0.5

Table 154e — OAI - OPAI - APAI — Prostate cancer - Cases

Age group (years)	Incidence 1990 Number ('000s)	Rate (per 100 000)	Prevalence 1990 Number ('000s)	Rate (per 100 000)	Avg. age at onset (years)	Average duration (years)	Deaths 1990 Number ('000s)	Rate (per 100 000)	Deaths 2000 (Projected) Number ('000s)	Rate (per 100 000)
Males										
0-4	0	0.2	0	0.3	2.5	3.9	0	0.1	0	0.1
5-14	0	0.2	1	0.8	10.0	3.9	0	0.1	0	0.1
15-44	0	0.1	1	0.5	29.7	3.9	0	0.0	0	0.1
45-59	3	8.7	12	34.2	52.3	3.9	1	3.5	2	3.7
60+	24	118.1	88	436.6	69.6	3.7	11	55.7	16	59.3
All ages	27	8.0	102	29.6	66.8	3.7	13	3.7	18	4.5
Females										
0-4	0	0	0	0	-	-	0	0	0	0
5-14	0	0	0	0	-	-	0	0	0	0
15-44	0	0	0	0	-	-	0	0	0	0
45-59	0	0	0	0	-	-	0	0	0	0
60+	0	0	0	0	-	-	0	0	0	0
All ages	0	0	0	0	-	-	0	0	0	0
Total	27	4.0	102	14.9	66.8	3.7	13	1.8	18	2.3

Table 154f — SSA - ASS - ASS — Prostate cancer - Cases

Age group (years)	Incidence 1990 Number ('000s)	Rate (per 100 000)	Prevalence 1990 Number ('000s)	Rate (per 100 000)	Avg. age at onset (years)	Average duration (years)	Deaths 1990 Number ('000s)	Rate (per 100 000)	Deaths 2000 (Projected) Number ('000s)	Rate (per 100 000)
Males										
0-4	0	0.0	0	0.0	-	-	0	0.0	0	0.0
5-14	0	0.0	0	0.0	-	-	0	0.0	0	0.0
15-44	0	0.4	1	1.4	29.4	3.5	0	0.2	0	0.2
45-59	8	41.4	30	146.0	52.2	3.5	4	21.8	6	21.2
60+	47	451.9	158	1 506.0	69.2	3.3	28	263.5	39	271.8
All ages	56	22.3	189	75.0	66.4	3.4	32	12.8	45	13.1
Females										
0-4	0	0	0	0	-	-	0	0	0	0
5-14	0	0	0	0	-	-	0	0	0	0
15-44	0	0	0	0	-	-	0	0	0	0
45-59	0	0	0	0	-	-	0	0	0	0
60+	0	0	0	0	-	-	0	0	0	0
All ages	0	0	0	0	-	-	0	0	0	0
Total	56	11.0	189	37.1	66.4	3.4	32	6.3	45	6.5

For epidemiological sources see Murray et al. 1996. For the methods used to estimate and project incidence, prevalence, and deaths see Murray and Lopez 1996a. See explanatory notes for definitions and caveats.

Table 154   **Cuadro 154**   **Tableau 154**
Prostate cancer   **Cáncer de próstata**   **Cancer de la prostate**

Cases   Casos   Cas

Table 154g   LAC - ALC - ALC   Prostate cancer - Cases

Age group (years)	Incidence 1990 Number ('000s)	Rate (per 100 000)	Prevalence 1990 Number ('000s)	Rate (per 100 000)	Avg. age at onset (years)	Average duration (years)	Deaths 1990 Number ('000s)	Rate (per 100 000)	Deaths 2000 (Projected) Number ('000s)	Rate (per 100 000)
Males										
0-4	0	0.0	0	0.0	2.5	4.2	0	0.0	0	0.0
5-14	0	0.0	0	0.1	10.0	4.2	0	0.0	0	0.0
15-44	0	0.4	2	1.7	29.8	4.2	0	0.1	0	0.1
45-59	4	18.2	17	75.8	52.3	4.2	1	5.7	2	5.7
60+	47	330.6	185	1 296.9	70.3	3.9	19	131.3	27	138.6
All ages	52	23.2	203	91.7	68.5	3.9	20	9.1	29	11.0
Females										
0-4	0	0	0	0	-	-	0	0	0	0
5-14	0	0	0	0	-	-	0	0	0	0
15-44	0	0	0	0	-	-	0	0	0	0
45-59	0	0	0	0	-	-	0	0	0	0
60+	0	0	0	0	-	-	0	0	0	0
All ages	0	0	0	0	-	-	0	0	0	0
Total	52	11.6	203	45.7	68.5	3.9	20	4.5	29	5.5

Table 154h   MEC - AOM - CMO   Prostate cancer - Cases

Age group (years)	Incidence 1990 Number ('000s)	Rate (per 100 000)	Prevalence 1990 Number ('000s)	Rate (per 100 000)	Avg. age at onset (years)	Average duration (years)	Deaths 1990 Number ('000s)	Rate (per 100 000)	Deaths 2000 (Projected) Number ('000s)	Rate (per 100 000)
Males										
0-4	0	0.0	0	0.0	2.5	3.9	0	0.0	0	0.0
5-14	0	0.1	0	0.3	10.0	3.9	0	0.0	0	0.0
15-44	0	0.2	1	0.8	29.8	3.9	0	0.1	0	0.1
45-59	2	7.7	7	30.0	52.3	3.9	1	3.1	1	3.0
60+	8	58.0	29	214.5	69.7	3.7	4	27.4	5	26.8
All ages	10	3.9	37	14.5	65.4	3.7	5	1.8	6	1.8
Females										
0-4	0	0	0	0	-	-	0	0	0	0
5-14	0	0	0	0	-	-	0	0	0	0
15-44	0	0	0	0	-	-	0	0	0	0
45-59	0	0	0	0	-	-	0	0	0	0
60+	0	0	0	0	-	-	0	0	0	0
All ages	0	0	0	0	-	-	0	0	0	0
Total	10	2.0	37	7.4	65.4	3.7	5	0.9	6	0.9

Table 154i   World - Mundo - Monde   Prostate cancer - Cases

Age group (years)	Incidence 1990 Number ('000s)	Rate (per 100 000)	Prevalence 1990 Number ('000s)	Rate (per 100 000)	Avg. age at onset (years)	Average duration (years)	Deaths 1990 Number ('000s)	Rate (per 100 000)	Deaths 2000 (Projected) Number ('000s)	Rate (per 100 000)
Males										
0-4	0	0.0	0	0.1	2.5	4.2	0	0.0	0	0.0
5-14	0	0.0	1	0.2	10.0	4.0	0	0.0	0	0.0
15-44	4	0.3	15	1.2	29.8	4.3	1	0.1	1	0.1
45-59	55	17.6	240	76.9	52.3	4.4	13	4.2	17	4.2
60+	621	283.9	2 626	1 199.8	70.7	4.2	179	81.7	235	85.2
All ages	680	25.6	2 883	108.6	68.9	4.2	193	7.3	253	8.2
Females										
0-4	0	0	0	0	-	-	0	0	0	0
5-14	0	0	0	0	-	-	0	0	0	0
15-44	0	0	0	0	-	-	0	0	0	0
45-59	0	0	0	0	-	-	0	0	0	0
60+	0	0	0	0	-	-	0	0	0	0
All ages	0	0	0	0	-	-	0	0	0	0
Total	680	12.9	2 883	54.7	68.9	4.2	193	3.7	253	4.1

For epidemiological sources see Murray et al. 1996. For the methods used to estimate and project incidence, prevalence, and deaths see Murray and Lopez 1996a. See explanatory notes for definitions and caveats.

Table 155 Bladder cancer	Cuadro 155 Cáncer de vesícula	Tableau 155 Cancer de la vessie
Cases	Casos	Cas

Table 155a EME - PEMC - EMBE — Bladder cancer - Cases

Age group (years)	Incidence 1990 Number ('000s)	Rate (per 100 000)	Prevalence 1990 Number ('000s)	Rate (per 100 000)	Avg. age at onset (years)	Average duration (years)	Deaths 1990 Number ('000s)	Rate (per 100 000)	Deaths 2000 (Projected) Number ('000s)	Rate (per 100 000)
Males										
0-4	0	0.5	0	1.1	2.5	4.9	0	0.0	0	0.0
5-14	0	0.3	1	1.5	10.0	4.9	0	0.0	0	0.0
15-44	4	2.4	22	11.8	29.9	4.9	0	0.1	0	0.1
45-59	30	44.8	141	213.0	52.4	4.8	3	4.2	3	4.2
60+	142	235.1	684	1 129.6	71.1	4.8	30	50.1	36	49.2
All ages	177	45.3	848	217.0	66.8	4.8	33	8.5	39	9.5
Females										
0-4	0	0.1	0	0.2	2.5	4.8	0	0.0	0	0.0
5-14	0	0.1	0	0.4	10.0	4.8	0	0.0	0	0.0
15-44	1	0.8	7	3.9	30.0	4.8	0	0.1	0	0.1
45-59	6	8.5	27	40.2	52.4	4.7	1	1.0	1	0.9
60+	40	47.7	168	199.0	72.4	4.2	13	14.8	14	14.3
All ages	48	11.7	203	49.8	68.6	4.3	13	3.3	15	3.4
Total	224	28.1	1 050	131.6	67.2	4.7	47	5.8	54	6.4

Table 155b FSE - PEAS - AESE — Bladder cancer - Cases

Age group (years)	Incidence 1990 Number ('000s)	Rate (per 100 000)	Prevalence 1990 Number ('000s)	Rate (per 100 000)	Avg. age at onset (years)	Average duration (years)	Deaths 1990 Number ('000s)	Rate (per 100 000)	Deaths 2000 (Projected) Number ('000s)	Rate (per 100 000)
Males										
0-4	0	1.5	0	2.8	2.5	4.8	0	0.2	0	0.2
5-14	0	0.6	1	2.7	10.0	4.8	0	0.1	0	0.1
15-44	1	1.8	6	8.4	29.8	4.7	0	0.2	0	0.2
45-59	14	50.6	62	230.4	52.2	4.6	2	8.7	3	10.8
60+	34	161.6	156	743.1	70.0	4.6	10	45.3	13	52.0
All ages	49	29.8	225	136.4	63.5	4.6	12	7.3	17	9.8
Females										
0-4	0	0.1	0	0.2	2.5	4.6	0	0.0	0	0.0
5-14	0	0.0	0	0.2	10.0	4.6	0	0.0	0	0.0
15-44	1	0.8	3	3.6	29.9	4.6	0	0.1	0	0.1
45-59	2	8.1	11	36.7	52.4	4.5	0	1.5	0	1.4
60+	9	23.9	35	95.7	71.5	4.0	3	8.8	4	8.9
All ages	12	6.5	49	26.9	65.3	4.1	4	2.1	4	2.3
Total	61	17.6	274	79.2	63.8	4.5	16	4.6	21	5.9

Table 155c India - India - Inde — Bladder cancer - Cases

Age group (years)	Incidence 1990 Number ('000s)	Rate (per 100 000)	Prevalence 1990 Number ('000s)	Rate (per 100 000)	Avg. age at onset (years)	Average duration (years)	Deaths 1990 Number ('000s)	Rate (per 100 000)	Deaths 2000 (Projected) Number ('000s)	Rate (per 100 000)
Males										
0-4	0	0.0	0	0.0	2.5	4.2	0	0.0	0	0.0
5-14	0	0.0	0	0.1	10.0	4.2	0	0.0	0	0.0
15-44	1	0.4	3	1.4	29.8	4.1	0	0.1	0	0.1
45-59	3	6.7	13	26.9	52.3	4.0	1	2.5	2	2.7
60+	9	29.1	35	117.2	69.7	4.0	4	13.3	5	14.5
All ages	13	2.9	51	11.5	62.8	4.0	5	1.2	7	1.4
Females										
0-4	0	0.0	0	0.1	2.5	4.0	0	0.0	0	0.0
5-14	0	0.0	0	0.2	10.0	4.0	0	0.0	0	0.0
15-44	0	0.1	1	0.5	29.8	4.0	0	0.0	0	0.0
45-59	1	1.8	3	7.2	52.4	4.0	0	0.7	0	0.7
60+	2	7.0	7	24.6	70.1	3.5	1	3.7	2	3.9
All ages	3	0.8	12	2.8	61.2	3.7	1	0.4	2	0.4
Total	16	1.9	62	7.3	62.5	4.0	7	0.8	9	0.9

For epidemiological sources see Murray et al. 1996. For the methods used to estimate and project incidence, prevalence, and deaths see Murray and Lopez 1996a. See explanatory notes for definitions and caveats.

Table 155
Bladder cancer

Cuadro 155
Cáncer de vesícula

Tableau 155
Cancer de la vessie

Cases

Casos

Cas

Table 155d   China - China - Chine

Bladder cancer - Cases

Age group (years)	Incidence 1990 Number ('000s)	Rate (per 100 000)	Prevalence 1990 Number ('000s)	Rate (per 100 000)	Avg. age at onset (years)	Average duration (years)	Deaths 1990 Number ('000s)	Rate (per 100 000)	Deaths 2000 (Projected) Number ('000s)	Rate (per 100 000)
Males										
0-4	0	0.0	0	0.1	2.5	4.5	0	0.0	0	0.0
5-14	0	0.0	0	0.2	10.0	4.5	0	0.0	0	0.0
15-44	3	0.8	11	3.7	29.9	4.4	1	0.2	1	0.3
45-59	7	9.8	30	41.6	52.3	4.3	2	2.7	3	3.3
60+	32	66.2	139	284.5	69.8	4.3	12	24.8	18	29.2
All ages	42	7.2	181	31.0	64.3	4.3	15	2.5	22	3.3
Females										
0-4	0	0.0	0	0.1	2.5	4.3	0	0.0	0	0.0
5-14	0	0.0	0	0.1	10.0	4.3	0	0.0	0	0.0
15-44	0	0.1	2	0.6	29.9	4.3	0	0.0	0	0.0
45-59	1	2.2	6	9.3	52.4	4.2	0	0.7	1	0.7
60+	8	14.6	28	54.8	70.6	3.8	3	6.6	5	7.4
All ages	9	1.7	36	6.6	65.7	3.9	4	0.7	6	0.9
Total	52	4.6	217	19.2	64.6	4.2	19	1.7	27	2.1

Table 155e   OAI - OPAI - APAI

Bladder cancer - Cases

Age group (years)	Incidence 1990 Number ('000s)	Rate (per 100 000)	Prevalence 1990 Number ('000s)	Rate (per 100 000)	Avg. age at onset (years)	Average duration (years)	Deaths 1990 Number ('000s)	Rate (per 100 000)	Deaths 2000 (Projected) Number ('000s)	Rate (per 100 000)
Males										
0-4	0	0.0	0	0.0	-	-	0	0.0	0	0.0
5-14	0	0.0	0	0.0	-	-	0	0.0	0	0.0
15-44	1	0.7	5	2.9	29.7	4.3	0	0.2	0	0.2
45-59	5	15.4	22	64.3	52.3	4.2	2	4.8	2	5.1
60+	15	72.4	62	304.7	69.6	4.2	6	29.1	9	30.9
All ages	21	6.1	88	25.7	63.2	4.2	8	2.3	11	2.8
Females										
0-4	0	0.1	0	0.2	2.5	4.2	0	0.0	0	0.0
5-14	0	0.1	0	0.3	10.0	4.2	0	0.0	0	0.0
15-44	0	0.3	2	1.2	29.8	4.2	0	0.1	0	0.1
45-59	1	3.4	5	14.1	52.3	4.1	0	1.1	0	1.1
60+	5	22.8	19	84.0	70.3	3.7	2	10.9	4	10.9
All ages	7	2.0	26	7.7	63.7	3.8	3	0.9	4	1.1
Total	28	4.1	114	16.7	63.3	4.1	11	1.6	16	1.9

Table 155f   SSA - ASS - ASS

Bladder cancer - Cases

Age group (years)	Incidence 1990 Number ('000s)	Rate (per 100 000)	Prevalence 1990 Number ('000s)	Rate (per 100 000)	Avg. age at onset (years)	Average duration (years)	Deaths 1990 Number ('000s)	Rate (per 100 000)	Deaths 2000 (Projected) Number ('000s)	Rate (per 100 000)
Males										
0-4	0	0.0	0	0.0	2.4	4.1	0	0.0	0	0.0
5-14	0	0.0	0	0.2	10.0	4.1	0	0.0	0	0.0
15-44	2	1.6	7	6.5	29.4	4.0	1	0.6	1	0.6
45-59	6	30.2	24	117.9	52.2	3.9	2	12.3	3	11.9
60+	12	115.4	48	453.8	69.2	3.9	6	55.7	8	57.5
All ages	20	7.9	79	31.1	60.5	3.9	9	3.6	12	3.6
Females										
0-4	0	0.0	0	0.0	-	-	0	0.0	0	0.0
5-14	0	0.0	0	0.0	-	-	0	0.0	0	0.0
15-44	2	1.6	7	6.2	29.5	3.9	0	0.4	0	0.3
45-59	3	14.4	12	55.4	52.2	3.9	1	6.0	2	5.6
60+	5	41.8	18	144.4	69.7	3.5	3	22.9	4	21.8
All ages	10	3.9	37	14.4	57.7	3.7	5	1.8	6	1.7
Total	30	5.9	116	22.7	59.5	3.8	14	2.7	18	2.6

For epidemiological sources see Murray et al. 1996. For the methods used to estimate and project incidence, prevalence, and deaths see Murray and Lopez 1996a. See explanatory notes for definitions and caveats.

Table 155   **Cuadro 155**   **Tableau 155**
Bladder cancer   **Cáncer de vesícula**   **Cancer de la vessie**

Cases   Casos   Cas

Table 155g   LAC - ALC - ALC   Bladder cancer - Cases

Age group (years)	Incidence 1990 Number ('000s)	Rate (per 100 000)	Prevalence 1990 Number ('000s)	Rate (per 100 000)	Avg. age at onset (years)	Average duration (years)	Deaths 1990 Number ('000s)	Rate (per 100 000)	Deaths 2000 (Projected) Number ('000s)	Rate (per 100 000)
Males										
0-4	0	0.1	0	0.2	2.5	4.6	0	0.0	0	0.0
5-14	0	0.2	0	0.9	10.0	4.6	0	0.0	0	0.0
15-44	1	1.0	5	4.5	29.8	4.4	0	0.2	0	0.2
45-59	4	20.2	19	87.6	52.3	4.3	1	5.0	2	5.0
60+	14	97.0	61	425.4	70.3	4.4	5	33.8	7	35.5
All ages	19	8.8	85	38.4	63.5	4.4	6	2.8	9	3.3
Females										
0-4	0	0.1	0	0.1	2.5	4.4	0	0.0	0	0.0
5-14	0	0.1	0	0.3	10.0	4.4	0	0.0	0	0.0
15-44	0	0.4	2	1.6	29.9	4.4	0	0.1	0	0.1
45-59	1	5.0	5	21.6	52.4	4.3	0	1.3	0	1.3
60+	4	24.7	16	94.6	71.1	3.8	2	10.6	3	10.7
All ages	6	2.6	23	10.2	64.1	4.0	2	1.0	3	1.1
Total	25	5.7	108	24.3	63.7	4.3	8	1.9	12	2.2

Table 155h   MEC - AOM - CMO   Bladder cancer - Cases

Age group (years)	Incidence 1990 Number ('000s)	Rate (per 100 000)	Prevalence 1990 Number ('000s)	Rate (per 100 000)	Avg. age at onset (years)	Average duration (years)	Deaths 1990 Number ('000s)	Rate (per 100 000)	Deaths 2000 (Projected) Number ('000s)	Rate (per 100 000)
Males										
0-4	0	0.1	0	0.2	2.5	4.4	0	0.0	0	0.0
5-14	0	0.2	1	1.1	10.0	4.4	0	0.1	0	0.1
15-44	3	2.5	12	10.5	29.8	4.3	1	0.7	1	0.7
45-59	8	33.7	31	140.4	52.3	4.2	2	10.5	3	10.4
60+	11	83.0	48	349.3	69.7	4.2	5	33.4	6	32.7
All ages	22	8.5	92	35.8	58.0	4.2	8	3.0	11	3.2
Females										
0-4	0	0.1	0	0.1	2.5	4.2	0	0.0	0	0.0
5-14	0	0.1	0	0.6	10.0	4.2	0	0.0	0	0.0
15-44	1	0.6	3	2.7	29.8	4.2	0	0.2	0	0.2
45-59	2	7.6	7	31.5	52.3	4.1	1	2.5	1	2.2
60+	2	16.2	9	59.6	70.4	3.7	1	7.7	1	7.0
All ages	5	2.0	20	7.9	57.2	3.9	2	0.8	2	0.8
Total	27	5.3	111	22.1	57.9	4.2	10	1.9	13	2.0

Table 155i   World - Mundo - Monde   Bladder cancer - Cases

Age group (years)	Incidence 1990 Number ('000s)	Rate (per 100 000)	Prevalence 1990 Number ('000s)	Rate (per 100 000)	Avg. age at onset (years)	Average duration (years)	Deaths 1990 Number ('000s)	Rate (per 100 000)	Deaths 2000 (Projected) Number ('000s)	Rate (per 100 000)
Males										
0-4	0	0.1	1	0.3	2.5	4.4	0	0.0	0	0.0
5-14	1	0.1	3	0.6	10.0	4.4	0	0.0	0	0.0
15-44	16	1.3	70	5.6	29.8	4.4	3	0.3	4	0.3
45-59	77	24.6	343	109.7	52.3	4.3	16	5.1	22	5.4
60+	269	123.0	1 231	562.7	70.1	4.4	77	35.2	102	36.9
All ages	363	13.7	1 648	62.1	63.2	4.3	96	3.6	128	4.1
Females										
0-4	0	0.1	0	0.1	2.5	4.2	0	0.0	0	0.0
5-14	0	0.1	1	0.2	10.0	4.2	0	0.0	0	0.0
15-44	6	0.5	25	2.1	29.8	4.3	1	0.1	1	0.1
45-59	18	5.7	77	24.7	52.4	4.3	4	1.4	5	1.3
60+	76	28.1	301	111.8	71.2	3.9	29	10.6	35	10.5
All ages	100	3.8	405	15.5	63.4	3.9	34	1.3	42	1.4
Total	463	8.8	2 053	39.0	63.3	4.2	131	2.5	170	2.8

For epidemiological sources see Murray et al. 1996. For the methods used to estimate and project incidence, prevalence, and deaths see Murray and Lopez 1996a. See explanatory notes for definitions and caveats.

Table 156
Lymphomas and multiple myeloma
Cases

Cuadro 156
Linfomas y mieloma múltiple
Casos

Tableau 156
Lymphomes et myélome multiple
Cas

Table 156a   EME - PEMC - EMBE — Lymphomas and multiple myeloma - Cases

Age group (years)	Incidence 1990 Number ('000s)	Rate (per 100 000)	Prevalence 1990 Number ('000s)	Rate (per 100 000)	Avg. age at onset (years)	Average duration (years)	Deaths 1990 Number ('000s)	Rate (per 100 000)	Deaths 2000 (Projected) Number ('000s)	Rate (per 100 000)
Males										
0-4	1	2.2	1	4.1	2.5	4.7	0	0.2	0	0.2
5-14	2	3.1	8	14.5	10.0	4.6	0	0.4	0	0.4
15-44	23	12.4	103	56.0	29.9	4.5	4	2.3	4	2.3
45-59	22	33.4	91	138.1	52.4	4.1	7	10.9	8	10.7
60+	55	91.3	192	317.8	71.1	3.5	30	49.2	34	46.9
All ages	102	26.2	396	101.3	56.5	3.9	42	10.6	47	11.3
Females										
0-4	0	0.8	0	1.5	2.5	4.5	0	0.2	0	0.1
5-14	1	2.3	5	10.8	10.0	4.8	0	0.2	0	0.2
15-44	14	7.6	62	34.6	30.0	4.6	2	1.2	2	1.2
45-59	14	20.6	58	85.9	52.4	4.2	4	6.5	5	5.8
60+	53	62.9	178	210.1	72.4	3.3	31	36.6	34	34.5
All ages	82	20.2	304	74.6	61.0	3.7	38	9.2	40	9.4
Total	185	23.1	699	87.7	58.5	3.8	79	9.9	87	10.4

Table 156b   FSE - PEAS - AESE — Lymphomas and multiple myeloma - Cases

Age group (years)	Incidence 1990 Number ('000s)	Rate (per 100 000)	Prevalence 1990 Number ('000s)	Rate (per 100 000)	Avg. age at onset (years)	Average duration (years)	Deaths 1990 Number ('000s)	Rate (per 100 000)	Deaths 2000 (Projected) Number ('000s)	Rate (per 100 000)
Males										
0-4	1	4.5	1	7.9	2.5	4.4	0	1.1	0	1.0
5-14	1	5.3	6	22.7	10.0	4.3	0	1.4	0	1.4
15-44	7	8.9	28	37.2	29.8	4.2	2	2.7	2	2.8
45-59	6	23.4	24	90.0	52.2	3.9	3	9.8	4	12.1
60+	7	32.5	22	106.0	70.0	3.3	4	19.7	5	21.3
All ages	22	13.3	82	49.7	46.7	3.8	9	5.6	12	6.9
Females										
0-4	0	2.1	0	3.5	2.5	4.2	0	0.7	0	0.7
5-14	1	2.6	3	11.5	10.0	4.5	0	0.5	0	0.5
15-44	4	5.8	19	24.8	29.9	4.3	1	1.6	1	1.6
45-59	4	12.1	14	46.9	52.4	3.9	1	5.0	2	4.7
60+	7	17.9	20	56.0	71.5	3.1	4	11.4	5	10.9
All ages	15	8.5	57	31.2	51.3	3.7	7	3.9	7	4.0
Total	37	10.8	139	40.1	48.6	3.8	16	4.8	19	5.4

Table 156c   India - India - Inde — Lymphomas and multiple myeloma - Cases

Age group (years)	Incidence 1990 Number ('000s)	Rate (per 100 000)	Prevalence 1990 Number ('000s)	Rate (per 100 000)	Avg. age at onset (years)	Average duration (years)	Deaths 1990 Number ('000s)	Rate (per 100 000)	Deaths 2000 (Projected) Number ('000s)	Rate (per 100 000)
Males										
0-4	1	1.9	2	2.6	2.5	3.4	1	1.1	1	1.2
5-14	2	1.7	6	5.6	10.0	3.3	1	1.0	1	1.0
15-44	5	2.4	16	8.0	29.8	3.3	3	1.5	4	1.6
45-59	4	9.3	13	28.1	52.3	3.0	3	6.2	4	6.6
60+	5	17.3	13	44.9	69.7	2.6	4	13.3	5	14.5
All ages	17	3.9	50	11.4	43.6	3.0	11	2.6	15	2.9
Females										
0-4	0	0.4	0	0.5	2.5	3.2	0	0.2	0	0.3
5-14	0	0.4	1	1.4	10.0	3.4	0	0.2	0	0.2
15-44	2	1.1	7	3.6	29.8	3.3	1	0.6	1	0.6
45-59	2	5.3	7	16.2	52.4	3.0	2	3.5	2	3.4
60+	5	15.8	11	39.7	70.1	2.5	4	12.5	5	12.9
All ages	10	2.3	27	6.6	53.4	2.9	7	1.6	9	1.8
Total	27	3.2	77	9.1	47.1	3.0	18	2.1	24	2.4

For epidemiological sources see Murray et al. 1996. For the methods used to estimate and project incidence, prevalence, and deaths see Murray and Lopez 1996a. See explanatory notes for definitions and caveats.

Table 156
Lymphomas and multiple myeloma
Cases

Cuadro 156
Linfomas y mieloma múltiple
Casos

Tableau 156
Lymphomes et myélome multiple
Cas

Table 156d — China - China - Chine — Lymphomas and multiple myeloma - Cases

Age group (years)	Incidence 1990 Number ('000s)	Rate (per 100 000)	Prevalence 1990 Number ('000s)	Rate (per 100 000)	Avg. age at onset (years)	Average duration (years)	Deaths 1990 Number ('000s)	Rate (per 100 000)	Deaths 2000 (Projected) Number ('000s)	Rate (per 100 000)
Males										
0-4	0	0.0	0	0.0	-	-	0	0.0	0	0.0
5-14	2	2.0	7	7.6	10.0	3.8	1	0.9	1	0.9
15-44	7	2.2	25	8.3	29.9	3.7	3	1.0	3	1.0
45-59	6	8.6	22	29.6	52.3	3.4	3	4.8	6	5.7
60+	11	22.6	32	66.1	69.8	2.9	8	15.7	11	18.2
All ages	26	4.5	87	14.8	50.8	3.3	15	2.6	21	3.2
Females										
0-4	0	0.0	0	0.0	-	-	0	0.0	0	0.0
5-14	0	0.0	0	0.0	-	-	0	0.0	0	0.0
15-44	3	1.0	11	3.8	29.9	3.8	1	0.5	1	0.5
45-59	5	7.9	18	27.2	52.4	3.5	3	4.3	4	4.5
60+	5	9.3	14	26.2	70.6	2.8	3	6.7	5	7.6
All ages	13	2.3	42	7.6	54.2	3.3	8	1.4	10	1.7
Total	39	3.4	128	11.3	51.9	3.3	23	2.0	31	2.4

Table 156e — OAI - OPAI - APAI — Lymphomas and multiple myeloma - Cases

Age group (years)	Incidence 1990 Number ('000s)	Rate (per 100 000)	Prevalence 1990 Number ('000s)	Rate (per 100 000)	Avg. age at onset (years)	Average duration (years)	Deaths 1990 Number ('000s)	Rate (per 100 000)	Deaths 2000 (Projected) Number ('000s)	Rate (per 100 000)
Males										
0-4	2	4.6	3	6.8	2.5	3.7	1	2.1	1	2.1
5-14	5	5.4	17	19.8	10.0	3.7	2	2.6	2	2.5
15-44	5	3.4	19	12.0	29.7	3.6	3	1.7	4	1.9
45-59	3	9.9	11	32.6	52.3	3.3	2	5.9	3	6.2
60+	9	47.0	27	132.7	69.6	2.8	7	33.9	10	36.2
All ages	25	7.2	77	22.4	42.3	3.3	15	4.3	20	4.9
Females										
0-4	1	2.1	1	3.0	2.5	3.6	0	1.1	0	1.1
5-14	2	2.0	6	7.6	10.0	3.8	1	0.9	1	0.8
15-44	3	1.9	11	7.0	29.8	3.6	2	1.0	2	1.0
45-59	2	5.6	6	18.5	52.3	3.4	1	3.3	1	3.1
60+	8	37.1	23	100.9	70.3	2.7	6	27.7	9	27.7
All ages	16	4.7	48	14.1	50.4	3.1	10	3.0	14	3.4
Total	41	6.0	125	18.3	45.5	3.2	25	3.6	33	4.1

Table 156f — SSA - ASS - ASS — Lymphomas and multiple myeloma - Cases

Age group (years)	Incidence 1990 Number ('000s)	Rate (per 100 000)	Prevalence 1990 Number ('000s)	Rate (per 100 000)	Avg. age at onset (years)	Average duration (years)	Deaths 1990 Number ('000s)	Rate (per 100 000)	Deaths 2000 (Projected) Number ('000s)	Rate (per 100 000)
Males										
0-4	2	4.5	3	5.8	2.4	3.2	1	2.8	2	2.8
5-14	7	9.6	21	30.6	10.0	3.2	4	6.0	5	5.7
15-44	4	3.9	13	12.2	29.4	3.1	3	2.5	4	2.6
45-59	3	15.8	9	45.4	52.2	2.9	2	11.1	3	10.8
60+	7	68.2	18	169.6	69.2	2.5	6	54.5	8	56.2
All ages	23	9.2	64	25.3	36.7	2.9	16	6.4	22	6.4
Females										
0-4	2	3.7	2	4.6	2.4	3.1	1	2.4	2	2.6
5-14	6	7.9	18	26.0	10.0	3.3	3	4.8	4	4.2
15-44	3	2.7	9	8.4	29.5	3.1	1	1.0	1	0.9
45-59	2	8.2	5	23.7	52.2	2.9	1	5.7	2	5.3
60+	4	33.5	10	80.3	69.7	2.4	3	27.4	5	26.1
All ages	16	6.3	45	17.3	33.0	3.0	10	4.0	13	3.8
Total	39	7.7	109	21.3	35.2	2.9	26	5.2	35	5.1

For epidemiological sources see Murray et al. 1996. For the methods used to estimate and project incidence, prevalence, and deaths see Murray and Lopez 1996a. See explanatory notes for definitions and caveats.

Table 156
Lymphomas and multiple myeloma
Cases

Cuadro 156
Linfomas y mieloma múltiple
Casos

Tableau 156
Lymphomes et myélome multiple
Cas

Table 156g   LAC - ALC - ALC   Lymphomas and multiple myeloma - Cases

Age group (years)	Incidence 1990 Number ('000s)	Rate (per 100 000)	Prevalence 1990 Number ('000s)	Rate (per 100 000)	Avg. age at onset (years)	Average duration (years)	Deaths 1990 Number ('000s)	Rate (per 100 000)	Deaths 2000 (Projected) Number ('000s)	Rate (per 100 000)
Males										
0-4	1	3.9	2	6.3	2.5	4.0	0	1.4	0	1.4
5-14	3	5.6	12	22.2	10.0	4.0	1	2.2	1	2.1
15-44	5	4.9	20	18.9	29.8	3.9	2	2.0	3	2.1
45-59	4	15.9	13	56.4	52.3	3.6	2	8.2	2	8.1
60+	5	34.7	15	104.9	70.3	3.0	3	23.2	5	24.2
All ages	18	7.9	61	27.3	40.7	3.6	9	4.0	12	4.4
Females										
0-4	1	2.2	1	3.3	2.5	3.8	0	0.9	0	1.0
5-14	2	4.0	8	16.3	10.0	4.1	1	1.4	1	1.2
15-44	3	2.8	12	11.1	29.9	3.9	1	1.1	1	1.1
45-59	3	11.1	9	39.9	52.4	3.6	1	5.7	2	5.5
60+	6	33.8	17	98.4	71.1	2.9	4	23.7	6	23.7
All ages	14	6.2	47	21.0	46.9	3.5	7	3.3	10	3.6
Total	31	7.1	107	24.1	43.4	3.5	16	3.6	21	4.0

Table 156h   MEC - AOM - CMO   Lymphomas and multiple myeloma - Cases

Age group (years)	Incidence 1990 Number ('000s)	Rate (per 100 000)	Prevalence 1990 Number ('000s)	Rate (per 100 000)	Avg. age at onset (years)	Average duration (years)	Deaths 1990 Number ('000s)	Rate (per 100 000)	Deaths 2000 (Projected) Number ('000s)	Rate (per 100 000)
Males										
0-4	1	1.7	1	2.5	2.5	3.7	0	0.8	0	0.8
5-14	2	3.7	9	13.4	10.0	3.7	1	1.8	1	1.7
15-44	3	3.0	12	10.8	29.8	3.6	2	1.5	2	1.6
45-59	2	6.9	5	22.8	52.3	3.3	1	4.1	1	4.0
60+	3	20.7	8	58.4	69.7	2.8	2	14.9	3	14.7
All ages	11	4.2	35	13.7	37.3	3.4	6	2.4	8	2.4
Females										
0-4	0	1.0	1	1.4	2.5	3.6	0	0.5	0	0.5
5-14	2	2.6	6	9.8	10.0	3.8	1	1.1	1	1.0
15-44	1	1.3	5	4.8	29.8	3.6	1	0.7	1	0.6
45-59	1	2.8	2	9.5	52.3	3.3	0	1.7	0	1.5
60+	2	11.9	5	32.4	70.4	2.7	1	8.9	2	8.0
All ages	6	2.4	19	7.6	37.8	3.3	3	1.4	4	1.3
Total	17	3.3	54	10.7	37.5	3.4	10	1.9	12	1.9

Table 156i   World - Mundo - Monde   Lymphomas and multiple myeloma - Cases

Age group (years)	Incidence 1990 Number ('000s)	Rate (per 100 000)	Prevalence 1990 Number ('000s)	Rate (per 100 000)	Avg. age at onset (years)	Average duration (years)	Deaths 1990 Number ('000s)	Rate (per 100 000)	Deaths 2000 (Projected) Number ('000s)	Rate (per 100 000)
Males										
0-4	8	2.6	12	3.8	2.5	3.7	4	1.2	4	1.3
5-14	23	4.2	85	15.5	10.0	3.7	11	2.0	13	2.0
15-44	59	4.7	237	18.9	29.8	4.0	22	1.7	26	1.8
45-59	51	16.2	188	60.3	52.3	3.7	23	7.5	31	7.8
60+	103	46.9	328	149.8	70.5	3.2	64	29.0	81	29.5
All ages	244	9.2	851	32.1	48.8	3.6	123	4.6	155	5.0
Females										
0-4	4	1.4	6	1.9	2.5	3.5	2	0.7	3	0.9
5-14	13	2.5	48	9.2	10.0	3.7	6	1.1	7	1.1
15-44	33	2.8	135	11.3	29.9	4.1	10	0.9	12	0.8
45-59	32	10.3	120	38.7	52.4	3.7	14	4.6	18	4.4
60+	89	33.2	278	103.1	71.7	3.1	57	21.3	69	20.5
All ages	172	6.6	587	22.5	53.6	3.5	90	3.5	108	3.5
Total	416	7.9	1 438	27.3	50.8	3.5	214	4.1	263	4.3

For epidemiological sources see Murray et al. 1996. For the methods used to estimate and project incidence, prevalence, and deaths see Murray and Lopez 1996a. See explanatory notes for definitions and caveats.

Table 157	Cuadro 157	Tableau 157
Leukaemia	Leucemia	Leucémie
Cases	Casos	Cas

Table 157a EME - PEMC - EMBE — Leukaemia - Cases

Age group (years)	Incidence 1990 Number ('000s)	Rate (per 100 000)	Prevalence 1990 Number ('000s)	Rate (per 100 000)	Avg. age at onset (years)	Average duration (years)	Deaths 1990 Number ('000s)	Rate (per 100 000)	Deaths 2000 (Projected) Number ('000s)	Rate (per 100 000)
Males										
0-4	2	9.3	2	8.8	2.5	2.4	0	1.4	0	1.1
5-14	2	4.0	5	10.2	10.0	2.6	1	1.7	1	1.5
15-44	7	3.5	27	14.9	29.9	4.2	4	2.3	4	2.2
45-59	8	12.1	39	58.7	52.4	4.8	4	6.5	5	6.4
60+	30	49.5	147	243.2	71.1	4.9	22	35.5	25	34.1
All ages	49	12.6	221	56.7	56.5	4.6	31	8.0	35	8.4
Females										
0-4	2	7.9	2	7.8	2.5	2.5	0	1.3	0	1.1
5-14	2	3.7	5	10.4	10.0	2.8	1	1.2	1	1.1
15-44	5	2.5	20	11.3	30.0	4.5	3	1.6	3	1.5
45-59	5	7.5	24	36.1	52.4	4.8	3	4.7	3	4.2
00+	23	27.0	112	132.5	72.4	4.9	19	22.4	21	21.3
All ages	36	8.9	164	40.3	57.3	4.6	26	6.4	28	6.4
Total	85	10.7	385	48.3	56.8	4.6	57	7.2	62	7.4

Table 157b FSE - PEAS - AESE — Leukaemia - Cases

Age group (years)	Incidence 1990 Number ('000s)	Rate (per 100 000)	Prevalence 1990 Number ('000s)	Rate (per 100 000)	Avg. age at onset (years)	Average duration (years)	Deaths 1990 Number ('000s)	Rate (per 100 000)	Deaths 2000 (Projected) Number ('000s)	Rate (per 100 000)
Males										
0-4	1	9.8	1	8.6	2.5	2.2	0	3.0	0	2.9
5-14	1	5.4	3	12.8	10.0	2.4	1	2.8	1	2.8
15-44	3	3.6	10	13.7	29.8	3.8	2	2.6	2	2.7
45-59	4	13.3	16	58.0	52.2	4.4	2	8.3	3	10.2
60+	6	30.5	28	135.3	70.0	4.4	5	23.5	7	26.2
All ages	16	9.4	59	35.8	47.3	3.9	10	6.2	13	7.6
Females										
0-4	1	7.3	1	6.6	2.5	2.3	0	2.3	0	2.4
5-14	1	4.3	3	11.2	10.0	2.6	1	2.0	0	1.8
15-44	2	2.7	8	10.9	29.9	4.1	1	1.9	1	1.8
45-59	2	8.1	11	35.2	52.4	4.4	2	5.6	2	5.3
60+	5	14.9	24	66.0	71.5	4.4	5	12.8	5	12.4
All ages	12	6.6	47	25.8	49.2	4.0	9	4.8	9	4.8
Total	27	7.9	106	30.5	48.1	4.0	19	5.5	22	6.1

Table 157c India - India - Inde — Leukaemia - Cases

Age group (years)	Incidence 1990 Number ('000s)	Rate (per 100 000)	Prevalence 1990 Number ('000s)	Rate (per 100 000)	Avg. age at onset (years)	Average duration (years)	Deaths 1990 Number ('000s)	Rate (per 100 000)	Deaths 2000 (Projected) Number ('000s)	Rate (per 100 000)
Males										
0-4	2	2.8	1	1.8	2.5	1.7	1	2.0	1	2.2
5-14	2	2.2	4	3.8	10.0	1.8	2	1.8	2	1.8
15-44	3	1.5	8	4.0	29.8	2.6	3	1.3	4	1.4
45-59	2	3.8	5	11.1	52.3	2.9	2	3.2	2	3.4
60+	2	6.9	6	20.6	69.7	3.0	2	6.3	2	6.8
All ages	11	2.5	24	5.5	33.0	2.4	9	2.1	11	2.2
Females										
0-4	1	1.4	1	1.0	2.5	1.7	1	1.0	1	1.3
5-14	1	1.4	3	2.6	10.0	1.9	1	1.1	1	1.0
15-44	2	1.4	7	3.7	29.8	2.8	2	1.2	3	1.2
45-59	2	3.5	5	10.2	52.4	2.9	1	3.1	2	3.0
60+	2	5.4	5	15.9	70.1	3.0	1	5.1	2	5.2
All ages	8	1.9	19	4.7	36.3	2.6	7	1.6	8	1.7
Total	19	2.2	44	5.1	34.3	2.5	16	1.9	19	2.0

For epidemiological sources see Murray et al. 1996. For the methods used to estimate and project incidence, prevalence, and deaths see Murray and Lopez 1996a. See explanatory notes for definitions and caveats.

Table 157	Cuadro 157	Tableau 157
Leukaemia	Leucemia	Leucémie

Cases   Casos   Cas

Table 157d China - China - Chine   Leukaemia - Cases

Age group (years)	Incidence 1990 Number ('000s)	Rate (per 100 000)	Prevalence 1990 Number ('000s)	Rate (per 100 000)	Avg. age at onset (years)	Average duration (years)	Deaths 1990 Number ('000s)	Rate (per 100 000)	Deaths 2000 (Projected) Number ('000s)	Rate (per 100 000)
Males										
0-4	6	9.1	4	7.1	2.5	1.9	3	4.8	3	5.2
5-14	7	7.6	15	15.8	10.0	2.1	5	5.2	6	5.3
15-44	18	5.7	57	18.5	29.9	3.2	14	4.6	16	5.1
45-59	8	11.2	30	41.0	52.3	3.7	6	8.4	10	10.0
60+	7	14.8	27	54.9	69.8	3.7	6	12.5	9	14.7
All ages	46	7.8	133	22.7	33.7	3.0	34	5.8	44	6.7
Females										
0-4	6	10.0	5	8.0	2.5	2.0	3	5.4	4	6.4
5-14	4	4.5	9	10.3	10.0	2.3	3	2.9	3	2.8
15-44	17	6.2	60	21.0	29.9	3.4	14	4.9	15	5.0
45-59	7	10.4	24	37.9	52.4	3.6	5	8.3	8	8.6
60+	8	15.2	29	56.3	70.6	3.7	7	13.8	10	15.4
All ages	42	7.6	127	23.2	35.4	3.2	32	5.8	40	6.3
Total	88	7.7	260	22.9	34.5	3.1	66	5.8	84	6.5

Table 157e OAI - OPAI - APAI   Leukaemia - Cases

Age group (years)	Incidence 1990 Number ('000s)	Rate (per 100 000)	Prevalence 1990 Number ('000s)	Rate (per 100 000)	Avg. age at onset (years)	Average duration (years)	Deaths 1990 Number ('000s)	Rate (per 100 000)	Deaths 2000 (Projected) Number ('000s)	Rate (per 100 000)
Males										
0-4	4	9.7	3	7.2	2.5	1.8	3	5.8	2	5.7
5-14	8	9.8	16	19.4	10.0	2.0	6	7.1	6	6.9
15-44	4	2.7	13	8.2	29.7	3.0	4	2.2	5	2.5
45-59	1	4.2	5	14.3	52.3	3.4	1	3.2	2	3.4
60+	4	21.8	15	75.9	69.6	3.5	4	18.9	6	20.1
All ages	23	6.6	53	15.4	26.6	2.5	17	5.0	20	5.0
Females										
0-4	4	10.5	3	8.0	2.5	1.9	3	6.3	3	6.7
5-14	6	7.6	13	16.4	10.0	2.1	4	5.2	4	4.8
15-44	3	2.0	10	6.6	29.8	3.2	3	1.7	3	1.7
45-59	1	3.6	4	12.2	52.3	3.4	1	2.9	1	2.8
60+	4	18.0	14	62.6	70.3	3.5	4	16.6	5	16.5
All ages	19	5.6	45	13.4	27.3	2.6	14	4.2	17	4.2
Total	42	6.1	98	14.4	26.9	2.6	31	4.6	37	4.6

Table 157f SSA - ASS - ASS   Leukaemia - Cases

Age group (years)	Incidence 1990 Number ('000s)	Rate (per 100 000)	Prevalence 1990 Number ('000s)	Rate (per 100 000)	Avg. age at onset (years)	Average duration (years)	Deaths 1990 Number ('000s)	Rate (per 100 000)	Deaths 2000 (Projected) Number ('000s)	Rate (per 100 000)
Males										
0-4	0	0.6	0	0.4	2.4	1.5	0	0.5	0	0.5
5-14	1	1.3	1	2.1	10.0	1.6	1	1.1	1	1.0
15-44	1	1.0	2	2.4	29.4	2.4	1	0.9	1	0.9
45-59	1	2.6	1	7.0	52.2	2.6	0	2.3	1	2.3
60+	2	19.9	6	53.5	69.2	2.7	2	18.5	3	19.1
All ages	5	1.9	11	4.4	43.9	2.4	4	1.7	6	1.7
Females										
0-4	1	1.3	0	0.8	2.4	1.6	0	1.1	1	1.2
5-14	2	2.5	3	4.4	10.0	1.8	1	2.1	2	1.9
15-44	1	1.0	3	2.4	29.5	2.5	1	0.5	1	0.5
45-59	1	3.9	2	10.3	52.2	2.6	1	3.5	1	3.3
60+	2	13.4	5	36.0	69.7	2.7	2	12.9	2	12.3
All ages	6	2.3	13	5.0	35.7	2.3	5	1.9	6	1.8
Total	11	2.1	24	4.7	39.4	2.3	9	1.8	12	1.8

For epidemiological sources see Murray et al. 1996. For the methods used to estimate and project incidence, prevalence, and deaths see Murray and Lopez 1996a. See explanatory notes for definitions and caveats.

Table 157	Cuadro 157	Tableau 157
Leukaemia	Leucemia	Leucémie
Cases	Casos	Cas

Table 157g — LAC - ALC - ALC — Leukaemia - Cases

Age group (years)	Incidence 1990 Number ('000s)	Rate (per 100 000)	Prevalence 1990 Number ('000s)	Rate (per 100 000)	Avg. age at onset (years)	Average duration (years)	Deaths 1990 Number ('000s)	Rate (per 100 000)	Deaths 2000 (Projected) Number ('000s)	Rate (per 100 000)
Males										
0-4	2	5.3	1	4.3	2.5	2.0	1	2.5	1	2.4
5-14	3	5.9	7	12.9	10.0	2.2	2	3.8	2	3.6
15-44	2	2.3	8	7.8	29.8	3.4	2	1.8	2	1.9
45-59	1	5.1	4	19.6	52.3	3.9	1	3.6	1	3.5
60+	2	15.1	8	59.2	70.3	3.9	2	12.4	3	13.1
All ages	10	4.6	29	13.0	30.7	3.0	7	3.2	9	3.3
Females										
0-4	1	4.3	1	3.6	2.5	2.1	1	2.1	1	2.1
5-14	3	5.2	6	12.4	10.0	2.4	2	3.0	2	2.8
15-44	2	1.6	6	5.7	29.9	3.6	1	1.2	2	1.2
45-59	1	4.2	4	16.0	52.4	3.9	1	3.2	1	3.1
60+	2	13.1	9	51.4	71.1	3.9	2	11.7	3	11.8
All ages	9	3.9	26	11.5	33.0	3.1	6	2.7	7	2.8
Total	19	4.3	54	12.3	31.7	3.1	13	3.0	16	3.1

Table 157h — MEC - AOM - CMO — Leukaemia - Cases

Age group (years)	Incidence 1990 Number ('000s)	Rate (per 100 000)	Prevalence 1990 Number ('000s)	Rate (per 100 000)	Avg. age at onset (years)	Average duration (years)	Deaths 1990 Number ('000s)	Rate (per 100 000)	Deaths 2000 (Projected) Number ('000s)	Rate (per 100 000)
Males										
0-4	1	2.4	1	1.8	2.5	1.8	1	1.4	1	1.4
5-14	3	4.4	6	8.8	10.0	2.0	2	3.2	3	3.1
15-44	2	1.9	7	5.9	29.8	3.0	2	1.6	2	1.6
45-59	1	3.8	3	13.2	52.3	3.4	1	3.0	1	3.0
60+	2	14.8	7	51.5	69.7	3.5	2	12.8	2	12.6
All ages	9	3.5	23	9.0	31.6	2.7	7	2.7	9	2.7
Females										
0-4	1	2.7	1	2.1	2.5	1.9	1	1.6	1	1.8
5-14	3	5.6	7	12.0	10.0	2.1	2	3.8	3	3.4
15-44	1	1.4	5	4.4	29.8	3.2	1	1.1	2	1.1
45-59	1	2.7	2	9.1	52.3	3.4	0	2.2	1	2.0
60+	2	13.5	7	47.0	70.4	3.5	2	12.4	2	11.2
All ages	9	3.5	22	9.0	29.8	2.7	7	2.7	8	2.5
Total	18	3.5	45	9.0	30.7	2.7	14	2.7	17	2.6

Table 157i — World - Mundo - Monde — Leukaemia - Cases

Age group (years)	Incidence 1990 Number ('000s)	Rate (per 100 000)	Prevalence 1990 Number ('000s)	Rate (per 100 000)	Avg. age at onset (years)	Average duration (years)	Deaths 1990 Number ('000s)	Rate (per 100 000)	Deaths 2000 (Projected) Number ('000s)	Rate (per 100 000)
Males										
0-4	18	5.6	14	4.4	2.5	1.9	9	2.8	9	2.7
5-14	28	5.1	58	10.6	10.0	2.0	19	3.5	21	3.4
15-44	40	3.2	133	10.6	29.8	3.2	31	2.5	37	2.5
45-59	25	8.2	103	33.0	52.3	3.8	17	5.5	24	6.0
60+	56	25.7	245	112.0	70.1	3.9	44	20.0	56	20.3
All ages	168	6.3	554	20.9	37.4	3.1	120	4.5	147	4.8
Females										
0-4	17	5.4	14	4.4	2.5	1.9	9	2.8	10	3.0
5-14	22	4.3	50	9.5	10.0	2.2	14	2.7	15	2.5
15-44	34	2.8	119	9.9	29.8	3.4	26	2.2	29	2.1
45-59	19	6.3	76	24.6	52.4	3.8	15	4.7	19	4.6
60+	48	17.7	204	75.9	71.2	4.0	42	15.4	51	15.0
All ages	140	5.4	463	17.7	38.1	3.2	105	4.0	123	4.0
Total	308	5.9	1 017	19.3	37.7	3.1	226	4.3	270	4.4

For epidemiological sources see Murray et al. 1996. For the methods used to estimate and project incidence, prevalence, and deaths see Murray and Lopez 1996a. See explanatory notes for definitions and caveats.

Table 158
Diabetes mellitus

Cuadro 158
Diabetes mellitus

Tableau 158
Diabète sucré

Cases

Casos

Cas

Table 158a   EME - PEMC - EMBE — Diabetes mellitus - Cases

Age group (years)	Incidence 1990 Number ('000s)	Rate (per 100 000)	Prevalence 1990 Number ('000s)	Rate (per 100 000)	Avg. age at onset (years)	Average duration (years)	Deaths 1990 Number ('000s)	Rate (per 100 000)	Deaths 2000 (Projected) Number ('000s)	Rate (per 100 000)
Males										
0-4	3	11.0	7	27	2.5	63.6	0	0.1	0	0.1
5-14	4	8.0	50	94	10.0	57.5	0	0.0	0	0.0
15-44	113	61.6	1 900	1 032	30.0	39.5	3	1.4	2	1.3
45-59	408	616.9	4 240	6 411	52.3	20.6	7	11.0	7	9.2
60+	567	936.4	10 573	17 463	70.7	9.0	47	77.9	53	73.3
All ages	1 096	280.6	16 771	4 295	59.2	16.8	57	14.6	63	15.2
Females										
0-4	3	10.0	6	25	2.5	69.6	0	0.1	0	0.1
5-14	6	11.0	53	104	10.0	63.8	0	0.1	0	0.1
15-44	109	60.8	1 898	1 059	29.9	45.2	2	0.9	1	0.7
45-59	404	595.9	4 332	6 389	52.3	24.9	5	7.5	5	5.7
60+	692	818.0	14 790	17 490	72.4	10.2	81	96.1	96	98.3
All ages	1 213	297.7	21 079	5 175	61.5	18.6	88	21.6	102	23.7
Total	2 308	289.3	37 850	4 744	60.4	17.8	145	18.2	164	19.6

Table 158b   FSE - PEAS - AESE — Diabetes mellitus - Cases

Age group (years)	Incidence 1990 Number ('000s)	Rate (per 100 000)	Prevalence 1990 Number ('000s)	Rate (per 100 000)	Avg. age at onset (years)	Average duration (years)	Deaths 1990 Number ('000s)	Rate (per 100 000)	Deaths 2000 (Projected) Number ('000s)	Rate (per 100 000)
Males										
0-4	1	7.0	2	15	2.5	19.5	0	0.1	0	0.1
5-14	2	7.0	12	43	10.0	32.0	0	0.1	0	0.0
15-44	31	41.2	495	649	29.6	32.9	1	1.6	1	1.3
45-59	118	436.1	1 130	4 191	52.1	16.2	2	9.0	2	7.8
60+	161	768.9	2 336	11 142	69.6	7.3	7	35.7	9	34.6
All ages	313	189.4	3 975	2 404	58.4	13.4	11	6.8	12	7.2
Females										
0-4	1	7.0	2	15	2.5	21.6	0	0.2	0	0.1
5-14	2	7.0	11	43	10.0	36.7	0	0.1	0	0.1
15-44	32	42.2	498	665	30.0	39.9	1	1.2	1	0.9
45-59	130	433.0	1 326	4 419	52.3	20.9	3	8.4	2	6.8
60+	356	977.3	5 199	14 284	71.1	8.6	16	43.0	17	41.1
All ages	520	287.4	7 036	3 889	63.6	13.7	19	10.6	20	10.7
Total	833	240.6	11 011	3 180	61.6	13.6	30	8.8	32	9.0

Table 158c   India - India - Inde — Diabetes mellitus - Cases

Age group (years)	Incidence 1990 Number ('000s)	Rate (per 100 000)	Prevalence 1990 Number ('000s)	Rate (per 100 000)	Avg. age at onset (years)	Average duration (years)	Deaths 1990 Number ('000s)	Rate (per 100 000)	Deaths 2000 (Projected) Number ('000s)	Rate (per 100 000)
Males										
0-4	4	7.0	3	5.6	2.5	0.97	2	3.5	2	3.8
5-14	7	7.0	7	7.0	10.0	5.27	4	4.3	3	2.8
15-44	96	47.7	1 364	680.4	29.7	32.98	5	2.3	4	1.8
45-59	345	725.2	3 068	6 448.9	52.2	16.89	10	20.9	10	16.4
60+	283	949.2	4 795	16 109.5	69.1	7.35	28	94.5	29	77.6
All ages	734	167.1	9 238	2 102.4	55.1	15.11	49	11.2	48	9.4
Females										
0-4	4	7.0	3	5.6	2.5	0.97	2	3.6	2	4.0
5-14	7	7.0	7	7.0	10.0	5.26	4	4.4	3	2.8
15-44	87	47.7	1 236	674.7	29.7	34.08	4	2.2	3	1.4
45-59	329	714.1	2 956	6 425.8	52.2	17.93	11	23.3	10	17.4
60+	272	941.3	4 645	16 058.5	69.5	7.49	34	116.2	39	101.4
All ages	699	170.4	8 847	2 157.2	55.4	15.66	55	13.3	58	12.0
Total	1 433	168.7	18 085	2 128.9	55.3	15.38	104	12.2	106	10.6

For epidemiological sources see McKeigue and King 1996. For the methods used to estimate and project incidence, prevalence, and deaths see Murray and Lopez 1996a. See explanatory notes for definitions and caveats.

Table 158 — Diabetes mellitus
Cuadro 158 — Diabetes mellitus
Tableau 158 — Diabète sucré

Cases — Casos — Cas

Table 158d — China - China - Chine — Diabetes mellitus - Cases

Age group (years)	Incidence 1990 Number ('000s)	Rate (per 100 000)	Prevalence 1990 Number ('000s)	Rate (per 100 000)	Avg. age at onset (years)	Average duration (years)	Deaths 1990 Number ('000s)	Rate (per 100 000)	Deaths 2000 (Projected) Number ('000s)	Rate (per 100 000)
Males										
0-4	1	2.0	2	2.8	2.5	2.8	0	0.4	0	0.4
5-14	2	2.0	5	4.8	10.0	13.1	0	0.4	0	0.2
15-44	46	15.2	665	217.2	30.0	34.5	3	1.1	3	1.0
45-59	169	233.1	1 504	2 069.2	52.3	18.0	6	7.9	6	6.2
60+	198	403.5	3 074	6 276.8	69.6	8.0	17	35.0	17	29.0
All ages	417	71.2	5 250	897.1	57.7	15.0	27	4.6	27	4.2
Females										
0-4	1	2.0	2	2.8	2.5	2.8	0	0.4	0	0.4
5-14	2	2.0	4	4.8	10.0	13.5	0	0.4	0	0.2
15-44	41	14.6	577	203.1	30.5	36.2	3	1.0	2	0.7
45-59	151	235.0	1 343	2 086.0	52.3	19.7	6	9.7	7	7.2
60+	179	347.0	3 087	5 975.7	70.8	8.5	23	45.4	27	42.3
All ages	375	68.4	5 014	914.1	58.4	16.1	33	6.0	36	5.8
Total	792	69.8	10 264	905.3	58.0	15.5	60	5.3	64	5.0

Table 158e — OAI - OPAI - APAI — Diabetes mellitus - Cases

Age group (years)	Incidence 1990 Number ('000s)	Rate (per 100 000)	Prevalence 1990 Number ('000s)	Rate (per 100 000)	Avg. age at onset (years)	Average duration (years)	Deaths 1990 Number ('000s)	Rate (per 100 000)	Deaths 2000 (Projected) Number ('000s)	Rate (per 100 000)
Males										
0-4	1	2.0	1	1.9	2.5	1.2	0	0.7	0	0.6
5-14	2	2.0	2	2.5	10.0	6.4	1	0.9	1	0.6
15-44	77	47.7	1 084	674.1	29.7	31.9	3	1.9	3	1.6
45-59	241	706.2	2 133	6 247.4	52.1	16.1	6	18.5	7	14.7
60+	179	885.0	3 035	15 020.0	69.1	7.2	15	76.6	18	64.1
All ages	499	145.5	6 255	1 823.8	54.5	15.3	26	7.6	28	7.0
Females										
0-4	1	2.0	1	1.9	2.5	1.2	0	0.7	0	0.7
5-14	2	2.0	2	2.5	10.0	6.5	1	0.9	0	0.6
15-44	76	47.7	1 070	670.5	29.7	33.5	3	1.6	2	1.1
45-59	244	695.0	2 186	6 231.1	52.2	17.6	7	19.3	7	14.2
60+	202	893.3	3 482	15 363.9	69.8	7.6	22	98.8	28	86.5
All ages	525	154.6	6 741	1 985.2	55.5	16.0	33	9.6	38	9.4
Total	1 024	150.0	12 996	1 904.1	55.0	15.6	59	8.6	66	8.2

Table 158f — SSA - ASS - ASS — Diabetes mellitus - Cases

Age group (years)	Incidence 1990 Number ('000s)	Rate (per 100 000)	Prevalence 1990 Number ('000s)	Rate (per 100 000)	Avg. age at onset (years)	Average duration (years)	Deaths 1990 Number ('000s)	Rate (per 100 000)	Deaths 2000 (Projected) Number ('000s)	Rate (per 100 000)
Males										
0-4	1	2.0	1	1.1	2.4	0.61	0	0.8	1	0.8
5-14	1	2.0	1	1.3	10.0	2.95	1	2.0	1	1.4
15-44	22	20.9	300	289.5	29.4	29.54	1	0.9	1	0.7
45-59	77	377.7	646	3 179.1	52.1	15.65	2	10.4	2	8.0
60+	54	514.1	874	8 320.9	69.0	7.10	5	49.2	6	39.3
All ages	155	61.4	1 822	722.0	54.1	14.41	10	4.0	11	3.1
Females										
0-4	1	2.0	1	1.1	2.4	0.61	0	1.0	1	1.0
5-14	1	2.0	1	1.3	10.0	2.99	1	2.0	1	1.4
15-44	22	20.9	307	288.7	29.5	30.66	0	0.4	0	0.3
45-59	82	372.9	700	3 162.9	52.2	16.40	3	11.8	2	8.4
60+	73	572.6	1 099	8 635.4	69.4	7.25	8	65.7	9	52.2
All ages	180	69.8	2 107	816.8	55.8	14.27	13	5.2	14	4.0
Total	335	65.6	3 929	769.9	55.0	14.33	23	4.6	24	3.5

For epidemiological sources see McKeigue and King 1996. For the methods used to estimate and project incidence, prevalence, and deaths see Murray and Lopez 1996a. See explanatory notes for definitions and caveats.

Table 158
Diabetes mellitus

Cuadro 158
Diabetes mellitus

Tableau 158
Diabète sucré

Cases

Casos

Cas

Table 158g   LAC - ALC - ALC   Diabetes mellitus - Cases

Age group (years)	Incidence 1990 Number ('000s)	Rate (per 100 000)	Prevalence 1990 Number ('000s)	Rate (per 100 000)	Avg. age at onset (years)	Average duration (years)	Deaths 1990 Number ('000s)	Rate (per 100 000)	Deaths 2000 (Projected) Number ('000s)	Rate (per 100 000)
Males										
0-4	1	5.0	2	5.7	2.5	1.7	0	1.2	0	1.2
5-14	3	5.0	4	8.3	10.0	8.9	1	1.4	1	1.0
15-44	64	61.8	926	888.2	29.7	33.8	3	2.9	3	2.5
45-59	189	849.3	1 715	7 706.8	52.2	17.4	8	34.9	9	28.3
60+	154	1 084.6	2 726	19 155.5	69.6	7.9	23	164.6	28	142.0
All ages	412	185.8	5 373	2 424.5	54.8	16.3	35	15.9	41	15.4
Females										
0-4	1	5.0	2	5.7	2.5	1.7	0	1.2	0	1.1
5-14	3	5.0	4	8.3	10.0	9.0	1	1.2	0	0.9
15-44	63	60.5	895	859.6	29.8	35.8	4	3.4	3	2.5
45-59	195	836.0	1 786	7 645.5	52.2	19.6	11	45.3	11	34.2
60+	159	942.2	3 172	18 856.7	70.4	8.7	38	227.2	48	202.4
All ages	421	188.9	5 859	2 630.9	55.3	17.8	53	24.0	63	23.4
Total	832	187.4	11 232	2 527.9	55.0	17.1	89	20.0	103	19.4

Table 158h   MEC - AOM - CMO   Diabetes mellitus - Cases

Age group (years)	Incidence 1990 Number ('000s)	Rate (per 100 000)	Prevalence 1990 Number ('000s)	Rate (per 100 000)	Avg. age at onset (years)	Average duration (years)	Deaths 1990 Number ('000s)	Rate (per 100 000)	Deaths 2000 (Projected) Number ('000s)	Rate (per 100 000)
Males										
0-4	3	7.0	3	6.6	2.5	1.2	1	2.2	1	2.2
5-14	5	7.0	6	8.7	10.0	6.6	2	3.0	2	2.1
15-44	85	74.2	1 210	1 062.7	29.8	33.0	3	3.0	4	2.4
45-59	248	1 108.2	2 219	9 936.0	52.1	16.6	7	29.2	7	22.8
60+	143	1 051.1	2 981	21 840.3	69.1	7.4	15	110.1	17	91.1
All ages	483	188.4	6 420	2 503.9	52.6	16.6	28	10.9	31	9.2
Females										
0-4	3	7.0	3	6.6	2.5	1.2	1	2.2	1	2.1
5-14	4	7.0	5	8.7	10.0	6.7	2	3.0	2	2.1
15-44	80	74.2	1 131	1 054.8	29.8	34.5	3	2.6	2	1.8
45-59	234	1 049.1	2 137	9 586.7	52.1	18.2	7	31.0	7	22.5
60+	151	976.2	3 261	21 108.5	69.8	7.9	21	135.5	24	111.0
All ages	471	191.1	6 537	2 650.0	53.3	17.4	33	13.6	36	11.1
Total	954	189.7	12 957	2 575.5	52.9	17.0	61	12.2	67	10.1

Table 158i   World - Mundo - Monde   Diabetes mellitus - Cases

Age group (years)	Incidence 1990 Number ('000s)	Rate (per 100 000)	Prevalence 1990 Number ('000s)	Rate (per 100 000)	Avg. age at onset (years)	Average duration (years)	Deaths 1990 Number ('000s)	Rate (per 100 000)	Deaths 2000 (Projected) Number ('000s)	Rate (per 100 000)
Males										
0-4	15	4.8	20	6.2	2.5	7.3	4	1.4	5	1.4
5-14	26	4.6	87	15.7	10.0	13.4	10	1.7	7	1.2
15-44	534	42.7	7 946	635.7	29.8	33.9	22	1.8	22	1.5
45-59	1 794	574.4	16 654	5 331.6	52.2	17.7	48	15.4	50	12.5
60+	1 739	794.6	30 396	13 888.4	69.7	8.0	159	72.7	176	64.0
All ages	4 108	154.8	55 103	2 076.5	56.0	15.4	244	9.2	261	8.4
Females										
0-4	15	4.7	19	6.0	2.5	7.8	4	1.4	5	1.4
5-14	26	4.9	88	16.7	10.0	14.3	9	1.8	7	1.2
15-44	510	42.6	7 612	635.1	29.9	36.4	19	1.6	15	1.1
45-59	1 769	568.8	16 766	5 390.1	52.2	20.1	51	16.6	51	12.6
60+	2 084	774.0	38 736	14 388.4	71.0	8.8	244	90.6	288	85.5
All ages	4 403	168.5	63 220	2 418.8	57.4	16.3	328	12.5	366	11.9
Total	8 512	161.6	118 323	2 246.4	56.7	15.9	571	10.8	627	10.2

For epidemiological sources see McKeigue and King 1996. For the methods used to estimate and project incidence, prevalence, and deaths see Murray and Lopez 1996a. See explanatory notes for definitions and caveats.

Table 159
Diabetes mellitus

Cuadro 159
Diabetes mellitus

Tableau 159
Diabète sucré

Diabetic foot   Pie diabético   Pied diabétique

Table 159a   EME - PEMC - EMBE   Diabetes mellitus - Diabetic foot

Age group (years)	Incidence 1990 Number ('000s)	Rate (per 100 000)	Prevalence 1990 Number ('000s)	Rate (per 100 000)	Avg. age at onset (years)	Average duration (years)	Deaths 1990 Number ('000s)	Rate (per 100 000)	Deaths 2000 (Projected) Number ('000s)	Rate (per 100 000)
Males										
0-4	0	0	0	0.0	-	-	-	-	-	-
5-14	0	0	0	0.0	-	-	-	-	-	-
15-44	76	41	13	7.0	29.9	0.17	-	-	-	-
45-59	202	306	34	52.0	52.4	0.17	-	-	-	-
60+	516	853	88	145.0	71.1	0.17	-	-	-	-
All ages	795	203	135	34.6	62.4	0.17	-	-	-	-
Females										
0-4	0	0	0	0.0	-	-	-	-	-	-
5-14	0	0	0	0.0	-	-	-	-	-	-
15-44	74	41	13	7.0	30.0	0.17	-	-	-	-
45-59	207	306	35	52.0	52.4	0.17	-	-	-	-
60+	711	841	121	143.0	72.4	0.17	-	-	-	-
All ages	993	244	169	41.4	65.1	0.17	-	-	-	-
Total	1 787	224	304	38.1	63.9	0.17	-	-	-	-

Table 159b   FSE - PEAS - AESE   Diabetes mellitus - Diabetic foot

Age group (years)	Incidence 1990 Number ('000s)	Rate (per 100 000)	Prevalence 1990 Number ('000s)	Rate (per 100 000)	Avg. age at onset (years)	Average duration (years)	Deaths 1990 Number ('000s)	Rate (per 100 000)	Deaths 2000 (Projected) Number ('000s)	Rate (per 100 000)
Males										
0-4	0	0	0	0.0	-	-	-	-	-	-
5-14	0	0	0	0.0	-	-	-	-	-	-
15-44	22	29	4	5.0	29.8	0.17	-	-	-	-
45-59	56	206	9	35.0	52.2	0.17	-	-	-	-
60+	113	541	19	92.0	70.0	0.17	-	-	-	-
All ages	191	116	33	19.7	60.1	0.17	-	-	-	-
Females										
0-4	0	0	0	0.0	-	-	-	-	-	-
5-14	0	0	0	0.0	-	-	-	-	-	-
15-44	22	29	4	5.0	29.8	0.17	-	-	-	-
45-59	62	206	11	35.0	52.2	0.17	-	-	-	-
60+	218	600	37	102.0	70.0	0.17	-	-	-	-
All ages	302	167	51	28.4	63.4	0.17	-	-	-	-
Total	494	143	84	24.2	62.1	0.17	-	-	-	-

Table 159c   India - India - Inde   Diabetes mellitus - Diabetic foot

Age group (years)	Incidence 1990 Number ('000s)	Rate (per 100 000)	Prevalence 1990 Number ('000s)	Rate (per 100 000)	Avg. age at onset (years)	Average duration (years)	Deaths 1990 Number ('000s)	Rate (per 100 000)	Deaths 2000 (Projected) Number ('000s)	Rate (per 100 000)
Males										
0-4	0	0	0	0.0	-	-	-	-	-	-
5-14	0	0	0	0.0	-	-	-	-	-	-
15-44	71	35	12	6.0	29.8	0.17	-	-	-	-
45-59	157	329	27	56.0	52.3	0.17	-	-	-	-
60+	256	859	43	146.0	69.7	0.17	-	-	-	-
All ages	483	110	82	18.7	58.2	0.17	-	-	-	-
Females										
0-4	0	0	0	0.0	-	-	-	-	-	-
5-14	0	0	0	0.0	-	-	-	-	-	-
15-44	65	35	11	6.0	29.8	0.17	-	-	-	-
45-59	154	335	26	57.0	52.4	0.17	-	-	-	-
60+	248	859	42	146.0	70.1	0.17	-	-	-	-
All ages	467	114	79	19.4	58.7	0.17	-	-	-	-
Total	950	112	162	19.0	58.4	0.17	-	-	-	-

For epidemiological sources see McKeigue and King 1996. For the methods used to estimate and project incidence, prevalence, and deaths see Murray and Lopez 1996a. See explanatory notes for definitions and caveats.

Table 159
Diabetes mellitus

Cuadro 159
Diabetes mellitus

Tableau 159
Diabète sucré

Diabetic foot

Pie diabético

Pied diabétique

Table 159d   China - China - Chine   Diabetes mellitus - Diabetic foot

Age group (years)	Incidence 1990 Number ('000s)	Rate (per 100 000)	Prevalence 1990 Number ('000s)	Rate (per 100 000)	Avg. age at onset (years)	Average duration (years)	Deaths 1990 Number ('000s)	Rate (per 100 000)	Deaths 2000 (Projected) Number ('000s)	Rate (per 100 000)
Males										
0-4	0	0	0	0.0	-	-	-	-	-	-
5-14	0	0	0	0.0	-	-	-	-	-	-
15-44	36	12	6	2.0	29.9	0.17	-	-	-	-
45-59	73	100	12	17.0	52.3	0.17	-	-	-	-
60+	150	306	25	52.0	69.8	0.17	-	-	-	-
All ages	259	44	44	7.5	59.3	0.17	-	-	-	-
Females										
0-4	0	0	0	0.0	-	-	-	-	-	-
5-14	0	0	0	0.0	-	-	-	-	-	-
15-44	33	12	6	2.0	29.9	0.17	-	-	-	-
45-59	64	100	11	17.0	52.4	0.17	-	-	-	-
60+	152	294	26	50.0	70.6	0.17	-	-	-	-
All ages	250	46	42	7.7	60.5	0.17	-	-	-	-
Total	508	45	86	7.6	59.9	0.17	-	-	-	-

Table 159e   OAI - OPAI - APAI   Diabetes mellitus - Diabetic foot

Age group (years)	Incidence 1990 Number ('000s)	Rate (per 100 000)	Prevalence 1990 Number ('000s)	Rate (per 100 000)	Avg. age at onset (years)	Average duration (years)	Deaths 1990 Number ('000s)	Rate (per 100 000)	Deaths 2000 (Projected) Number ('000s)	Rate (per 100 000)
Males										
0-4	0	0	0	0.0	-	-	-	-	-	-
5-14	0	0	0	0.0	-	-	-	-	-	-
15-44	57	35	10	6.0	29.7	0.17	-	-	-	-
45-59	108	318	18	54.0	52.3	0.17	-	-	-	-
60+	162	800	27	136.0	69.6	0.17	-	-	-	-
All ages	327	95	56	16.2	56.9	0.17	-	-	-	-
Females										
0-4	0	0	0	0.0	-	-	-	-	-	-
5-14	0	0	0	0.0	-	-	-	-	-	-
15-44	56	35	10	6.0	29.8	0.17	-	-	-	-
45-59	111	318	19	54.0	52.3	0.17	-	-	-	-
60+	187	824	32	140.0	70.3	0.17	-	-	-	-
All ages	354	104	60	17.7	58.2	0.17	-	-	-	-
Total	681	100	116	17.0	57.6	0.17	-	-	-	-

Table 159f   SSA - ASS - ASS   Diabetes mellitus - Diabetic foot

Age group (years)	Incidence 1990 Number ('000s)	Rate (per 100 000)	Prevalence 1990 Number ('000s)	Rate (per 100 000)	Avg. age at onset (years)	Average duration (years)	Deaths 1990 Number ('000s)	Rate (per 100 000)	Deaths 2000 (Projected) Number ('000s)	Rate (per 100 000)
Males										
0-4	0	0	0	0.0	-	-	-	-	-	-
5-14	0	0	0	0.0	-	-	-	-	-	-
15-44	12	12	2	2.0	29.4	0.17	-	-	-	-
45-59	32	159	5	27.0	52.2	0.17	-	-	-	-
60+	48	453	8	77.0	69.2	0.17	-	-	-	-
All ages	92	36	16	6.2	58.0	0.17	-	-	-	-
Females										
0-4	0	0	0	0.0	-	-	-	-	-	-
5-14	0	0	0	0.0	-	-	-	-	-	-
15-44	13	12	2	2.0	29.5	0.17	-	-	-	-
45-59	35	159	6	27.0	52.2	0.17	-	-	-	-
60+	59	465	10	79.0	69.7	0.17	-	-	-	-
All ages	107	41	18	7.0	59.2	0.17	-	-	-	-
Total	199	39	34	6.6	58.6	0.17	-	-	-	-

For epidemiological sources see McKeigue and King 1996. For the methods used to estimate and project incidence, prevalence, and deaths see Murray and Lopez 1996a. See explanatory notes for definitions and caveats.

Table 159	Cuadro 159	Tableau 159
Diabetes mellitus	Diabetes mellitus	Diabète sucré
Diabetic foot	Pie diabético	Pied diabétique

Table 159g   LAC - ALC - ALC

Diabetes mellitus - Diabetic foot

Age group (years)	Incidence 1990 Number ('000s)	Rate (per 100 000)	Prevalence 1990 Number ('000s)	Rate (per 100 000)	Avg. age at onset (years)	Average duration (years)	Deaths 1990 Number ('000s)	Rate (per 100 000)	Deaths 2000 (Projected) Number ('000s)	Rate (per 100 000)
Males										
0-4	0	0	0	0.0	-	-	-	-	-	-
5-14	0	0	0	0.0	-	-	-	-	-	-
15-44	46	44	8	7.5	29.8	0.17	-	-	-	-
45-59	88	394	15	67.0	52.3	0.17	-	-	-	-
60+	146	1 027	25	174.7	70.3	0.17	-	-	-	-
All ages	280	126	48	21.5	58.0	0.17	-	-	-	-
Females										
0-4	0	0	0	0.0	-	-	-	-	-	-
5-14	0	0	0	0.0	-	-	-	-	-	-
15-44	46	44	8	7.5	29.9	0.17	-	-	-	-
45-59	91	392	16	66.6	52.4	0.17	-	-	-	-
60+	177	1 052	30	178.9	71.1	0.17	-	-	-	-
All ages	314	141	53	24.0	59.7	0.17	-	-	-	-
Total	594	134	101	22.7	58.9	0.17	-	-	-	-

Table 159h   MEC - AOM - CMO

Diabetes mellitus - Diabetic foot

Age group (years)	Incidence 1990 Number ('000s)	Rate (per 100 000)	Prevalence 1990 Number ('000s)	Rate (per 100 000)	Avg. age at onset (years)	Average duration (years)	Deaths 1990 Number ('000s)	Rate (per 100 000)	Deaths 2000 (Projected) Number ('000s)	Rate (per 100 000)
Males										
0-4	0	0	0	0.0	-	-	-	-	-	-
5-14	0	0	0	0.0	-	-	-	-	-	-
15-44	60	53	10	9.0	29.8	0.17	-	-	-	-
45-59	113	506	19	86.0	52.3	0.17	-	-	-	-
60+	159	1 165	27	198.0	69.7	0.17	-	-	-	-
All ages	332	130	56	22.0	56.5	0.17	-	-	-	-
Females										
0-4	0	0	0	0.0	-	-	-	-	-	-
5-14	0	0	0	0.0	-	-	-	-	-	-
15-44	57	53	10	9.0	29.8	0.17	-	-	-	-
45-59	109	488	19	83.0	52.3	0.17	-	-	-	-
60+	175	1 135	30	193.0	70.4	0.17	-	-	-	-
All ages	341	138	58	23.5	57.9	0.17	-	-	-	-
Total	673	134	114	22.8	57.2	0.17	-	-	-	-

Table 159i   World - Mundo - Monde

Diabetes mellitus - Diabetic foot

Age group (years)	Incidence 1990 Number ('000s)	Rate (per 100 000)	Prevalence 1990 Number ('000s)	Rate (per 100 000)	Avg. age at onset (years)	Average duration (years)	Deaths 1990 Number ('000s)	Rate (per 100 000)	Deaths 2000 (Projected) Number ('000s)	Rate (per 100 000)
Males										
0-4	0	0	0	0.0	-	-	-	-	-	-
5-14	0	0	0	0.0	-	-	-	-	-	-
15-44	380	30	65	5.2	29.8	0.17	-	-	-	-
45-59	829	265	141	45.1	52.3	0.17	-	-	-	-
60+	1 550	708	263	120.4	70.1	0.17	-	-	-	-
All ages	2 758	104	469	17.7	58.8	0.17	-	-	-	-
Females										
0-4	0	0	0	0.0	-	-	-	-	-	-
5-14	0	0	0	0.0	-	-	-	-	-	-
15-44	365	30	62	5.2	29.8	0.17	-	-	-	-
45-59	835	268	142	45.6	52.3	0.17	-	-	-	-
60+	1 928	716	328	121.8	71.0	0.17	-	-	-	-
All ages	3 128	120	532	20.3	60.4	0.17	-	-	-	-
Total	5 887	112	1 001	19.0	59.7	0.17	-	-	-	-

For epidemiological sources see McKeigue and King 1996. For the methods used to estimate and project incidence, prevalence, and deaths see Murray and Lopez 1996a. See explanatory notes for definitions and caveats.

Table 160	Cuadro 160	Tableau 160
Diabetes mellitus	**Diabetes mellitus**	**Diabète sucré**

Neuropathy · Neuropatía · Neuropathie

Table 160a EME - PEMC - EMBE — Diabetes mellitus - Neuropathy

Age group (years)	Incidence 1990 Number ('000s)	Rate (per 100 000)	Prevalence 1990 Number ('000s)	Rate (per 100 000)	Avg. age at onset (years)	Average duration (years)	Deaths 1990 Number ('000s)	Rate (per 100 000)	Deaths 2000 (Projected) Number ('000s)	Rate (per 100 000)
Males										
0-4	-	-	0	0	-	-	0	0	0	0
5-14	-	-	0	0	-	-	0	0	0	0
15-44	-	-	332	180	-	-	0	0	0	0
45-59	-	-	833	1 259	-	-	0	0	0	0
60+	-	-	2 108	3 482	-	-	0	0	0	0
All ages	-	-	3 273	838	-	-	0	0	0	0
Females										
0-4	-	-	0	0	-	-	0	0	0	0
5-14	-	-	0	0	-	-	0	0	0	0
15-44	-	-	325	182	-	-	0	0	0	0
45-59	-	-	853	1 258	-	-	0	0	0	0
60+	-	-	2 959	3 500	-	-	0	0	0	0
All ages	-	-	4 138	1 016	-	-	0	0	0	0
Total	-	-	7 411	929	-	-	0	0	0	0

Table 160b FSE - PEAS - AESE — Diabetes mellitus - Neuropathy

Age group (years)	Incidence 1990 Number ('000s)	Rate (per 100 000)	Prevalence 1990 Number ('000s)	Rate (per 100 000)	Avg. age at onset (years)	Average duration (years)	Deaths 1990 Number ('000s)	Rate (per 100 000)	Deaths 2000 (Projected) Number ('000s)	Rate (per 100 000)
Males										
0-4	-	-	0	0	-	-	0	0	0	0
5-14	-	-	0	0	-	-	0	0	0	0
15-44	-	-	92	120	-	-	0	0	0	0
45-59	-	-	226	838	-	-	0	0	0	0
60+	-	-	465	2 220	-	-	0	0	0	0
All ages	-	-	783	474	-	-	0	0	0	0
Females										
0-4	-	-	0	0	-	-	0	0	0	0
5-14	-	-	0	0	-	-	0	0	0	0
15-44	-	-	90	120	-	-	0	0	0	0
45-59	-	-	253	842	-	-	0	0	0	0
60+	-	-	895	2 459	-	-	0	0	0	0
All ages	-	-	1 238	684	-	-	0	0	0	0
Total	-	-	2 021	584	-	-	0	0	0	0

Table 160c India - India - Inde — Diabetes mellitus - Neuropathy

Age group (years)	Incidence 1990 Number ('000s)	Rate (per 100 000)	Prevalence 1990 Number ('000s)	Rate (per 100 000)	Avg. age at onset (years)	Average duration (years)	Deaths 1990 Number ('000s)	Rate (per 100 000)	Deaths 2000 (Projected) Number ('000s)	Rate (per 100 000)
Males										
0-4	-	-	0	0	-	-	0	0	0	0
5-14	-	-	0	0	-	-	0	0	0	0
15-44	-	-	283	141	-	-	0	0	0	0
45-59	-	-	638	1 341	-	-	0	0	0	0
60+	-	-	1 048	3 519	-	-	0	0	0	0
All ages	-	-	1 968	448	-	-	0	0	0	0
Females										
0-4	-	-	0	0	-	-	0	0	0	0
5-14	-	-	0	0	-	-	0	0	0	0
15-44	-	-	258	141	-	-	0	0	0	0
45-59	-	-	617	1 340	-	-	0	0	0	0
60+	-	-	1 019	3 522	-	-	0	0	0	0
All ages	-	-	1 894	462	-	-	0	0	0	0
Total	-	-	3 862	455	-	-	0	0	0	0

For epidemiological sources see McKeigue and King 1996. For the methods used to estimate and project incidence, prevalence, and deaths see Murray and Lopez 1996a. See explanatory notes for definitions and caveats.

Table 160
Diabetes mellitus

Cuadro 160
Diabetes mellitus

Tableau 160
Diabète sucré

Neuropathy

Neuropatía

Neuropathie

Table 160d — China - China - Chine — Diabetes mellitus - Neuropathy

Age group (years)	Incidence 1990 Number ('000s)	Rate (per 100 000)	Prevalence 1990 Number ('000s)	Rate (per 100 000)	Avg. age at onset (years)	Average duration (years)	Deaths 1990 Number ('000s)	Rate (per 100 000)	Deaths 2000 (Projected) Number ('000s)	Rate (per 100 000)
Males										
0-4	-	-	0	0	-	-	0	0	0	0
5-14	-	-	0	0	-	-	0	0	0	0
15-44	-	-	127	42	-	-	0	0	0	0
45-59	-	-	306	421	-	-	0	0	0	0
60+	-	-	617	1 260	-	-	0	0	0	0
All ages	-	-	1 050	180	-	-	0	0	0	0
Females										
0-4	-	-	0	0	-	-	0	0	0	0
5-14	-	-	0	0	-	-	0	0	0	0
15-44	-	-	110	39	-	-	0	0	0	0
45-59	-	-	270	419	-	-	0	0	0	0
60+	-	-	620	1 201	-	-	0	0	0	0
All ages	-	-	1 000	182	-	-	0	0	0	0
Total	-	-	2 051	181	-	-	0	0	0	0

Table 160e — OAI - OPAI - APAI — Diabetes mellitus - Neuropathy

Age group (years)	Incidence 1990 Number ('000s)	Rate (per 100 000)	Prevalence 1990 Number ('000s)	Rate (per 100 000)	Avg. age at onset (years)	Average duration (years)	Deaths 1990 Number ('000s)	Rate (per 100 000)	Deaths 2000 (Projected) Number ('000s)	Rate (per 100 000)
Males										
0-4	-	-	0	0	-	-	0	0	0	0
5-14	-	-	0	0	-	-	0	0	0	0
15-44	-	-	226	140	-	-	0	0	0	0
45-59	-	-	444	1 300	-	-	0	0	0	0
60+	-	-	664	3 283	-	-	0	0	0	0
All ages	-	-	1 333	389	-	-	0	0	0	0
Females										
0-4	-	-	0	0	-	-	0	0	0	0
5-14	-	-	0	0	-	-	0	0	0	0
15-44	-	-	225	141	-	-	0	0	0	0
45-59	-	-	456	1 301	-	-	0	0	0	0
60+	-	-	766	3 380	-	-	0	0	0	0
All ages	-	-	1 447	426	-	-	0	0	0	0
Total	-	-	2 781	407	-	-	0	0	0	0

Table 160f — SSA - ASS - ASS — Diabetes mellitus - Neuropathy

Age group (years)	Incidence 1990 Number ('000s)	Rate (per 100 000)	Prevalence 1990 Number ('000s)	Rate (per 100 000)	Avg. age at onset (years)	Average duration (years)	Deaths 1990 Number ('000s)	Rate (per 100 000)	Deaths 2000 (Projected) Number ('000s)	Rate (per 100 000)
Males										
0-4	-	-	0	0	-	-	0	0	0	0
5-14	-	-	0	0	-	-	0	0	0	0
15-44	-	-	62	60	-	-	0	0	0	0
45-59	-	-	134	661	-	-	0	0	0	0
60+	-	-	192	1 827	-	-	0	0	0	0
All ages	-	-	389	154	-	-	0	0	0	0
Females										
0-4	-	-	0	0	-	-	0	0	0	0
5-14	-	-	0	0	-	-	0	0	0	0
15-44	-	-	64	61	-	-	0	0	0	0
45-59	-	-	146	659	-	-	0	0	0	0
60+	-	-	242	1 900	-	-	0	0	0	0
All ages	-	-	452	175	-	-	0	0	0	0
Total	-	-	841	165	-	-	0	0	0	0

For epidemiological sources see McKeigue and King 1996. For the methods used to estimate and project incidence, prevalence, and deaths see Murray and Lopez 1996a. See explanatory notes for definitions and caveats.

Table 160
Diabetes mellitus

Cuadro 160
Diabetes mellitus

Tableau 160
Diabète sucré

Neuropathy

Neuropatía

Neuropathie

Table 160g   LAC - ALC - ALC

Diabetes mellitus - Neuropathy

Age group (years)	Incidence 1990 Number ('000s)	Incidence 1990 Rate (per 100 000)	Prevalence 1990 Number ('000s)	Prevalence 1990 Rate (per 100 000)	Avg. age at onset (years)	Average duration (years)	Deaths 1990 Number ('000s)	Deaths 1990 Rate (per 100 000)	Deaths 2000 (Projected) Number ('000s)	Deaths 2000 (Projected) Rate (per 100 000)
Males										
0-4	-	-	0	0	-	-	0	0	0	0
5-14	-	-	0	0	-	-	0	0	0	0
15-44	-	-	187	179	-	-	0	0	0	0
45-59	-	-	359	1 613	-	-	0	0	0	0
60+	-	-	598	4 204	-	-	0	0	0	0
All ages	-	-	1 144	516	-	-	0	0	0	0
Females										
0-4	-	-	0	0	-	-	0	0	0	0
5-14	-	-	0	0	-	-	0	0	0	0
15-44	-	-	187	180	-	-	0	0	0	0
45-59	-	-	374	1 602	-	-	0	0	0	0
60+	-	-	724	4 306	-	-	0	0	0	0
All ages	-	-	1 286	577	-	-	0	0	0	0
Total	-	-	2 430	547	-	-	0	0	0	0

Table 160h   MEC - AOM - CMO

Diabetes mellitus - Neuropathy

Age group (years)	Incidence 1990 Number ('000s)	Incidence 1990 Rate (per 100 000)	Prevalence 1990 Number ('000s)	Prevalence 1990 Rate (per 100 000)	Avg. age at onset (years)	Average duration (years)	Deaths 1990 Number ('000s)	Deaths 1990 Rate (per 100 000)	Deaths 2000 (Projected) Number ('000s)	Deaths 2000 (Projected) Rate (per 100 000)
Males										
0-4	-	-	0	0	-	-	0	0	0	0
5-14	-	-	0	0	-	-	0	0	0	0
15-44	-	-	251	221	-	-	0	0	0	0
45-59	-	-	461	2 063	-	-	0	0	0	0
60+	-	-	650	4 760	-	-	0	0	0	0
All ages	-	-	1 362	531	-	-	0	0	0	0
Females										
0-4	-	-	0	0	-	-	0	0	0	0
5-14	-	-	0	0	-	-	0	0	0	0
15-44	-	-	237	221	-	-	0	0	0	0
45-59	-	-	446	1 999	-	-	0	0	0	0
60+	-	-	717	4 640	-	-	0	0	0	0
All ages	-	-	1 399	567	-	-	0	0	0	0
Total	-	-	2 761	549	-	-	0	0	0	0

Table 160i   World - Mundo - Monde

Diabetes mellitus - Neuropathy

Age group (years)	Incidence 1990 Number ('000s)	Incidence 1990 Rate (per 100 000)	Prevalence 1990 Number ('000s)	Prevalence 1990 Rate (per 100 000)	Avg. age at onset (years)	Average duration (years)	Deaths 1990 Number ('000s)	Deaths 1990 Rate (per 100 000)	Deaths 2000 (Projected) Number ('000s)	Deaths 2000 (Projected) Rate (per 100 000)
Males										
0-4	-	-	0	0	-	-	0	0	0	0
5-14	-	-	0	0	-	-	0	0	0	0
15-44	-	-	1 560	125	-	-	0	0	0	0
45-59	-	-	3 400	1 089	-	-	0	0	0	0
60+	-	-	6 342	2 898	-	-	0	0	0	0
All ages	-	-	11 302	426	-	-	0	0	0	0
Females										
0-4	-	-	0	0	-	-	0	0	0	0
5-14	-	-	0	0	-	-	0	0	0	0
15-44	-	-	1 498	125	-	-	0	0	0	0
45-59	-	-	3 414	1 098	-	-	0	0	0	0
60+	-	-	7 943	2 950	-	-	0	0	0	0
All ages	-	-	12 854	492	-	-	0	0	0	0
Total	-	-	24 157	459	-	-	0	0	0	0

For epidemiological sources see McKeigue and King 1996. For the methods used to estimate and project incidence, prevalence, and deaths see Murray and Lopez 1996a. See explanatory notes for definitions and caveats.

Table 161	Cuadro 161	Tableau 161
Diabetes mellitus	**Diabetes mellitus**	**Diabète sucré**

Retinopathy - blindness • Retinopatía - ceguera • Rétinopathie - cécité

Table 161a   EME - PEMC - EMBE
Diabetes mellitus - Retinopathy - blindness

Age group (years)	Incidence 1990 Number ('000s)	Rate (per 100 000)	Prevalence 1990 Number ('000s)	Rate (per 100 000)	Avg. age at onset (years)	Average duration (years)	Deaths 1990 Number ('000s)	Rate (per 100 000)	Deaths 2000 (Projected) Number ('000s)	Rate (per 100 000)
Males										
0-4	0	0.0	0	0	-	-	0	0	0	0
5-14	0	0.0	0	0	-	-	0	0	0	0
15-44	8	4.1	109	59	29.9	35.9	0	0	0	0
45-59	17	25.6	196	297	52.4	17.1	0	0	0	0
60+	42	69.9	562	928	71.0	6.8	0	0	0	0
All ages	67	17.2	867	222	61.4	12.7	0	0	0	0
Females										
0-4	0	0.0	0	0	-	-	0	0	0	0
5-14	0	0.0	0	0	-	-	0	0	0	0
15-44	8	4.2	107	59	30.0	42.3	0	0	0	0
45-59	17	25.6	201	297	52.4	22.0	0	0	0	0
60+	59	70.0	785	928	72.3	8.5	0	0	0	0
All ages	84	20.7	1 093	268	64.2	14.3	0	0	0	0
Total	151	19.0	1 960	246	63.0	13.6	0	0	0	0

Table 161b   FSE - PEAS - AESE
Diabetes mellitus - Retinopathy - blindness

Age group (years)	Incidence 1990 Number ('000s)	Rate (per 100 000)	Prevalence 1990 Number ('000s)	Rate (per 100 000)	Avg. age at onset (years)	Average duration (years)	Deaths 1990 Number ('000s)	Rate (per 100 000)	Deaths 2000 (Projected) Number ('000s)	Rate (per 100 000)
Males										
0-4	0	0.0	0	0	-	-	0	0	0	0
5-14	0	0.0	0	0	-	-	0	0	0	0
15-44	2	2.6	21	28	29.8	29.0	0	0	0	0
45-59	5	16.8	43	159	52.2	12.9	0	0	0	0
60+	10	49.0	81	385	70.0	5.5	0	0	0	0
All ages	17	10.2	145	88	60.3	10.2	0	0	0	0
Females										
0-4	0	0.0	0	0	-	-	0	0	0	0
5-14	0	0.0	0	0	-	-	0	0	0	0
15-44	2	2.7	21	28	29.8	29.1	0	0	0	0
45-59	5	17.7	48	159	52.2	12.8	0	0	0	0
60+	21	57.1	146	400	70.0	5.3	0	0	0	0
All ages	28	15.6	214	118	63.7	8.4	0	0	0	0
Total	45	13.0	359	104	62.4	9.1	0	0	0	0

Table 161c   India - India - Inde
Diabetes mellitus - Retinopathy - blindness

Age group (years)	Incidence 1990 Number ('000s)	Rate (per 100 000)	Prevalence 1990 Number ('000s)	Rate (per 100 000)	Avg. age at onset (years)	Average duration (years)	Deaths 1990 Number ('000s)	Rate (per 100 000)	Deaths 2000 (Projected) Number ('000s)	Rate (per 100 000)
Males										
0-4	0	0.0	0	0	-	-	0	0	0	0
5-14	0	0.0	0	0	-	-	0	0	0	0
15-44	5	2.7	86	43	29.8	31.1	0	0	0	0
45-59	12	25.8	124	261	52.3	14.3	0	0	0	0
60+	19	64.4	194	651	69.6	5.6	0	0	0	0
All ages	37	8.4	404	92	57.9	12.2	0	0	0	0
Females										
0-4	0	0.0	0	0	-	-	0	0	0	0
5-14	0	0.0	0	0	-	-	0	0	0	0
15-44	5	2.7	79	43	29.8	33.0	0	0	0	0
45-59	12	25.7	123	268	52.3	15.8	0	0	0	0
60+	19	64.2	199	688	70.0	5.8	0	0	0	0
All ages	35	8.6	401	98	58.4	12.9	0	0	0	0
Total	72	8.5	805	95	58.1	12.6	0	0	0	0

For epidemiological sources see McKeigue and King 1996. For the methods used to estimate and project incidence, prevalence, and deaths see Murray and Lopez 1996a. See explanatory notes for definitions and caveats.

Table 161
Diabetes mellitus

Cuadro 161
Diabetes mellitus

Tableau 161
Diabète sucré

Retinopathy - blindness

Retinopatía - ceguera

Rétinopathie - cécité

Table 161d   China - China - Chine   Diabetes mellitus - Retinopathy - blindness

Age group (years)	Incidence 1990 Number ('000s)	Rate (per 100 000)	Prevalence 1990 Number ('000s)	Rate (per 100 000)	Avg. age at onset (years)	Average duration (years)	Deaths 1990 Number ('000s)	Rate (per 100 000)	Deaths 2000 (Projected) Number ('000s)	Rate (per 100 000)
Males										
0-4	0	0.0	0	0	-	-	0	0	0	0
5-14	0	0.0	0	0	-	-	0	0	0	0
15-44	3	0.9	43	14	29.9	33.1	0	0	0	0
45-59	6	8.3	60	82	52.3	14.8	0	0	0	0
60+	12	25.1	112	228	69.8	5.8	0	0	0	0
All ages	21	3.6	214	37	59.6	11.9	0	0	0	0
Females										
0-4	0	0.0	0	0	-	-	0	0	0	0
5-14	0	0.0	0	0	-	-	0	0	0	0
15-44	2	0.8	42	15	29.9	36.1	0	0	0	0
45-59	5	8.3	54	84	52.4	17.1	0	0	0	0
60+	12	23.9	131	254	70.6	6.6	0	0	0	0
All ages	20	3.7	228	41	61.0	12.8	0	0	0	0
Total	41	3.6	442	39	60.3	12.3	0	0	0	0

Table 161e   OAI - OPAI - APAI   Diabetes mellitus - Retinopathy - blindness

Age group (years)	Incidence 1990 Number ('000s)	Rate (per 100 000)	Prevalence 1990 Number ('000s)	Rate (per 100 000)	Avg. age at onset (years)	Average duration (years)	Deaths 1990 Number ('000s)	Rate (per 100 000)	Deaths 2000 (Projected) Number ('000s)	Rate (per 100 000)
Males										
0-4	0	0.0	0	0	-	-	0	0	0	0
5-14	0	0.0	0	0	-	-	0	0	0	0
15-44	4	2.7	69	43	29.7	29.6	0	0	0	0
45-59	9	25.0	85	249	52.3	13.3	0	0	0	0
60+	12	60.1	119	591	69.6	5.4	0	0	0	0
All ages	25	7.3	274	80	56.8	12.3	0	0	0	0
Females										
0-4	0	0.0	0	0	-	-	0	0	0	0
5-14	0	0.0	0	0	-	-	0	0	0	0
15-44	4	2.7	69	43	29.8	32.2	0	0	0	0
45-59	9	24.9	90	257	52.3	15.2	0	0	0	0
60+	14	61.5	149	658	70.3	5.9	0	0	0	0
All ages	27	7.9	308	91	58.0	13.1	0	0	0	0
Total	52	7.6	582	85	57.4	12.7	0	0	0	0

Table 161f   SSA - ASS - ASS   Diabetes mellitus - Retinopathy - blindness

Age group (years)	Incidence 1990 Number ('000s)	Rate (per 100 000)	Prevalence 1990 Number ('000s)	Rate (per 100 000)	Avg. age at onset (years)	Average duration (years)	Deaths 1990 Number ('000s)	Rate (per 100 000)	Deaths 2000 (Projected) Number ('000s)	Rate (per 100 000)
Males										
0-4	0	0.0	0	0	-	-	0	0	0	0
5-14	0	0.0	0	0	-	-	0	0	0	0
15-44	1	1.2	13	13	29.4	25.4	0	0	0	0
45-59	3	12.7	22	107	52.2	12.5	0	0	0	0
60+	3	33.3	32	305	69.2	5.3	0	0	0	0
All ages	7	2.9	67	27	56.6	11.2	0	0	0	0
Females										
0-4	0	0.0	0	0	-	-	0	0	0	0
5-14	0	0.0	0	0	-	-	0	0	0	0
15-44	1	1.2	15	14	29.5	27.4	0	0	0	0
45-59	3	12.7	24	110	52.2	13.6	0	0	0	0
60+	4	34.5	41	325	69.7	5.5	0	0	0	0
All ages	8	3.3	81	31	58.0	11.4	0	0	0	0
Total	16	3.1	148	29	57.3	11.3	0	0	0	0

For epidemiological sources see McKeigue and King 1996. For the methods used to estimate and project incidence, prevalence, and deaths see Murray and Lopez 1996a. See explanatory notes for definitions and caveats.

Table 161 · Cuadro 161 · Tableau 161
Diabetes mellitus · Diabetes mellitus · Diabète sucré

Retinopathy - blindness · Retinopatía - ceguera · Rétinopathie - cécité

Table 161g LAC - ALC - ALC

Diabetes mellitus - Retinopathy - blindness

Age group (years)	Incidence 1990 Number ('000s)	Rate (per 100 000)	Prevalence 1990 Number ('000s)	Rate (per 100 000)	Avg. age at onset (years)	Average duration (years)	Deaths 1990 Number ('000s)	Rate (per 100 000)	Deaths 2000 (Projected) Number ('000s)	Rate (per 100 000)
Males										
0-4	0	0.0	0	0	-	-	0	0	0	0
5-14	0	0.0	0	0	-	-	0	0	0	0
15-44	4	3.5	54	51	29.8	32.2	0	0	0	0
45-59	7	30.9	70	314	52.3	15.2	0	0	0	0
60+	11	76.7	118	832	70.3	6.1	0	0	0	0
All ages	22	9.7	242	109	57.5	13.5	0	0	0	0
Females										
0-4	0	0.0	0	0	-	-	0	0	0	0
5-14	0	0.0	0	0	-	-	0	0	0	0
15-44	4	3.4	55	53	29.8	36.1	0	0	0	0
45-59	7	30.6	76	324	52.4	17.9	0	0	0	0
60+	13	75.4	162	963	71.0	7.1	0	0	0	0
All ages	23	10.5	292	131	59.0	14.8	0	0	0	0
Total	45	10.1	534	120	58.3	14.2	0	0	0	0

Table 161h MEC - AOM - CMO

Diabetes mellitus - Retinopathy - blindness

Age group (years)	Incidence 1990 Number ('000s)	Rate (per 100 000)	Prevalence 1990 Number ('000s)	Rate (per 100 000)	Avg. age at onset (years)	Average duration (years)	Deaths 1990 Number ('000s)	Rate (per 100 000)	Deaths 2000 (Projected) Number ('000s)	Rate (per 100 000)
Males										
0-4	0	0.0	0	0	-	-	0	0	0	0
5-14	0	0.0	0	0	-	-	0	0	0	0
15-44	5	4.3	66	58	29.8	31.2	0	0	0	0
45-59	9	39.7	85	380	52.3	13.9	0	0	0	0
60+	12	87.4	123	900	69.7	5.5	0	0	0	0
All ages	26	10.0	274	107	56.1	13.2	0	0	0	0
Females										
0-4	0	0.0	0	0	-	-	0	0	0	0
5-14	0	0.0	0	0	-	-	0	0	0	0
15-44	5	4.2	62	58	29.8	33.8	0	0	0	0
45-59	9	38.3	86	385	52.3	15.9	0	0	0	0
60+	13	84.4	149	967	70.4	6.1	0	0	0	0
All ages	26	10.6	297	121	57.4	14.1	0	0	0	0
Total	52	10.3	571	114	56.7	13.7	0	0	0	0

Table 161i World - Mundo - Monde

Diabetes mellitus - Retinopathy - blindness

Age group (years)	Incidence 1990 Number ('000s)	Rate (per 100 000)	Prevalence 1990 Number ('000s)	Rate (per 100 000)	Avg. age at onset (years)	Average duration (years)	Deaths 1990 Number ('000s)	Rate (per 100 000)	Deaths 2000 (Projected) Number ('000s)	Rate (per 100 000)
Males										
0-4	0	0.0	0	0	-	-	0	0	0	0
5-14	0	0.0	0	0	-	-	0	0	0	0
15-44	32	2.5	461	37	29.8	32.0	0	0	0	0
45-59	67	21.3	685	219	52.3	14.8	0	0	0	0
60+	123	56.0	1 341	613	70.2	6.0	0	0	0	0
All ages	221	8.3	2 487	94	58.9	12.4	0	0	0	0
Females										
0-4	0	0.0	0	0	-	-	0	0	0	0
5-14	0	0.0	0	0	-	-	0	0	0	0
15-44	30	2.5	448	37	29.8	35.4	0	0	0	0
45-59	67	21.6	703	226	52.3	17.3	0	0	0	0
60+	155	57.6	1 763	655	71.1	7.0	0	0	0	0
All ages	253	9.7	2 914	111	61.0	13.1	0	0	0	0
Total	474	9.0	5 401	103	60.0	12.8	0	0	0	0

For epidemiological sources see McKeigue and King 1996. For the methods used to estimate and project incidence, prevalence, and deaths see Murray and Lopez 1996a. See explanatory notes for definitions and caveats.

Table 162
Diabetes mellitus

Cuadro 162
Diabetes mellitus

Tableau 162
Diabète sucré

Amputation
Amputación
Amputation

Table 162a — EME - PEMC - EMBE — Diabetes mellitus - Amputation

Age group (years)	Incidence 1990 Number ('000s)	Rate (per 100 000)	Prevalence 1990 Number ('000s)	Rate (per 100 000)	Avg. age at onset (years)	Average duration (years)	Deaths 1990 Number ('000s)	Rate (per 100 000)	Deaths 2000 (Projected) Number ('000s)	Rate (per 100 000)
Males										
0-4	0	0.0	0	0	-	-	0	0	0	0
5-14	0	0.0	0	0	-	-	0	0	0	0
15-44	8	4.1	113	61	29.9	41.3	0	0	0	0
45-59	17	25.6	204	308	52.4	21.3	0	0	0	0
60+	42	69.2	632	1 044	71.0	9.2	0	0	0	0
All ages	66	17.0	949	243	61.6	15.9	0	0	0	0
Females										
0-4	0	0.0	0	0	-	-	0	0	0	0
5-14	0	0.0	0	0	-	-	0	0	0	0
15-44	8	4.2	114	63	30.0	47.0	0	0	0	0
45-59	17	25.5	214	316	52.4	25.9	0	0	0	0
60+	59	69.2	993	1 174	72.3	10.8	0	0	0	0
All ages	83	20.5	1 320	324	64.3	17.2	0	0	0	0
Total	150	18.8	2 269	284	63.1	16.6	0	0	0	0

Table 162b — FSE - PEAS - AESE — Diabetes mellitus - Amputation

Age group (years)	Incidence 1990 Number ('000s)	Rate (per 100 000)	Prevalence 1990 Number ('000s)	Rate (per 100 000)	Avg. age at onset (years)	Average duration (years)	Deaths 1990 Number ('000s)	Rate (per 100 000)	Deaths 2000 (Projected) Number ('000s)	Rate (per 100 000)
Males										
0-4	0	0.0	0	0	-	-	0	0	0	0
5-14	0	0.0	0	0	-	-	0	0	0	0
15-44	2	2.6	28	37	29.8	29.0	0	0	0	0
45-59	5	16.7	46	171	52.2	12.9	0	0	0	0
60+	9	44.4	82	393	70.0	5.5	0	0	0	0
All ages	16	9.6	157	95	59.9	10.6	0	0	0	0
Females										
0-4	0	0.0	0	0	-	-	0	0	0	0
5-14	0	0.0	0	0	-	-	0	0	0	0
15-44	2	2.7	30	40	29.9	42.0	0	0	0	0
45-59	5	17.6	62	208	52.4	21.5	0	0	0	0
60+	21	56.8	272	746	71.5	8.6	0	0	0	0
All ages	28	15.4	364	201	64.9	13.4	0	0	0	0
Total	44	12.6	521	150	63.1	12.4	0	0	0	0

Table 162c — India - India - Inde — Diabetes mellitus - Amputation

Age group (years)	Incidence 1990 Number ('000s)	Rate (per 100 000)	Prevalence 1990 Number ('000s)	Rate (per 100 000)	Avg. age at onset (years)	Average duration (years)	Deaths 1990 Number ('000s)	Rate (per 100 000)	Deaths 2000 (Projected) Number ('000s)	Rate (per 100 000)
Males										
0-4	0	0.0	0	0	-	-	0	0	0	0
5-14	0	0.0	0	0	-	-	0	0	0	0
15-44	5	2.7	80	40	29.8	36.9	0	0	0	0
45-59	12	25.7	126	265	52.3	18.2	0	0	0	0
60+	19	64.0	258	866	69.6	7.7	0	0	0	0
All ages	37	8.4	464	106	57.9	15.5	0	0	0	0
Females										
0-4	0	0.0	0	0	-	-	0	0	0	0
5-14	0	0.0	0	0	-	-	0	0	0	0
15-44	5	2.7	73	40	29.8	38.7	0	0	0	0
45-59	12	25.6	123	267	52.3	19.4	0	0	0	0
60+	18	63.7	253	873	70.0	7.9	0	0	0	0
All ages	35	8.6	448	109	58.4	16.1	0	0	0	0
Total	72	8.5	913	107	58.2	15.8	0	0	0	0

For epidemiological sources see McKeigue and King 1996. For the methods used to estimate and project incidence, prevalence, and deaths see Murray and Lopez 1996a. See explanatory notes for definitions and caveats.

Table 162
Diabetes mellitus

Cuadro 162
Diabetes mellitus

Tableau 162
Diabète sucré

Amputation

Amputación

Amputation

Table 162d — China - China - Chine — Diabetes mellitus - Amputation

Age group (years)	Incidence 1990 Number ('000s)	Rate (per 100 000)	Prevalence 1990 Number ('000s)	Rate (per 100 000)	Avg. age at onset (years)	Average duration (years)	Deaths 1990 Number ('000s)	Rate (per 100 000)	Deaths 2000 (Projected) Number ('000s)	Rate (per 100 000)
Males										
0-4	0	0.0	0	0	-	-	0	0	0	0
5-14	0	0.0	0	0	-	-	0	0	0	0
15-44	3	0.9	40	13	29.9	38.6	0	0	0	0
45-59	6	8.3	62	86	52.3	19.0	0	0	0	0
60+	12	25.1	162	330	69.8	8.2	0	0	0	0
All ages	21	3.6	263	45	59.7	15.2	0	0	0	0
Females										
0-4	0	0.0	0	0	-	-	0	0	0	0
5-14	0	0.0	0	0	-	-	0	0	0	0
15-44	2	0.8	34	12	29.9	41.4	0	0	0	0
45-59	5	8.3	55	85	52.4	21.2	0	0	0	0
60+	12	23.8	176	340	70.6	9.0	0	0	0	0
All ages	20	3.6	265	48	61.0	16.0	0	0	0	0
Total	41	3.6	529	47	60.3	15.6	0	0	0	0

Table 162e — OAI - OPAI - APAI — Diabetes mellitus - Amputation

Age group (years)	Incidence 1990 Number ('000s)	Rate (per 100 000)	Prevalence 1990 Number ('000s)	Rate (per 100 000)	Avg. age at onset (years)	Average duration (years)	Deaths 1990 Number ('000s)	Rate (per 100 000)	Deaths 2000 (Projected) Number ('000s)	Rate (per 100 000)
Males										
0-4	0	0.0	0	0	-	-	0	0	0	0
5-14	0	0.0	0	0	-	-	0	0	0	0
15-44	4	2.7	64	40	29.7	35.6	0	0	0	0
45-59	9	24.9	87	256	52.3	17.3	0	0	0	0
60+	12	59.7	162	801	69.6	7.5	0	0	0	0
All ages	25	7.3	313	91	56.7	15.7	0	0	0	0
Females										
0-4	0	0.0	0	0	-	-	0	0	0	0
5-14	0	0.0	0	0	-	-	0	0	0	0
15-44	4	2.7	63	40	29.8	38.0	0	0	0	0
45-59	9	24.9	91	259	52.3	19.1	0	0	0	0
60+	14	61.0	191	844	70.3	8.0	0	0	0	0
All ages	27	7.9	345	102	58.0	16.4	0	0	0	0
Total	52	7.6	658	96	57.4	16.1	0	0	0	0

Table 162f — SSA - ASS - ASS — Diabetes mellitus - Amputation

Age group (years)	Incidence 1990 Number ('000s)	Rate (per 100 000)	Prevalence 1990 Number ('000s)	Rate (per 100 000)	Avg. age at onset (years)	Average duration (years)	Deaths 1990 Number ('000s)	Rate (per 100 000)	Deaths 2000 (Projected) Number ('000s)	Rate (per 100 000)
Males										
0-4	0	0.0	0	0	-	-	0	0	0	0
5-14	0	0.0	0	0	-	-	0	0	0	0
15-44	1	1.2	17	17	29.4	32.8	0	0	0	0
45-59	3	12.7	25	124	52.2	16.8	0	0	0	0
60+	3	33.2	46	434	69.2	7.5	0	0	0	0
All ages	7	2.9	88	35	56.6	15.0	0	0	0	0
Females										
0-4	0	0.0	0	0	-	-	0	0	0	0
5-14	0	0.0	0	0	-	-	0	0	0	0
15-44	1	1.2	18	17	29.5	34.5	0	0	0	0
45-59	3	12.6	27	124	52.2	17.8	0	0	0	0
60+	4	34.4	56	443	69.7	7.7	0	0	0	0
All ages	8	3.3	102	39	58.0	15.0	0	0	0	0
Total	16	3.1	190	37	57.3	15.0	0	0	0	0

For epidemiological sources see McKeigue and King 1996. For the methods used to estimate and project incidence, prevalence, and deaths see Murray and Lopez 1996a. See explanatory notes for definitions and caveats.

Table 162
Diabetes mellitus

Cuadro 162
Diabetes mellitus

Tableau 162
Diabète sucré

Amputation   Amputación   Amputation

Table 162g   LAC - ALC - ALC   Diabetes mellitus - Amputation

Age group (years)	Incidence 1990 Number ('000s)	Rate (per 100 000)	Prevalence 1990 Number ('000s)	Rate (per 100 000)	Avg. age at onset (years)	Average duration (years)	Deaths 1990 Number ('000s)	Rate (per 100 000)	Deaths 2000 (Projected) Number ('000s)	Rate (per 100 000)
Males										
0-4	0	0.0	0	0.0	-	-	0	0	0	0
5-14	0	0.0	0	0.0	-	-	0	0	0	0
15-44	4	3.5	55	52.4	29.8	38.1	0	0	0	0
45-59	7	30.8	72	325.6	52.3	19.3	0	0	0	0
60+	11	75.9	156	1 098.6	70.3	8.5	0	0	0	0
All ages	21	9.6	283	127.9	57.5	17.1	0	0	0	0
Females										
0-4	0	0.0	0	0.0	-	-	0	0	0	0
5-14	0	0.0	0	0.0	-	-	0	0	0	0
15-44	4	3.4	53	50.9	29.8	41.7	0	0	0	0
45-59	7	30.5	76	324.5	52.4	22.2	0	0	0	0
60+	13	74.6	199	1 183.2	71.0	9.5	0	0	0	0
All ages	23	10.4	328	147.2	59.0	18.4	0	0	0	0
Total	45	10.0	611	137.6	58.3	17.7	0	0	0	0

Table 162h   MEC - AOM - CMO   Diabetes mellitus - Amputation

Age group (years)	Incidence 1990 Number ('000s)	Rate (per 100 000)	Prevalence 1990 Number ('000s)	Rate (per 100 000)	Avg. age at onset (years)	Average duration (years)	Deaths 1990 Number ('000s)	Rate (per 100 000)	Deaths 2000 (Projected) Number ('000s)	Rate (per 100 000)
Males										
0-4	0	0.0	0	0	-	-	0	0	0	0
5-14	0	0.0	0	0	-	-	0	0	0	0
15-44	5	4.2	72	63	29.8	36.9	0	0	0	0
45-59	9	39.6	91	408	52.3	17.8	0	0	0	0
60+	12	86.4	168	1 233	69.7	7.7	0	0	0	0
All ages	25	9.9	331	129	56.1	16.8	0	0	0	0
Females										
0-4	0	0.0	0	0	-	-	0	0	0	0
5-14	0	0.0	0	0	-	-	0	0	0	0
15-44	5	4.2	67	63	29.8	39.2	0	0	0	0
45-59	9	38.2	90	402	52.3	19.7	0	0	0	0
60+	13	83.5	193	1 246	70.4	8.3	0	0	0	0
All ages	26	10.5	349	142	57.4	17.4	0	0	0	0
Total	51	10.2	680	135	56.7	17.1	0	0	0	0

Table 162i   World - Mundo - Monde   Diabetes mellitus - Amputation

Age group (years)	Incidence 1990 Number ('000s)	Rate (per 100 000)	Prevalence 1990 Number ('000s)	Rate (per 100 000)	Avg. age at onset (years)	Average duration (years)	Deaths 1990 Number ('000s)	Rate (per 100 000)	Deaths 2000 (Projected) Number ('000s)	Rate (per 100 000)
Males										
0-4	0	0.0	0	0	-	-	0	0	0	0
5-14	0	0.0	0	0	-	-	0	0	0	0
15-44	32	2.5	469	37	29.8	37.1	0	0	0	0
45-59	66	21.3	715	229	52.3	18.4	0	0	0	0
60+	121	55.1	1 666	761	70.1	8.0	0	0	0	0
All ages	219	8.2	2 849	107	58.5	15.4	0	0	0	0
Females										
0-4	0	0.0	0	0	-	-	0	0	0	0
5-14	0	0.0	0	0	-	-	0	0	0	0
15-44	30	2.5	452	38	29.8	40.6	0	0	0	0
45-59	67	21.5	738	237	52.4	21.5	0	0	0	0
60+	154	57.0	2 332	866	71.1	9.2	0	0	0	0
All ages	251	9.6	3 521	135	60.2	16.3	0	0	0	0
Total	470	8.9	6 371	121	59.4	15.9	0	0	0	0

For epidemiological sources see McKeigue and King 1996. For the methods used to estimate and project incidence, prevalence, and deaths see Murray and Lopez 1996a. See explanatory notes for definitions and caveats.

Table 163 — **Cuadro 163** — **Tableau 163**
Unipolar major depression — **Depresión mayor unipolar** — **Dépression unipolaire majeure**

Depressive episodes — Episodios depresivos — Episodes dépressifs

Table 163a — EME - PEMC - EMBE — Unipolar major depression - Depressive episodes

Age group (years)	Incidence 1990 Number ('000s)	Rate (per 100 000)	Prevalence 1990 Number ('000s)	Rate (per 100 000)	Avg. age at onset (years)	Average duration (years)	Deaths 1990 Number ('000s)	Rate (per 100 000)	Deaths 2000 (Projected) Number ('000s)	Rate (per 100 000)
Males										
0-4	0	0	0	0	-	-	0	0	0	0
5-14	0	0	0	0	-	-	0	0	0	0
15-44	4 488	2 438	2 481	1 348	31.9	0.56	0	0	0	0
45-59	1 295	1 958	742	1 122	52.4	0.56	0	0	0	0
60+	595	983	351	579	68.0	0.56	0	0	0	0
All ages	6 378	1 633	3 574	915	39.4	0.56	0	0	0	0
Females										
0-4	0	0	0	0	-	-	0	0	0	0
5-14	0	0	0	0	-	-	0	0	0	0
15-44	8 256	4 607	4 565	2 547	32.1	0.56	0	0	0	0
45-59	2 408	3 551	1 379	2 033	52.4	0.56	0	0	0	0
60+	1 457	1 723	849	1 004	69.3	0.56	0	0	0	0
All ages	12 120	2 976	6 793	1 668	40.6	0.56	0	0	0	0
Total	18 499	2 319	10 367	1 299	40.2	0.56	0	0	0	0

Table 163b — FSE - PEAS - AESE — Unipolar major depression - Depressive episodes

Age group (years)	Incidence 1990 Number ('000s)	Rate (per 100 000)	Prevalence 1990 Number ('000s)	Rate (per 100 000)	Avg. age at onset (years)	Average duration (years)	Deaths 1990 Number ('000s)	Rate (per 100 000)	Deaths 2000 (Projected) Number ('000s)	Rate (per 100 000)
Males										
0-4	0	0	0	0	-	-	0	0	0	0
5-14	0	0	0	0	-	-	0	0	0	0
15-44	1 854	2 430	1 068	1 400	31.8	0.59	0	0	0	0
45-59	528	1 957	318	1 180	52.2	0.59	0	0	0	0
60+	216	1 029	134	640	67.1	0.59	0	0	0	0
All ages	2 597	1 571	1 520	920	38.9	0.59	0	0	0	0
Females										
0-4	0	0	0	0	-	-	0	0	0	0
5-14	0	0	0	0	-	-	0	0	0	0
15-44	3 447	4 599	1 987	2 650	32.0	0.59	0	0	0	0
45-59	1 065	3 548	637	2 123	52.4	0.59	0	0	0	0
60+	646	1 775	396	1 088	68.6	0.59	0	0	0	0
All ages	5 158	2 851	3 020	1 669	40.8	0.59	0	0	0	0
Total	7 755	2 240	4 540	1 311	40.2	0.59	0	0	0	0

Table 163c — India - India - Inde — Unipolar major depression - Depressive episodes

Age group (years)	Incidence 1990 Number ('000s)	Rate (per 100 000)	Prevalence 1990 Number ('000s)	Rate (per 100 000)	Avg. age at onset (years)	Average duration (years)	Deaths 1990 Number ('000s)	Rate (per 100 000)	Deaths 2000 (Projected) Number ('000s)	Rate (per 100 000)
Males										
0-4	0	0	0	0	-	-	0	0	0	0
5-14	0	0	0	0	-	-	0	0	0	0
15-44	4 867	2 427	2 977	1 485	31.8	0.62	0	0	0	0
45-59	930	1 955	597	1 254	52.3	0.63	0	0	0	0
60+	311	1 043	207	695	66.8	0.63	0	0	0	0
All ages	6 107	1 390	3 781	860	36.7	0.62	0	0	0	0
Females										
0-4	0	0	0	0	-	-	0	0	0	0
5-14	0	0	0	0	-	-	0	0	0	0
15-44	8 374	4 570	5 122	2 795	31.9	0.62	0	0	0	0
45-59	1 630	3 543	1 045	2 270	52.4	0.63	0	0	0	0
60+	544	1 881	361	1 247	67.3	0.62	0	0	0	0
All ages	10 548	2 572	6 527	1 592	36.9	0.62	0	0	0	0
Total	16 655	1 961	10 308	1 213	36.8	0.62	0	0	0	0

For epidemiological sources see Üstün et al. 1996. For the methods used to estimate and project incidence, prevalence, and deaths see Murray and Lopez 1996a. See explanatory notes for definitions and caveats.

Table 163
Unipolar major depression

Depressive episodes

Cuadro 163
Depresión mayor unipolar

Episodios depresivos

Tableau 163
Dépression unipolaire majeure

Episodes dépressifs

Table 163d China - China - Chine Unipolar major depression - Depressive episodes

Age group (years)	Incidence 1990 Number ('000s)	Rate (per 100 000)	Prevalence 1990 Number ('000s)	Rate (per 100 000)	Avg. age at onset (years)	Average duration (years)	Deaths 1990 Number ('000s)	Rate (per 100 000)	Deaths 2000 (Projected) Number ('000s)	Rate (per 100 000)
Males										
0-4	0	0	0	0	-	-	0	0	0	0
5-14	0	0	0	0	-	-	0	0	0	0
15-44	7 451	2 433	4 648	1 517	31.9	0.64	0	0	0	0
45-59	1 421	1 955	926	1 274	52.3	0.64	0	0	0	0
60+	509	1 039	345	704	66.9	0.64	0	0	0	0
All ages	9 381	1 603	5 919	1 011	36.9	0.64	0	0	0	0
Females										
0-4	0	0	0	0	-	-	0	0	0	0
5-14	0	0	0	0	-	-	0	0	0	0
15-44	13 023	4 584	8 128	2 861	32.0	0.64	0	0	0	0
45-59	2 281	3 541	1 490	2 314	52.4	0.64	0	0	0	0
60+	951	1 841	641	1 241	67.8	0.64	0	0	0	0
All ages	16 255	2 964	10 260	1 870	37.0	0.64	0	0	0	0
Total	25 635	2 261	16 178	1 427	36.9	0.64	0	0	0	0

Table 163e OAI - OPAI - APAI Unipolar major depression - Depressive episodes

Age group (years)	Incidence 1990 Number ('000s)	Rate (per 100 000)	Prevalence 1990 Number ('000s)	Rate (per 100 000)	Avg. age at onset (years)	Average duration (years)	Deaths 1990 Number ('000s)	Rate (per 100 000)	Deaths 2000 (Projected) Number ('000s)	Rate (per 100 000)
Males										
0-4	0	0	0	0	-	-	0	0	0	0
5-14	0	0	0	0	-	-	0	0	0	0
15-44	3 900	2 425	2 386	1 484	31.8	0.62	0	0	0	0
45-59	668	1 955	429	1 258	52.3	0.63	0	0	0	0
60+	213	1 052	142	702	66.8	0.63	0	0	0	0
All ages	4 781	1 394	2 957	862	36.2	0.62	0	0	0	0
Females										
0-4	0	0	0	0	-	-	0	0	0	0
5-14	0	0	0	0	-	-	0	0	0	0
15-44	7 297	4 572	4 464	2 797	31.9	0.62	0	0	0	0
45-59	1 243	3 543	797	2 271	52.3	0.63	0	0	0	0
60+	424	1 872	281	1 240	67.5	0.63	0	0	0	0
All ages	8 965	2 640	5 542	1 632	36.4	0.62	0	0	0	0
Total	13 745	2 014	8 499	1 245	36.3	0.62	0	0	0	0

Table 163f SSA - ASS - ASS Unipolar major depression - Depressive episodes

Age group (years)	Incidence 1990 Number ('000s)	Rate (per 100 000)	Prevalence 1990 Number ('000s)	Rate (per 100 000)	Avg. age at onset (years)	Average duration (years)	Deaths 1990 Number ('000s)	Rate (per 100 000)	Deaths 2000 (Projected) Number ('000s)	Rate (per 100 000)
Males										
0-4	0	0	0	0	-	-	0	0	0	0
5-14	0	0	0	0	-	-	0	0	0	0
15-44	2 493	2 402	1 561	1 504	31.5	0.64	0	0	0	0
45-59	397	1 956	261	1 284	52.2	0.64	0	0	0	0
60+	112	1 071	77	730	66.5	0.64	0	0	0	0
All ages	3 002	1 190	1 898	752	35.5	0.64	0	0	0	0
Females										
0-4	0	0	0	0	-	-	0	0	0	0
5-14	0	0	0	0	-	-	0	0	0	0
15-44	4 816	4 532	3 014	2 837	31.7	0.64	0	0	0	0
45-59	783	3 541	514	2 324	52.2	0.64	0	0	0	0
60+	245	1 923	166	1 306	66.9	0.64	0	0	0	0
All ages	5 844	2 265	3 694	1 432	35.9	0.64	0	0	0	0
Total	8 846	1 734	5 593	1 096	35.8	0.64	0	0	0	0

For epidemiological sources see Üstün et al. 1996. For the methods used to estimate and project incidence, prevalence, and deaths see Murray and Lopez 1996a. See explanatory notes for definitions and caveats.

Table 163 | **Cuadro 163** | **Tableau 163**
Unipolar major depression | **Depresión mayor unipolar** | **Dépression unipolaire majeure**

Depressive episodes | Episodios depresivos | Episodes dépressifs

Table 163g LAC - ALC - ALC Unipolar major depression - Depressive episodes

Age group (years)	Incidence 1990 Number ('000s)	Rate (per 100 000)	Prevalence 1990 Number ('000s)	Rate (per 100 000)	Avg. age at onset (years)	Average duration (years)	Deaths 1990 Number ('000s)	Rate (per 100 000)	Deaths 2000 (Projected) Number ('000s)	Rate (per 100 000)
Males										
0-4	0	0	0	0	-	-	0	0	0	0
5-14	0	0	0	0	-	-	0	0	0	0
15-44	2 534	2 430	1 520	1 457	31.8	0.61	0	0	0	0
45-59	435	1 956	273	1 227	52.3	0.61	0	0	0	0
60+	145	1 016	94	659	67.4	0.61	0	0	0	0
All ages	3 114	1 405	1 886	851	36.3	0.61	0	0	0	0
Females										
0-4	0	0	0	0	-	-	0	0	0	0
5-14	0	0	0	0	-	-	0	0	0	0
15-44	4 770	4 583	2 863	2 751	32.0	0.61	0	0	0	0
45-59	828	3 545	519	2 221	52.4	0.61	0	0	0	0
60+	304	1 809	196	1 166	68.1	0.61	0	0	0	0
All ages	5 902	2 651	3 578	1 607	36.7	0.61	0	0	0	0
Total	9 016	2 029	5 465	1 230	36.6	0.61	0	0	0	0

Table 163h MEC - AOM - CMO Unipolar major depression - Depressive episodes

Age group (years)	Incidence 1990 Number ('000s)	Rate (per 100 000)	Prevalence 1990 Number ('000s)	Rate (per 100 000)	Avg. age at onset (years)	Average duration (years)	Deaths 1990 Number ('000s)	Rate (per 100 000)	Deaths 2000 (Projected) Number ('000s)	Rate (per 100 000)
Males										
0-4	0	0	0	0	-	-	0	0	0	0
5-14	0	0	0	0	-	-	0	0	0	0
15-44	2 768	2 430	1 694	1 487	31.9	0.62	0	0	0	0
45-59	437	1 955	280	1 254	52.3	0.63	0	0	0	0
60+	143	1 045	95	694	66.9	0.62	0	0	0	0
All ages	3 347	1 306	2 069	807	36.1	0.62	0	0	0	0
Females										
0-4	0	0	0	0	-	-	0	0	0	0
5-14	0	0	0	0	-	-	0	0	0	0
15-44	4 910	4 580	3 004	2 802	32.0	0.62	0	0	0	0
45-59	790	3 543	506	2 270	52.4	0.63	0	0	0	0
60+	287	1 860	190	1 230	67.6	0.62	0	0	0	0
All ages	5 987	2 427	3 701	1 500	36.4	0.62	0	0	0	0
Total	9 334	1 855	5 769	1 147	36.3	0.62	0	0	0	0

Table 163i World - Mundo - Monde Unipolar major depression - Depressive episodes

Age group (years)	Incidence 1990 Number ('000s)	Rate (per 100 000)	Prevalence 1990 Number ('000s)	Rate (per 100 000)	Avg. age at onset (years)	Average duration (years)	Deaths 1990 Number ('000s)	Rate (per 100 000)	Deaths 2000 (Projected) Number ('000s)	Rate (per 100 000)
Males										
0-4	0	0	0	0	-	-	0	0	0	0
5-14	0	0	0	0	-	-	0	0	0	0
15-44	30 354	2 429	18 335	1 467	31.8	0.62	0	0	0	0
45-59	6 110	1 956	3 826	1 225	52.3	0.61	0	0	0	0
60+	2 243	1 025	1 444	660	67.2	0.61	0	0	0	0
All ages	38 708	1 459	23 605	890	37.1	0.61	0	0	0	0
Females										
0-4	0	0	0	0	-	-	0	0	0	0
5-14	0	0	0	0	-	-	0	0	0	0
15-44	54 892	4 580	33 148	2 766	32.0	0.62	0	0	0	0
45-59	11 027	3 545	6 886	2 214	52.4	0.61	0	0	0	0
60+	4 859	1 805	3 081	1 144	68.2	0.60	0	0	0	0
All ages	70 778	2 708	43 114	1 650	37.6	0.61	0	0	0	0
Total	109 486	2 079	66 720	1 267	37.4	0.61	0	0	0	0

For epidemiological sources see Üstün et al. 1996. For the methods used to estimate and project incidence, prevalence, and deaths see Murray and Lopez 1996a. See explanatory notes for definitions and caveats.

Table 164	Cuadro 164	Tableau 164
Bipolar disorder	**Trastorno bipolar**	**Trouble bipolaire**

Cases   Casos   Cas

Table 164a   EME - PEMC - EMBE   Bipolar disorder - Cases

Age group (years)	Incidence 1990 Number ('000s)	Rate (per 100 000)	Prevalence 1990 Number ('000s)	Rate (per 100 000)	Avg. age at onset (years)	Average duration (years)	Deaths 1990 Number ('000s)	Rate (per 100 000)	Deaths 2000 (Projected) Number ('000s)	Rate (per 100 000)
Males										
0-4	0	0	0	0	-	-	0	0.0	0	0.0
5-14	0	0	0	0	-	-	0	0.0	0	0.0
15-44	896	487	993	540	30.9	1.1	0	0.0	0	0.0
45-59	103	155	140	211	52.4	1.2	0	0.0	0	0.0
60+	62	103	76	125	69.4	1.2	0	0.2	0	0.2
All ages	1 061	272	1 208	309	35.2	1.1	0	0.0	0	0.0
Females										
0-4	0	0	0	0	-	-	0	0.0	0	0.0
5-14	0	0	0	0	-	-	0	0.0	0	0.0
15-44	873	487	968	540	31.0	1.2	0	0.0	0	0.0
45-59	104	154	141	208	52.4	1.1	0	0.1	0	0.0
60+	85	100	100	118	70.6	1.2	0	0.3	0	0.3
All ages	1 061	261	1 209	297	36.3	1.2	0	0.1	0	0.1
Total	2 123	266	2 418	303	35.7	1.1	1	0.1	1	0.1

Table 164b   FSE - PEAS - AESE   Bipolar disorder - Cases

Age group (years)	Incidence 1990 Number ('000s)	Rate (per 100 000)	Prevalence 1990 Number ('000s)	Rate (per 100 000)	Avg. age at onset (years)	Average duration (years)	Deaths 1990 Number ('000s)	Rate (per 100 000)	Deaths 2000 (Projected) Number ('000s)	Rate (per 100 000)
Males										
0-4	0	0	0	0	-	-	0	0.0	0	0.0
5-14	0	0	0	0	-	-	0	0.0	0	0.0
15-44	371	487	444	582	30.8	1.2	0	0.3	0	0.2
45-59	42	155	64	237	52.2	1.3	0	0.8	0	0.7
60+	22	103	30	143	68.3	1.2	1	4.6	1	5.0
All ages	435	263	538	326	34.7	1.2	1	0.8	2	1.0
Females										
0-4	0	0	0	0	-	-	0	0.0	0	0.0
5-14	0	0	0	0	-	-	0	0.0	0	0.0
15-44	365	487	438	584	31.0	1.2	0	0.2	0	0.1
45-59	46	154	69	230	52.4	1.2	0	0.7	0	0.6
60+	36	100	48	133	69.8	1.3	4	11.6	5	12.7
All ages	448	247	555	307	36.4	1.2	5	2.5	6	2.9
Total	882	255	1 094	316	35.6	1.2	6	1.7	7	2.0

Table 164c   India - India - Inde   Bipolar disorder - Cases

Age group (years)	Incidence 1990 Number ('000s)	Rate (per 100 000)	Prevalence 1990 Number ('000s)	Rate (per 100 000)	Avg. age at onset (years)	Average duration (years)	Deaths 1990 Number ('000s)	Rate (per 100 000)	Deaths 2000 (Projected) Number ('000s)	Rate (per 100 000)
Males										
0-4	0	0	0	0	-	-	0	0.0	0	0.0
5-14	0	0	0	0	-	-	0	0.0	0	0.0
15-44	977	487	1 300	648	30.8	1.4	0	0.1	0	0.1
45-59	74	155	128	269	52.3	1.4	0	0.3	0	0.3
60+	31	103	49	164	68.0	1.4	1	2.4	1	2.0
All ages	1 081	246	1 476	336	33.3	1.4	1	0.2	1	0.2
Females										
0-4	0	0	0	0	-	-	0	0.0	0	0.0
5-14	0	0	0	0	-	-	0	0.0	0	0.0
15-44	892	487	1 192	651	30.8	1.4	0	0.1	0	0.0
45-59	71	154	122	266	52.4	1.4	0	0.2	0	0.1
60+	29	100	46	160	68.4	1.4	1	4.3	2	3.9
All ages	992	242	1 361	332	33.4	1.4	1	0.3	2	0.4
Total	2 073	244	2 837	334	33.4	1.4	2	0.3	3	0.3

For epidemiological sources see Üstün et al. 1996. For the methods used to estimate and project incidence, prevalence, and deaths see Murray and Lopez 1996a. See explanatory notes for definitions and caveats.

Table 164
Bipolar disorder

Cuadro 164
Trastorno bipolar

Tableau 164
Trouble bipolaire

Cases

Casos

Cas

Table 164d — China - China - Chine — Bipolar disorder - Cases

Age group (years)	Incidence 1990 Number ('000s)	Rate (per 100 000)	Prevalence 1990 Number ('000s)	Rate (per 100 000)	Avg. age at onset (years)	Average duration (years)	Deaths 1990 Number ('000s)	Rate (per 100 000)	Deaths 2000 (Projected) Number ('000s)	Rate (per 100 000)
Males										
0-4	0	0	0	0	-	-	0	0.0	0	0.0
5-14	0	0	0	0	-	-	0	0.0	0	0.0
15-44	1 492	487	2 054	671	30.9	1.4	0	0.1	0	0.0
45-59	113	155	202	278	52.3	1.4	0	0.1	0	0.1
60+	50	103	83	169	68.1	1.5	0	1.0	1	0.8
All ages	1 655	283	2 339	400	33.5	1.4	1	0.1	1	0.1
Females										
0-4	0	0	0	0	-	-	0	0.0	0	0.0
5-14	0	0	0	0	-	-	0	0.0	0	0.0
15-44	1 383	487	1 907	671	30.9	1.4	0	0.0	0	0.0
45-59	99	154	178	276	52.4	1.5	0	0.2	0	0.1
60+	52	100	84	162	68.9	1.5	1	2.7	2	2.7
All ages	1 534	280	2 168	395	33.6	1.4	2	0.3	2	0.3
Total	3 189	281	4 508	398	33.5	1.4	2	0.2	3	0.2

Table 164e — OAI - OPAI - APAI — Bipolar disorder - Cases

Age group (years)	Incidence 1990 Number ('000s)	Rate (per 100 000)	Prevalence 1990 Number ('000s)	Rate (per 100 000)	Avg. age at onset (years)	Average duration (years)	Deaths 1990 Number ('000s)	Rate (per 100 000)	Deaths 2000 (Projected) Number ('000s)	Rate (per 100 000)
Males										
0-4	0	0	0	0	-	-	0	0.0	0	0.0
5-14	0	0	0	0	-	-	0	0.0	0	0.0
15-44	783	487	1 042	648	30.8	1.4	0	0.1	0	0.1
45-59	53	155	92	270	52.3	1.4	0	0.3	0	0.3
60+	21	103	33	164	68.0	1.4	0	1.9	0	1.7
All ages	857	250	1 167	340	33.0	1.4	1	0.2	1	0.2
Females										
0-4	0	0	0	0	-	-	0	0.0	0	0.0
5-14	0	0	0	0	-	-	0	0.0	0	0.0
15-44	777	487	1 035	648	30.8	1.4	0	0.0	0	0.0
45-59	54	154	93	265	52.3	1.4	0	0.2	0	0.2
60+	23	100	36	158	68.6	1.4	1	3.5	1	3.3
All ages	854	251	1 163	343	33.2	1.4	1	0.3	1	0.3
Total	1 711	251	2 330	341	33.1	1.4	2	0.2	2	0.2

Table 164f — SSA - ASS - ASS — Bipolar disorder - Cases

Age group (years)	Incidence 1990 Number ('000s)	Rate (per 100 000)	Prevalence 1990 Number ('000s)	Rate (per 100 000)	Avg. age at onset (years)	Average duration (years)	Deaths 1990 Number ('000s)	Rate (per 100 000)	Deaths 2000 (Projected) Number ('000s)	Rate (per 100 000)
Males										
0-4	0	0	0	0	-	-	0	0.0	0	0.0
5-14	0	0	0	0	-	-	0	0.0	0	0.0
15-44	505	487	694	669	30.5	1.4	0	0.1	0	0.1
45-59	31	155	58	286	52.2	1.5	0	0.3	0	0.3
60+	11	103	18	175	67.6	1.5	0	2.0	0	1.6
All ages	548	217	770	305	32.5	1.4	0	0.1	0	0.1
Females										
0-4	0	0	0	0	-	-	0	0.0	0	0.0
5-14	0	0	0	0	-	-	0	0.0	0	0.0
15-44	517	487	712	670	30.6	1.4	0	0.0	0	0.0
45-59	34	154	64	291	52.2	1.5	0	0.2	0	0.1
60+	13	100	22	172	68.1	1.5	0	3.8	1	3.2
All ages	564	219	798	309	32.7	1.5	1	0.2	1	0.2
Total	1 112	218	1 568	307	32.6	1.4	1	0.2	1	0.1

For epidemiological sources see Üstün et al. 1996. For the methods used to estimate and project incidence, prevalence, and deaths see Murray and Lopez 1996a. See explanatory notes for definitions and caveats.

Table 164	Cuadro 164	Tableau 164
Bipolar disorder	Trastorno bipolar	Trouble bipolaire
Cases	Casos	Cas

Table 164g LAC - ALC - ALC — Bipolar disorder - Cases

Age group (years)	Incidence 1990 Number ('000s)	Rate (per 100 000)	Prevalence 1990 Number ('000s)	Rate (per 100 000)	Avg. age at onset (years)	Average duration (years)	Deaths 1990 Number ('000s)	Rate (per 100 000)	Deaths 2000 (Projected) Number ('000s)	Rate (per 100 000)
Males										
0-4	0	0	0	0	-	-	0	0.0	0	0.0
5-14	0	0	0	0	-	-	0	0.0	0	0.0
15-44	508	487	654	627	30.8	1.3	0	0.1	0	0.0
45-59	34	155	57	256	52.3	1.3	0	0.2	0	0.2
60+	15	103	22	154	68.6	1.4	0	1.2	0	1.1
All ages	557	251	733	331	33.1	1.3	0	0.1	0	0.1
Females										
0-4	0	0	0	0	-	-	0	0.0	0	0.0
5-14	0	0	0	0	-	-	0	0.0	0	0.0
15-44	507	487	653	628	30.9	1.3	0	0.1	0	0.0
45-59	36	154	59	253	52.4	1.3	0	0.2	0	0.2
60+	17	100	25	147	69.4	1.4	0	2.0	0	2.0
All ages	560	251	737	331	33.4	1.3	0	0.2	1	0.2
Total	1 117	251	1 470	331	33.3	1.3	1	0.2	1	0.2

Table 164h MEC - AOM - CMO — Bipolar disorder - Cases

Age group (years)	Incidence 1990 Number ('000s)	Rate (per 100 000)	Prevalence 1990 Number ('000s)	Rate (per 100 000)	Avg. age at onset (years)	Average duration (years)	Deaths 1990 Number ('000s)	Rate (per 100 000)	Deaths 2000 (Projected) Number ('000s)	Rate (per 100 000)
Males										
0-4	0	0	0	0	-	-	0	0.0	0	0.0
5-14	0	0	0	0	-	-	0	0.0	0	0.0
15-44	555	487	739	649	30.9	1.4	0	0.1	0	0.1
45-59	35	155	60	269	52.3	1.4	0	0.3	0	0.2
60+	14	103	22	164	68.1	1.4	0	1.7	0	1.4
All ages	603	235	821	320	33.0	1.4	0	0.1	0	0.1
Females										
0-4	0	0	0	0	-	-	0	0.0	0	0.0
5-14	0	0	0	0	-	-	0	0.0	0	0.0
15-44	522	487	696	649	30.9	1.4	0	0.1	0	0.0
45-59	34	154	59	265	52.4	1.4	0	0.3	0	0.2
60+	15	100	24	158	68.8	1.4	0	2.4	0	2.1
All ages	572	232	780	316	33.2	1.4	1	0.2	1	0.2
Total	1 175	234	1 601	318	33.1	1.4	1	0.2	1	0.2

Table 164i World - Mundo - Monde — Bipolar disorder - Cases

Age group (years)	Incidence 1990 Number ('000s)	Rate (per 100 000)	Prevalence 1990 Number ('000s)	Rate (per 100 000)	Avg. age at onset (years)	Average duration (years)	Deaths 1990 Number ('000s)	Rate (per 100 000)	Deaths 2000 (Projected) Number ('000s)	Rate (per 100 000)
Males										
0-4	0	0	0	0	-	-	0	0.0	0	0.0
5-14	0	0	0	0	-	-	0	0.0	0	0.0
15-44	6 087	487	7 920	634	30.8	1.4	1	0.1	1	0.1
45-59	484	155	801	256	52.3	1.3	1	0.3	1	0.2
60+	225	103	333	152	68.5	1.3	3	1.5	4	1.4
All ages	6 797	256	9 054	341	33.6	1.4	5	0.2	5	0.2
Females										
0-4	0	0	0	0	-	-	0	0.0	0	0.0
5-14	0	0	0	0	-	-	0	0.0	0	0.0
15-44	5 837	487	7 601	634	30.9	1.4	1	0.0	0	0.0
45-59	478	154	786	253	52.4	1.3	1	0.2	1	0.2
60+	269	100	385	143	69.5	1.3	9	3.4	11	3.4
All ages	6 585	252	8 771	336	34.0	1.4	10	0.4	13	0.4
Total	13 381	254	17 826	338	33.8	1.4	15	0.3	18	0.3

For epidemiological sources see Üstün et al. 1996. For the methods used to estimate and project incidence, prevalence, and deaths see Murray and Lopez 1996a. See explanatory notes for definitions and caveats.

Table 165	Cuadro 165	Tableau 165
Schizophrenia	Esquizofrenia	Schizophrénie
Cases	Casos	Cas

Table 165a   EME - PEMC - EMBE   Schizophrenia - Cases

Age group (years)	Incidence 1990 Number ('000s)	Rate (per 100 000)	Prevalence 1990 Number ('000s)	Rate (per 100 000)	Avg. age at onset (years)	Average duration (years)	Deaths 1990 Number ('000s)	Rate (per 100 000)	Deaths 2000 (Projected) Number ('000s)	Rate (per 100 000)
Males										
0-4	0	0	0	0	-	-	0	0.0	0	0.0
5-14	0	0	0	0	-	-	0	0.0	0	0.0
15-44	82	45	1 978	1 075	20.5	52.4	0	0.2	0	0.2
45-59	0	0	870	1 316	-	-	1	1.0	1	0.8
60+	0	0	758	1 252	-	-	4	7.2	5	7.0
All ages	82	21	3 606	924	20.5	52.4	5	1.4	6	1.5
Females										
0-4	0	0	0	0	-	-	0	0.0	0	0.0
5-14	0	0	0	0	-	-	0	0.0	0	0.0
15-44	80	45	1 597	891	24.9	53.7	0	0.0	0	0.0
45-59	0	0	900	1 328	-	-	0	0.3	0	0.3
60+	0	0	1 060	1 254	-	-	7	8.4	9	9.0
All ages	80	20	3 557	873	24.9	53.7	7	1.8	9	2.1
Total	162	20	7 164	898	22.7	53.0	13	1.6	15	1.8

Table 165b   FSE - PEAS - AESE   Schizophrenia - Cases

Age group (years)	Incidence 1990 Number ('000s)	Rate (per 100 000)	Prevalence 1990 Number ('000s)	Rate (per 100 000)	Avg. age at onset (years)	Average duration (years)	Deaths 1990 Number ('000s)	Rate (per 100 000)	Deaths 2000 (Projected) Number ('000s)	Rate (per 100 000)
Males										
0-4	0	0	0	0	-	-	0	0.0	0	0.0
5-14	0	0	0	0	-	-	0	0.0	0	0.0
15-44	29	39	694	910	20.5	45.8	0	0.6	0	0.5
45-59	0	0	296	1 097	-	-	1	2.2	1	1.9
60+	0	0	211	1 008	-	-	1	5.5	1	5.8
All ages	29	18	1 201	726	20.5	45.8	2	1.3	2	1.4
Females										
0-4	0	0	0	0	-	-	0	0.0	0	0.0
5-14	0	0	0	0	-	-	0	0.0	0	0.0
15-44	28	38	567	757	24.9	50.3	0	0.2	0	0.2
45-59	0	0	338	1 126	-	-	0	0.9	0	0.7
60+	0	0	383	1 054	-	-	2	4.7	2	4.9
All ages	28	16	1 289	712	24.9	50.3	2	1.2	2	1.3
Total	58	17	2 490	719	22.7	48.0	4	1.3	5	1.3

Table 165c   India - India - Inde   Schizophrenia - Cases

Age group (years)	Incidence 1990 Number ('000s)	Rate (per 100 000)	Prevalence 1990 Number ('000s)	Rate (per 100 000)	Avg. age at onset (years)	Average duration (years)	Deaths 1990 Number ('000s)	Rate (per 100 000)	Deaths 2000 (Projected) Number ('000s)	Rate (per 100 000)
Males										
0-4	0	0	0	0	-	-	0	0.0	0	0.0
5-14	0	0	0	0	-	-	0	0.0	0	0.0
15-44	46	23	1 075	536	20.5	46.5	0	0.2	0	0.2
45-59	0	0	309	649	-	-	1	1.4	1	1.1
60+	0	0	179	601	-	-	1	4.7	1	3.9
All ages	46	10	1 562	356	20.5	46.5	2	0.6	3	0.5
Females										
0-4	0	0	0	0	-	-	0	0.0	0	0.0
5-14	0	0	0	0	-	-	0	0.0	0	0.0
15-44	41	23	810	442	24.7	44.7	0	0.1	0	0.1
45-59	0	0	304	660	-	-	0	0.6	0	0.5
60+	0	0	176	607	-	-	2	5.8	2	5.2
All ages	41	10	1 289	314	24.7	44.7	2	0.5	2	0.5
Total	87	10	2 851	336	22.5	45.6	5	0.5	5	0.5

For epidemiological sources see Regier et al. 1996. For the methods used to estimate and project incidence, prevalence, and deaths see Murray and Lopez 1996a. See explanatory notes for definitions and caveats.

Table 165
Schizophrenia

Cuadro 165
Esquizofrenia

Tableau 165
Schizophrénie

Cases

Casos

Cas

Table 165d — China - China - Chine — Schizophrenia - Cases

Age group (years)	Incidence 1990 Number ('000s)	Rate (per 100 000)	Prevalence 1990 Number ('000s)	Rate (per 100 000)	Avg. age at onset (years)	Average duration (years)	Deaths 1990 Number ('000s)	Rate (per 100 000)	Deaths 2000 (Projected) Number ('000s)	Rate (per 100 000)
Males										
0-4	0	0	0	0	-	-	0	0.0	0	0.0
5-14	0	0	0	0	-	-	0	0.0	0	0.0
15-44	69	23	1 649	538	20.5	48.5	6	2.0	5	1.7
45-59	0	0	475	654	-	-	1	1.0	1	0.8
60+	0	0	297	606	-	-	3	6.5	3	5.6
All ages	69	12	2 421	414	20.5	48.5	10	1.7	9	1.4
Females										
0-4	0	0	0	0	-	-	0	0.0	0	0.0
5-14	0	0	0	0	-	-	0	0.0	0	0.0
15-44	64	22	1 265	445	24.8	47.6	3	0.9	2	0.6
45-59	0	0	427	663	-	-	1	1.5	1	1.1
60+	0	0	317	613	-	-	2	3.5	2	3.3
All ages	64	12	2 009	366	24.8	47.6	5	1.0	5	0.8
Total	133	12	4 430	391	22.6	48.1	15	1.4	15	1.1

Table 165e — OAI - OPAI - APAI — Schizophrenia - Cases

Age group (years)	Incidence 1990 Number ('000s)	Rate (per 100 000)	Prevalence 1990 Number ('000s)	Rate (per 100 000)	Avg. age at onset (years)	Average duration (years)	Deaths 1990 Number ('000s)	Rate (per 100 000)	Deaths 2000 (Projected) Number ('000s)	Rate (per 100 000)
Males										
0-4	0	0	0	0	-	-	0	0.0	0	0.0
5-14	0	0	0	0	-	-	0	0.0	0	0.0
15-44	62	39	1 461	908	20.5	45.2	1	0.4	1	0.3
45-59	0	0	375	1 098	-	-	1	2.5	1	1.9
60+	0	0	204	1 008	-	-	1	7.1	2	6.1
All ages	62	18	2 039	595	20.5	45.2	3	0.8	3	0.8
Females										
0-4	0	0	0	0	-	-	0	0.0	0	0.0
5-14	0	0	0	0	-	-	0	0.0	0	0.0
15-44	61	38	1 198	750	24.7	44.4	0	0.1	0	0.1
45-59	0	0	393	1 119	-	-	0	1.0	0	0.8
60+	0	0	232	1 025	-	-	2	8.6	3	7.7
All ages	61	18	1 822	537	24.7	44.4	3	0.7	3	0.8
Total	124	18	3 861	566	22.6	44.8	5	0.8	6	0.8

Table 165f — SSA - ASS - ASS — Schizophrenia - Cases

Age group (years)	Incidence 1990 Number ('000s)	Rate (per 100 000)	Prevalence 1990 Number ('000s)	Rate (per 100 000)	Avg. age at onset (years)	Average duration (years)	Deaths 1990 Number ('000s)	Rate (per 100 000)	Deaths 2000 (Projected) Number ('000s)	Rate (per 100 000)
Males										
0-4	0	0.0	0	0	-	-	0	0.0	0	0.0
5-14	0	0.0	0	0	-	-	0	0.0	0	0.0
15-44	12	11.9	274	264	20.3	39.7	0	0.3	0	0.2
45-59	0	0.0	64	317	-	-	0	1.1	0	0.8
60+	0	0.0	30	289	-	-	0	2.5	0	2.0
All ages	12	4.9	369	146	20.3	39.7	1	0.3	1	0.2
Females										
0-4	0	0.0	0	0	-	-	0	0.0	0	0.0
5-14	0	0.0	0	0	-	-	0	0.0	0	0.0
15-44	12	11.5	231	218	24.5	39.3	0	0.1	0	0.0
45-59	0	0.0	72	327	-	-	0	0.5	0	0.4
60+	0	0.0	38	296	-	-	0	3.3	0	2.7
All ages	12	4.8	341	132	24.5	39.3	1	0.2	1	0.2
Total	25	4.8	710	139	22.4	39.5	1	0.3	1	0.2

For epidemiological sources see Regier et al. 1996. For the methods used to estimate and project incidence, prevalence, and deaths see Murray and Lopez 1996a. See explanatory notes for definitions and caveats.

ERRATA

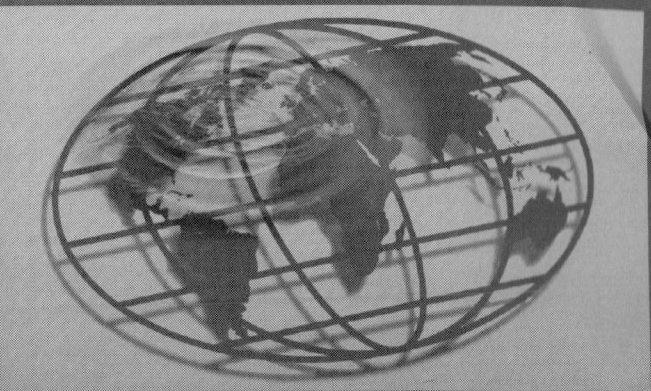

GLOBAL HEALTH STATISTICS

Christopher J. L. Murray
Alan D. Lopez

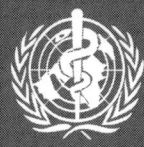

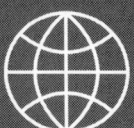

WORLD HEALTH
ORGANIZATION

HARVARD SCHOOL OF
PUBLIC HEALTH

WORLD
BANK

le 96	Cuadro 96	Tableau 96
cariasis	Ascaridiasis	Ascaridose
ognitive impairment	Obstrucción Intestinal	Obstruction intestinale

Table 96a — EME - PEMC - EMBE — Ascariasis - Cognitive impairment

Age group (years)	Incidence 1990 Number ('000s)	Rate (per 100 000)	Prevalence 1990 Number ('000s)	Rate (per 100 000)	Avg. age at onset (years)	Average duration (years)	Deaths 1990 Number ('000s)	Rate (per 100 000)	Deaths 2000 (Projected) Number ('000s)	Rate (per 100 000)
Males										
0-4	0	0	0	0	-	-	0	0	0	0
5-14	0	0	0	0	-	-	0	0	0	0
15-44	0	0	0	0	-	-	0	0	0	0
45-59	0	0	0	0	-	-	0	0	0	0
60+	0	0	0	0	-	-	0	0	0	0
All ages	0	0	0	0	-	-	0	0	0	0
Females										
0-4	0	0	0	0	-	-	0	0	0	0
5-14	0	0	0	0	-	-	0	0	0	0
15-44	0	0	0	0	-	-	0	0	0	0
45-59	0	0	0	0	-	-	0	0	0	0
60+	0	0	0	0	-	-	0	0	0	0
All ages	0	0	0	0	-	-	0	0	0	0
Total	0	0	0	0	-	-	0	0	0	0

Table 96b — FSE - PEAS - AESE — Ascariasis - Cognitive impairment

Age group (years)	Incidence 1990 Number ('000s)	Rate (per 100 000)	Prevalence 1990 Number ('000s)	Rate (per 100 000)	Avg. age at onset (years)	Average duration (years)	Deaths 1990 Number ('000s)	Rate (per 100 000)	Deaths 2000 (Projected) Number ('000s)	Rate (per 100 000)
Males										
0-4	0	0	0	0	-	-	0	0	0	0
5-14	0	0	0	0	-	-	0	0	0	0
15-44	0	0	0	0	-	-	0	0	0	0
45-59	0	0	0	0	-	-	0	0	0	0
60+	0	0	0	0	-	-	0	0	0	0
All ages	0	0	0	0	-	-	0	0	0	0
Females										
0-4	0	0	0	0	-	-	0	0	0	0
5-14	0	0	0	0	-	-	0	0	0	0
15-44	0	0	0	0	-	-	0	0	0	0
45-59	0	0	0	0	-	-	0	0	0	0
60+	0	0	0	0	-	-	0	0	0	0
All ages	0	0	0	0	-	-	0	0	0	0
Total	0	0	0	0	-	-	0	0	0	0

Table 96c — India - India - Inde — Ascariasis - Cognitive impairment

Age group (years)	Incidence 1990 Number ('000s)	Rate (per 100 000)	Prevalence 1990 Number ('000s)	Rate (per 100 000)	Avg. age at onset (years)	Average duration (years)	Deaths 1990 Number ('000s)	Rate (per 100 000)	Deaths 2000 (Projected) Number ('000s)	Rate (per 100 000)
Males										
0-4	3	5.0	7	12	2.5	58.4	0	0	0	0
5-14	77	75.7	422	415	10.0	57.5	0	0	0	0
15-44	0	0.0	1 567	782	-	-	0	0	0	0
45-59	0	0.0	372	782	-	-	0	0	0	0
60+	0	0.0	233	782	-	-	0	0	0	0
All ages	80	18.2	2 601	592	9.7	57.5	0	0	0	0
Females										
0-4	3	5.0	7	12	2.5	59.4	0	0	0	0
5-14	72	75.7	395	415	10.0	59.1	0	0	0	0
15-44	0	0.0	1 432	782	-	-	0	0	0	0
45-59	0	0.0	360	782	-	-	0	0	0	0
60+	0	0.0	226	782	-	-	0	0	0	0
All ages	75	18.3	2 420	590	9.7	59.1	0	0	0	0
Total	155	18.2	5 021	591	9.7	58.3	0	0	0	0

For epidemiological sources see Bundy et al. 1996. See explanatory notes for definitions and caveats.

Table 96	Cuadro 96	Tableau 96
Ascariasis	**Ascaridiasis**	**Ascaridose**

Cognitive impairment	Obstrucción Intestinal	Obstruction intestinale

Table 96d   China - China - Chine

Ascariasis - Cognitive impairment

Age group (years)	Incidence 1990 Number ('000s)	Rate (per 100 000)	Prevalence 1990 Number ('000s)	Rate (per 100 000)	Avg. age at onset (years)	Average duration (years)	Deaths 1990 Number ('000s)	Rate (per 100 000)	Deaths 2000 (Projected) Number ('000s)	Rate (per 100 000)
Males										
0-4	11	18	27	45	2.5	63.7	0	0	0	0
5-14	254	262	1 403	1 447	10.0	59.9	0	0	0	0
15-44	0	0	8 303	2 711	-	-	0	0	0	0
45-59	0	0	1 970	2 711	-	-	0	0	0	0
60+	0	0	1 328	2 711	-	-	0	0	0	0
All ages	265	45	13 031	2 227	9.7	60.1	0	0	0	0
Females										
0-4	10	18	26	45	2.5	66.6	0	0	0	0
5-14	237	262	1 308	1 447	10.0	63.2	0	0	0	0
15-44	0	0	7 700	2 711	-	-	0	0	0	0
45-59	0	0	1 746	2 711	-	-	0	0	0	0
60ı	0	0	1 400	2 711	-	-	0	0	0	0
All ages	247	45	12 180	2 221	9.7	63.4	0	0	0	0
Total	513	45	25 211	2 224	9.7	61.7	0	0	0	0

Table 96e   OAI - OPAI - APAI

Ascariasis - Cognitive impairment

Age group (years)	Incidence 1990 Number ('000s)	Rate (per 100 000)	Prevalence 1990 Number ('000s)	Rate (per 100 000)	Avg. age at onset (years)	Average duration (years)	Deaths 1990 Number ('000s)	Rate (per 100 000)	Deaths 2000 (Projected) Number ('000s)	Rate (per 100 000)
Males										
0-4	7	16	17	39	2.5	58.3	0	0	0	0
5-14	196	233	1 079	1 283	10.0	56.2	0	0	0	0
15-44	0	0	3 875	2 409	-	-	0	0	0	0
45-59	0	0	822	2 409	-	-	0	0	0	0
60+	0	0	487	2 409	-	-	0	0	0	0
All ages	203	59	6 280	1 831	9.7	56.3	0	0	0	0
Females										
0-4	7	16	17	40	2.5	61.6	0	0	0	0
5-14	187	233	1 030	1 284	10.0	59.2	0	0	0	0
15-44	0	0	3 845	2 409	-	-	0	0	0	0
45-59	0	0	845	2 409	-	-	0	0	0	0
60+	0	0	546	2 409	-	-	0	0	0	0
All ages	194	57	6 283	1 850	9.7	59.3	0	0	0	0
Total	397	58	12 563	1 841	9.7	57.7	0	0	0	0

Table 96f   SSA - ASS - ASS

Ascariasis - Cognitive impairment

Age group (years)	Incidence 1990 Number ('000s)	Rate (per 100 000)	Prevalence 1990 Number ('000s)	Rate (per 100 000)	Avg. age at onset (years)	Average duration (years)	Deaths 1990 Number ('000s)	Rate (per 100 000)	Deaths 2000 (Projected) Number ('000s)	Rate (per 100 000)
Males										
0-4	2	4.0	5	10	2.4	47.7	0	0	0	0
5-14	36	51.9	201	285	10.0	49.3	0	0	0	0
15-44	0	0.0	559	539	-	-	0	0	0	0
45-59	0	0.0	109	539	-	-	0	0	0	0
60+	0	0.0	57	539	-	-	0	0	0	0
All ages	38	15.2	930	369	9.6	49.2	0	0	0	0
Females										
0-4	2	4.0	5	10	2.5	50.8	0	0	0	0
5-14	36	51.9	199	286	10.0	52.0	0	0	0	0
15-44	0	0.0	572	539	-	-	0	0	0	0
45-59	0	0.0	119	539	-	-	0	0	0	0
60+	0	0.0	69	539	-	-	0	0	0	0
All ages	38	14.8	964	374	9.6	51.9	0	0	0	0
Total	76	15.0	1 894	371	9.6	50.6	0	0	0	0

For epidemiological sources see Bundy et al. 1996. See explanatory notes for definitions and caveats.

Table 164
Schizophrenia

Cuadro 164
Esquizofrenia

Tableau 164
Schizophrénie

Cases

Casos

Cas

Table 165g   LAC - ALC - ALC   Schizophrenia - Cases

Age group (years)	Incidence 1990 Number ('000s)	Rate (per 100 000)	Prevalence 1990 Number ('000s)	Rate (per 100 000)	Avg. age at onset (years)	Average duration (years)	Deaths 1990 Number ('000s)	Rate (per 100 000)	Deaths 2000 (Projected) Number ('000s)	Rate (per 100 000)
Males										
0-4	0	0	0	0	-	-	0	0.0	0	0.0
5-14	0	0	0	0	-	-	0	0.0	0	0.0
15-44	40	39	949	910	20.5	47.8	0	0.4	0	0.3
45-59	0	0	244	1 096	-	-	1	2.7	1	2.2
60+	0	0	143	1 003	-	-	1	7.5	1	6.6
All ages	40	18	1 335	603	20.5	47.8	2	0.9	2	0.9
Females										
0-4	0	0	0	0	-	-	0	0.0	0	0.0
5-14	0	0	0	0	-	-	0	0.0	0	0.0
15-44	40	38	783	753	24.8	47.8	0	0.2	0	0.1
45-59	0	0	261	1 119	-	-	0	1.0	0	0.8
60+	0	0	176	1 047	-	-	1	7.0	2	6.6
All ages	40	18	1 221	548	24.8	47.8	2	0.7	2	0.7
Total	80	18	2 556	575	22.6	47.8	4	0.8	4	0.8

Table 165h   MEC - AOM - CMO   Schizophrenia - Cases

Age group (years)	Incidence 1990 Number ('000s)	Rate (per 100 000)	Prevalence 1990 Number ('000s)	Rate (per 100 000)	Avg. age at onset (years)	Average duration (years)	Deaths 1990 Number ('000s)	Rate (per 100 000)	Deaths 2000 (Projected) Number ('000s)	Rate (per 100 000)
Males										
0-4	0	0	0	0	-	-	0	0.0	0	0.0
5-14	0	0	0	0	-	-	0	0.0	0	0.0
15-44	44	38	1 038	911	20.5	46.9	0	0.3	0	0.2
45-59	0	0	246	1 104	-	-	0	2.2	1	1.7
60+	0	0	139	1 017	-	-	1	6.9	1	5.9
All ages	44	17	1 423	555	20.5	46.9	2	0.7	2	0.6
Females										
0-4	0	0	0	0	-	-	0	0.0	0	0.0
5-14	0	0	0	0	-	-	0	0.0	0	0.0
15-44	41	38	807	753	24.8	45.7	0	0.3	0	0.2
45-59	0	0	250	1 121	-	-	1	2.6	1	1.9
60+	0	0	159	1 031	-	-	1	6.4	1	5.4
All ages	41	17	1 217	493	24.8	45.7	2	0.8	2	0.6
Total	85	17	2 640	525	22.6	46.3	4	0.7	4	0.6

Table 165i   World - Mundo - Monde   Schizophrenia - Cases

Age group (years)	Incidence 1990 Number ('000s)	Rate (per 100 000)	Prevalence 1990 Number ('000s)	Rate (per 100 000)	Avg. age at onset (years)	Average duration (years)	Deaths 1990 Number ('000s)	Rate (per 100 000)	Deaths 2000 (Projected) Number ('000s)	Rate (per 100 000)
Males										
0-4	0	0	0	0	-	-	0	0.0	0	0.0
5-14	0	0	0	0	-	-	0	0.0	0	0.0
15-44	385	31	9 117	729	20.5	47.8	9	0.7	8	0.6
45-59	0	0	2 879	922	-	-	5	1.5	5	1.2
60+	0	0	1 961	896	-	-	14	6.3	16	5.7
All ages	385	15	13 957	526	20.5	47.8	28	1.0	29	0.9
Females										
0-4	0	0	0	0	-	-	0	0.0	0	0.0
5-14	0	0	0	0	-	-	0	0.0	0	0.0
15-44	367	31	7 258	606	24.8	47.8	4	0.3	3	0.2
45-59	0	0	2 945	947	-	-	3	1.0	3	0.8
60+	0	0	2 541	944	-	-	17	6.3	21	6.1
All ages	367	14	12 745	488	24.8	47.8	24	0.9	27	0.9
Total	753	14	26 702	507	22.6	47.8	51	1.0	56	0.9

For epidemiological sources see Ustun et al. 1996. For the methods used to estimate and project incidence, prevalence, and deaths see Murray and Lopez 1996a. See explanatory notes for definitions and caveats.

Table 160   **Cuadro 160**   **Tableau 160**
Diabetes mellitus   **Diabetes mellitus**   **Diabète sucré**

Neuropathy   Neuropatía   Neuropathie

Table 160a   **EME - PEMC - EMBE**   Diabetes mellitus - Neuropathy

Age group (years)	Incidence 1990 Number ('000s)	Rate (per 100 000)	Prevalence 1990 Number ('000s)	Rate (per 100 000)	Avg. age at onset (years)	Average duration (years)	Deaths 1990 Number ('000s)	Rate (per 100 000)	Deaths 2000 (Projected) Number ('000s)	Rate (per 100 000)
Males										
0-4	-	-	0	0	-	-	0	0	0	0
5-14	-	-	0	0	-	-	0	0	0	0
15-44	-	-	332	180	-	-	0	0	0	0
45-59	-	-	833	1 259	-	-	0	0	0	0
60+	-	-	2 108	3 482	-	-	0	0	0	0
All ages	-	-	3 273	838	-	-	0	0	0	0
Females										
0-4	-	-	0	0	-	-	0	0	0	0
5-14	-	-	0	0	-	-	0	0	0	0
15-44	-	-	325	182	-	-	0	0	0	0
45-59	-	-	853	1 258	-	-	0	0	0	0
60+	-	-	2 959	3 500	-	-	0	0	0	0
All ages	-	-	4 138	1 016	-	-	0	0	0	0
Total	-	-	7 411	929	-	-	0	0	0	0

Table 160b   **FSE - PEAS - AESE**   Diabetes mellitus - Neuropathy

Age group (years)	Incidence 1990 Number ('000s)	Rate (per 100 000)	Prevalence 1990 Number ('000s)	Rate (per 100 000)	Avg. age at onset (years)	Average duration (years)	Deaths 1990 Number ('000s)	Rate (per 100 000)	Deaths 2000 (Projected) Number ('000s)	Rate (per 100 000)
Males										
0-4	-	-	0	0	-	-	0	0	0	0
5-14	-	-	0	0	-	-	0	0	0	0
15-44	-	-	92	120	-	-	0	0	0	0
45-59	-	-	226	838	-	-	0	0	0	0
60+	-	-	465	2 220	-	-	0	0	0	0
All ages	-	-	783	474	-	-	0	0	0	0
Females										
0-4	-	-	0	0	-	-	0	0	0	0
5-14	-	-	0	0	-	-	0	0	0	0
15-44	-	-	90	120	-	-	0	0	0	0
45-59	-	-	253	842	-	-	0	0	0	0
60+	-	-	895	2 459	-	-	0	0	0	0
All ages	-	-	1 238	684	-	-	0	0	0	0
Total	-	-	2 021	584	-	-	0	0	0	0

Table 160c   **India - India - Inde**   Diabetes mellitus - Neuropathy

Age group (years)	Incidence 1990 Number ('000s)	Rate (per 100 000)	Prevalence 1990 Number ('000s)	Rate (per 100 000)	Avg. age at onset (years)	Average duration (years)	Deaths 1990 Number ('000s)	Rate (per 100 000)	Deaths 2000 (Projected) Number ('000s)	Rate (per 100 000)
Males										
0-4	-	-	0	0	-	-	0	0	0	0
5-14	-	-	0	0	-	-	0	0	0	0
15-44	-	-	283	141	-	-	0	0	0	0
45-59	-	-	638	1 341	-	-	0	0	0	0
60+	-	-	1 048	3 519	-	-	0	0	0	0
All ages	-	-	1 968	448	-	-	0	0	0	0
Females										
0-4	-	-	0	0	-	-	0	0	0	0
5-14	-	-	0	0	-	-	0	0	0	0
15-44	-	-	258	141	-	-	0	0	0	0
45-59	-	-	617	1 340	-	-	0	0	0	0
60+	-	-	1 019	3 522	-	-	0	0	0	0
All ages	-	-	1 894	462	-	-	0	0	0	0
Total	-	-	3 862	455	-	-	0	0	0	0

For epidemiological sources see McKeigue and King 1996. For the methods used to estimate and project incidence, prevalence, and deaths see Murray and Lopez 1996a. See explanatory notes for definitions and caveats.

Table 166
Epilepsy

Cuadro 166
Epilepsia

Tableau 166
Epilepsie

Cases

Casos

Cas

Table 166a — EME - PEMC - EMBE — Epilepsy - Cases

Age group (years)	Incidence 1990 Number ('000s)	Rate (per 100 000)	Prevalence 1990 Number ('000s)	Rate (per 100 000)	Avg. age at onset (years)	Average duration (years)	Deaths 1990 Number ('000s)	Rate (per 100 000)	Deaths 2000 (Projected) Number ('000s)	Rate (per 100 000)
Males										
0-4	24	90	38	145	2.5	6.7	0	0.4	0	0.3
5-14	48	90	254	477	10.0	9.9	0	0.2	0	0.2
15-44	87	47	958	521	29.9	11.1	2	1.1	2	0.9
45-59	39	60	484	732	52.4	11.0	1	1.4	1	1.2
60+	43	72	435	719	71.1	5.2	1	2.2	1	2.0
All ages	241	62	2 170	556	34.3	9.3	4	1.1	4	1.0
Females										
0-4	21	85	34	137	2.5	7.8	0	0.3	0	0.3
5-14	45	89	260	514	10.0	11.3	0	0.2	0	0.1
15-44	73	41	916	511	30.0	11.9	1	0.6	1	0.4
45-59	40	60	516	762	52.4	11.4	0	0.7	0	0.5
60+	84	99	614	726	72.4	4.6	1	1.5	1	1.5
All ages	264	65	2 341	575	41.3	9.1	3	0.7	3	0.6
Total	504	63	4 511	565	38.0	9.2	7	0.9	7	0.8

Table 166b — FSE - PEAS - AESE — Epilepsy - Cases

Age group (years)	Incidence 1990 Number ('000s)	Rate (per 100 000)	Prevalence 1990 Number ('000s)	Rate (per 100 000)	Avg. age at onset (years)	Average duration (years)	Deaths 1990 Number ('000s)	Rate (per 100 000)	Deaths 2000 (Projected) Number ('000s)	Rate (per 100 000)
Males										
0-4	66	478	53	387	2.5	2.7	0	0.8	0	0.7
5-14	49	178	261	955	10.0	9.5	0	0.9	0	0.7
15-44	81	107	854	1 120	29.8	8.0	2	2.3	1	1.9
45-59	48	178	252	935	52.2	4.0	1	3.0	1	2.6
60+	50	239	134	637	70.0	2.1	1	4.5	1	4.4
All ages	294	178	1 554	940	30.9	5.4	4	2.3	4	2.1
Females										
0-4	18	140	32	240	2.5	8.1	0	0.5	0	0.5
5-14	37	139	231	873	10.0	9.6	0	0.6	0	0.5
15-44	37	50	432	576	30.0	7.0	1	1.4	1	1.1
45-59	30	99	164	546	52.4	5.6	0	1.4	0	1.1
60+	36	100	185	507	71.5	3.7	1	2.6	1	2.5
All ages	158	88	1 042	576	35.9	6.7	3	1.4	2	1.3
Total	453	131	2 597	750	32.7	5.9	6	1.9	6	1.7

Table 166c — India - India - Inde — Epilepsy - Cases

Age group (years)	Incidence 1990 Number ('000s)	Rate (per 100 000)	Prevalence 1990 Number ('000s)	Rate (per 100 000)	Avg. age at onset (years)	Average duration (years)	Deaths 1990 Number ('000s)	Rate (per 100 000)	Deaths 2000 (Projected) Number ('000s)	Rate (per 100 000)
Males										
0-4	279	466	263	440	2.5	1.8	1	0.8	1	0.9
5-14	111	109	469	461	10.0	5.5	1	0.9	1	0.6
15-44	153	77	1 271	634	29.8	7.4	3	1.6	3	1.2
45-59	53	112	186	392	52.3	2.5	1	3.0	1	2.3
60+	98	329	132	442	69.7	1.3	2	5.7	2	4.6
All ages	695	158	2 320	528	23.0	3.6	8	1.7	7	1.4
Females										
0-4	226	398	261	460	2.5	2.4	1	1.0	1	1.2
5-14	104	110	421	442	10.0	10.4	1	0.6	0	0.4
15-44	49	27	1 185	647	29.8	17.1	3	1.4	2	1.0
45-59	9	20	182	396	52.4	5.3	0	1.0	0	0.8
60+	29	100	128	444	70.1	3.9	1	3.6	1	3.1
All ages	417	102	2 178	531	13.4	6.3	5	1.3	5	1.0
Total	1 112	131	4 498	529	19.4	4.6	13	1.5	12	1.2

For epidemiological sources see Reynolds et al. 1996. For the methods used to estimate and project incidence, prevalence, and deaths see Murray and Lopez 1996a. See explanatory notes for definitions and caveats.

Table 166	Cuadro 166	Tableau 166
Epilepsy	Epilepsia	Epilepsie
Cases	Casos	Cas

Table 166d   China - China - Chine — Epilepsy - Cases

Age group (years)	Incidence 1990 Number ('000s)	Rate (per 100 000)	Prevalence 1990 Number ('000s)	Rate (per 100 000)	Avg. age at onset (years)	Average duration (years)	Deaths 1990 Number ('000s)	Rate (per 100 000)	Deaths 2000 (Projected) Number ('000s)	Rate (per 100 000)
Males										
0-4	210	349	200	332	2.5	1.6	0	0.3	0	0.4
5-14	164	169	427	440	10.0	3.7	0	0.3	0	0.2
15-44	213	70	1 465	478	29.9	6.0	5	1.5	3	1.0
45-59	116	159	334	460	52.3	2.7	1	1.0	1	0.8
60+	89	182	200	408	69.8	1.9	1	1.9	1	1.6
All ages	793	135	2 626	449	26.3	3.4	7	1.2	6	0.8
Females										
0-4	173	299	198	342	2.5	1.9	0	0.3	0	0.3
5-14	171	189	411	455	10.0	4.1	0	0.2	0	0.1
15-44	144	51	1 371	482	29.9	9.1	3	1.2	2	0.8
45-59	32	50	314	488	52.4	6.1	1	1.0	1	0.7
60+	52	100	176	340	70.6	2.6	1	1.9	1	1.7
All ages	572	104	2 471	450	20.6	4.7	5	1.0	4	0.7
Total	1 365	120	5 097	450	23.9	3.9	12	1.1	10	0.8

Table 166e   OAI - OPAI - APAI — Epilepsy - Cases

Age group (years)	Incidence 1990 Number ('000s)	Rate (per 100 000)	Prevalence 1990 Number ('000s)	Rate (per 100 000)	Avg. age at onset (years)	Average duration (years)	Deaths 1990 Number ('000s)	Rate (per 100 000)	Deaths 2000 (Projected) Number ('000s)	Rate (per 100 000)
Males										
0-4	170	389	127	290	2.5	1.1	0	0.6	0	0.6
5-14	288	343	543	647	10.0	3.0	1	0.8	0	0.6
15-44	160	99	1 067	664	29.7	5.6	2	1.5	3	1.3
45-59	81	238	226	662	52.3	2.5	1	3.1	1	2.5
60+	60	299	101	499	69.6	1.4	1	4.3	1	3.6
All ages	760	222	2 064	602	21.7	2.9	5	1.6	5	1.3
Females										
0-4	126	299	129	308	2.5	1.8	0	0.6	0	0.6
5-14	213	265	528	658	10.0	4.6	1	0.6	0	0.5
15-44	105	66	1 067	669	29.8	8.9	2	1.0	1	0.7
45-59	26	74	234	667	52.3	6.0	0	1.1	0	0.9
60+	32	139	111	489	70.3	2.6	1	2.5	1	2.2
All ages	500	147	2 069	609	18.2	4.7	3	1.0	3	0.8
Total	1 260	185	4 134	606	20.3	3.7	9	1.3	9	1.1

Table 166f   SSA - ASS - ASS — Epilepsy - Cases

Age group (years)	Incidence 1990 Number ('000s)	Rate (per 100 000)	Prevalence 1990 Number ('000s)	Rate (per 100 000)	Avg. age at onset (years)	Average duration (years)	Deaths 1990 Number ('000s)	Rate (per 100 000)	Deaths 2000 (Projected) Number ('000s)	Rate (per 100 000)
Males										
0-4	273	575	271	570	2.4	1.4	0	0.4	0	0.4
5-14	231	328	406	577	10.0	2.0	1	0.8	1	0.6
15-44	114	110	454	438	29.4	3.6	2	1.7	2	1.3
45-59	28	137	88	435	52.2	2.8	1	3.1	1	2.4
60+	28	263	51	481	69.2	1.6	0	4.5	1	3.6
All ages	673	267	1 270	503	14.4	2.0	4	1.5	4	1.1
Females										
0-4	267	567	273	580	2.4	1.6	0	0.5	0	0.5
5-14	153	219	403	578	10.0	3.1	0	0.7	0	0.5
15-44	75	71	464	437	29.5	5.9	1	0.6	1	0.4
45-59	11	50	98	444	52.2	6.0	0	1.0	0	0.7
60+	18	139	62	484	69.7	2.8	0	2.7	0	2.2
All ages	523	203	1 300	504	11.8	2.8	2	0.7	2	0.5
Total	1 196	234	2 570	504	13.3	2.4	6	1.1	6	0.8

For epidemiological sources see Reynolds et al. 1996. For the methods used to estimate and project incidence, prevalence, and deaths see Murray and Lopez 1996a. See explanatory notes for definitions and caveats.

Table 166	Cuadro 166	Tableau 166
Epilepsy	Epilepsia	Epilepsie
Cases	Casos	Cas

Table 166g   LAC - ALC - ALC   Epilepsy - Cases

Age group (years)	Incidence 1990 Number ('000s)	Rate (per 100 000)	Prevalence 1990 Number ('000s)	Rate (per 100 000)	Avg. age at onset (years)	Average duration (years)	Deaths 1990 Number ('000s)	Rate (per 100 000)	Deaths 2000 (Projected) Number ('000s)	Rate (per 100 000)
Males										
0-4	172	598	100	350	2.5	0.82	0	0.9	0	0.9
5-14	243	466	418	802	10.0	2.64	1	1.2	1	0.9
15-44	186	178	1 053	1 010	29.8	5.14	1	1.4	1	1.1
45-59	88	396	230	1 035	52.3	2.33	0	2.2	1	1.8
60+	82	576	105	737	70.3	1.16	0	2.5	0	2.2
All ages	771	348	1 907	861	24.4	2.65	3	1.4	3	1.2
Females										
0-4	130	468	105	378	2.5	1.27	0	0.8	0	0.7
5-14	191	377	411	811	10.0	3.41	0	0.9	0	0.6
15-44	114	109	791	760	29.9	6.83	2	1.6	1	1.1
45-59	14	60	153	654	52.4	6.73	0	1.3	0	1.0
60+	25	149	110	655	71.1	3.50	0	1.5	0	1.3
All ages	474	213	1 569	705	17.2	3.75	3	1.3	3	1.0
Total	1 244	280	3 476	782	21.6	3.06	6	1.4	6	1.1

Table 166h   MEC - AOM - CMO   Epilepsy - Cases

Age group (years)	Incidence 1990 Number ('000s)	Rate (per 100 000)	Prevalence 1990 Number ('000s)	Rate (per 100 000)	Avg. age at onset (years)	Average duration (years)	Deaths 1990 Number ('000s)	Rate (per 100 000)	Deaths 2000 (Projected) Number ('000s)	Rate (per 100 000)
Males										
0-4	246	597	198	480	2.5	1.2	1	1.4	1	1.4
5-14	182	278	366	561	10.0	2.2	1	1.8	1	1.3
15-44	97	85	350	307	29.8	3.2	2	1.8	2	1.4
45-59	22	100	70	312	52.3	2.8	1	2.6	1	2.0
60+	29	210	41	303	69.7	1.3	1	3.8	1	3.1
All ages	575	224	1 024	400	14.7	1.9	5	1.9	5	1.5
Females										
0-4	237	597	191	480	2.5	1.1	0	1.1	1	1.1
5-14	190	306	347	560	10.0	3.1	1	1.7	1	1.2
15-44	24	22	318	296	29.9	9.3	2	1.7	2	1.2
45-59	6	29	67	301	52.3	8.9	0	1.7	0	1.3
60+	7	44	46	298	70.4	4.2	0	1.9	0	1.6
All ages	464	188	969	393	8.6	2.5	4	1.6	4	1.2
Total	1 039	207	1 994	396	12.0	2.2	9	1.8	9	1.4

Table 166i   World - Mundo - Monde   Epilepsy - Cases

Age group (years)	Incidence 1990 Number ('000s)	Rate (per 100 000)	Prevalence 1990 Number ('000s)	Rate (per 100 000)	Avg. age at onset (years)	Average duration (years)	Deaths 1990 Number ('000s)	Rate (per 100 000)	Deaths 2000 (Projected) Number ('000s)	Rate (per 100 000)
Males										
0-4	1 439	448	1 250	389	2.5	1.5	2	0.7	2	0.7
5-14	1 316	239	3 145	571	10.0	3.4	5	0.8	4	0.6
15-44	1 091	87	7 472	598	29.8	6.0	19	1.5	17	1.2
45-59	476	152	1 871	599	52.3	3.4	7	2.1	7	1.7
60+	479	219	1 198	547	69.9	1.9	7	3.3	8	2.8
All ages	4 801	181	14 936	563	22.4	3.3	40	1.5	38	1.2
Females										
0-4	1 198	387	1 223	395	2.5	1.9	2	0.7	2	0.7
5-14	1 104	210	3 014	573	10.0	4.8	3	0.7	3	0.5
15-44	621	52	6 543	546	29.8	9.1	14	1.1	11	0.8
45-59	169	54	1 729	556	52.4	7.4	3	1.1	3	0.8
60+	282	105	1 431	532	71.2	3.6	6	2.1	7	2.0
All ages	3 373	129	13 939	533	18.2	4.6	28	1.1	26	0.9
Total	8 173	155	28 875	548	20.7	3.8	68	1.3	65	1.0

For epidemiological sources see Reynolds et al. 1996. For the methods used to estimate and project incidence, prevalence, and deaths see Murray and Lopez 1996a. See explanatory notes for definitions and caveats.

Table 167   **Cuadro 167**   **Tableau 167**
Alcohol use   **Uso de alcohol**   **Usage d'alcool**
Alcohol dependence syndrome   Síndrome de dependencia del alcohol   Syndrome de dépendance alcoolique

Table 167a   EME - PEMC - EMBE   Alcohol use - Alcohol dependence syndrome

Age group (years)	Incidence 1990 Number ('000s)	Rate (per 100 000)	Prevalence 1990 Number ('000s)	Rate (per 100 000)	Avg. age at onset (years)	Average duration (years)	Deaths 1990 Number ('000s)	Rate (per 100 000)	Deaths 2000 (Projected) Number ('000s)	Rate (per 100 000)
Males										
0-4	0	0	0	0	-	-	0	0.0	0	0.0
5-14	0	0	0	0	-	-	0	0.0	0	0.0
15-44	7 546	4 100	11 978	6 507	28.9	1.7	3	1.6	3	1.5
45-59	1 314	1 986	2 372	3 586	52.4	1.6	5	7.7	5	6.4
60+	492	813	909	1 501	72.0	1.5	4	7.2	4	6.1
All ages	9 352	2 395	15 259	3 908	34.5	1.6	12	3.2	12	2.9
Females										
0-4	0	0	0	0	-	-	0	0.0	0	0.0
5-14	0	0	0	0	-	-	0	0.0	0	0.0
15-44	1 364	761	2 169	1 210	28.8	1.7	1	0.4	1	0.3
45-59	222	327	406	599	52.4	1.6	1	1.9	1	1.4
60+	147	174	258	305	73.0	1.5	1	1.5	1	1.3
All ages	1 733	426	2 833	696	35.6	1.6	3	0.8	3	0.7
Total	11 085	1 389	18 092	2 268	34.6	1.6	16	2.0	15	1.8

Table 167b   FSE - PEAS - AESE   Alcohol use - Alcohol dependence syndrome

Age group (years)	Incidence 1990 Number ('000s)	Rate (per 100 000)	Prevalence 1990 Number ('000s)	Rate (per 100 000)	Avg. age at onset (years)	Average duration (years)	Deaths 1990 Number ('000s)	Rate (per 100 000)	Deaths 2000 (Projected) Number ('000s)	Rate (per 100 000)
Males										
0-4	0	0	0	0	-	-	0	0.0	0	0.0
5-14	0	0	0	0	-	-	0	0.0	0	0.0
15-44	2 910	3 815	4 608	6 041	28.9	1.7	1	1.9	1	1.5
45-59	521	1 931	940	3 486	52.2	1.6	2	9.2	3	8.0
60+	163	778	307	1 464	70.7	1.5	3	12.8	3	11.6
All ages	3 594	2 174	5 855	3 542	34.2	1.6	7	4.0	7	3.9
Females										
0-4	0	0	0	0	-	-	0	0.0	0	0.0
5-14	0	0	0	0	-	-	0	0.0	0	0.0
15-44	409	546	653	871	28.3	1.7	0	0.3	0	0.2
45-59	30	100	68	225	52.4	1.6	0	1.6	0	1.3
60+	25	68	42	116	72.2	1.5	1	2.2	1	2.0
All ages	464	256	762	421	32.2	1.7	2	0.8	1	0.8
Total	4 058	1 172	6 618	1 911	33.9	1.6	8	2.4	8	2.2

Table 167c   India - India - Inde   Alcohol use - Alcohol dependence syndrome

Age group (years)	Incidence 1990 Number ('000s)	Rate (per 100 000)	Prevalence 1990 Number ('000s)	Rate (per 100 000)	Avg. age at onset (years)	Average duration (years)	Deaths 1990 Number ('000s)	Rate (per 100 000)	Deaths 2000 (Projected) Number ('000s)	Rate (per 100 000)
Males										
0-4	0	0.0	0	0.0	-	-	0	0.0	0	0.0
5-14	0	0.0	0	0.0	-	-	0	0.0	0	0.0
15-44	1 622	808.7	2 584	1 288.5	28.1	1.7	2	1.0	2	0.8
45-59	128	268.7	244	512.6	52.3	1.6	2	4.0	2	3.1
60+	29	97.1	56	188.6	69.8	1.5	1	3.5	1	2.7
All ages	1 778	404.7	2 884	656.3	30.5	1.7	5	1.1	5	1.0
Females										
0-4	0	0.0	0	0.0	-	-	0	0.0	0	0.0
5-14	0	0.0	0	0.0	-	-	0	0.0	0	0.0
15-44	157	85.5	250	136.7	27.6	1.7	0	0.1	0	0.0
45-59	9	20.0	19	40.5	52.4	1.6	0	0.2	0	0.2
60+	1	2.2	2	6.3	72.1	1.5	0	0.6	0	0.5
All ages	166	40.6	271	66.1	29.1	1.7	0	0.1	0	0.1
Total	1 945	228.9	3 155	371.4	30.4	1.7	5	0.6	5	0.5

For epidemiological sources see Lopez et al. 1996. For the methods used to estimate and project incidence, prevalence, and deaths see Murray and Lopez 1996a. See explanatory notes for definitions and caveats.

Table 167	Cuadro 167	Tableau 167
Alcohol use	**Uso de alcohol**	**Usage d'alcool**
Alcohol dependence syndrome	Síndrome de dependencia del alcohol	Syndrome de dépendance alcoolique

Table 167d China - China - Chine Alcohol use - Alcohol dependence syndrome

Age group (years)	Incidence 1990 Number ('000s)	Rate (per 100 000)	Prevalence 1990 Number ('000s)	Rate (per 100 000)	Avg. age at onset (years)	Average duration (years)	Deaths 1990 Number ('000s)	Rate (per 100 000)	Deaths 2000 (Projected) Number ('000s)	Rate (per 100 000)
Males										
0-4	0	0.0	0	0.0	-	-	0	0.0	0	0.0
5-14	0	0.0	0	0.0	-	-	0	0.0	0	0.0
15-44	2 875	938.6	4 595	1 500.1	27.9	1.7	3	0.9	3	0.8
45-59	253	347.8	466	641.4	52.3	1.6	1	1.5	1	1.2
60+	62	127.1	120	244.7	70.7	1.5	1	1.2	1	0.9
All ages	3 190	545.1	5 181	885.3	30.7	1.7	4	0.7	4	0.7
Females										
0-4	0	0.0	0	0.0	-	-	0	0.0	0	0.0
5-14	0	0.0	0	0.0	-	-	0	0.0	0	0.0
15-44	228	80.1	365	128.5	27.6	1.7	0	0.1	0	0.0
45-59	10	15.0	21	32.2	52.4	1.6	0	0.2	0	0.2
60+	1	1.9	3	5.0	72.6	1.5	0	0.3	0	0.3
All ages	238	43.4	388	70.8	28.8	1.7	0	0.1	0	0.1
Total	3 428	302.4	5 569	491.2	30.5	1.7	5	0.4	5	0.4

Table 167e OAI - OPAI - APAI Alcohol use - Alcohol dependence syndrome

Age group (years)	Incidence 1990 Number ('000s)	Rate (per 100 000)	Prevalence 1990 Number ('000s)	Rate (per 100 000)	Avg. age at onset (years)	Average duration (years)	Deaths 1990 Number ('000s)	Rate (per 100 000)	Deaths 2000 (Projected) Number ('000s)	Rate (per 100 000)
Males										
0-4	0	0	0	0	-	-	0	0.0	0	0.0
5-14	0	0	0	0	-	-	0	0.0	0	0.0
15-44	3 665	2 279	5 865	3 647	27.4	1.7	2	1.1	2	0.9
45-59	226	662	433	1 268	52.3	1.6	2	6.3	2	5.0
60+	62	305	113	561	70.7	1.5	1	5.4	1	4.3
All ages	3 952	1 152	6 411	1 869	29.5	1.7	5	1.4	5	1.3
Females										
0-4	0	0	0	0	-	-	0	0.0	0	0.0
5-14	0	0	0	0	-	-	0	0.0	0	0.0
15-44	305	191	488	305	27.4	1.7	0	0.1	0	0.0
45-59	11	30	24	68	52.3	1.6	0	0.6	0	0.4
60+	3	11	5	21	72.2	1.5	0	1.0	0	0.9
All ages	318	94	516	152	28.6	1.7	1	0.2	1	0.1
Total	4 270	626	6 928	1 015	29.4	1.7	5	0.8	6	0.7

Table 167f SSA - ASS - ASS Alcohol use - Alcohol dependence syndrome

Age group (years)	Incidence 1990 Number ('000s)	Rate (per 100 000)	Prevalence 1990 Number ('000s)	Rate (per 100 000)	Avg. age at onset (years)	Average duration (years)	Deaths 1990 Number ('000s)	Rate (per 100 000)	Deaths 2000 (Projected) Number ('000s)	Rate (per 100 000)
Males										
0-4	0	0	0	0	-	-	0	0.0	0	0.0
5-14	0	0	0	0	-	-	0	0.0	0	0.0
15-44	3 005	2 896	4 760	4 587	27.9	1.6	1	1.0	1	0.7
45-59	209	1 030	398	1 957	52.2	1.6	1	6.4	1	4.9
60+	30	285	63	597	70.6	1.5	1	10.3	1	8.2
All ages	3 244	1 286	5 220	2 069	29.9	1.6	3	1.3	4	1.0
Females										
0-4	0	0	0	0	-	-	0	0.0	0	0.0
5-14	0	0	0	0	-	-	0	0.0	0	0.0
15-44	706	664	1 132	1 065	26.5	1.6	0	0.2	0	0.1
45-59	31	140	61	278	52.2	1.6	1	2.8	1	2.0
60+	13	99	22	171	69.7	1.5	1	4.0	1	3.1
All ages	749	290	1 215	471	28.3	1.6	1	0.5	1	0.4
Total	3 993	783	6 435	1 261	29.6	1.6	5	0.9	5	0.7

For epidemiological sources see Lopez et al. 1996. For the methods used to estimate and project incidence, prevalence, and deaths see Murray and Lopez 1996a. See explanatory notes for definitions and caveats.

Table 167	Cuadro 167	Tableau 167
Alcohol use	**Uso de alcohol**	**Usage d'alcool**
Alcohol dependence syndrome	Síndrome de dependencia del alcohol	Syndrome de dépendance alcoolique

Table 167g   LAC - ALC - ALC   Alcohol use - Alcohol dependence syndrome

Age group (years)	Incidence 1990 Number ('000s)	Rate (per 100 000)	Prevalence 1990 Number ('000s)	Rate (per 100 000)	Avg. age at onset (years)	Average duration (years)	Deaths 1990 Number ('000s)	Rate (per 100 000)	Deaths 2000 (Projected) Number ('000s)	Rate (per 100 000)
Males										
0-4	0	0	0	0	-	-	0	0.0	0	0.0
5-14	0	0	0	0	-	-	0	0.0	0	0.0
15-44	6 919	6 634	10 992	10 541	28.5	1.7	4	3.9	4	3.4
45-59	773	3 473	1 368	6 151	52.3	1.6	4	16.5	4	13.4
60+	339	2 384	583	4 096	70.8	1.5	2	16.5	3	13.7
All ages	8 031	3 624	12 944	5 841	32.6	1.6	10	4.5	11	4.2
Females										
0-4	0	0	0	0	-	-	0	0.0	0	0.0
5-14	0	0	0	0	-	-	0	0.0	0	0.0
15-44	647	622	1 036	996	27.5	1.7	1	0.5	1	0.4
45-59	28	120	60	255	52.4	1.6	0	1.8	0	1.4
60+	17	102	29	171	71.5	1.5	0	1.8	0	1.5
All ages	692	311	1 125	505	29.6	1.7	1	0.6	1	0.5
Total	8 723	1 963	14 068	3 166	32.3	1.6	11	2.5	12	2.3

Table 167h   MEC - AOM - CMO   Alcohol use - Alcohol dependence syndrome

Age group (years)	Incidence 1990 Number ('000s)	Rate (per 100 000)	Prevalence 1990 Number ('000s)	Rate (per 100 000)	Avg. age at onset (years)	Average duration (years)	Deaths 1990 Number ('000s)	Rate (per 100 000)	Deaths 2000 (Projected) Number ('000s)	Rate (per 100 000)
Males										
0-4	0	0.0	0	0	-	-	0	0.0	0	0.0
5-14	0	0.0	0	0	-	-	0	0.0	0	0.0
15-44	488	428.2	774	679	28.8	1.7	0	0.2	0	0.2
45-59	30	134.7	60	267	52.3	1.6	0	1.1	0	0.9
60+	10	70.7	17	127	70.8	1.5	0	1.1	0	0.9
All ages	527	205.7	851	332	30.9	1.7	1	0.3	1	0.2
Females										
0-4	0	0.0	0	0	-	-	0	0.0	0	0.0
5-14	0	0.0	0	0	-	-	0	0.0	0	0.0
15-44	54	50.3	87	81	26.9	1.7	0	0.0	0	0.0
45-59	2	8.0	4	17	52.3	1.6	0	0.2	0	0.1
60+	1	7.7	2	13	71.4	1.5	0	0.3	0	0.2
All ages	57	23.1	93	38	28.6	1.7	0	0.0	0	0.0
Total	584	116.1	943	188	30.7	1.7	1	0.1	1	0.1

Table 167i   World - Mundo - Monde   Alcohol use - Alcohol dependence syndrome

Age group (years)	Incidence 1990 Number ('000s)	Rate (per 100 000)	Prevalence 1990 Number ('000s)	Rate (per 100 000)	Avg. age at onset (years)	Average duration (years)	Deaths 1990 Number ('000s)	Rate (per 100 000)	Deaths 2000 (Projected) Number ('000s)	Rate (per 100 000)
Males										
0-4	0	0	0	0	-	-	0	0.0	0	0.0
5-14	0	0	0	0	-	-	0	0.0	0	0.0
15-44	29 029	2 322	46 155	3 693	28.4	1.7	16	1.3	16	1.1
45-59	3 453	1 105	6 281	2 011	52.3	1.6	18	5.7	19	4.6
60+	1 187	542	2 168	991	71.2	1.5	13	6.1	14	5.1
All ages	33 669	1 269	54 604	2 058	32.3	1.6	47	1.8	49	1.6
Females										
0-4	0	0	0	0	-	-	0	0.0	0	0.0
5-14	0	0	0	0	-	-	0	0.0	0	0.0
15-44	3 869	323	6 179	516	27.9	1.7	2	0.2	2	0.1
45-59	342	110	662	213	52.4	1.6	3	1.0	3	0.8
60+	207	77	362	134	72.6	1.5	4	1.3	4	1.1
All ages	4 417	169	7 203	276	31.8	1.7	9	0.3	9	0.3
Total	38 086	723	61 807	1 173	32.3	1.6	56	1.1	57	0.9

For epidemiological sources see Lopez et al. 1996. For the methods used to estimate and project incidence, prevalence, and deaths see Murray and Lopez 1996a. See explanatory notes for definitions and caveats.

Table 168
Dementia

Cuadro 168
Demencia

Tableau 168
Démence

Cases

Casos

Cas

Table 168a — EME - PEMC - EMBE — Dementia - Cases

Age group (years)	Incidence 1990 Number ('000s)	Rate (per 100 000)	Prevalence 1990 Number ('000s)	Rate (per 100 000)	Avg. age at onset (years)	Average duration (years)	Deaths 1990 Number ('000s)	Rate (per 100 000)	Deaths 2000 (Projected) Number ('000s)	Rate (per 100 000)
Males										
0-4	1	5.5	3	11	2.5	29.5	1	2.2	0	1.6
5-14	0	0.9	11	21	10.0	40.1	0	0.4	0	0.3
15-44	2	0.9	56	31	29.9	31.7	1	0.5	1	0.4
45-59	27	40.6	147	222	55.0	18.4	2	3.3	2	2.8
60+	335	553.3	2 357	3 893	79.0	6.4	31	51.9	37	50.8
All ages	365	93.6	2 574	659	76.6	7.5	35	9.0	40	9.8
Females										
0-4	1	5.5	3	11	2.5	31.0	1	2.1	0	1.6
5-14	0	0.9	11	21	10.0	42.5	0	0.3	0	0.2
15-44	2	0.9	55	31	30.0	34.4	1	0.3	0	0.2
45-59	28	40.6	148	219	55.2	21.3	2	2.4	1	1.8
60+	563	665.2	4 291	5 074	79.4	7.3	55	65.5	68	69.7
All ages	593	145.7	4 507	1 107	77.9	8.1	58	14.3	70	16.4
Total	959	120.2	7 082	888	77.4	7.8	94	11.7	111	13.2

Table 168b — FSE - PEAS - AESE — Dementia - Cases

Age group (years)	Incidence 1990 Number ('000s)	Rate (per 100 000)	Prevalence 1990 Number ('000s)	Rate (per 100 000)	Avg. age at onset (years)	Average duration (years)	Deaths 1990 Number ('000s)	Rate (per 100 000)	Deaths 2000 (Projected) Number ('000s)	Rate (per 100 000)
Males										
0-4	1	5.5	1	10	2.5	27.7	0	2.2	0	2.0
5-14	0	0.9	6	21	10.0	37.3	0	0.6	0	0.5
15-44	1	0.9	23	31	29.8	28.5	0	0.4	0	0.4
45-59	11	39.7	58	215	54.9	16.0	0	1.5	0	1.3
60+	96	459.2	663	3 162	77.6	5.9	4	19.8	6	22.0
All ages	109	65.7	751	455	74.4	7.2	5	3.2	7	3.9
Females										
0-4	1	5.5	1	11	2.5	30.0	0	1.9	0	1.8
5-14	0	0.9	6	21	10.0	41.1	0	0.4	0	0.3
15-44	1	0.9	23	31	29.9	32.8	0	0.4	0	0.3
45-59	12	40.7	67	223	55.0	19.5	0	1.2	0	1.0
60+	214	589.2	1 513	4 158	79.3	6.5	11	30.4	14	33.0
All ages	228	126.2	1 610	890	77.5	7.4	12	6.6	14	7.7
Total	337	97.3	2 362	682	76.5	7.3	17	5.0	21	5.9

Table 168c — India - India - Inde — Dementia - Cases

Age group (years)	Incidence 1990 Number ('000s)	Rate (per 100 000)	Prevalence 1990 Number ('000s)	Rate (per 100 000)	Avg. age at onset (years)	Average duration (years)	Deaths 1990 Number ('000s)	Rate (per 100 000)	Deaths 2000 (Projected) Number ('000s)	Rate (per 100 000)
Males										
0-4	3	5.6	6	11	2.5	26.0	0	0.5	0	0.6
5-14	1	0.8	22	21	10.0	37.3	0	0.1	0	0.1
15-44	2	0.8	59	30	29.8	29.0	1	0.4	1	0.3
45-59	14	29.9	79	166	55.1	15.9	1	2.2	1	1.7
60+	104	348.2	740	2 485	76.3	6.1	9	28.6	9	24.5
All ages	124	28.2	906	206	70.8	8.3	11	2.4	11	2.2
Females										
0-4	3	5.6	6	11	2.5	26.2	1	1.2	1	1.3
5-14	1	0.8	20	21	10.0	38.0	0	0.2	0	0.1
15-44	2	0.8	54	30	29.8	30.0	1	0.4	1	0.3
45-59	14	30.1	77	168	55.1	17.0	1	1.9	1	1.5
60+	107	370.6	769	2 658	76.8	6.2	9	29.8	11	27.4
All ages	127	30.9	926	226	71.6	8.4	11	2.7	13	2.7
Total	250	29.5	1 833	216	71.2	8.3	22	2.6	24	2.4

For epidemiological sources see Ritchie et al. 1996. For the methods used to estimate and project incidence, prevalence, and deaths see Murray and Lopez 1996a. See explanatory notes for definitions and caveats.

Table 168 | **Cuadro 168** | **Tableau 168**
Dementia | **Demencia** | **Démence**

Cases | Casos | Cas

Table 168d   China - China - Chine — Dementia - Cases

Age group (years)	Incidence 1990 Number ('000s)	Rate (per 100 000)	Prevalence 1990 Number ('000s)	Rate (per 100 000)	Avg. age at onset (years)	Average duration (years)	Deaths 1990 Number ('000s)	Rate (per 100 000)	Deaths 2000 (Projected) Number ('000s)	Rate (per 100 000)
Males										
0-4	3	5.6	6	11	2.5	28.2	0	0.8	0	0.8
5-14	1	0.8	21	21	10.0	38.6	0	0.2	0	0.2
15-44	3	0.8	91	30	29.9	29.8	1	0.3	1	0.2
45-59	22	30.0	122	167	55.1	16.1	1	1.7	1	1.3
60+	174	355.8	1 247	2 546	76.5	6.2	8	16.9	9	14.6
All ages	203	34.7	1 487	254	72.1	8.0	11	1.9	12	1.8
Females										
0-4	3	5.6	6	11	2.5	28.9	0	0.7	0	0.8
5-14	1	0.8	19	21	10.0	40.0	0	0.1	0	0.1
15-44	2	0.8	84	30	29.9	31.4	1	0.3	1	0.2
45-59	19	30.3	109	169	55.1	17.9	1	1.9	1	1.5
60+	209	404.9	1 518	2 939	77.6	6.5	13	25.5	16	25.3
All ages	235	42.9	1 737	317	74.0	8.1	16	2.9	19	3.0
Total	438	38.6	3 224	284	73.1	8.1	27	2.4	30	2.4

Table 168e   OAI - OPAI - APAI — Dementia - Cases

Age group (years)	Incidence 1990 Number ('000s)	Rate (per 100 000)	Prevalence 1990 Number ('000s)	Rate (per 100 000)	Avg. age at onset (years)	Average duration (years)	Deaths 1990 Number ('000s)	Rate (per 100 000)	Deaths 2000 (Projected) Number ('000s)	Rate (per 100 000)
Males										
0-4	2	5.5	5	10	2.5	26.2	0	0.5	0	0.5
5-14	1	0.9	18	21	10.0	36.8	0	0.1	0	0.1
15-44	1	0.9	49	31	29.7	28.3	1	0.3	1	0.3
45-59	14	40.0	74	217	54.9	15.5	1	2.5	1	2.0
60+	87	432.6	603	2 985	77.3	5.2	6	30.6	7	26.9
All ages	106	30.8	749	218	71.6	7.5	8	2.3	9	2.3
Females										
0-4	2	5.5	4	10	2.5	27.2	0	1.2	0	1.1
5-14	1	0.9	17	21	10.0	38.0	0	0.2	0	0.2
15-44	1	0.9	49	31	29.8	29.8	0	0.3	0	0.2
45-59	14	40.4	77	220	55.0	17.0	1	2.4	1	1.8
60+	111	489.8	770	3 399	78.1	6.1	8	33.9	10	31.7
All ages	130	38.2	918	270	73.3	8.1	10	2.8	12	3.0
Total	235	34.5	1 666	244	72.5	7.8	18	2.6	21	2.6

Table 168f   SSA - ASS - ASS — Dementia - Cases

Age group (years)	Incidence 1990 Number ('000s)	Rate (per 100 000)	Prevalence 1990 Number ('000s)	Rate (per 100 000)	Avg. age at onset (years)	Average duration (years)	Deaths 1990 Number ('000s)	Rate (per 100 000)	Deaths 2000 (Projected) Number ('000s)	Rate (per 100 000)
Males										
0-4	1	2.1	2	3.9	2.4	22.0	0	0.3	0	0.3
5-14	0	0.3	6	8.0	10.0	33.0	0	0.1	0	0.1
15-44	0	0.3	12	11.5	29.4	26.0	0	0.3	0	0.2
45-59	3	14.9	16	78.9	55.0	14.6	0	2.2	0	1.7
60+	18	170.8	126	1 195.6	76.0	5.9	3	27.4	3	22.7
All ages	23	8.9	161	63.8	68.5	8.4	4	1.5	4	1.3
Females										
0-4	3	5.7	5	10.6	2.4	23.1	0	0.7	0	0.7
5-14	1	1.1	16	22.9	10.0	34.3	0	0.2	0	0.1
15-44	1	1.1	38	36.0	29.5	27.2	0	0.1	0	0.1
45-59	3	15.0	24	107.7	55.0	15.6	1	2.3	0	1.7
60+	49	384.5	168	1 320.0	76.7	6.1	3	26.2	4	21.7
All ages	57	22.1	251	97.3	70.0	8.3	4	1.7	5	1.4
Total	80	15.6	412	80.8	69.6	8.3	8	1.6	9	1.3

For epidemiological sources see Ritchie et al. 1996. For the methods used to estimate and project incidence, prevalence, and deaths see Murray and Lopez 1996a. See explanatory notes for definitions and caveats.

Table 168   **Cuadro 168**   **Tableau 168**
Dementia   **Demencia**   **Démence**

Cases   Casos   Cas

Table 168g   LAC - ALC - ALC   Dementia - Cases

Age group (years)	Incidence 1990 Number ('000s)	Rate (per 100 000)	Prevalence 1990 Number ('000s)	Rate (per 100 000)	Avg. age at onset (years)	Average duration (years)	Deaths 1990 Number ('000s)	Rate (per 100 000)	Deaths 2000 (Projected) Number ('000s)	Rate (per 100 000)
Males										
0-4	2	5.5	3	10	2.5	27.4	1	2.1	1	1.9
5-14	0	0.9	11	21	10.0	38.2	0	0.8	0	0.6
15-44	1	0.9	32	31	29.8	29.8	0	0.3	0	0.3
45-59	13	59.0	108	487	60.5	14.0	0	2.0	1	1.6
60+	136	957.0	889	6 250	79.7	5.4	2	14.4	3	13.0
All ages	152	68.7	1 044	471	76.7	6.6	4	1.7	4	1.6
Females										
0-4	2	5.5	3	10	2.5	28.6	1	2.2	1	2.1
5-14	0	0.9	11	21	10.0	39.7	0	0.6	0	0.4
15-44	1	0.9	32	31	29.8	31.6	0	0.4	0	0.3
45-59	9	40.7	52	222	55.0	18.7	0	1.5	0	1.2
60+	93	552.3	652	3 873	78.9	6.3	3	15.0	3	14.3
All ages	105	47.3	749	336	74.9	8.1	4	1.9	5	1.8
Total	258	58.0	1 793	404	76.0	7.2	8	1.8	9	1.7

Table 168h   MEC - AOM - CMO   Dementia - Cases

Age group (years)	Incidence 1990 Number ('000s)	Rate (per 100 000)	Prevalence 1990 Number ('000s)	Rate (per 100 000)	Avg. age at onset (years)	Average duration (years)	Deaths 1990 Number ('000s)	Rate (per 100 000)	Deaths 2000 (Projected) Number ('000s)	Rate (per 100 000)
Males										
0-4	2	5.6	4	11	2.5	26.5	0	0.4	0	0.4
5-14	0	0.7	13	20	10.0	37.7	0	0.1	0	0.1
15-44	1	0.7	30	26	29.8	29.1	0	0.3	0	0.2
45-59	2	11.2	17	78	55.1	15.8	0	2.0	0	1.6
60+	19	138.4	135	987	76.8	6.1	3	25.4	4	22.3
All ages	25	9.7	200	78	65.1	10.2	4	1.7	5	1.6
Females										
0-4	2	5.6	4	11	2.5	27.2	0	0.9	0	0.9
5-14	0	0.7	13	20	10.0	38.9	0	0.2	0	0.1
15-44	1	0.7	26	24	22.5	34.0	0	0.3	0	0.2
45-59	1	5.7	12	52	54.0	17.9	0	2.0	0	1.5
60+	24	154.2	171	1 106	77.7	6.3	4	25.8	5	22.6
All ages	28	11.5	226	91	68.4	9.7	5	2.1	6	1.9
Total	53	10.6	425	85	66.9	9.9	10	1.9	11	1.7

Table 168i   World - Mundo - Monde   Dementia - Cases

Age group (years)	Incidence 1990 Number ('000s)	Rate (per 100 000)	Prevalence 1990 Number ('000s)	Rate (per 100 000)	Avg. age at onset (years)	Average duration (years)	Deaths 1990 Number ('000s)	Rate (per 100 000)	Deaths 2000 (Projected) Number ('000s)	Rate (per 100 000)
Males										
0-4	16	5.1	31	10	2.5	26.8	3	0.9	3	0.8
5-14	4	0.8	107	19	10.0	37.7	1	0.3	1	0.2
15-44	10	0.8	353	28	29.8	29.5	4	0.3	4	0.3
45-59	106	33.9	621	199	55.7	16.3	7	2.3	7	1.8
60+	970	443.1	6 760	3 089	78.0	6.0	67	30.6	78	28.2
All ages	1 106	41.7	7 872	297	74.0	7.6	83	3.1	93	3.0
Females										
0-4	17	5.6	33	11	2.5	27.2	4	1.2	4	1.1
5-14	5	0.9	112	21	10.0	38.5	1	0.2	1	0.2
15-44	10	0.9	362	30	29.3	31.2	4	0.3	3	0.2
45-59	101	32.6	566	182	55.1	18.7	6	2.0	6	1.5
60+	1 370	508.9	9 852	3 660	78.6	6.7	106	39.3	131	38.8
All ages	1 504	57.5	10 924	418	75.6	8.0	121	4.6	145	4.7
Total	2 610	49.5	18 796	357	75.0	7.9	203	3.9	237	3.9

For epidemiological sources see Ritchie et al. 1996. For the methods used to estimate and project incidence, prevalence, and deaths see Murray and Lopez 1996a. See explanatory notes for definitions and caveats.

Table 169
Parkinson disease

Cuadro 169
Enfermedad de Parkinson

Tableau 169
Maladie de Parkinson

Cases

Casos

Cas

Table 169a   EME - PEMC - EMBE   Parkinson disease - Cases

Age group (years)	Incidence 1990 Number ('000s)	Rate (per 100 000)	Prevalence 1990 Number ('000s)	Rate (per 100 000)	Avg. age at onset (years)	Average duration (years)	Deaths 1990 Number ('000s)	Rate (per 100 000)	Deaths 2000 (Projected) Number ('000s)	Rate (per 100 000)
Males										
0-4	0	0	0	0	-	-	0	0.0	0	0.0
5-14	0	0	0	0	-	-	0	0.0	0	0.0
15-44	0	0	0	0	-	-	0	0.0	0	0.0
45-59	13	20	97	146	52.4	23.0	0	0.3	0	0.2
60+	46	75	647	1 068	71.0	10.7	15	24.5	18	24.4
All ages	59	15	744	190	66.8	13.5	15	3.9	18	4.3
Females										
0-4	0	0	0	0	-	-	0	0.0	0	0.0
5-14	0	0	0	0	-	-	0	0.0	0	0.0
15-44	0	0	0	0	-	-	0	0.0	0	0.0
45-59	14	20	100	148	52.4	27.5	0	0.2	0	0.2
60+	64	75	1 005	1 188	72.3	12.4	14	16.7	17	17.9
All ages	77	19	1 105	271	68.8	15.0	14	3.5	18	4.1
Total	136	17	1 849	232	67.9	14.4	29	3.7	35	4.2

Table 169b   FSE - PEAS - AESE   Parkinson disease - Cases

Age group (years)	Incidence 1990 Number ('000s)	Rate (per 100 000)	Prevalence 1990 Number ('000s)	Rate (per 100 000)	Avg. age at onset (years)	Average duration (years)	Deaths 1990 Number ('000s)	Rate (per 100 000)	Deaths 2000 (Projected) Number ('000s)	Rate (per 100 000)
Males										
0-4	0	0.0	0	0	-	-	0	0.0	0	0.0
5-14	0	0.0	0	0	-	-	0	0.0	0	0.0
15-44	0	0.0	0	0	-	-	0	0.0	0	0.0
45-59	4	14.0	27	100	52.2	19.7	0	0.4	0	0.3
60+	11	52.9	146	698	70.0	9.6	3	12.4	4	13.9
All ages	15	9.0	173	105	65.5	12.2	3	1.6	4	2.1
Females										
0-4	0	0.0	0	0	-	-	0	0.0	0	0.0
5-14	0	0.0	0	0	-	-	0	0.0	0	0.0
15-44	0	0.0	0	0	-	-	0	0.0	0	0.0
45-59	4	14.0	31	103	52.4	25.1	0	0.3	0	0.2
60+	19	52.8	288	792	71.5	11.4	4	11.4	5	12.2
All ages	23	12.9	319	176	68.1	13.9	4	2.3	5	2.7
Total	38	11.1	493	142	67.1	13.2	7	2.0	9	2.4

Table 169c   India - India - Inde   Parkinson disease - Cases

Age group (years)	Incidence 1990 Number ('000s)	Rate (per 100 000)	Prevalence 1990 Number ('000s)	Rate (per 100 000)	Avg age at onset (years)	Average duration (years)	Deaths 1990 Number ('000s)	Rate (per 100 000)	Deaths 2000 (Projected) Number ('000s)	Rate (per 100 000)
Males										
0-4	0	0.0	0	0	-	-	0	0.0	0	0.0
5-14	0	0.0	0	0	-	-	0	0.0	0	0.0
15-44	0	0.0	0	0	-	-	0	0.0	0	0.0
45-59	5	10.0	35	73	52.4	20.8	0	0.3	0	0.2
60+	11	37.9	146	490	70.1	9.5	4	13.8	4	11.8
All ages	16	3.6	180	41	64.8	12.8	4	1.0	4	0.9
Females										
0-4	0	0.0	0	0	-	-	0	0.0	0	0.0
5-14	0	0.0	0	0	-	-	0	0.0	0	0.0
15-44	0	0.0	0	0	-	-	0	0.0	0	0.0
45-59	6	13.0	43	94	52.3	19.0	0	0.1	0	0.1
60+	14	49.2	174	601	69.6	8.9	2	6.6	2	6.0
All ages	20	4.9	217	53	64.5	11.9	2	0.5	2	0.5
Total	36	4.3	397	47	64.6	12.3	6	0.7	7	0.7

For the methods used to estimate and project incidence, prevalence, and deaths see Murray and Lopez 1996a. See explanatory notes for definitions and caveats.

Table 169 — **Cuadro 169** — **Tableau 169**
Parkinson disease — **Enfermedad de Parkinson** — **Maladie de Parkinson**

Cases — Casos — Cas

Table 169d China - China - Chine — Parkinson disease - Cases

Age group (years)	Incidence 1990 Number ('000s)	Rate (per 100 000)	Prevalence 1990 Number ('000s)	Rate (per 100 000)	Avg. age at onset (years)	Average duration (years)	Deaths 1990 Number ('000s)	Rate (per 100 000)	Deaths 2000 (Projected) Number ('000s)	Rate (per 100 000)
Males										
0-4	0	0.0	0	0	-	-	0	0.0	0	0.0
5-14	0	0.0	0	0	-	-	0	0.0	0	0.0
15-44	0	0.0	0	0	-	-	0	0.0	0	0.0
45-59	4	5.5	29	40	52.3	19.0	0	0.1	0	0.1
60+	10	20.9	118	240	69.8	8.2	3	5.7	3	5.0
All ages	14	2.4	146	25	64.9	11.2	3	0.5	3	0.5
Females										
0-4	0	0.0	0	0	-	-	0	0.0	0	0.0
5-14	0	0.0	0	0	-	-	0	0.0	0	0.0
15-44	0	0.0	0	0	-	-	0	0.0	0	0.0
45-59	3	4.9	23	36	52.4	22.7	0	0.2	0	0.1
60+	10	18.7	126	245	70.6	10.4	2	4.4	3	4.4
All ages	13	2.3	150	27	66.1	13.5	2	0.4	3	0.5
Total	27	2.4	296	26	65.5	12.3	5	0.5	6	0.5

Table 169e OAI - OPAI - APAI — Parkinson disease - Cases

Age group (years)	Incidence 1990 Number ('000s)	Rate (per 100 000)	Prevalence 1990 Number ('000s)	Rate (per 100 000)	Avg. age at onset (years)	Average duration (years)	Deaths 1990 Number ('000s)	Rate (per 100 000)	Deaths 2000 (Projected) Number ('000s)	Rate (per 100 000)
Males										
0-4	0	0.0	0	0	-	-	0	0.0	0	0.0
5-14	0	0.0	0	0	-	-	0	0.0	0	0.0
15-44	0	0.0	0	0	-	-	0	0.0	0	0.0
45-59	4	13.0	32	93	52.3	18.4	0	0.3	0	0.2
60+	10	49.2	121	599	69.6	8.8	2	11.9	3	10.5
All ages	14	4.2	153	45	64.3	11.8	3	0.7	3	0.7
Females										
0-4	0	0.0	0	0	-	-	0	0.0	0	0.0
5-14	0	0.0	0	0	-	-	0	0.0	0	0.0
15-44	0	0.0	0	0	-	-	0	0.0	0	0.0
45-59	4	10.0	25	73	52.3	20.7	0	0.1	0	0.1
60+	9	37.8	113	498	70.3	9.7	1	5.9	2	5.5
All ages	12	3.6	138	41	65.1	12.9	1	0.4	2	0.5
Total	26	3.9	291	43	64.6	12.3	4	0.6	5	0.6

Table 169f SSA - ASS - ASS — Parkinson disease - Cases

Age group (years)	Incidence 1990 Number ('000s)	Rate (per 100 000)	Prevalence 1990 Number ('000s)	Rate (per 100 000)	Avg. age at onset (years)	Average duration (years)	Deaths 1990 Number ('000s)	Rate (per 100 000)	Deaths 2000 (Projected) Number ('000s)	Rate (per 100 000)
Males										
0-4	0	0.0	0	0	-	-	0	0.0	0	0.0
5-14	0	0.0	0	0	-	-	0	0.0	0	0.0
15-44	0	0.0	0	0	-	-	0	0.0	0	0.0
45-59	2	11.1	16	79	52.2	17.4	0	0.2	0	0.2
60+	4	42.2	53	501	69.2	8.5	1	11.6	1	9.6
All ages	7	2.7	69	27	63.5	11.5	1	0.5	1	0.4
Females										
0-4	0	0.0	0	0	-	-	0	0.0	0	0.0
5-14	0	0.0	0	0	-	-	0	0.0	0	0.0
15-44	0	0.0	0	0	-	-	0	0.0	0	0.0
45-59	2	8.8	14	63	52.2	19.0	0	0.2	0	0.1
60+	4	33.3	54	421	69.7	9.1	1	6.0	1	4.9
All ages	6	2.4	68	26	64.2	12.3	1	0.3	1	0.3
Total	13	2.5	136	27	63.8	11.9	2	0.4	2	0.3

For the methods used to estimate and project incidence, prevalence, and deaths see Murray and Lopez 1996a. See explanatory notes for definitions and caveats.

Table 169
Parkinson disease

Cuadro 169
Enfermedad de Parkinson

Tableau 169
Maladie de Parkinson

Cases

Casos

Cas

Table 169g LAC - ALC - ALC — Parkinson disease - Cases

Age group (years)	Incidence 1990 Number ('000s)	Rate (per 100 000)	Prevalence 1990 Number ('000s)	Rate (per 100 000)	Avg. age at onset (years)	Average duration (years)	Deaths 1990 Number ('000s)	Rate (per 100 000)	Deaths 2000 (Projected) Number ('000s)	Rate (per 100 000)
Males										
0-4	0	0.0	0	0	-	-	0	0.0	0	0.0
5-14	0	0.0	0	0	-	-	0	0.0	0	0.0
15-44	0	0.0	0	0	-	-	0	0.0	0	0.0
45-59	2	7.0	11	51	52.3	21.1	0	0.1	0	0.1
60+	3	24.5	42	296	70.3	9.9	1	7.1	1	6.6
All ages	5	2.3	53	24	64.7	13.4	1	0.5	1	0.5
Females										
0-4	0	0.0	0	0	-	-	0	0.0	0	0.0
5-14	0	0.0	0	0	-	-	0	0.0	0	0.0
15-44	0	0.0	0	0	-	-	0	0.0	0	0.0
45-59	1	5.4	9	40	52.4	22.9	0	0.1	0	0.1
60+	3	19.0	44	259	71.1	10.0	1	4.3	1	4.2
All ages	4	2.0	53	24	65.8	13.6	1	0.3	1	0.4
Total	9	2.1	106	24	65.2	13.5	2	0.4	2	0.4

Table 169h MEC - AOM - CMO — Parkinson disease - Cases

Age group (years)	Incidence 1990 Number ('000s)	Rate (per 100 000)	Prevalence 1990 Number ('000s)	Rate (per 100 000)	Avg. age at onset (years)	Average duration (years)	Deaths 1990 Number ('000s)	Rate (per 100 000)	Deaths 2000 (Projected) Number ('000s)	Rate (per 100 000)
Males										
0-4	0	0.0	0	0	-	-	0	0.0	0	0.0
5-14	0	0.0	0	0	-	-	0	0.0	0	0.0
15-44	0	0.0	0	0	-	-	0	0.0	0	0.0
45-59	3	12.3	21	93	52.3	18.8	0	0.3	0	0.2
60+	7	49.2	82	604	69.7	8.9	2	12.0	2	10.5
All ages	9	3.7	103	40	64.6	11.8	2	0.7	2	0.6
Females										
0-4	0	0.0	0	0	-	-	0	0.0	0	0.0
5-14	0	0.0	0	0	-	-	0	0.0	0	0.0
15-44	0	0.0	0	0	-	-	0	0.0	0	0.0
45-59	2	10.0	16	73	52.3	21.1	0	0.2	0	0.1
60+	6	37.8	77	502	70.4	9.8	1	6.0	1	5.2
All ages	8	3.3	94	38	65.4	12.9	1	0.4	1	0.4
Total	18	3.5	197	39	65.0	12.3	3	0.5	3	0.5

Table 169i World - Mundo - Monde — Parkinson disease - Cases

Age group (years)	Incidence 1990 Number ('000s)	Rate (per 100 000)	Prevalence 1990 Number ('000s)	Rate (per 100 000)	Avg. age at onset (years)	Average duration (years)	Deaths 1990 Number ('000s)	Rate (per 100 000)	Deaths 2000 (Projected) Number ('000s)	Rate (per 100 000)
Males										
0-4	0	0.0	0	0	-	-	0	0.0	0	0.0
5-14	0	0.0	0	0	-	-	0	0.0	0	0.0
15-44	0	0.0	0	0	-	-	0	0.0	0	0.0
45-59	37	11.8	268	86	52.3	20.6	1	0.2	1	0.2
60+	103	46.9	1 355	619	70.4	9.8	31	14.0	36	13.1
All ages	139	5.3	1 622	61	65.6	12.6	31	1.2	37	1.2
Females										
0-4	0	0.0	0	0	-	-	0	0.0	0	0.0
5-14	0	0.0	0	0	-	-	0	0.0	0	0.0
15-44	0	0.0	0	0	-	-	0	0.0	0	0.0
45-59	36	11.5	263	84	52.4	23.7	1	0.2	1	0.1
60+	128	47.7	1 881	699	71.4	11.2	26	9.7	32	9.6
All ages	164	6.3	2 143	82	67.3	14.0	27	1.0	33	1.1
Total	304	5.8	3 766	71	66.5	13.4	58	1.1	70	1.1

For the methods used to estimate and project incidence, prevalence, and deaths see Murray and Lopez 1996a. See explanatory notes for definitions and caveats.

Table 170
Multiple sclerosis

Cuadro 170
Esclerosis múltiple

Tableau 170
Sclérose en plaques

Cases

Casos

Cas

Table 170a EME - PEMC - EMBE — Multiple sclerosis - Cases

Age group (years)	Incidence 1990 Number ('000s)	Rate (per 100 000)	Prevalence 1990 Number ('000s)	Rate (per 100 000)	Avg. age at onset (years)	Average duration (years)	Deaths 1990 Number ('000s)	Rate (per 100 000)	Deaths 2000 (Projected) Number ('000s)	Rate (per 100 000)
Males										
0-4	0	0.0	0	0	-	-	0	0.0	0	0.0
5-14	0	0.0	0	0	-	-	0	0.0	0	0.0
15-44	6	3.5	83	45	31.4	34.7	0	0.2	0	0.2
45-59	0	0.7	63	95	52.4	19.4	1	1.1	1	0.9
60+	0	0.2	45	75	64.8	12.1	1	1.7	1	1.5
All ages	7	1.8	191	49	33.3	33.4	2	0.6	2	0.5
Females										
0-4	0	0.0	0	0	-	-	0	0.0	0	0.0
5-14	0	0.0	0	0	-	-	0	0.0	0	0.0
15-44	8	4.5	111	62	30.8	37.9	1	0.3	0	0.3
45-59	1	1.0	83	122	52.4	21.9	1	1.6	1	1.2
60+	0	0.0	77	91	-	-	2	2.0	2	1.8
All ages	9	2.2	271	66	32.5	36.6	3	0.8	3	0.7
Total	16	2.0	461	58	32.8	35.2	6	0.7	5	0.6

Table 170b FSE - PEAS - AESE — Multiple sclerosis - Cases

Age group (years)	Incidence 1990 Number ('000s)	Rate (per 100 000)	Prevalence 1990 Number ('000s)	Rate (per 100 000)	Avg. age at onset (years)	Average duration (years)	Deaths 1990 Number ('000s)	Rate (per 100 000)	Deaths 2000 (Projected) Number ('000s)	Rate (per 100 000)
Males										
0-4	0	0.0	0	0	-	-	0	0.0	0	0.0
5-14	0	0.0	0	0	-	-	0	0.0	0	0.0
15-44	3	3.5	34	45	31.3	31.2	0	0.5	0	0.4
45-59	0	0.7	26	95	52.2	17.0	0	1.6	0	1.4
60+	0	0.2	16	77	64.8	10.7	1	3.9	1	3.9
All ages	3	1.7	76	46	33.1	30.0	2	1.0	2	1.0
Females										
0-4	0	0.0	0	0	-	-	0	0.0	0	0.0
5-14	0	0.0	0	0	-	-	0	0.0	0	0.0
15-44	3	4.5	46	62	30.8	36.1	1	0.8	0	0.6
45-59	0	1.0	37	122	52.4	20.3	1	1.9	1	1.5
60+	0	0.0	34	93	-	-	2	4.3	2	4.3
All ages	4	2.1	117	65	32.6	34.8	3	1.5	3	1.5
Total	7	1.9	192	56	32.8	32.7	4	1.3	4	1.3

Table 170c India - India - Inde — Multiple sclerosis - Cases

Age group (years)	Incidence 1990 Number ('000s)	Rate (per 100 000)	Prevalence 1990 Number ('000s)	Rate (per 100 000)	Avg. age at onset (years)	Average duration (years)	Deaths 1990 Number ('000s)	Rate (per 100 000)	Deaths 2000 (Projected) Number ('000s)	Rate (per 100 000)
Males										
0-4	0	0.0	0	0	-	-	0	0.0	0	0.0
5-14	0	0.0	0	0	-	-	0	0.0	0	0.0
15-44	7	3.5	89	45	31.3	31.8	0	0.2	0	0.2
45-59	0	0.7	45	95	52.3	17.2	1	1.1	1	0.9
60+	0	0.2	23	77	64.7	10.2	1	1.8	1	1.4
All ages	7	1.7	157	36	32.5	31.0	1	0.3	1	0.3
Females										
0-4	0	0.0	25	0	-	-	0	0.0	0	0.0
5-14	0	0.0	90	0	-	-	0	0.0	0	0.0
15-44	8	4.5	142	61	30.6	33.2	0	0.3	0	0.2
45-59	0	1.0	56	122	52.4	18.0	1	1.4	1	1.0
60+	0	0.0	28	96	-	-	1	2.2	1	1.9
All ages	9	2.1	341	83	31.8	32.4	2	0.4	2	0.4
Total	16	1.9	498	59	32.1	31.7	3	0.4	3	0.3

For the methods used to estimate and project incidence, prevalence, and deaths see Murray and Lopez 1996a. See explanatory notes for definitions and caveats.

Table 170
Multiple sclerosis

Cuadro 170
Esclerosis múltiple

Tableau 170
Sclérose en plaques

Cases

Casos

Cas

Table 170d — China - China - Chine — Multiple sclerosis - Cases

Age group (years)	Incidence 1990 Number ('000s)	Rate (per 100 000)	Prevalence 1990 Number ('000s)	Rate (per 100 000)	Avg. age at onset (years)	Average duration (years)	Deaths 1990 Number ('000s)	Rate (per 100 000)	Deaths 2000 (Projected) Number ('000s)	Rate (per 100 000)
Males										
0-4	0	0.0	0	0	-	-	0	0.0	0	0.0
5-14	0	0.0	0	0	-	-	0	0.0	0	0.0
15-44	11	3.5	137	45	31.4	32.7	1	0.2	1	0.2
45-59	1	0.7	69	95	52.3	17.5	1	1.1	1	0.9
60+	0	0.2	38	77	64.7	10.4	1	1.7	1	1.4
All ages	11	1.9	244	42	32.6	31.8	2	0.4	2	0.3
Females										
0-4	0	0.0	0	0	-	-	0	0.0	0	0.0
5-14	0	0.0	0	0	-	-	0	0.0	0	0.0
15-44	13	4.5	175	62	30.7	34.7	1	0.3	1	0.2
45-59	1	1.0	79	122	52.4	18.9	1	1.6	1	1.2
60+	0	0.0	49	95	-	-	1	2.1	1	1.9
All ages	14	2.5	302	55	31.7	33.9	3	0.5	3	0.5
Total	25	2.2	546	48	32.1	33.0	5	0.5	5	0.4

Table 170e — OAI - OPAI - APAI — Multiple sclerosis - Cases

Age group (years)	Incidence 1990 Number ('000s)	Rate (per 100 000)	Prevalence 1990 Number ('000s)	Rate (per 100 000)	Avg. age at onset (years)	Average duration (years)	Deaths 1990 Number ('000s)	Rate (per 100 000)	Deaths 2000 (Projected) Number ('000s)	Rate (per 100 000)
Males										
0-4	0	0.0	0	0	-	-	0	0.0	0	0.0
5-14	0	0.0	0	0	-	-	0	0.0	0	0.0
15-44	6	3.5	71	44	31.2	31.0	0	0.2	0	0.1
45-59	0	0.7	32	95	52.3	16.7	0	1.0	0	0.8
60+	0	0.2	16	77	64.7	10.0	0	1.5	0	1.2
All ages	6	1.7	119	35	32.3	30.3	1	0.3	1	0.3
Females										
0-4	0	0.0	0	0	-	-	0	0.0	0	0.0
5-14	0	0.0	0	0	-	-	0	0.0	0	0.0
15-44	7	4.5	97	61	30.6	32.9	0	0.2	0	0.1
45-59	0	1.0	43	122	52.3	17.9	0	1.4	0	1.0
60+	0	0.0	22	95	-	-	0	1.9	1	1.6
All ages	8	2.2	162	48	31.6	32.2	1	0.4	1	0.3
Total	13	2.0	281	41	31.9	31.4	2	0.3	2	0.3

Table 170f — SSA - ASS - ASS — Multiple sclerosis - Cases

Age group (years)	Incidence 1990 Number ('000s)	Rate (per 100 000)	Prevalence 1990 Number ('000s)	Rate (per 100 000)	Avg. age at onset (years)	Average duration (years)	Deaths 1990 Number ('000s)	Rate (per 100 000)	Deaths 2000 (Projected) Number ('000s)	Rate (per 100 000)
Males										
0-4	0	0.0	0	0	-	-	0	0.0	0	0.0
5-14	0	0.0	0	0	-	-	0	0.0	0	0.0
15-44	4	3.5	45	43	30.9	28.5	0	0.2	0	0.1
45-59	0	0.7	19	95	52.2	15.8	0	1.1	0	0.9
60+	0	0.2	8	78	64.7	9.6	0	1.8	0	1.4
All ages	4	1.5	72	29	31.9	27.9	1	0.2	1	0.2
Females										
0-4	0	0.0	0	0	-	-	0	0.0	0	0.0
5-14	0	0.0	0	0	-	-	0	0.0	0	0.0
15-44	5	4.5	63	60	30.3	30.1	0	0.1	0	0.1
45-59	0	1.0	27	122	52.2	16.6	0	1.7	0	1.2
60+	0	0.0	12	96	-	-	0	2.3	0	1.8
All ages	5	2.0	103	40	31.3	29.5	1	0.3	1	0.2
Total	9	1.7	175	34	31.5	28.8	1	0.3	1	0.2

For the methods used to estimate and project incidence, prevalence, and deaths see Murray and Lopez 1996a. See explanatory notes for definitions and caveats.

Table 170
Multiple sclerosis

Cuadro 170
Esclerosis múltiple

Tableau 170
Sclérose en plaques

Cases   Casos   Cas

Table 170g   LAC - ALC - ALC   Multiple sclerosis - Cases

Age group (years)	Incidence 1990		Prevalence 1990		Avg. age at onset (years)	Average duration (years)	Deaths 1990		Deaths 2000 (Projected)	
	Number ('000s)	Rate (per 100 000)	Number ('000s)	Rate (per 100 000)			Number ('000s)	Rate (per 100 000)	Number ('000s)	Rate (per 100 000)
Males										
0-4	0	0.0	0	0	-	-	0	0.0	0	0.0
5-14	0	0.0	0	0	-	-	0	0.0	0	0.0
15-44	4	3.5	47	45	31.3	32.7	0	0.2	0	0.2
45-59	0	0.7	21	95	52.3	18.1	0	1.0	0	0.8
60+	0	0.2	11	76	64.8	11.0	0	1.6	0	1.4
All ages	4	1.7	78	35	32.4	31.9	1	0.3	1	0.3
Females										
0-4	0	0.0	0	0	-	-	0	0.0	0	0.0
5-14	0	0.0	0	0	-	-	0	0.0	0	0.0
15-44	5	4.5	64	61	30.7	34.8	0	0.2	0	0.2
45-59	0	1.0	29	122	52.4	19.5	0	1.5	0	1.2
60+	0	0.0	16	94	-	-	0	2.0	0	1.7
All ages	5	2.2	108	49	31.7	34.1	1	0.4	1	0.4
Total	9	2.0	187	42	32.0	33.1	2	0.4	2	0.3

Table 170h   MEC - AOM - CMO   Multiple sclerosis - Cases

Age group (years)	Incidence 1990		Prevalence 1990		Avg. age at onset (years)	Average duration (years)	Deaths 1990		Deaths 2000 (Projected)	
	Number ('000s)	Rate (per 100 000)	Number ('000s)	Rate (per 100 000)			Number ('000s)	Rate (per 100 000)	Number ('000s)	Rate (per 100 000)
Males										
0-4	0	0.0	0	0	-	-	0	0.0	0	0.0
5-14	0	0.0	0	0	-	-	0	0.0	0	0.0
15-44	4	3.5	51	45	31.3	31.8	0	0.2	0	0.1
45-59	0	0.7	21	95	52.3	17.0	0	1.0	0	0.8
60+	0	0.2	11	77	64.7	10.2	0	1.5	0	1.2
All ages	4	1.6	83	32	32.3	31.1	1	0.2	1	0.2
Females										
0-4	0	0.0	0	0	-	-	0	0.0	0	0.0
5-14	0	0.0	0	0	-	-	0	0.0	0	0.0
15-44	5	4.5	66	61	30.7	33.7	0	0.2	0	0.1
45-59	0	1.0	27	122	52.3	18.3	0	1.4	0	1.1
60+	0	0.0	15	95	-	-	0	1.9	0	1.5
All ages	5	2.1	108	44	31.7	33.0	1	0.3	1	0.3
Total	9	1.8	190	38	31.9	32.2	1	0.3	2	0.2

Table 170i   World - Mundo - Monde   Multiple sclerosis - Cases

Age group (years)	Incidence 1990		Prevalence 1990		Avg. age at onset (years)	Average duration (years)	Deaths 1990		Deaths 2000 (Projected)	
	Number ('000s)	Rate (per 100 000)	Number ('000s)	Rate (per 100 000)			Number ('000s)	Rate (per 100 000)	Number ('000s)	Rate (per 100 000)
Males										
0-4	0	0.0	0	0.0	-	-	0	0.0	0	0.0
5-14	0	0.0	0	0.0	-	-	0	0.0	0	0.0
15-44	44	3.5	557	44.6	31.3	32.1	3	0.2	3	0.2
45-59	2	0.7	296	94.7	52.3	17.6	4	1.1	4	0.9
60+	0	0.2	168	76.5	64.7	10.8	4	1.9	4	1.6
All ages	46	1.7	1 020	38.4	32.6	31.2	10	0.4	11	0.3
Females										
0-4	0	0.0	25	8.2	-	-	0	0.0	0	0.0
5-14	0	0.0	90	17.2	-	-	0	0.0	0	0.0
15-44	54	4.5	764	63.7	30.7	34.3	3	0.3	3	0.2
45-59	3	1.0	380	122.3	52.4	19.3	5	1.5	5	1.2
60+	0	0.0	252	93.5	-	-	6	2.4	7	2.1
All ages	58	2.2	1 511	57.8	31.8	33.5	15	0.6	15	0.5
Total	104	2.0	2 532	48.1	32.2	32.5	25	0.5	25	0.4

For the methods used to estimate and project incidence, prevalence, and deaths see Murray and Lopez 1996a. See explanatory notes for definitions and caveats.

Table 171
Drug use
Dysfunctional and harmful
drug use

Cuadro 171
Uso de drogas
Uso disfuncional y dañino
de drogas

Tableau 171
Usage de drogues
Usage disfonctionnel et nocif
de drogues

Table 171a EME - PEMC - EMBE — Drug use - Dysfunctional and harmful drug use

Age group (years)	Incidence 1990 Number ('000s)	Rate (per 100 000)	Prevalence 1990 Number ('000s)	Rate (per 100 000)	Avg. age at onset (years)	Average duration (years)	Deaths 1990 Number ('000s)	Rate (per 100 000)	Deaths 2000 (Projected) Number ('000s)	Rate (per 100 000)
Males										
0-4	-	-	3	11.4	-	-	0	0.0	0	0.0
5-14	-	-	297	556.7	-	-	0	0.0	0	0.0
15-44	-	-	2 550	1 385.4	-	-	3	1.6	2	1.4
45-59	-	-	120	181.4	-	-	0	0.1	0	0.1
60+	-	-	30	49.5	-	-	0	0.1	0	0.1
All ages	-	-	3 000	768.3	-	-	3	0.8	3	0.6
Females										
0-4	-	-	1	4.0	-	-	0	0.0	0	0.0
5-14	-	-	99	195.3	-	-	0	0.0	0	0.0
15-44	-	-	850	474.3	-	-	1	0.3	0	0.3
45-59	-	-	40	59.0	-	-	0	0.1	0	0.0
60+	-	-	10	11.8	-	-	0	0.1	0	0.0
All ages	-	-	1 000	245.5	-	-	1	0.2	1	0.1
Total	-	-	4 000	501.4	-	-	4	0.5	3	0.4

Table 171b FSE - PEAS - AESE — Drug use - Dysfunctional and harmful drug use

Age group (years)	Incidence 1990 Number ('000s)	Rate (per 100 000)	Prevalence 1990 Number ('000s)	Rate (per 100 000)	Avg. age at onset (years)	Average duration (years)	Deaths 1990 Number ('000s)	Rate (per 100 000)	Deaths 2000 (Projected) Number ('000s)	Rate (per 100 000)
Males										
0-4	-	-	1	8.7	-	-	0	0	0	0
5-14	-	-	119	434.4	-	-	0	0	0	0
15-44	-	-	1 020	1 337.2	-	-	0	0	0	0
45-59	-	-	48	178.0	-	-	0	0	0	0
60+	-	-	12	57.2	-	-	0	0	0	0
All ages	-	-	1 200	725.9	-	-	0	0	0	0
Females										
0-4	-	-	0	2.3	-	-	0	0	0	0
5-14	-	-	30	112.4	-	-	0	0	0	0
15-44	-	-	255	340.2	-	-	0	0	0	0
45-59	-	-	12	40.0	-	-	0	0	0	0
60+	-	-	3	8.2	-	-	0	0	0	0
All ages	-	-	300	165.8	-	-	0	0	0	0
Total	-	-	1 500	433.2	-	-	0	0	0	0

Table 171c India - India - Inde — Drug use - Dysfunctional and harmful drug use

Age group (years)	Incidence 1990 Number ('000s)	Rate (per 100 000)	Prevalence 1990 Number ('000s)	Rate (per 100 000)	Avg. age at onset (years)	Average duration (years)	Deaths 1990 Number ('000s)	Rate (per 100 000)	Deaths 2000 (Projected) Number ('000s)	Rate (per 100 000)
Males										
0-4	-	-	0	0.3	-	-	0	0.0	0	0.0
5-14	-	-	18	17.5	-	-	0	0.0	0	0.0
15-44	-	-	153	76.3	-	-	0	0.1	0	0.1
45-59	-	-	7	15.1	-	-	0	0.0	0	0.0
60+	-	-	2	6.0	-	-	0	0.0	0	0.0
All ages	-	-	180	41.0	-	-	0	0.0	0	0.0
Females										
0-4	-	-	0	0.0	-	-	0	0.0	0	0.0
5-14	-	-	2	2.1	-	-	0	0.0	0	0.0
15-44	-	-	17	9.3	-	-	0	0.0	0	0.0
45-59	-	-	1	1.7	-	-	0	0.0	0	0.0
60+	-	-	0	0.7	-	-	0	0.0	0	0.0
All ages	-	-	20	4.9	-	-	0	0.0	0	0.0
Total	-	-	200	23.5	-	-	0	0.0	0	0.0

For epidemiological sources see Donoghoe et al. 1996. For the methods used to estimate and project incidence, prevalence, and deaths see Murray and Lopez 1996a. See explanatory notes for definitions and caveats.

Table 171
Drug use
Dysfunctional and harmful drug use

Cuadro 171
Uso de drogas
Uso disfuncional y dañino de drogas

Tableau 171
Usage de drogues
Usage disfonctionnel et nocif de drogues

Table 171d **China - China - Chine** Drug use - Dysfunctional and harmful drug use

Age group (years)	Incidence 1990 Number ('000s)	Rate (per 100 000)	Prevalence 1990 Number ('000s)	Rate (per 100 000)	Avg. age at onset (years)	Average duration (years)	Deaths 1990 Number ('000s)	Rate (per 100 000)	Deaths 2000 (Projected) Number ('000s)	Rate (per 100 000)
Males										
0-4	-	-	0	0.7	-	-	0	0.0	0	0.0
5-14	-	-	45	46.0	-	-	0	0.0	0	0.0
15-44	-	-	383	125.1	-	-	0	0.1	0	0.1
45-59	-	-	18	24.8	-	-	0	0.0	0	0.0
60+	-	-	5	9.2	-	-	0	0.0	0	0.0
All ages	-	-	450	77.1	-	-	0	0.1	0	0.0
Females										
0-4	-	-	0	0.1	-	-	0	0.0	0	0.0
5-14	-	-	5	5.5	-	-	0	0.0	0	0.0
15-44	-	-	43	15.0	-	-	0	0.0	0	0.0
45-59	-	-	2	3.1	-	-	0	0.0	0	0.0
60+	-	-	1	1.0	-	-	0	0.0	0	0.0
All ages	-	-	50	9.1	-	-	0	0.0	0	0.0
Total	-	-	500	44.2	-	-	0	0.0	0	0.0

Table 171e **OAI - OPAI - APAI** Drug use - Dysfunctional and harmful drug use

Age group (years)	Incidence 1990 Number ('000s)	Rate (per 100 000)	Prevalence 1990 Number ('000s)	Rate (per 100 000)	Avg. age at onset (years)	Average duration (years)	Deaths 1990 Number ('000s)	Rate (per 100 000)	Deaths 2000 (Projected) Number ('000s)	Rate (per 100 000)
Males										
0-4	-	-	2	5.1	-	-	0	0.0	0	0.0
5-14	-	-	223	265.1	-	-	0	0.0	0	0.0
15-44	-	-	1 913	1 189.2	-	-	1	0.9	1	0.7
45-59	-	-	90	263.6	-	-	0	0.2	0	0.2
60+	-	-	23	111.3	-	-	0	0.2	0	0.2
All ages	-	-	2 250	656.0	-	-	2	0.4	2	0.4
Females										
0-4	-	-	0	0.6	-	-	0	0.0	0	0.0
5-14	-	-	25	30.9	-	-	0	0.0	0	0.0
15-44	-	-	213	133.1	-	-	0	0.1	0	0.1
45-59	-	-	10	28.5	-	-	0	0.0	0	0.0
60+	-	-	3	11.0	-	-	0	0.0	0	0.0
All ages	-	-	250	73.6	-	-	0	0.0	0	0.0
Total	-	-	2 500	366.3	-	-	2	0.2	2	0.2

Table 171f **SSA - ASS - ASS** Drug use - Dysfunctional and harmful drug use

Age group (years)	Incidence 1990 Number ('000s)	Rate (per 100 000)	Prevalence 1990 Number ('000s)	Rate (per 100 000)	Avg. age at onset (years)	Average duration (years)	Deaths 1990 Number ('000s)	Rate (per 100 000)	Deaths 2000 (Projected) Number ('000s)	Rate (per 100 000)
Males										
0-4	-	-	1	1.9	-	-	0	0.0	0	0.0
5-14	-	-	89	126.8	-	-	0	0.0	0	0.0
15-44	-	-	765	737.2	-	-	1	0.6	1	0.4
45-59	-	-	36	177.3	-	-	0	0.1	0	0.1
60+	-	-	9	85.6	-	-	0	0.2	0	0.2
All ages	-	-	900	356.7	-	-	1	0.3	1	0.2
Females										
0-4	-	-	0	0.2	-	-	0	0.0	0	0.0
5-14	-	-	10	14.2	-	-	0	0.0	0	0.0
15-44	-	-	85	80.0	-	-	0	0.0	0	0.0
45-59	-	-	4	18.1	-	-	0	0.0	0	0.0
60+	-	-	1	7.9	-	-	0	0.0	0	0.0
All ages	-	-	100	38.8	-	-	0	0.0	0	0.0
Total	-	-	1 000	196.0	-	-	1	0.1	1	0.1

For epidemiological sources see Donoghoe et al. 1996. For the methods used to estimate and project incidence, prevalence, and deaths see Murray and Lopez 1996a. See explanatory notes for definitions and caveats.

Table 171 | **Cuadro 171** | **Tableau 171**

Drug use | **Uso de drogas** | **Usage de drogues**

Dysfunctional and harmful drug use | Uso disfuncional y dañino de drogas | Usage disfonctionnel et nocif de drogues

Table 171g LAC - ALC - ALC — Drug use - Dysfunctional and harmful drug use

Age group (years)	Incidence 1990 Number ('000s)	Rate (per 100 000)	Prevalence 1990 Number ('000s)	Rate (per 100 000)	Avg. age at onset (years)	Average duration (years)	Deaths 1990 Number ('000s)	Rate (per 100 000)	Deaths 2000 (Projected) Number ('000s)	Rate (per 100 000)
Males										
0-4	-	-	2	6.8	-	-	0	0.0	0	0.0
5-14	-	-	193	370.4	-	-	0	0.0	0	0.0
15-44	-	-	1 658	1 589.4	-	-	1	1.1	1	0.9
45-59	-	-	78	350.6	-	-	0	0.3	0	0.2
60+	-	-	20	137.0	-	-	0	0.3	0	0.3
All ages	-	-	1 950	879.9	-	-	1	0.6	1	0.5
Females										
0-4	-	-	1	3.8	-	-	0	0.0	0	0.0
5-14	-	-	104	204.9	-	-	0	0.0	0	0.0
15-44	-	-	893	857.5	-	-	1	0.6	1	0.4
45-59	-	-	42	179.8	-	-	0	0.1	0	0.1
60+	-	-	11	62.4	-	-	0	0.2	0	0.1
All ages	-	-	1 050	471.5	-	-	1	0.3	1	0.2
Total	-	-	3 000	675.2	-	-	2	0.4	2	0.4

Table 171h MEC - AOM - CMO — Drug use - Dysfunctional and harmful drug use

Age group (years)	Incidence 1990 Number ('000s)	Rate (per 100 000)	Prevalence 1990 Number ('000s)	Rate (per 100 000)	Avg. age at onset (years)	Average duration (years)	Deaths 1990 Number ('000s)	Rate (per 100 000)	Deaths 2000 (Projected) Number ('000s)	Rate (per 100 000)
Males										
0-4	-	-	2	5.5	-	-	0	0.0	0	0.0
5-14	-	-	223	340.9	-	-	0	0.0	0	0.0
15-44	-	-	1 913	1 679.2	-	-	1	1.3	1	1.0
45-59	-	-	90	402.9	-	-	0	0.3	0	0.2
60+	-	-	23	164.8	-	-	0	0.4	0	0.3
All ages	-	-	2 250	877.6	-	-	2	0.6	2	0.5
Females										
0-4	-	-	0	0.6	-	-	0	0.0	0	0.0
5-14	-	-	25	39.9	-	-	0	0.0	0	0.0
15-44	-	-	213	198.2	-	-	0	0.1	0	0.1
45-59	-	-	10	44.9	-	-	0	0.0	0	0.0
60+	-	-	3	16.2	-	-	0	0.0	0	0.0
All ages	-	-	250	101.3	-	-	0	0.1	0	0.0
Total	-	-	2 500	496.9	-	-	2	0.3	2	0.3

Table 171i World - Mundo - Monde — Drug use - Dysfunctional and harmful drug use

Age group (years)	Incidence 1990 Number ('000s)	Rate (per 100 000)	Prevalence 1990 Number ('000s)	Rate (per 100 000)	Avg. age at onset (years)	Average duration (years)	Deaths 1990 Number ('000s)	Rate (per 100 000)	Deaths 2000 (Projected) Number ('000s)	Rate (per 100 000)
Males										
0-4	-	-	12	3.8	-	-	0	0.0	0	0.0
5-14	-	-	1 206	218.8	-	-	0	0.0	0	0.0
15-44	-	-	10 354	828.4	-	-	8	0.6	7	0.5
45-59	-	-	487	156.0	-	-	0	0.1	0	0.1
60+	-	-	122	55.7	-	-	0	0.1	0	0.1
All ages	-	-	12 181	459.0	-	-	9	0.3	8	0.3
Females										
0-4	-	-	3	1.0	-	-	0	0.0	0	0.0
5-14	-	-	299	56.9	-	-	0	0.0	0	0.0
15-44	-	-	2 567	214.2	-	-	2	0.1	1	0.1
45-59	-	-	121	38.8	-	-	0	0.0	0	0.0
60+	-	-	30	11.2	-	-	0	0.0	0	0.0
All ages	-	-	3 020	115.6	-	-	2	0.1	2	0.1
Total	-	-	15 201	288.6	-	-	11	0.2	10	0.2

For epidemiological sources see Donoghoe et al. 1996. For the methods used to estimate and project incidence, prevalence, and deaths see Murray and Lopez 1996a. See explanatory notes for definitions and caveats.

Table 172	Cuadro 172	Tableau 172
Post-traumatic stress disorder	**Trastorno de estrés post-traumático**	**Troubles anxieux post-traumatiques**
Cases	Casos	Cas

Table 172a   EME - PEMC - EMBE   Post-traumatic stress disorder - Cases

Age group (years)	Incidence 1990 Number ('000s)	Rate (per 100 000)	Prevalence 1990 Number ('000s)	Rate (per 100 000)	Avg. age at onset (years)	Average duration (years)	Deaths 1990 Number ('000s)	Rate (per 100 000)	Deaths 2000 (Projected) Number ('000s)	Rate (per 100 000)
Males										
0-4	26	100	38	144	2.5	2.5	0	0	0	0
5-14	53	100	129	242	10.0	2.5	0	0	0	0
15-44	184	100	459	249	29.9	2.5	0	0	0	0
45-59	33	50	96	146	52.4	2.5	0	0	0	0
60+	12	20	42	69	71.1	2.5	0	0	0	0
All ages	308	79	764	196	28.2	2.5	0	0	0	0
Females										
0-4	43	170	61	245	2.5	2.5	0	0	0	0
5-14	86	169	208	411	10.0	2.5	0	0	0	0
15-44	303	169	758	423	30.0	2.5	0	0	0	0
45-59	54	80	159	234	52.4	2.5	0	0	0	0
60+	25	30	83	98	72.4	2.5	0	0	0	0
All ages	511	125	1 270	312	28.8	2.5	0	0	0	0
Total	819	103	2 034	255	28.6	2.5	0	0	0	0

Table 172b   FSE - PEAS - AESE   Post-traumatic stress disorder - Cases

Age group (years)	Incidence 1990 Number ('000s)	Rate (per 100 000)	Prevalence 1990 Number ('000s)	Rate (per 100 000)	Avg. age at onset (years)	Average duration (years)	Deaths 1990 Number ('000s)	Rate (per 100 000)	Deaths 2000 (Projected) Number ('000s)	Rate (per 100 000)
Males										
0-4	14	100	20	144	2.5	2.5	0	0	0	0
5-14	27	100	66	242	10.0	2.5	0	0	0	0
15-44	76	100	192	252	29.8	2.5	0	0	0	0
45-59	13	50	41	150	52.2	2.5	0	0	0	0
60+	4	20	15	72	70.0	2.5	0	0	0	0
All ages	135	82	334	202	26.5	2.5	0	0	0	0
Females										
0-4	22	170	32	245	2.5	2.5	0	0	0	0
5-14	45	169	109	412	10.0	2.5	0	0	0	0
15-44	127	169	319	426	29.9	2.5	0	0	0	0
45-59	24	80	71	236	52.4	2.5	0	0	0	0
60+	11	30	37	102	71.5	2.5	0	0	0	0
All ages	229	126	568	314	27.7	2.5	0	0	0	0
Total	364	105	903	261	27.2	2.5	0	0	0	0

Table 172c   India - India - Inde   Post-traumatic stress disorder - Cases

Age group (years)	Incidence 1990 Number ('000s)	Rate (per 100 000)	Prevalence 1990 Number ('000s)	Rate (per 100 000)	Avg. age at onset (years)	Average duration (years)	Deaths 1990 Number ('000s)	Rate (per 100 000)	Deaths 2000 (Projected) Number ('000s)	Rate (per 100 000)
Males										
0-4	60	100	87	146	2.5	2.5	0	0	0	0
5-14	102	100	248	244	10.0	2.5	0	0	0	0
15-44	200	100	506	252	29.8	2.5	0	0	0	0
45-59	24	50	70	148	52.3	2.5	0	0	0	0
60+	6	20	22	73	69.7	2.5	0	0	0	0
All ages	391	89	933	212	22.5	2.5	0	0	0	0
Females										
0-4	96	170	141	249	2.5	2.5	0	0	0	0
5-14	161	169	396	416	10.0	2.5	0	0	0	0
15-44	310	169	781	426	29.8	2.5	0	0	0	0
45-59	37	80	110	238	52.4	2.5	0	0	0	0
60+	9	30	32	109	70.1	2.5	0	0	0	0
All ages	613	149	1 459	356	22.2	2.5	0	0	0	0
Total	1 004	118	2 393	282	22.3	2.5	0	0	0	0

For epidemiological sources see de L'Horne et al. 1996. For the methods used to estimate and project incidence, prevalence, and deaths see Murray and Lopez 1996a. See explanatory notes for definitions and caveats.

Table 172 Post-traumatic stress disorder Cases	Cuadro 172 Trastorno de estrés post-traumático Casos	Tableau 172 Troubles anxieux post-traumatiques Cas

Table 172d China - China - Chine — Post-traumatic stress disorder - Cases

Age group (years)	Incidence 1990 Number ('000s)	Rate (per 100 000)	Prevalence 1990 Number ('000s)	Rate (per 100 000)	Avg. age at onset (years)	Average duration (years)	Deaths 1990 Number ('000s)	Rate (per 100 000)	Deaths 2000 (Projected) Number ('000s)	Rate (per 100 000)
Males										
0-4	60	100	87	145	2.5	2.5	0	0	0	0
5-14	97	100	235	243	10.0	2.5	0	0	0	0
15-44	306	100	769	251	29.9	2.5	0	0	0	0
45-59	36	50	107	147	52.3	2.5	0	0	0	0
60+	10	20	36	73	69.8	2.5	0	0	0	0
All ages	509	87	1 234	211	25.2	2.5	0	0	0	0
Females										
0-4	98	170	142	245	2.5	2.5	0	0	0	0
5-14	153	169	373	412	10.0	2.5	0	0	0	0
15-44	481	169	1 211	426	29.9	2.5	0	0	0	0
45-59	51	80	153	237	52.4	2.5	0	0	0	0
60+	15	30	55	106	70.6	2.5	0	0	0	0
All ages	799	146	1 933	352	25.0	2.5	0	0	0	0
Total	1 308	115	3 167	279	25.1	2.5	0	0	0	0

Table 172e OAI - OPAI - APAI — Post-traumatic stress disorder - Cases

Age group (years)	Incidence 1990 Number ('000s)	Rate (per 100 000)	Prevalence 1990 Number ('000s)	Rate (per 100 000)	Avg. age at onset (years)	Average duration (years)	Deaths 1990 Number ('000s)	Rate (per 100 000)	Deaths 2000 (Projected) Number ('000s)	Rate (per 100 000)
Males										
0-4	44	100	64	146	2.5	2.5	0	0	0	0
5-14	84	100	205	244	10.0	2.5	0	0	0	0
15-44	160	100	404	251	29.7	2.5	0	0	0	0
45-59	17	50	51	148	52.3	2.5	0	0	0	0
60+	4	20	15	73	69.6	2.5	0	0	0	0
All ages	309	90	738	215	22.3	2.5	0	0	0	0
Females										
0-4	71	170	103	246	2.5	2.5	0	0	0	0
5-14	136	169	332	413	10.0	2.5	0	0	0	0
15-44	270	169	680	426	29.8	2.5	0	0	0	0
45-59	28	80	84	239	52.3	2.5	0	0	0	0
60+	7	30	24	108	70.3	2.5	0	0	0	0
All ages	512	151	1 223	360	22.5	2.5	0	0	0	0
Total	821	120	1 961	287	22.4	2.5	0	0	0	0

Table 172f SSA - ASS - ASS — Post-traumatic stress disorder - Cases

Age group (years)	Incidence 1990 Number ('000s)	Rate (per 100 000)	Prevalence 1990 Number ('000s)	Rate (per 100 000)	Avg. age at onset (years)	Average duration (years)	Deaths 1990 Number ('000s)	Rate (per 100 000)	Deaths 2000 (Projected) Number ('000s)	Rate (per 100 000)
Males										
0-4	47	100	70	148	2.4	2.5	0	0	0	0
5-14	70	100	175	249	10.0	2.5	0	0	0	0
15-44	104	100	265	255	29.4	2.5	0	0	0	0
45-59	10	50	31	152	52.2	2.5	0	0	0	0
60+	2	20	8	76	69.2	2.5	0	0	0	0
All ages	233	92	549	217	19.4	2.5	0	0	0	0
Females										
0-4	80	170	118	250	2.4	2.5	0	0	0	0
5-14	118	169	294	421	10.0	2.5	0	0	0	0
15-44	180	169	457	430	29.5	2.5	0	0	0	0
45-59	18	80	54	243	52.2	2.5	0	0	0	0
60+	4	30	14	112	69.7	2.5	0	0	0	0
All ages	399	155	937	363	19.7	2.5	0	0	0	0
Total	633	124	1 486	291	19.6	2.5	0	0	0	0

For epidemiological sources see de L'Horne et al. 1996. For the methods used to estimate and project incidence, prevalence, and deaths see Murray and Lopez 1996a. See explanatory notes for definitions and caveats.

Table 172
Post-traumatic stress disorder
Cases

Cuadro 172
Trastorno de estrés post-traumático
Casos

Tableau 172
Troubles anxieux post-traumatiques
Cas

Table 172g   LAC - ALC - ALC   Post-traumatic stress disorder - Cases

Age group (years)	Incidence 1990 Number ('000s)	Rate (per 100 000)	Prevalence 1990 Number ('000s)	Rate (per 100 000)	Avg. age at onset (years)	Average duration (years)	Deaths 1990 Number ('000s)	Rate (per 100 000)	Deaths 2000 (Projected) Number ('000s)	Rate (per 100 000)
Males										
0-4	29	100	42	145	2.5	2.5	0	0	0	0
5-14	52	100	127	244	10.0	2.5	0	0	0	0
15-44	104	100	263	252	29.8	2.5	0	0	0	0
45-59	11	50	33	147	52.3	2.5	0	0	0	0
60+	3	20	10	71	70.3	2.5	0	0	0	0
All ages	199	90	475	214	22.5	2.5	0	0	0	0
Females										
0-4	47	170	68	246	2.5	2.5	0	0	0	0
5-14	86	169	210	413	10.0	2.5	0	0	0	0
15-44	176	169	445	427	29.9	2.5	0	0	0	0
45-59	19	80	56	238	52.4	2.5	0	0	0	0
60+	5	30	18	104	71.1	2.5	0	0	0	0
All ages	333	149	795	357	22.8	2.5	0	0	0	0
Total	531	120	1 270	286	22.7	2.5	0	0	0	0

Table 172h   MEC - AOM - CMO   Post-traumatic stress disorder - Cases

Age group (years)	Incidence 1990 Number ('000s)	Rate (per 100 000)	Prevalence 1990 Number ('000s)	Rate (per 100 000)	Avg. age at onset (years)	Average duration (years)	Deaths 1990 Number ('000s)	Rate (per 100 000)	Deaths 2000 (Projected) Number ('000s)	Rate (per 100 000)
Males										
0-4	41	100	60	146	2.5	2.5	0	0	0	0
5-14	65	100	160	245	10.0	2.5	0	0	0	0
15-44	114	100	287	252	29.8	2.5	0	0	0	0
45-59	11	50	33	148	52.3	2.5	0	0	0	0
60+	3	20	10	73	69.7	2.5	0	0	0	0
All ages	234	91	550	214	21.0	2.5	0	0	0	0
Females										
0-4	67	170	97	245	2.5	2.5	0	0	0	0
5-14	105	169	257	415	10.0	2.5	0	0	0	0
15-44	181	169	458	427	29.8	2.5	0	0	0	0
45-59	18	80	53	238	52.4	2.5	0	0	0	0
60+	5	30	17	108	70.4	2.5	0	0	0	0
All ages	376	153	882	357	21.0	2.5	0	0	0	0
Total	610	121	1 432	285	21.0	2.5	0	0	0	0

Table 172i   World - Mundo - Monde   Post-traumatic stress disorder - Cases

Age group (years)	Incidence 1990 Number ('000s)	Rate (per 100 000)	Prevalence 1990 Number ('000s)	Rate (per 100 000)	Avg. age at onset (years)	Average duration (years)	Deaths 1990 Number ('000s)	Rate (per 100 000)	Deaths 2000 (Projected) Number ('000s)	Rate (per 100 000)
Males										
0-4	321	100	468	146	2.5	2.5	0	0	0	0
5-14	550	100	1 346	244	10.0	2.5	0	0	0	0
15-44	1 247	100	3 145	252	29.8	2.5	0	0	0	0
45-59	156	50	461	148	52.3	2.5	0	0	0	0
60+	44	20	157	72	70.1	2.5	0	0	0	0
All ages	2 317	87	5 577	210	23.6	2.5	0	0	0	0
Females										
0-4	525	170	763	247	2.5	2.5	0	0	0	0
5-14	890	169	2 178	414	10.0	2.5	0	0	0	0
15-44	2 029	169	5 109	426	29.8	2.5	0	0	0	0
45-59	248	80	738	237	52.4	2.5	0	0	0	0
60+	81	30	280	104	71.2	2.5	0	0	0	0
All ages	3 772	144	9 067	347	23.7	2.5	0	0	0	0
Total	6 090	116	14 644	278	23.7	2.5	0	0	0	0

For epidemiological sources see de L'Horne et al. 1996. For the methods used to estimate and project incidence, prevalence, and deaths see Murray and Lopez 1996a. See explanatory notes for definitions and caveats.

Table 173	Cuadro 173	Tableau 173
Obsessive-compulsive disorders	Trastornos obsesivo-compulsivos	Troubles obsessionnels et compulsifs
Cases	Casos	Cas

Table 173a   EME - PEMC - EMBE   Obsessive-compulsive disorders - Cases

Age group (years)	Incidence 1990 Number ('000s)	Rate (per 100 000)	Prevalence 1990 Number ('000s)	Rate (per 100 000)	Avg. age at onset (years)	Average duration (years)	Deaths 1990 Number ('000s)	Rate (per 100 000)	Deaths 2000 (Projected) Number ('000s)	Rate (per 100 000)
Males										
0-4	0	0	0	0	-	-	0	0	0	0
5-14	239	447	323	606	10.0	1.6	0	0	0	0
15-44	1 777	965	2 763	1 501	29.9	1.6	0	0	0	0
45-59	204	308	400	604	52.4	1.6	0	0	0	0
60+	193	318	363	600	71.1	1.6	0	0	0	0
All ages	2 412	618	3 850	986	33.1	1.6	0	0	0	0
Females										
0-4	0	0	0	0	-	-	0	0	0	0
5-14	302	595	409	807	10.0	1.6	0	0	0	0
15-44	2 301	1 284	3 579	1 997	30.0	1.6	0	0	0	0
45-59	369	545	674	994	52.4	1.6	0	0	0	0
60+	361	427	589	696	72.4	1.6	0	0	0	0
All ages	3 333	818	5 251	1 289	35.3	1.6	0	0	0	0
Total	5 745	720	9 101	1 141	34.4	1.6	0	0	0	0

Table 173b   FSE - PEAS - AESE   Obsessive-compulsive disorders - Cases

Age group (years)	Incidence 1990 Number ('000s)	Rate (per 100 000)	Prevalence 1990 Number ('000s)	Rate (per 100 000)	Avg. age at onset (years)	Average duration (years)	Deaths 1990 Number ('000s)	Rate (per 100 000)	Deaths 2000 (Projected) Number ('000s)	Rate (per 100 000)
Males										
0-4	0	0	0	0	-	-	0	0	0	0
5-14	122	447	166	606	10.0	1.6	0	0	0	0
15-44	736	965	1 145	1 501	29.8	1.6	0	0	0	0
45-59	83	308	164	609	52.2	1.6	0	0	0	0
60+	67	318	125	598	70.0	1.6	0	0	0	0
All ages	1 009	610	1 600	968	31.9	1.6	0	0	0	0
Females										
0-4	0	0	0	0	-	-	0	0	0	0
5-14	157	595	213	807	10.0	1.6	0	0	0	0
15-44	962	1 284	1 497	1 997	29.9	1.6	0	0	0	0
45-59	163	545	299	996	52.4	1.6	0	0	0	0
60+	156	427	254	698	71.5	1.6	0	0	0	0
All ages	1 439	795	2 263	1 251	34.8	1.6	0	0	0	0
Total	2 447	707	3 863	1 116	33.6	1.6	0	0	0	0

Table 173c   India - India - Inde   Obsessive-compulsive disorders - Cases

Age group (years)	Incidence 1990 Number ('000s)	Rate (per 100 000)	Prevalence 1990 Number ('000s)	Rate (per 100 000)	Avg. age at onset (years)	Average duration (years)	Deaths 1990 Number ('000s)	Rate (per 100 000)	Deaths 2000 (Projected) Number ('000s)	Rate (per 100 000)
Males										
0-4	0	0	0	0	-	-	0	0	0	0
5-14	455	447	616	605	10.0	1.6	0	0	0	0
15-44	1 936	965	3 009	1 500	29.8	1.6	0	0	0	0
45-59	147	308	289	607	52.3	1.6	0	0	0	0
60+	95	318	178	598	69.7	1.6	0	0	0	0
All ages	2 632	599	4 092	931	29.1	1.6	0	0	0	0
Females										
0-4	0	0	0	0	-	-	0	0	0	0
5-14	567	595	767	805	10.0	1.6	0	0	0	0
15-44	2 353	1 284	3 657	1 996	29.8	1.6	0	0	0	0
45-59	251	545	459	997	52.4	1.6	0	0	0	0
60+	124	427	203	700	70.1	1.6	0	0	0	0
All ages	3 294	803	5 086	1 240	29.6	1.6	0	0	0	0
Total	5 926	698	9 177	1 080	29.4	1.6	0	0	0	0

For epidemiological sources see Andrews 1996. For the methods used to estimate and project incidence, prevalence, and deaths see Murray and Lopez 1996a. See explanatory notes for definitions and caveats.

Table 173	Cuadro 173	Tableau 173
Obsessive-compulsive disorders	**Trastornos obsesivo-compulsivos**	**Troubles obsessionnels et compulsifs**
Cases	Casos	Cas

Table 173d   China - China - Chine   Obsessive-compulsive disorders - Cases

Age group (years)	Incidence 1990 Number ('000s)	Rate (per 100 000)	Prevalence 1990 Number ('000s)	Rate (per 100 000)	Avg. age at onset (years)	Average duration (years)	Deaths 1990 Number ('000s)	Rate (per 100 000)	Deaths 2000 (Projected) Number ('000s)	Rate (per 100 000)
Males										
0-4	0	0	0	0	-	-	0	0	0	0
5-14	434	447	588	606	10.0	1.6	0	0	0	0
15-44	2 957	965	4 598	1 501	29.9	1.6	0	0	0	0
45-59	224	308	440	606	52.3	1.6	0	0	0	0
60+	156	318	293	598	69.8	1.6	0	0	0	0
All ages	3 771	644	5 919	1 011	30.6	1.6	0	0	0	0
Females										
0-4	0	0	0	0	-	-	0	0	0	0
5-14	538	595	729	806	10.0	1.6	0	0	0	0
15-44	3 647	1 284	5 673	1 997	29.9	1.6	0	0	0	0
45-59	351	545	641	996	52.4	1.6	0	0	0	0
60+	221	427	361	699	70.6	1.6	0	0	0	0
All ages	4 757	867	7 405	1 350	31.2	1.6	0	0	0	0
Total	8 527	752	13 324	1 175	30.9	1.6	0	0	0	0

Table 173e   OAI - OPAI - APAI   Obsessive-compulsive disorders - Cases

Age group (years)	Incidence 1990 Number ('000s)	Rate (per 100 000)	Prevalence 1990 Number ('000s)	Rate (per 100 000)	Avg. age at onset (years)	Average duration (years)	Deaths 1990 Number ('000s)	Rate (per 100 000)	Deaths 2000 (Projected) Number ('000s)	Rate (per 100 000)
Males										
0-4	0	0	0	0	-	-	0	0	0	0
5-14	376	447	509	606	10.0	1.6	0	0	0	0
15-44	1 553	965	2 413	1 500	29.7	1.6	0	0	0	0
45-59	105	308	208	608	52.3	1.6	0	0	0	0
60+	64	318	121	598	69.6	1.6	0	0	0	0
All ages	2 098	612	3 250	948	28.5	1.6	0	0	0	0
Females										
0-4	0	0	0	0	-	-	0	0	0	0
5-14	477	595	647	806	10.0	1.6	0	0	0	0
15-44	2 049	1 284	3 186	1 996	29.8	1.6	0	0	0	0
45-59	191	545	350	998	52.3	1.6	0	0	0	0
60+	97	427	159	700	70.3	1.6	0	0	0	0
All ages	2 815	829	4 341	1 278	29.4	1.6	0	0	0	0
Total	4 913	720	7 591	1 112	29.0	1.6	0	0	0	0

Table 173f   SSA - ASS - ASS   Obsessive-compulsive disorders - Cases

Age group (years)	Incidence 1990 Number ('000s)	Rate (per 100 000)	Prevalence 1990 Number ('000s)	Rate (per 100 000)	Avg. age at onset (years)	Average duration (years)	Deaths 1990 Number ('000s)	Rate (per 100 000)	Deaths 2000 (Projected) Number ('000s)	Rate (per 100 000)
Males										
0-4	0	0	0	0	-	-	0	0	0	0
5-14	314	447	424	604	10.0	1.6	0	0	0	0
15-44	1 002	965	1 554	1 498	29.4	1.6	0	0	0	0
45-59	63	308	124	611	52.2	1.6	0	0	0	0
60+	33	318	63	597	69.2	1.6	0	0	0	0
All ages	1 412	560	2 165	858	27.0	1.6	0	0	0	0
Females										
0-4	0	0	0	0	-	-	0	0	0	0
5-14	416	595	561	804	10.0	1.6	0	0	0	0
15-44	1 364	1 284	2 118	1 993	29.5	1.6	0	0	0	0
45-59	120	545	221	1 001	52.2	1.6	0	0	0	0
60+	54	427	89	702	69.7	1.6	0	0	0	0
All ages	1 955	758	2 990	1 159	27.9	1.6	0	0	0	0
Total	3 367	660	5 155	1 010	27.5	1.6	0	0	0	0

For epidemiological sources see Andrews 1996. For the methods used to estimate and project incidence, prevalence, and deaths see Murray and Lopez 1996a. See explanatory notes for definitions and caveats.

Table 173
Obsessive-compulsive disorders
Cases

Cuadro 173
Trastornos obsesivo-compulsivos
Casos

Tableau 173
Troubles obsessionnels et compulsifs
Cas

Table 173g   LAC - ALC - ALC — Obsessive-compulsive disorders - Cases

Age group (years)	Incidence 1990 Number ('000s)	Rate (per 100 000)	Prevalence 1990 Number ('000s)	Rate (per 100 000)	Avg. age at onset (years)	Average duration (years)	Deaths 1990 Number ('000s)	Rate (per 100 000)	Deaths 2000 (Projected) Number ('000s)	Rate (per 100 000)
Males										
0-4	0	0	0	0	-	-	0	0	0	0
5-14	233	447	316	606	10.0	1.6	0	0	0	0
15-44	1 007	965	1 565	1 501	29.8	1.6	0	0	0	0
45-59	69	308	135	606	52.3	1.6	0	0	0	0
60+	45	318	85	599	70.3	1.6	0	0	0	0
All ages	1 354	611	2 101	948	28.9	1.6	0	0	0	0
Females										
0-4	0	0	0	0	-	-	0	0	0	0
5-14	302	595	409	806	10.0	1.6	0	0	0	0
15-44	1 336	1 284	2 078	1 996	29.8	1.6	0	0	0	0
45-59	127	545	233	996	52.4	1.6	0	0	0	0
60+	72	427	118	699	71.1	1.6	0	0	0	0
All ages	1 837	825	2 837	1 274	29.7	1.6	0	0	0	0
Total	3 191	718	4 938	1 111	29.4	1.6	0	0	0	0

Table 173h   MEC - AOM - CMO — Obsessive-compulsive disorders - Cases

Age group (years)	Incidence 1990 Number ('000s)	Rate (per 100 000)	Prevalence 1990 Number ('000s)	Rate (per 100 000)	Avg. age at onset (years)	Average duration (years)	Deaths 1990 Number ('000s)	Rate (per 100 000)	Deaths 2000 (Projected) Number ('000s)	Rate (per 100 000)
Males										
0-4	0	0	0	0	-	-	0	0	0	0
5-14	292	447	396	606	10.0	1.6	0	0	0	0
15-44	1 099	965	1 709	1 501	29.8	1.6	0	0	0	0
45-59	69	308	136	607	52.3	1.6	0	0	0	0
60+	43	318	82	598	69.7	1.6	0	0	0	0
All ages	1 504	587	2 322	906	28.1	1.6	0	0	0	0
Females										
0-4	0	0	0	0	-	-	0	0	0	0
5-14	369	595	500	806	10.0	1.6	0	0	0	0
15-44	1 376	1 284	2 140	1 996	29.8	1.6	0	0	0	0
45-59	121	545	222	997	52.4	1.6	0	0	0	0
60+	66	427	108	700	70.4	1.6	0	0	0	0
All ages	1 933	784	2 971	1 204	28.8	1.6	0	0	0	0
Total	3 437	683	5 293	1 052	28.5	1.6	0	0	0	0

Table 173i   World - Mundo - Monde — Obsessive-compulsive disorders - Cases

Age group (years)	Incidence 1990 Number ('000s)	Rate (per 100 000)	Prevalence 1990 Number ('000s)	Rate (per 100 000)	Avg. age at onset (years)	Average duration (years)	Deaths 1990 Number ('000s)	Rate (per 100 000)	Deaths 2000 (Projected) Number ('000s)	Rate (per 100 000)
Males										
0-4	0	0	0	0	-	-	0	0	0	0
5-14	2 466	447	3 338	606	10.0	1.6	0	0	0	0
15-44	12 066	965	18 756	1 501	29.8	1.6	0	0	0	0
45-59	963	308	1 895	607	52.3	1.6	0	0	0	0
60+	697	318	1 310	599	70.1	1.6	0	0	0	0
All ages	16 191	610	25 299	953	29.9	1.6	0	0	0	0
Females										
0-4	0	0	0	0	-	-	0	0	0	0
5-14	3 128	595	4 235	806	10.0	1.6	0	0	0	0
15-44	15 390	1 284	23 928	1 996	29.8	1.6	0	0	0	0
45-59	1 694	545	3 100	997	52.4	1.6	0	0	0	0
60+	1 150	427	1 880	698	71.2	1.6	0	0	0	0
All ages	21 362	817	33 143	1 268	30.9	1.6	0	0	0	0
Total	37 553	713	58 442	1 110	30.5	1.6	0	0	0	0

For epidemiological sources see Andrews 1996. For the methods used to estimate and project incidence, prevalence, and deaths see Murray and Lopez 1996a. See explanatory notes for definitions and caveats.

Table 174	Cuadro 174	Tableau 174
Panic disorder	Trastorno de pánico	Trouble d'angoisse
Cases	Casos	Cas

Table 174a   EME - PEMC - EMBE   Panic disorder - Cases

Age group (years)	Incidence 1990 Number ('000s)	Rate (per 100 000)	Prevalence 1990 Number ('000s)	Rate (per 100 000)	Avg. age at onset (years)	Average duration (years)	Deaths 1990 Number ('000s)	Rate (per 100 000)	Deaths 2000 (Projected) Number ('000s)	Rate (per 100 000)
Males										
0-4	0	0.0	0	0	-	-	0	0	0	0
5-14	137	257.5	96	181	10.0	0.75	0	0	0	0
15-44	990	537.9	736	400	29.9	0.75	0	0	0	0
45-59	356	537.9	267	404	52.4	0.75	0	0	0	0
60+	4	6.5	12	20	71.1	0.75	0	0	0	0
All ages	1 487	380.8	1 112	285	33.6	0.75	0	0	0	0
Females										
0-4	0	0.0	0	0	-	-	0	0	0	0
5-14	137	269.5	96	189	10.0	0.75	0	0	0	0
15-44	2 110	1 177.7	1 560	870	30.0	0.75	0	0	0	0
45-59	576	849.5	441	650	52.4	0.75	0	0	0	0
60+	235	277.5	194	230	72.4	0.76	0	0	0	0
All ages	3 058	750.7	2 291	562	36.6	0.75	0	0	0	0
Total	4 545	569.7	3 402	426	35.6	0.75	0	0	0	0

Table 174b   FSE - PEAS - AESE   Panic disorder - Cases

Age group (years)	Incidence 1990 Number ('000s)	Rate (per 100 000)	Prevalence 1990 Number ('000s)	Rate (per 100 000)	Avg. age at onset (years)	Average duration (years)	Deaths 1990 Number ('000s)	Rate (per 100 000)	Deaths 2000 (Projected) Number ('000s)	Rate (per 100 000)
Males										
0-4	0	0.0	0	0	-	-	0	0	0	0
5-14	70	257.5	49	181	10.0	0.75	0	0	0	0
15-44	410	537.9	305	400	29.8	0.75	0	0	0	0
45-59	145	537.9	109	404	52.2	0.75	0	0	0	0
60+	1	6.5	5	22	70.0	0.75	0	0	0	0
All ages	627	379.4	468	283	32.8	0.75	0	0	0	0
Females										
0-4	0	0.0	0	0	-	-	0	0	0	0
5-14	71	269.5	50	189	10.0	0.75	0	0	0	0
15-44	883	1 177.7	652	870	29.9	0.75	0	0	0	0
45-59	255	849.5	195	650	52.4	0.75	0	0	0	0
60+	101	277.6	84	231	71.5	0.75	0	0	0	0
All ages	1 310	724.0	982	543	36.4	0.75	0	0	0	0
Total	1 937	559.5	1 450	419	35.3	0.75	0	0	0	0

Table 174c   India - India - Inde   Panic disorder - Cases

Age group (years)	Incidence 1990 Number ('000s)	Rate (per 100 000)	Prevalence 1990 Number ('000s)	Rate (per 100 000)	Avg. age at onset (years)	Average duration (years)	Deaths 1990 Number ('000s)	Rate (per 100 000)	Deaths 2000 (Projected) Number ('000s)	Rate (per 100 000)
Males										
0-4	0	0.0	0	0	-	-	0	0	0	0
5-14	262	257.5	184	181	10.0	0.75	0	0	0	0
15-44	1 079	537.9	801	400	29.8	0.75	0	0	0	0
45-59	256	537.9	192	404	52.3	0.75	0	0	0	0
60+	2	6.5	7	23	69.7	0.75	0	0	0	0
All ages	1 598	363.8	1 184	270	30.2	0.75	0	0	0	0
Females										
0-4	0	0.0	0	0	-	-	0	0	0	0
5-14	257	269.5	180	189	10.0	0.75	0	0	0	0
15-44	2 158	1 177.7	1 594	870	29.8	0.75	0	0	0	0
45-59	391	849.5	299	650	52.4	0.75	0	0	0	0
60+	80	277.6	68	234	70.1	0.75	0	0	0	0
All ages	2 886	703.7	2 141	522	32.2	0.75	0	0	0	0
Total	4 484	527.9	3 325	391	31.5	0.75	0	0	0	0

For epidemiological sources see Andrews 1996. For the methods used to estimate and project incidence, prevalence, and deaths see Murray and Lopez 1996a. See explanatory notes for definitions and caveats.

Table 174
Panic disorder

Cuadro 174
Trastorno de pánico

Tableau 174
Trouble d'angoisse

Cases

Casos

Cas

Table 174d   China - China - Chine   Panic disorder - Cases

Age group (years)	Incidence 1990 Number ('000s)	Rate (per 100 000)	Prevalence 1990 Number ('000s)	Rate (per 100 000)	Avg. age at onset (years)	Average duration (years)	Deaths 1990 Number ('000s)	Rate (per 100 000)	Deaths 2000 (Projected) Number ('000s)	Rate (per 100 000)
Males										
0-4	0	0.0	0	0	-	-	0	0	0	0
5-14	250	257.5	175	181	10.0	0.75	0	0	0	0
15-44	1 647	537.9	1 224	400	29.9	0.75	0	0	0	0
45-59	391	537.9	294	404	52.3	0.75	0	0	0	0
60+	3	6.5	11	23	69.8	0.75	0	0	0	0
All ages	2 291	391.6	1 705	291	31.6	0.75	0	0	0	0
Females										
0-4	0	0.0	0	0	-	-	0	0	0	0
5-14	244	269.5	171	189	10.0	0.75	0	0	0	0
15-44	3 346	1 177.7	2 472	870	29.9	0.75	0	0	0	0
45-59	547	849.5	419	650	52.4	0.75	0	0	0	0
60+	143	277.6	120	233	70.6	0.75	0	0	0	0
All ages	4 280	780.3	3 182	580	33.0	0.75	0	0	0	0
Total	6 571	579.6	4 887	431	32.5	0.75	0	0	0	0

Table 174e   OAI - OPAI - APAI   Panic disorder - Cases

Age group (years)	Incidence 1990 Number ('000s)	Rate (per 100 000)	Prevalence 1990 Number ('000s)	Rate (per 100 000)	Avg. age at onset (years)	Average duration (years)	Deaths 1990 Number ('000s)	Rate (per 100 000)	Deaths 2000 (Projected) Number ('000s)	Rate (per 100 000)
Males										
0-4	0	0.0	0	0	-	-	0	0	0	0
5-14	216	257.5	152	181	10.0	0.75	0	0	0	0
15-44	865	537.9	643	400	29.7	0.75	0	0	0	0
45-59	184	537.9	138	404	52.3	0.75	0	0	0	0
60+	1	6.5	5	23	69.6	0.75	0	0	0	0
All ages	1 266	369.3	937	273	29.7	0.75	0	0	0	0
Females										
0-4	0	0.0	0	0	-	-	0	0	0	0
5-14	216	269.5	152	189	10.0	0.75	0	0	0	0
15-44	1 880	1 177.7	1 389	870	29.8	0.75	0	0	0	0
45-59	298	849.6	228	650	52.3	0.75	0	0	0	0
60+	63	277.6	53	234	70.3	0.75	0	0	0	0
All ages	2 457	723.6	1 821	536	31.8	0.75	0	0	0	0
Total	3 723	545.5	2 759	404	31.1	0.75	0	0	0	0

Table 174f   SSA - ASS - ASS   Panic disorder - Cases

Age group (years)	Incidence 1990 Number ('000s)	Rate (per 100 000)	Prevalence 1990 Number ('000s)	Rate (per 100 000)	Avg. age at onset (years)	Average duration (years)	Deaths 1990 Number ('000s)	Rate (per 100 000)	Deaths 2000 (Projected) Number ('000s)	Rate (per 100 000)
Males										
0-4	0	0.0	0	0	-	-	0	0	0	0
5-14	181	257.6	127	181	10.0	0.75	0	0	0	0
15-44	558	537.9	414	399	29.4	0.75	0	0	0	0
45-59	109	538.0	82	404	52.2	0.75	0	0	0	0
60+	1	6.5	3	24	69.2	0.75	0	0	0	0
All ages	849	336.5	626	248	28.2	0.75	0	0	0	0
Females										
0-4	0	0.0	0	0	-	-	0	0	0	0
5-14	188	269.5	132	189	10.0	0.75	0	0	0	0
15-44	1 252	1 177.8	924	869	29.5	0.75	0	0	0	0
45-59	188	849.6	144	650	52.2	0.75	0	0	0	0
60+	35	277.7	30	236	69.7	0.75	0	0	0	0
All ages	1 663	644.7	1 229	477	30.7	0.75	0	0	0	0
Total	2 512	492.3	1 855	364	29.9	0.75	0	0	0	0

For epidemiological sources see Andrews 1996. For the methods used to estimate and project incidence, prevalence, and deaths see Murray and Lopez 1996a. See explanatory notes for definitions and caveats.

Table 174
Panic disorder

Cuadro 174
Trastorno de pánico

Tableau 174
Trouble d'angoisse

Cases

Casos

Cas

Table 174g　　　**LAC - ALC - ALC**　　　　　　　　　　　　　Panic disorder - Cases

Age group (years)	Incidence 1990 Number ('000s)	Rate (per 100 000)	Prevalence 1990 Number ('000s)	Rate (per 100 000)	Avg. age at onset (years)	Average duration (years)	Deaths 1990 Number ('000s)	Rate (per 100 000)	Deaths 2000 (Projected) Number ('000s)	Rate (per 100 000)
Males										
0-4	0	0.0	0	0	-	-	0	0	0	0
5-14	134	257.5	94	181	10.0	0.75	0	0	0	0
15-44	561	537.9	417	400	29.8	0.75	0	0	0	0
45-59	120	537.9	90	404	52.3	0.75	0	0	0	0
60+	1	6.5	3	22	70.3	0.75	0	0	0	0
All ages	816	368.1	604	273	29.9	0.75	0	0	0	0
Females										
0-4	0	0.0	0	0	-	-	0	0	0	0
5-14	137	269.5	96	189	10.0	0.75	0	0	0	0
15-44	1 226	1 177.7	906	870	29.8	0.75	0	0	0	0
45-59	198	849.5	152	650	52.4	0.75	0	0	0	0
60+	47	277.6	39	232	71.1	0.75	0	0	0	0
All ages	1 608	722.0	1 193	536	32.1	0.75	0	0	0	0
Total	2 423	545.5	1 797	404	31.4	0.75	0	0	0	0

Table 174h　　　**MEC - AOM - CMO**　　　　　　　　　　　　　Panic disorder - Cases

Age group (years)	Incidence 1990 Number ('000s)	Rate (per 100 000)	Prevalence 1990 Number ('000s)	Rate (per 100 000)	Avg. age at onset (years)	Average duration (years)	Deaths 1990 Number ('000s)	Rate (per 100 000)	Deaths 2000 (Projected) Number ('000s)	Rate (per 100 000)
Males										
0-4	0	0.0	0	0	-	-	0	0	0	0
5-14	168	257.5	118	181	10.0	0.75	0	0	0	0
15-44	613	537.9	455	400	29.8	0.75	0	0	0	0
45-59	120	537.9	90	404	52.3	0.75	0	0	0	0
60+	1	6.5	3	23	69.7	0.75	0	0	0	0
All ages	902	351.8	667	260	29.1	0.75	0	0	0	0
Females										
0-4	0	0.0	0	0	-	-	0	0	0	0
5-14	167	269.5	117	189	10.0	0.75	0	0	0	0
15-44	1 263	1 177.7	933	870	29.8	0.75	0	0	0	0
45-59	189	849.5	145	650	52.4	0.75	0	0	0	0
60+	43	277.6	36	234	70.4	0.75	0	0	0	0
All ages	1 662	673.7	1 231	499	31.4	0.75	0	0	0	0
Total	2 564	509.7	1 898	377	30.6	0.75	0	0	0	0

Table 174i　　　**World - Mundo - Monde**　　　　　　　　　　　　　Panic disorder - Cases

Age group (years)	Incidence 1990 Number ('000s)	Rate (per 100 000)	Prevalence 1990 Number ('000s)	Rate (per 100 000)	Avg. age at onset (years)	Average duration (years)	Deaths 1990 Number ('000s)	Rate (per 100 000)	Deaths 2000 (Projected) Number ('000s)	Rate (per 100 000)
Males										
0-4	0	0.0	0	0	-	-	0	0	0	0
5-14	1 420	257.5	996	181	10.0	0.75	0	0	0	0
15-44	6 723	537.9	4 995	400	29.8	0.75	0	0	0	0
45-59	1 680	537.9	1 263	404	52.3	0.75	0	0	0	0
60+	14	6.5	48	22	70.1	0.75	0	0	0	0
All ages	9 837	370.7	7 303	275	30.8	0.75	0	0	0	0
Females										
0-4	0	0.0	0	0		-	0	0	0	0
5-14	1 416	269.5	994	189	10.0	0.75	0	0	0	0
15-44	14 117	1 177.8	10 429	870	29.8	0.75	0	0	0	0
45-59	2 643	849.6	2 022	650	52.4	0.75	0	0	0	0
60+	747	277.6	625	232	71.2	0.75	0	0	0	0
All ages	18 923	724.0	14 070	538	33.1	0.75	0	0	0	0
Total	28 760	546.0	21 373	406	32.3	0.75	0	0	0	0

For epidemiological sources see Andrews 1996. For the methods used to estimate and project incidence, prevalence, and deaths see Murray and Lopez 1996a. See explanatory notes for definitions and caveats.

Table 175	Cuadro 175	Tableau 175
Glaucoma	Glaucoma	Glaucome
Blindness	Ceguera	Cécité

Table 175a EME - PEMC - EMBE · Glaucoma - Blindness

Age group (years)	Incidence 1990 Number ('000s)	Rate (per 100 000)	Prevalence 1990 Number ('000s)	Rate (per 100 000)	Avg. age at onset (years)	Average duration (years)	Deaths 1990 Number ('000s)	Rate (per 100 000)	Deaths 2000 (Projected) Number ('000s)	Rate (per 100 000)
Males										
0-4	0	0.0	0	0.0	-	-	0	0	0	0
5-14	0	0.0	0	0.0	-	-	0	0	0	0
15-44	0	0.1	2	1.1	29.9	32.6	0	0	0	0
45-59	2	3.6	18	27.2	52.4	16.1	0	0	0	0
60+	6	9.3	54	89.6	71.1	6.4	0	0	0	0
All ages	8	2.1	74	19.0	64.9	9.7	0	0	0	0
Females										
0-4	0	0.0	0	0.0	-	-	0	0	0	0
5-14	0	0.0	0	0.0	-	-	0	0	0	0
15-44	0	0.0	1	0.4	30.0	39.9	0	0	0	0
45-59	2	3.4	17	25.2	52.4	21.0	0	0	0	0
60+	8	9.0	90	106.3	72.4	8.2	0	0	0	0
All ages	10	2.4	108	26.5	67.6	11.3	0	0	0	0
Total	18	2.3	182	22.8	66.4	10.6	0	0	0	0

Table 175b FSE - PEAS - AESE · Glaucoma - Blindness

Age group (years)	Incidence 1990 Number ('000s)	Rate (per 100 000)	Prevalence 1990 Number ('000s)	Rate (per 100 000)	Avg. age at onset (years)	Average duration (years)	Deaths 1990 Number ('000s)	Rate (per 100 000)	Deaths 2000 (Projected) Number ('000s)	Rate (per 100 000)
Males										
0-4	0	0.0	0	0.0	-	-	0	0	0	0
5-14	0	0.0	0	0.0	-	-	0	0	0	0
15-44	0	0.0	0	0.3	29.8	25.0	0	0	0	0
45-59	1	2.4	4	15.6	52.2	12.4	0	0	0	0
60+	3	13.7	19	90.1	70.0	5.4	0	0	0	0
All ages	4	2.1	23	14.1	66.5	6.8	0	0	0	0
Females										
0-4	0	0.0	0	0.0	-	-	0	0	0	0
5-14	0	0.0	0	0.0	-	-	0	0	0	0
15-44	0	0.1	1	1.1	29.9	35.6	0	0	0	0
45-59	1	4.5	10	34.0	52.4	18.0	0	0	0	0
60+	4	9.9	40	110.4	71.5	7.0	0	0	0	0
All ages	5	2.8	51	28.3	65.8	10.3	0	0	0	0
Total	9	2.5	75	21.5	66.1	8.9	0	0	0	0

Table 175c India - India - Inde · Glaucoma - Blindness

Age group (years)	Incidence 1990 Number ('000s)	Rate (per 100 000)	Prevalence 1990 Number ('000s)	Rate (per 100 000)	Avg. age at onset (years)	Average duration (years)	Deaths 1990 Number ('000s)	Rate (per 100 000)	Deaths 2000 (Projected) Number ('000s)	Rate (per 100 000)
Males										
0-4	0	0.0	0	0.0	-	-	0	0	0	0
5-14	0	0.0	0	0.0	-	-	0	0	0	0
15-44	2	1.2	31	15.7	29.8	26.1	0	0	0	0
45-59	37	78.4	260	545.8	52.3	13.2	0	0	0	0
60+	35	117.5	353	1 186.9	69.6	5.2	0	0	0	0
All ages	75	17.0	644	146.7	59.7	9.8	0	0	0	0
Females										
0-4	0	0.0	0	0.0	-	-	0	0	0	0
5-14	0	0.0	0	0.0	-	-	0	0	0	0
15-44	1	0.5	11	6.0	29.8	28.0	0	0	0	0
45-59	25	53.4	173	376.3	52.3	14.7	0	0	0	0
60+	34	117.5	313	1 081.8	70.0	5.6	0	0	0	0
All ages	59	14.5	497	121.2	62.1	9.7	0	0	0	0
Total	134	15.8	1 142	134.4	60.8	9.8	0	0	0	0

For the methods used to estimate and project incidence, prevalence, and deaths see Murray and Lopez 1996a. See explanatory notes for definitions and caveats.

Table 175	Cuadro 175	Tableau 175
Glaucoma	Glaucoma	Glaucome
Blindness	Ceguera	Cécité

Table 175d — China - China - Chine — Glaucoma - Blindness

Age group (years)	Incidence 1990 Number ('000s)	Rate (per 100 000)	Prevalence 1990 Number ('000s)	Rate (per 100 000)	Avg. age at onset (years)	Average duration (years)	Deaths 1990 Number ('000s)	Rate (per 100 000)	Deaths 2000 (Projected) Number ('000s)	Rate (per 100 000)
Males										
0-4	0	0.0	0	0.0	-	-	0	0.4	0	0.4
5-14	0	0.0	0	0.0	-	-	0	0.0	0	0.0
15-44	2	0.5	21	7.0	29.9	29.2	0	0.1	0	0.1
45-59	20	27.3	143	196.4	52.3	13.6	1	1.0	1	0.8
60+	35	71.7	284	579.2	69.7	5.2	2	4.7	2	3.8
All ages	56	9.7	448	76.5	62.5	8.8	4	0.6	4	0.5
Females										
0-4	0	0.0	0	0.0	-	-	0	0.4	0	0.5
5-14	0	0.0	0	0.0	-	-	0	0.0	0	0.0
15-44	4	1.6	63	22.2	29.9	32.6	0	0.0	0	0.0
45-59	49	76.2	369	572.4	52.4	15.9	1	0.9	1	0.7
60+	50	97.6	638	1 235.6	70.6	6.0	2	3.5	2	3.3
All ages	104	19.0	1 070	195.1	60.3	11.8	3	0.5	3	0.5
Total	160	14.2	1 518	133.9	61.0	10.8	6	0.6	7	0.5

Table 175e — OAI - OPAI - APAI — Glaucoma - Blindness

Age group (years)	Incidence 1990 Number ('000s)	Rate (per 100 000)	Prevalence 1990 Number ('000s)	Rate (per 100 000)	Avg. age at onset (years)	Average duration (years)	Deaths 1990 Number ('000s)	Rate (per 100 000)	Deaths 2000 (Projected) Number ('000s)	Rate (per 100 000)
Males										
0-4	0	0.0	0	0.0	-	-	0	0	0	0
5-14	0	0.0	0	0.0	-	-	0	0	0	0
15-44	1	0.6	13	8.0	29.7	24.5	0	0	0	0
45-59	18	52.0	120	350.6	52.3	12.3	0	0	0	0
60+	21	102.2	175	865.4	69.6	5.0	0	0	0	0
All ages	39	11.5	307	89.6	60.8	8.8	0	0	0	0
Females										
0-4	0	0.0	0	0.0	-	-	0	0	0	0
5-14	0	0.0	0	0.0	-	-	0	0	0	0
15-44	3	1.8	38	23.7	29.8	27.4	0	0	0	0
45-59	41	116.8	291	830.1	52.3	14.2	0	0	0	0
60+	31	135.8	378	1 669.5	70.3	5.6	0	0	0	0
All ages	75	22.0	708	208.4	58.8	11.2	0	0	0	0
Total	114	16.7	1 015	148.7	59.5	10.4	0	0	0	0

Table 175f — SSA - ASS - ASS — Glaucoma - Blindness

Age group (years)	Incidence 1990 Number ('000s)	Rate (per 100 000)	Prevalence 1990 Number ('000s)	Rate (per 100 000)	Avg. age at onset (years)	Average duration (years)	Deaths 1990 Number ('000s)	Rate (per 100 000)	Deaths 2000 (Projected) Number ('000s)	Rate (per 100 000)
Males										
0-4	0	0.0	0	0.0	-	-	0	0	0	0
5-14	0	0.0	0	0.0	-	-	0	0	0	0
15-44	0	0.1	1	1.1	29.4	18.0	0	0	0	0
45-59	14	68.3	86	422.6	52.2	11.0	0	0	0	0
60+	43	412.4	252	2 395.5	69.1	4.8	0	0	0	0
All ages	57	22.7	339	134.2	64.9	6.3	0	0	0	0
Females										
0-4	0	0.0	0	0.0	-	-	0	0	0	0
5-14	0	0.0	0	0.0	-	-	0	0	0	0
15-44	0	0.2	2	1.9	29.5	20.2	0	0	0	0
45-59	20	92.5	132	597.0	52.2	12.4	0	0	0	0
60+	58	456.5	382	2 999.8	69.5	5.2	0	0	0	0
All ages	79	30.5	516	200.0	64.9	7.1	0	0	0	0
Total	136	26.7	855	167.5	64.9	6.8	0	0	0	0

For the methods used to estimate and project incidence, prevalence, and deaths see Murray and Lopez 1996a. See explanatory notes for definitions and caveats.

Table 175	Cuadro 175	Tableau 175
Glaucoma	Glaucoma	Glaucome
Blindness	Ceguera	Cécité

Table 175g — LAC - ALC - ALC — Glaucoma - Blindness

Age group (years)	Incidence 1990 Number ('000s)	Rate (per 100 000)	Prevalence 1990 Number ('000s)	Rate (per 100 000)	Avg. age at onset (years)	Average duration (years)	Deaths 1990 Number ('000s)	Rate (per 100 000)	Deaths 2000 (Projected) Number ('000s)	Rate (per 100 000)
Males										
0-4	0	0.0	0	0.0	-	-	0	0	0	0
5-14	0	0.0	0	0.0	-	-	0	0	0	0
15-44	0	0.1	1	0.9	29.8	27.6	0	0	0	0
45-59	2	10.8	16	74.0	52.3	14.1	0	0	0	0
60+	7	46.9	49	344.0	70.3	5.6	0	0	0	0
All ages	9	4.1	66	29.9	65.3	8.0	0	0	0	0
Females										
0-4	0	0.0	0	0.0	-	-	0	0	0	0
5-14	0	0.0	0	0.0	-	-	0	0	0	0
15-44	0	0.2	2	2.1	29.9	31.5	0	0	0	0
45-59	4	18.3	31	131.0	52.4	16.7	0	0	0	0
60+	9	53.8	84	501.3	71.1	6.4	0	0	0	0
All ages	13	6.0	117	52.6	64.7	10.0	0	0	0	0
Total	23	5.1	183	41.3	64.9	9.2	0	0	0	0

Table 175h — MEC - AOM - CMO — Glaucoma - Blindness

Age group (years)	Incidence 1990 Number ('000s)	Rate (per 100 000)	Prevalence 1990 Number ('000s)	Rate (per 100 000)	Avg. age at onset (years)	Average duration (years)	Deaths 1990 Number ('000s)	Rate (per 100 000)	Deaths 2000 (Projected) Number ('000s)	Rate (per 100 000)
Males										
0-4	0	0.0	0	0.0	-	-	0	0	0	0
5-14	0	0.0	0	0.0	-	-	0	0	0	0
15-44	0	0.0	1	0.6	29.8	26.9	0	0	0	0
45-59	4	19.3	29	128.1	52.3	12.8	0	0	0	0
60+	7	49.4	53	385.7	69.7	5.1	0	0	0	0
All ages	11	4.3	82	32.0	62.8	8.2	0	0	0	0
Females										
0-4	0	0.0	0	0.0	-	-	0	0	0	0
5-14	0	0.0	0	0.0	-	-	0	0	0	0
15-44	0	0.1	2	1.6	29.8	29.6	0	0	0	0
45-59	7	30.4	47	210.6	52.3	14.8	0	0	0	0
60+	8	53.8	85	547.7	70.4	5.8	0	0	0	0
All ages	15	6.2	133	54.0	62.0	10.0	0	0	0	0
Total	26	5.2	215	42.8	62.3	9.2	0	0	0	0

Table 175i — World - Mundo - Monde — Glaucoma - Blindness

Age group (years)	Incidence 1990 Number ('000s)	Rate (per 100 000)	Prevalence 1990 Number ('000s)	Rate (per 100 000)	Avg. age at onset (years)	Average duration (years)	Deaths 1990 Number ('000s)	Rate (per 100 000)	Deaths 2000 (Projected) Number ('000s)	Rate (per 100 000)
Males										
0-4	0	0.0	0	0.0	-	-	0	0.1	0	0.1
5-14	0	0.0	0	0.0	-	-	0	0.0	0	0.0
15-44	5	0.4	71	5.7	29.8	26.7	0	0.0	0	0.0
45-59	99	31.5	675	216.1	52.3	12.9	1	0.2	1	0.2
60+	156	71.3	1 238	565.8	69.6	5.1	2	1.1	2	0.8
All ages	260	9.8	1 984	74.8	62.2	8.5	4	0.1	4	0.1
Females										
0-4	0	0.0	0	0.0	-	-	0	0.1	0	0.1
5-14	0	0.0	0	0.0	-	-	0	0.0	0	0.0
15-44	9	0.7	119	10.0	29.8	30.2	0	0.0	0	0.0
45-59	150	48.2	1 070	344.0	52.3	14.8	1	0.2	1	0.2
60+	202	75.0	2 011	746.8	70.2	5.7	2	0.7	2	0.6
All ages	360	13.8	3 200	122.4	61.8	10.1	3	0.1	3	0.1
Total	620	11.8	5 184	98.4	62.0	9.4	6	0.1	7	0.1

For the methods used to estimate and project incidence, prevalence, and deaths see Murray and Lopez 1996a. See explanatory notes for definitions and caveats.

Table 176	Cuadro 176	Tableau 176
Cataracts	Cataratas	Cataractes

| Blindness | Ceguera | Cécité |

Table 176a — EME - PEMC - EMBE — Cataracts - Blindness

Age group (years)	Incidence 1990 Number ('000s)	Rate (per 100 000)	Prevalence 1990 Number ('000s)	Rate (per 100 000)	Avg. age at onset (years)	Average duration (years)	Deaths 1990 Number ('000s)	Rate (per 100 000)	Deaths 2000 (Projected) Number ('000s)	Rate (per 100 000)
Males										
0-4	1	2.3	1	4.1	2.5	2.08	0	0	0	0
5-14	0	0.1	0	0.3	10.0	0.50	0	0	0	0
15-44	2	1.2	1	0.6	29.9	0.50	0	0	0	0
45-59	11	17.0	5	8.2	52.4	0.50	0	0	0	0
60+	67	110.0	33	54.4	71.1	0.50	0	0	0	0
All ages	81	20.7	41	10.4	66.8	0.51	0	0	0	0
Females										
0-4	1	2.3	1	4.1	2.5	2.09	0	0	0	0
5-14	0	0.1	0	0.3	10.0	0.50	0	0	0	0
15-44	2	1.2	1	0.6	30.0	0.50	0	0	0	0
45-59	11	16.0	5	7.8	52.4	0.50	0	0	0	0
60+	79	94.0	40	47.2	72.4	0.50	0	0	0	0
All ages	93	22.9	47	11.7	68.6	0.51	0	0	0	0
Total	174	21.8	88	11.1	67.8	0.51	0	0	0	0

Table 176b — FSE - PEAS - AESE — Cataracts - Blindness

Age group (years)	Incidence 1990 Number ('000s)	Rate (per 100 000)	Prevalence 1990 Number ('000s)	Rate (per 100 000)	Avg. age at onset (years)	Average duration (years)	Deaths 1990 Number ('000s)	Rate (per 100 000)	Deaths 2000 (Projected) Number ('000s)	Rate (per 100 000)
Males										
0-4	1	4.8	1	7.6	2.5	1.95	0	0	0	0
5-14	0	0.3	0	1.0	10.0	0.75	0	0	0	0
15-44	2	2.0	1	1.5	29.8	0.75	0	0	0	0
45-59	7	27.0	5	19.6	52.2	0.75	0	0	0	0
60+	43	204.9	32	154.4	70.0	0.75	0	0	0	0
All ages	52	31.7	40	24.2	65.4	0.76	0	0	0	0
Females										
0-4	1	4.9	1	7.9	2.5	1.95	0	0	0	0
5-14	0	0.3	0	1.0	10.0	0.75	0	0	0	0
15-44	1	2.0	1	1.5	29.9	0.75	0	0	0	0
45-59	7	24.0	5	17.3	52.4	0.75	0	0	0	0
60+	53	145.0	40	108.6	71.5	0.75	0	0	0	0
All ages	62	34.4	47	26.1	67.5	0.76	0	0	0	0
Total	115	33.1	87	25.2	66.6	0.76	0	0	0	0

Table 176c — India - India - Inde — Cataracts - Blindness

Age group (years)	Incidence 1990 Number ('000s)	Rate (per 100 000)	Prevalence 1990 Number ('000s)	Rate (per 100 000)	Avg. age at onset (years)	Average duration (years)	Deaths 1990 Number ('000s)	Rate (per 100 000)	Deaths 2000 (Projected) Number ('000s)	Rate (per 100 000)
Males										
0-4	4	6.3	6	10.0	2.5	3.4	0	0	0	0
5-14	0	0.3	7	6.7	10.0	3.1	0	0	0	0
15-44	81	40.5	127	63.3	29.8	1.7	0	0	0	0
45-59	454	954.7	763	1 603.3	52.3	1.9	0	0	0	0
60+	878	2 949.5	1 482	4 978.2	69.4	1.6	0	0	0	0
All ages	1 417	322.6	2 384	542.6	61.5	1.7	0	0	0	0
Females										
0-4	4	6.7	6	10.5	2.5	3.3	0	0	0	0
5-14	0	0.4	7	7.0	10.0	3.1	0	0	0	0
15-44	75	41.0	127	69.4	29.8	1.8	0	0	0	0
45-59	412	895.1	762	1 656.9	52.3	2.1	0	0	0	0
60+	964	3 332.3	1 807	6 246.6	69.7	1.8	0	0	0	0
All ages	1 455	354.7	2 709	660.5	62.5	1.9	0	0	0	0
Total	2 872	338.1	5 093	599.5	62.0	1.8	0	0	0	0

For epidemiological sources see Negrel et al. 1996. For the methods used to estimate and project incidence, prevalence, and deaths see Murray and Lopez 1996a. See explanatory notes for definitions and caveats.

Table 176	Cuadro 176	Tableau 176
Cataracts	Cataratas	Cataractes

| Blindness | Ceguera | Cécité |

Table 176d — China - China - Chine — Cataracts - Blindness

Age group (years)	Incidence 1990 Number ('000s)	Rate (per 100 000)	Prevalence 1990 Number ('000s)	Rate (per 100 000)	Avg. age at onset (years)	Average duration (years)	Deaths 1990 Number ('000s)	Rate (per 100 000)	Deaths 2000 (Projected) Number ('000s)	Rate (per 100 000)
Males										
0-4	3	4.2	4	6.6	2.5	3.1	0	0.7	0	0.7
5-14	0	0.2	4	3.8	10.0	2.8	0	0.0	0	0.0
15-44	31	10.0	48	15.7	29.9	1.6	0	0.0	0	0.0
45-59	149	204.4	216	296.9	52.3	1.6	1	1.5	1	1.2
60+	469	957.0	715	1 460.1	69.7	1.5	2	4.0	2	3.2
All ages	651	111.2	987	168.6	63.6	1.5	3	0.6	4	0.5
Females										
0-4	2	3.8	4	6.4	2.5	3.7	0	0.0	0	0.0
5-14	0	0.2	4	4.3	10.0	3.2	0	0.0	0	0.0
15-44	26	9.0	48	16.8	29.9	2.0	0	0.1	0	0.1
45-59	125	194.4	214	332.5	52.4	2.0	1	1.2	1	0.9
60+	473	914.9	887	1 716.9	70.5	1.8	1	2.5	1	2.2
All ages	626	114.1	1 157	210.9	65.0	1.9	2	0.4	2	0.4
Total	1 276	112.6	2 143	189.1	64.3	1.7	6	0.5	6	0.5

Table 176e — OAI - OPAI - APAI — Cataracts - Blindness

Age group (years)	Incidence 1990 Number ('000s)	Rate (per 100 000)	Prevalence 1990 Number ('000s)	Rate (per 100 000)	Avg. age at onset (years)	Average duration (years)	Deaths 1990 Number ('000s)	Rate (per 100 000)	Deaths 2000 (Projected) Number ('000s)	Rate (per 100 000)
Males										
0-4	2	3.6	3	5.9	2.5	3.5	0	0.0	0	0.0
5-14	0	0.2	3	3.9	10.0	3.2	0	0.0	0	0.0
15-44	35	22.0	60	37.2	29.7	1.8	0	0.0	0	0.0
45-59	216	633.4	360	1 055.5	52.2	1.9	0	0.0	0	0.0
60+	418	2 069.1	694	3 436.6	69.4	1.6	0	0.2	0	0.2
All ages	671	195.8	1 121	326.7	61.6	1.7	0	0.0	0	0.0
Females										
0-4	1	3.2	2	5.7	2.5	4.3	0	0.1	0	0.1
5-14	0	0.2	4	4.6	10.0	3.7	0	0.0	0	0.0
15-44	32	20.0	59	37.1	29.8	2.0	0	0.0	0	0.0
45-59	195	554.4	358	1 019.9	52.3	2.1	0	0.0	0	0.0
60+	452	1 995.0	846	3 731.6	70.1	1.8	0	0.0	0	0.0
All ages	680	200.3	1 269	373.6	63.0	1.9	0	0.0	0	0.0
Total	1 351	198.0	2 389	350.1	62.3	1.8	0	0.0	0	0.0

Table 176f — SSA - ASS - ASS — Cataracts - Blindness

Age group (years)	Incidence 1990 Number ('000s)	Rate (per 100 000)	Prevalence 1990 Number ('000s)	Rate (per 100 000)	Avg. age at onset (years)	Average duration (years)	Deaths 1990 Number ('000s)	Rate (per 100 000)	Deaths 2000 (Projected) Number ('000s)	Rate (per 100 000)
Males										
0-4	3	6.5	6	12	2.4	5.8	0	0	0	0
5-14	0	0.3	10	14	10.0	5.8	0	0	0	0
15-44	23	22.0	76	73	29.4	3.8	0	0	0	0
45-59	139	683.1	496	2 441	52.1	4.8	0	0	0	0
60+	216	2 051.6	855	8 134	68.7	3.4	0	0	0	0
All ages	380	150.8	1 441	571	59.7	4.0	0	0	0	0
Females										
0-4	3	6.3	5	12	2.4	6.2	0	0	0	0
5-14	0	0.3	10	14	10.0	6.3	0	0	0	0
15-44	19	18.0	77	72	29.5	4.9	0	0	0	0
45-59	112	508.6	492	2 224	52.2	6.4	0	0	0	0
60+	228	1 793.3	1 038	8 156	69.2	3.8	0	0	0	0
All ages	363	140.8	1 622	629	61.3	4.7	0	0	0	0
Total	744	145.7	3 063	600	60.5	4.3	0	0	0	0

For epidemiological sources see Negrel et al. 1996. For the methods used to estimate and project incidence, prevalence, and deaths see Murray and Lopez 1996a. See explanatory notes for definitions and caveats.

Table 176	Cuadro 176	Tableau 176
Cataracts	Cataratas	Cataractes

Blindness	Ceguera	Cécité

Table 176g LAC - ALC - ALC   Cataracts - Blindness

Age group (years)	Incidence 1990 Number ('000s)	Rate (per 100 000)	Prevalence 1990 Number ('000s)	Rate (per 100 000)	Avg. age at onset (years)	Average duration (years)	Deaths 1990 Number ('000s)	Rate (per 100 000)	Deaths 2000 (Projected) Number ('000s)	Rate (per 100 000)
Males										
0-4	5	17.1	7	23.6	2.5	2.3	0	0	0	0
5-14	0	0.1	5	8.6	10.0	2.2	0	0	0	0
15-44	12	11.7	17	15.9	29.8	1.4	0	0	0	0
45-59	62	279.0	84	377.2	52.3	1.5	0	0	0	0
60+	298	2 092.1	399	2 802.1	70.1	1.3	0	0	0	0
All ages	377	170.1	511	230.4	65.0	1.4	0	0	0	0
Females										
0-4	5	17.1	7	23.8	2.5	2.4	0	0	0	0
5-14	0	0.9	5	10.3	10.0	2.2	0	0	0	0
15-44	12	11.7	17	16.0	29.9	1.4	0	0	0	0
45-59	61	259.1	83	353.8	52.4	1.5	0	0	0	0
60+	355	2 108.9	489	2 903.7	70.9	1.3	0	0	0	0
All ages	433	194.3	600	269.3	66.3	1.4	0	0	0	0
Total	810	182.2	1 110	249.9	65.7	1.4	0	0	0	0

Table 176h MEC - AOM - CMO   Cataracts - Blindness

Age group (years)	Incidence 1990 Number ('000s)	Rate (per 100 000)	Prevalence 1990 Number ('000s)	Rate (per 100 000)	Avg. age at onset (years)	Average duration (years)	Deaths 1990 Number ('000s)	Rate (per 100 000)	Deaths 2000 (Projected) Number ('000s)	Rate (per 100 000)
Males										
0-4	2	5.9	4	8.9	2.5	2.9	0	0	0	0
5-14	0	0.3	3	5.1	10.0	2.8	0	0	0	0
15-44	24	21.0	37	32.9	29.8	1.7	0	0	0	0
45-59	155	692.0	259	1 157.9	52.3	1.9	0	0	0	0
60+	308	2 254.5	515	3 773.6	69.5	1.6	0	0	0	0
All ages	489	190.7	818	319.1	61.8	1.7	0	0	0	0
Females										
0-4	2	5.5	4	8.9	2.5	3.4	0	0	0	0
5-14	0	0.3	4	5.9	10.0	3.2	0	0	0	0
15-44	23	21.0	38	35.8	29.8	1.8	0	0	0	0
45-59	143	642.4	264	1 185.4	52.3	2.1	0	0	0	0
60+	334	2 160.4	631	4 086.4	70.2	1.8	0	0	0	0
All ages	502	203.4	941	381.5	63.0	1.9	0	0	0	0
Total	991	196.9	1 759	349.7	62.4	1.8	0	0	0	0

Table 176i World - Mundo - Monde   Cataracts - Blindness

Age group (years)	Incidence 1990 Number ('000s)	Rate (per 100 000)	Prevalence 1990 Number ('000s)	Rate (per 100 000)	Avg. age at onset (years)	Average duration (years)	Deaths 1990 Number ('000s)	Rate (per 100 000)	Deaths 2000 (Projected) Number ('000s)	Rate (per 100 000)
Males										
0-4	20	6.1	31	9.6	2.5	3.3	0	0.1	0	0.1
5-14	1	0.2	32	5.8	10.0	3.2	0	0.0	0	0.0
15-44	210	16.8	367	29.4	29.8	1.9	0	0.0	0	0.0
45-59	1 193	381.9	2 188	700.4	52.3	2.1	1	0.4	1	0.3
60+	2 696	1 231.6	4 725	2 159.1	69.5	1.7	2	0.9	2	0.7
All ages	4 119	155.2	7 342	276.7	62.2	1.8	4	0.1	4	0.1
Females										
0-4	18	6.0	30	9.6	2.5	3.6	0	0.0	0	0.0
5-14	2	0.3	33	6.3	10.0	3.2	0	0.0	0	0.0
15-44	190	15.9	368	30.7	29.8	2.1	0	0.0	0	0.0
45-59	1 066	342.6	2 184	702.0	52.3	2.5	1	0.2	1	0.2
60+	2 938	1 091.2	5 777	2 145.9	70.2	1.9	1	0.5	1	0.4
All ages	4 214	161.2	8 391	321.1	63.5	2.0	2	0.1	3	0.1
Total	8 333	158.2	15 734	298.7	62.8	1.9	6	0.1	6	0.1

For epidemiological sources see Negrel et al. 1996. For the methods used to estimate and project incidence, prevalence, and deaths see Murray and Lopez 1996a. See explanatory notes for definitions and caveats.

Table 177
Rheumatic heart disease

Cuadro 177
Cardiopatía reumática

Tableau 177
Cardiopathie rhumatismale

Congestive heart failure

Insuficiencia cardíaca congestiva

Insuffisance cardiaque congestive

Table 177a EME - PEMC - EMBE Rheumatic heart disease - Congestive heart failure

Age group (years)	Incidence 1990 Number ('000s)	Rate (per 100 000)	Prevalence 1990 Number ('000s)	Rate (per 100 000)	Avg. age at onset (years)	Average duration (years)	Deaths 1990 Number ('000s)	Rate (per 100 000)	Deaths 2000 (Projected) Number ('000s)	Rate (per 100 000)
Males										
0-4	0	0.0	0	0.0	-	-	0	0.0	0	0.0
5-14	0	0.0	0	0.1	10.0	6.3	0	0.0	0	0.0
15-44	1	0.5	4	2.3	34.2	6.2	0	0.3	0	0.2
45-59	2	3.0	9	13.3	52.4	5.7	1	1.6	1	1.6
60+	8	13.9	37	60.9	73.0	4.1	5	7.6	5	7.1
All ages	11	2.9	50	12.8	66.1	4.5	6	1.6	7	1.7
Females										
0-4	0	0.0	0	0.0	-	-	0	0.0	0	0.0
5-14	0	0.1	0	0.2	10.0	5.9	0	0.0	0	0.0
15-44	1	0.5	4	2.4	33.9	6.2	1	0.3	0	0.3
45-59	3	4.9	14	20.8	52.4	5.9	2	2.4	1	1.7
60+	21	25.2	95	112.8	74.5	4.3	12	14.1	12	12.4
All ages	26	6.3	114	28.0	70.0	4.6	14	3.5	14	3.2
Total	37	4.6	164	20.5	68.8	4.6	20	2.5	21	2.5

Table 177b FSE - PEAS - AESE Rheumatic heart disease - Congestive heart failure

Age group (years)	Incidence 1990 Number ('000s)	Rate (per 100 000)	Prevalence 1990 Number ('000s)	Rate (per 100 000)	Avg. age at onset (years)	Average duration (years)	Deaths 1990 Number ('000s)	Rate (per 100 000)	Deaths 2000 (Projected) Number ('000s)	Rate (per 100 000)
Males										
0-4	0	0.0	0	0.0	-	-	0	0.0	0	0.0
5-14	0	0.6	1	2.0	10.0	6.2	0	0.2	0	0.2
15-44	4	5.8	20	26.4	33.6	6.0	2	3.2	2	3.0
45-59	9	31.8	38	142.0	52.2	5.4	5	16.8	6	18.6
60+	2	10.0	21	99.5	69.5	4.1	3	15.4	4	15.2
All ages	15	9.2	80	48.3	48.7	5.4	10	6.2	12	7.0
Females										
0-4	0	0.0	0	0.0	-	-	0	0.0	0	0.0
5-14	0	0.6	1	2.0	10.0	6.3	0	0.2	0	0.1
15-44	3	4.1	14	18.1	34.9	6.2	2	2.2	1	1.9
45-59	12	40.4	52	172.1	52.4	5.8	6	19.5	6	17.0
60+	6	15.3	47	129.4	71.5	4.4	7	19.4	7	16.5
All ages	21	11.6	113	62.4	54.6	5.5	15	8.1	14	7.5
Total	36	10.5	193	55.6	52.1	5.4	25	7.2	26	7.3

Table 177c India - India - Inde Rheumatic heart disease - Congestive heart failure

Age group (years)	Incidence 1990 Number ('000s)	Rate (per 100 000)	Prevalence 1990 Number ('000s)	Rate (per 100 000)	Avg. age at onset (years)	Average duration (years)	Deaths 1990 Number ('000s)	Rate (per 100 000)	Deaths 2000 (Projected) Number ('000s)	Rate (per 100 000)
Males										
0-4	0	0.2	0	0.3	2.5	5.1	0	0.1	0	0.1
5-14	2	2.0	7	6.4	10.0	5.9	1	1.1	1	0.7
15-44	15	7.5	73	36.4	31.3	5.8	11	5.4	12	4.9
45-59	14	30.0	63	132.0	52.3	5.4	10	21.1	14	24.0
60+	5	17.9	38	126.4	68.9	4.0	7	22.9	9	24.8
All ages	37	8.4	180	41.0	43.6	5.4	29	6.6	36	7.1
Females										
0-4	0	0.2	0	0.4	2.5	5.0	0	0.1	0	0.1
5-14	3	3.0	9	9.6	10.0	5.9	2	1.8	1	1.0
15-44	21	11.3	100	54.5	31.3	5.8	15	8.2	14	6.0
45-59	21	44.9	91	198.5	52.3	5.5	15	31.6	16	28.7
60+	8	26.6	54	187.5	69.2	4.1	10	34.2	12	31.4
All ages	52	12.7	255	62.1	44.0	5.4	41	10.0	43	9.0
Total	89	10.4	435	51.2	43.9	5.4	70	8.2	80	8.0

For epidemiological sources see Michaud 1996. For the methods used to estimate and project incidence, prevalence, and deaths see Murray and Lopez 1996a. See explanatory notes for definitions and caveats.

Table 177
Rheumatic heart disease

Congestive heart failure

Cuadro 177
Cardiopatía reumática

Insuficiencia cardíaca congestiva

Tableau 177
Cardiopathie rhumatismale

Insuffisance cardiaque congestive

Table 177d China - China - Chine Rheumatic heart disease - Congestive heart failure

Age group (years)	Incidence 1990 Number ('000s)	Rate (per 100 000)	Prevalence 1990 Number ('000s)	Rate (per 100 000)	Avg. age at onset (years)	Average duration (years)	Deaths 1990 Number ('000s)	Rate (per 100 000)	Deaths 2000 (Projected) Number ('000s)	Rate (per 100 000)
Males										
0-4	0	0.0	0	0.0	-	-	0	0.0	0	0.0
5-14	2	2.0	6	6.5	10.0	6.7	1	0.7	0	0.4
15-44	26	8.3	138	44.9	30.7	6.6	17	5.5	15	4.6
45-59	20	28.0	99	136.7	52.3	5.9	13	17.5	20	21.0
60+	74	151.4	304	621.2	73.8	3.7	38	78.4	51	85.4
All ages	122	20.8	547	93.6	60.2	4.7	69	11.7	87	13.3
Females										
0-4	2	4.0	0	0.0	0.0	0.0	1	1.3	1	1.1
5-14	2	2.6	8	8.4	10.0	6.7	1	0.7	0	0.4
15-44	29	10.4	158	55.5	31.1	6.6	19	6.8	15	5.1
45-59	33	51.9	155	240.5	52.4	6.0	19	30.2	23	25.2
60+	91	176.9	407	788.1	74.4	3.9	54	104.0	66	102.3
All ages	159	29.0	727	132.6	59.7	4.9	94	17.1	105	16.8
Total	281	24.8	1 275	112.4	59.9	4.8	163	14.3	192	15.0

Table 177e OAI - OPAI - APAI Rheumatic heart disease - Congestive heart failure

Age group (years)	Incidence 1990 Number ('000s)	Rate (per 100 000)	Prevalence 1990 Number ('000s)	Rate (per 100 000)	Avg. age at onset (years)	Average duration (years)	Deaths 1990 Number ('000s)	Rate (per 100 000)	Deaths 2000 (Projected) Number ('000s)	Rate (per 100 000)
Males										
0-4	0	0.0	0	0.0	-	-	0	0.0	0	0.0
5-14	0	0.5	1	1.6	10.0	6.1	0	0.3	0	0.2
15-44	1	0.8	7	4.3	31.7	6.5	1	0.5	1	0.4
45-59	1	3.1	5	15.0	52.3	5.6	1	1.8	1	1.9
60+	7	34.3	27	132.6	73.8	3.7	3	15.0	4	15.7
All ages	10	2.8	40	11.7	63.2	4.4	5	1.3	6	1.5
Females										
0-4	0	0.0	0	0.0	-	-	0	0.0	0	0.0
5-14	1	0.8	2	2.4	10.0	6.1	0	0.4	0	0.2
15-44	2	1.2	11	6.6	32.3	6.6	1	0.6	1	0.5
45-59	1	4.2	7	21.1	52.3	5.9	1	2.4	1	2.0
60+	8	34.5	31	139.0	74.6	3.8	4	15.6	5	15.3
All ages	12	3.5	51	15.1	61.5	4.6	6	1.7	7	1.7
Total	21	3.1	92	13.4	62.3	4.5	10	1.5	13	1.6

Table 177f SSA - ASS - ASS Rheumatic heart disease - Congestive heart failure

Age group (years)	Incidence 1990 Number ('000s)	Rate (per 100 000)	Prevalence 1990 Number ('000s)	Rate (per 100 000)	Avg. age at onset (years)	Average duration (years)	Deaths 1990 Number ('000s)	Rate (per 100 000)	Deaths 2000 (Projected) Number ('000s)	Rate (per 100 000)
Males										
0-4	0	0.3	0	0.5	2.4	4.3	0	0.1	0	0.1
5-14	5	6.6	13	18.5	10.0	5.2	3	4.5	3	2.9
15-44	5	5.2	36	34.5	26.4	6.1	5	4.7	6	3.9
45-59	1	3.0	4	20.3	52.2	5.4	1	3.3	1	3.1
60+	0	3.0	2	18.1	69.2	3.9	0	3.3	0	3.3
All ages	11	4.4	55	21.8	21.9	5.6	9	3.6	10	2.8
Females										
0-4	0	0.5	0	0.8	2.4	4.4	0	0.1	0	0.1
5-14	7	9.9	19	27.8	10.0	5.3	4	6.9	4	4.1
15-44	8	7.8	55	51.6	26.5	6.1	4	3.7	4	2.6
45-59	1	4.5	7	30.5	52.2	5.5	1	5.0	1	4.3
60+	1	4.5	3	27.1	69.7	4.0	1	5.0	1	4.5
All ages	17	6.6	85	32.9	22.5	5.6	11	4.1	10	2.8
Total	28	5.5	140	27.4	22.2	5.6	20	3.8	19	2.8

For epidemiological sources see Michaud 1996. For the methods used to estimate and project incidence, prevalence, and deaths see Murray and Lopez 1996a. See explanatory notes for definitions and caveats.

Table 177
Rheumatic heart disease

Cuadro 177
Cardiopatía reumática

Tableau 177
Cardiopathie rhumatismale

Congestive heart failure

Insuficiencia cardíaca congestiva

Insuffisance cardiaque congestive

Table 177g LAC - ALC - ALC Rheumatic heart disease - Congestive heart failure

Age group (years)	Incidence 1990 Number ('000s)	Rate (per 100 000)	Prevalence 1990 Number ('000s)	Rate (per 100 000)	Avg. age at onset (years)	Average duration (years)	Deaths 1990 Number ('000s)	Rate (per 100 000)	Deaths 2000 (Projected) Number ('000s)	Rate (per 100 000)
Males										
0-4	0	0.2	0	0.3	2.5	5.1	0	0.1	0	0.1
5-14	1	1.6	3	5.3	10.0	6.7	0	0.7	0	0.5
15-44	2	1.7	11	10.6	30.0	6.5	1	0.8	1	0.8
45-59	1	3.9	4	20.1	52.3	5.9	1	2.8	1	2.8
60+	1	7.0	5	35.9	72.5	4.0	1	5.1	1	5.1
All ages	4	2.0	23	10.5	40.1	5.9	3	1.2	3	1.2
Females										
0-4	0	0.2	0	0.3	2.5	5.1	0	0.1	0	0.1
5-14	1	2.5	4	8.0	10.0	6.7	1	1.0	0	0.7
15-44	3	3.3	20	19.2	31.8	6.6	2	2.0	2	1.6
45-59	2	8.2	10	43.8	52.4	6.1	1	6.0	2	5.5
60+	2	10.6	10	60.1	72.5	4.3	1	8.9	2	8.2
All ages	8	3.8	44	19.9	41.9	6.0	6	2.5	6	2.3
Total	13	2.9	68	15.2	41.3	5.9	8	1.8	9	1.8

Table 177h MEC - AOM - CMO Rheumatic heart disease - Congestive heart failure

Age group (years)	Incidence 1990 Number ('000s)	Rate (per 100 000)	Prevalence 1990 Number ('000s)	Rate (per 100 000)	Avg. age at onset (years)	Average duration (years)	Deaths 1990 Number ('000s)	Rate (per 100 000)	Deaths 2000 (Projected) Number ('000s)	Rate (per 100 000)
Males										
0-4	0	0.3	0	0.6	2.5	5.1	0	0.1	0	0.1
5-14	5	8.4	16	25.0	10.0	5.9	3	4.3	3	3.0
15-44	7	6.6	52	46.1	27.0	6.6	6	5.5	7	4.8
45-59	1	4.1	6	29.0	52.3	5.9	1	4.1	1	4.2
60+	0	3.0	3	22.7	69.7	4.3	0	3.2	1	3.3
All ages	14	5.6	79	30.6	23.1	6.2	10	4.1	12	3.5
Females										
0-4	0	0.5	0	0.8	2.5	5.1	0	0.1	0	0.1
5-14	7	11.7	22	34.8	10.0	5.9	4	6.2	3	3.9
15-44	10	9.7	72	67.1	27.2	6.7	8	7.3	7	5.3
45-59	1	6.3	10	44.7	52.3	6.1	1	6.2	2	5.4
60+	1	4.5	5	34.2	70.4	4.4	1	4.9	1	4.4
All ages	20	8.1	109	44.2	24.0	6.2	14	5.6	13	4.1
Total	34	6.8	188	37.3	23.6	6.2	24	4.8	25	3.8

Table 177i World - Mundo - Monde Rheumatic heart disease - Congestive heart failure

Age group (years)	Incidence 1990 Number ('000s)	Rate (per 100 000)	Prevalence 1990 Number ('000s)	Rate (per 100 000)	Avg. age at onset (years)	Average duration (years)	Deaths 1990 Number ('000s)	Rate (per 100 000)	Deaths 2000 (Projected) Number ('000s)	Rate (per 100 000)
Males										
0-4	0	0.1	1	0.2	2.5	4.78	0	0.0	0	0.0
5-14	16	2.8	47	8.5	10.0	5.85	8	1.5	7	1.1
15-44	62	4.9	341	27.3	30.3	6.30	43	3.5	44	3.0
45-59	49	15.5	229	73.5	52.3	5.62	31	10.0	46	11.4
60+	99	45.1	437	199.4	73.3	3.80	58	26.3	76	27.6
All ages	225	8.5	1 054	39.7	52.5	5.02	141	5.3	173	5.6
Females										
0-4	3	0.9	1	0.3	0.4	0.87	1	0.3	1	0.2
5-14	21	4.1	64	12.3	10.0	5.84	12	2.3	9	1.5
15-44	78	6.5	433	36.1	30.4	6.33	51	4.3	45	3.2
45-59	75	24.2	346	111.3	52.4	5.82	46	14.8	52	13.0
60+	137	50.8	654	243.0	74.0	4.02	89	33.1	106	31.4
All ages	315	12.0	1 499	57.3	52.9	5.12	199	7.6	213	6.9
Total	540	10.2	2 553	48.5	52.7	5.08	340	6.5	385	6.3

For epidemiological sources see Michaud 1996. For the methods used to estimate and project incidence, prevalence, and deaths see Murray and Lopez 1996a. See explanatory notes for definitions and caveats.

Table 178
Ischaemic heart disease

Cuadro 178
Cardiopatía isquémica

Tableau 178
Cardiopathie ischémique

Acute myocardial infarction   Infarto agudo del miocardio   Infarctus aigu du myocarde

Table 178a   EME - PEMC - EMBE   Ischaemic heart disease - Acute myocardial infarction

Age group (years)	Incidence 1990 Number ('000s)	Rate (per 100 000)	Prevalence 1990 Number ('000s)	Rate (per 100 000)	Avg. age at onset (years)	Average duration (years)	Deaths 1990 Number ('000s)	Rate (per 100 000)	Deaths 2000 (Projected) Number ('000s)	Rate (per 100 000)
Males										
0-4	0	0	0	0.0	-	-	0	0.0	0	0.0
5-14	0	0	0	0.0	-	-	0	0.0	0	0.0
15-44	60	33	3	1.9	29.9	0.06	18	10.0	17	9.8
45-59	282	427	16	24.6	52.4	0.06	98	147.7	118	149.2
60+	857	1 415	49	81.6	71.1	0.06	713	1 177.8	804	1 113.7
All ages	1 199	307	69	17.7	64.6	0.06	829	212.4	940	228.8
Females										
0-4	0	0	0	0.0	-	-	0	0.0	0	0.0
5-14	0	0	0	0.0	-	-	0	0.0	0	0.0
15-44	17	10	1	0.6	30.0	0.06	5	2.7	4	2.5
45-59	78	115	5	6.6	52.4	0.06	29	42.1	25	30.3
60+	921	1 089	53	62.9	72.4	0.06	805	951.8	869	891.0
All ages	1 017	250	59	14.4	70.1	0.06	838	205.8	898	209.7
Total	2 216	278	128	16.0	67.2	0.06	1 668	209.0	1 838	219.0

Table 178b   FSE - PEAS - AESE   Ischaemic heart disease - Acute myocardial infarction

Age group (years)	Incidence 1990 Number ('000s)	Rate (per 100 000)	Prevalence 1990 Number ('000s)	Rate (per 100 000)	Avg. age at onset (years)	Average duration (years)	Deaths 1990 Number ('000s)	Rate (per 100 000)	Deaths 2000 (Projected) Number ('000s)	Rate (per 100 000)
Males										
0-4	0	0	0	0.0	-	-	0	0.0	0	0.0
5-14	0	0	0	0.0	-	-	0	0.0	0	0.0
15-44	61	79	3	4.6	29.8	0.06	24	31.1	21	28.4
45-59	243	902	14	52.0	52.2	0.06	99	365.6	127	405.7
60+	430	2 051	25	118.3	70.0	0.06	346	1 648.2	488	1 916.6
All ages	734	444	42	25.6	60.8	0.06	468	283.0	636	372.0
Females										
0-4	0	0	0	0.0	-	-	0	0.0	0	0.0
5-14	0	0	0	0.0	-	-	0	0.0	0	0.0
15-44	13	17	1	1.0	29.9	0.06	4	5.8	4	5.1
45-59	64	212	4	12.2	52.4	0.06	30	100.1	30	87.4
60+	641	1 760	37	101.6	71.5	0.06	525	1 441.8	645	1 566.3
All ages	717	396	41	22.9	69.1	0.06	559	309.1	678	363.0
Total	1 451	419	84	24.2	64.9	0.06	1 027	296.6	1 315	367.3

Table 178c   India - India - Inde   Ischaemic heart disease - Acute myocardial infarction

Age group (years)	Incidence 1990 Number ('000s)	Rate (per 100 000)	Prevalence 1990 Number ('000s)	Rate (per 100 000)	Avg. age at onset (years)	Average duration (years)	Deaths 1990 Number ('000s)	Rate (per 100 000)	Deaths 2000 (Projected) Number ('000s)	Rate (per 100 000)
Males										
0-4	0	0	0	0.0	-	-	0	0.0	0	0.0
5-14	0	0	0	0.0	-	-	0	0.0	0	0.0
15-44	41	21	2	1.2	29.8	0.06	13	6.7	17	7.0
45-59	267	561	15	32.4	52.3	0.06	111	233.1	159	266.0
60+	567	1 905	33	109.9	69.7	0.06	495	1 663.1	673	1 822.6
All ages	876	199	51	11.5	62.5	0.06	619	140.9	849	165.7
Females										
0-4	0	0	0	0.0	-	-	0	0.0	0	0.0
5-14	0	0	0	0.0	-	-	0	0.0	0	0.0
15-44	31	17	2	1.0	29.8	0.06	10	5.4	10	4.4
45-59	134	290	8	16.7	52.4	0.06	67	145.8	75	132.2
60+	543	1 878	31	108.3	70.1	0.06	479	1 655.5	657	1 689.1
All ages	708	173	41	10.0	65.0	0.06	556	135.5	743	153.7
Total	1 584	186	91	10.8	63.6	0.06	1 175	138.3	1 591	159.9

For epidemiological sources see Beaglehole et al. 1996. For the methods used to estimate and project incidence, prevalence, and deaths see Murray and Lopez 1996a. See explanatory notes for definitions and caveats.

Table 178
Ischaemic heart disease

Cuadro 178
Cardiopatía isquémica

Tableau 178
Cardiopathie ischémique

Acute myocardial infarction

Infarto agudo del miocardio

Infarctus aigu du myocarde

Table 178d   China - China - Chine   Ischaemic heart disease - Acute myocardial infarction

Age group (years)	Incidence 1990 Number ('000s)	Rate (per 100 000)	Prevalence 1990 Number ('000s)	Rate (per 100 000)	Avg. age at onset (years)	Average duration (years)	Deaths 1990 Number ('000s)	Rate (per 100 000)	Deaths 2000 (Projected) Number ('000s)	Rate (per 100 000)
Males										
0-4	0	0	0	0.0	-	-	0	0.0	0	0.0
5-14	0	0	0	0.0	-	-	0	0.0	0	0.0
15-44	50	16	3	0.9	29.9	0.06	21	6.7	23	7.2
45-59	133	183	8	10.5	52.3	0.06	53	72.5	85	86.9
60+	433	884	25	51.0	69.8	0.06	313	638.2	419	693.9
All ages	616	105	36	6.1	62.8	0.06	386	65.9	527	80.3
Females										
0-4	0	0	0	0.0	-	-	0	0.0	0	0.0
5-14	0	0	0	0.0	-	-	0	0.0	0	0.0
15-44	50	18	3	1.0	29.9	0.06	15	5.2	14	4.5
45-59	65	100	4	5.8	52.4	0.06	37	57.3	44	47.9
60+	383	742	22	42.8	70.6	0.06	325	628.7	409	635.3
All ages	498	91	29	5.2	64.1	0.06	377	68.7	467	74.7
Total	1 115	98	64	5.7	63.4	0.06	762	67.3	993	77.6

Table 178e   OAI - OPAI - APAI   Ischaemic heart disease - Acute myocardial infarction

Age group (years)	Incidence 1990 Number ('000s)	Rate (per 100 000)	Prevalence 1990 Number ('000s)	Rate (per 100 000)	Avg. age at onset (years)	Average duration (years)	Deaths 1990 Number ('000s)	Rate (per 100 000)	Deaths 2000 (Projected) Number ('000s)	Rate (per 100 000)
Males										
0-4	0	0	0	0.0	-	-	0	0.0	0	0.0
5-14	0	0	0	0.0	-	-	0	0.0	0	0.0
15-44	52	32	3	1.9	29.7	0.06	16	9.9	21	10.3
45-59	71	207	4	11.9	52.3	0.06	36	104.5	50	109.8
60+	239	1 183	14	68.3	69.6	0.06	182	898.6	259	935.2
All ages	362	106	21	6.1	60.5	0.06	233	68.0	331	81.7
Females										
0-4	0	0	0	0.0	-	-	0	0.0	0	0.0
5-14	0	0	0	0.0	-	-	0	0.0	0	0.0
15-44	38	24	2	1.4	29.8	0.06	10	6.4	11	5.7
45-59	36	102	2	5.9	52.3	0.06	24	69.0	27	56.7
60+	231	1 019	13	58.8	70.3	0.06	193	851.5	274	843.7
All ages	305	90	18	5.2	63.2	0.06	227	67.0	312	77.5
Total	667	98	38	5.6	61.7	0.06	461	67.5	643	79.6

Table 178f   SSA - ASS - ASS   Ischaemic heart disease - Acute myocardial infarction

Age group (years)	Incidence 1990 Number ('000s)	Rate (per 100 000)	Prevalence 1990 Number ('000s)	Rate (per 100 000)	Avg. age at onset (years)	Average duration (years)	Deaths 1990 Number ('000s)	Rate (per 100 000)	Deaths 2000 (Projected) Number ('000s)	Rate (per 100 000)
Males										
0-4	0	0	0	0.0	-	-	0	0.0	0	0.0
5-14	0	0	0	0.0	-	-	0	0.0	0	0.0
15-44	33	31	2	1.8	29.4	0.06	11	11.0	15	10.2
45-59	40	197	2	11.4	52.2	0.06	22	107.0	27	100.7
60+	73	692	4	39.9	69.2	0.06	59	561.6	83	575.1
All ages	145	58	8	3.3	55.6	0.06	92	36.5	124	36.2
Females										
0-4	0	0	0	0.0	-	-	0	0.0	0	0.0
5-14	0	0	0	0.0	-	-	0	0.0	0	0.0
15-44	30	28	2	1.6	29.5	0.06	5	4.8	5	3.8
45-59	34	153	2	8.9	52.2	0.06	23	103.8	26	89.0
60+	95	747	5	43.1	69.7	0.06	85	664.3	113	644.6
All ages	159	62	9	3.6	58.4	0.06	117	45.3	149	42.8
Total	304	60	18	3.4	57.0	0.06	209	40.9	273	39.5

For epidemiological sources see Beaglehole et al. 1996. For the methods used to estimate and project incidence, prevalence, and deaths see Murray and Lopez 1996a. See explanatory notes for definitions and caveats.

Table 178
Ischaemic heart disease

Cuadro 178
Cardiopatía isquémica

Tableau 178
Cardiopathie ischémique

Acute myocardial infarction

Infarto agudo del miocardio

Infarctus aigu du myocarde

Table 178g LAC - ALC - ALC — Ischaemic heart disease - Acute myocardial infarction

Age group (years)	Incidence 1990 Number ('000s)	Rate (per 100 000)	Prevalence 1990 Number ('000s)	Rate (per 100 000)	Avg. age at onset (years)	Average duration (years)	Deaths 1990 Number ('000s)	Rate (per 100 000)	Deaths 2000 (Projected) Number ('000s)	Rate (per 100 000)
Males										
0-4	0	0	0	0.0	-	-	0	0.0	0	0.0
5-14	0	0	0	0.0	-	-	0	0.0	0	0.0
15-44	34	33	2	1.9	29.8	0.06	11	10.4	14	10.7
45-59	78	352	5	20.3	52.3	0.06	34	153.5	47	153.1
60+	165	1 158	10	66.8	70.3	0.06	134	942.2	191	967.6
All ages	277	125	16	7.2	60.2	0.06	179	80.8	252	94.8
Females										
0-4	0	0	0	0.0	-	-	0	0.0	0	0.0
5-14	0	0	0	0.0	-	-	0	0.0	0	0.0
15-44	30	29	2	1.7	29.9	0.06	9	8.3	9	7.3
45-59	38	163	2	9.4	52.4	0.06	22	95.5	28	87.3
60+	163	967	9	55.8	71.1	0.06	138	820.3	195	828.6
All ages	231	104	13	6.0	62.6	0.06	169	75.8	233	87.0
Total	508	114	29	6.6	61.3	0.06	348	78.3	484	90.9

Table 178h MEC - AOM - CMO — Ischaemic heart disease - Acute myocardial infarction

Age group (years)	Incidence 1990 Number ('000s)	Rate (per 100 000)	Prevalence 1990 Number ('000s)	Rate (per 100 000)	Avg. age at onset (years)	Average duration (years)	Deaths 1990 Number ('000s)	Rate (per 100 000)	Deaths 2000 (Projected) Number ('000s)	Rate (per 100 000)
Males										
0-4	0	0	0	0.0	-	-	0	0	0	0
5-14	0	0	0	0.0	-	-	0	0	0	0
15-44	59	52	3	3.0	29.8	0.06	22	19	28	19
45-59	117	526	7	30.3	52.3	0.06	59	266	86	271
60+	287	2 100	17	121.1	69.7	0.06	238	1 745	348	1 868
All ages	464	181	27	10.4	60.2	0.06	319	124	462	139
Females										
0-4	0	0	0	0.0	-	-	0	0	0	0
5-14	0	0	0	0.0	-	-	0	0	0	0
15-44	39	37	2	2.1	29.8	0.06	15	14	16	11
45-59	59	265	3	15.3	52.3	0.06	34	154	42	135
60+	274	1 774	16	102.3	70.4	0.06	242	1 565	343	1604
All ages	373	151	21	8.7	63.2	0.06	291	118	401	124
Total	836	166	48	9.6	61.5	0.06	610	121	863	132

Table 178i World - Mundo - Monde — Ischaemic heart disease - Acute myocardial infarction

Age group (years)	Incidence 1990 Number ('000s)	Rate (per 100 000)	Prevalence 1990 Number ('000s)	Rate (per 100 000)	Avg. age at onset (years)	Average duration (years)	Deaths 1990 Number ('000s)	Rate (per 100 000)	Deaths 2000 (Projected) Number ('000s)	Rate (per 100 000)
Males										
0-4	0	0	0	0.0	-	-	0	0.0	0	0.0
5-14	0	0	0	0.0	-	-	0	0.0	0	0.0
15-44	391	31	23	1.8	29.8	0.06	136	10.9	156	10.8
45-59	1 232	394	71	22.7	52.3	0.06	511	163.5	699	173.5
60+	3 050	1 394	176	80.4	70.2	0.06	2 479	1 132.8	3 265	1 185.4
All ages	4 673	176	270	10.2	62.1	0.06	3 126	117.8	4 120	133.1
Females										
0-4	0	0	0	0.0	-	-	0	0.0	0	0.0
5-14	0	0	0	0.0	-	-	0	0.0	0	0.0
15-44	249	21	14	1.2	29.8	0.06	73	6.1	73	5.3
45-59	507	163	29	9.4	52.4	0.06	266	85.7	296	73.5
60+	3 251	1 208	188	69.7	71.2	0.06	2 791	1 036.6	3 506	1 040.3
All ages	4 007	153	231	8.8	66.2	0.06	3 134	119.9	3 881	126.7
Total	8 680	165	501	9.5	64.0	0.06	6 260	118.8	8 000	129.9

For epidemiological sources see Beaglehole et al. 1996. For the methods used to estimate and project incidence, prevalence, and deaths see Murray and Lopez 1996a. See explanatory notes for definitions and caveats.

Table 179
Ischaemic heart disease

Cuadro 179
Cardiopatía isquémica

Tableau 179
Cardiopathie ischémique

Angina pectoris

Angina de pecho

Angine de poitrine

Table 179a   EME - PEMC - EMBE   Ischaemic heart disease - Angina pectoris

Age group (years)	Incidence 1990 Number ('000s)	Rate (per 100 000)	Prevalence 1990 Number ('000s)	Rate (per 100 000)	Avg. age at onset (years)	Average duration (years)	Deaths 1990 Number ('000s)	Rate (per 100 000)	Deaths 2000 (Projected) Number ('000s)	Rate (per 100 000)
Males										
0-4	-	-	0	0	-	-	0	0	0	0
5-14	-	-	0	0	-	-	0	0	0	0
15-44	-	-	136	74	-	-	0	0	0	0
45-59	-	-	1 369	2 070	-	-	0	0	0	0
60+	-	-	4 170	6 887	-	-	0	0	0	0
All ages	-	-	5 675	1 453	-	-	0	0	0	0
Females										
0-4	-	-	0	0	-	-	0	0	0	0
5-14	-	-	0	0	-	-	0	0	0	0
15-44	-	-	43	24	-	-	0	0	0	0
45-59	-	-	325	479	-	-	0	0	0	0
60+	-	-	2 140	2 531	-	-	0	0	0	0
All ages	-	-	2 508	616	-	-	0	0	0	0
Total	-	-	8 183	1 026	-	-	0	0	0	0

Table 179b   FSE - PEAS - AESE   Ischaemic heart disease - Angina pectoris

Age group (years)	Incidence 1990 Number ('000s)	Rate (per 100 000)	Prevalence 1990 Number ('000s)	Rate (per 100 000)	Avg. age at onset (years)	Average duration (years)	Deaths 1990 Number ('000s)	Rate (per 100 000)	Deaths 2000 (Projected) Number ('000s)	Rate (per 100 000)
Males										
0-4	-	-	0	0	-	-	0	0	0	0
5-14	-	-	0	0	-	-	0	0	0	0
15-44	-	-	171	224	-	-	0	0	0	0
45-59	-	-	1 376	5 102	-	-	0	0	0	0
60+	-	-	2 309	11 014	-	-	0	0	0	0
All ages	-	-	3 856	2 333	-	-	0	0	0	0
Females										
0-4	-	-	0	0	-	-	0	0	0	0
5-14	-	-	0	0	-	-	0	0	0	0
15-44	-	-	33	45	-	-	0	0	0	0
45-59	-	-	342	1 141	-	-	0	0	0	0
60+	-	-	1 593	4 376	-	-	0	0	0	0
All ages	-	-	1 968	1 088	-	-	0	0	0	0
Total	-	-	5 824	1 682	-	-	0	0	0	0

Table 179c   India - India - Inde   Ischaemic heart disease - Angina pectoris

Age group (years)	Incidence 1990 Number ('000s)	Rate (per 100 000)	Prevalence 1990 Number ('000s)	Rate (per 100 000)	Avg. age at onset (years)	Average duration (years)	Deaths 1990 Number ('000s)	Rate (per 100 000)	Deaths 2000 (Projected) Number ('000s)	Rate (per 100 000)
Males										
0-4	-	-	0	0	-	-	0	0	0	0
5-14	-	-	0	0	-	-	0	0	0	0
15-44	-	-	107	54	-	-	0	0	0	0
45-59	-	-	1 287	2 705	-	-	0	0	0	0
60+	-	-	2 862	9 616	-	-	0	0	0	0
All ages	-	-	4 257	969	-	-	0	0	0	0
Females										
0-4	-	-	0	0	-	-	0	0	0	0
5-14	-	-	0	0	-	-	0	0	0	0
15-44	-	-	77	42	-	-	0	0	0	0
45-59	-	-	638	1 386	-	-	0	0	0	0
60+	-	-	1 639	5 665	-	-	0	0	0	0
All ages	-	-	2 353	574	-	-	0	0	0	0
Total	-	-	6 610	778	-	-	0	0	0	0

For epidemiological sources see Beaglehole et al. 1996. For the methods used to estimate and project incidence, prevalence, and deaths see Murray and Lopez 1996a. See explanatory notes for definitions and caveats.

Table 179　　　　　　　　　　　　　**Cuadro 179**　　　　　　　　　　　　　**Tableau 179**
Ischaemic heart disease　　　　　　**Cardiopatía isquémica**　　　　　　**Cardiopathie ischémique**

Angina pectoris　　　　　　　　　　　　Angina de pecho　　　　　　　　　　　　Angine de poitrine

Table 179d　　　China - China - Chine　　　　　　　　Ischaemic heart disease - Angina pectoris

Age group (years)	Incidence 1990 Number ('000s)	Rate (per 100 000)	Prevalence 1990 Number ('000s)	Rate (per 100 000)	Avg. age at onset (years)	Average duration (years)	Deaths 1990 Number ('000s)	Rate (per 100 000)	Deaths 2000 (Projected) Number ('000s)	Rate (per 100 000)
Males										
0-4	-	-	0	0	-	-	0	0	0	0
5-14	-	-	0	0	-	-	0	0	0	0
15-44	-	-	198	65	-	-	0	0	0	0
45-59	-	-	734	1 010	-	-	0	0	0	0
60+	-	-	1 955	3 991	-	-	0	0	0	0
All ages	-	-	2 887	493	-	-	0	0	0	0
Females										
0-4	-	-	0	0	-	-	0	0	0	0
5-14	-	-	0	0	-	-	0	0	0	0
15-44	-	-	129	46	-	-	0	0	0	0
45-59	-	-	419	651	-	-	0	0	0	0
60+	-	-	1 066	2 064	-	-	0	0	0	0
All ages	-	-	1 615	294	-	-	0	0	0	0
Total	-	-	4 502	397	-	-	0	0	0	0

Table 179e　　　OAI - OPAI - APAI　　　　　　　　Ischaemic heart disease - Angina pectoris

Age group (years)	Incidence 1990 Number ('000s)	Rate (per 100 000)	Prevalence 1990 Number ('000s)	Rate (per 100 000)	Avg. age at onset (years)	Average duration (years)	Deaths 1990 Number ('000s)	Rate (per 100 000)	Deaths 2000 (Projected) Number ('000s)	Rate (per 100 000)
Males										
0-4	-	-	0	0	-	-	0	0	0	0
5-14	-	-	0	0	-	-	0	0	0	0
15-44	-	-	128	80	-	-	0	0	0	0
45-59	-	-	432	1 264	-	-	0	0	0	0
60+	-	-	973	4 814	-	-	0	0	0	0
All ages	-	-	1 533	447	-	-	0	0	0	0
Females										
0-4	-	-	0	0	-	-	0	0	0	0
5-14	-	-	0	0	-	-	0	0	0	0
15-44	-	-	93	58	-	-	0	0	0	0
45-59	-	-	234	668	-	-	0	0	0	0
60+	-	-	562	2 482	-	-	0	0	0	0
All ages	-	-	889	262	-	-	0	0	0	0
Total	-	-	2 422	355	-	-	0	0	0	0

Table 179f　　　SSA - ASS - ASS　　　　　　　　Ischaemic heart disease - Angina pectoris

Age group (years)	Incidence 1990 Number ('000s)	Rate (per 100 000)	Prevalence 1990 Number ('000s)	Rate (per 100 000)	Avg. age at onset (years)	Average duration (years)	Deaths 1990 Number ('000s)	Rate (per 100 000)	Deaths 2000 (Projected) Number ('000s)	Rate (per 100 000)
Males										
0-4	-	-	0	0	-	-	0	0	0	0
5-14	-	-	0	0	-	-	0	0	0	0
15-44	-	-	81	78	-	-	0	0	0	0
45-59	-	-	231	1 137	-	-	0	0	0	0
60+	-	-	302	2 877	-	-	0	0	0	0
All ages	-	-	615	244	-	-	0	0	0	0
Females										
0-4	-	-	0	0	-	-	0	0	0	0
5-14	-	-	0	0	-	-	0	0	0	0
15-44	-	-	71	67	-	-	0	0	0	0
45-59	-	-	195	880	-	-	0	0	0	0
60+	-	-	257	2 018	-	-	0	0	0	0
All ages	-	-	522	202	-	-	0	0	0	0
Total	-	-	1 137	223	-	-	0	0	0	0

For epidemiological sources see Beaglehole et al. 1996. For the methods used to estimate and project incidence, prevalence, and deaths see Murray and Lopez 1996a. See explanatory notes for definitions and caveats.

Table 179
Ischaemic heart disease

Cuadro 179
Cardiopatía isquémica

Tableau 179
Cardiopathie ischémique

Angina pectoris

Angina de pecho

Angine de poitrine

Table 179g   LAC - ALC - ALC   Ischaemic heart disease - Angina pectoris

Age group (years)	Incidence 1990 Number ('000s)	Rate (per 100 000)	Prevalence 1990 Number ('000s)	Rate (per 100 000)	Avg. age at onset (years)	Average duration (years)	Deaths 1990 Number ('000s)	Rate (per 100 000)	Deaths 2000 (Projected) Number ('000s)	Rate (per 100 000)
Males										
0-4	-	-	0	0	-	-	0	0	0	0
5-14	-	-	0	0	-	-	0	0	0	0
15-44	-	-	91	88	-	-	0	0	0	0
45-59	-	-	435	1 955	-	-	0	0	0	0
60+	-	-	767	5 391	-	-	0	0	0	0
All ages	-	-	1 293	584	-	-	0	0	0	0
Females										
0-4	-	-	0	0	-	-	0	0	0	0
5-14	-	-	0	0	-	-	0	0	0	0
15-44	-	-	75	72	-	-	0	0	0	0
45-59	-	-	234	1 002	-	-	0	0	0	0
60+	-	-	419	2 488	-	-	0	0	0	0
All ages	-	-	727	327	-	-	0	0	0	0
Total	-	-	2 021	455	-	-	0	0	0	0

Table 179h   MEC - AOM - CMO   Ischaemic heart disease - Angina pectoris

Age group (years)	Incidence 1990 Number ('000s)	Rate (per 100 000)	Prevalence 1990 Number ('000s)	Rate (per 100 000)	Avg. age at onset (years)	Average duration (years)	Deaths 1990 Number ('000s)	Rate (per 100 000)	Deaths 2000 (Projected) Number ('000s)	Rate (per 100 000)
Males										
0-4	-	-	0	0	-	-	0	0	0	0
5-14	-	-	0	0	-	-	0	0	0	0
15-44	-	-	176	155	-	-	0	0	0	0
45-59	-	-	666	2 983	-	-	0	0	0	0
60+	-	-	1 207	8 840	-	-	0	0	0	0
All ages	-	-	2 049	799	-	-	0	0	0	0
Females										
0-4	-	-	0	0	-	-	0	0	0	0
5-14	-	-	0	0	-	-	0	0	0	0
15-44	-	-	98	92	-	-	0	0	0	0
45-59	-	-	347	1 555	-	-	0	0	0	0
60+	-	-	764	4 945	-	-	0	0	0	0
All ages	-	-	1 209	490	-	-	0	0	0	0
Total	-	-	3 258	648	-	-	0	0	0	0

Table 179i   World - Mundo - Monde   Ischaemic heart disease - Angina pectoris

Age group (years)	Incidence 1990 Number ('000s)	Rate (per 100 000)	Prevalence 1990 Number ('000s)	Rate (per 100 000)	Avg. age at onset (years)	Average duration (years)	Deaths 1990 Number ('000s)	Rate (per 100 000)	Deaths 2000 (Projected) Number ('000s)	Rate (per 100 000)
Males										
0-4	-	-	0	0	-	-	0	0	0	0
5-14	-	-	0	0	-	-	0	0	0	0
15-44	-	-	1 089	87	-	-	0	0	0	0
45-59	-	-	6 530	2 090	-	-	0	0	0	0
60+	-	-	14 545	6 646	-	-	0	0	0	0
All ages	-	-	22 164	835	-	-	0	0	0	0
Females										
0-4	-	-	0	0	-	-	0	0	0	0
5-14	-	-	0	0	-	-	0	0	0	0
15-44	-	-	619	52	-	-	0	0	0	0
45-59	-	-	2 734	879	-	-	0	0	0	0
60+	-	-	8 439	3 135	-	-	0	0	0	0
All ages	-	-	11 792	451	-	-	0	0	0	0
Total	-	-	33 957	645	-	-	0	0	0	0

For epidemiological sources see Beaglehole et al. 1996. For the methods used to estimate and project incidence, prevalence, and deaths see Murray and Lopez 1996a. See explanatory notes for definitions and caveats.

Table 180 — Cuadro 180 — Tableau 180
Ischaemic heart disease — Cardiopatía isquémica — Cardiopathie ischémique

Congestive heart failure — Insuficiencia cardíaca congestiva — Insuffisance cardiaque congestive

Table 180a EME - PEMC - EMBE — Ischaemic heart disease - Congestive heart failure

Age group (years)	Incidence 1990 Number ('000s)	Rate (per 100 000)	Prevalence 1990 Number ('000s)	Rate (per 100 000)	Avg. age at onset (years)	Average duration (years)	Deaths 1990 Number ('000s)	Rate (per 100 000)	Deaths 2000 (Projected) Number ('000s)	Rate (per 100 000)
Males										
0-4	0	0.0	0	0.0	-	-	-	-	-	-
5-14	0	0.0	0	0.0	-	-	-	-	-	-
15-44	9	4.9	53	28.6	29.9	6.9	-	-	-	-
45-59	42	63.8	193	292.2	52.4	5.0	-	-	-	-
60+	128	211.1	313	517.7	71.1	2.1	-	-	-	-
All ages	179	45.8	559	143.3	64.6	3.0	-	-	-	-
Females										
0-4	0	0.0	0	0.0	-	-	-	-	-	-
5-14	0	0.0	0	0.0	-	-	-	-	-	-
15-44	3	1.4	14	7.7	30.0	6.8	-	-	-	-
45-59	12	17.3	47	68.9	52.5	4.2	-	-	-	-
60+	138	163.0	173	205.0	72.4	1.2	-	-	-	-
All ages	152	37.3	234	57.4	70.2	1.5	-	-	-	-
Total	331	41.5	793	99.4	67.2	2.3	-	-	-	-

Table 180b FSE - PEAS - AESE — Ischaemic heart disease - Congestive heart failure

Age group (years)	Incidence 1990 Number ('000s)	Rate (per 100 000)	Prevalence 1990 Number ('000s)	Rate (per 100 000)	Avg. age at onset (years)	Average duration (years)	Deaths 1990 Number ('000s)	Rate (per 100 000)	Deaths 2000 (Projected) Number ('000s)	Rate (per 100 000)
Males										
0-4	0	0.0	0	0	-	-	-	-	-	-
5-14	0	0.0	0	0	-	-	-	-	-	-
15-44	9	11.9	51	67	29.8	7.0	-	-	-	-
45-59	36	134.6	165	611	52.2	5.1	-	-	-	-
60+	64	306.7	175	833	69.8	2.3	-	-	-	-
All ages	110	66.3	390	236	60.7	3.6	-	-	-	-
Females										
0-4	0	0.0	0	0	-	-	-	-	-	-
5-14	0	0.0	0	0	-	-	-	-	-	-
15-44	2	2.6	13	17	30.0	8.4	-	-	-	-
45-59	10	31.8	47	157	52.4	5.2	-	-	-	-
60+	96	263.9	157	432	71.4	1.6	-	-	-	-
All ages	108	59.4	217	120	69.0	2.0	-	-	-	-
Total	217	62.7	607	175	64.8	2.8	-	-	-	-

Table 180c India - India - Inde — Ischaemic heart disease - Congestive heart failure

Age group (years)	Incidence 1990 Number ('000s)	Rate (per 100 000)	Prevalence 1990 Number ('000s)	Rate (per 100 000)	Avg. age at onset (years)	Average duration (years)	Deaths 1990 Number ('000s)	Rate (per 100 000)	Deaths 2000 (Projected) Number ('000s)	Rate (per 100 000)
Males										
0-4	0	0.0	0	0	-	-	-	-	-	-
5-14	0	0.0	0	0	-	-	-	-	-	-
15-44	6	3.1	32	16	29.8	6.4	-	-	-	-
45-59	40	84.0	166	350	52.3	4.8	-	-	-	-
60+	85	285.6	188	632	69.5	2.0	-	-	-	-
All ages	131	29.9	387	88	62.4	3.0	-	-	-	-
Females										
0-4	0	0.0	0	0	-	-	-	-	-	-
5-14	0	0.0	0	0	-	-	-	-	-	-
15-44	5	2.6	28	15	29.8	7.3	-	-	-	-
45-59	20	43.5	85	184	52.4	4.6	-	-	-	-
60+	82	281.9	133	459	69.9	1.5	-	-	-	-
All ages	106	25.9	245	60	64.8	2.4	-	-	-	-
Total	237	27.9	632	74	63.5	2.7	-	-	-	-

For epidemiological sources see Beaglehole et al. 1996. For the methods used to estimate and project incidence, prevalence, and deaths see Murray and Lopez 1996a. See explanatory notes for definitions and caveats.

Table 180
Ischaemic heart disease

Cuadro 180
Cardiopatía isquémica

Tableau 180
Cardiopathie ischémique

Congestive heart failure

Insuficiencia cardíaca congestiva

Insuffisance cardiaque congestive

Table 180d China - China - Chine — Ischaemic heart disease - Congestive heart failure

Age group (years)	Incidence 1990 Number ('000s)	Rate (per 100 000)	Prevalence 1990 Number ('000s)	Rate (per 100 000)	Avg. age at onset (years)	Average duration (years)	Deaths 1990 Number ('000s)	Rate (per 100 000)	Deaths 2000 (Projected) Number ('000s)	Rate (per 100 000)
Males										
0-4	0	0.0	0	0	-	-	-	-	-	-
5-14	0	0.0	0	0	-	-	-	-	-	-
15-44	8	2.5	43	14	29.9	7.3	-	-	-	-
45-59	20	27.4	94	129	52.4	5.2	-	-	-	-
60+	65	133.0	145	296	69.7	2.0	-	-	-	-
All ages	93	15.8	282	48	62.7	3.2	-	-	-	-
Females										
0-4	0	0.0	0	0	-	-	-	-	-	-
5-14	0	0.0	0	0	-	-	-	-	-	-
15-44	8	2.7	49	17	29.9	8.3	-	-	-	-
45-59	10	15.0	50	78	52.4	5.1	-	-	-	-
60+	58	111.6	98	189	70.6	1.6	-	-	-	-
All ages	75	13.7	196	36	64.1	2.7	-	-	-	-
Total	168	14.8	479	42	63.4	3.0	-	-	-	-

Table 180e OAI - OPAI - APAI — Ischaemic heart disease - Congestive heart failure

Age group (years)	Incidence 1990 Number ('000s)	Rate (per 100 000)	Prevalence 1990 Number ('000s)	Rate (per 100 000)	Avg. age at onset (years)	Average duration (years)	Deaths 1990 Number ('000s)	Rate (per 100 000)	Deaths 2000 (Projected) Number ('000s)	Rate (per 100 000)
Males										
0-4	0	0.0	0	0	-	-	-	-	-	-
5-14	0	0.0	0	0	-	-	-	-	-	-
15-44	8	4.9	41	26	29.8	6.5	-	-	-	-
45-59	11	31.0	49	143	52.3	4.7	-	-	-	-
60+	36	178.0	62	308	69.5	1.6	-	-	-	-
All ages	54	15.9	152	44	60.4	2.9	-	-	-	-
Females										
0-4	0	0.0	0	0	-	-	-	-	-	-
5-14	0	0.0	0	0	-	-	-	-	-	-
15-44	6	3.5	34	21	29.8	7.4	-	-	-	-
45-59	5	15.3	26	75	52.4	4.6	-	-	-	-
60+	35	153.0	49	216	70.2	1.4	-	-	-	-
All ages	46	13.5	109	32	63.1	2.5	-	-	-	-
Total	100	14.7	261	38	61.7	2.7	-	-	-	-

Table 180f SSA - ASS - ASS — Ischaemic heart disease - Congestive heart failure

Age group (years)	Incidence 1990 Number ('000s)	Hate (per 100 000)	Prevalence 1990 Number ('000s)	Rate (per 100 000)	Avg. age at onset (years)	Average duration (years)	Deaths 1990 Number ('000s)	Rate (per 100 000)	Deaths 2000 (Projected) Number ('000s)	Rate (per 100 000)
Males										
0-4	0	0.0	0	0	-	-	-	-	-	-
5-14	0	0.0	0	0	-	-	-	-	-	-
15-44	5	4.7	23	23	29.4	5.7	-	-	-	-
45-59	6	29.6	25	121	52.2	4.2	-	-	-	-
60+	11	104.2	21	199	69.2	1.7	-	-	-	-
All ages	22	8.7	69	27	55.6	3.3	-	-	-	-
Females										
0-4	0	0.0	0	0	-	-	-	-	-	-
5-14	0	0.0	0	0	-	-	-	-	-	-
15-44	5	4.2	25	23	29.5	6.6	-	-	-	-
45-59	5	23.0	22	98	52.3	4.1	-	-	-	-
60+	14	112.6	20	158	69.7	1.3	-	-	-	-
All ages	24	9.3	67	26	58.4	2.9	-	-	-	-
Total	46	9.0	136	27	57.1	3.1	-	-	-	-

For epidemiological sources see Beaglehole et al. 1996. For the methods used to estimate and project incidence, prevalence, and deaths see Murray and Lopez 1996a. See explanatory notes for definitions and caveats.

Table 180   **Cuadro 180**   **Tableau 180**
Ischaemic heart disease   **Cardiopatía isquémica**   **Cardiopathie ischémique**

Congestive heart failure   Insuficiencia cardíaca congestiva   Insuffisance cardiaque congestive

Table 180g   LAC - ALC - ALC   Ischaemic heart disease - Congestive heart failure

Age group (years)	Incidence 1990 Number ('000s)	Rate (per 100 000)	Prevalence 1990 Number ('000s)	Rate (per 100 000)	Avg. age at onset (years)	Average duration (years)	Deaths 1990 Number ('000s)	Rate (per 100 000)	Deaths 2000 (Projected) Number ('000s)	Rate (per 100 000)
Males										
0-4	0	0.0	0	0	-	-	-	-	-	-
5-14	0	0.0	0	0	-	-	-	-	-	-
15-44	5	4.9	28	27	29.8	6.9	-	-	-	-
45-59	12	52.7	53	239	52.4	5.0	-	-	-	-
60+	25	173.8	56	393	70.2	2.0	-	-	-	-
All ages	42	18.8	137	62	60.2	3.5	-	-	-	-
Females										
0-4	0	0.0	0	0	-	-	-	-	-	-
5-14	0	0.0	0	0	-	-	-	-	-	-
15-44	5	4.3	28	27	29.9	7.8	-	-	-	-
45-59	6	24.4	28	122	52.4	4.9	-	-	-	-
60+	24	145.3	39	233	71.0	1.5	-	-	-	-
All ages	35	15.6	95	43	62.6	2.9	-	-	-	-
Total	76	17.2	233	52	61.3	3.2	-	-	-	-

Table 180h   MEC - AOM - CMO   Ischaemic heart disease - Congestive heart failure

Age group (years)	Incidence 1990 Number ('000s)	Rate (per 100 000)	Prevalence 1990 Number ('000s)	Rate (per 100 000)	Avg. age at onset (years)	Average duration (years)	Deaths 1990 Number ('000s)	Rate (per 100 000)	Deaths 2000 (Projected) Number ('000s)	Rate (per 100 000)
Males										
0-4	0	0.0	0	0	-	-	-	-	-	-
5-14	0	0.0	0	0	-	-	-	-	-	-
15-44	9	7.8	46	41	29.9	6.4	-	-	-	-
45-59	18	78.9	76	339	52.3	4.6	-	-	-	-
60+	44	321.1	86	630	69.6	1.8	-	-	-	-
All ages	70	27.4	208	81	60.2	3.1	-	-	-	-
Females										
0-4	0	0.0	0	0	-	-	-	-	-	-
5-14	0	0.0	0	0	-	-	-	-	-	-
15-44	6	5.5	35	33	29.9	7.4	-	-	-	-
45-59	9	39.8	40	181	52.4	4.6	-	-	-	-
60+	41	267.9	58	378	70.3	1.3	-	-	-	-
All ages	56	22.8	134	54	63.2	2.5	-	-	-	-
Total	127	25.2	342	68	61.6	2.8	-	-	-	-

Table 180i   World - Mundo - Monde   Ischaemic heart disease - Congestive heart failure

Age group (years)	Incidence 1990 Number ('000s)	Rate (per 100 000)	Prevalence 1990 Number ('000s)	Rate (per 100 000)	Avg. age at onset (years)	Average duration (years)	Deaths 1990 Number ('000s)	Rate (per 100 000)	Deaths 2000 (Projected) Number ('000s)	Rate (per 100 000)
Males										
0-4	0	0.0	0	0.0	-	-	-	-	-	-
5-14	0	0.0	0	0.0	-	-	-	-	-	-
15-44	59	4.7	319	25.5	29.8	6.7	-	-	-	-
45-59	184	59.0	821	262.7	52.3	4.9	-	-	-	-
60+	458	209.1	1 046	478.0	70.1	2.0	-	-	-	-
All ages	701	26.4	2 185	82.3	61.4	3.1	-	-	-	-
Females										
0-4	0	0.0	0	0.0	-	-	-	-	-	-
5-14	0	0.0	0	0.0	-	-	-	-	-	-
15-44	37	3.1	224	18.7	29.9	7.5	-	-	-	-
45-59	76	24.4	346	111.1	52.4	4.7	-	-	-	-
60+	488	181.3	727	270.2	71.1	1.4	-	-	-	-
All ages	601	23.0	1 297	49.6	64.6	2.4	-	-	-	-
Total	1 302	24.7	3 482	66.1	62.9	2.8	-	-	-	-

For epidemiological sources see Beaglehole et al. 1996. For the methods used to estimate and project incidence, prevalence, and deaths see Murray and Lopez 1996a. See explanatory notes for definitions and caveats.

Table 181
Cerebrovascular disease

First-ever stroke

Cuadro 181
Enfermedad cerebrovascular

Primer accidente cerebrovascular

Tableau 181
Maladie cérébrovasculaire

Premier accident vasculaire cérébral

Table 181a   EME - PEMC - EMBE   Cerebrovascular disease - First-ever stroke

Age group (years)	Incidence 1990 Number ('000s)	Rate (per 100 000)	Prevalence 1990 Number ('000s)	Rate (per 100 000)	Avg. age at onset (years)	Average duration (years)	Deaths 1990 Number ('000s)	Rate (per 100 000)	Deaths 2000 (Projected) Number ('000s)	Rate (per 100 000)
Males										
0-4	0	1.1	0	0	2.5	0.0	0	1.1	0	1.0
5-14	0	0.3	0	0	10.0	0.0	0	0.3	0	0.3
15-44	37	19.9	483	262	29.9	27.5	8	4.1	7	3.9
45-59	79	119.6	780	1 179	52.4	14.5	24	36.9	29	37.2
60+	465	767.4	3 259	5 382	73.5	5.6	289	477.6	331	458.3
All ages	581	148.8	4 521	1 158	67.8	8.2	322	82.3	368	89.5
Females										
0-4	0	0.8	0	0	2.5	0.0	0	0.8	0	0.7
5-14	0	0.2	0	0	10.0	0.0	0	0.2	0	0.2
15-44	29	16.0	389	217	30.0	31.5	5	3.0	5	2.7
45-59	69	101.9	708	1 044	52.4	17.3	15	22.7	14	16.8
60+	603	712.9	3 849	4 551	76.3	5.1	446	526.9	484	496.1
All ages	701	172.1	4 946	1 214	72.0	7.4	467	114.6	502	117.3
Total	1 282	160.7	9 467	1 187	70.1	7.8	788	98.8	870	103.7

Table 181b   FSE - PEAS - AESE   Cerebrovascular disease - First-ever stroke

Age group (years)	Incidence 1990 Number ('000s)	Rate (per 100 000)	Prevalence 1990 Number ('000s)	Rate (per 100 000)	Avg. age at onset (years)	Average duration (years)	Deaths 1990 Number ('000s)	Rate (per 100 000)	Deaths 2000 (Projected) Number ('000s)	Rate (per 100 000)
Males										
0-4	0	0.9	0	0	2.5	0.0	0	0.9	0	0.9
5-14	0	0.3	0	0	10.0	0.0	0	0.3	0	0.3
15-44	22	28.4	239	314	29.7	16.2	8	9.9	7	9.1
45-59	61	226.8	376	1 395	52.2	7.7	37	135.5	46	148.5
60+	282	1 343.9	1 259	6 005	72.0	3.6	195	928.6	276	1 084.1
All ages	365	220.6	1 874	1 134	66.1	5.0	239	144.6	329	192.7
Females										
0-4	0	0.6	0	0	2.5	0.0	0	0.6	0	0.6
5-14	0	0.3	0	0	10.0	0.0	0	0.3	0	0.2
15-44	22	29.5	298	398	29.9	25.0	4	5.0	3	4.4
45-59	56	187.4	501	1 670	52.4	10.8	25	83.1	25	73.3
60+	444	1 219.7	1 714	4 710	75.1	3.1	371	1 019.5	451	1 096.2
All ages	522	288.7	2 513	1 389	70.7	4.8	400	221.0	480	256.7
Total	887	256.2	4 388	1 267	68.8	4.9	639	184.5	809	226.1

Table 181c   India - India - Inde   Cerebrovascular disease - First-ever stroke

Age group (years)	Incidence 1990 Number ('000s)	Rate (per 100 000)	Prevalence 1990 Number ('000s)	Rate (per 100 000)	Avg. age at onset (years)	Average duration (years)	Deaths 1990 Number ('000s)	Rate (per 100 000)	Deaths 2000 (Projected) Number ('000s)	Rate (per 100 000)
Males										
0-4	3	5.5	0	0	2.5	0.0	3	5.5	3	5.8
5-14	2	1.6	0	0	10.0	0.0	2	1.6	1	1.1
15-44	21	10.4	240	120	29.8	17.5	5	2.6	7	2.7
45-59	58	122.6	360	756	52.3	7.8	32	67.4	45	75.7
60+	221	741.9	797	2 677	71.6	3.1	185	620.9	251	680.2
All ages	305	69.4	1 397	318	64.0	4.9	227	51.7	307	60.0
Females										
0-4	3	6.0	0	0	2.5	0.0	3	6.0	3	5.5
5-14	2	2.1	0	0	10.0	0.0	2	2.1	1	1.4
15-44	25	13.8	278	151	29.8	18.1	6	3.5	6	2.6
45-59	47	102.7	360	782	52.3	9.2	20	43.4	23	39.7
60+	221	765.4	696	2 407	72.3	2.6	189	652.6	258	663.4
All ages	299	73.0	1 334	325	64.3	4.9	220	53.8	291	60.2
Total	604	71.1	2 731	321	64.2	4.9	448	52.7	598	60.1

For epidemiological sources see Bonita et al. 1996. For the methods used to estimate and project incidence, prevalence, and deaths see Murray and Lopez 1996a. See explanatory notes for definitions and caveats.

Table 181
Cerebrovascular disease

Cuadro 181
Enfermedad cerebrovascular

Tableau 181
Maladie cérébrovasculaire

First-ever stroke   Primer accidente cerebrovascular   Premier accident vasculaire cérébral

Table 181d   China - China - Chine   Cerebrovascular disease - First-ever stroke

Age group (years)	Incidence 1990 Number ('000s)	Rate (per 100 000)	Prevalence 1990 Number ('000s)	Rate (per 100 000)	Avg. age at onset (years)	Average duration (years)	Deaths 1990 Number ('000s)	Rate (per 100 000)	Deaths 2000 (Projected) Number ('000s)	Rate (per 100 000)
Males										
0-4	2	3.8	0	0	2.5	0.0	2	3.8	2	3.9
5-14	2	1.7	0	0	10.0	0.0	2	1.7	1	1.1
15-44	82	26.9	977	319	29.9	18.1	25	8.2	28	8.8
45-59	156	214.8	1 025	1 410	52.3	7.5	98	134.3	154	157.8
60+	654	1 335.7	2 272	4 639	71.6	3.0	545	1 112.2	728	1 206.3
All ages	897	153.2	4 274	730	64.1	5.1	672	114.8	914	139.3
Females										
0-4	2	3.1	0	0	2.5	0.0	2	3.1	2	2.7
5-14	1	0.7	0	0	10.0	0.0	1	0.7	0	0.4
15-44	78	27.4	958	337	29.9	19.0	19	6.6	17	5.6
45-59	113	174.9	812	1 261	52.4	7.4	71	110.5	85	93.6
60+	557	1 077.9	1 330	2 574	74.2	2.0	509	984.3	633	981.9
All ages	750	136.7	3 100	565	66.1	4.6	601	109.5	737	118.0
Total	1 647	145.2	7 374	650	65.0	4.9	1 272	112.2	1 650	128.9

Table 181e   OAI - OPAI - APAI   Cerebrovascular disease - First-ever stroke

Age group (years)	Incidence 1990 Number ('000s)	Rate (per 100 000)	Prevalence 1990 Number ('000s)	Rate (per 100 000)	Avg. age at onset (years)	Average duration (years)	Deaths 1990 Number ('000s)	Rate (per 100 000)	Deaths 2000 (Projected) Number ('000s)	Rate (per 100 000)
Males										
0-4	4	9.2	0	0	2.5	0.0	4	9.2	4	9.1
5-14	8	9.9	0	0	10.0	0.0	8	9.9	6	7.3
15-44	35	22.0	342	213	29.7	13.4	16	10.2	19	9.5
45-59	45	132.1	273	800	52.2	6.9	29	85.7	41	89.5
60+	162	803.0	532	2 634	71.9	2.8	133	655.8	189	680.2
All ages	255	74.3	1 148	335	59.5	4.9	190	55.5	259	64.0
Females										
0-4	4	8.6	0	0	2.5	0.0	4	8.6	3	7.6
5-14	6	7.9	0	0	10.0	0.0	6	7.9	4	5.3
15-44	32	20.0	337	211	29.8	16.2	11	6.6	11	5.2
45-59	45	127.6	318	908	52.3	8.2	24	67.2	26	56.1
60+	183	807.3	517	2 281	74.1	2.3	156	686.8	219	673.7
All ages	269	79.4	1 172	345	62.8	4.8	200	58.8	264	65.4
Total	524	76.8	2 320	340	61.2	4.9	390	57.2	523	64.7

Table 181f   SSA - ASS - ASS   Cerebrovascular disease - First-ever stroke

Age group (years)	Incidence 1990 Number ('000s)	Rate (per 100 000)	Prevalence 1990 Number ('000s)	Rate (per 100 000)	Avg. age at onset (years)	Average duration (years)	Deaths 1990 Number ('000s)	Rate (per 100 000)	Deaths 2000 (Projected) Number ('000s)	Rate (per 100 000)
Males										
0-4	2	4.0	0	0	2.4	0.0	2	4.0	3	4.0
5-14	6	8.8	0	0	10.0	0.0	6	8.8	6	6.4
15-44	32	30.9	207	200	29.4	7.1	23	22.2	28	19.9
45-59	38	186.5	125	613	52.1	3.8	32	157.1	39	148.8
60+	111	1 052.9	288	2 744	71.2	2.4	89	846.6	125	867.8
All ages	189	74.8	620	246	57.6	3.4	152	60.2	201	58.7
Females										
0-4	2	4.6	0	0	2.4	0.0	2	4.6	3	4.1
5-14	6	8.8	0	0	10.0	0.0	6	8.8	6	5.9
15-44	31	29.5	168	158	31.3	6.3	13	12.6	14	9.5
45-59	60	272.0	246	1 111	52.2	4.8	44	197.7	50	171.5
60+	180	1 410.1	310	2 432	73.1	1.5	166	1 303.0	222	1 269.9
All ages	279	108.3	724	281	62.0	2.7	231	89.7	294	84.5
Total	468	91.7	1 344	263	60.2	3.0	383	75.1	496	71.7

For epidemiological sources see Bonita et al. 1996. For the methods used to estimate and project incidence, prevalence, and deaths see Murray and Lopez 1996a. See explanatory notes for definitions and caveats.

Table 181
Cerebrovascular disease

Cuadro 181
Enfermedad cerebrovascular

Tableau 181
Maladie cérébrovasculaire

First-ever stroke

Primer accidente cerebrovascular

Premier accident vasculaire cérébral

Table 181g LAC - ALC - ALC — Cerebrovascular disease - First-ever stroke

Age group (years)	Incidence 1990 Number ('000s)	Rate (per 100 000)	Prevalence 1990 Number ('000s)	Rate (per 100 000)	Avg. age at onset (years)	Average duration (years)	Deaths 1990 Number ('000s)	Rate (per 100 000)	Deaths 2000 (Projected) Number ('000s)	Rate (per 100 000)
Males										
0-4	0	1.1	0	0	2.5	0.0	0	1.1	0	1.1
5-14	1	1.1	0	0	10.0	0.0	1	1.1	1	0.9
15-44	23	22.0	233	224	29.8	14.2	9	8.9	12	9.0
45-59	33	147.3	190	854	52.3	7.0	23	104.1	32	103.9
60+	118	828.4	471	3 307	72.7	3.5	88	618.7	125	635.7
All ages	174	78.7	894	403	62.9	5.6	121	54.8	170	63.9
Females										
0-4	0	1.0	0	0	2.5	0.0	0	1.0	0	0.9
5-14	1	1.1	0	0	10.0	0.0	1	1.1	0	0.8
15-44	20	19.2	183	175	29.8	12.3	11	10.3	11	8.9
45-59	29	122.8	157	673	52.4	6.9	20	83.9	25	77.3
60+	125	740.1	409	2 432	74.7	2.9	96	571.6	135	573.8
All ages	174	78.1	749	336	65.6	4.6	127	57.1	172	64.4
Total	348	78.4	1 643	370	64.2	5.1	249	56.0	342	64.2

Table 181h MEC - AOM - CMO — Cerebrovascular disease - First-ever stroke

Age group (years)	Incidence 1990 Number ('000s)	Rate (per 100 000)	Prevalence 1990 Number ('000s)	Rate (per 100 000)	Avg. age at onset (years)	Average duration (years)	Deaths 1990 Number ('000s)	Rate (per 100 000)	Deaths 2000 (Projected) Number ('000s)	Rate (per 100 000)
Males										
0-4	2	4.6	0	0	2.5	0.0	2	4.6	2	4.6
5-14	5	8.1	0	0	10.0	0.0	5	8.1	5	6.2
15-44	23	20.0	241	212	29.8	15.7	8	6.7	9	6.3
45-59	27	120.1	180	804	52.3	8.0	16	73.2	24	74.5
60+	95	696.5	397	2 911	72.3	3.5	67	493.9	99	528.4
All ages	152	59.2	819	319	59.4	6.0	99	38.4	139	41.7
Females										
0-4	1	3.7	0	0	2.5	0.0	1	3.7	2	3.4
5-14	5	7.6	0	0	10.0	0.0	5	7.6	4	5.4
15-44	20	18.4	220	205	29.8	17.4	5	4.8	5	3.8
45-59	26	117.5	189	846	52.3	8.6	15	65.5	18	57.9
60+	112	724.0	378	2 448	74.3	2.8	87	563.6	123	575.7
All ages	164	66.4	787	319	62.9	5.4	113	45.8	152	47.3
Total	316	62.8	1 606	319	61.2	5.7	212	42.1	291	44.5

Table 181i World - Mundo - Monde — Cerebrovascular disease - First-ever stroke

Age group (years)	Incidence 1990 Number ('000s)	Rate (per 100 000)	Prevalence 1990 Number ('000s)	Rate (per 100 000)	Avg. age at onset (years)	Average duration (years)	Deaths 1990 Number ('000s)	Rate (per 100 000)	Deaths 2000 (Projected) Number ('000s)	Rate (per 100 000)
Males										
0-4	14	4.4	0	0	2.5	0.0	14	4.4	15	4.4
5-14	24	4.4	0	0	10.0	0.0	24	4.4	20	3.3
15-44	275	22.0	2 963	237	29.8	17.2	102	8.1	117	8.1
45-59	497	159.2	3 307	1 059	52.3	8.7	291	93.2	411	102.2
60+	2 107	962.9	9 275	4 238	72.3	3.8	1 590	726.7	2 123	770.9
All ages	2 917	109.9	15 546	586	63.0	5.5	2 022	76.2	2 687	86.8
Females										
0-4	13	4.2	0	0	2.5	0.0	13	4.2	12	3.8
5-14	21	3.9	0	0	10.0	0.0	21	3.9	17	2.8
15-44	257	21.4	2 831	236	30.0	18.9	74	6.2	72	5.1
45-59	445	143.1	3 291	1 058	52.4	10.1	233	74.9	266	66.0
60+	2 424	900.3	9 202	3 418	74.8	3.3	2 019	749.8	2 526	749.4
All ages	3 159	120.9	15 326	586	65.9	5.0	2 359	90.3	2 893	94.4
Total	6 077	115.4	30 872	586	64.5	5.2	4 381	83.2	5 580	90.6

For epidemiological sources see Bonita et al. 1996. For the methods used to estimate and project incidence, prevalence, and deaths see Murray and Lopez 1996a. See explanatory notes for definitions and caveats.

Table 182
Inflammatory heart diseases

Myocarditis

Cuadro 182
Enfermedades inflamatorias del corazón

Miocarditis

Tableau 182
Maladies cardiaques inflammatoires

Myocardite

Table 182a EME - PEMC - EMBE · Inflammatory heart diseases - Myocarditis

Age group (years)	Incidence 1990 Number ('000s)	Rate (per 100 000)	Prevalence 1990 Number ('000s)	Rate (per 100 000)	Avg. age at onset (years)	Average duration (years)	Deaths 1990 Number ('000s)	Rate (per 100 000)	Deaths 2000 (Projected) Number ('000s)	Rate (per 100 000)
Males										
0-4	0	0.9	0	1.6	2.5	4.0	0	0.3	0	0.2
5-14	0	0.0	1	1.0	10.0	4.0	0	0.1	0	0.1
15-44	0	0.2	2	0.8	29.9	4.0	0	0.1	0	0.1
45-59	0	0.3	1	1.2	52.4	3.8	0	0.2	0	0.2
60+	0	0.5	1	1.7	71.1	3.2	0	0.3	0	0.2
All ages	1	0.3	4	1.1	38.2	3.8	1	0.2	1	0.1
Females										
0-4	0	1.1	0	1.9	2.5	4.0	0	0.3	0	0.2
5-14	0	0.0	1	1.1	10.0	4.0	0	0.1	0	0.0
15-44	0	0.2	1	0.7	30.0	4.0	0	0.1	0	0.1
45-59	0	0.3	1	0.9	52.4	3.9	0	0.1	0	0.1
60+	0	0.5	2	1.9	72.4	3.3	0	0.3	0	0.3
All ages	1	0.3	4	1.1	42.1	3.7	1	0.1	1	0.1
Total	2	0.3	9	1.1	40.2	3.8	1	0.2	1	0.1

Table 182b FSE - PEAS - AESE · Inflammatory heart diseases - Myocarditis

Age group (years)	Incidence 1990 Number ('000s)	Rate (per 100 000)	Prevalence 1990 Number ('000s)	Rate (per 100 000)	Avg. age at onset (years)	Average duration (years)	Deaths 1990 Number ('000s)	Rate (per 100 000)	Deaths 2000 (Projected) Number ('000s)	Rate (per 100 000)
Males										
0-4	0	0.8	0	1.4	2.5	3.9	0	0.2	0	0.2
5-14	0	0.0	0	0.8	10.0	4.0	0	0.1	0	0.1
15-44	0	0.4	1	1.5	29.8	3.9	0	0.2	0	0.2
45-59	0	0.7	1	2.4	52.2	3.7	0	0.4	0	0.4
60+	0	0.6	1	2.4	70.0	3.1	0	0.3	0	0.4
All ages	1	0.4	3	1.6	37.9	3.7	0	0.2	0	0.3
Females										
0-4	0	1.0	0	1.7	2.5	4.0	0	0.3	0	0.2
5-14	0	0.0	0	1.0	10.0	4.0	0	0.0	0	0.0
15-44	0	0.3	1	1.1	29.9	4.0	0	0.2	0	0.1
45-59	0	0.6	1	2.1	52.4	3.9	0	0.3	0	0.3
60+	0	0.7	1	2.7	71.5	3.3	0	0.4	0	0.4
All ages	1	0.4	3	1.6	43.8	3.7	0	0.2	0	0.2
Total	2	0.4	6	1.6	41.0	3.7	1	0.2	1	0.2

Table 182c India - India - Inde · Inflammatory heart diseases - Myocarditis

Age group (years)	Incidence 1990 Number ('000s)	Rate (per 100 000)	Prevalence 1990 Number ('000s)	Rate (per 100 000)	Avg. age at onset (years)	Average duration (years)	Deaths 1990 Number ('000s)	Rate (per 100 000)	Deaths 2000 (Projected) Number ('000s)	Rate (per 100 000)
Males										
0-4	2	3.4	3	5.3	2.5	3.2	1	1.1	1	1.2
5-14	0	0.0	3	2.7	10.0	3.3	0	0.1	0	0.0
15-44	1	0.3	2	0.8	29.8	3.3	0	0.2	0	0.1
45-59	0	0.6	1	1.6	52.3	3.2	0	0.3	0	0.4
60+	0	1.5	1	4.4	69.7	2.7	0	0.8	0	0.9
All ages	3	0.7	10	2.2	20.2	3.1	1	0.3	2	0.3
Females										
0-4	1	2.5	2	4.0	2.5	3.2	1	1.7	1	1.5
5-14	1	1.0	4	4.2	10.0	3.3	1	0.8	0	0.5
15-44	0	0.1	1	0.6	29.8	3.3	0	0.1	0	0.1
45-59	0	0.6	1	1.6	52.4	3.2	0	0.3	0	0.3
60+	0	1.0	1	3.1	70.1	2.7	0	0.6	0	0.6
All ages	3	0.7	9	2.2	17.1	3.2	2	0.5	2	0.4
Total	6	0.7	19	2.2	18.7	3.1	3	0.4	4	0.4

For epidemiological sources see Lozano et al. 1996. For the methods used to estimate and project incidence, prevalence, and deaths see Murray and Lopez 1996a. See explanatory notes for definitions and caveats.

Table 182
Inflammatory heart diseases

Myocarditis

Cuadro 182
Enfermedades inflamatorias del corazón

Miocarditis

Tableau 182
Maladies cardiaques inflammatoires

Myocardite

Table 182d — China - China - Chine — Inflammatory heart diseases - Myocarditis

Age group (years)	Incidence 1990 Number ('000s)	Rate (per 100 000)	Prevalence 1990 Number ('000s)	Rate (per 100 000)	Avg. age at onset (years)	Average duration (years)	Deaths 1990 Number ('000s)	Rate (per 100 000)	Deaths 2000 (Projected) Number ('000s)	Rate (per 100 000)
Males										
0-4	1	2.0	2	3.4	2.5	3.9	0	0.6	0	0.6
5-14	0	0.0	2	2.1	10.0	4.0	0	0.0	0	0.0
15-44	1	0.2	2	0.7	29.9	4.0	0	0.1	0	0.1
45-59	0	0.3	1	0.9	52.3	3.8	0	0.1	0	0.2
60+	0	1.0	2	3.3	69.8	3.1	0	0.5	0	0.5
All ages	2	0.4	8	1.4	26.0	3.7	1	0.2	1	0.2
Females										
0-4	1	2.2	2	3.8	2.5	3.9	0	0.6	0	0.5
5-14	0	0.0	2	2.3	10.0	4.0	0	0.1	0	0.1
15-44	0	0.1	2	0.6	29.9	4.0	0	0.1	0	0.1
45-59	0	0.3	1	1.0	52.4	3.8	0	0.1	0	0.1
60+	0	0.6	1	2.2	70.6	3.2	0	0.3	0	0.3
All ages	2	0.4	8	1.4	21.9	3.8	1	0.2	1	0.1
Total	5	0.4	16	1.4	24.0	3.8	2	0.2	2	0.2

Table 182e — OAI - OPAI - APAI — Inflammatory heart diseases - Myocarditis

Age group (years)	Incidence 1990 Number ('000s)	Rate (per 100 000)	Prevalence 1990 Number ('000s)	Rate (per 100 000)	Avg. age at onset (years)	Average duration (years)	Deaths 1990 Number ('000s)	Rate (per 100 000)	Deaths 2000 (Projected) Number ('000s)	Rate (per 100 000)
Males										
0-4	5	12.0	9	20.5	2.5	3.8	1	3.0	1	2.9
5-14	0	0.0	10	12.5	10.0	4.0	0	0.4	0	0.3
15-44	1	0.4	3	1.8	29.7	3.9	0	0.3	0	0.2
45-59	0	0.5	1	1.9	52.3	3.7	0	0.3	0	0.3
60+	0	1.5	1	5.1	69.6	3.1	0	0.7	0	0.7
All ages	6	1.9	24	7.0	9.8	3.8	2	0.7	2	0.6
Females										
0-4	7	15.5	11	26.5	2.5	3.9	2	3.9	1	3.3
5-14	0	0.0	13	16.1	10.0	4.0	2	2.3	1	1.4
15-44	0	0.2	2	1.1	29.8	3.9	0	0.2	0	0.1
45-59	0	0.4	0	1.4	52.3	3.8	0	0.2	0	0.2
60+	0	0.9	0	1.4	70.3	3.1	0	0.5	0	0.5
All ages	7	2.1	27	7.8	6.4	3.8	4	1.1	3	0.7
Total	13	2.0	50	7.4	8.0	3.8	6	0.9	5	0.7

Table 182f — SSA - ASS - ASS — Inflammatory heart diseases - Myocarditis

Age group (years)	Incidence 1990 Number ('000s)	Rate (per 100 000)	Prevalence 1990 Number ('000s)	Rate (per 100 000)	Avg. age at onset (years)	Average duration (years)	Deaths 1990 Number ('000s)	Rate (per 100 000)	Deaths 2000 (Projected) Number ('000s)	Rate (per 100 000)
Males										
0-4	3	5.7	5	9.5	2.4	3.6	1	1.4	1	1.4
5-14	0	0.0	4	6.0	10.0	3.9	0	0.2	0	0.1
15-44	0	0.3	1	1.2	29.4	3.9	0	0.2	0	0.2
45-59	0	0.7	0	2.4	52.2	3.7	0	0.4	0	0.4
60+	0	3.0	1	9.7	69.2	3.0	0	1.5	0	1.5
All ages	3	1.4	12	4.6	12.9	3.6	1	0.5	2	0.5
Females										
0-4	5	10.5	8	17.7	2.4	3.7	1	2.6	1	2.2
5-14	0	0.0	8	11.0	10.0	3.9	1	1.7	1	1.0
15-44	0	0.2	1	1.0	29.5	3.9	0	0.1	0	0.1
45-59	0	0.8	1	2.6	52.2	3.7	0	0.4	0	0.3
60+	0	2.1	1	7.2	69.7	3.1	0	1.1	0	1.1
All ages	6	2.2	19	7.2	8.2	3.6	3	1.0	3	0.8
Total	9	1.8	30	5.9	10.0	3.6	4	0.8	4	0.6

For epidemiological sources see Lozano et al. 1996. For the methods used to estimate and project incidence, prevalence, and deaths see Murray and Lopez 1996a. See explanatory notes for definitions and caveats.

Table 182
Inflammatory heart diseases

Myocarditis

Cuadro 182
Enfermedades inflamatorias del corazón

Miocarditis

Tableau 182
Maladies cardiaques inflammatoires

Myocardite

Table 182g   LAC - ALC - ALC — Inflammatory heart diseases - Myocarditis

Age group (years)	Incidence 1990 Number ('000s)	Rate (per 100 000)	Prevalence 1990 Number ('000s)	Rate (per 100 000)	Avg. age at onset (years)	Average duration (years)	Deaths 1990 Number ('000s)	Rate (per 100 000)	Deaths 2000 (Projected) Number ('000s)	Rate (per 100 000)
Males										
0-4	1	2.3	1	3.9	2.5	3.9	0	0.6	0	0.6
5-14	0	0.0	1	2.4	10.0	4.0	0	0.0	0	0.0
15-44	0	0.2	1	0.6	29.8	3.9	0	0.1	0	0.1
45-59	0	0.3	0	1.1	52.3	3.8	0	0.2	0	0.2
60+	0	1.2	1	4.0	70.3	3.1	0	0.6	0	0.6
All ages	1	0.5	4	1.7	20.8	3.8	0	0.2	0	0.2
Females										
0-4	1	2.7	1	4.6	2.5	3.9	0	0.7	0	0.6
5-14	0	0.0	1	2.8	10.0	4.0	0	0.2	0	0.2
15-44	0	0.1	1	0.5	29.9	4.0	0	0.1	0	0.1
45-59	0	0.3	0	1.0	52.4	3.8	0	0.2	0	0.1
60+	0	0.7	0	2.5	71.1	3.2	0	0.4	0	0.4
All ages	1	0.5	4	1.8	16.8	3.8	0	0.2	0	0.2
Total	2	0.5	8	1.7	18.8	3.8	1	0.2	1	0.2

Table 182h   MEC - AOM - CMO — Inflammatory heart diseases - Myocarditis

Age group (years)	Incidence 1990 Number ('000s)	Rate (per 100 000)	Prevalence 1990 Number ('000s)	Rate (per 100 000)	Avg. age at onset (years)	Average duration (years)	Deaths 1990 Number ('000s)	Rate (per 100 000)	Deaths 2000 (Projected) Number ('000s)	Rate (per 100 000)
Males										
0-4	6	14.0	10	23.8	2.5	3.8	1	3.5	2	3.5
5-14	0	0.0	9	14.5	10.0	4.0	0	0.3	0	0.2
15-44	0	0.4	2	1.8	29.8	3.9	0	0.3	0	0.2
45-59	0	0.7	1	2.5	52.3	3.7	0	0.4	0	0.4
60+	0	2.0	1	6.8	69.7	3.1	0	1.1	0	1.2
All ages	7	2.6	23	8.9	8.3	3.8	2	0.9	3	0.8
Females										
0-4	7	17.5	12	29.8	2.5	3.8	2	4.4	2	3.9
5-14	0	0.0	11	18.2	10.0	4.0	1	2.0	1	1.3
15-44	0	0.3	2	1.6	29.8	4.0	0	0.2	0	0.2
45-59	0	0.6	0	2.1	52.3	3.8	0	0.3	0	0.3
60+	0	1.3	1	4.6	70.4	3.2	0	0.7	0	0.7
All ages	8	3.1	26	10.5	6.3	3.8	3	1.4	3	1.0
Total	14	2.8	49	9.7	7.2	3.8	6	1.1	6	0.9

Table 182i   World - Mundo - Monde — Inflammatory heart diseases - Myocarditis

Age group (years)	Incidence 1990 Number ('000s)	Rate (per 100 000)	Prevalence 1990 Number ('000s)	Rate (per 100 000)	Avg. age at onset (years)	Average duration (years)	Deaths 1990 Number ('000s)	Rate (per 100 000)	Deaths 2000 (Projected) Number ('000s)	Rate (per 100 000)
Males										
0-4	18	5.6	30	9.4	2.5	3.7	5	1.5	5	1.5
5-14	0	0.0	31	5.6	10.0	3.8	1	0.1	1	0.1
15-44	3	0.3	13	1.0	29.8	3.8	2	0.2	2	0.1
45-59	1	0.4	5	1.5	52.3	3.7	1	0.2	1	0.2
60+	2	1.1	8	3.7	70.1	3.1	1	0.7	2	0.7
All ages	25	0.9	87	3.3	22.1	3.6	10	0.4	11	0.4
Females										
0-4	22	7.2	38	12.2	2.5	3.7	6	2.0	6	1.8
5-14	1	0.2	40	7.6	10.0	3.9	5	1.0	4	0.6
15-44	2	0.2	10	0.8	29.8	3.9	1	0.1	1	0.1
45-59	1	0.4	4	1.4	52.4	3.7	1	0.2	1	0.2
60+	2	0.8	7	2.6	71.2	3.2	1	0.5	2	0.5
All ages	29	1.1	99	3.8	20.5	3.7	14	0.5	13	0.4
Total	54	1.0	186	3.5	21.3	3.7	24	0.4	24	0.4

For epidemiological sources see Lozano et al. 1996. For the methods used to estimate and project incidence, prevalence, and deaths see Murray and Lopez 1996a. See explanatory notes for definitions and caveats.

Table 183
Inflammatory heart diseases

Pericarditis

Cuadro 183
Enfermedades inflamatorias del corazón

Pericarditis

Tableau 183
Maladies cardiaques inflammatoires

Péricardite

Table 183a — EME - PEMC - EMBE — Inflammatory heart diseases - Pericarditis

Age group (years)	Incidence 1990 Number ('000s)	Rate (per 100 000)	Prevalence 1990 Number ('000s)	Rate (per 100 000)	Avg. age at onset (years)	Average duration (years)	Deaths 1990 Number ('000s)	Rate (per 100 000)	Deaths 2000 (Projected) Number ('000s)	Rate (per 100 000)
Males										
0-4	1	5.0	0	0.4	2.5	0.08	0	0.0	0	0.0
5-14	0	0.2	0	0.0	10.0	0.08	0	0.0	0	0.0
15-44	8	4.2	1	0.3	29.9	0.08	0	0.0	0	0.0
45-59	11	16.5	1	1.4	52.4	0.08	0	0.1	0	0.1
60+	30	49.0	2	4.1	71.1	0.08	0	0.3	0	0.3
All ages	50	12.7	4	1.1	58.6	0.08	0	0.1	0	0.1
Females										
0-4	1	5.0	0	0.4	2.5	0.08	0	0.0	0	0.0
5-14	0	0.2	0	0.0	10.0	0.08	0	0.0	0	0.0
15-44	10	5.6	1	0.5	30.0	0.08	0	0.0	0	0.0
45-59	4	6.0	0	0.5	52.4	0.08	0	0.0	0	0.0
60+	53	63.0	4	5.3	72.4	0.08	0	0.4	0	0.4
All ages	69	16.9	6	1.4	63.7	0.08	0	0.1	0	0.1
Total	119	14.9	10	1.2	61.6	0.08	1	0.1	1	0.1

Table 183b — FSE - PEAS - AESE — Inflammatory heart diseases - Pericarditis

Age group (years)	Incidence 1990 Number ('000s)	Rate (per 100 000)	Prevalence 1990 Number ('000s)	Rate (per 100 000)	Avg. age at onset (years)	Average duration (years)	Deaths 1990 Number ('000s)	Rate (per 100 000)	Deaths 2000 (Projected) Number ('000s)	Rate (per 100 000)
Males										
0-4	1	5.0	0	0.4	2.5	0.08	0	0.0	0	0.0
5-14	0	0.0	0	0.0	10.0	0.08	0	0.0	0	0.0
15-44	6	8.0	1	0.7	29.8	0.08	0	0.0	0	0.0
45-59	9	32.0	1	2.7	52.2	0.08	0	0.1	0	0.1
60+	14	65.1	1	5.4	70.0	0.08	0	0.4	0	0.5
All ages	29	17.6	2	1.5	54.7	0.08	0	0.1	0	0.1
Females										
0-4	1	5.0	0	0.4	2.5	0.08	0	0.0	0	0.0
5-14	0	0.0	0	0.0	10.0	0.08	0	0.0	0	0.0
15-44	7	9.0	1	0.7	29.9	0.08	0	0.0	0	0.0
45-59	4	12.0	0	1.0	52.4	0.08	0	0.0	0	0.0
60+	30	83.1	3	7.0	71.5	0.08	0	0.5	0	0.6
All ages	41	22.8	3	1.9	61.9	0.08	0	0.1	0	0.1
Total	70	20.3	6	1.7	58.9	0.08	0	0.1	0	0.1

Table 183c — India - India - Inde — Inflammatory heart diseases - Pericarditis

Age group (years)	Incidence 1990 Number ('000s)	Rate (per 100 000)	Prevalence 1990 Number ('000s)	Rate (per 100 000)	Avg. age at onset (years)	Average duration (years)	Deaths 1990 Number ('000s)	Rate (per 100 000)	Deaths 2000 (Projected) Number ('000s)	Rate (per 100 000)
Males										
0-4	18	30.0	2	3.0	2.5	0.10	0	0.2	0	0.2
5-14	7	6.5	1	0.6	10.0	0.10	0	0.1	0	0.0
15-44	11	5.5	1	0.5	29.8	0.10	0	0.0	0	0.0
45-59	13	27.0	1	2.7	52.3	0.10	0	0.2	0	0.2
60+	14	46.1	1	4.6	69.7	0.10	0	0.4	0	0.4
All ages	62	14.1	6	1.4	33.3	0.10	0	0.1	1	0.1
Females										
0-4	3	4.5	0	0.4	2.5	0.10	0	0.1	0	0.1
5-14	25	26.0	2	2.6	10.0	0.10	0	0.2	0	0.1
15-44	17	9.3	2	0.9	29.8	0.10	0	0.1	0	0.1
45-59	4	9.0	0	0.9	52.4	0.10	0	0.1	0	0.1
60+	8	27.0	1	2.7	70.1	0.10	0	0.2	0	0.2
All ages	56	13.7	6	1.4	27.1	0.10	0	0.1	0	0.1
Total	118	13.9	12	1.4	30.3	0.10	1	0.1	1	0.1

For epidemiological sources see Lozano et al. 1996. For the methods used to estimate and project incidence, prevalence, and deaths see Murray and Lopez 1996a. See explanatory notes for definitions and caveats.

Table 183	Cuadro 183	Tableau 183
Inflammatory heart diseases	**Enfermedades inflamatorias del corazón**	**Maladies cardiaques inflammatoires**
Pericarditis	Pericarditis	Péricardite

Table 183d   China - China - Chine   Inflammatory heart diseases - Pericarditis

Age group (years)	Incidence 1990 Number ('000s)	Rate (per 100 000)	Prevalence 1990 Number ('000s)	Rate (per 100 000)	Avg. age at onset (years)	Average duration (years)	Deaths 1990 Number ('000s)	Rate (per 100 000)	Deaths 2000 (Projected) Number ('000s)	Rate (per 100 000)
Males										
0-4	10	16.5	1	1.4	2.5	0.08	0	0.1	0	0.1
5-14	1	1.5	0	0.1	10.0	0.08	0	0.0	0	0.0
15-44	12	4.0	1	0.3	29.9	0.08	0	0.0	0	0.0
45-59	9	13.0	1	1.1	52.3	0.08	0	0.1	0	0.1
60+	17	35.0	1	2.9	69.8	0.08	0	0.2	0	0.2
All ages	50	8.6	4	0.7	41.7	0.08	0	0.1	0	0.1
Females										
0-4	2	4.0	0	0.3	2.5	0.08	0	0.0	0	0.0
5-14	3	3.0	0	0.2	10.0	0.08	0	0.0	0	0.0
15-44	23	8.0	2	0.7	29.9	0.08	0	0.1	0	0.0
45-59	4	5.5	0	0.5	52.4	0.08	0	0.0	0	0.0
60+	8	16.0	1	1.3	70.6	0.08	0	0.1	0	0.1
All ages	40	7.2	3	0.6	37.5	0.08	0	0.0	0	0.0
Total	90	7.9	7	0.7	39.9	0.08	1	0.1	1	0.0

Table 183e   OAI - OPAI - APAI   Inflammatory heart diseases - Pericarditis

Age group (years)	Incidence 1990 Number ('000s)	Rate (per 100 000)	Prevalence 1990 Number ('000s)	Rate (per 100 000)	Avg. age at onset (years)	Average duration (years)	Deaths 1990 Number ('000s)	Rate (per 100 000)	Deaths 2000 (Projected) Number ('000s)	Rate (per 100 000)
Males										
0-4	35	81.0	4	8.0	2.5	0.10	0	0.6	0	0.6
5-14	29	35.0	3	3.5	10.0	0.10	0	0.3	0	0.2
15-44	15	9.3	1	0.9	29.7	0.10	0	0.1	0	0.1
45-59	8	22.0	1	2.2	52.3	0.10	0	0.2	0	0.2
60+	9	45.1	1	4.5	69.6	0.10	0	0.3	0	0.3
All ages	96	28.1	10	2.8	19.2	0.10	1	0.2	1	0.2
Females										
0-4	10	23.0	1	2.3	2.5	0.10	0	0.2	0	0.1
5-14	56	70.0	6	6.9	10.0	0.10	0	0.5	0	0.3
15-44	20	12.5	2	1.2	29.8	0.10	0	0.1	0	0.1
45-59	2	7.0	0	0.7	52.3	0.10	0	0.0	0	0.0
60+	5	20.0	0	2.0	70.3	0.10	0	0.1	0	0.1
All ages	93	27.3	9	2.7	17.5	0.10	1	0.2	1	0.1
Total	189	27.7	19	2.8	18.4	0.10	1	0.2	1	0.2

Table 183f   SSA - ASS - ASS   Inflammatory heart diseases - Pericarditis

Age group (years)	Incidence 1990 Number ('000s)	Rate (per 100 000)	Prevalence 1990 Number ('000s)	Rate (per 100 000)	Avg. age at onset (years)	Average duration (years)	Deaths 1990 Number ('000s)	Rate (per 100 000)	Deaths 2000 (Projected) Number ('000s)	Rate (per 100 000)
Males										
0-4	18	38.0	2	3.8	2.4	0.10	0	0.3	0	0.3
5-14	10	14.0	1	1.4	10.0	0.10	0	0.1	0	0.1
15-44	7	7.0	1	0.7	29.4	0.10	0	0.1	0	0.0
45-59	7	32.0	1	3.2	52.2	0.10	0	0.3	0	0.2
60+	8	80.1	1	7.9	69.2	0.10	0	0.6	0	0.6
All ages	50	19.8	5	2.0	25.5	0.10	0	0.2	0	0.1
Females										
0-4	7	15.0	1	1.5	2.4	0.10	0	0.1	0	0.1
5-14	36	52.0	4	5.2	10.0	0.10	0	0.4	0	0.2
15-44	13	12.0	1	1.2	29.5	0.10	0	0.1	0	0.0
45-59	2	10.0	0	1.0	52.2	0.10	0	0.1	0	0.1
60+	7	55.1	1	5.5	69.7	0.10	0	0.4	0	0.4
All ages	65	25.3	6	2.5	20.8	0.10	0	0.2	0	0.1
Total	115	22.6	11	2.2	22.9	0.10	1	0.2	1	0.1

For epidemiological sources see Lozano et al. 1996. For the methods used to estimate and project incidence, prevalence, and deaths see Murray and Lopez 1996a. See explanatory notes for definitions and caveats.

Table 183
Inflammatory heart diseases
Pericarditis

Cuadro 183
Enfermedades inflamatorias del corazón
Pericarditis

Tableau 183
Maladies cardiaques inflammatoires
Péricardite

Table 183g   LAC - ALC - ALC   Inflammatory heart diseases - Pericarditis

Age group (years)	Incidence 1990 Number ('000s)	Rate (per 100 000)	Prevalence 1990 Number ('000s)	Rate (per 100 000)	Avg. age at onset (years)	Average duration (years)	Deaths 1990 Number ('000s)	Rate (per 100 000)	Deaths 2000 (Projected) Number ('000s)	Rate (per 100 000)
Males										
0-4	4	15.0	0	1.5	2.5	0.10	0	0.1	0	0.1
5-14	2	4.0	0	0.4	10.0	0.10	0	0.0	0	0.0
15-44	4	3.5	0	0.3	29.8	0.10	0	0.0	0	0.0
45-59	3	15.0	0	1.5	52.3	0.10	0	0.1	0	0.1
60+	5	32.0	0	3.2	70.3	0.10	0	0.3	0	0.3
All ages	18	8.1	2	0.8	35.4	0.10	0	0.1	0	0.1
Females										
0-4	1	4.5	0	0.4	2.5	0.10	0	0.0	0	0.0
5-14	4	7.8	0	0.8	10.0	0.10	0	0.1	0	0.0
15-44	7	7.0	1	0.7	29.9	0.10	0	0.1	0	0.0
45-59	1	4.0	0	0.4	52.4	0.10	0	0.0	0	0.0
60+	3	15.0	0	1.5	71.1	0.10	0	0.1	0	0.1
All ages	16	7.2	2	0.7	30.7	0.10	0	0.1	0	0.0
Total	34	7.6	3	0.8	33.2	0.10	0	0.1	0	0.1

Table 183h   MEC - AOM - CMO   Inflammatory heart diseases - Pericarditis

Age group (years)	Incidence 1990 Number ('000s)	Rate (per 100 000)	Prevalence 1990 Number ('000s)	Rate (per 100 000)	Avg. age at onset (years)	Average duration (years)	Deaths 1990 Number ('000s)	Rate (per 100 000)	Deaths 2000 (Projected) Number ('000s)	Rate (per 100 000)
Males										
0-4	40	96	4	9.5	2.5	0.10	0	0.7	0	0.7
5-14	19	29	2	2.9	10.0	0.10	0	0.2	0	0.2
15-44	11	10	1	0.9	29.8	0.10	0	0.1	0	0.1
45-59	7	30	1	3.0	52.3	0.10	0	0.2	0	0.2
60+	9	65	1	6.4	69.7	0.10	0	0.5	0	0.5
All ages	85	33	8	3.3	18.6	0.10	1	0.3	1	0.2
Females										
0-4	10	25	1	2.5	2.5	0.10	0	0.2	0	0.2
5-14	39	63	4	6.3	10.0	0.10	0	0.5	0	0.3
15-44	18	17	2	1.7	29.8	0.10	0	0.1	0	0.1
45-59	2	10	0	1.0	52.3	0.10	0	0.1	0	0.1
60+	4	28	0	2.8	70.4	0.10	0	0.2	0	0.2
All ages	74	30	7	3.0	18.7	0.10	1	0.2	1	0.2
Total	158	31	16	3.1	18.6	0.10	1	0.2	1	0.2

Table 183i   World - Mundo - Monde   Inflammatory heart diseases - Pericarditis

Age group (years)	Incidence 1990 Number ('000s)	Rate (per 100 000)	Prevalence 1990 Number ('000s)	Rate (per 100 000)	Avg. age at onset (years)	Average duration (years)	Deaths 1990 Number ('000s)	Rate (per 100 000)	Deaths 2000 (Projected) Number ('000s)	Rate (per 100 000)
Males										
0-4	127	39.6	12	3.9	2.5	0.09	1	0.3	1	0.3
5-14	68	12.4	7	1.2	10.0	0.09	1	0.1	0	0.1
15-44	74	5.9	7	0.6	29.8	0.09	1	0.0	1	0.0
45-59	66	21.1	6	1.9	52.3	0.09	0	0.1	1	0.2
60+	105	48.1	9	4.3	70.1	0.09	1	0.3	1	0.3
All ages	441	16.6	42	1.6	36.4	0.09	3	0.1	4	0.1
Females										
0-4	35	11.2	3	1.1	2.5	0.09	0	0.1	0	0.1
5-14	163	31.0	16	3.1	10.0	0.09	1	0.2	1	0.1
15-44	115	9.6	11	0.9	29.8	0.09	1	0.1	1	0.0
45-59	23	7.5	2	0.7	52.4	0.09	0	0.0	0	0.0
60+	118	43.8	10	3.8	71.2	0.09	0	0.1	0	0.1
All ages	453	17.4	43	1.6	35.0	0.09	3	0.1	2	0.1
Total	894	17.0	84	1.6	35.7	0.09	6	0.1	6	0.1

For epidemiological sources see Lozano et al. 1996. For the methods used to estimate and project incidence, prevalence, and deaths see Murray and Lopez 1996a. See explanatory notes for definitions and caveats.

Table 184
Inflammatory heart diseases

Endocarditis

Cuadro 184
Enfermedades inflamatorias del corazón

Endocarditis

Tableau 184
Maladies cardiaques inflammatoires

Endocardite

Table 184a EME - PEMC - EMBE   Inflammatory heart diseases - Endocarditis

Age group (years)	Incidence 1990 Number ('000s)	Rate (per 100 000)	Prevalence 1990 Number ('000s)	Rate (per 100 000)	Avg. age at onset (years)	Average duration (years)	Deaths 1990 Number ('000s)	Rate (per 100 000)	Deaths 2000 (Projected) Number ('000s)	Rate (per 100 000)
Males										
0-4	1	5.0	2	7.7	2.5	3.0	0	0.1	0	0.0
5-14	2	4.5	7	13.2	10.0	3.0	0	0.0	0	0.0
15-44	59	32.0	162	87.9	29.9	3.0	0	0.2	0	0.2
45-59	21	32.0	63	95.4	52.4	2.9	0	0.5	0	0.5
60+	18	30.0	53	87.6	71.1	2.5	1	1.5	1	1.4
All ages	102	26.1	287	73.5	41.1	2.9	2	0.4	2	0.4
Females										
0-4	1	3.5	1	5.1	2.5	2.6	0	0.1	0	0.0
5-14	2	4.0	5	9.8	10.0	2.6	0	0.0	0	0.0
15-44	54	30.0	130	72.7	30.0	2.6	0	0.1	0	0.1
45-59	20	30.0	53	78.4	52.4	2.6	0	0.2	0	0.2
60+	25	30.0	63	74.3	72.4	2.2	2	1.9	2	1.7
All ages	102	25.1	252	62.0	44.3	2.5	2	0.5	2	0.5
Total	204	25.6	540	67.6	42.7	2.7	4	0.5	4	0.5

Table 184b FSE - PEAS - AESE   Inflammatory heart diseases - Endocarditis

Age group (years)	Incidence 1990 Number ('000s)	Rate (per 100 000)	Prevalence 1990 Number ('000s)	Rate (per 100 000)	Avg. age at onset (years)	Average duration (years)	Deaths 1990 Number ('000s)	Rate (per 100 000)	Deaths 2000 (Projected) Number ('000s)	Rate (per 100 000)
Males										
0-4	1	5.5	1	8.5	2.5	3.0	0	0.0	0	0.0
5-14	1	5.0	4	14.6	10.0	3.0	0	0.0	0	0.0
15-44	27	35.2	73	96.1	29.8	3.0	0	0.4	0	0.4
45-59	9	35.2	28	103.8	52.2	2.8	0	1.1	0	1.2
60+	7	33.0	20	95.4	70.0	2.4	0	2.1	1	2.4
All ages	45	27.4	126	76.5	39.6	2.8	1	0.6	1	0.8
Females										
0-4	1	3.9	1	5.6	2.5	2.6	0	0.0	0	0.0
5-14	1	4.4	3	10.8	10.0	2.6	0	0.0	0	0.0
15-44	25	33.0	60	79.8	29.9	2.6	0	0.2	0	0.2
45-59	10	33.0	26	85.7	52.4	2.5	0	0.5	0	0.4
60+	12	33.0	29	80.7	71.5	2.2	1	2.5	1	2.8
All ages	48	26.7	118	65.5	44.1	2.5	1	0.7	1	0.8
Total	94	27.0	245	70.7	41.9	2.6	2	0.7	3	0.8

Table 184c India - India - Inde   Inflammatory heart diseases - Endocarditis

Age group (years)	Incidence 1990 Number ('000s)	Rate (per 100 000)	Prevalence 1990 Number ('000s)	Rate (per 100 000)	Avg. age at onset (years)	Average duration (years)	Deaths 1990 Number ('000s)	Rate (per 100 000)	Deaths 2000 (Projected) Number ('000s)	Rate (per 100 000)
Males										
0-4	5	9.0	8	13.0	2.5	2.6	0	0.7	0	0.8
5-14	8	8.1	22	21.8	10.0	2.8	1	0.9	1	0.5
15-44	115	57.5	314	156.6	29.8	2.9	2	0.9	2	0.8
45-59	27	57.5	81	170.3	52.3	2.8	1	1.7	1	2.0
60+	16	54.0	47	159.2	69.7	2.4	1	2.4	1	2.6
All ages	172	39.2	472	107.5	35.3	2.9	5	1.1	5	1.0
Females										
0-4	4	6.3	5	8.5	2.5	2.2	0	0.8	0	0.7
5-14	7	7.2	16	16.4	10.0	2.5	1	1.2	1	0.7
15-44	99	53.9	235	128.3	29.8	2.6	2	1.1	2	0.8
45-59	25	53.9	64	139.3	52.4	2.5	1	1.3	1	1.2
60+	16	54.0	40	138.4	70.1	2.2	1	1.9	1	2.0
All ages	150	36.5	360	87.7	36.2	2.5	5	1.2	4	0.9
Total	322	37.9	832	97.9	35.7	2.7	10	1.1	10	1.0

For epidemiological sources see Lozano et al. 1996. For the methods used to estimate and project incidence, prevalence, and deaths see Murray and Lopez 1996a. See explanatory notes for definitions and caveats.

Table 184
Inflammatory heart diseases

Endocarditis

Cuadro 184
Enfermedades inflamatorias
del corazón
Endocarditis

Tableau 184
Maladies cardiaques
inflammatoires
Endocardite

Table 184d   China - China - Chine   Inflammatory heart diseases - Endocarditis

Age group (years)	Incidence 1990 Number ('000s)	Rate (per 100 000)	Prevalence 1990 Number ('000s)	Rate (per 100 000)	Avg. age at onset (years)	Average duration (years)	Deaths 1990 Number ('000s)	Rate (per 100 000)	Deaths 2000 (Projected) Number ('000s)	Rate (per 100 000)
Males										
0-4	4	6.0	5	8.8	2.5	2.7	0	0.4	0	0.4
5-14	5	5.4	14	14.5	10.0	2.8	0	0.3	0	0.1
15-44	118	38.4	320	104.6	29.9	3.0	2	0.6	2	0.5
45-59	28	38.4	83	113.6	52.3	2.8	1	0.8	1	0.9
60+	18	36.0	52	106.2	69.8	2.4	1	1.3	1	1.4
All ages	172	29.4	474	81.1	36.4	2.9	4	0.6	4	0.6
Females										
0-4	2	4.2	3	5.8	2.5	2.3	0	0.3	0	0.2
5-14	4	4.8	10	10.9	10.0	2.5	0	0.1	0	0.1
15-44	102	36.0	243	85.7	29.9	2.6	2	0.7	2	0.5
45-59	23	36.0	60	92.9	52.4	2.5	0	0.6	0	0.5
60+	19	36.0	48	92.2	70.6	2.2	0	0.9	1	0.9
All ages	151	27.5	364	66.4	37.4	2.5	3	0.6	3	0.5
Total	323	28.5	839	74.0	36.9	2.7	7	0.6	7	0.5

Table 184e   OAI - OPAI - APAI   Inflammatory heart diseases - Endocarditis

Age group (years)	Incidence 1990 Number ('000s)	Rate (per 100 000)	Prevalence 1990 Number ('000s)	Rate (per 100 000)	Avg. age at onset (years)	Average duration (years)	Deaths 1990 Number ('000s)	Rate (per 100 000)	Deaths 2000 (Projected) Number ('000s)	Rate (per 100 000)
Males										
0-4	3	6.5	4	9.4	2.5	2.6	1	2.1	1	2.1
5-14	5	5.8	13	15.5	10.0	2.8	4	4.4	2	3.0
15-44	67	41.6	182	112.9	29.7	2.9	3	1.7	3	1.5
45-59	14	41.6	42	122.7	52.3	2.8	0	1.4	1	1.5
60+	8	39.0	23	114.6	69.6	2.4	0	1.9	1	2.0
All ages	97	28.2	264	76.9	34.5	2.9	8	2.4	8	1.9
Females										
0-4	2	4.6	3	6.2	2.5	2.3	1	1.7	1	1.5
5-14	4	5.2	9	11.8	10.0	2.4	3	3.2	2	1.9
15-44	62	39.0	148	92.5	29.8	2.5	2	1.4	2	1.1
45-59	14	39.0	35	100.4	52.3	2.5	0	0.9	0	0.7
60+	9	39.0	23	99.7	70.3	2.2	0	1.3	0	1.3
All ages	91	26.7	217	64.0	35.6	2.5	6	1.8	5	1.3
Total	187	27.5	481	70.5	35.0	2.7	14	2.1	13	1.6

Table 184f   SSA - ASS - ASS   Inflammatory heart diseases - Endocarditis

Age group (years)	Incidence 1990 Number ('000s)	Rate (per 100 000)	Prevalence 1990 Number ('000s)	Rate (per 100 000)	Avg. age at onset (years)	Average duration (years)	Deaths 1990 Number ('000s)	Rate (per 100 000)	Deaths 2000 (Projected) Number ('000s)	Rate (per 100 000)
Males										
0-4	4	8.0	5	11.4	2.4	2.4	0	1.0	1	1.0
5-14	5	7.2	13	19.1	10.0	2.7	1	1.7	1	1.1
15-44	53	51.1	143	138.3	29.4	2.9	1	1.0	1	0.9
45-59	10	51.1	31	151.0	52.2	2.8	0	2.2	1	2.1
60+	5	48.0	15	141.1	69.2	2.4	0	4.2	1	4.3
All ages	77	30.7	208	82.3	32.5	2.8	4	1.4	4	1.2
Females										
0-4	3	5.6	3	7.4	2.4	2.2	1	1.2	1	1.0
5-14	4	6.4	10	14.4	10.0	2.4	2	2.4	1	1.4
15-44	51	48.0	120	113.4	29.5	2.5	1	1.0	1	0.7
45-59	11	48.0	27	123.5	52.2	2.5	0	1.6	0	1.3
60+	6	48.0	16	122.8	69.7	2.2	0	3.9	1	3.7
All ages	75	29.0	177	68.6	33.9	2.5	4	1.7	4	1.2
Total	152	29.8	385	75.4	33.2	2.6	8	1.6	8	1.2

For epidemiological sources see Lozano et al. 1996. For the methods used to estimate and project incidence, prevalence, and deaths see Murray and Lopez 1996a. See explanatory notes for definitions and caveats.

Table 184
Inflammatory heart diseases

Endocarditis

Cuadro 184
Enfermedades inflamatorias del corazón

Endocarditis

Tableau 184
Maladies cardiaques inflammatoires

Endocardite

Table 184g   LAC - ALC - ALC   Inflammatory heart diseases - Endocarditis

Age group (years)	Incidence 1990 Number ('000s)	Rate (per 100 000)	Prevalence 1990 Number ('000s)	Rate (per 100 000)	Avg. age at onset (years)	Average duration (years)	Deaths 1990 Number ('000s)	Rate (per 100 000)	Deaths 2000 (Projected) Number ('000s)	Rate (per 100 000)
Males										
0-4	3	10.0	4	15	2.5	2.7	0	0.4	0	0.4
5-14	4	7.0	11	21	10.0	2.9	0	0.5	0	0.4
15-44	44	42.0	120	115	29.8	3.0	1	0.5	1	0.5
45-59	9	42.0	28	125	52.3	2.8	0	0.9	0	0.9
60+	6	40.0	17	118	70.3	2.5	0	1.5	0	1.5
All ages	65	29.5	179	81	34.2	2.9	1	0.6	2	0.6
Females										
0-4	2	8.5	3	12	2.5	2.4	0	0.3	0	0.3
5-14	3	6.0	8	16	10.0	2.5	0	0.3	0	0.2
15-44	40	38.0	94	91	29.8	2.6	1	0.7	1	0.6
45-59	9	38.0	23	98	52.4	2.5	0	0.7	0	0.6
60+	6	35.0	15	91	71.1	2.2	0	1.0	0	1.0
All ages	60	26.8	144	65	35.1	2.5	1	0.6	1	0.5
Total	125	28.1	323	73	34.7	2.7	3	0.6	3	0.5

Table 184h   MEC - AOM - CMO   Inflammatory heart diseases - Endocarditis

Age group (years)	Incidence 1990 Number ('000s)	Rate (per 100 000)	Prevalence 1990 Number ('000s)	Rate (per 100 000)	Avg. age at onset (years)	Average duration (years)	Deaths 1990 Number ('000s)	Rate (per 100 000)	Deaths 2000 (Projected) Number ('000s)	Rate (per 100 000)
Males										
0-4	3	7.5	4	10.9	2.5	2.6	1	2.5	1	2.5
5-14	4	6.7	12	18.2	10.0	2.8	2	3.7	2	2.6
15-44	55	47.9	149	130.8	29.8	3.0	2	1.7	2	1.5
45-59	11	47.9	32	142.1	52.3	2.8	0	2.0	1	2.0
60+	7	48.0	19	140.5	69.7	2.4	0	2.9	1	3.1
All ages	79	31.0	216	84.3	34.0	2.9	6	2.4	7	2.1
Females										
0-4	2	5.3	3	7.1	2.5	2.3	1	2.0	1	1.7
5-14	4	6.0	9	13.7	10.0	2.5	2	2.9	1	1.8
15-44	48	45.0	115	107.1	29.8	2.6	2	2.0	2	1.5
45-59	10	45.0	26	116.2	52.3	2.5	0	1.4	0	1.2
60+	7	45.0	18	115.5	70.4	2.2	0	1.9	0	1.9
All ages	71	28.8	170	68.9	35.1	2.5	5	2.2	5	1.6
Total	150	29.9	386	76.8	34.5	2.7	12	2.3	12	1.9

Table 184i   World - Mundo - Monde   Inflammatory heart diseases - Endocarditis

Age group (years)	Incidence 1990 Number ('000s)	Rate (per 100 000)	Prevalence 1990 Number ('000s)	Rate (per 100 000)	Avg. age at onset (years)	Average duration (years)	Deaths 1990 Number ('000s)	Rate (per 100 000)	Deaths 2000 (Projected) Number ('000s)	Rate (per 100 000)
Males										
0-4	24	7.4	35	10.8	2.5	2.6	3	1.0	4	1.1
5-14	35	6.4	96	17.5	10.0	2.8	9	1.6	7	1.1
15-44	537	42.9	1 463	117.1	29.8	3.0	12	0.9	12	0.9
45-59	130	41.8	387	123.8	52.3	2.8	4	1.2	5	1.3
60+	84	38.4	246	112.6	70.1	2.4	4	1.8	5	1.9
All ages	810	30.5	2 227	83.9	36.1	2.9	32	1.2	34	1.1
Females										
0-4	16	5.3	22	7.2	2.5	2.3	3	0.9	3	0.8
5-14	30	5.7	69	13.2	10.0	2.5	7	1.4	5	0.9
15-44	480	40.1	1 146	95.6	29.8	2.6	11	0.9	10	0.7
45-59	121	39.0	314	101.0	52.4	2.5	2	0.8	3	0.7
60+	99	36.9	251	93.3	71.2	2.2	3	1.3	4	1.3
All ages	747	28.6	1 803	69.0	37.8	2.5	27	1.1	25	0.8
Total	1 557	29.6	4 031	76.5	36.9	2.7	59	1.1	59	1.0

For epidemiological sources see Lozano et al. 1996. For the methods used to estimate and project incidence, prevalence, and deaths see Murray and Lopez 1996a. See explanatory notes for definitions and caveats.

Table 185
Inflammatory heart diseases

Cardiomyopathy

Cuadro 185
Enfermedades inflamatorias del corazón

Cardiomiopatia

Tableau 185
Maladies cardiaques inflammatoires

Cardiomyopathie

Table 185a   EME - PEMC - EMBE   Inflammatory heart diseases - Cardiomyopathy

Age group (years)	Incidence 1990 Number ('000s)	Rate (per 100 000)	Prevalence 1990 Number ('000s)	Rate (per 100 000)	Avg. age at onset (years)	Average duration (years)	Deaths 1990 Number ('000s)	Rate (per 100 000)	Deaths 2000 (Projected) Number ('000s)	Rate (per 100 000)
Males										
0-4	1	3.7	2	6.4	2.5	4.0	0	1.0	0	0.8
5-14	0	0.0	2	3.8	10.0	4.0	0	0.2	0	0.1
15-44	7	3.8	24	13.1	29.9	4.0	4	2.0	3	1.8
45-59	12	18.3	38	58.0	52.4	3.8	6	8.7	7	8.8
60+	42	68.9	142	234.7	71.1	3.2	21	34.8	24	32.7
All ages	62	15.8	208	53.4	61.7	3.4	31	7.9	34	8.3
Females										
0-4	1	4.7	2	8.1	2.5	4.0	0	1.2	0	1.0
5-14	0	0.0	2	4.9	10.0	4.0	0	0.2	0	0.1
15-44	2	1.3	8	4.5	30.0	4.0	1	0.7	1	0.6
45-59	5	7.0	15	22.0	52.4	3.9	2	3.4	2	2.4
60+	51	60.7	174	205.5	72.4	3.3	25	30.0	27	27.8
All ages	60	14.6	201	49.4	67.8	3.4	29	7.2	30	7.1
Total	121	15.2	410	51.3	64.7	3.4	60	7.5	64	7.7

Table 185b   FSE - PEAS - AESE   Inflammatory heart diseases - Cardiomyopathy

Age group (years)	Incidence 1990 Number ('000s)	Rate (per 100 000)	Prevalence 1990 Number ('000s)	Rate (per 100 000)	Avg. age at onset (years)	Average duration (years)	Deaths 1990 Number ('000s)	Rate (per 100 000)	Deaths 2000 (Projected) Number ('000s)	Rate (per 100 000)
Males										
0-4	0	3.0	1	5.2	2.5	3.9	0	0.7	0	0.8
5-14	0	0.0	1	3.1	10.0	4.0	0	0.2	0	0.2
15-44	6	7.6	20	26.4	29.8	3.9	3	4.0	3	3.7
45-59	10	37.0	31	115.9	52.2	3.7	5	17.2	6	19.0
60+	19	90.8	66	314.3	70.0	3.1	10	47.5	14	55.7
All ages	35	21.3	119	71.9	57.6	3.4	18	10.7	23	13.5
Females										
0-4	1	4.0	1	6.9	2.5	4.0	0	1.1	0	1.0
5-14	0	0.0	1	4.2	10.0	4.0	0	0.2	0	0.1
15-44	2	2.2	6	7.8	29.9	4.0	1	1.2	1	1.0
45-59	5	15.5	14	48.0	52.4	3.9	2	7.2	2	6.3
60+	29	80.8	100	273.6	71.5	3.3	15	40.7	18	44.2
All ages	36	20.0	122	67.3	66.2	3.4	18	10.0	21	11.4
Total	71	20.6	241	69.5	61.9	3.4	36	10.3	44	12.4

Table 185c   India - India - Inde   Inflammatory heart diseases - Cardiomyopathy

Age group (years)	Incidence 1990 Number ('000s)	Rate (per 100 000)	Prevalence 1990 Number ('000s)	Rate (per 100 000)	Avg. age at onset (years)	Average duration (years)	Deaths 1990 Number ('000s)	Rate (per 100 000)	Deaths 2000 (Projected) Number ('000s)	Rate (per 100 000)
Males										
0-4	5	8.8	8	14.0	2.5	3.2	2	2.7	2	2.9
5-14	0	0.0	7	7.1	10.0	3.3	1	1.3	1	0.8
15-44	10	5.1	31	15.3	29.8	3.3	6	2.9	6	2.6
45-59	18	37.8	48	101.3	52.3	3.2	9	19.9	13	22.6
60+	28	93.9	82	275.7	69.6	2.7	16	54.8	22	60.2
All ages	61	14.0	177	40.2	52.1	3.0	34	7.8	45	8.7
Females										
0-4	3	5.6	5	8.9	2.5	3.2	2	4.2	2	3.7
5-14	3	3.4	12	12.3	10.0	3.3	2	1.8	1	1.0
15-44	7	4.0	24	13.1	29.8	3.3	5	2.6	4	1.8
45-59	16	34.0	42	90.9	52.4	3.2	8	17.7	9	16.1
60+	31	108.8	91	315.8	70.0	2.7	18	61.2	24	62.0
All ages	61	14.8	174	42.4	53.9	3.0	35	8.6	41	8.4
Total	122	14.4	351	41.3	53.0	3.0	70	8.2	85	8.6

For epidemiological sources see Lozano et al. 1996. For the methods used to estimate and project incidence, prevalence, and deaths see Murray and Lopez 1996a. See explanatory notes for definitions and caveats.

Table 185
Inflammatory heart diseases

Cardiomyopathy

Cuadro 185
Enfermedades inflamatorias del corazón

Cardiomiopatia

Tableau 185
Maladies cardiaques inflammatoires

Cardiomyopathie

Table 185d — China - China - Chine — Inflammatory heart diseases - Cardiomyopathy

Age group (years)	Incidence 1990 Number ('000s)	Rate (per 100 000)	Prevalence 1990 Number ('000s)	Rate (per 100 000)	Avg. age at onset (years)	Average duration (years)	Deaths 1990 Number ('000s)	Rate (per 100 000)	Deaths 2000 (Projected) Number ('000s)	Rate (per 100 000)
Males										
0-4	3	4.8	5	8.2	2.5	3.9	1	1.6	1	1.6
5-14	0	0.0	5	5.0	10.0	4.0	0	0.4	0	0.2
15-44	11	3.5	38	12.3	29.9	4.0	5	1.7	5	1.5
45-59	13	17.8	41	56.0	52.3	3.8	6	8.6	10	10.2
60+	30	61.9	101	206.8	73.8	3.1	15	31.2	20	34.0
All ages	57	9.7	189	32.4	57.0	3.4	28	4.8	36	5.6
Females										
0-4	3	4.8	5	8.2	2.5	3.9	1	1.5	1	1.3
5-14	0	0.0	5	5.0	10.0	4.0	0	0.2	0	0.1
15-44	10	3.6	36	12.6	29.9	4.0	5	1.9	4	1.3
45-59	11	17.4	35	55.0	52.4	3.8	5	8.3	6	6.9
60+	32	62.0	109	210.4	70.6	3.2	16	31.4	20	31.7
All ages	56	10.3	189	34.5	56.2	3.5	28	5.1	32	5.1
Total	113	10.0	379	33.4	56.6	3.5	56	5.0	68	5.3

Table 185e — OAI - OPAI - APAI — Inflammatory heart diseases - Cardiomyopathy

Age group (years)	Incidence 1990 Number ('000s)	Rate (per 100 000)	Prevalence 1990 Number ('000s)	Rate (per 100 000)	Avg. age at onset (years)	Average duration (years)	Deaths 1990 Number ('000s)	Rate (per 100 000)	Deaths 2000 (Projected) Number ('000s)	Rate (per 100 000)
Males										
0-4	16	37.0	28	63	2.5	3.8	3	7.6	3	7.5
5-14	10	11.5	57	68	10.0	4.0	5	6.3	4	4.3
15-44	16	9.8	66	41	29.7	3.9	8	5.1	9	4.5
45-59	12	34.0	37	110	52.3	3.7	6	16.3	8	17.1
60+	19	92.8	64	315	69.6	3.1	9	47.0	14	48.9
All ages	72	21.0	251	73	35.0	3.7	32	9.3	37	9.2
Females										
0-4	18	43.0	31	73	2.5	3.9	4	9.4	3	8.0
5-14	2	2.0	40	50	10.0	4.0	4	4.8	2	2.9
15-44	11	7.2	43	27	29.8	3.9	6	3.5	5	2.6
45-59	9	24.5	28	80	52.3	3.8	4	11.8	5	9.7
60+	21	92.8	71	311	70.3	3.1	10	45.8	15	45.2
All ages	61	17.9	213	63	38.4	3.6	28	8.2	30	7.5
Total	133	19.4	464	68	36.5	3.6	60	8.8	67	8.4

Table 185f — SSA - ASS - ASS — Inflammatory heart diseases - Cardiomyopathy

Age group (years)	Incidence 1990 Number ('000s)	Rate (per 100 000)	Prevalence 1990 Number ('000s)	Rate (per 100 000)	Avg. age at onset (years)	Average duration (years)	Deaths 1990 Number ('000s)	Rate (per 100 000)	Deaths 2000 (Projected) Number ('000s)	Rate (per 100 000)
Males										
0-4	7	15.5	12	26	2.4	3.6	2	3.6	2	3.5
5-14	2	2.5	16	23	10.0	3.9	2	2.4	2	1.6
15-44	8	7.8	30	29	29.4	3.9	4	4.0	5	3.6
45-59	11	56.4	35	172	52.2	3.7	5	25.2	6	23.7
60+	21	197.0	68	649	69.2	3.0	10	94.9	14	96.9
All ages	49	19.6	161	64	46.7	3.4	23	9.0	29	8.5
Females										
0-4	13	28.5	23	48	2.4	3.7	3	6.3	3	5.5
5-14	2	2.3	25	36	10.0	3.9	2	3.5	2	2.1
15-44	7	6.5	26	24	29.5	3.9	3	2.5	3	1.8
45-59	10	46.9	32	144	52.2	3.7	5	20.8	5	17.8
60+	32	255.2	105	827	69.6	3.1	15	121.0	20	115.0
All ages	65	25.1	211	82	47.2	3.4	28	10.9	33	9.6
Total	114	22.4	372	73	46.9	3.4	51	9.9	63	9.0

For epidemiological sources see Lozano et al. 1996. For the methods used to estimate and project incidence, prevalence, and deaths see Murray and Lopez 1996a. See explanatory notes for definitions and caveats.

Table 185
Inflammatory heart diseases
Cardiomyopathy

Cuadro 185
Enfermedades inflamatorias del corazón
Cardiomiopatia

Tableau 185
Maladies cardiaques inflammatoires
Cardiomyopathie

Table 185g LAC - ALC - ALC   Inflammatory heart diseases - Cardiomyopathy

Age group (years)	Incidence 1990 Number ('000s)	Rate (per 100 000)	Prevalence 1990 Number ('000s)	Rate (per 100 000)	Avg. age at onset (years)	Average duration (years)	Deaths 1990 Number ('000s)	Rate (per 100 000)	Deaths 2000 (Projected) Number ('000s)	Rate (per 100 000)
Males										
0-4	1	4.4	2	7.1	2.5	3.2	0	1.4	0	1.4
5-14	0	0.1	2	3.7	10.0	3.3	0	0.7	0	0.5
15-44	3	3.2	10	9.6	29.8	3.3	2	1.9	2	1.8
45-59	4	20.0	12	54.0	52.3	3.2	2	10.8	3	10.8
60+	9	62.9	26	183.2	70.3	2.7	5	36.3	7	37.3
All ages	18	8.1	52	23.5	53.5	3.0	10	4.7	14	5.2
Females										
0-4	1	5.0	2	8.0	2.5	3.3	0	1.7	0	1.5
5-14	0	0.0	2	4.1	10.0	3.3	0	0.5	0	0.3
15-44	3	3.3	10	9.8	29.8	3.3	2	2.0	2	1.6
45-59	4	16.0	10	43.9	52.4	3.2	2	8.6	3	7.9
60+	10	58.0	29	169.5	71.1	2.8	6	33.8	8	34.0
All ages	18	8.2	53	23.9	54.3	3.0	10	4.7	13	5.0
Total	36	8.2	105	23.7	53.9	3.0	21	4.7	27	5.1

Table 185h MEC - AOM - CMO   Inflammatory heart diseases - Cardiomyopathy

Age group (years)	Incidence 1990 Number ('000s)	Rate (per 100 000)	Prevalence 1990 Number ('000s)	Rate (per 100 000)	Avg. age at onset (years)	Average duration (years)	Deaths 1990 Number ('000s)	Rate (per 100 000)	Deaths 2000 (Projected) Number ('000s)	Rate (per 100 000)
Males										
0-4	18	43.0	30	73	2.5	3.8	4	8.9	4	8.9
5-14	3	4.5	37	56	10.0	4.0	3	5.3	3	3.8
15-44	12	10.8	47	41	29.8	3.9	6	5.0	7	4.5
45-59	11	49.9	35	158	52.3	3.7	5	22.6	7	23.1
60+	19	142.5	66	483	69.7	3.1	10	70.7	14	75.6
All ages	64	24.8	215	84	37.4	3.6	28	10.7	36	10.7
Females										
0-4	19	49.0	33	83	2.5	3.8	4	10.6	4	9.4
5-14	0	0.0	32	51	10.0	4.0	3	4.3	2	2.7
15-44	12	10.8	42	39	29.8	4.0	5	4.7	5	3.5
45-59	9	38.8	28	125	52.3	3.8	4	18.1	5	15.8
60+	20	127.6	67	434	70.4	3.2	10	63.7	14	64.6
All ages	59	24.1	201	82	37.6	3.6	26	10.5	30	9.4
Total	123	24.4	416	83	37.5	3.6	53	10.6	66	10.1

Table 185i World - Mundo - Monde   Inflammatory heart diseases - Cardiomyopathy

Age group (years)	Incidence 1990 Number ('000s)	Rate (per 100 000)	Prevalence 1990 Number ('000s)	Rate (per 100 000)	Avg. age at onset (years)	Average duration (years)	Deaths 1990 Number ('000s)	Rate (per 100 000)	Deaths 2000 (Projected) Number ('000s)	Rate (per 100 000)
Males										
0-4	52	16.2	88	27	2.5	3.6	12	3.7	13	3.9
5-14	14	2.6	126	23	10.0	3.8	13	2.3	10	1.5
15-44	73	5.9	264	21	29.8	3.8	37	3.0	40	2.7
45-59	92	29.3	278	89	52.3	3.6	44	14.1	61	15.1
60+	187	85.4	615	281	71.0	3.0	97	44.2	129	47.0
All ages	418	15.8	1 372	52	50.9	3.4	202	7.6	253	8.2
Females										
0-4	60	19.4	101	33	2.5	3.7	15	4.9	15	4.5
5-14	6	1.2	118	22	10.0	3.8	11	2.1	8	1.3
15-44	55	4.6	195	16	29.8	3.8	27	2.3	25	1.8
45-59	68	21.7	205	66	52.4	3.7	33	10.5	37	9.2
60+	227	84.4	745	277	71.2	3.2	117	43.5	148	44.0
All ages	416	15.9	1 364	52	53.2	3.4	204	7.8	233	7.6
Total	834	15.8	2 736	52	52.1	3.4	407	7.7	486	7.9

For epidemiological sources see Lozano et al. 1996. For the methods used to estimate and project incidence, prevalence, and deaths see Murray and Lopez 1996a. See explanatory notes for definitions and caveats.

Table 186
Chronic obstructive pulmonary disease
Symptomatic cases

Cuadro 186
Enfermedad pulmonar obtructiva crónica
Casos sintomáticos

Tableau 186
Maladie pulmonaire obstructive chronique
Cas symptomatiques

Table 186a   EME - PEMC - EMBE   Chronic obstructive pulmonary disease - Symptomatic cases

Age group (years)	Incidence 1990 Number ('000s)	Rate (per 100 000)	Prevalence 1990 Number ('000s)	Rate (per 100 000)	Avg. age at onset (years)	Average duration (years)	Deaths 1990 Number ('000s)	Rate (per 100 000)	Deaths 2000 (Projected) Number ('000s)	Rate (per 100 000)
Males										
0-4	0	0.0	0	0	-	-	0	0.0	0	0.0
5-14	0	0.0	0	0	-	-	0	0.0	0	0.0
15-44	10	5.5	137	75	29.9	26.1	1	0.4	1	0.4
45-59	60	91.4	463	700	52.4	11.0	8	12.0	9	11.0
60+	366	604.7	2 126	3 511	70.7	5.1	148	244.1	174	240.6
All ages	437	111.8	2 726	698	67.2	6.4	156	40.1	183	44.6
Females										
0-4	0	0.0	0	0	-	-	0	0.0	0	0.0
5-14	0	0.0	0	0	-	-	0	0.0	0	0.0
15-44	5	2.9	71	40	30.0	26.9	0	0.2	0	0.2
45-59	35	51.8	267	394	52.5	11.6	5	6.7	6	7.1
60+	193	227.7	1 207	1 428	72.3	5.4	83	98.0	103	105.4
All ages	233	57.2	1 545	379	68.4	6.8	88	21.6	109	25.4
Total	670	83.9	4 271	535	67.6	6.6	244	30.6	292	34.8

Table 186b   FSE - PEAS - AESE   Chronic obstructive pulmonary disease - Symptomatic cases

Age group (years)	Incidence 1990 Number ('000s)	Rate (per 100 000)	Prevalence 1990 Number ('000s)	Rate (per 100 000)	Avg. age at onset (years)	Average duration (years)	Deaths 1990 Number ('000s)	Rate (per 100 000)	Deaths 2000 (Projected) Number ('000s)	Rate (per 100 000)
Males										
0-4	0	0.0	0	0	-	-	0	0.0	0	0.0
5-14	0	0.0	0	0	-	-	0	0.0	0	0.0
15-44	11	15.0	154	202	29.8	24.6	1	1.1	1	1.2
45-59	64	235.7	485	1 800	52.2	10.3	8	30.9	13	40.4
60+	67	321.0	576	2 745	69.8	4.9	39	187.3	73	285.4
All ages	142	86.1	1 215	735	58.7	8.9	48	29.3	86	50.4
Females										
0-4	0	0.0	0	0	-	-	0	0.0	0	0.0
5-14	0	0.0	0	0	-	-	0	0.0	0	0.0
15-44	5	7.0	71	95	30.0	26.4	0	0.5	0	0.5
45-59	11	37.9	116	387	52.4	11.3	2	6.6	3	8.4
60+	71	195.5	437	1 201	71.4	5.2	29	78.9	48	117.0
All ages	88	48.5	625	345	66.5	7.3	31	17.2	51	27.5
Total	230	66.4	1 839	531	61.7	8.3	80	23.0	138	38.4

Table 186c   India - India - Inde   Chronic obstructive pulmonary disease - Symptomatic cases

Age group (years)	Incidence 1990 Number ('000s)	Rate (per 100 000)	Prevalence 1990 Number ('000s)	Rate (per 100 000)	Avg. age at onset (years)	Average duration (years)	Deaths 1990 Number ('000s)	Rate (per 100 000)	Deaths 2000 (Projected) Number ('000s)	Rate (per 100 000)
Males										
0-4	0	0	0	0	-	-	0	0.0	0	0.0
5-14	0	0	0	0	-	-	0	0.0	0	0.0
15-44	22	11	297	148	29.8	25.0	2	0.8	2	0.8
45-59	85	180	652	1 371	52.3	10.5	11	23.4	18	29.4
60+	145	488	970	3 257	69.4	4.8	68	229.3	103	278.1
All ages	253	57	1 918	437	60.2	8.5	81	18.4	122	23.9
Females										
0-4	0	0	0	0	-	-	0	0.0	0	0.0
5-14	0	0	0	0	-	-	0	0.0	0	0.0
15-44	21	12	286	156	29.8	25.4	2	0.8	2	0.8
45-59	65	140	524	1 139	52.4	10.8	9	19.5	13	22.1
60+	81	280	599	2 072	69.9	4.9	42	146.3	68	175.2
All ages	167	41	1 409	344	58.0	9.8	53	12.9	83	17.1
Total	419	49	3 328	392	59.3	9.0	134	15.7	205	20.6

For epidemiological sources see Gakidou et al. 1996b. For the methods used to estimate and project incidence, prevalence, and deaths see Murray and Lopez 1996a. See explanatory notes for definitions and caveats.

Table 186
Chronic obstructive
pulmonary disease
Symptomatic cases

Cuadro 186
Enfermedad pulmonar
obtructiva crónica
Casos sintomáticos

Tableau 186
Maladie pulmonaire
obstructive chronique
Cas symptomatiques

Table 186d — China - China - Chine — Chronic obstructive pulmonary disease - Symptomatic cases

Age group (years)	Incidence 1990 Number ('000s)	Rate (per 100 000)	Prevalence 1990 Number ('000s)	Rate (per 100 000)	Avg. age at onset (years)	Average duration (years)	Deaths 1990 Number ('000s)	Rate (per 100 000)	Deaths 2000 (Projected) Number ('000s)	Rate (per 100 000)
Males										
0-4	0	0	0	0	-	-	0	0.0	0	0.0
5-14	0	0	0	0	-	-	0	0.0	0	0.0
15-44	168	55	2 281	745	29.9	25.5	10	3.3	12	3.8
45-59	433	596	3 627	4 991	52.3	10.7	62	85.3	95	97.0
60+	1 501	3 064	9 403	19 197	68.1	5.0	661	1 349.1	828	1 373.0
All ages	2 101	359	15 311	2 616	61.8	7.8	733	125.2	935	142.5
Females										
0-4	0	0	0	0	-	-	0	0.0	0	0.0
5-14	0	0	0	0	-	-	0	0.0	0	0.0
15-44	126	44	1 711	602	29.9	26.1	8	2.8	10	3.3
45-59	322	499	2 678	4 159	52.3	11.1	44	67.9	63	68.7
60+	1 365	2 641	8 631	16 704	69.1	5.2	634	1 226.4	777	1 205.7
All ages	1 812	330	13 020	2 374	63.4	7.7	685	124.9	849	136.1
Total	3 913	345	28 331	2 499	62.5	7.8	1 418	125.1	1 785	139.4

Table 186e — OAI - OPAI - APAI — Chronic obstructive pulmonary disease - Symptomatic cases

Age group (years)	Incidence 1990 Number ('000s)	Rate (per 100 000)	Prevalence 1990 Number ('000s)	Rate (per 100 000)	Avg. age at onset (years)	Average duration (years)	Deaths 1990 Number ('000s)	Rate (per 100 000)	Deaths 2000 (Projected) Number ('000s)	Rate (per 100 000)
Males										
0-4	0	0.0	0	0	-	-	0	0.0	0	0.0
5-14	0	0.0	0	0	-	-	0	0.0	0	0.0
15-44	14	8.9	192	120	29.8	24.6	1	0.6	1	0.6
45-59	32	94.3	267	781	52.3	10.3	5	13.5	6	13.9
60+	91	448.0	532	2 630	69.4	4.8	38	188.2	59	213.5
All ages	137	39.9	990	289	61.3	8.1	44	12.7	67	16.5
Females										
0-4	0	0.0	0	0	-	-	0	0.0	0	0.0
5-14	0	0.0	0	0	-	-	0	0.0	0	0.0
15-44	10	6.2	133	84	29.8	25.2	1	0.5	1	0.4
45-59	14	39.4	133	379	52.4	10.7	2	6.6	3	7.0
60+	60	264.0	341	1 506	70.2	4.9	24	107.0	40	123.4
All ages	84	24.6	607	179	62.5	8.3	27	8.0	44	11.0
Total	221	32.3	1 598	234	61.7	8.2	71	10.4	111	13.8

Table 186f — SSA - ASS - ASS — Chronic obstructive pulmonary disease - Symptomatic cases

Age group (years)	Incidence 1990 Number ('000s)	Rate (per 100 000)	Prevalence 1990 Number ('000s)	Rate (per 100 000)	Avg. age at onset (years)	Average duration (years)	Deaths 1990 Number ('000s)	Rate (per 100 000)	Deaths 2000 (Projected) Number ('000s)	Rate (per 100 000)
Males										
0-4	0	0	0	0	-	-	0	0.0	0	0.0
5-14	0	0	0	0	-	-	0	0.0	0	0.0
15-44	29	28	355	342	29.4	18.4	4	3.8	5	3.5
45-59	50	248	361	1 775	52.2	7.7	13	61.6	15	56.7
60+	87	826	398	3 787	68.9	3.6	43	411.7	67	468.2
All ages	167	66	1 113	441	56.9	7.4	60	23.7	87	25.5
Females										
0-4	0	0	0	0	-	-	0	0.0	0	0.0
5-14	0	0	0	0	-	-	0	0.0	0	0.0
15-44	14	13	173	163	29.5	18.8	1	1.1	1	1.0
45-59	32	145	220	994	52.3	7.8	8	34.3	11	37.7
60+	53	418	249	1 956	69.5	3.7	27	211.6	47	267.7
All ages	99	39	642	249	58.2	7.2	36	13.9	59	17.0
Total	266	52	1 755	344	57.4	7.3	95	18.7	147	21.2

For epidemiological sources see Gakidou et al. 1996b. For the methods used to estimate and project incidence, prevalence, and deaths see Murray and Lopez 1996a. See explanatory notes for definitions and caveats.

Table 186	Cuadro 186	Tableau 186
Chronic obstructive	**Enfermedad pulmonar**	**Maladie pulmonaire**
pulmonary disease	**obtructiva crónica**	**obstructive chronique**
Symptomatic cases	Casos sintomáticos	Cas symptomatiques

Table 186g LAC - ALC - ALC Chronic obstructive pulmonary disease - Symptomatic cases

Age group (years)	Incidence 1990 Number ('000s)	Rate (per 100 000)	Prevalence 1990 Number ('000s)	Rate (per 100 000)	Avg. age at onset (years)	Average duration (years)	Deaths 1990 Number ('000s)	Rate (per 100 000)	Deaths 2000 (Projected) Number ('000s)	Rate (per 100 000)
Males										
0-4	0	0	0	0	-	-	0	0.0	0	0.0
5-14	0	0	0	0	-	-	0	0.0	0	0.0
15-44	12	12	169	162	29.8	25.3	1	0.9	1	0.9
45-59	28	124	231	1 037	52.3	10.7	4	17.7	5	17.4
60+	65	459	411	2 889	70.1	4.9	29	202.0	46	234.0
All ages	105	48	811	366	60.7	8.9	34	15.2	53	19.8
Females										
0-4	0	0	0	0	-	-	0	0.0	0	0.0
5-14	0	0	0	0	-	-	0	0.0	0	0.0
15-44	12	11	159	153	29.9	25.9	1	0.8	1	0.8
45-59	17	74	166	711	52.4	11.1	3	12.1	5	16.7
60+	43	254	280	1 664	70.9	5.1	19	115.8	36	150.8
All ages	72	32	605	272	59.7	10.0	23	10.4	42	15.7
Total	177	40	1 416	319	60.3	9.3	57	12.8	95	17.8

Table 186h MEC - AOM - CMO Chronic obstructive pulmonary disease - Symptomatic cases

Age group (years)	Incidence 1990 Number ('000s)	Rate (per 100 000)	Prevalence 1990 Number ('000s)	Rate (per 100 000)	Avg. age at onset (years)	Average duration (years)	Deaths 1990 Number ('000s)	Rate (per 100 000)	Deaths 2000 (Projected) Number ('000s)	Rate (per 100 000)
Males										
0-4	0	0	0	0	-	-	0	0.0	0	0.0
5-14	0	0	0	0	-	-	0	0.0	0	0.0
15-44	17	15	228	200	29.8	15.9	1	1.1	2	1.1
45-59	7	33	36	160	52.3	3.5	6	28.2	10	31.5
60+	88	646	427	3 131	69.4	4.8	30	217.9	55	293.5
All ages	112	44	691	269	62.4	6.4	37	14.5	66	19.9
Females										
0-4	0	0	0	0	-	-	0	0.0	0	0.0
5-14	0	0	0	0	-	-	0	0.0	0	0.0
15-44	14	13	184	172	29.9	25.6	1	0.9	1	0.8
45-59	24	108	212	953	52.4	10.8	4	16.2	6	18.9
60+	44	282	301	1 946	70.3	5.0	21	135.5	39	182.2
All ages	81	33	697	283	58.2	10.2	26	10.4	46	14.3
Total	193	38	1 388	276	60.6	8.0	63	12.5	112	17.1

Table 186i World - Mundo - Monde Chronic obstructive pulmonary disease - Symptomatic cases

Age group (years)	Incidence 1990 Number ('000s)	Rate (per 100 000)	Prevalence 1990 Number ('000s)	Rate (per 100 000)	Avg. age at onset (years)	Average duration (years)	Deaths 1990 Number ('000s)	Rate (per 100 000)	Deaths 2000 (Projected) Number ('000s)	Rate (per 100 000)
Males										
0-4	0	0	0	0	-	-	0	0.0	0	0.0
5-14	0	0	0	0	-	-	0	0.0	0	0.0
15-44	284	23	3 812	305	29.8	24.1	20	1.6	25	1.7
45-59	760	243	6 121	1 959	52.3	10.4	117	37.4	171	42.3
60+	2 410	1 101	14 842	6 781	68.8	5.0	1 056	482.5	1 405	510.1
All ages	3 454	130	24 775	934	62.0	7.7	1 193	45.0	1 600	51.7
Females										
0-4	0	0	0	0	-	-	0	0.0	0	0.0
5-14	0	0	0	0	-	-	0	0.0	0	0.0
15-44	207	17	2 789	233	29.9	25.5	14	1.2	17	1.2
45-59	520	167	4 317	1 388	52.3	10.9	76	24.3	110	27.2
60+	1 909	709	12 045	4 474	69.7	5.2	879	326.5	1 158	343.4
All ages	2 635	101	19 151	733	63.1	7.9	969	37.1	1 284	41.9
Total	6 089	116	43 926	834	62.5	7.8	2 162	41.0	2 884	46.8

For epidemiological sources see Gakidou et al. 1996b. For the methods used to estimate and project incidence, prevalence, and deaths see Murray and Lopez 1996a. See explanatory notes for definitions and caveats.

Table 187	Cuadro 187	Tableau 187
Asthma	Asma	Asthme

Cases | Casos | Cas

Table 187a   EME - PEMC - EMBE   Asthma - Cases

Age group (years)	Incidence 1990 Number ('000s)	Incidence 1990 Rate (per 100 000)	Prevalence 1990 Number ('000s)	Prevalence 1990 Rate (per 100 000)	Avg. age at onset (years)	Average duration (years)	Deaths 1990 Number ('000s)	Deaths 1990 Rate (per 100 000)	Deaths 2000 (Projected) Number ('000s)	Deaths 2000 (Projected) Rate (per 100 000)
Males										
0-4	400	1 518	559	2 119	3.0	3.1	0	0.2	0	0.2
5-14	440	824	1 628	3 051	10.0	3.6	0	0.3	0	0.3
15-44	625	339	3 655	1 986	30.5	5.8	1	0.7	1	0.6
45-59	265	401	1 526	2 307	52.4	4.8	1	2.1	2	1.9
60+	244	402	1 197	1 976	71.1	3.7	8	12.5	9	12.1
All ages	1 973	505	8 564	2 193	28.3	4.4	10	2.7	12	2.8
Females										
0-4	250	996	348	1 388	3.0	3.1	0	0.2	0	0.1
5-14	285	562	1 033	2 038	10.1	3.7	0	0.2	0	0.2
15-44	581	324	3 177	1 773	30.9	5.9	1	0.6	1	0.6
45-59	249	368	1 485	2 190	52.4	5.0	1	2.0	2	2.1
60+	256	303	1 312	1 551	72.4	3.9	9	10.7	11	11.4
All ages	1 621	398	7 354	1 806	32.8	4.6	12	2.9	14	3.3
Total	3 594	451	15 919	1 995	30.3	4.5	22	2.8	26	3.1

Table 187b   FSE - PEAS - AESE   Asthma - Cases

Age group (years)	Incidence 1990 Number ('000s)	Incidence 1990 Rate (per 100 000)	Prevalence 1990 Number ('000s)	Prevalence 1990 Rate (per 100 000)	Avg. age at onset (years)	Average duration (years)	Deaths 1990 Number ('000s)	Deaths 1990 Rate (per 100 000)	Deaths 2000 (Projected) Number ('000s)	Deaths 2000 (Projected) Rate (per 100 000)
Males										
0-4	168	1 219	234	1 698	3.0	3.1	0	0.2	0	0.2
5-14	181	663	672	2 457	10.0	3.6	0	0.3	0	0.3
15-44	234	307	1 319	1 730	31.2	5.8	0	0.6	0	0.6
45-59	108	401	620	2 300	52.2	4.7	1	2.1	1	2.8
60+	84	402	416	1 982	70.0	3.6	2	10.6	4	16.0
All ages	776	469	3 261	1 973	27.3	4.3	3	2.0	5	3.2
Females										
0-4	105	799	146	1 111	3.0	3.1	0	0.1	0	0.1
5-14	119	451	433	1 637	10.1	3.7	0	0.2	0	0.2
15-44	221	295	1 171	1 562	31.7	5.9	0	0.5	0	0.5
45-59	110	368	655	2 182	52.3	4.9	1	2.0	1	2.5
60+	110	303	568	1 561	71.5	3.8	3	9.4	5	13.3
All ages	666	368	2 972	1 643	33.3	4.6	4	2.5	7	3.6
Total	1 442	416	6 233	1 800	30.1	4.4	8	2.3	12	3.4

Table 187c   India - India - Inde   Asthma - Cases

Age group (years)	Incidence 1990 Number ('000s)	Incidence 1990 Rate (per 100 000)	Prevalence 1990 Number ('000s)	Prevalence 1990 Rate (per 100 000)	Avg. age at onset (years)	Average duration (years)	Deaths 1990 Number ('000s)	Deaths 1990 Rate (per 100 000)	Deaths 2000 (Projected) Number ('000s)	Deaths 2000 (Projected) Rate (per 100 000)
Males										
0-4	543	908	801	1 340	3.0	3.8	0	0.4	0	0.3
5-14	507	498	2 302	2 263	10.0	4.7	1	0.7	1	0.6
15-44	410	204	3 033	1 512	30.3	7.1	1	0.7	2	0.7
45-59	115	242	818	1 720	52.3	5.6	2	4.0	3	5.0
60+	72	243	430	1 446	69.7	3.9	6	21.3	10	25.9
All ages	1 648	375	7 385	1 681	18.3	5.0	11	2.4	15	3.0
Females										
0-4	336	593	503	888	3.0	4.1	0	0.3	0	0.2
5-14	323	339	1 511	1 586	10.1	5.0	1	0.6	0	0.4
15-44	357	195	2 574	1 405	30.7	7.5	1	0.7	1	0.6
45-59	102	222	800	1 738	52.3	6.0	2	4.1	3	4.6
60+	53	182	360	1 244	70.1	4.1	5	18.1	8	21.5
All ages	1 171	285	5 748	1 402	20.7	5.6	9	2.2	13	2.7
Total	2 818	332	13 133	1 546	19.3	5.2	20	2.3	28	2.8

For epidemiological sources see Mahapatra et al. 1996a. For the methods used to estimate and project incidence, prevalence, and deaths see Murray and Lopez 1996a. See explanatory notes for definitions and caveats.

Table 187	Cuadro 187	Tableau 187
Asthma	Asma	Asthme

Cases   Casos   Cas

Table 187d   China - China - Chine   Asthma - Cases

Age group (years)	Incidence 1990 Number ('000s)	Rate (per 100 000)	Prevalence 1990 Number ('000s)	Rate (per 100 000)	Avg. age at onset (years)	Average duration (years)	Deaths 1990 Number ('000s)	Rate (per 100 000)	Deaths 2000 (Projected) Number ('000s)	Rate (per 100 000)
Males										
0-4	910	1 511	1 359	2 256	3.0	3.9	0	0.5	0	0.4
5-14	794	818	3 605	3 717	10.0	4.7	1	0.7	1	0.5
15-44	1 034	338	7 644	2 496	30.4	7.2	3	0.8	3	0.9
45-59	290	398	2 067	2 844	52.3	5.7	3	4.6	5	5.2
60+	196	400	1 189	2 428	69.8	4.0	12	24.7	15	25.1
All ages	3 224	551	15 864	2 711	22.0	5.3	19	3.2	24	3.7
Females										
0-4	574	991	855	1 476	3.0	3.9	0	0.3	0	0.2
5-14	506	560	2 243	2 481	10.1	4.7	0	0.3	0	0.2
15-44	916	323	6 214	2 187	30.9	7.2	2	0.7	2	0.8
45-59	236	366	1 743	2 706	52.3	5.8	3	4.3	4	4.4
60+	156	302	1 006	1 947	70.6	4.1	11	20.8	13	20.0
All ages	2 388	435	12 061	2 199	24.5	5.6	16	2.9	19	3.1
Total	5 612	495	27 925	2 463	23.1	5.4	35	3.1	43	3.4

Table 187e   OAI - OPAI - APAI   Asthma - Cases

Age group (years)	Incidence 1990 Number ('000s)	Rate (per 100 000)	Prevalence 1990 Number ('000s)	Rate (per 100 000)	Avg. age at onset (years)	Average duration (years)	Deaths 1990 Number ('000s)	Rate (per 100 000)	Deaths 2000 (Projected) Number ('000s)	Rate (per 100 000)
Males										
0-4	333	760	550	1 256	3.0	6.5	0	0.3	0	0.2
5-14	348	414	2 263	2 693	10.0	8.0	1	0.8	1	0.7
15-44	272	169	3 310	2 058	30.3	10.5	2	1.4	3	1.3
45-59	68	200	759	2 223	52.3	7.7	2	4.9	2	5.0
60+	41	201	386	1 910	69.6	4.9	5	24.2	7	26.8
All ages	1 062	310	7 268	2 119	18.0	8.0	10	2.8	13	3.2
Females										
0-4	209	498	345	822	3.0	6.5	0	0.2	0	0.1
5-14	226	282	1 432	1 785	10.1	8.1	0	0.6	0	0.4
15-44	258	162	2 740	1 717	30.7	10.7	2	1.0	2	1.0
45-59	65	184	736	2 098	52.2	8.1	2	4.3	2	4.6
60+	34	151	357	1 575	70.3	5.1	5	20.2	7	22.6
All ages	792	233	5 610	1 652	21.0	8.4	8	2.4	12	2.9
Total	1 854	272	12 878	1 887	19.3	8.2	18	2.6	25	3.1

Table 187f   SSA - ASS - ASS   Asthma - Cases

Age group (years)	Incidence 1990 Number ('000s)	Rate (per 100 000)	Prevalence 1990 Number ('000s)	Rate (per 100 000)	Avg. age at onset (years)	Average duration (years)	Deaths 1990 Number ('000s)	Rate (per 100 000)	Deaths 2000 (Projected) Number ('000s)	Rate (per 100 000)
Males										
0-4	566	1 192	826	1 741	2.9	3.7	0	0.6	0	0.4
5-14	463	660	2 112	3 006	10.0	4.6	1	1.0	1	0.8
15-44	281	270	2 075	2 000	29.9	6.8	2	2.0	3	1.8
45-59	65	321	461	2 272	52.2	5.4	1	6.4	2	5.9
60+	34	322	200	1 903	69.2	3.8	3	31.6	5	35.9
All ages	1 409	558	5 675	2 249	14.5	4.7	8	3.1	10	3.0
Females										
0-4	459	975	672	1 428	2.9	3.7	0	0.3	0	0.2
5-14	390	559	1 735	2 485	10.1	4.6	0	0.6	0	0.4
15-44	341	321	2 310	2 174	30.4	6.9	1	1.0	1	0.9
45-59	81	366	599	2 709	52.2	5.6	1	5.0	2	5.5
60+	38	302	249	1 955	69.7	4.0	3	22.6	5	28.2
All ages	1 310	508	5 564	2 157	17.2	4.9	6	2.2	8	2.4
Total	2 718	533	11 239	2 203	15.8	4.8	13	2.6	19	2.7

For epidemiological sources see Mahapatra et al. 1996a. For the methods used to estimate and project incidence, prevalence, and deaths see Murray and Lopez 1996a. See explanatory notes for definitions and caveats.

Table 187	Cuadro 187	Tableau 187
Asthma	Asma	Asthme

Cases	Casos	Cas

Table 187g LAC - ALC - ALC — Asthma - Cases

Age group (years)	Incidence 1990 Number ('000s)	Rate (per 100 000)	Prevalence 1990 Number ('000s)	Rate (per 100 000)	Avg. age at onset (years)	Average duration (years)	Deaths 1990 Number ('000s)	Rate (per 100 000)	Deaths 2000 (Projected) Number ('000s)	Rate (per 100 000)
Males										
0-4	348	1 212	518	1 802	3.0	3.9	0	0.4	0	0.3
5-14	344	660	1 561	2 995	10.0	4.7	0	0.7	0	0.6
15-44	283	271	2 090	2 004	30.4	7.1	1	1.1	1	1.1
45-59	71	321	507	2 280	52.3	5.7	1	4.1	1	4.0
60+	46	322	275	1 934	70.3	4.1	3	22.3	5	25.5
All ages	1 092	493	4 951	2 234	18.3	5.1	6	2.6	8	3.1
Females										
0-4	281	1 015	418	1 510	3.0	3.9	0	0.3	0	0.2
5-14	293	577	1 294	2 550	10.1	4.7	0	0.5	0	0.4
15-44	271	261	1 931	1 855	31.2	7.2	1	0.9	1	0.8
45-59	83	356	574	2 456	52.4	5.8	1	4.7	2	6.5
60+	67	401	390	2 319	71.1	4.2	4	23.1	7	29.8
All ages	996	447	4 606	2 068	21.5	5.2	6	2.8	10	3.9
Total	2 088	470	9 557	2 151	19.9	5.2	12	2.7	19	3.5

Table 187h MEC - AOM - CMO — Asthma - Cases

Age group (years)	Incidence 1990 Number ('000s)	Rate (per 100 000)	Prevalence 1990 Number ('000s)	Rate (per 100 000)	Avg. age at onset (years)	Average duration (years)	Deaths 1990 Number ('000s)	Rate (per 100 000)	Deaths 2000 (Projected) Number ('000s)	Rate (per 100 000)
Males										
0-4	312	759	515	1 250	3.0	6.5	0	0.2	0	0.2
5-14	270	414	1 760	2 694	10.0	8.1	0	0.6	0	0.5
15-44	193	169	2 348	2 062	30.4	10.7	1	0.9	1	0.9
45-59	45	200	499	2 232	52.3	7.9	1	3.9	1	4.3
60+	27	201	265	1 938	69.7	5.1	3	19.6	5	26.3
All ages	848	331	5 386	2 101	16.2	8.0	5	2.0	8	2.4
Females										
0-4	197	496	324	816	3.0	3.9	0	0.2	0	0.1
5-14	175	282	1 107	1 785	10.1	4.7	0	0.4	0	0.4
15-44	174	162	1 845	1 721	31.2	7.2	1	0.6	1	0.5
45-59	41	184	471	2 111	52.4	5.8	1	3.5	1	4.1
60+	23	151	247	1 597	71.1	4.2	3	16.9	5	22.4
All ages	610	247	3 993	1 619	19.0	5.2	4	1.8	7	2.2
Total	1 458	290	9 380	1 865	17.4	6.8	9	1.9	15	2.3

Table 187i World - Mundo - Monde — Asthma - Cases

Age group (years)	Incidence 1990 Number ('000s)	Rate (per 100 000)	Prevalence 1990 Number ('000s)	Rate (per 100 000)	Avg. age at onset (years)	Average duration (years)	Deaths 1990 Number ('000s)	Rate (per 100 000)	Deaths 2000 (Projected) Number ('000s)	Rate (per 100 000)
Males										
0-4	3 580	1 114	5 361	1 669	3.0	4.2	1	0.4	1	0.3
5-14	3 347	607	15 905	2 885	10.0	5.1	4	0.7	4	0.6
15-44	3 332	267	25 474	2 038	30.4	7.2	12	1.0	14	1.0
45-59	1 027	329	7 257	2 323	52.3	5.6	12	3.8	17	4.2
60+	744	340	4 357	1 991	70.2	3.9	42	19.4	60	21.8
All ages	12 031	453	58 355	2 199	20.9	5.4	71	2.7	96	3.1
Females										
0-4	2 411	780	3 612	1 168	3.0	4.0	1	0.2	1	0.2
5-14	2 317	441	10 787	2 053	10.1	4.9	2	0.4	2	0.3
15-44	3 120	260	21 961	1 832	30.9	7.2	9	0.8	10	0.7
45-59	967	311	7 062	2 270	52.3	5.7	11	3.6	16	4.0
60+	739	274	4 488	1 667	71.3	4.0	42	15.8	62	18.4
All ages	9 553	366	47 909	1 833	24.1	5.4	66	2.5	91	3.0
Total	21 584	410	106 264	2 017	22.3	5.4	137	2.6	187	3.0

For epidemiological sources see Mahapatra et al. 1996a. For the methods used to estimate and project incidence, prevalence, and deaths see Murray and Lopez 1996a. See explanatory notes for definitions and caveats.

Table 188   **Cuadro 188**   **Tableau 188**
Peptic ulcer   **Ulcera péptica**   **Ulcère peptique**

Cases   Casos   Cas

Table 188a   EME - PEMC - EMBE   Peptic ulcer - Cases

Age group (years)	Incidence 1990 Number ('000s)	Rate (per 100 000)	Prevalence 1990 Number ('000s)	Rate (per 100 000)	Avg. age at onset (years)	Average duration (years)	Deaths 1990 Number ('000s)	Rate (per 100 000)	Deaths 2000 (Projected) Number ('000s)	Rate (per 100 000)
Males										
0-4	1	2.0	1	3.9	2.5	6.2	0	0.1	0	0.0
5-14	5	10.0	19	35.5	10.0	6.3	0	0.0	0	0.0
15-44	245	133.1	1 203	653.4	29.9	6.0	1	0.3	1	0.3
45-59	210	317.0	1 042	1 575.6	52.4	5.6	2	2.7	2	2.8
60+	104	171.2	695	1 147.6	71.1	3.9	14	22.4	18	24.3
All ages	564	144.5	2 960	757.9	45.6	5.5	16	4.1	20	5.0
Females										
0-4	1	2.0	1	3.8	2.5	6.1	0	0.0	0	0.0
5-14	3	6.0	11	22.5	10.0	6.2	0	0.0	0	0.0
15-44	152	84.6	746	416.3	30.0	6.1	0	0.1	0	0.1
45-59	135	199.0	689	1 016.5	52.4	6.0	1	0.9	1	0.9
60+	90	106.3	598	706.6	72.4	4.1	14	17.0	17	17.2
All ages	380	93.3	2 045	502.1	47.8	5.6	15	3.7	18	4.1
Total	944	118.4	5 005	627.3	46.5	5.5	31	3.9	38	4.5

Table 188b   FSE - PEAS - AESE   Peptic ulcer - Cases

Age group (years)	Incidence 1990 Number ('000s)	Rate (per 100 000)	Prevalence 1990 Number ('000s)	Rate (per 100 000)	Avg. age at onset (years)	Average duration (years)	Deaths 1990 Number ('000s)	Rate (per 100 000)	Deaths 2000 (Projected) Number ('000s)	Rate (per 100 000)
Males										
0-4	0	2.0	1	3.9	2.5	6.1	0	0.0	0	0.0
5-14	3	10.0	181	660.6	10.0	6.2	0	0.0	0	0.0
15-44	102	133.1	504	660.6	29.8	6.1	1	1.6	1	1.3
45-59	85	316.8	439	1 627.9	52.2	5.7	3	11.3	4	12.2
60+	36	171.0	271	1 290.8	70.0	3.9	6	26.4	8	29.7
All ages	226	136.6	1 395	843.7	44.4	5.6	10	5.9	12	7.2
Females										
0-4	0	2.0	1	3.9	2.5	6.1	0	0.0	0	0.0
5-14	2	6.0	6	22.4	10.0	6.2	0	0.0	0	0.0
15-44	63	84.6	314	419.5	29.9	6.2	0	0.3	0	0.2
45-59	60	198.9	310	1 034.5	52.4	6.0	1	2.0	1	2.0
60+	39	106.3	274	751.7	71.5	4.1	4	10.2	4	10.6
All ages	164	90.5	905	500.2	47.7	5.6	5	2.5	5	2.8
Total	390	112.5	2 300	664.2	45.8	5.6	14	4.1	18	4.9

Table 188c   India - India - Inde   Peptic ulcer - Cases

Age group (years)	Incidence 1990 Number ('000s)	Rate (per 100 000)	Prevalence 1990 Number ('000s)	Rate (per 100 000)	Avg. age at onset (years)	Average duration (years)	Deaths 1990 Number ('000s)	Rate (per 100 000)	Deaths 2000 (Projected) Number ('000s)	Rate (per 100 000)
Males										
0-4	3	5.0	6	9.4	2.5	5.7	0	0.2	0	0.1
5-14	20	20.0	73	72.0	10.0	6.1	0	0.1	0	0.1
15-44	446	222.6	2 178	1 086.4	29.7	5.9	5	2.6	5	1.8
45-59	296	622.8	1 432	3 010.8	52.3	5.5	8	17.4	9	15.7
60+	109	365.4	720	2 419.5	69.7	3.6	13	44.7	16	43.5
All ages	875	199.1	4 410	1 003.6	41.8	5.5	27	6.2	30	5.9
Females										
0-4	1	2.0	2	3.7	2.5	5.6	0	0.4	0	0.2
5-14	10	10.0	33	34.8	10.0	6.1	0	0.4	0	0.2
15-44	204	111.4	994	542.7	29.8	5.9	4	2.0	3	1.3
45-59	145	316.3	686	1 490.8	52.3	5.4	4	9.3	4	7.3
60+	53	182.1	327	1 132.0	70.1	3.5	7	23.9	9	22.5
All ages	413	100.7	2 043	498.2	42.3	5.4	15	3.8	16	3.3
Total	1 288	151.6	6 453	759.6	42.0	5.5	42	5.0	46	4.6

For epidemiological sources see Mahapatra et al. 1996b. For the methods used to estimate and project incidence, prevalence, and deaths see Murray and Lopez 1996a. See explanatory notes for definitions and caveats.

Table 188	Cuadro 188	Tableau 188
Peptic ulcer	Ulcera péptica	Ulcère peptique
Cases	Casos	Cas

Table 188d — China - China - Chine — Peptic ulcer - Cases

Age group (years)	Incidence 1990 Number ('000s)	Rate (per 100 000)	Prevalence 1990 Number ('000s)	Rate (per 100 000)	Avg. age at onset (years)	Average duration (years)	Deaths 1990 Number ('000s)	Rate (per 100 000)	Deaths 2000 (Projected) Number ('000s)	Rate (per 100 000)
Males										
0-4	1	2.0	2	3.8	2.5	6.0	0	0.5	0	0.3
5-14	7	7.0	25	25.7	10.0	6.2	0	0.1	0	0.0
15-44	250	81.7	1 223	399.3	29.9	6.0	2	0.6	1	0.4
45-59	173	238.3	831	1 144.1	52.3	5.5	3	4.1	3	3.5
60+	69	139.9	452	922.4	69.8	3.6	13	27.4	16	27.0
All ages	500	85.4	2 534	432.9	42.8	5.5	19	3.2	21	3.2
Females										
0-4	1	1.0	1	1.9	2.5	5.9	0	0.6	0	0.3
5-14	4	4.0	13	14.3	10.0	6.1	0	0.1	0	0.0
15-44	133	46.9	651	229.1	29.9	5.9	1	0.3	1	0.2
45-59	88	137.1	415	643.9	52.4	5.4	2	2.4	2	1.8
60+	41	79.7	252	486.9	70.6	3.6	12	22.3	14	21.7
All ages	267	48.7	1 331	242.7	43.3	5.4	14	2.6	16	2.6
Total	767	67.6	3 865	340.9	43.0	5.5	33	2.9	38	3.0

Table 188e — OAI - OPAI - APAI — Peptic ulcer - Cases

Age group (years)	Incidence 1990 Number ('000s)	Rate (per 100 000)	Prevalence 1990 Number ('000s)	Rate (per 100 000)	Avg. age at onset (years)	Average duration (years)	Deaths 1990 Number ('000s)	Rate (per 100 000)	Deaths 2000 (Projected) Number ('000s)	Rate (per 100 000)
Males										
0-4	1	2.0	1	3.4	2.5	5.8	0	0.4	0	0.3
5-14	6	7.0	22	25.6	10.0	6.1	0	0.3	0	0.2
15-44	131	81.7	640	397.9	29.7	5.9	1	0.8	1	0.7
45-59	81	238.3	389	1 140.0	52.3	5.4	3	9.0	4	8.3
60+	28	139.9	187	927.5	69.6	3.6	10	47.3	13	46.9
All ages	248	72.2	1 240	361.4	41.1	5.5	14	4.2	18	4.6
Females										
0-4	0	1.0	1	1.9	2.5	5.8	0	0.3	0	0.2
5-14	3	4.0	11	14.3	10.0	6.1	0	0.3	0	0.2
15-44	75	46.9	364	228.3	29.8	5.9	1	0.4	1	0.3
45-59	48	137.1	225	642.0	52.3	5.3	1	3.6	1	3.0
60+	18	79.7	111	491.0	70.3	3.6	7	30.8	10	29.4
All ages	145	42.6	713	210.0	41.8	5.4	9	2.7	12	2.9
Total	392	57.5	1 953	286.1	41.4	5.5	24	3.5	30	3.7

Table 188f — SSA - ASS - ASS — Peptic ulcer - Cases

Age group (years)	Incidence 1990 Number ('000s)	Rate (per 100 000)	Prevalence 1990 Number ('000s)	Rate (per 100 000)	Avg. age at onset (years)	Average duration (years)	Deaths 1990 Number ('000s)	Rate (per 100 000)	Deaths 2000 (Projected) Number ('000s)	Rate (per 100 000)
Males										
0-4	0	1.0	1	1.8	2.4	5.4	0	0.0	0	0.0
5-14	4	5.0	12	17.5	10.0	6.0	0	0.0	0	0.0
15-44	54	51.9	260	250.9	29.4	5.7	3	2.9	3	2.1
45-59	32	158.8	152	749.5	52.2	5.3	2	11.2	3	10.3
60+	10	95.5	66	631.0	69.2	3.6	3	25.8	3	24.2
All ages	100	39.7	492	195.0	39.9	5.4	8	3.2	9	2.7
Females										
0-4	0	1.0	1	1.8	2.4	5.4	0	0.0	0	0.0
5-14	3	4.0	10	14.2	10.0	6.0	0	0.0	0	0.0
15-44	47	43.9	226	212.4	29.5	5.7	1	0.6	1	0.4
45-59	29	133.2	136	616.9	52.2	5.2	1	6.3	2	5.2
60+	10	79.7	63	491.5	69.7	3.5	3	25.3	4	22.9
All ages	90	34.7	435	168.8	40.8	5.3	5	2.0	6	1.8
Total	190	37.2	927	181.8	40.3	5.4	13	2.6	15	2.2

For epidemiological sources see Mahapatra et al. 1996b. For the methods used to estimate and project incidence, prevalence, and deaths see Murray and Lopez 1996a. See explanatory notes for definitions and caveats.

Table 188
Peptic ulcer

Cuadro 188
Ulcera péptica

Tableau 188
Ulcère peptique

Cases

Casos

Cas

Table 188g LAC - ALC - ALC Peptic ulcer - Cases

Age group (years)	Incidence 1990 Number ('000s)	Rate (per 100 000)	Prevalence 1990 Number ('000s)	Rate (per 100 000)	Avg. age at onset (years)	Average duration (years)	Deaths 1990 Number ('000s)	Rate (per 100 000)	Deaths 2000 (Projected) Number ('000s)	Rate (per 100 000)
Males										
0-4	1	2.0	1	3.7	2.5	5.7	0	0.1	0	0.1
5-14	4	7.0	13	25.6	10.0	6.1	0	0.1	0	0.1
15-44	85	81.7	405	388.7	29.8	5.7	1	0.8	1	0.7
45-59	53	238.4	248	1 113.0	52.3	5.3	1	6.0	2	5.9
60+	20	140.0	118	829.3	70.3	3.5	4	31.3	6	32.0
All ages	162	73.3	785	354.4	41.6	5.3	7	3.0	9	3.4
Females										
0-4	0	1.0	1	1.9	2.5	5.8	0	0.2	0	0.1
5-14	2	4.0	7	14.3	10.0	6.1	0	0.1	0	0.0
15-44	49	46.9	238	228.7	29.8	5.9	0	0.4	0	0.3
45-59	32	137.1	150	643.7	52.4	5.5	1	2.9	1	2.5
60+	13	79.7	81	482.3	71.1	3.7	4	21.8	5	21.4
All ages	97	43.4	477	214.4	42.5	5.5	5	2.2	6	2.4
Total	259	58.3	1 263	284.2	41.9	5.4	11	2.6	15	2.9

Table 188h MEC - AOM - CMO Peptic ulcer - Cases

Age group (years)	Incidence 1990 Number ('000s)	Rate (per 100 000)	Prevalence 1990 Number ('000s)	Rate (per 100 000)	Avg. age at onset (years)	Average duration (years)	Deaths 1990 Number ('000s)	Rate (per 100 000)	Deaths 2000 (Projected) Number ('000s)	Rate (per 100 000)
Males										
0-4	1	2.0	2	3.8	2.5	5.8	0	0.0	0	0.0
5-14	5	7.0	17	25.7	10.0	6.2	0	0.2	0	0.1
15-44	93	81.7	454	398.8	29.8	5.9	1	0.7	1	0.6
45-59	53	238.3	255	1 141.5	52.3	5.5	1	5.6	2	5.3
60+	19	139.9	126	924.3	69.7	3.6	2	14.9	3	14.3
All ages	171	66.6	854	333.0	40.6	5.5	4	1.7	5	1.6
Females										
0-4	0	1.0	1	1.9	2.5	5.7	0	0.1	0	0.0
5-14	2	4.0	9	14.3	10.0	6.1	0	0.1	0	0.0
15-44	50	46.9	245	228.7	29.8	5.9	0	0.3	0	0.2
45-59	31	137.1	143	642.6	52.3	5.4	0	1.9	0	1.6
60+	12	79.7	76	489.4	70.4	3.6	1	6.6	1	6.1
All ages	96	38.9	474	192.0	41.5	5.4	2	0.7	2	0.7
Total	267	53.0	1 327	263.8	40.9	5.5	6	1.2	7	1.1

Table 188i World - Mundo - Monde Peptic ulcer - Cases

Age group (years)	Incidence 1990 Number ('000s)	Rate (per 100 000)	Prevalence 1990 Number ('000s)	Rate (per 100 000)	Avg. age at onset (years)	Average duration (years)	Deaths 1990 Number ('000s)	Rate (per 100 000)	Deaths 2000 (Projected) Number ('000s)	Rate (per 100 000)
Males										
0-4	8	2.4	14	4.5	2.5	5.8	1	0.2	0	0.1
5-14	53	9.6	362	65.6	10.0	6.2	1	0.1	0	0.1
15-44	1 406	112.5	6 868	549.5	29.8	5.9	15	1.2	14	0.9
45-59	984	315.1	4 789	1 533.1	52.3	5.5	24	7.7	29	7.2
60+	394	180.0	2 635	1 204.2	70.1	3.7	65	29.5	83	30.1
All ages	2 845	107.2	14 668	552.8	42.7	5.5	105	3.9	126	4.1
Females										
0-4	4	1.3	8	2.5	2.5	5.7	1	0.2	0	0.1
5-14	28	5.4	101	19.2	10.0	6.1	1	0.1	0	0.1
15-44	773	64.5	3 779	315.3	29.8	6.0	7	0.6	6	0.4
45-59	569	182.8	2 755	885.8	52.4	5.6	11	3.5	11	2.8
60+	276	102.6	1 781	661.4	71.2	3.8	51	19.1	64	18.9
All ages	1 650	63.1	8 424	322.3	44.1	5.5	71	2.7	82	2.7
Total	4 496	85.4	23 092	438.4	43.2	5.5	175	3.3	208	3.4

For epidemiological sources see Mahapatra et al. 1996b. For the methods used to estimate and project incidence, prevalence, and deaths see Murray and Lopez 1996a. See explanatory notes for definitions and caveats.

Table 189	Cuadro 189	Tableau 189
Cirrhosis of the liver	**Cirrosis hepática**	**Cirrhose du foie**
Symptomatic cases	Casos sintomáticos	Cas symtpomatiques

Table 189a — EME - PEMC - EMBE — Cirrhosis of the liver - Symptomatic cases

Age group (years)	Incidence 1990 Number ('000s)	Rate (per 100 000)	Prevalence 1990 Number ('000s)	Rate (per 100 000)	Avg. age at onset (years)	Average duration (years)	Deaths 1990 Number ('000s)	Rate (per 100 000)	Deaths 2000 (Projected) Number ('000s)	Rate (per 100 000)
Males										
0-4	0	0.6	0	1.3	2.5	10.3	0	0.1	0	0.1
5-14	0	0.0	1	1.5	10.0	10.4	0	0.0	0	0.0
15-44	15	7.9	103	55.8	29.9	10.0	10	5.3	9	5.2
45-59	51	76.6	275	415.4	52.4	8.8	26	39.4	33	41.0
60+	46	75.3	439	724.2	71.0	6.0	41	68.3	49	68.4
All ages	111	28.4	817	209.3	57.0	7.8	77	19.8	91	22.2
Females										
0-4	0	0.4	0	0.9	2.5	10.4	0	0.1	0	0.1
5-14	0	0.0	1	1.0	10.0	10.4	0	0.0	0	0.0
15-44	5	2.9	37	20.8	30.0	10.2	4	2.0	3	2.0
45-59	18	26.0	97	143.0	52.4	9.3	9	13.6	11	13.2
60+	34	39.9	286	338.7	72.4	6.5	27	31.4	29	29.3
All ages	57	13.9	421	103.4	62.1	7.7	39	9.7	43	10.0
Total	168	21.0	1 238	155.2	58.7	7.8	117	14.6	134	15.9

Table 189b — FSE - PEAS - AESE — Cirrhosis of the liver - Symptomatic cases

Age group (years)	Incidence 1990 Number ('000s)	Rate (per 100 000)	Prevalence 1990 Number ('000s)	Rate (per 100 000)	Avg. age at onset (years)	Average duration (years)	Deaths 1990 Number ('000s)	Rate (per 100 000)	Deaths 2000 (Projected) Number ('000s)	Rate (per 100 000)
Males										
0-4	0	1.9	1	4.1	2.5	10.2	0	0.4	0	0.3
5-14	0	0.0	1	4.8	10.0	10.3	0	0.1	0	0.1
15-44	6	8.5	46	60.1	29.8	9.7	4	5.7	4	4.7
45-59	25	90.9	130	481.4	52.2	8.1	12	45.7	15	49.4
60+	17	82.9	171	816.6	69.9	5.6	16	75.7	20	80.1
All ages	49	29.4	349	211.0	55.3	7.5	33	19.7	39	23.1
Females										
0-4	0	1.5	0	3.2	2.5	10.3	0	0.3	0	0.2
5-14	0	0.0	1	3.8	10.0	10.4	0	0.2	0	0.1
15-44	2	3.1	17	22.4	29.9	10.1	2	2.1	1	1.7
45-59	10	34.2	55	183.1	52.4	9.0	5	17.4	6	16.6
60+	15	41.9	136	373.8	71.5	6.2	12	33.7	13	32.8
All ages	28	15.5	209	115.6	60.6	7.6	19	10.6	21	11.0
Total	77	22.1	558	161.2	57.2	7.5	52	15.0	60	16.8

Table 189c — India - India - Inde — Cirrhosis of the liver - Symptomatic cases

Age group (years)	Incidence 1990 Number ('000s)	Rate (per 100 000)	Prevalence 1990 Number ('000s)	Rate (per 100 000)	Avg. age at onset (years)	Average duration (years)	Deaths 1990 Number ('000s)	Rate (per 100 000)	Deaths 2000 (Projected) Number ('000s)	Rate (per 100 000)
Males										
0-4	7	11.3	14	23	2.5	9.5	1	2.1	1	1.4
5-14	0	0.0	29	28	10.0	10.2	1	1.0	1	0.5
15-44	35	17.5	257	128	29.9	9.8	24	11.9	21	8.3
45-59	79	167.1	433	911	52.3	8.3	41	85.7	46	77.2
60+	41	137.7	425	1 429	69.6	5.6	41	136.8	49	132.5
All ages	162	36.9	1 159	264	49.8	8.0	108	24.5	117	22.8
Females										
0-4	9	15.5	18	32	2.5	9.4	2	2.9	1	1.9
5-14	0	0.0	37	39	10.0	10.2	2	2.0	1	1.1
15-44	13	7.0	105	57	29.8	9.9	10	5.4	8	3.5
45-59	28	60.7	154	336	52.4	8.6	15	31.6	14	24.7
60+	17	58.2	163	564	70.0	5.7	16	53.9	20	50.4
All ages	66	16.2	477	116	45.9	8.2	44	10.6	44	9.1
Total	229	26.9	1 636	193	48.6	8.1	151	17.8	161	16.1

For epidemiological sources see Gakidou et al. 1996a. For the methods used to estimate and project incidence, prevalence, and deaths see Murray and Lopez 1996a. See explanatory notes for definitions and caveats.

Table 189   **Cuadro 189**   **Tableau 189**
Cirrhosis of the liver   **Cirrosis hepática**   **Cirrhose du foie**

Symptomatic cases   Casos sintomáticos   Cas symtpomatiques

Table 189d   China - China - Chine   Cirrhosis of the liver - Symptomatic cases

Age group (years)	Incidence 1990 Number ('000s)	Rate (per 100 000)	Prevalence 1990 Number ('000s)	Rate (per 100 000)	Avg. age at onset (years)	Average duration (years)	Deaths 1990 Number ('000s)	Rate (per 100 000)	Deaths 2000 (Projected) Number ('000s)	Rate (per 100 000)
Males										
0-4	7	12.0	15	26	2.5	10.2	2	2.8	1	1.5
5-14	0	0.0	30	31	10.0	10.3	1	0.6	0	0.3
15-44	39	12.8	294	96	29.9	9.9	28	9.1	24	7.4
45-59	71	97.7	395	543	52.3	8.4	37	51.3	43	44.0
60+	72	147.4	591	1 206	69.7	5.6	56	114.7	65	107.3
All ages	190	32.4	1 324	226	52.4	7.7	123	21.1	133	20.2
Females										
0-4	3	4.8	6	10	2.5	9.9	1	0.9	0	0.5
5-14	0	0.0	11	12	10.0	10.4	1	0.7	0	0.3
15-44	12	4.1	90	32	29.9	10.0	8	3.0	6	2.1
45-59	34	52.9	182	282	52.4	8.8	17	26.5	18	19.8
60+	50	97.3	395	764	70.6	5.9	37	71.9	42	65.0
All ages	99	18.0	683	125	57.6	7.5	64	11.6	67	10.7
Total	288	25.4	2 007	177	54.2	7.6	187	16.5	200	15.6

Table 189e   OAI - OPAI - APAI   Cirrhosis of the liver - Symptomatic cases

Age group (years)	Incidence 1990 Number ('000s)	Rate (per 100 000)	Prevalence 1990 Number ('000s)	Rate (per 100 000)	Avg. age at onset (years)	Average duration (years)	Deaths 1990 Number ('000s)	Rate (per 100 000)	Deaths 2000 (Projected) Number ('000s)	Rate (per 100 000)
Males										
0-4	5	11.3	10	23	2.5	9.6	1	2.3	1	1.5
5-14	0	0.0	24	28	10.0	10.2	1	1.5	1	0.8
15-44	27	16.9	199	124	29.9	9.7	19	11.8	20	9.6
45-59	73	212.7	385	1 128	52.3	8.1	37	107.4	46	99.9
60+	38	186.5	380	1 880	69.5	5.5	37	183.2	48	173.8
All ages	142	41.5	998	291	50.9	7.8	95	27.6	115	28.4
Females										
0-4	3	8.0	7	17	2.5	9.7	1	1.6	0	1.0
5-14	0	0.0	16	20	10.0	10.2	1	1.4	1	0.8
15-44	6	3.7	47	30	29.8	9.8	5	3.1	5	2.4
45-59	23	64.3	117	334	52.4	8.5	11	31.9	12	26.5
60+	24	104.6	191	842	70.3	5.8	18	81.5	24	73.0
All ages	55	16.3	379	112	54.6	7.6	36	10.7	42	10.5
Total	198	29.0	1 377	202	51.9	7.7	131	19.2	157	19.4

Table 189f   SSA - ASS - ASS   Cirrhosis of the liver - Symptomatic cases

Age group (years)	Incidence 1990 Number ('000s)	Rate (per 100 000)	Prevalence 1990 Number ('000s)	Rate (per 100 000)	Avg. age at onset (years)	Average duration (years)	Deaths 1990 Number ('000s)	Rate (per 100 000)	Deaths 2000 (Projected) Number ('000s)	Rate (per 100 000)
Males										
0-4	0	0.0	0	0.0	-	-	0	0.0	0	0.0
5-14	2	3.1	8	11.5	10.0	9.8	1	1.1	1	0.6
15-44	8	7.9	63	61.2	29.4	9.3	6	6.1	6	4.4
45-59	15	72.2	79	390.6	52.2	7.9	8	37.3	9	34.3
60+	11	108.1	92	877.2	69.2	5.4	9	84.0	11	77.7
All ages	36	14.4	243	96.3	49.9	7.5	24	9.3	27	7.9
Females										
0-4	0	0.0	0	0.0	-	-	0	0.0	0	0.0
5-14	1	1.7	4	6.2	10.0	9.9	0	0.6	0	0.4
15-44	4	3.3	29	26.9	29.5	9.5	2	1.7	2	1.2
45-59	6	27.0	33	148.8	52.3	8.2	3	14.1	3	11.6
60+	7	53.3	51	402.2	69.7	5.6	5	38.4	6	33.6
All ages	17	6.8	117	45.4	51.6	7.5	10	4.0	11	3.2
Total	54	10.5	360	70.6	50.5	7.5	34	6.6	39	5.6

For epidemiological sources see Gakidou et al. 1996a. For the methods used to estimate and project incidence, prevalence, and deaths see Murray and Lopez 1996a. See explanatory notes for definitions and caveats.

Table 189
Cirrhosis of the liver

Symptomatic cases

Cuadro 189
Cirrosis hepática

Casos sintomáticos

Tableau 189
Cirrhose du foie

Cas symptomatiques

Table 189g — LAC - ALC - ALC — Cirrhosis of the liver - Symptomatic cases

Age group (years)	Incidence 1990 Number ('000s)	Rate (per 100 000)	Prevalence 1990 Number ('000s)	Rate (per 100 000)	Avg. age at onset (years)	Average duration (years)	Deaths 1990 Number ('000s)	Rate (per 100 000)	Deaths 2000 (Projected) Number ('000s)	Rate (per 100 000)
Males										
0-4	1	5.0	3	10.4	2.5	9.8	0	1.0	0	0.7
5-14	0	0.0	7	12.5	10.0	10.3	0	0.5	0	0.3
15-44	17	16.3	122	117.2	29.8	9.8	12	11.3	13	9.9
45-59	32	144.8	177	796.5	52.3	8.5	17	75.0	23	73.5
60+	15	104.1	164	1 151.4	70.3	5.8	16	109.6	21	107.1
All ages	66	29.6	473	213.4	49.4	8.3	45	20.1	57	21.4
Females										
0-4	1	4.0	2	8.8	2.5	9.9	0	0.8	0	0.5
5-14	0	0.0	5	10.5	10.0	10.3	0	0.5	0	0.3
15-44	5	4.8	38	36.2	29.9	10.0	4	3.5	4	2.9
45-59	11	45.1	58	247.5	52.4	8.9	5	23.3	7	20.4
60+	9	55.9	84	496.8	71.1	6.1	8	46.9	10	43.3
All ages	26	11.7	187	83.9	52.7	8.1	17	7.8	21	7.8
Total	92	20.6	660	148.5	50.4	8.2	62	14.0	78	14.6

Table 189h — MEC - AOM - CMO — Cirrhosis of the liver - Symptomatic cases

Age group (years)	Incidence 1990 Number ('000s)	Rate (per 100 000)	Prevalence 1990 Number ('000s)	Rate (per 100 000)	Avg. age at onset (years)	Average duration (years)	Deaths 1990 Number ('000s)	Rate (per 100 000)	Deaths 2000 (Projected) Number ('000s)	Rate (per 100 000)
Males										
0-4	2	4.3	4	8.9	2.5	9.6	0	0.8	0	0.5
5-14	1	1.2	10	15.4	10.0	10.3	1	1.5	1	0.9
15-44	6	5.4	49	42.6	29.9	9.8	5	4.1	5	3.2
45-59	17	76.0	89	399.4	52.3	8.2	8	37.4	11	35.5
60+	14	103.1	119	869.9	69.7	5.6	11	82.7	15	78.8
All ages	40	15.5	270	105.4	51.9	7.6	26	10.0	32	9.5
Females										
0-4	1	3.3	3	6.8	2.5	9.6	0	0.6	0	0.4
5-14	4	5.8	19	30.2	10.0	10.3	2	2.9	1	1.8
15-44	2	2.0	30	28.3	29.9	9.9	3	2.7	3	2.0
45-59	11	49.6	57	254.9	52.4	8.6	5	23.8	6	20.2
60+	12	80.2	100	647.1	70.4	5.8	9	60.9	12	55.5
All ages	31	12.4	209	84.5	51.0	7.8	20	8.0	23	7.0
Total	70	14.0	479	95.2	51.5	7.7	45	9.0	54	8.3

Table 189i — World - Mundo - Monde — Cirrhosis of the liver - Symptomatic cases

Age group (years)	Incidence 1990 Number ('000s)	Rate (per 100 000)	Prevalence 1990 Number ('000s)	Rate (per 100 000)	Avg. age at onset (years)	Average duration (years)	Deaths 1990 Number ('000s)	Rate (per 100 000)	Deaths 2000 (Projected) Number ('000s)	Rate (per 100 000)
Males										
0-4	23	7.0	47	15	2.5	9.8	5	1.4	3	0.8
5-14	3	0.5	109	20	10.0	9.9	5	0.9	3	0.5
15-44	154	12.3	1 133	91	29.9	9.8	107	8.6	101	7.0
45-59	362	115.9	1 963	628	52.3	8.3	186	59.4	226	56.0
60+	254	116.1	2 381	1 088	69.9	5.7	227	103.6	279	101.2
All ages	795	30.0	5 633	212	52.0	7.8	529	20.0	611	19.7
Females										
0-4	18	5.7	37	12	2.5	9.6	3	1.1	2	0.6
5-14	5	0.9	94	18	10.0	10.2	6	1.2	4	0.7
15-44	49	4.1	393	33	29.8	9.9	37	3.1	32	2.3
45-59	140	45.0	753	242	52.4	8.7	71	22.9	77	19.1
60+	168	62.5	1 406	522	70.9	6.0	132	49.1	155	46.1
All ages	380	14.5	2 682	103	54.9	7.7	250	9.5	271	8.8
Total	1 175	22.3	8 315	158	52.9	7.8	779	14.8	882	14.3

For epidemiological sources see Gakidou et al. 1996a. For the methods used to estimate and project incidence, prevalence, and deaths see Murray and Lopez 1996a. See explanatory notes for definitions and caveats.

Table 190　**Cuadro 190**　**Tableau 190**
Appendicitis　**Apendicitis**　**Appendicite**

Episodes　Episodios　Episodes

Table 190a　EME - PEMC - EMBE　Appendicitis - Episodes

Age group (years)	Incidence 1990 Number ('000s)	Rate (per 100 000)	Prevalence 1990 Number ('000s)	Rate (per 100 000)	Avg. age at onset (years)	Average duration (years)	Deaths 1990 Number ('000s)	Rate (per 100 000)	Deaths 2000 (Projected) Number ('000s)	Rate (per 100 000)
Males										
0-4	8	30	0	1.2	2.5	0.04	0	0.0	0	0.0
5-14	100	187	4	7.5	11.2	0.04	0	0.1	0	0.0
15-44	319	173	13	6.9	26.8	0.04	0	0.0	0	0.0
45-59	52	79	2	3.1	52.1	0.04	0	0.2	0	0.2
60+	40	67	2	2.7	71.1	0.04	1	0.9	1	0.9
All ages	519	133	21	5.3	29.4	0.04	1	0.2	1	0.2
Females										
0-4	8	30	0	1.2	2.5	0.04	0	0.0	0	0.0
5-14	79	155	3	6.2	10.7	0.04	0	0.0	0	0.0
15-44	226	126	9	5.1	26.2	0.04	0	0.0	0	0.0
45-59	41	60	2	2.4	52.2	0.04	0	0.1	0	0.1
60+	43	50	2	2.0	71.7	0.04	1	0.6	1	0.6
All ages	396	97	16	3.9	30.2	0.04	1	0.2	1	0.2
Total	915	115	37	4.6	29.8	0.04	1	0.2	2	0.2

Table 190b　FSE - PEAS - AESE　Appendicitis - Episodes

Age group (years)	Incidence 1990 Number ('000s)	Rate (per 100 000)	Prevalence 1990 Number ('000s)	Rate (per 100 000)	Avg. age at onset (years)	Average duration (years)	Deaths 1990 Number ('000s)	Rate (per 100 000)	Deaths 2000 (Projected) Number ('000s)	Rate (per 100 000)
Males										
0-4	4	30	0	1.2	2.5	0.04	0	0.0	0	0.0
5-14	51	187	2	7.5	11.2	0.04	0	0.0	0	0.0
15-44	133	174	5	7.0	26.7	0.04	0	0.1	0	0.1
45-59	21	79	1	3.1	51.9	0.04	0	0.3	0	0.3
60+	14	66	1	2.7	70.0	0.04	0	1.1	0	1.2
All ages	223	135	9	5.4	27.8	0.04	0	0.2	0	0.3
Females										
0-4	4	30	0	1.2	2.5	0.04	0	0.0	0	0.0
5-14	41	155	2	6.2	10.7	0.04	0	0.0	0	0.0
15-44	95	126	4	5.1	26.2	0.04	0	0.1	0	0.0
45-59	18	60	1	2.4	52.1	0.04	0	0.1	0	0.1
60+	18	51	1	2.0	70.8	0.04	0	0.5	0	0.5
All ages	176	97	7	3.9	29.4	0.04	0	0.2	0	0.2
Total	399	115	16	4.6	28.5	0.04	1	0.2	1	0.2

Table 190c　India - India - Inde　Appendicitis - Episodes

Age group (years)	Incidence 1990 Number ('000s)	Rate (per 100 000)	Prevalence 1990 Number ('000s)	Rate (per 100 000)	Avg. age at onset (years)	Average duration (years)	Deaths 1990 Number ('000s)	Rate (per 100 000)	Deaths 2000 (Projected) Number ('000s)	Rate (per 100 000)
Males										
0-4	8	13	0	0.5	2.5	0.04	0	0.4	0	0.3
5-14	85	84	3	3.0	11.2	0.04	2	1.7	1	0.8
15-44	156	78	6	2.8	26.7	0.04	4	2.2	4	1.4
45-59	17	35	1	1.3	51.9	0.04	1	1.1	1	1.0
60+	9	30	0	1.1	69.8	0.04	0	1.2	0	1.1
All ages	275	63	10	2.3	24.1	0.04	7	1.6	6	1.1
Females										
0-4	8	13	0	0.5	2.5	0.04	0	0.4	0	0.3
5-14	66	69	2	2.5	10.7	0.04	1	1.5	1	0.8
15-44	104	57	4	2.1	26.1	0.04	3	1.6	2	1.0
45-59	12	27	0	1.0	52.0	0.04	0	0.8	0	0.6
60+	7	23	0	0.8	69.6	0.04	0	0.9	0	0.8
All ages	197	48	7	1.8	23.1	0.04	5	1.3	4	0.8
Total	472	56	17	2.0	23.7	0.04	12	1.5	10	1.0

For epidemiological sources see Ashley et al. 1996. For the methods used to estimate and project incidence, prevalence, and deaths see Murray and Lopez 1996a. See explanatory notes for definitions and caveats.

Table 190
Appendicitis

Cuadro 190
Apendicitis

Tableau 190
Appendicite

Episodes

Episodios

Episodes

Table 190d China - China - Chine — Appendicitis - Episodes

Age group (years)	Incidence 1990 Number ('000s)	Rate (per 100 000)	Prevalence 1990 Number ('000s)	Rate (per 100 000)	Avg. age at onset (years)	Average duration (years)	Deaths 1990 Number ('000s)	Rate (per 100 000)	Deaths 2000 (Projected) Number ('000s)	Rate (per 100 000)
Males										
0-4	8	14	0	0.5	2.5	0.04	0	0.2	0	0.1
5-14	82	85	3	3.3	11.2	0.04	1	1.5	1	0.7
15-44	241	79	9	3.0	26.8	0.04	4	1.5	3	0.9
45-59	26	36	1	1.4	52.0	0.04	1	0.7	1	0.6
60+	15	30	1	1.2	69.7	0.04	0	0.9	1	0.9
All ages	372	64	14	2.5	26.3	0.04	7	1.2	5	0.7
Females										
0-4	8	14	0	0.5	2.5	0.04	0	0.2	0	0.1
5-14	63	70	2	2.7	10.7	0.04	1	1.2	1	0.6
15-44	163	57	6	2.2	26.2	0.04	3	1.0	2	0.6
45-59	18	27	1	1.1	52.1	0.04	0	0.5	0	0.4
60+	12	23	0	0.9	70.1	0.04	0	0.7	0	0.6
All ages	264	48	10	1.9	25.5	0.04	5	0.9	3	0.5
Total	636	56	25	2.2	25.9	0.04	12	1.0	8	0.6

Table 190e OAI - OPAI - APAI — Appendicitis - Episodes

Age group (years)	Incidence 1990 Number ('000s)	Rate (per 100 000)	Prevalence 1990 Number ('000s)	Rate (per 100 000)	Avg. age at onset (years)	Average duration (years)	Deaths 1990 Number ('000s)	Rate (per 100 000)	Deaths 2000 (Projected) Number ('000s)	Rate (per 100 000)
Males										
0-4	6	14	0	0.5	2.5	0.04	0	0.3	0	0.2
5-14	71	84	3	3.1	11.2	0.04	2	2.6	1	1.4
15-44	126	79	5	2.9	26.7	0.04	3	1.8	3	1.3
45-59	12	36	0	1.3	52.0	0.04	0	1.0	0	0.9
60+	6	30	0	1.1	70.2	0.04	0	1.1	0	1.0
All ages	221	65	8	2.4	23.7	0.04	6	1.7	5	1.1
Females										
0-4	6	14	0	0.5	2.5	0.04	0	0.3	0	0.2
5-14	56	70	2	2.6	10.7	0.04	2	2.1	1	1.3
15-44	63	39	2	1.4	26.1	0.04	2	1.1	2	0.8
45-59	10	27	0	1.0	52.1	0.04	0	0.7	0	0.6
60+	5	23	0	0.8	70.3	0.04	0	0.8	0	0.7
All ages	139	41	5	1.5	22.4	0.04	4	1.2	3	0.8
Total	360	53	13	1.9	23.2	0.04	10	1.4	8	1.0

Table 190f SSA - ASS - ASS — Appendicitis - Episodes

Age group (years)	Incidence 1990 Number ('000s)	Rate (per 100 000)	Prevalence 1990 Number ('000s)	Rate (per 100 000)	Avg. age at onset (years)	Average duration (years)	Deaths 1990 Number ('000s)	Rate (per 100 000)	Deaths 2000 (Projected) Number ('000s)	Rate (per 100 000)
Males										
0-4	7	13.8	0	0.5	2.4	0.04	0	0.4	0	0.3
5-14	60	86.0	2	3.3	11.1	0.04	4	5.2	3	2.9
15-44	84	81.4	3	3.2	26.4	0.04	4	3.7	4	2.6
45-59	7	36.3	0	1.4	51.9	0.04	0	2.0	0	1.8
60+	3	30.6	0	1.2	69.5	0.04	0	1.9	0	1.8
All ages	162	64.2	6	2.5	21.7	0.04	8	3.3	7	2.2
Females										
0-4	4	9.3	0	0.4	2.4	0.04	0	0.4	0	0.3
5-14	33	47.8	1	1.9	10.7	0.04	3	4.4	2	2.6
15-44	42	39.9	2	1.5	25.8	0.04	1	1.4	1	0.9
45-59	4	18.6	0	0.7	52.0	0.04	0	1.5	0	1.3
60+	2	15.8	0	0.6	69.4	0.04	0	1.5	0	1.3
All ages	86	33.4	3	1.3	21.0	0.04	5	2.1	5	1.3
Total	248	48.7	10	1.9	21.5	0.04	14	2.7	12	1.7

For epidemiological sources see Ashley et al. 1996. For the methods used to estimate and project incidence, prevalence, and deaths see Murray and Lopez 1996a. See explanatory notes for definitions and caveats.

Table 190
Appendicitis

Cuadro 190
Apendicitis

Tableau 190
Appendicite

Episodes

Episodios

Episodes

Table 190g   LAC - ALC - ALC   Appendicitis - Episodes

Age group (years)	Incidence 1990 Number ('000s)	Rate (per 100 000)	Prevalence 1990 Number ('000s)	Rate (per 100 000)	Avg. age at onset (years)	Average duration (years)	Deaths 1990 Number ('000s)	Rate (per 100 000)	Deaths 2000 (Projected) Number ('000s)	Rate (per 100 000)
Males										
0-4	5	18	0	0.7	2.5	0.04	0	0.1	0	0.1
5-14	59	113	2	4.5	11.2	0.04	0	0.6	0	0.4
15-44	109	105	4	4.1	26.7	0.04	0	0.5	0	0.4
45-59	10	45	0	1.8	52.0	0.04	0	0.3	0	0.3
60+	6	40	0	1.6	71.0	0.04	0	0.8	0	0.7
All ages	189	85	7	3.4	23.9	0.04	1	0.5	1	0.4
Females										
0-4	5	18	0	0.7	2.5	0.04	0	0.1	0	0.1
5-14	47	93	2	3.7	10.7	0.04	0	0.4	0	0.3
15-44	80	77	3	3.0	26.1	0.04	0	0.3	0	0.2
45-59	8	36	0	1.4	52.1	0.04	0	0.2	0	0.2
60+	5	30	0	1.2	71.1	0.04	0	0.5	0	0.5
All ages	146	65	6	2.6	23.4	0.04	1	0.3	1	0.2
Total	335	75	13	3.0	23.7	0.04	2	0.4	2	0.3

Table 190h   MEC - AOM - CMO   Appendicitis - Episodes

Age group (years)	Incidence 1990 Number ('000s)	Rate (per 100 000)	Prevalence 1990 Number ('000s)	Rate (per 100 000)	Avg. age at onset (years)	Average duration (years)	Deaths 1990 Number ('000s)	Rate (per 100 000)	Deaths 2000 (Projected) Number ('000s)	Rate (per 100 000)
Males										
0-4	7	16	0	0.6	2.5	0.04	0	0.2	0	0.1
5-14	66	101	3	3.8	11.2	0.04	1	1.6	1	0.9
15-44	107	94	4	3.6	26.7	0.04	1	1.2	1	0.9
45-59	10	43	0	1.6	52.0	0.04	0	0.7	0	0.6
60+	5	36	0	1.4	70.2	0.04	0	0.9	0	0.8
All ages	195	76	7	2.9	22.9	0.04	3	1.1	2	0.7
Females										
0-4	6	16	0	0.6	2.5	0.04	0	0.2	0	0.1
5-14	52	84	2	3.2	10.7	0.04	1	1.3	1	0.8
15-44	74	69	3	2.6	26.1	0.04	1	0.8	1	0.5
45-59	7	33	0	1.2	52.1	0.04	0	0.5	0	0.4
60+	4	28	0	1.0	70.3	0.04	0	0.6	0	0.6
All ages	144	58	5	2.2	22.1	0.04	2	0.8	2	0.5
Total	339	67	13	2.5	22.6	0.04	5	0.9	4	0.6

Table 190i   World - Mundo - Monde   Appendicitis - Episodes

Age group (years)	Incidence 1990 Number ('000s)	Rate (per 100 000)	Prevalence 1990 Number ('000s)	Rate (per 100 000)	Avg. age at onset (years)	Average duration (years)	Deaths 1990 Number ('000s)	Rate (per 100 000)	Deaths 2000 (Projected) Number ('000s)	Rate (per 100 000)
Males										
0-4	53	16	2	0.6	2.5	0.04	1	0.3	1	0.2
5-14	575	104	22	4.0	11.2	0.04	10	1.9	7	1.1
15-44	1 277	102	49	4.0	26.7	0.04	18	1.4	15	1.0
45-59	155	50	6	1.9	52.0	0.04	2	0.7	3	0.7
60+	98	45	4	1.7	70.5	0.04	2	1.0	3	1.0
All ages	2 157	81	83	3.1	25.8	0.04	33	1.2	27	0.9
Females										
0-4	48	16	2	0.6	2.5	0.04	1	0.3	1	0.2
5-14	438	83	17	3.2	10.7	0.04	8	1.6	6	1.0
15-44	847	71	33	2.7	26.1	0.04	10	0.9	8	0.6
45-59	118	38	5	1.5	52.1	0.04	2	0.5	2	0.4
60+	96	36	4	1.4	71.0	0.04	2	0.7	2	0.6
All ages	1 547	59	60	2.3	25.8	0.04	23	0.9	18	0.6
Total	3 704	70	143	2.7	25.8	0.04	56	1.1	46	0.7

For epidemiological sources see Ashley et al. 1996. For the methods used to estimate and project incidence, prevalence, and deaths see Murray and Lopez 1996a. See explanatory notes for definitions and caveats.

Table 191	Cuadro 191	Tableau 191
Nephritis and nephrosis	**Nefritis y nefrosis**	**Néphrite et néphrose**

Acute glomerulonephritis　　　　　Glomérulo nefritis aguda　　　　　Glomerulonéphrite aiguë

Table 191a   EME - PEMC - EMBE　　　　　Nephritis and nephrosis - Acute glomerulonephritis

Age group (years)	Incidence 1990 Number ('000s)	Rate (per 100 000)	Prevalence 1990 Number ('000s)	Rate (per 100 000)	Avg. age at onset (years)	Average duration (years)	Deaths 1990 Number ('000s)	Rate (per 100 000)	Deaths 2000 (Projected) Number ('000s)	Rate (per 100 000)
Males										
0-4	2	7.0	2	5.9	2.5	1.0	-	-	-	-
5-14	1	1.0	1	1.7	10.0	1.2	-	-	-	-
15-44	1	0.5	2	1.0	29.9	2.1	-	-	-	-
45-59	0	0.3	1	1.0	52.4	3.1	-	-	-	-
60+	1	1.2	2	2.6	71.1	2.1	-	-	-	-
All ages	4	1.1	7	1.7	23.6	1.6	-	-	-	-
Females										
0-4	3	10.0	2	8.4	2.6	1.0	-	-	-	-
5-14	0	0.2	1	1.2	10.0	1.2	-	-	-	-
15-44	0	0.2	1	0.4	30.0	2.1	-	-	-	-
45-59	0	0.2	0	0.6	52.5	3.1	-	-	-	-
60+	1	1.0	2	2.2	72.4	2.1	-	-	-	-
All ages	4	1.0	6	1.4	22.1	1.4	-	-	-	-
Total	8	1.0	12	1.5	22.9	1.5	-	-	-	-

Table 191b   FSE - PEAS - AESE　　　　　Nephritis and nephrosis - Acute glomerulonephritis

Age group (years)	Incidence 1990 Number ('000s)	Rate (per 100 000)	Prevalence 1990 Number ('000s)	Rate (per 100 000)	Avg. age at onset (years)	Average duration (years)	Deaths 1990 Number ('000s)	Rate (per 100 000)	Deaths 2000 (Projected) Number ('000s)	Rate (per 100 000)
Males										
0-4	0	2.0	0	1.7	2.5	1.0	-	-	-	-
5-14	1	3.0	1	3.2	10.0	1.2	-	-	-	-
15-44	2	2.0	3	4.0	29.8	2.1	-	-	-	-
45-59	0	0.6	1	2.5	52.2	3.0	-	-	-	-
60+	0	0.6	0	1.5	70.0	2.0	-	-	-	-
All ages	3	1.8	5	3.1	24.6	1.8	-	-	-	-
Females										
0-4	0	2.0	0	1.7	2.5	1.0	-	-	-	-
5-14	1	3.0	1	3.2	10.0	1.2	-	-	-	-
15-44	1	2.0	3	4.0	29.9	2.1	-	-	-	-
45-59	0	0.5	1	2.3	52.4	3.1	-	-	-	-
60+	0	0.3	0	0.8	71.5	2.1	-	-	-	-
All ages	3	1.6	5	2.8	24.5	1.8	-	-	-	-
Total	6	1.7	10	2.9	24.6	1.8	-	-	-	-

Table 191c   India - India - Inde　　　　　Nephritis and nephrosis - Acute glomerulonephritis

Age group (years)	Incidence 1990 Number ('000s)	Rate (per 100 000)	Prevalence 1990 Number ('000s)	Rate (per 100 000)	Avg. age at onset (years)	Average duration (years)	Deaths 1990 Number ('000s)	Rate (per 100 000)	Deaths 2000 (Projected) Number ('000s)	Rate (per 100 000)
Males										
0-4	5	8.0	4	6.6	2.5	0.99	-	-	-	-
5-14	15	15.0	16	15.5	10.0	1.19	-	-	-	-
15-44	2	1.0	6	3.0	29.8	2.05	-	-	-	-
45-59	0	1.0	1	2.4	52.3	2.40	-	-	-	-
60+	1	2.0	1	4.5	69.7	2.06	-	-	-	-
All ages	23	5.3	28	6.4	12.6	1.27	-	-	-	-
Females										
0-4	5	8.0	4	6.6	2.5	0.99	-	-	-	-
5-14	19	20.0	19	20.5	10.0	1.18	-	-	-	-
15-44	2	1.0	6	3.2	29.8	2.04	-	-	-	-
45-59	0	0.8	1	2.6	52.4	3.11	-	-	-	-
60+	0	1.3	1	3.0	70.1	2.03	-	-	-	-
All ages	26	6.4	31	7.6	11.5	1.24	-	-	-	-
Total	49	5.8	59	7.0	12.0	1.25	-	-	-	-

For epidemiological sources see Orzeszyna et al. 1996. For the methods used to estimate and project incidence, prevalence, and deaths see Murray and Lopez 1996a. See explanatory notes for definitions and caveats.

Table 191
Nephritis and nephrosis

Acute glomerulonephritis

Cuadro 191
Nefritis y nefrosis

Glomérulo nefritis aguda

Tableau 191
Néphrite et néphrose

Glomerulonéphrite aiguë

Table 191d   China - China - Chine   Nephritis and nephrosis - Acute glomerulonephritis

Age group (years)	Incidence 1990 Number ('000s)	Rate (per 100 000)	Prevalence 1990 Number ('000s)	Rate (per 100 000)	Avg. age at onset (years)	Average duration (years)	Deaths 1990 Number ('000s)	Rate (per 100 000)	Deaths 2000 (Projected) Number ('000s)	Rate (per 100 000)
Males										
0-4	3	5.0	2	4.1	2.5	1.0	-	-	-	-
5-14	6	6.0	6	6.4	10.0	1.2	-	-	-	-
15-44	12	4.0	24	8.0	29.9	2.1	-	-	-	-
45-59	1	1.5	5	6.5	52.4	3.8	-	-	-	-
60+	1	1.8	4	7.2	69.8	3.2	-	-	-	-
All ages	23	3.9	41	7.1	23.9	1.9	-	-	-	-
Females										
0-4	6	10.0	5	8.3	2.5	1.0	-	-	-	-
5-14	5	5.0	5	5.9	10.0	1.2	-	-	-	-
15-44	11	4.0	22	7.8	29.9	2.1	-	-	-	-
45-59	1	0.8	3	4.4	52.4	4.0	-	-	-	-
60+	1	1.0	2	4.6	70.6	3.8	-	-	-	-
All ages	23	4.1	37	6.8	20.4	1.7	-	-	-	-
Total	46	4.0	79	6.9	22.1	1.8	-	-	-	-

Table 191e   OAI - OPAI - APAI   Nephritis and nephrosis - Acute glomerulonephritis

Age group (years)	Incidence 1990 Number ('000s)	Rate (per 100 000)	Prevalence 1990 Number ('000s)	Rate (per 100 000)	Avg. age at onset (years)	Average duration (years)	Deaths 1990 Number ('000s)	Rate (per 100 000)	Deaths 2000 (Projected) Number ('000s)	Rate (per 100 000)
Males										
0-4	2	5.0	2	4.1	2.5	1.0	-	-	-	-
5-14	11	13.0	11	13.3	10.0	1.2	-	-	-	-
15-44	2	1.0	4	2.8	29.8	2.1	-	-	-	-
45-59	1	2.0	2	5.8	52.3	3.3	-	-	-	-
60+	1	3.0	2	9.9	69.6	2.8	-	-	-	-
All ages	16	4.7	21	6.2	15.0	1.4	-	-	-	-
Females										
0-4	3	8.0	3	6.6	2.5	1.0	-	-	-	-
5-14	8	10.0	9	10.6	10.0	1.2	-	-	-	-
15-44	8	5.0	16	10.1	29.8	2.1	-	-	-	-
45-59	0	1.0	2	4.9	52.4	3.2	-	-	-	-
60+	0	1.8	1	5.1	70.3	2.5	-	-	-	-
All ages	20	5.9	30	8.9	18.6	1.6	-	-	-	-
Total	36	5.3	52	7.6	17.0	1.5	-	-	-	-

Table 191f   SSA - ASS - ASS   Nephritis and nephrosis - Acute glomerulonephritis

Age group (years)	Incidence 1990 Number ('000s)	Rate (per 100 000)	Prevalence 1990 Number ('000s)	Rate (per 100 000)	Avg. age at onset (years)	Average duration (years)	Deaths 1990 Number ('000s)	Rate (per 100 000)	Deaths 2000 (Projected) Number ('000s)	Rate (per 100 000)
Males										
0-4	9	20.0	8	16.3	2.5	1.0	-	-	-	-
5-14	23	33.0	24	34.4	10.0	1.2	-	-	-	-
15-44	3	3.0	8	8.0	29.4	2.0	-	-	-	-
45-59	0	2.0	1	6.7	52.2	3.0	-	-	-	-
60+	0	3.0	1	7.0	69.2	2.0	-	-	-	-
All ages	37	14.5	42	16.7	10.7	1.2	-	-	-	-
Females										
0-4	16	35.0	13	28.6	2.5	1.0	-	-	-	-
5-14	23	33.0	25	35.8	10.0	1.2	-	-	-	-
15-44	3	3.0	8	7.9	29.5	2.0	-	-	-	-
45-59	0	1.5	1	5.3	52.3	3.2	-	-	-	-
60+	0	2.5	1	6.8	69.7	2.4	-	-	-	-
All ages	43	16.8	49	18.9	9.3	1.2	-	-	-	-
Total	80	15.6	91	17.9	10.0	1.2	-	-	-	-

For epidemiological sources see Orzeszyna et al. 1996. For the methods used to estimate and project incidence, prevalence, and deaths see Murray and Lopez 1996a. See explanatory notes for definitions and caveats.

Table 191
Nephritis and nephrosis

Cuadro 191
Nefritis y nefrosis

Tableau 191
Néphrite et néphrose

Acute glomerulonephritis

Glomérulo nefritis aguda

Glomerulonéphrite aiguë

Table 191g   LAC - ALC - ALC   Nephritis and nephrosis - Acute glomerulonephritis

Age group (years)	Incidence 1990 Number ('000s)	Rate (per 100 000)	Prevalence 1990 Number ('000s)	Rate (per 100 000)	Avg. age at onset (years)	Average duration (years)	Deaths 1990 Number ('000s)	Rate (per 100 000)	Deaths 2000 (Projected) Number ('000s)	Rate (per 100 000)
Males										
0-4	1	5.0	1	4.1	2.5	1.0	-	-	-	-
5-14	2	4.0	2	4.4	10.0	1.2	-	-	-	-
15-44	3	3.0	6	6.0	29.8	2.1	-	-	-	-
45-59	0	1.0	1	4.2	52.4	3.4	-	-	-	-
60+	0	2.5	1	7.9	70.3	2.9	-	-	-	-
All ages	7	3.3	12	5.3	21.4	1.7	-	-	-	-
Females										
0-4	3	10.0	2	8.3	2.5	1.0	-	-	-	-
5-14	4	8.0	4	8.8	10.0	1.2	-	-	-	-
15-44	3	3.0	6	6.2	29.9	2.1	-	-	-	-
45-59	0	1.0	1	4.1	52.4	3.4	-	-	-	-
60+	0	1.5	1	4.8	71.1	2.8	-	-	-	-
All ages	10	4.7	15	6.7	16.4	1.5	-	-	-	-
Total	18	4.0	27	6.0	18.4	1.6	-	-	-	-

Table 191h   MEC - AOM - CMO   Nephritis and nephrosis - Acute glomerulonephritis

Age group (years)	Incidence 1990 Number ('000s)	Rate (per 100 000)	Prevalence 1990 Number ('000s)	Rate (per 100 000)	Avg. age at onset (years)	Average duration (years)	Deaths 1990 Number ('000s)	Rate (per 100 000)	Deaths 2000 (Projected) Number ('000s)	Rate (per 100 000)
Males										
0-4	2	5.0	2	4.1	2.5	0.99	-	-	-	-
5-14	5	8.0	5	8.4	10.0	1.18	-	-	-	-
15-44	1	1.0	3	2.4	29.9	2.04	-	-	-	-
45-59	0	1.1	1	3.4	52.3	3.08	-	-	-	-
60+	0	1.4	0	3.3	69.7	2.02	-	-	-	-
All ages	9	3.5	11	4.3	13.3	1.32	-	-	-	-
Females										
0-4	3	7.0	2	5.8	2.5	0.99	-	-	-	-
5-14	7	11.0	7	11.5	10.0	1.18	-	-	-	-
15-44	2	2.0	5	4.4	29.9	2.04	-	-	-	-
45-59	0	1.0	1	3.6	52.4	3.11	-	-	-	-
60+	0	1.1	0	2.7	70.4	2.05	-	-	-	-
All ages	12	4.9	15	6.2	13.4	1.34	-	-	-	-
Total	21	4.2	26	5.3	13.4	1.33	-	-	-	-

Table 191i   World - Mundo - Monde   Nephritis and nephrosis - Acute glomerulonephritis

Age group (years)	Incidence 1990 Number ('000s)	Rate (per 100 000)	Prevalence 1990 Number ('000s)	Rate (per 100 000)	Avg. age at onset (years)	Average duration (years)	Deaths 1990 Number ('000s)	Rate (per 100 000)	Deaths 2000 (Projected) Number ('000s)	Rate (per 100 000)
Males										
0-4	25	7.8	21	6.4	2.5	0.99	-	-	-	-
5-14	64	11.6	67	12.1	10.0	1.18	-	-	-	-
15-44	26	2.1	57	4.6	29.8	2.10	-	-	-	-
45-59	3	1.1	12	3.9	52.3	3.27	-	-	-	-
60+	4	1.7	11	5.0	70.0	2.52	-	-	-	-
All ages	122	4.6	168	6.3	15.7	1.44	-	-	-	-
Females										
0-4	38	12.4	32	10.2	2.5	0.99	-	-	-	-
5-14	66	12.6	71	13.6	10.0	1.18	-	-	-	-
15-44	31	2.6	67	5.6	29.8	2.08	-	-	-	-
45-59	2	0.7	10	3.2	52.4	3.37	-	-	-	-
60+	3	1.1	9	3.2	71.0	2.53	-	-	-	-
All ages	142	5.4	189	7.2	14.4	1.39	-	-	-	-
Total	264	5.0	357	6.8	15.0	1.41	-	-	-	-

For epidemiological sources see Orzeszyna et al. 1996. For the methods used to estimate and project incidence, prevalence, and deaths see Murray and Lopez 1996a. See explanatory notes for definitions and caveats.

Table 192
Nephritis and nephrosis

Cuadro 192
Nefritis y nefrosis

Tableau 192
Néphrite et néphrose

End-stage renal disease   Enfermedad renal terminal   Maladie rénale terminale

Table 192a   EME - PEMC - EMBE   Nephritis and nephrosis - End-stage renal disease

Age group (years)	Incidence 1990 Number ('000s)	Rate (per 100 000)	Prevalence 1990 Number ('000s)	Rate (per 100 000)	Avg. age at onset (years)	Average duration (years)	Deaths 1990 Number ('000s)	Rate (per 100 000)	Deaths 2000 (Projected) Number ('000s)	Rate (per 100 000)
Males										
0-4	6	21.0	10	39	2.6	12.6	0	1.2	0	0.9
5-14	0	0.2	29	54	10.0	15.8	0	0.1	0	0.1
15-44	7	4.0	102	56	29.9	11.7	1	0.7	1	0.6
45-59	3	4.0	28	43	52.4	4.7	3	4.6	3	3.8
60+	36	60.0	55	90	71.1	1.5	34	56.3	39	54.1
All ages	52	13.3	225	58	56.9	4.3	39	9.9	44	10.6
Females										
0-4	5	20.0	9	38	2.6	12.9	0	0.8	0	0.6
5-14	1	2.0	31	61	10.0	15.9	0	0.1	0	0.1
15-44	2	1.2	65	36	30.0	11.8	1	0.4	1	0.3
45-59	3	4.5	20	30	52.5	4.8	2	2.9	2	2.2
60+	42	50.0	64	76	72.4	1.5	38	45.4	46	47.4
All ages	53	13.1	190	47	61.8	3.4	41	10.1	49	11.4
Total	105	13.2	415	52	59.4	3.9	80	10.0	92	11.0

Table 192b   FSE - PEAS - AESE   Nephritis and nephrosis - End-stage renal disease

Age group (years)	Incidence 1990 Number ('000s)	Rate (per 100 000)	Prevalence 1990 Number ('000s)	Rate (per 100 000)	Avg. age at onset (years)	Average duration (years)	Deaths 1990 Number ('000s)	Rate (per 100 000)	Deaths 2000 (Projected) Number ('000s)	Rate (per 100 000)
Males										
0-4	1	8.5	2	16	2.5	10.5	0	0.5	0	0.4
5-14	1	2.0	8	29	10.0	12.7	0	0.4	0	0.3
15-44	8	10.0	68	89	29.8	9.8	2	2.9	2	2.4
45-59	3	11.0	25	93	52.3	4.5	3	10.8	3	9.4
60+	5	23.0	8	36	70.0	1.3	5	25.2	6	24.9
All ages	17	10.4	110	67	42.5	6.6	11	6.4	11	6.5
Females										
0-4	1	10.0	2	19	2.5	12.2	0	0.4	0	0.4
5-14	2	7.5	15	57	10.0	15.0	0	0.3	0	0.2
15-44	5	7.0	71	95	30.0	11.3	1	1.9	1	1.4
45-59	2	8.0	22	74	52.4	4.5	2	7.0	2	5.8
60+	5	14.0	8	22	71.5	1.3	5	14.9	6	14.0
All ages	16	8.9	119	66	41.8	7.6	9	5.0	9	4.7
Total	33	9.6	229	66	42.2	7.1	20	5.7	20	5.6

Table 192c   India - India - Inde   Nephritis and nephrosis - End-stage renal disease

Age group (years)	Incidence 1990 Number ('000s)	Rate (per 100 000)	Prevalence 1990 Number ('000s)	Rate (per 100 000)	Avg. age at onset (years)	Average duration (years)	Deaths 1990 Number ('000s)	Rate (per 100 000)	Deaths 2000 (Projected) Number ('000s)	Rate (per 100 000)
Males										
0-4	15	25.0	26	43	2.5	7.76	2	3.3	2	3.6
5-14	24	24.0	141	139	10.0	11.39	6	6.2	4	4.1
15-44	6	3.0	196	98	29.8	9.19	5	2.6	5	2.0
45-59	12	25.0	38	79	52.3	2.77	9	19.9	9	15.6
60+	24	80.0	16	53	69.6	0.63	25	82.8	25	67.7
All ages	81	18.4	416	95	33.8	6.13	48	10.8	46	8.9
Females										
0-4	13	23.0	23	41	2.5	8.47	1	1.9	1	2.1
5-14	21	22.0	126	132	10.0	12.03	10	10.4	7	6.6
15-44	15	8.0	256	140	29.8	9.68	7	3.6	5	2.3
45-59	7	15.0	34	74	52.4	3.01	7	15.6	7	11.9
60+	19	65.0	13	46	70.0	0.68	18	63.6	22	56.1
All ages	74	18.1	452	110	31.7	7.23	43	10.5	42	8.7
Total	155	18.3	868	102	32.8	6.66	91	10.7	88	8.8

For epidemiological sources see Orzeszyna et al. 1996. For the methods used to estimate and project incidence, prevalence, and deaths see Murray and Lopez 1996a. See explanatory notes for definitions and caveats.

Table 192
Nephritis and nephrosis

Cuadro 192
Nefritis y nefrosis

Tableau 192
Néphrite et néphrose

End-stage renal disease · Enfermedad renal terminal · Maladie rénale terminale

Table 192d China - China - Chine — Nephritis and nephrosis - End-stage renal disease

Age group (years)	Incidence 1990 Number ('000s)	Rate (per 100 000)	Prevalence 1990 Number ('000s)	Rate (per 100 000)	Avg. age at onset (years)	Average duration (years)	Deaths 1990 Number ('000s)	Rate (per 100 000)	Deaths 2000 (Projected) Number ('000s)	Rate (per 100 000)
Males										
0-4	13	22.0	24	40	2.5	9.33	1	2.1	1	2.2
5-14	10	10.0	88	90	10.0	11.63	2	1.7	1	1.1
15-44	35	11.5	369	121	29.9	8.66	17	5.5	13	4.2
45-59	9	12.0	55	75	52.4	3.43	10	13.2	10	10.3
60+	26	54.0	26	53	69.8	0.92	28	56.9	28	47.1
All ages	93	15.9	561	96	37.4	6.38	57	9.8	55	8.3
Females										
0-4	17	30.0	32	55	2.5	9.90	2	3.1	2	3.4
5-14	7	8.0	95	105	10.0	11.74	1	1.2	1	0.8
15-44	24	8.5	278	98	29.9	9.84	12	4.2	9	2.9
45-59	6	9.0	33	52	52.4	3.26	7	10.2	7	7.7
60+	20	38.0	19	37	70.6	0.93	20	38.9	24	36.7
All ages	74	13.5	458	83	34.1	7.17	42	7.6	42	6.7
Total	167	14.8	1 019	90	35.9	6.73	99	8.7	97	7.5

Table 192e OAI - OPAI - APAI — Nephritis and nephrosis - End-stage renal disease

Age group (years)	Incidence 1990 Number ('000s)	Rate (per 100 000)	Prevalence 1990 Number ('000s)	Rate (per 100 000)	Avg. age at onset (years)	Average duration (years)	Deaths 1990 Number ('000s)	Rate (per 100 000)	Deaths 2000 (Projected) Number ('000s)	Rate (per 100 000)
Males										
0-4	12	28.0	24	54	2.5	8.80	1	2.8	1	2.7
5-14	17	20.0	117	139	10.0	11.67	4	5.0	3	3.5
15-44	14	9.0	221	137	29.8	9.06	6	4.0	7	3.2
45-59	7	20.0	32	93	52.3	3.17	7	21.0	8	16.6
60+	24	119.9	18	90	69.6	0.72	22	109.9	26	92.9
All ages	75	21.7	411	120	35.9	6.35	41	12.0	44	10.9
Females										
0-4	13	30.0	23	55	2.5	9.26	1	2.6	1	2.5
5-14	16	20.0	120	150	10.0	11.43	3	3.7	2	2.5
15-44	7	4.2	155	97	29.8	8.50	6	4.1	6	2.8
45-59	11	30.0	37	106	52.4	3.20	8	21.6	8	16.2
60+	25	109.9	21	91	70.3	0.78	26	114.2	33	102.2
All ages	71	20.8	356	105	38.1	5.79	44	13.0	50	12.3
Total	145	21.3	767	112	36.9	6.08	85	12.5	94	11.6

Table 192f SSA - ASS - ASS — Nephritis and nephrosis - End-stage renal disease

Age group (years)	Incidence 1990 Number ('000s)	Rate (per 100 000)	Prevalence 1990 Number ('000s)	Rate (per 100 000)	Avg. age at onset (years)	Average duration (years)	Deaths 1990 Number ('000s)	Rate (per 100 000)	Deaths 2000 (Projected) Number ('000s)	Rate (per 100 000)
Males										
0-4	47	99.8	81	171	2.5	8.18	5	11.2	7	11.1
5-14	45	64.7	335	476	10.0	12.00	8	10.9	7	7.4
15-44	5	5.0	303	292	29.4	8.93	9	8.6	9	6.4
45-59	7	35.0	25	121	52.2	2.73	7	32.3	7	24.7
60+	11	100.0	7	63	69.2	0.59	17	159.2	18	126.7
All ages	116	45.8	750	297	15.8	8.69	45	17.9	48	14.1
Females										
0-4	38	79.9	64	137	2.5	8.30	5	9.6	6	9.7
5-14	35	49.8	260	372	10.0	12.06	7	9.4	6	6.2
15-44	6	6.0	256	241	29.5	9.00	5	4.6	4	2.9
45-59	9	39.9	30	134	52.3	2.75	8	35.5	8	25.8
60+	13	100.0	9	68	69.7	0.63	14	110.1	15	87.6
All ages	100	38.9	619	240	19.7	8.19	38	14.7	39	11.2
Total	216	42.3	1 369	268	17.6	8.46	83	16.3	87	12.6

For epidemiological sources see Orzeszyna et al. 1996. For the methods used to estimate and project incidence, prevalence, and deaths see Murray and Lopez 1996a. See explanatory notes for definitions and caveats.

Table 192	Cuadro 192	Tableau 192
Nephritis and nephrosis	**Nefritis y nefrosis**	**Néphrite et néphrose**
End-stage renal disease	Enfermedad renal terminal	Maladie rénale terminale

Table 192g   LAC - ALC - ALC   Nephritis and nephrosis - End-stage renal disease

Age group (years)	Incidence 1990 Number ('000s)	Rate (per 100 000)	Prevalence 1990 Number ('000s)	Rate (per 100 000)	Avg. age at onset (years)	Average duration (years)	Deaths 1990 Number ('000s)	Rate (per 100 000)	Deaths 2000 (Projected) Number ('000s)	Rate (per 100 000)
Males										
0-4	11	40.0	21	73	2.5	11.06	1	3.5	1	3.3
5-14	16	29.9	117	224	10.0	14.46	1	1.7	1	1.3
15-44	1	1.0	148	142	29.8	10.46	3	2.5	3	2.1
45-59	4	20.0	19	86	52.4	3.65	3	14.6	4	11.8
60+	10	70.0	10	69	70.3	0.93	12	81.8	14	71.4
All ages	43	19.2	315	142	27.0	9.14	19	8.8	22	8.3
Females										
0-4	15	54.9	28	102	2.5	11.60	1	2.9	1	2.7
5-14	21	40.9	158	312	10.0	14.64	1	1.7	1	1.2
15-44	5	5.0	237	227	29.9	10.62	4	3.7	3	2.6
45-59	3	13.0	20	87	52.4	3.82	3	14.5	4	11.2
60+	10	60.0	11	65	71.1	1.03	11	64.3	14	58.5
All ages	54	24.4	454	204	23.5	19.84	20	8.8	22	8.3
Total	97	21.8	769	173	25.1	15.14	39	8.8	44	8.3

Table 192h   MEC - AOM - CMO   Nephritis and nephrosis - End-stage renal disease

Age group (years)	Incidence 1990 Number ('000s)	Rate (per 100 000)	Prevalence 1990 Number ('000s)	Rate (per 100 000)	Avg. age at onset (years)	Average duration (years)	Deaths 1990 Number ('000s)	Rate (per 100 000)	Deaths 2000 (Projected) Number ('000s)	Rate (per 100 000)
Males										
0-4	16	40.0	29	71	2.5	10.21	1	3.2	2	3.2
5-14	20	29.9	143	219	10.0	13.89	2	2.7	2	1.9
15-44	8	7.0	210	185	29.9	10.09	4	3.6	4	2.8
45-59	4	18.0	21	95	52.3	3.38	4	17.0	4	13.3
60+	9	65.0	7	54	69.7	0.78	10	73.9	12	62.2
All ages	57	22.2	411	160	22.9	9.50	21	8.2	23	7.0
Females										
0-4	16	40.0	29	73	2.5	10.38	1	2.7	1	2.7
5-14	19	29.9	136	219	10.0	13.76	3	4.2	2	2.9
15-44	12	11.1	233	218	29.9	10.13	5	4.3	4	2.8
45-59	2	10.0	19	84	52.4	3.42	3	14.2	3	10.6
60+	6	40.0	6	36	70.4	0.85	7	42.1	7	34.9
All ages	55	22.2	423	171	20.7	10.11	18	7.3	18	5.7
Total	112	22.2	834	166	21.8	9.80	39	7.8	42	6.3

Table 192i   World - Mundo - Monde   Nephritis and nephrosis - End-stage renal disease

Age group (years)	Incidence 1990 Number ('000s)	Rate (per 100 000)	Prevalence 1990 Number ('000s)	Rate (per 100 000)	Avg. age at onset (years)	Average duration (years)	Deaths 1990 Number ('000s)	Rate (per 100 000)	Deaths 2000 (Projected) Number ('000s)	Rate (per 100 000)
Males										
0-4	122	38.1	217	68	2.5	9.08	13	3.9	15	4.3
5-14	132	24.0	976	177	10.0	12.39	23	4.1	18	2.9
15-44	85	6.8	1 617	129	29.8	9.31	48	3.8	44	3.0
45-59	49	15.6	243	78	52.3	3.28	46	14.7	47	11.8
60+	145	66.2	146	67	70.1	0.96	153	69.7	169	61.2
All ages	533	20.1	3 199	121	31.6	7.20	281	10.6	293	9.5
Females										
0-4	118	38.2	212	68	2.5	9.60	11	3.4	13	3.8
5-14	121	23.1	941	179	10.0	12.73	24	4.6	19	3.1
15-44	76	6.4	1 552	129	29.8	9.87	40	3.4	33	2.3
45-59	43	13.7	216	69	52.4	3.33	40	12.8	40	9.8
60+	140	51.9	150	56	71.0	1.03	140	51.8	167	49.7
All ages	498	19.1	3 070	117	32.0	8.51	255	9.7	271	8.8
Total	1 031	19.6	6 270	119	31.8	7.83	536	10.2	563	9.1

For epidemiological sources see Orzeszyna et al. 1996. For the methods used to estimate and project incidence, prevalence, and deaths see Murray and Lopez 1996a. See explanatory notes for definitions and caveats.

Table 193
Benign prostatic hypertrophy
Symptomatic cases

Cuadro 193
Hipertrofia prostática benigna
Casos sintomáticos

Tableau 193
Hypertrophie bénigne de la prostate
Cas symptomatiques

Table 193a EME - PEMC - EMBE — Benign prostatic hypertrophy - Symptomatic cases

Age group (years)	Incidence 1990 Number ('000s)	Rate (per 100 000)	Prevalence 1990 Number ('000s)	Rate (per 100 000)	Avg. age at onset (years)	Average duration (years)	Deaths 1990 Number ('000s)	Rate (per 100 000)	Deaths 2000 (Projected) Number ('000s)	Rate (per 100 000)
Males										
0-4	0	0	0	0	-	-	0	0.0	0	0.0
5-14	0	0	0	0	-	-	0	0.0	0	0.0
15-44	0	0	0	0	-	-	0	0.0	0	0.0
45-59	1 001	1 513	2 586	3 910	55.0	2.8	0	0.0	0	0.0
60+	1 626	2 685	4 965	8 200	70.0	2.3	4	6.1	4	6.1
All ages	2 626	673	7 551	1 934	64.3	2.5	4	1.0	4	1.1
Females										
0-4	0	0	0	0	-	-	0	0	0	0
5-14	0	0	0	0	-	-	0	0	0	0
15-44	0	0	0	0	-	-	0	0	0	0
45-59	0	0	0	0	-	-	0	0	0	0
60+	0	0	0	0	-	-	0	0	0	0
All ages	0	0	0	0	-	-	0	0	0	0
Total	2 626	329	7 551	946	64.3	2.5	4	0.5	4	0.5

Table 193b FSE - PEAS - AESE — Benign prostatic hypertrophy - Symptomatic cases

Age group (years)	Incidence 1990 Number ('000s)	Rate (per 100 000)	Prevalence 1990 Number ('000s)	Rate (per 100 000)	Avg. age at onset (years)	Average duration (years)	Deaths 1990 Number ('000s)	Rate (per 100 000)	Deaths 2000 (Projected) Number ('000s)	Rate (per 100 000)
Males										
0-4	0	0	0	0	-	-	0	0.0	0	0.0
5-14	0	0	0	0	-	-	0	0.0	0	0.0
15-44	0	0	0	0	-	-	0	0.0	0	0.0
45-59	512	1 900	1 314	4 870	55.0	2.7	0	0.6	0	0.5
60+	629	3 000	1 908	9 100	70.0	2.2	6	29.3	8	32.7
All ages	1 141	690	3 221	1 948	63.3	2.4	6	3.8	8	5.0
Females										
0-4	0	0	0	0	-	-	0	0	0	0
5-14	0	0	0	0	-	-	0	0	0	0
15-44	0	0	0	0	-	-	0	0	0	0
45-59	0	0	0	0	-	-	0	0	0	0
60+	0	0	0	0	-	-	0	0	0	0
All ages	0	0	0	0	-	-	0	0	0	0
Total	1 141	330	3 221	930	63.3	2.4	6	1.8	8	2.4

Table 193c India - India - Inde — Benign prostatic hypertrophy - Symptomatic cases

Age group (years)	Incidence 1990 Number ('000s)	Rate (per 100 000)	Prevalence 1990 Number ('000s)	Rate (per 100 000)	Avg. age at onset (years)	Average duration (years)	Deaths 1990 Number ('000s)	Rate (per 100 000)	Deaths 2000 (Projected) Number ('000s)	Rate (per 100 000)
Males										
0-4	0	0	0	0	-	-	0	0.0	0	0.0
5-14	0	0	0	0	-	-	0	0.0	0	0.0
15-44	0	0	0	0	-	-	0	0.0	0	0.0
45-59	572	1 202	4 258	8 952	55.0	16.2	0	0.2	0	0.2
60+	171	576	6 905	23 197	70.0	7.2	11	36.3	11	29.7
All ages	743	169	11 163	2 541	58.5	14.1	11	2.5	11	2.2
Females										
0-4	0	0	0	0	-	-	0	0	0	0
5-14	0	0	0	0	-	-	0	0	0	0
15-44	0	0	0	0	-	-	0	0	0	0
45-59	0	0	0	0	-	-	0	0	0	0
60+	0	0	0	0	-	-	0	0	0	0
All ages	0	0	0	0	-	-	0	0	0	0
Total	743	87	11 163	1 314	58.5	14.1	11	1.3	11	1.1

For the methods used to estimate and project incidence, prevalence, and deaths see Murray and Lopez 1996a. See explanatory notes for definitions and caveats.

Table 193	Cuadro 193	Tableau 193
Benign prostatic hypertrophy	**Hipertrofia prostática benigna**	**Hypertrophie bénigne de la prostate**
Symptomatic cases	Casos sintomáticos	Cas symptomatiques

Table 193d China - China - Chine — Benign prostatic hypertrophy - Symptomatic cases

Age group (years)	Incidence 1990 Number ('000s)	Rate (per 100 000)	Prevalence 1990 Number ('000s)	Rate (per 100 000)	Avg. age at onset (years)	Average duration (years)	Deaths 1990 Number ('000s)	Rate (per 100 000)	Deaths 2000 (Projected) Number ('000s)	Rate (per 100 000)
Males										
0-4	0	0	0	0	-	-	0	0.0	0	0.0
5-14	0	0	0	0	-	-	0	0.0	0	0.0
15-44	0	0	0	0	-	-	0	0.0	0	0.0
45-59	879	1 209	6 615	9 102	55.0	16.1	0	0.3	0	0.2
60+	275	561	11 345	23 163	70.0	7.0	6	12.5	7	10.9
All ages	1 153	197	17 960	3 069	58.6	13.9	7	1.2	7	1.1
Females										
0-4	0	0	0	0	-	-	0	0	0	0
5-14	0	0	0	0	-	-	0	0	0	0
15-44	0	0	0	0	-	-	0	0	0	0
45-59	0	0	0	0	-	-	0	0	0	0
60+	0	0	0	0	-	-	0	0	0	0
All ages	0	0	0	0	-	-	0	0	0	0
Total	1 153	102	17 960	1 584	58.6	13.9	7	0.6	7	0.6

Table 193e OAI - OPAI - APAI — Benign prostatic hypertrophy - Symptomatic cases

Age group (years)	Incidence 1990 Number ('000s)	Rate (per 100 000)	Prevalence 1990 Number ('000s)	Rate (per 100 000)	Avg. age at onset (years)	Average duration (years)	Deaths 1990 Number ('000s)	Rate (per 100 000)	Deaths 2000 (Projected) Number ('000s)	Rate (per 100 000)
Males										
0-4	0	0	0	0	-	-	0	0.0	0	0.0
5-14	0	0	0	0	-	-	0	0.0	0	0.0
15-44	0	0	0	0	-	-	0	0.0	0	0.0
45-59	420	1 231	3 151	9 230	55.0	17.3	0	0.0	0	0.0
60+	107	529	4 717	23 343	70.0	7.4	1	3.0	1	2.7
All ages	527	154	7 868	2 294	58.0	15.2	1	0.2	1	0.2
Females										
0-4	0	0	0	0	-	-	0	0	0	0
5-14	0	0	0	0	-	-	0	0	0	0
15-44	0	0	0	0	-	-	0	0	0	0
45-59	0	0	0	0	-	-	0	0	0	0
60+	0	0	0	0	-	-	0	0	0	0
All ages	0	0	0	0	-	-	0	0	0	0
Total	527	77	7 868	1 153	58.0	15.2	1	0.1	1	0.1

Table 193f SSA - ASS - ASS — Benign prostatic hypertrophy - Symptomatic cases

Age group (years)	Incidence 1990 Number ('000s)	Rate (per 100 000)	Prevalence 1990 Number ('000s)	Rate (per 100 000)	Avg. age at onset (years)	Average duration (years)	Deaths 1990 Number ('000s)	Rate (per 100 000)	Deaths 2000 (Projected) Number ('000s)	Rate (per 100 000)
Males										
0-4	0	0	0	0	-	-	0	0.0	0	0.0
5-14	0	0	0	0	-	-	0	0.0	0	0.0
15-44	0	0	0	0	-	-	0	0.0	0	0.0
45-59	376	1 850	2 831	13 938	55.0	18.5	0	0.0	0	0.0
60+	52	497	3 360	31 977	70.0	4.9	0	4.5	1	3.8
All ages	428	170	6 191	2 453	56.8	16.8	0	0.2	1	0.2
Females										
0-4	0	0	0	0	-	-	0	0	0	0
5-14	0	0	0	0	-	-	0	0	0	0
15-44	0	0	0	0	-	-	0	0	0	0
45-59	0	0	0	0	-	-	0	0	0	0
60+	0	0	0	0	-	-	0	0	0	0
All ages	0	0	0	0	-	-	0	0	0	0
Total	428	84	6 191	1 213	56.8	16.8	0	0.1	1	0.1

For the methods used to estimate and project incidence, prevalence, and deaths see Murray and Lopez 1996a. See explanatory notes for definitions and caveats.

Table 193
Benign prostatic hypertrophy
Symptomatic cases

Cuadro 193
Hipertrofia prostática benigna
Casos sintomáticos

Tableau 193
Hypertrophie bénigne de la prostate
Cas symptomatiques

Table 193g   LAC - ALC - ALC   Benign prostatic hypertrophy - Symptomatic cases

Age group (years)	Incidence 1990		Prevalence 1990		Avg. age at onset (years)	Average duration (years)	Deaths 1990		Deaths 2000 (Projected)	
	Number ('000s)	Rate (per 100 000)	Number ('000s)	Rate (per 100 000)			Number ('000s)	Rate (per 100 000)	Number ('000s)	Rate (per 100 000)
Males										
0-4	0	0	0	0	-	-	0	0.0	0	0.0
5-14	0	0	0	0	-	-	0	0.0	0	0.0
15-44	0	0	0	0	-	-	0	0.0	0	0.0
45-59	344	1 545	2 611	11 734	55.0	19.2	0	0.2	0	0.2
60+	49	346	3 759	26 417	70.0	7.8	2	13.1	2	11.8
All ages	393	177	6 370	2 874	56.9	17.7	2	0.9	2	0.9
Females										
0-4	0	0	0	0	-	-	0	0	0	0
5-14	0	0	0	0	-	-	0	0	0	0
15-44	0	0	0	0	-	-	0	0	0	0
45-59	0	0	0	0	-	-	0	0	0	0
60+	0	0	0	0	-	-	0	0	0	0
All ages	0	0	0	0	-	-	0	0	0	0
Total	393	88	6 370	1 434	56.9	17.7	2	0.4	2	0.4

Table 193h   MEC - AOM - CMO   Benign prostatic hypertrophy - Symptomatic cases

Age group (years)	Incidence 1990		Prevalence 1990		Avg. age at onset (years)	Average duration (years)	Deaths 1990		Deaths 2000 (Projected)	
	Number ('000s)	Rate (per 100 000)	Number ('000s)	Rate (per 100 000)			Number ('000s)	Rate (per 100 000)	Number ('000s)	Rate (per 100 000)
Males										
0-4	0	0	0	0	-	-	0	0.0	0	0.0
5-14	0	0	0	0	-	-	0	0.0	0	0.0
15-44	0	0	0	0	-	-	0	0.0	0	0.0
45-59	398	1 780	2 725	12 200	55.0	16.1	0	0.4	0	0.3
60+	100	732	3 822	28 000	70.0	4.3	2	11.1	2	9.6
All ages	498	194	6 547	2 554	58.0	13.7	2	0.6	2	0.6
Females										
0-4	0	0	0	0	-	-	0	0	0	0
5-14	0	0	0	0	-	-	0	0	0	0
15-44	0	0	0	0	-	-	0	0	0	0
45-59	0	0	0	0	-	-	0	0	0	0
60+	0	0	0	0	-	-	0	0	0	0
All ages	0	0	0	0	-	-	0	0	0	0
Total	498	99	6 547	1 301	58.0	13.7	2	0.3	2	0.3

Table 193i   World - Mundo - Monde   Benign prostatic hypertrophy - Symptomatic cases

Age group (years)	Incidence 1990		Prevalence 1990		Avg. age at onset (years)	Average duration (years)	Deaths 1990		Deaths 2000 (Projected)	
	Number ('000s)	Rate (per 100 000)	Number ('000s)	Rate (per 100 000)			Number ('000s)	Rate (per 100 000)	Number ('000s)	Rate (per 100 000)
Males										
0-4	0	0	0	0	-	-	0	0.0	0	0.0
5-14	0	0	0	0	-	-	0	0.0	0	0.0
15-44	0	0	0	0	-	-	0	0.0	0	0.0
45-59	4 501	1 441	26 090	8 352	55.0	12.2	1	0.2	1	0.2
60+	3 009	1 375	40 782	18 634	70.0	3.4	31	14.3	36	12.9
All ages	7 510	283	66 872	2 520	61.0	8.6	32	1.2	37	1.2
Females										
0-4	0	0	0	0	-	-	0	0	0	0
5-14	0	0	0	0	-	-	0	0	0	0
15-44	0	0	0	0	-	-	0	0	0	0
45-59	0	0	0	0	-	-	0	0	0	0
60+	0	0	0	0	-	-	0	0	0	0
All ages	0	0	0	0	-	-	0	0	0	0
Total	7 510	143	66 872	1 270	61.0	8.6	32	0.6	37	0.6

For the methods used to estimate and project incidence, prevalence, and deaths see Murray and Lopez 1996a. See explanatory notes for definitions and caveats.

Table 194
Rheumatoid arthritis

Cuadro 194
Artritis reumatoide

Tableau 194
Arthrite rhumatoïde

Cases

Casos

Cas

Table 194a   EME - PEMC - EMBE   Rheumatoid arthritis - Cases

Age group (years)	Incidence 1990 Number ('000s)	Rate (per 100 000)	Prevalence 1990 Number ('000s)	Rate (per 100 000)	Avg. age at onset (years)	Average duration (years)	Deaths 1990 Number ('000s)	Rate (per 100 000)	Deaths 2000 (Projected) Number ('000s)	Rate (per 100 000)
Males										
0-4	0	0.0	0	0	-	-	0	0.0	0	0.0
5-14	0	0.0	0	0	-	-	0	0.0	0	0.0
15-44	29	15.9	180	98	29.9	8.2	0	0.0	0	0.0
45-59	70	105.6	352	533	52.4	7.4	0	0.3	0	0.3
60+	107	177.9	734	1 226	71.1	5.3	2	3.1	2	2.8
All ages	206	52.8	1 266	325	58.9	6.5	2	0.5	2	0.6
Females										
0-4	0	0.0	0	0	-	-	0	0.0	0	0.0
5-14	2	4.2	7	15	10.0	8.4	0	0.0	0	0.0
15-44	167	93.3	1 037	579	29.9	8.3	0	0.0	0	0.0
45-59	121	177.9	784	1 157	52.4	7.8	0	0.7	0	0.5
60+	326	395.5	2 212	2 682	72.3	5.7	6	7.7	8	7.7
All ages	616	152.0	4 041	997	56.7	6.8	7	1.7	8	1.9
Total	822	103.4	5 307	667	57.2	6.7	9	1.1	10	1.2

Table 194b   FSE - PEAS - AESE   Rheumatoid arthritis - Cases

Age group (years)	Incidence 1990 Number ('000s)	Rate (per 100 000)	Prevalence 1990 Number ('000s)	Rate (per 100 000)	Avg. age at onset (years)	Average duration (years)	Deaths 1990 Number ('000s)	Rate (per 100 000)	Deaths 2000 (Projected) Number ('000s)	Rate (per 100 000)
Males										
0-4	0	0.0	0	0	-	-	0	0.0	0	0.0
5-14	0	0.0	0	0	-	-	0	0.0	0	0.0
15-44	34	45.1	210	275	29.8	8.0	0	0.0	0	0.0
45-59	24	87.5	151	561	52.2	6.9	0	0.1	0	0.1
60+	31	146.2	210	1 007	70.0	5.0	0	0.5	0	0.5
All ages	89	53.6	571	346	49.6	6.7	0	0.1	0	0.1
Females										
0-4	0	0.0	0	0	-	-	0	0.0	0	0.0
5-14	2	5.7	5	20	10.0	8.4	0	0.0	0	0.0
15-44	108	143.7	668	891	29.9	8.2	0	0.0	0	0.0
45-59	75	248.5	500	1 665	52.4	7.6	0	0.4	0	0.3
60+	89	247.7	729	2 037	71.5	5.5	0	1.1	0	1.1
All ages	273	151.1	1 902	1 055	49.4	7.2	1	0.3	1	0.3
Total	361	104.5	2 473	716	49.5	7.0	1	0.2	1	0.2

Table 194c   India - India - Inde   Rheumatoid arthritis - Cases

Age group (years)	Incidence 1990 Number ('000s)	Rate (per 100 000)	Prevalence 1990 Number ('000s)	Rate (per 100 000)	Avg. age at onset (years)	Average duration (years)	Deaths 1990 Number ('000s)	Rate (per 100 000)	Deaths 2000 (Projected) Number ('000s)	Rate (per 100 000)
Males										
0-4	0	0.0	0	0.0	-	-	0	0.0	0	0.0
5-14	0	0.0	0	0.0	-	-	0	0.0	0	0.0
15-44	16	8.1	99	49.3	29.8	8.0	0	0.0	0	0.0
45-59	6	12.0	40	84.6	52.3	7.1	0	0.1	0	0.1
60+	4	13.0	31	103.6	69.7	4.9	1	2.5	1	2.0
All ages	26	5.9	170	38.7	40.7	7.4	1	0.2	1	0.2
Females										
0-4	0	0.0	0	0.0	-	-	0	0.0	0	0.0
5-14	1	1.5	5	5.3	10.0	8.3	0	0.0	0	0.0
15-44	31	17.0	194	105.9	29.8	8.1	0	0.1	0	0.0
45-59	25	53.8	140	305.3	52.4	7.3	1	1.2	1	0.9
60+	17	57.8	130	452.6	70.1	5.1	0	0.9	0	0.8
All ages	74	18.0	470	114.6	45.9	7.1	1	0.2	1	0.2
Total	100	11.7	640	75.3	44.7	7.2	2	0.2	2	0.2

For epidemiological sources see Symmons 1996. For the methods used to estimate and project incidence, prevalence, and deaths see Murray and Lopez 1996a. See explanatory notes for definitions and caveats.

Table 194
Rheumatoid arthritis

Cuadro 194
Artritis reumatoide

Tableau 194
Arthrite rhumatoïde

Cases

Casos

Cas

Table 194d China - China - Chine   Rheumatoid arthritis - Cases

Age group (years)	Incidence 1990 Number ('000s)	Rate (per 100 000)	Prevalence 1990 Number ('000s)	Rate (per 100 000)	Avg. age at onset (years)	Average duration (years)	Deaths 1990 Number ('000s)	Rate (per 100 000)	Deaths 2000 (Projected) Number ('000s)	Rate (per 100 000)
Males										
0-4	0	0.0	0	0	-	-	0	0.0	0	0.0
5-14	0	0.0	0	0	-	-	0	0.0	0	0.0
15-44	39	12.8	239	78	29.9	8.1	0	0.0	0	0.0
45-59	74	101.5	364	500	52.3	7.1	0	0.1	0	0.1
60+	51	104.3	399	817	69.8	5.0	1	1.5	1	1.3
All ages	164	28.0	1 002	171	52.4	6.7	1	0.1	1	0.1
Females										
0-4	0	0.0	0	0	-	-	0	0.0	0	0.0
5-14	3	2.9	9	10	10.0	8.4	0	0.0	0	0.0
15-44	80	28.0	500	176	29.9	8.2	0	0.1	0	0.0
45-59	129	200.3	646	1 003	52.4	7.4	0	0.1	0	0.1
60+	143	278.5	1 026	2 000	70.6	5.2	1	1.3	1	1.3
All ages	354	64.6	2 181	398	54.3	6.7	1	0.2	1	0.2
Total	518	45.7	3 183	281	53.7	6.7	2	0.2	2	0.2

Table 194e OAI - OPAI - APAI   Rheumatoid arthritis - Cases

Age group (years)	Incidence 1990 Number ('000s)	Rate (per 100 000)	Prevalence 1990 Number ('000s)	Rate (per 100 000)	Avg. age at onset (years)	Average duration (years)	Deaths 1990 Number ('000s)	Rate (per 100 000)	Deaths 2000 (Projected) Number ('000s)	Rate (per 100 000)
Males										
0-4	0	0.0	0	0.0	-	-	0	0.0	0	0.0
5-14	0	0.0	0	0.0	-	-	0	0.0	0	0.0
15-44	1	0.9	9	5.5	29.7	8.0	0	0.0	0	0.0
45-59	12	36.5	56	164.5	52.3	6.9	0	0.2	0	0.2
60+	46	228.4	247	1 228.3	69.6	4.9	0	0.7	0	0.5
All ages	60	17.5	312	91.0	65.0	5.4	0	0.1	0	0.1
Females										
0-4	0	0.0	0	0.0	-	-	0	0.0	0	0.0
5-14	1	1.1	3	4.0	10.0	8.3	0	0.0	0	0.0
15-44	23	14.4	143	89.8	29.8	8.1	0	0.0	0	0.0
45-59	20	55.9	107	304.3	52.3	7.2	0	0.4	0	0.3
60+	88	391.3	486	2 160.9	70.3	5.1	0	1.4	0	1.2
All ages	132	38.7	739	217.7	60.0	6.0	0	0.1	1	0.1
Total	191	28.1	1 051	154.0	61.6	5.8	1	0.1	1	0.1

Table 194f SSA - ASS - ASS   Rheumatoid arthritis - Cases

Age group (years)	Incidence 1990 Number ('000s)	Rate (per 100 000)	Prevalence 1990 Number ('000s)	Rate (per 100 000)	Avg. age at onset (years)	Average duration (years)	Deaths 1990 Number ('000s)	Rate (per 100 000)	Deaths 2000 (Projected) Number ('000s)	Rate (per 100 000)
Males										
0-4	0	0.0	0	0.0	-	-	0	0.0	0	0.0
5-14	0	0.0	0	0.0	-	-	0	0.0	0	0.0
15-44	7	6.7	42	40.2	29.4	7.7	0	0.0	0	0.0
45-59	4	21.5	24	120.2	52.2	6.7	0	0.2	0	0.2
60+	3	27.5	21	200.7	69.2	4.8	0	1.2	0	1.0
All ages	14	5.6	87	34.6	44.5	6.8	0	0.1	0	0.1
Females										
0-4	0	0.0	0	0.0	-	-	0	0.0	0	0.0
5-14	1	1.5	4	5.1	10.0	8.1	0	0.0	0	0.0
15-44	17	16.2	106	100.0	29.5	7.8	0	0.0	0	0.0
45-59	12	53.8	66	300.3	52.2	7.0	0	0.3	0	0.2
60+	7	53.8	55	431.3	69.7	5.0	0	0.6	0	0.5
All ages	37	14.3	231	89.5	43.4	7.0	0	0.1	0	0.0
Total	51	10.0	318	62.3	43.9	7.0	0	0.1	0	0.0

For epidemiological sources see Symmons 1996. For the methods used to estimate and project incidence, prevalence, and deaths see Murray and Lopez 1996a. See explanatory notes for definitions and caveats.

Table 194
Rheumatoid arthritis

Cuadro 194
Artritis reumatoide

Tableau 194
Arthrite rhumatoïde

Cases

Casos

Cas

Table 194g LAC - ALC - ALC — Rheumatoid arthritis - Cases

Age group (years)	Incidence 1990 Number ('000s)	Rate (per 100 000)	Prevalence 1990 Number ('000s)	Rate (per 100 000)	Avg. age at onset (years)	Average duration (years)	Deaths 1990 Number ('000s)	Rate (per 100 000)	Deaths 2000 (Projected) Number ('000s)	Rate (per 100 000)
Males										
0-4	0	0.0	0	0	-	-	0	0.0	0	0.0
5-14	0	0.0	0	0	-	-	0	0.0	0	0.0
15-44	34	32.7	208	199	29.8	8.1	0	0.0	0	0.0
45-59	27	121.7	148	667	52.3	7.2	0	0.2	0	0.1
60+	19	131.3	144	1 024	70.3	5.1	0	2.6	0	2.3
All ages	80	36.0	501	226	46.9	7.1	0	0.2	1	0.2
Females										
0-4	0	0.0	0	0	-	-	0	0.0	0	0.0
5-14	3	5.7	10	20	10.0	8.3	0	0.0	0	0.0
15-44	152	146.2	940	903	29.8	8.2	0	0.1	0	0.1
45-59	73	314.0	459	1 967	52.4	7.5	0	0.6	0	0.5
60+	53	316.9	427	2 573	71.1	5.4	1	4.2	1	3.8
All ages	281	126.3	1 837	826	43.1	7.5	1	0.4	1	0.4
Total	361	81.2	2 337	526	44.0	7.4	1	0.3	2	0.3

Table 194h MEC - AOM - CMO — Rheumatoid arthritis - Cases

Age group (years)	Incidence 1990 Number ('000s)	Rate (per 100 000)	Prevalence 1990 Number ('000s)	Rate (per 100 000)	Avg. age at onset (years)	Average duration (years)	Deaths 1990 Number ('000s)	Rate (per 100 000)	Deaths 2000 (Projected) Number ('000s)	Rate (per 100 000)
Males										
0-4	0	0.0	0	0.0	-	-	0	0.0	0	0
5-14	0	0.0	0	0.0	-	-	0	0.0	0	0
15-44	5	4.0	28	24.7	29.8	8.1	0	0.0	0	0
45-59	2	10.0	13	59.9	52.3	7.0	0	0.1	0	0
60+	2	12.0	12	90.6	69.7	5.0	0	0.1	0	0
All ages	8	3.3	54	21.0	43.4	7.9	0	0.0	0	0
Females										
0-4	0	0.0	0	0.0	-	-	0	0.0	0	0
5-14	1	1.5	3	5.3	10.0	8.3	0	0.0	0	0
15-44	17	16.3	109	102.1	29.8	8.1	0	0.0	0	0
45-59	16	69.7	83	373.3	52.3	7.3	0	0.1	0	0
60+	12	75.6	90	588.2	70.4	5.2	0	0.0	0	0
All ages	46	18.5	286	116.1	47.2	7.1	0	0.0	0	0
Total	54	10.7	340	67.6	46.6	7.5	0	0.0	0	0

Table 194i World - Mundo - Monde — Rheumatoid arthritis - Cases

Age group (years)	Incidence 1990 Number ('000s)	Rate (per 100 000)	Prevalence 1990 Number ('000s)	Rate (per 100 000)	Avg. age at onset (years)	Average duration (years)	Deaths 1990 Number ('000s)	Rate (per 100 000)	Deaths 2000 (Projected) Number ('000s)	Rate (per 100 000)
Males										
0-4	0	0.0	0	0.0	-	-	0	0.0	0	0.0
5-14	0	0.0	0	0.0	-	-	0	0.0	0	0.0
15-44	166	13.3	1 014	81.1	29.8	8.1	0	0.0	0	0.0
45-59	219	70.1	1 150	368.1	52.3	7.2	1	0.2	1	0.1
60+	261	119.2	1 799	821.9	70.3	5.1	4	1.9	4	1.6
All ages	646	24.4	3 963	149.3	53.8	6.6	5	0.2	5	0.2
Females										
0-4	0	0.0	0	0.0	-	-	0	0.0	0	0.0
5-14	13	2.6	47	9.0	10.0	8.3	0	0.0	0	0.0
15-44	595	49.7	3 698	308.5	29.9	8.2	0	0.0	0	0.0
45-59	469	150.9	2 786	895.6	52.4	7.5	2	0.5	1	0.4
60+	733	272.4	5 155	1 915.0	71.4	5.5	9	3.3	10	3.1
All ages	1 812	69.3	11 686	447.1	52.3	6.8	11	0.4	12	0.4
Total	2 458	46.7	15 649	297.1	52.7	6.8	16	0.3	18	0.3

For epidemiological sources see Symmons 1996. For the methods used to estimate and project incidence, prevalence, and deaths see Murray and Lopez 1996a. See explanatory notes for definitions and caveats.

Table 195	Cuadro 195	Tableau 195
Osteoarthritis	Osteoartritis	Ostéoarthrite
Hip	Cadera	Hanche

Table 195a   EME - PEMC - EMBE   Osteoarthritis - Hip

Age group (years)	Incidence 1990 Number ('000s)	Rate (per 100 000)	Prevalence 1990 Number ('000s)	Rate (per 100 000)	Avg. age at onset (years)	Average duration (years)	Deaths 1990 Number ('000s)	Rate (per 100 000)	Deaths 2000 (Projected) Number ('000s)	Rate (per 100 000)
Males										
0-4	0	0.0	0	0	-	-	0	0	0	0
5-14	0	0.0	0	0	-	-	0	0	0	0
15-44	25	13.5	370	201	29.9	44.8	0	0	0	0
45-59	151	228.1	1 390	2 101	52.3	24.5	0	0	0	0
60+	43	71.5	2 766	4 621	71.0	11.3	0	0	0	0
All ages	218	56.1	4 526	1 161	53.4	24.2	0	0	0	0
Females										
0-4	0	0.0	0	0	-	-	0	0	0	0
5-14	0	0.0	0	0	-	-	0	0	0	0
15-44	11	6.0	161	90	30.0	50.0	0	0	0	0
45-59	120	177.3	1 022	1 508	52.4	28.8	0	0	0	0
60+	8	9.7	2 441	2 960	72.4	12.7	0	0	0	0
All ages	139	34.3	3 625	895	51.8	29.5	0	0	0	0
Total	357	45.0	8 151	1 025	52.8	26.3	0	0	0	0

Table 195b   FSE - PEAS - AESE   Osteoarthritis - Hip

Age group (years)	Incidence 1990 Number ('000s)	Rate (per 100 000)	Prevalence 1990 Number ('000s)	Rate (per 100 000)	Avg. age at onset (years)	Average duration (years)	Deaths 1990 Number ('000s)	Rate (per 100 000)	Deaths 2000 (Projected) Number ('000s)	Rate (per 100 000)
Males										
0-4	0	0	0	0	-	-	0	0	0	0
5-14	0	0	0	0	-	-	0	0	0	0
15-44	21	27	305	400	29.7	39.2	0	0	0	0
45-59	7	25	267	991	52.2	20.8	0	0	0	0
60+	32	154	569	2 726	69.9	10.1	0	0	0	0
All ages	59	36	1 141	691	53.9	21.4	0	0	0	0
Females										
0-4	0	0	0	0	-	-	0	0	0	0
5-14	0	0	0	0	-	-	0	0	0	0
15-44	10	13	150	200	29.9	46.8	0	0	0	0
45-59	24	81	300	1 000	52.4	26.1	0	0	0	0
60+	28	79	906	2 529	71.5	11.8	0	0	0	0
All ages	63	35	1 356	752	57.5	22.9	0	0	0	0
Total	122	35	2 497	723	55.8	22.2	0	0	0	0

Table 195c   India - India - Inde   Osteoarthritis - Hip

Age group (years)	Incidence 1990 Number ('000s)	Rate (per 100 000)	Prevalence 1990 Number ('000s)	Rate (per 100 000)	Avg. age at onset (years)	Average duration (years)	Deaths 1990 Number ('000s)	Rate (per 100 000)	Deaths 2000 (Projected) Number ('000s)	Rate (per 100 000)
Males										
0-4	0	0.0	0	0	-	-	0	0	0	0
5-14	0	0.0	0	0	-	-	0	0	0	0
15-44	0	0.0	0	0	-	-	0	0	0	0
45-59	32	67.8	236	497	52.3	21.0	0	0	0	0
60+	51	170.3	793	2 672	69.6	9.8	0	0	0	0
All ages	83	18.8	1 029	234	62.9	14.2	0	0	0	0
Females										
0-4	0	0.0	0	0	-	-	0	0	0	0
5-14	0	0.0	0	0	-	-	0	0	0	0
15-44	0	0.0	0	0	-	-	0	0	0	0
45-59	0	0.0	0	0	-	-	0	0	0	0
60+	35	122.2	356	1 236	70.0	10.2	0	0	0	0
All ages	35	8.6	356	87	70.0	10.2	0	0	0	0
Total	118	13.9	1 386	163	65.0	13.0	0	0	0	0

For epidemiological sources see Symmons 1996. For the methods used to estimate and project incidence, prevalence, and deaths see Murray and Lopez 1996a. See explanatory notes for definitions and caveats.

Table 195
Osteoarthritis

Cuadro 195
Osteoartritis

Tableau 195
Ostéoarthrite

Hip   Cadera   Hanche

Table 195d   China - China - Chine   Osteoarthritis - Hip

Age group (years)	Incidence 1990 Number ('000s)	Rate (per 100 000)	Prevalence 1990 Number ('000s)	Rate (per 100 000)	Avg. age at onset (years)	Average duration (years)	Deaths 1990 Number ('000s)	Rate (per 100 000)	Deaths 2000 (Projected) Number ('000s)	Rate (per 100 000)
Males										
0-4	0	0	0	0	-	-	0	0	0	0
5-14	0	0	0	0	-	-	0	0	0	0
15-44	0	0	0	0	-	-	0	0	0	0
45-59	49	68	364	501	52.2	20.3	0	0	0	0
60+	85	175	1 339	2 741	69.5	9.7	0	0	0	0
All ages	135	23	1 703	291	63.2	13.6	0	0	0	0
Females										
0-4	0	0	0	0	-	-	0	0	0	0
5-14	0	0	0	0	-	-	0	0	0	0
15-44	0	0	0	0	-	-	0	0	0	0
45-59	0	0	0	0	-	-	0	0	0	0
60+	63	124	677	1 320	70.3	10.5	0	0	0	0
All ages	63	12	677	123	70.3	10.5	0	0	0	0
Total	198	17	2 380	210	65.4	12.6	0	0	0	0

Table 195e   OAI - OPAI - APAI   Osteoarthritis - Hip

Age group (years)	Incidence 1990 Number ('000s)	Rate (per 100 000)	Prevalence 1990 Number ('000s)	Rate (per 100 000)	Avg. age at onset (years)	Average duration (years)	Deaths 1990 Number ('000s)	Rate (per 100 000)	Deaths 2000 (Projected) Number ('000s)	Rate (per 100 000)
Males										
0-4	0	0.0	0	0	-	-	0	0	0	0
5-14	0	0.0	0	0	-	-	0	0	0	0
15-44	0	0.0	0	0	-	-	0	0	0	0
45-59	23	68.4	170	498	52.2	20.3	0	0	0	0
60+	34	166.8	531	2 637	69.5	9.7	0	0	0	0
All ages	57	16.6	701	204	62.4	14.1	0	0	0	0
Females										
0-4	0	0.0	0	0	-	-	0	0	0	0
5-14	0	0.0	0	0	-	-	0	0	0	0
15-44	0	0.0	0	0	-	-	0	0	0	0
45-59	0	0.0	0	0	-	-	0	0	0	0
60+	27	121.2	283	1 257	70.3	10.5	0	0	0	0
All ages	27	8.0	283	83	70.3	10.5	0	0	0	0
Total	84	12.3	983	144	65.0	12.9	0	0	0	0

Table 195f   SSA - ASS - ASS   Osteoarthritis - Hip

Age group (years)	Incidence 1990 Number ('000s)	Rate (per 100 000)	Prevalence 1990 Number ('000s)	Rate (per 100 000)	Avg. age at onset (years)	Average duration (years)	Deaths 1990 Number ('000s)	Rate (per 100 000)	Deaths 2000 (Projected) Number ('000s)	Rate (per 100 000)
Males										
0-4	0	0	0	0	-	-	0	0	0	0
5-14	0	0	0	0	-	-	0	0	0	0
15-44	0	0	0	0	-	-	0	0	0	0
45-59	0	0	0	0	-	-	0	0	0	0
60+	30	284	278	2 648	69.1	9.4	0	0	0	0
All ages	30	12	278	110	69.1	9.4	0	0	0	0
Females										
0-4	0	0	0	0	-	-	0	0	0	0
5-14	0	0	0	0	-	-	0	0	0	0
15-44	0	0	0	0	-	-	0	0	0	0
45-59	30	137	220	997	52.2	20.5	0	0	0	0
60+	12	96	378	2 986	69.7	9.8	0	0	0	0
All ages	42	16	599	232	57.2	17.5	0	0	0	0
Total	72	14	876	172	62.1	14.1	0	0	0	0

For epidemiological sources see Symmons 1996. For the methods used to estimate and project incidence, prevalence, and deaths see Murray and Lopez 1996a. See explanatory notes for definitions and caveats.

Table 195	Cuadro 195	Tableau 195
Osteoarthritis	Osteoartritis	Ostéoarthrite
Hip	Cadera	Hanche

Table 195g   LAC - ALC - ALC   Osteoarthritis - Hip

Age group (years)	Incidence 1990		Prevalence 1990		Avg. age at onset (years)	Average duration (years)	Deaths 1990		Deaths 2000 (Projected)	
	Number ('000s)	Rate (per 100 000)	Number ('000s)	Rate (per 100 000)			Number ('000s)	Rate (per 100 000)	Number ('000s)	Rate (per 100 000)
Males										
0-4	0	0	0	0	-	-	0	0	0	0
5-14	0	0	0	0	-	-	0	0	0	0
15-44	49	47	732	702	29.8	41.5	0	0	0	0
45-59	166	747	1 559	7 006	52.2	22.5	0	0	0	0
60+	91	648	2 743	19 441	69.9	10.7	0	0	0	0
All ages	307	139	5 033	2 272	53.9	22.0	0	0	0	0
Females										
0-4	0	0	0	0	-	-	0	0	0	0
5-14	0	0	0	0	-	-	0	0	0	0
15-44	35	34	521	500	29.8	44.6	0	0	0	0
45-59	125	533	1 170	5 009	52.3	24.9	0	0	0	0
60+	80	481	2 397	14 434	70.8	11.5	0	0	0	0
All ages	239	108	4 088	1 838	55.2	23.3	0	0	0	0
Total	546	123	9 121	2 055	54.4	22.6	0	U	0	0

Table 195h   MEC - AOM - CMO   Osteoarthritis - Hip

Age group (years)	Incidence 1990		Prevalence 1990		Avg. age at onset (years)	Average duration (years)	Deaths 1990		Deaths 2000 (Projected)	
	Number ('000s)	Rate (per 100 000)	Number ('000s)	Rate (per 100 000)			Number ('000s)	Rate (per 100 000)	Number ('000s)	Rate (per 100 000)
Males										
0-4	0	0.0	0	0	-	-	0	0	0	0
5-14	0	0.0	0	0	-	-	0	0	0	0
15-44	0	0.0	0	0	-	-	0	0	0	0
45-59	15	67.8	111	496	52.3	20.8	0	0	0	0
60+	23	170.3	365	2 686	69.7	9.9	0	0	0	0
All ages	38	14.9	476	186	62.8	14.2	0	0	0	0
Females										
0-4	0	0.0	0	0	-	-	0	0	0	0
5-14	0	0.0	0	0	-	-	0	0	0	0
15-44	0	0.0	0	0	-	-	0	0	0	0
45-59	0	0.0	0	0	-	-	0	0	0	0
60+	19	122.1	197	1 281	70.4	10.6	0	0	0	0
All ages	19	7.6	197	80	70.4	10.6	0	0	0	0
Total	57	11.3	672	134	65.3	13.0	0	0	0	0

Table 195i   World - Mundo - Monde   Osteoarthritis - Hip

Age group (years)	Incidence 1990		Prevalence 1990		Avg. age at onset (years)	Average duration (years)	Deaths 1990		Deaths 2000 (Projected)	
	Number ('000s)	Rate (per 100 000)	Number ('000s)	Rate (per 100 000)			Number ('000s)	Rate (per 100 000)	Number ('000s)	Rate (per 100 000)
Males										
0-4	0	0.0	0	0	-	-	0	0	0	0
5-14	0	0.0	0	0	-	-	0	0	0	0
15-44	95	7.6	1 407	113	29.8	41.8	0	0	0	0
45-59	444	142.1	4 097	1 312	52.2	22.6	0	0	0	0
60+	389	177.6	9 383	4 287	69.8	10.1	0	0	0	0
All ages	927	34.9	14 887	561	57.3	19.4	0	0	0	0
Females										
0-4	0	0.0	0	0	-	-	0	0	0	0
5-14	0	0.0	0	0	-	-	0	0	0	0
15-44	56	4.6	832	69	29.9	46.1	0	0	0	0
45-59	299	96.2	2 713	872	52.3	26.1	0	0	0	0
60+	273	101.4	7 635	2 836	70.6	10.9	0	0	0	0
All ages	628	24.0	11 180	428	58.3	21.3	0	0	0	0
Total	1 555	29.5	26 066	495	57.7	20.1	0	0	0	0

For epidemiological sources see Symmons 1996. For the methods used to estimate and project incidence, prevalence, and deaths see Murray and Lopez 1996a. See explanatory notes for definitions and caveats.

Table 196   **Cuadro 196**   **Tableau 196**
Osteoarthritis   **Osteoartritis**   **Ostéoarthrite**

Knee   Rodilla   Genou

Table 196a   **EME - PEMC - EMBE**   Osteoarthritis - Knee

Age group (years)	Incidence 1990 Number ('000s)	Rate (per 100 000)	Prevalence 1990 Number ('000s)	Rate (per 100 000)	Avg. age at onset (years)	Average duration (years)	Deaths 1990 Number ('000s)	Rate (per 100 000)	Deaths 2000 (Projected) Number ('000s)	Rate (per 100 000)
Males										
0-4	0	0	0	0	-	-	0	0	0	0
5-14	0	0	0	0	-	-	0	0	0	0
15-44	70	38	1 044	567	29.9	44.8	0	0	0	0
45-59	183	277	2 117	3 200	52.3	24.5	0	0	0	0
60+	168	280	5 045	8 427	70.9	11.4	0	0	0	0
All ages	421	108	8 205	2 105	56.0	22.6	0	0	0	0
Females										
0-4	0	0	0	0	-	-	0	0	0	0
5-14	0	0	0	0	-	-	0	0	0	0
15-44	96	53	1 435	801	29.9	50.0	0	0	0	0
45-59	345	509	3 695	5 450	52.3	28.9	0	0	0	0
60+	566	686	14 847	18 003	71.9	13.1	0	0	0	0
All ages	1 007	248	19 977	4 930	61.2	22.0	0	0	0	0
Total	1 428	180	28 182	3 545	59.7	22.2	0	0	0	0

Table 196b   **FSE - PEAS - AESE**   Osteoarthritis - Knee

Age group (years)	Incidence 1990 Number ('000s)	Rate (per 100 000)	Prevalence 1990 Number ('000s)	Rate (per 100 000)	Avg. age at onset (years)	Average duration (years)	Deaths 1990 Number ('000s)	Rate (per 100 000)	Deaths 2000 (Projected) Number ('000s)	Rate (per 100 000)
Males										
0-4	0	0	0	0	-	-	0	0	0	0
5-14	0	0	0	0	-	-	0	0	0	0
15-44	133	175	1 989	2 608	29.6	39.3	0	0	0	0
45-59	120	446	2 294	8 505	52.1	20.9	0	0	0	0
60+	94	451	3 358	16 090	69.7	10.2	0	0	0	0
All ages	348	210	7 641	4 625	48.2	25.1	0	0	0	0
Females										
0-4	0	0	0	0	-	-	0	0	0	0
5-14	0	0	0	0	-	-	0	0	0	0
15-44	105	140	1 575	2 101	29.8	46.9	0	0	0	0
45-59	246	820	3 122	10 404	52.2	26.2	0	0	0	0
60+	294	820	9 413	26 289	70.9	12.2	0	0	0	0
All ages	644	357	14 109	7 824	57.1	23.2	0	0	0	0
Total	992	287	21 751	6 294	54.0	23.8	0	0	0	0

Table 196c   **India - India - Inde**   Osteoarthritis - Knee

Age group (years)	Incidence 1990 Number ('000s)	Rate (per 100 000)	Prevalence 1990 Number ('000s)	Rate (per 100 000)	Avg. age at onset (years)	Average duration (years)	Deaths 1990 Number ('000s)	Rate (per 100 000)	Deaths 2000 (Projected) Number ('000s)	Rate (per 100 000)
Males										
0-4	0	0	0	0	-	-	0	0	0	0
5-14	0	0	0	0	-	-	0	0	0	0
15-44	51	26	757	378	29.7	39.9	0	0	0	0
45-59	89	187	1 019	2 143	52.3	21.0	0	0	0	0
60+	60	201	1 643	5 535	69.6	9.8	0	0	0	0
All ages	200	46	3 419	778	51.7	22.5	0	0	0	0
Females										
0-4	0	0	0	0	-	-	0	0	0	0
5-14	0	0	0	0	-	-	0	0	0	0
15-44	66	36	971	530	29.7	41.7	0	0	0	0
45-59	159	346	1 678	3 647	52.3	22.5	0	0	0	0
60+	163	564	3 473	12 047	69.8	10.3	0	0	0	0
All ages	387	94	6 121	1 493	55.8	20.7	0	0	0	0
Total	587	69	9 541	1 123	54.4	21.3	0	0	0	0

For epidemiological sources see Symmons 1996. For the methods used to estimate and project incidence, prevalence, and deaths see Murray and Lopez 1996a. See explanatory notes for definitions and caveats.

Table 196	Cuadro 196	Tableau 196
Osteoarthritis	Osteoartritis	Ostéoarthrite
Knee	Rodilla	Genou

Table 196d — China - China - Chine — Osteoarthritis - Knee

Age group (years)	Incidence 1990 Number ('000s)	Rate (per 100 000)	Prevalence 1990 Number ('000s)	Rate (per 100 000)	Avg. age at onset (years)	Average duration (years)	Deaths 1990 Number ('000s)	Rate (per 100 000)	Deaths 2000 (Projected) Number ('000s)	Rate (per 100 000)
Males										
0-4	0	0	0	0	-	-	0	0	0	0
5-14	0	0	0	0	-	-	0	0	0	0
15-44	45	15	675	220	29.9	41.2	0	0	0	0
45-59	104	143	1 091	1 502	52.3	21.4	0	0	0	0
60+	314	643	4 397	9 001	69.4	10.0	0	0	0	0
All ages	464	79	6 163	1 053	61.7	15.6	0	0	0	0
Females										
0-4	0	0	0	0	-	-	0	0	0	0
5-14	0	0	0	0	-	-	0	0	0	0
15-44	135	48	2 023	712	29.9	44.2	0	0	0	0
45-59	307	477	3 223	5 005	52.3	23.9	0	0	0	0
60+	350	682	8 208	16 004	70.2	11.0	0	0	0	0
All ages	792	145	13 454	2 455	56.4	21.7	0	0	0	0
Total	1 256	111	19 617	1 731	58.3	19.4	0	0	0	0

Table 196e — OAI - OPAI - APAI — Osteoarthritis - Knee

Age group (years)	Incidence 1990 Number ('000s)	Rate (per 100 000)	Prevalence 1990 Number ('000s)	Rate (per 100 000)	Avg. age at onset (years)	Average duration (years)	Deaths 1990 Number ('000s)	Rate (per 100 000)	Deaths 2000 (Projected) Number ('000s)	Rate (per 100 000)
Males										
0-4	0	0	0	0	-	-	0	0	0	0
5-14	0	0	0	0	-	-	0	0	0	0
15-44	57	35	837	520	29.7	38.8	0	0	0	0
45-59	196	575	1 810	5 302	52.1	20.4	0	0	0	0
60+	121	600	3 127	15 544	69.3	9.9	0	0	0	0
All ages	374	109	5 773	1 684	54.3	19.8	0	0	0	0
Females										
0-4	0	0	0	0	-	-	0	0	0	0
5-14	0	0	0	0	-	-	0	0	0	0
15-44	77	48	1 135	711	29.7	41.5	0	0	0	0
45-59	247	704	2 353	6 705	52.2	22.5	0	0	0	0
60+	114	506	3 887	17 300	70.0	10.6	0	0	0	0
All ages	437	129	7 375	2 173	52.9	22.7	0	0	0	0
Total	811	119	13 149	1 927	53.5	21.4	0	0	0	0

Table 196f — SSA - ASS - ASS — Osteoarthritis - Knee

Age group (years)	Incidence 1990 Number ('000s)	Rate (per 100 000)	Prevalence 1990 Number ('000s)	Rate (per 100 000)	Avg. age at onset (years)	Average duration (years)	Deaths 1990 Number ('000s)	Rate (per 100 000)	Deaths 2000 (Projected) Number ('000s)	Rate (per 100 000)
Males										
0-4	0	0	0	0	-	-	0	0	0	0
5-14	0	0	0	0	-	-	0	0	0	0
15-44	41	39	588	567	29.4	35.0	0	0	0	0
45-59	57	280	650	3 201	52.1	19.1	0	0	0	0
60+	33	314	870	8 303	69.1	9.4	0	0	0	0
All ages	131	52	2 109	836	49.3	21.6	0	0	0	0
Females										
0-4	0	0	0	0	-	-	0	0	0	0
5-14	0	0	0	0	-	-	0	0	0	0
15-44	59	55	852	802	29.4	37.2	0	0	0	0
45-59	114	516	1 206	5 451	52.1	20.6	0	0	0	0
60+	109	864	2 282	18 001	69.2	10.0	0	0	0	0
All ages	282	109	4 339	1 683	54.0	20.0	0	0	0	0
Total	413	81	6 448	1 264	52.5	20.5	0	0	0	0

For epidemiological sources see Symmons 1996. For the methods used to estimate and project incidence, prevalence, and deaths see Murray and Lopez 1996a. See explanatory notes for definitions and caveats.

Table 196 — Cuadro 196 — Tableau 196
Osteoarthritis — Osteoartritis — Ostéoarthrite

Knee — Rodilla — Genou

Table 196g   LAC - ALC - ALC   Osteoarthritis - Knee

Age group (years)	Incidence 1990 Number ('000s)	Rate (per 100 000)	Prevalence 1990 Number ('000s)	Rate (per 100 000)	Avg. age at onset (years)	Average duration (years)	Deaths 1990 Number ('000s)	Rate (per 100 000)	Deaths 2000 (Projected) Number ('000s)	Rate (per 100 000)
Males										
0-4	0	0	0	0	-	-	0	0	0	0
5-14	0	0	0	0	-	-	0	0	0	0
15-44	60	57	889	852	29.8	41.5	0	0	0	0
45-59	92	416	1 069	4 803	52.2	22.4	0	0	0	0
60+	61	430	1 757	12 454	70.1	10.6	0	0	0	0
All ages	213	96	3 714	1 677	51.0	24.4	0	0	0	0
Females										
0-4	0	0	0	0	-	-	0	0	0	0
5-14	0	0	0	0	-	-	0	0	0	0
15-44	66	64	990	951	29.8	44.6	0	0	0	0
45-59	188	807	1 871	8 010	52.2	24.9	0	0	0	0
60+	182	1 096	4 435	26 705	70.3	11.8	0	0	0	0
All ages	437	196	7 296	3 279	56.3	22.4	0	0	0	0
Total	650	146	11 010	2 480	54.6	23.1	0	0	0	0

Table 196h   MEC - AOM - CMO   Osteoarthritis - Knee

Age group (years)	Incidence 1990 Number ('000s)	Rate (per 100 000)	Prevalence 1990 Number ('000s)	Rate (per 100 000)	Avg. age at onset (years)	Average duration (years)	Deaths 1990 Number ('000s)	Rate (per 100 000)	Deaths 2000 (Projected) Number ('000s)	Rate (per 100 000)
Males										
0-4	0	0	0	0	-	-	0	0	0	0
5-14	0	0	0	0	-	-	0	0	0	0
15-44	29	25	430	378	29.8	40.0	0	0	0	0
45-59	42	186	476	2 130	52.3	20.8	0	0	0	0
60+	27	201	752	5 534	69.6	9.9	0	0	0	0
All ages	98	38	1 658	647	50.5	23.4	0	0	0	0
Females										
0-4	0	0	0	0	-	-	0	0	0	0
5-14	0	0	0	0	-	-	0	0	0	0
15-44	38	36	568	530	29.8	42.6	0	0	0	0
45-59	77	345	810	3 633	52.3	23.0	0	0	0	0
60+	83	542	1 842	12 003	70.1	10.7	0	0	0	0
All ages	198	80	3 220	1 306	55.4	21.6	0	0	0	0
Total	296	59	4 878	970	53.8	22.2	0	0	0	0

Table 196i   World - Mundo - Monde   Osteoarthritis - Knee

Age group (years)	Incidence 1990 Number ('000s)	Rate (per 100 000)	Prevalence 1990 Number ('000s)	Rate (per 100 000)	Avg. age at onset (years)	Average duration (years)	Deaths 1990 Number ('000s)	Rate (per 100 000)	Deaths 2000 (Projected) Number ('000s)	Rate (per 100 000)
Males										
0-4	0	0	0	0	-	-	0	0	0	0
5-14	0	0	0	0	-	-	0	0	0	0
15-44	486	39	7 209	577	29.7	40.2	0	0	0	0
45-59	884	283	10 526	3 370	52.2	21.6	0	0	0	0
60+	877	401	20 948	9 572	69.8	10.3	0	0	0	0
All ages	2 247	85	38 684	1 458	54.2	21.2	0	0	0	0
Females										
0-4	0	0	0	0	-	-	0	0	0	0
5-14	0	0	0	0	-	-	0	0	0	0
15-44	641	53	9 548	797	29.8	44.2	0	0	0	0
45-59	1 685	542	17 957	5 773	52.2	24.8	0	0	0	0
60+	1 860	691	48 387	17 973	70.7	11.8	0	0	0	0
All ages	4 185	160	75 892	2 904	57.0	22.0	0	0	0	0
Total	6 433	122	114 576	2 175	56.0	21.7	0	0	0	0

For epidemiological sources see Symmons 1996. For the methods used to estimate and project incidence, prevalence, and deaths see Murray and Lopez 1996a. See explanatory notes for definitions and caveats.

Table 197
Abdominal wall defect
Cases

Cuadro 197
Defecto de la pared abdominal
Casos

Tableau 197
Anomalie de la paroi abdominale
Cas

Table 197a EME - PEMC - EMBE Abdominal wall defect - Cases

Age group (years)	Incidence 1990 Number ('000s)	Rate (per 100 000)	Prevalence 1990 Number ('000s)	Rate (per 100 000)	Avg. age at onset (years)	Average duration (years)	Deaths 1990 Number ('000s)	Rate (per 100 000)	Deaths 2000 (Projected) Number ('000s)	Rate (per 100 000)
Males										
0-4	1	2.0	0	0.0	0.0	0.01	0	0.6	0	0.7
5-14	0	0.0	0	0.0	-	-	0	0.0	0	0.0
15-44	0	0.0	0	0.0	-	-	0	0.0	0	0.0
45-59	0	0.0	0	0.0	-	-	0	0.0	0	0.0
60+	0	0.0	0	0.0	-	-	0	0.0	0	0.0
All ages	1	0.1	0	0.0	0.0	0.01	0	0.0	0	0.0
Females										
0-4	1	4.0	0	0.0	0.0	0.01	0	1.2	0	1.2
5-14	0	0.0	0	0.0	-	-	0	0.0	0	0.0
15-44	0	0.0	0	0.0	-	-	0	0.0	0	0.0
45-59	0	0.0	0	0.0	-	-	0	0.0	0	0.0
60+	0	0.0	0	0.0	-	-	0	0.0	0	0.0
All ages	1	0.2	0	0.0	0.0	0.01	0	0.1	0	0.1
Total	2	0.2	0	0.0	0.0	0.01	0	0.1	1	0.1

Table 197b FSE - PEAS - AESE Abdominal wall defect - Cases

Age group (years)	Incidence 1990 Number ('000s)	Rate (per 100 000)	Prevalence 1990 Number ('000s)	Rate (per 100 000)	Avg. age at onset (years)	Average duration (years)	Deaths 1990 Number ('000s)	Rate (per 100 000)	Deaths 2000 (Projected) Number ('000s)	Rate (per 100 000)
Males										
0-4	0	2.0	0	0.0	0.0	0.01	0	0.6	0	1.0
5-14	0	0.0	0	0.0	-	-	0	0.0	0	0.0
15-44	0	0.0	0	0.0	-	-	0	0.0	0	0.0
45-59	0	0.0	0	0.0	-	-	0	0.0	0	0.0
60+	0	0.0	0	0.0	-	-	0	0.0	0	0.0
All ages	0	0.2	0	0.0	0.0	0.01	0	0.0	0	0.1
Females										
0-4	1	4.5	0	0.0	0.0	0.01	0	1.3	0	1.9
5-14	0	0.0	0	0.0	-	-	0	0.0	0	0.0
15-44	0	0.0	0	0.0	-	-	0	0.0	0	0.0
45-59	0	0.0	0	0.0	-	-	0	0.0	0	0.0
60+	0	0.0	0	0.0	-	-	0	0.0	0	0.0
All ages	1	0.3	0	0.0	0.0	0.01	0	0.1	0	0.1
Total	1	0.2	0	0.0	0.0	0.01	0	0.1	0	0.1

Table 197c India - India - Inde Abdominal wall defect - Cases

Age group (years)	Incidence 1990 Number ('000s)	Rate (per 100 000)	Prevalence 1990 Number ('000s)	Rate (per 100 000)	Avg. age at onset (years)	Average duration (years)	Deaths 1990 Number ('000s)	Rate (per 100 000)	Deaths 2000 (Projected) Number ('000s)	Rate (per 100 000)
Males										
0-4	1	1.3	0	0.0	0.0	0.01	1	1.2	1	1.5
5-14	0	0.0	0	0.0	-	-	0	0.0	0	0.0
15-44	0	0.0	0	0.0	-	-	0	0.0	0	0.0
45-59	0	0.0	0	0.0	-	-	0	0.0	0	0.0
60+	0	0.0	0	0.0	-	-	0	0.0	0	0.0
All ages	1	0.2	0	0.0	0.0	0.01	1	0.2	1	0.2
Females										
0-4	1	1.1	0	0.0	0.0	0.01	1	1.0	1	1.3
5-14	0	0.0	0	0.0	-	-	0	0.0	0	0.0
15-44	0	0.0	0	0.0	-	-	0	0.0	0	0.0
45-59	0	0.0	0	0.0	-	-	0	0.0	0	0.0
60+	0	0.0	0	0.0	-	-	0	0.0	0	0.0
All ages	1	0.2	0	0.0	0.0	0.01	1	0.1	1	0.1
Total	1	0.2	0	0.0	0.0	0.01	1	0.1	2	0.2

For epidemiological sources see Shibuya and Murray 1996c. For the methods used to estimate and project incidence, prevalence, and deaths see Murray and Lopez 1996a. See explanatory notes for definitions and caveats.

Table 197	Cuadro 197	Tableau 197
Abdominal wall defect	**Defecto de la pared abdominal**	**Anomalie de la paroi abdominale**
Cases	Casos	Cas

Table 197d   China - China - Chine   Abdominal wall defect - Cases

Age group (years)	Incidence 1990 Number ('000s)	Rate (per 100 000)	Prevalence 1990 Number ('000s)	Rate (per 100 000)	Avg. age at onset (years)	Average duration (years)	Deaths 1990 Number ('000s)	Rate (per 100 000)	Deaths 2000 (Projected) Number ('000s)	Rate (per 100 000)
Males										
0-4	1	1.6	0	0.0	0.0	0.01	0	0.6	0	0.7
5-14	0	0.0	0	0.0	-	-	0	0.0	0	0.0
15-44	0	0.0	0	0.0	-	-	0	0.0	0	0.0
45-59	0	0.0	0	0.0	-	-	0	0.0	0	0.0
60+	0	0.0	0	0.0	-	-	0	0.0	0	0.0
All ages	1	0.2	0	0.0	0.0	0.01	0	0.1	0	0.1
Females										
0-4	1	1.3	0	0.0	0.0	0.01	0	0.5	0	0.6
5-14	0	0.0	0	0.0	-	-	0	0.0	0	0.0
15-44	0	0.0	0	0.0	-	-	0	0.0	0	0.0
45-59	0	0.0	0	0.0	-	-	0	0.0	0	0.0
60+	0	0.0	0	0.0	-	-	0	0.0	0	0.0
All ages	1	0.1	0	0.0	0.0	0.01	0	0.1	0	0.1
Total	2	0.1	0	0.0	0.0	0.01	1	0.1	1	0.1

Table 197e   OAI - OPAI - APAI   Abdominal wall defect - Cases

Age group (years)	Incidence 1990 Number ('000s)	Rate (per 100 000)	Prevalence 1990 Number ('000s)	Rate (per 100 000)	Avg. age at onset (years)	Average duration (years)	Deaths 1990 Number ('000s)	Rate (per 100 000)	Deaths 2000 (Projected) Number ('000s)	Rate (per 100 000)
Males										
0-4	1	1.4	0	0.0	0.0	0.01	0	1.0	0	1.1
5-14	0	0.0	0	0.0	-	-	0	0.0	0	0.0
15-44	0	0.0	0	0.0	-	-	0	0.0	0	0.0
45-59	0	0.0	0	0.0	-	-	0	0.0	0	0.0
60+	0	0.0	0	0.0	-	-	0	0.0	0	0.0
All ages	1	0.2	0	0.0	0.0	0.01	0	0.1	0	0.1
Females										
0-4	0	0.9	0	0.0	0.0	0.01	0	0.7	0	0.7
5-14	0	0.0	0	0.0	-	-	0	0.0	0	0.0
15-44	0	0.0	0	0.0	-	-	0	0.0	0	0.0
45-59	0	0.0	0	0.0	-	-	0	0.0	0	0.0
60+	0	0.0	0	0.0	-	-	0	0.0	0	0.0
All ages	0	0.1	0	0.0	0.0	0.01	0	0.1	0	0.1
Total	1	0.1	0	0.0	0.0	0.01	1	0.1	1	0.1

Table 197f   SSA - ASS - ASS   Abdominal wall defect - Cases

Age group (years)	Incidence 1990 Number ('000s)	Rate (per 100 000)	Prevalence 1990 Number ('000s)	Rate (per 100 000)	Avg. age at onset (years)	Average duration (years)	Deaths 1990 Number ('000s)	Rate (per 100 000)	Deaths 2000 (Projected) Number ('000s)	Rate (per 100 000)
Males										
0-4	0	0.5	0	0.0	0.0	0.01	0	0.4	0	0.5
5-14	0	0.0	0	0.0	-	-	0	0.0	0	0.0
15-44	0	0.0	0	0.0	-	-	0	0.0	0	0.0
45-59	0	0.0	0	0.0	-	-	0	0.0	0	0.0
60+	0	0.0	0	0.0	-	-	0	0.0	0	0.0
All ages	0	0.1	0	0.0	0.0	0.01	0	0.1	0	0.1
Females										
0-4	0	0.5	0	0.0	0.0	0.01	0	0.4	0	0.5
5-14	0	0.0	0	0.0	-	-	0	0.0	0	0.0
15-44	0	0.0	0	0.0	-	-	0	0.0	0	0.0
45-59	0	0.0	0	0.0	-	-	0	0.0	0	0.0
60+	0	0.0	0	0.0	-	-	0	0.0	0	0.0
All ages	0	0.1	0	0.0	0.0	0.01	0	0.1	0	0.1
Total	0	0.1	0	0.0	0.0	0.01	0	0.1	1	0.1

For epidemiological sources see Shibuya and Murray 1996c. For the methods used to estimate and project incidence, prevalence, and deaths see Murray and Lopez 1996a. See explanatory notes for definitions and caveats.

Table 197	Cuadro 197	Tableau 197
Abdominal wall defect	Defecto de la pared abdominal	Anomalie de la paroi abdominale
Cases	Casos	Cas

Table 197g — LAC - ALC - ALC — Abdominal wall defect - Cases

Age group (years)	Incidence 1990 Number ('000s)	Rate (per 100 000)	Prevalence 1990 Number ('000s)	Rate (per 100 000)	Avg. age at onset (years)	Average duration (years)	Deaths 1990 Number ('000s)	Rate (per 100 000)	Deaths 2000 (Projected) Number ('000s)	Rate (per 100 000)
Males										
0-4	1	2.2	0	0.0	0.0	0.01	0	0.9	0	1.0
5-14	0	0.0	0	0.0	-	-	0	0.0	0	0.0
15-44	0	0.0	0	0.0	-	-	0	0.0	0	0.0
45-59	0	0.0	0	0.0	-	-	0	0.0	0	0.0
60+	0	0.0	0	0.0	-	-	0	0.0	0	0.0
All ages	1	0.3	0	0.0	0.0	0.01	0	0.1	0	0.1
Females										
0-4	1	2.3	0	0.0	0.0	0.01	0	0.9	0	1.0
5-14	0	0.0	0	0.0	-	-	0	0.0	0	0.0
15-44	0	0.0	0	0.0	-	-	0	0.0	0	0.0
45-59	0	0.0	0	0.0	-	-	0	0.0	0	0.0
60+	0	0.0	0	0.0	-	-	0	0.0	0	0.0
All ages	1	0.3	0	0.0	0.0	0.01	0	0.1	0	0.1
Total	1	0.3	0	0.0	0.0	0.01	1	0.1	1	0.1

Table 197h — MEC - AOM - CMO — Abdominal wall defect - Cases

Age group (years)	Incidence 1990 Number ('000s)	Rate (per 100 000)	Prevalence 1990 Number ('000s)	Rate (per 100 000)	Avg. age at onset (years)	Average duration (years)	Deaths 1990 Number ('000s)	Rate (per 100 000)	Deaths 2000 (Projected) Number ('000s)	Rate (per 100 000)
Males										
0-4	1	2.0	0	0.0	0.0	0.01	1	1.4	1	1.6
5-14	0	0.0	0	0.0	-	-	0	0.0	0	0.0
15-44	0	0.0	0	0.0	-	-	0	0.0	0	0.0
45-59	0	0.0	0	0.0	-	-	0	0.0	0	0.0
60+	0	0.0	0	0.0	-	-	0	0.0	0	0.0
All ages	1	0.3	0	0.0	0.0	0.01	1	0.2	1	0.2
Females										
0-4	0	1.1	0	0.0	0.0	0.01	0	0.8	0	0.9
5-14	0	0.0	0	0.0	-	-	0	0.0	0	0.0
15-44	0	0.0	0	0.0	-	-	0	0.0	0	0.0
45-59	0	0.0	0	0.0	-	-	0	0.0	0	0.0
60+	0	0.0	0	0.0	-	-	0	0.0	0	0.0
All ages	0	0.2	0	0.0	0.0	0.01	0	0.1	0	0.1
Total	1	0.3	0	0.0	0.0	0.01	1	0.2	1	0.2

Table 197i — World - Mundo - Monde — Abdominal wall defect - Cases

Age group (years)	Incidence 1990 Number ('000s)	Rate (per 100 000)	Prevalence 1990 Number ('000s)	Rate (per 100 000)	Avg. age at onset (years)	Average duration (years)	Deaths 1990 Number ('000s)	Rate (per 100 000)	Deaths 2000 (Projected) Number ('000s)	Rate (per 100 000)
Males										
0-4	5	1.5	0	0.0	0.0	0.01	3	0.9	3	1.0
5-14	0	0.0	0	0.0	-	-	0	0.0	0	0.0
15-44	0	0.0	0	0.0	-	-	0	0.0	0	0.0
45-59	0	0.0	0	0.0	-	-	0	0.0	0	0.0
60+	0	0.0	0	0.0	-	-	0	0.0	0	0.0
All ages	5	0.2	0	0.0	0.0	0.01	3	0.1	3	0.1
Females										
0-4	5	1.5	0	0.0	0.0	0.01	2	0.8	3	0.9
5-14	0	0.0	0	0.0	-	-	0	0.0	0	0.0
15-44	0	0.0	0	0.0	-	-	0	0.0	0	0.0
45-59	0	0.0	0	0.0	-	-	0	0.0	0	0.0
60+	0	0.0	0	0.0	-	-	0	0.0	0	0.0
All ages	5	0.2	0	0.0	0.0	0.01	2	0.1	3	0.1
Total	9	0.2	0	0.0	0.0	0.01	5	0.1	6	0.1

For epidemiological sources see Shibuya and Murray 1996c. For the methods used to estimate and project incidence, prevalence, and deaths see Murray and Lopez 1996a. See explanatory notes for definitions and caveats.

Table 198	Cuadro 198	Tableau 198
Anencephaly	Anencefalia	Anencéphalie

Cases   Casos   Cas

Table 198a — EME - PEMC - EMBE — Anencephaly - Cases

Age group (years)	Incidence 1990 Number ('000s)	Rate (per 100 000)	Prevalence 1990 Number ('000s)	Rate (per 100 000)	Avg. age at onset (years)	Average duration (years)	Deaths 1990 Number ('000s)	Rate (per 100 000)	Deaths 2000 (Projected) Number ('000s)	Rate (per 100 000)
Males										
0-4	1	4.0	0	0	0.0	0.01	1	4.0	1	4.8
5-14	0	0.0	0	0	-	-	0	0.0	0	0.0
15-44	0	0.0	0	0	-	-	0	0.0	0	0.0
45-59	0	0.0	0	0	-	-	0	0.0	0	0.0
60+	0	0.0	0	0	-	-	0	0.0	0	0.0
All ages	1	0.3	0	0	0.0	0.01	1	0.3	1	0.3
Females										
0-4	2	6.2	0	0	0.0	0.01	2	6.2	2	6.4
5-14	0	0.0	0	0	-	-	0	0.0	0	0.0
15-44	0	0.0	0	0	-	-	0	0.0	0	0.0
45-59	0	0.0	0	0	-	-	0	0.0	0	0.0
60+	0	0.0	0	0	-	-	0	0.0	0	0.0
All ages	2	0.4	0	0	0.0	0.01	2	0.4	2	0.4
Total	3	0.3	0	0	0.0	0.01	3	0.3	3	0.4

Table 198b — FSE - PEAS - AESE — Anencephaly - Cases

Age group (years)	Incidence 1990 Number ('000s)	Rate (per 100 000)	Prevalence 1990 Number ('000s)	Rate (per 100 000)	Avg. age at onset (years)	Average duration (years)	Deaths 1990 Number ('000s)	Rate (per 100 000)	Deaths 2000 (Projected) Number ('000s)	Rate (per 100 000)
Males										
0-4	0	2.2	0	0	0.0	0.01	0	2.2	0	3.5
5-14	0	0.0	0	0	-	-	0	0.0	0	0.0
15-44	0	0.0	0	0	-	-	0	0.0	0	0.0
45-59	0	0.0	0	0	-	-	0	0.0	0	0.0
60+	0	0.0	0	0	-	-	0	0.0	0	0.0
All ages	0	0.2	0	0	0.0	0.01	0	0.2	0	0.3
Females										
0-4	0	3.6	0	0	0.0	0.01	0	3.6	1	5.0
5-14	0	0.0	0	0	-	-	0	0.0	0	0.0
15-44	0	0.0	0	0	-	-	0	0.0	0	0.0
45-59	0	0.0	0	0	-	-	0	0.0	0	0.0
60+	0	0.0	0	0	-	-	0	0.0	0	0.0
All ages	0	0.3	0	0	0.0	0.01	0	0.3	1	0.3
Total	1	0.2	0	0	0.0	0.01	1	0.2	1	0.3

Table 198c — India - India - Inde — Anencephaly - Cases

Age group (years)	Incidence 1990 Number ('000s)	Rate (per 100 000)	Prevalence 1990 Number ('000s)	Rate (per 100 000)	Avg. age at onset (years)	Average duration (years)	Deaths 1990 Number ('000s)	Rate (per 100 000)	Deaths 2000 (Projected) Number ('000s)	Rate (per 100 000)
Males										
0-4	18	30.7	0	0	0.0	0.01	18	30.7	22	38.7
5-14	0	0.0	0	0	-	-	0	0.0	0	0.0
15-44	0	0.0	0	0	-	-	0	0.0	0	0.0
45-59	0	0.0	0	0	-	-	0	0.0	0	0.0
60+	0	0.0	0	0	-	-	0	0.0	0	0.0
All ages	18	4.2	0	0	0.0	0.01	18	4.2	22	4.3
Females										
0-4	28	48.7	0	0	0.0	0.01	28	48.7	33	61.0
5-14	0	0.0	0	0	-	-	0	0.0	0	0.0
15-44	0	0.0	0	0	-	-	0	0.0	0	0.0
45-59	0	0.0	0	0	-	-	0	0.0	0	0.0
60+	0	0.0	0	0	-	-	0	0.0	0	0.0
All ages	28	6.7	0	0	0.0	0.01	28	6.7	33	6.8
Total	46	5.4	0	0	0.0	0.01	46	5.4	55	5.5

For epidemiological sources see Shibuya and Murray 1996c. For the methods used to estimate and project incidence, prevalence, and deaths see Murray and Lopez 1996a. See explanatory notes for definitions and caveats.

Table 198
Anencephaly

Cuadro 198
Anencefalia

Tableau 198
Anencéphalie

Cases

Casos

Cas

Table 198d China - China - Chine   Anencephaly - Cases

Age group (years)	Incidence 1990 Number ('000s)	Rate (per 100 000)	Prevalence 1990 Number ('000s)	Rate (per 100 000)	Avg. age at onset (years)	Average duration (years)	Deaths 1990 Number ('000s)	Rate (per 100 000)	Deaths 2000 (Projected) Number ('000s)	Rate (per 100 000)
Males										
0-4	15	25.0	0	0	0.0	0.01	15	25.0	17	29.1
5-14	0	0.0	0	0	-	-	0	0.0	0	0.0
15-44	0	0.0	0	0	-	-	0	0.0	0	0.0
45-59	0	0.0	0	0	-	-	0	0.0	0	0.0
60+	0	0.0	0	0	-	-	0	0.0	0	0.0
All ages	15	2.6	0	0	0.0	0.01	15	2.6	17	2.6
Females										
0-4	24	41.3	0	0	0.0	0.01	24	41.3	26	47.4
5-14	0	0.0	0	0	-	-	0	0.0	0	0.0
15-44	0	0.0	0	0	-	-	0	0.0	0	0.0
45-59	0	0.0	0	0	-	-	0	0.0	0	0.0
60+	0	0.0	0	0	-	-	0	0.0	0	0.0
All ages	24	4.4	0	0	0.0	0.01	24	4.4	26	4.2
Total	39	3.4	0	0	0.0	0.01	39	3.4	44	3.4

Table 198e OAI - OPAI - APAI   Anencephaly - Cases

Age group (years)	Incidence 1990 Number ('000s)	Rate (per 100 000)	Prevalence 1990 Number ('000s)	Rate (per 100 000)	Avg. age at onset (years)	Average duration (years)	Deaths 1990 Number ('000s)	Rate (per 100 000)	Deaths 2000 (Projected) Number ('000s)	Rate (per 100 000)
Males										
0-4	8	17.4	0	0	0.0	0.01	8	17.4	9	19.3
5-14	0	0.0	0	0	-	-	0	0.0	0	0.0
15-44	0	0.0	0	0	-	-	0	0.0	0	0.0
45-59	0	0.0	0	0	-	-	0	0.0	0	0.0
60+	0	0.0	0	0	-	-	0	0.0	0	0.0
All ages	8	2.2	0	0	0.0	0.01	8	2.2	9	2.1
Females										
0-4	12	28.0	0	0	0.0	0.01	12	28.0	13	30.2
5-14	0	0.0	0	0	-	-	0	0.0	0	0.0
15-44	0	0.0	0	0	-	-	0	0.0	0	0.0
45-59	0	0.0	0	0	-	-	0	0.0	0	0.0
60+	0	0.0	0	0	-	-	0	0.0	0	0.0
All ages	12	3.5	0	0	0.0	0.01	12	3.5	13	3.2
Total	19	2.8	0	0	0.0	0.01	19	2.8	21	2.6

Table 198f SSA - ASS - ASS   Anencephaly - Cases

Age group (years)	Incidence 1990 Number ('000s)	Rate (per 100 000)	Prevalence 1990 Number ('000s)	Rate (per 100 000)	Avg. age at onset (years)	Average duration (years)	Deaths 1990 Number ('000s)	Rate (per 100 000)	Deaths 2000 (Projected) Number ('000s)	Rate (per 100 000)
Males										
0-4	5	9.6	0	0	0.0	0.01	5	9.6	7	11.0
5-14	0	0.0	0	0	-	-	0	0.0	0	0.0
15-44	0	0.0	0	0	-	-	0	0.0	0	0.0
45-59	0	0.0	0	0	-	-	0	0.0	0	0.0
60+	0	0.0	0	0	-	-	0	0.0	0	0.0
All ages	5	1.8	0	0	0.0	0.01	5	1.8	7	2.1
Females										
0-4	7	15.9	0	0	0.0	0.01	7	15.9	12	18.1
5-14	0	0.0	0	0	-	-	0	0.0	0	0.0
15-44	0	0.0	0	0	-	-	0	0.0	0	0.0
45-59	0	0.0	0	0	-	-	0	0.0	0	0.0
60+	0	0.0	0	0	-	-	0	0.0	0	0.0
All ages	7	2.9	0	0	0.0	0.01	7	2.9	12	3.3
Total	12	2.4	0	0	0.0	0.01	12	2.4	19	2.7

For epidemiological sources see Shibuya and Murray 1996c. For the methods used to estimate and project incidence, prevalence, and deaths see Murray and Lopez 1996a. See explanatory notes for definitions and caveats.

Table 198
Anencephaly

Cuadro 198
Anencefalia

Tableau 198
Anencéphalie

Cases

Casos

Cas

Table 198g LAC - ALC - ALC Anencephaly - Cases

Age group (years)	Incidence 1990 Number ('000s)	Rate (per 100 000)	Prevalence 1990 Number ('000s)	Rate (per 100 000)	Avg. age at onset (years)	Average duration (years)	Deaths 1990 Number ('000s)	Rate (per 100 000)	Deaths 2000 (Projected) Number ('000s)	Rate (per 100 000)
Males										
0-4	3	11.7	0	0	0.0	0.01	3	11.7	4	12.7
5-14	0	0.0	0	0	-	-	0	0.0	0	0.0
15-44	0	0.0	0	0	-	-	0	0.0	0	0.0
45-59	0	0.0	0	0	-	-	0	0.0	0	0.0
60+	0	0.0	0	0	-	-	0	0.0	0	0.0
All ages	3	1.5	0	0	0.0	0.01	3	1.5	4	1.4
Females										
0-4	5	18.8	0	0	0.0	0.01	5	18.8	6	20.2
5-14	0	0.0	0	0	-	-	0	0.0	0	0.0
15-44	0	0.0	0	0	-	-	0	0.0	0	0.0
45-59	0	0.0	0	0	-	-	0	0.0	0	0.0
60+	0	0.0	0	0	-	-	0	0.0	0	0.0
All ages	5	2.3	0	0	0.0	0.01	5	2.3	6	2.1
Total	9	1.9	0	0	0.0	0.01	9	1.9	9	1.8

Table 198h MEC - AOM - CMO Anencephaly - Cases

Age group (years)	Incidence 1990 Number ('000s)	Rate (per 100 000)	Prevalence 1990 Number ('000s)	Rate (per 100 000)	Avg. age at onset (years)	Average duration (years)	Deaths 1990 Number ('000s)	Rate (per 100 000)	Deaths 2000 (Projected) Number ('000s)	Rate (per 100 000)
Males										
0-4	8	18.5	0	0	0.0	0.01	8	18.5	10	20.8
5-14	0	0.0	0	0	-	-	0	0.0	0	0.0
15-44	0	0.0	0	0	-	-	0	0.0	0	0.0
45-59	0	0.0	0	0	-	-	0	0.0	0	0.0
60+	0	0.0	0	0	-	-	0	0.0	0	0.0
All ages	8	3.0	0	0	0.0	0.01	8	3.0	10	3.1
Females										
0-4	12	29.7	0	0	0.0	0.01	12	29.7	16	33.0
5-14	0	0.0	0	0	-	-	0	0.0	0	0.0
15-44	0	0.0	0	0	-	-	0	0.0	0	0.0
45-59	0	0.0	0	0	-	-	0	0.0	0	0.0
60+	0	0.0	0	0	-	-	0	0.0	0	0.0
All ages	12	4.8	0	0	0.0	0.01	12	4.8	16	4.9
Total	19	3.9	0	0	0.0	0.01	19	3.9	26	4.0

Table 198i World - Mundo - Monde Anencephaly - Cases

Age group (years)	Incidence 1990 Number ('000s)	Rate (per 100 000)	Prevalence 1990 Number ('000s)	Rate (per 100 000)	Avg. age at onset (years)	Average duration (years)	Deaths 1990 Number ('000s)	Rate (per 100 000)	Deaths 2000 (Projected) Number ('000s)	Rate (per 100 000)
Males										
0-4	58	18.0	1	0.2	0.0	0.01	58	18.0	72	20.7
5-14	0	0.0	0	0.0	-	-	0	0.0	0	0.0
15-44	0	0.0	0	0.0	-	-	0	0.0	0	0.0
45-59	0	0.0	0	0.0	-	-	0	0.0	0	0.0
60+	0	0.0	0	0.0	-	-	0	0.0	0	0.0
All ages	58	2.2	1	0.0	0.0	0.01	58	2.2	72	2.3
Females										
0-4	90	29.0	1	0.3	0.0	0.01	90	29.0	108	32.8
5-14	0	0.0	0	0.0	-	-	0	0.0	0	0.0
15-44	0	0.0	0	0.0	-	-	0	0.0	0	0.0
45-59	0	0.0	0	0.0	-	-	0	0.0	0	0.0
60+	0	0.0	0	0.0	-	-	0	0.0	0	0.0
All ages	90	3.4	1	0.0	0.0	0.01	90	3.4	108	3.5
Total	148	2.8	1	0.0	0.0	0.01	148	2.8	180	2.9

For epidemiological sources see Shibuya and Murray 1996c. For the methods used to estimate and project incidence, prevalence, and deaths see Murray and Lopez 1996a. See explanatory notes for definitions and caveats.

Table 199
Anorectal atresia

Cuadro 199
Atresia anorectal

Tableau 199
Atrésie anorectale

Cases

Casos

Cas

Table 199a EME - PEMC - EMBE Anorectal atresia - Cases

Age group (years)	Incidence 1990 Number ('000s)	Rate (per 100 000)	Prevalence 1990 Number ('000s)	Rate (per 100 000)	Avg. age at onset (years)	Average duration (years)	Deaths 1990 Number ('000s)	Rate (per 100 000)	Deaths 2000 (Projected) Number ('000s)	Rate (per 100 000)
Males										
0-4	1	2.7	0	1.3	0.0	0.50	0	0.1	0	0.2
5-14	0	0.0	0	0.0	-	-	0	0.0	0	0.0
15-44	0	0.0	0	0.0	-	-	0	0.0	0	0.0
45-59	0	0.0	0	0.0	-	-	0	0.0	0	0.0
60+	0	0.0	0	0.0	-	-	0	0.0	0	0.0
All ages	1	0.2	0	0.1	0.0	0.50	0	0.0	0	0.0
Females										
0-4	1	3.7	0	1.8	0.0	0.50	0	0.2	0	0.2
5-14	0	0.0	0	0.0	-	-	0	0.0	0	0.0
15-44	0	0.0	0	0.0	-	-	0	0.0	0	0.0
45-59	0	0.0	0	0.0	-	-	0	0.0	0	0.0
60+	0	0.0	0	0.0	-	-	0	0.0	0	0.0
All ages	1	0.2	0	0.1	0.0	0.50	0	0.0	0	0.0
Total	2	0.2	1	0.1	0.0	0.50	0	0.0	0	0.0

Table 199b FSE - PEAS - AESE Anorectal atresia - Cases

Age group (years)	Incidence 1990 Number ('000s)	Rate (per 100 000)	Prevalence 1990 Number ('000s)	Rate (per 100 000)	Avg. age at onset (years)	Average duration (years)	Deaths 1990 Number ('000s)	Rate (per 100 000)	Deaths 2000 (Projected) Number ('000s)	Rate (per 100 000)
Males										
0-4	0	3.5	0	2	0.0	0.50	0	0.2	0	0.3
5-14	0	0.0	0	0	-	-	0	0.0	0	0.0
15-44	0	0.0	0	0	-	-	0	0.0	0	0.0
45-59	0	0.0	0	0	-	-	0	0.0	0	0.0
60+	0	0.0	0	0	-	-	0	0.0	0	0.0
All ages	0	0.3	0	0	0.0	0.50	0	0.0	0	0.0
Females										
0-4	0	2.9	0	1	0.0	0.50	0	0.1	0	0.2
5-14	0	0.0	0	0	-	-	0	0.0	0	0.0
15-44	0	0.0	0	0	-	-	0	0.0	0	0.0
45-59	0	0.0	0	0	-	-	0	0.0	0	0.0
60+	0	0.0	0	0	-	-	0	0.0	0	0.0
All ages	0	0.2	0	0	0.0	0.50	0	0.0	0	0.0
Total	1	0.2	0	0	0.0	0.50	0	0.0	0	0.0

Table 199c India - India - Inde Anorectal atresia - Cases

Age group (years)	Incidence 1990 Number ('000s)	Rate (per 100 000)	Prevalence 1990 Number ('000s)	Rate (per 100 000)	Avg. age at onset (years)	Average duration (years)	Deaths 1990 Number ('000s)	Rate (per 100 000)	Deaths 2000 (Projected) Number ('000s)	Rate (per 100 000)
Males										
0-4	1	1.5	0	0.1	0.0	0.10	0	0.6	0	0.7
5-14	0	0.0	0	0.0	-	-	0	0.0	0	0.0
15-44	0	0.0	0	0.0	-	-	0	0.0	0	0.0
45-59	0	0.0	0	0.0	-	-	0	0.0	0	0.0
60+	0	0.0	0	0.0	-	-	0	0.0	0	0.0
All ages	1	0.2	0	0.0	0.0	0.10	0	0.1	0	0.1
Females										
0-4	1	1.3	0	0.1	0.0	0.10	0	0.5	0	0.6
5-14	0	0.0	0	0.0	-	-	0	0.0	0	0.0
15-44	0	0.0	0	0.0	-	-	0	0.0	0	0.0
45-59	0	0.0	0	0.0	-	-	0	0.0	0	0.0
60+	0	0.0	0	0.0	-	-	0	0.0	0	0.0
All ages	1	0.2	0	0.0	0.0	0.10	0	0.1	0	0.1
Total	2	0.2	0	0.0	0.0	0.10	1	0.1	1	0.1

For epidemiological sources see Shibuya and Murray 1996c. For the methods used to estimate and project incidence, prevalence, and deaths see Murray and Lopez 1996a. See explanatory notes for definitions and caveats.

Table 199	Cuadro 199	Tableau 199
Anorectal atresia	**Atresia anorectal**	**Atrésie anorectale**
Cases	Casos	Cas

Table 199d   China - China - Chine   Anorectal atresia - Cases

Age group (years)	Incidence 1990 Number ('000s)	Rate (per 100 000)	Prevalence 1990 Number ('000s)	Rate (per 100 000)	Avg. age at onset (years)	Average duration (years)	Deaths 1990 Number ('000s)	Rate (per 100 000)	Deaths 2000 (Projected) Number ('000s)	Rate (per 100 000)
Males										
0-4	1	1.4	0	0.3	0.0	0.20	0	0.1	0	0.2
5-14	0	0.0	0	0.0	-	-	0	0.0	0	0.0
15-44	0	0.0	0	0.0	-	-	0	0.0	0	0.0
45-59	0	0.0	0	0.0	-	-	0	0.0	0	0.0
60+	0	0.0	0	0.0	-	-	0	0.0	0	0.0
All ages	1	0.1	0	0.0	0.0	0.20	0	0.0	0	0.0
Females										
0-4	1	1.1	0	0.2	0.0	0.20	0	0.1	0	0.1
5-14	0	0.0	0	0.0	-	-	0	0.0	0	0.0
15-44	0	0.0	0	0.0	-	-	0	0.0	0	0.0
45-59	0	0.0	0	0.0	-	-	0	0.0	0	0.0
60+	0	0.0	0	0.0	-	-	0	0.0	0	0.0
All ages	1	0.1	0	0.0	0.0	0.20	0	0.0	0	0.0
Total	1	0.1	0	0.0	0.0	0.20	0	0.0	0	0.0

Table 199e   OAI - OPAI - APAI   Anorectal atresia - Cases

Age group (years)	Incidence 1990 Number ('000s)	Rate (per 100 000)	Prevalence 1990 Number ('000s)	Rate (per 100 000)	Avg. age at onset (years)	Average duration (years)	Deaths 1990 Number ('000s)	Rate (per 100 000)	Deaths 2000 (Projected) Number ('000s)	Rate (per 100 000)
Males										
0-4	1	1.6	0	0.3	0.0	0.20	0	0.3	0	0.4
5-14	0	0.0	0	0.0	-	-	0	0.0	0	0.0
15-44	0	0.0	0	0.0	-	-	0	0.0	0	0.0
45-59	0	0.0	0	0.0	-	-	0	0.0	0	0.0
60+	0	0.0	0	0.0	-	-	0	0.0	0	0.0
All ages	1	0.2	0	0.0	0.0	0.20	0	0.0	0	0.0
Females										
0-4	0	1.1	0	0.2	0.0	0.20	0	0.2	0	0.2
5-14	0	0.0	0	0.0	-	-	0	0.0	0	0.0
15-44	0	0.0	0	0.0	-	-	0	0.0	0	0.0
45-59	0	0.0	0	0.0	-	-	0	0.0	0	0.0
60+	0	0.0	0	0.0	-	-	0	0.0	0	0.0
All ages	0	0.1	0	0.0	0.0	0.20	0	0.0	0	0.0
Total	1	0.2	0	0.0	0.0	0.20	0	0.0	0	0.0

Table 199f   SSA - ASS - ASS   Anorectal atresia - Cases

Age group (years)	Incidence 1990 Number ('000s)	Rate (per 100 000)	Prevalence 1990 Number ('000s)	Rate (per 100 000)	Avg. age at onset (years)	Average duration (years)	Deaths 1990 Number ('000s)	Rate (per 100 000)	Deaths 2000 (Projected) Number ('000s)	Rate (per 100 000)
Males										
0-4	0	0.6	0	0.1	0.0	0.10	0	0.2	0	0.3
5-14	0	0.0	0	0.0	-	-	0	0.0	0	0.0
15-44	0	0.0	0	0.0	-	-	0	0.0	0	0.0
45-59	0	0.0	0	0.0	-	-	0	0.0	0	0.0
60+	0	0.0	0	0.0	-	-	0	0.0	0	0.0
All ages	0	0.1	0	0.0	0.0	0.10	0	0.0	0	0.0
Females										
0-4	0	0.5	0	0.1	0.0	0.10	0	0.2	0	0.3
5-14	0	0.0	0	0.0	-	-	0	0.0	0	0.0
15-44	0	0.0	0	0.0	-	-	0	0.0	0	0.0
45-59	0	0.0	0	0.0	-	-	0	0.0	0	0.0
60+	0	0.0	0	0.0	-	-	0	0.0	0	0.0
All ages	0	0.1	0	0.0	0.0	0.10	0	0.0	0	0.0
Total	1	0.1	0	0.0	0.0	0.10	0	0.0	0	0.0

For epidemiological sources see Shibuya and Murray 1996c. For the methods used to estimate and project incidence, prevalence, and deaths see Murray and Lopez 1996a. See explanatory notes for definitions and caveats.

Table 199
Anorectal atresia

Cuadro 199
Atresia anorectal

Tableau 199
Atrésie anorectale

Cases

Casos

Cas

Table 199g **LAC - ALC - ALC** Anorectal atresia - Cases

Age group (years)	Incidence 1990 Number ('000s)	Rate (per 100 000)	Prevalence 1990 Number ('000s)	Rate (per 100 000)	Avg. age at onset (years)	Average duration (years)	Deaths 1990 Number ('000s)	Rate (per 100 000)	Deaths 2000 (Projected) Number ('000s)	Rate (per 100 000)
Males										
0-4	1	2.6	0	0.5	0.0	0.20	0	0.3	0	0.3
5-14	0	0.0	0	0.0	-	-	0	0.0	0	0.0
15-44	0	0.0	0	0.0	-	-	0	0.0	0	0.0
45-59	0	0.0	0	0.0	-	-	0	0.0	0	0.0
60+	0	0.0	0	0.0	-	-	0	0.0	0	0.0
All ages	1	0.3	0	0.1	0.0	0.20	0	0.0	0	0.0
Females										
0-4	1	2.7	0	0.5	0.0	0.20	0	0.3	0	0.3
5-14	0	0.0	0	0.0	-	-	0	0.0	0	0.0
15-44	0	0.0	0	0.0	-	-	0	0.0	0	0.0
45-59	0	0.0	0	0.0	-	-	0	0.0	0	0.0
60+	0	0.0	0	0.0	-	-	0	0.0	0	0.0
All ages	1	0.3	0	0.1	0.0	0.20	0	0.0	0	0.0
Total	2	0.3	0	0.1	0.0	0.20	0	0.0	0	0.0

Table 199h **MEC - AOM - CMO** Anorectal atresia - Cases

Age group (years)	Incidence 1990 Number ('000s)	Rate (per 100 000)	Prevalence 1990 Number ('000s)	Rate (per 100 000)	Avg. age at onset (years)	Average duration (years)	Deaths 1990 Number ('000s)	Rate (per 100 000)	Deaths 2000 (Projected) Number ('000s)	Rate (per 100 000)
Males										
0-4	1	2.2	0	0.4	0.0	0.20	0	0.4	0	0.5
5-14	0	0.0	0	0.0	-	-	0	0.0	0	0.0
15-44	0	0.0	0	0.0	-	-	0	0.0	0	0.0
45-59	0	0.0	0	0.0	-	-	0	0.0	0	0.0
60+	0	0.0	0	0.0	-	-	0	0.0	0	0.0
All ages	1	0.4	0	0.1	0.0	0.20	0	0.1	0	0.1
Females										
0-4	1	1.3	0	0.3	0.0	0.20	0	0.3	0	0.3
5-14	0	0.0	0	0.0	-	-	0	0.0	0	0.0
15-44	0	0.0	0	0.0	-	-	0	0.0	0	0.0
45-59	0	0.0	0	0.0	-	-	0	0.0	0	0.0
60+	0	0.0	0	0.0	-	-	0	0.0	0	0.0
All ages	1	0.2	0	0.0	0.0	0.20	0	0.0	0	0.0
Total	1	0.3	0	0.1	0.0	0.20	0	0.1	0	0.1

Table 199i **World - Mundo - Monde** Anorectal atresia - Cases

Age group (years)	Incidence 1990 Number ('000s)	Rate (per 100 000)	Prevalence 1990 Number ('000s)	Rate (per 100 000)	Avg. age at onset (years)	Average duration (years)	Deaths 1990 Number ('000s)	Rate (per 100 000)	Deaths 2000 (Projected) Number ('000s)	Rate (per 100 000)
Males										
0-4	6	1.7	1	0.4	0.0	0.20	1	0.3	1	0.4
5-14	0	0.0	0	0.0	-	-	0	0.0	0	0.0
15-44	0	0.0	0	0.0	-	-	0	0.0	0	0.0
45-59	0	0.0	0	0.0	-	-	0	0.0	0	0.0
60+	0	0.0	0	0.0	-	-	0	0.0	0	0.0
All ages	6	0.2	1	0.1	0.0	0.24	1	0.0	1	0.0
Females										
0-4	5	1.5	1	0.4	0.0	0.20	1	0.3	1	0.3
5-14	0	0.0	0	0.0	-	-	0	0.0	0	0.0
15-44	0	0.0	0	0.0	-	-	0	0.0	0	0.0
45-59	0	0.0	0	0.0	-	-	0	0.0	0	0.0
60+	0	0.0	0	0.0	-	-	0	0.0	0	0.0
All ages	5	0.2	1	0.0	0.0	0.24	1	0.0	1	0.0
Total	10	0.2	3	0.0	0.0	0.24	2	0.0	2	0.0

For epidemiological sources see Shibuya and Murray 1996c. For the methods used to estimate and project incidence, prevalence, and deaths see Murray and Lopez 1996a. See explanatory notes for definitions and caveats.

Table 200
Cleft lip

Cuadro 200
Labio leporino

Tableau 200
Bec de lièvre

Cases

Casos

Cas

Table 200a EME - PEMC - EMBE Cleft lip - Cases

Age group (years)	Incidence 1990 Number ('000s)	Rate (per 100 000)	Prevalence 1990 Number ('000s)	Rate (per 100 000)	Avg. age at onset (years)	Average duration (years)	Deaths 1990 Number ('000s)	Rate (per 100 000)	Deaths 2000 (Projected) Number ('000s)	Rate (per 100 000)
Males										
0-4	6	22.2	28	105	0.0	68.1	0	0.9	0	1.1
5-14	0	0.0	55	104	-	-	0	0.0	0	0.0
15-44	0	0.0	191	104	-	-	0	0.0	0	0.0
45-59	0	0.0	69	104	-	-	0	0.0	0	0.0
60+	0	0.0	63	104	-	-	0	0.0	0	0.0
All ages	6	1.5	406	104	0.0	68.1	0	0.1	0	0.1
Females										
0-4	4	16.3	19	76	0.0	73.8	0	1.0	0	1.1
5-14	0	0.0	38	76	-	-	0	0.0	0	0.0
15-44	0	0.0	136	76	-	-	0	0.0	0	0.0
45-59	0	0.0	51	76	-	-	0	0.0	0	0.0
60+	0	0.0	64	76	-	-	0	0.0	0	0.0
All ages	4	1.0	309	76	0.0	73.8	0	0.1	0	0.1
Total	10	1.2	715	90	0.0	70.4	0	0.1	1	0.1

Table 200b FSE - PEAS - AESE Cleft lip - Cases

Age group (years)	Incidence 1990 Number ('000s)	Rate (per 100 000)	Prevalence 1990 Number ('000s)	Rate (per 100 000)	Avg. age at onset (years)	Average duration (years)	Deaths 1990 Number ('000s)	Rate (per 100 000)	Deaths 2000 (Projected) Number ('000s)	Rate (per 100 000)
Males										
0-4	3	22.2	14	105	0.0	62.8	0	1.5	0	2.4
5-14	0	0.0	28	104	-	-	0	0.0	0	0.0
15-44	0	0.0	79	104	-	-	0	0.0	0	0.0
45-59	0	0.0	28	104	-	-	0	0.0	0	0.0
60+	0	0.0	22	104	-	-	0	0.0	0	0.0
All ages	3	1.8	172	104	0.0	62.8	0	0.1	0	0.2
Females										
0-4	2	16.1	10	76	0.0	70.7	0	1.0	0	1.4
5-14	0	0.0	20	76	-	-	0	0.0	0	0.0
15-44	0	0.0	57	76	-	-	0	0.0	0	0.0
45-59	0	0.0	23	76	-	-	0	0.0	0	0.0
60+	0	0.0	28	76	-	-	0	0.0	0	0.0
All ages	2	1.2	137	76	0.0	70.7	0	0.1	0	0.1
Total	5	1.5	309	89	0.0	66.0	0	0.1	0	0.1

Table 200c India - India - Inde Cleft lip - Cases

Age group (years)	Incidence 1990 Number ('000s)	Rate (per 100 000)	Prevalence 1990 Number ('000s)	Rate (per 100 000)	Avg. age at onset (years)	Average duration (years)	Deaths 1990 Number ('000s)	Rate (per 100 000)	Deaths 2000 (Projected) Number ('000s)	Rate (per 100 000)
Males										
0-4	14	23.4	62	104	0.0	58.8	1	1.2	1	1.5
5-14	0	0.0	106	104	-	-	0	0.0	0	0.0
15-44	0	0.0	208	104	-	-	0	0.0	0	0.0
45-59	0	0.0	49	104	-	-	0	0.0	0	0.0
60+	0	0.0	31	104	-	-	0	0.0	0	0.0
All ages	14	3.2	457	104	0.0	58.8	1	0.2	1	0.2
Females										
0-4	10	17.1	43	76	0.0	59.7	1	0.8	1	0.9
5-14	0	0.0	72	75	-	-	0	0.0	0	0.0
15-44	0	0.0	138	75	-	-	0	0.0	0	0.0
45-59	0	0.0	35	75	-	-	0	0.0	0	0.0
60+	0	0.0	22	75	-	-	0	0.0	0	0.0
All ages	10	2.4	309	75	0.0	59.7	0	0.1	1	0.1
Total	24	2.8	766	90	0.0	59.1	1	0.1	1	0.1

For epidemiological sources see Shibuya and Murray 1996c. For the methods used to estimate and project incidence, prevalence, and deaths see Murray and Lopez 1996a. See explanatory notes for definitions and caveats.

Table 200
Cleft lip

Cuadro 200
Labio leporino

Tableau 200
Bec de lièvre

Cases

Casos

Cas

Table 200d China - China - Chine

Cleft lip - Cases

Age group (years)	Incidence 1990 Number ('000s)	Rate (per 100 000)	Prevalence 1990 Number ('000s)	Rate (per 100 000)	Avg. age at onset (years)	Average duration (years)	Deaths 1990 Number ('000s)	Rate (per 100 000)	Deaths 2000 (Projected) Number ('000s)	Rate (per 100 000)
Males										
0-4	22	37.3	95	158	0.0	64.1	0	0.7	1	0.9
5-14	0	0.0	153	158	-	-	0	0.0	0	0.0
15-44	0	0.0	485	158	-	-	0	0.0	0	0.0
45-59	0	0.0	115	158	-	-	0	0.0	0	0.0
60+	0	0.0	77	158	-	-	0	0.0	0	0.0
All ages	22	3.8	926	158	0.0	64.1	0	0.1	1	0.1
Females										
0-4	22	37.8	92	158	0.0	66.9	0	0.5	0	0.5
5-14	0	0.0	143	158	-	-	0	0.0	0	0.0
15-44	0	0.0	449	158	-	-	0	0.0	0	0.0
45-59	0	0.0	102	158	-	-	0	0.0	0	0.0
60+	0	0.0	82	158	-	-	0	0.0	0	0.0
All ages	22	4.0	868	158	0.0	66.9	0	0.1	0	0.0
Total	44	3.9	1 794	158	0.0	65.5	1	0.1	1	0.1

Table 200e OAI - OPAI - APAI

Cleft lip - Cases

Age group (years)	Incidence 1990 Number ('000s)	Rate (per 100 000)	Prevalence 1990 Number ('000s)	Rate (per 100 000)	Avg. age at onset (years)	Average duration (years)	Deaths 1990 Number ('000s)	Rate (per 100 000)	Deaths 2000 (Projected) Number ('000s)	Rate (per 100 000)
Males										
0-4	10	22.6	46	105	0.0	60.6	1	1.1	1	1.3
5-14	0	0.0	88	105	-	-	0	0.0	0	0.0
15-44	0	0.0	168	105	-	-	0	0.0	0	0.0
45-59	0	0.0	36	105	-	-	0	0.0	0	0.0
60+	0	0.0	21	105	-	-	0	0.0	0	0.0
All ages	10	2.9	359	105	0.0	60.6	1	0.1	1	0.1
Females										
0-4	7	16.6	32	77	0.0	64.5	0	0.6	0	0.6
5-14	0	0.0	62	77	-	-	0	0.0	0	0.0
15-44	0	0.0	123	77	-	-	0	0.0	0	0.0
45-59	0	0.0	27	77	-	-	0	0.0	0	0.0
60+	0	0.0	17	77	-	-	0	0.0	0	0.0
All ages	7	2.1	261	77	0.0	64.5	0	0.1	0	0.1
Total	17	2.5	620	91	0.0	62.2	1	0.1	1	0.1

Table 200f SSA - ASS - ASS

Cleft lip - Cases

Age group (years)	Incidence 1990 Number ('000s)	Rate (per 100 000)	Prevalence 1990 Number ('000s)	Rate (per 100 000)	Avg. age at onset (years)	Average duration (years)	Deaths 1990 Number ('000s)	Rate (per 100 000)	Deaths 2000 (Projected) Number ('000s)	Rate (per 100 000)
Males										
0-4	12	24.6	49	104	0.0	51.1	0	0.4	0	0.5
5-14	0	0.0	73	104	-	-	0	0.0	0	0.0
15-44	0	0.0	108	104	-	-	0	0.0	0	0.0
45-59	0	0.0	21	104	-	-	0	0.0	0	0.0
60+	0	0.0	11	104	-	-	0	0.0	0	0.0
All ages	12	4.6	262	104	0.0	51.1	0	0.1	0	0.1
Females										
0-4	9	18.7	37	79	0.0	54.1	0	0.3	0	0.4
5-14	0	0.0	55	79	-	-	0	0.0	0	0.0
15-44	0	0.0	84	79	-	-	0	0.0	0	0.0
45-59	0	0.0	18	79	-	-	0	0.0	0	0.0
60+	0	0.0	10	79	-	-	0	0.0	0	0.0
All ages	9	3.4	204	79	0.0	54.1	0	0.1	0	0.1
Total	20	4.0	466	91	0.0	52.4	0	0.1	1	0.1

For epidemiological sources see Shibuya and Murray 1996c. For the methods used to estimate and project incidence, prevalence, and deaths see Murray and Lopez 1996a. See explanatory notes for definitions and caveats.

Table 200
Cleft lip

Cuadro 200
Labio leporino

Tableau 200
Bec de lièvre

Cases

Casos

Cas

Table 200g **LAC - ALC - ALC** Cleft lip - Cases

Age group (years)	Incidence 1990 Number ('000s)	Rate (per 100 000)	Prevalence 1990 Number ('000s)	Rate (per 100 000)	Avg. age at onset (years)	Average duration (years)	Deaths 1990 Number ('000s)	Rate (per 100 000)	Deaths 2000 (Projected) Number ('000s)	Rate (per 100 000)
Males										
0-4	8	29.5	39	134	0.0	63.4	0	1.2	0	1.4
5-14	0	0.0	70	134	-	-	0	0.0	0	0.0
15-44	0	0.0	140	134	-	-	0	0.0	0	0.0
45-59	0	0.0	30	134	-	-	0	0.0	0	0.0
60+	0	0.0	19	134	-	-	0	0.0	0	0.0
All ages	8	3.8	297	134	0.0	63.4	0	0.2	0	0.1
Females										
0-4	6	21.8	28	100	0.0	67.3	0	1.0	0	1.0
5-14	0	0.0	51	100	-	-	0	0.0	0	0.0
15-44	0	0.0	104	100	-	-	0	0.0	0	0.0
45-59	0	0.0	23	100	-	-	0	0.0	0	0.0
60+	0	0.0	17	100	-	-	0	0.0	0	0.0
All ages	6	2.7	222	100	0.0	67.3	0	0.1	0	0.1
Total	15	3.3	519	117	0.0	65.0	1	0.1	1	0.1

Table 200h **MEC - AOM - CMO** Cleft lip - Cases

Age group (years)	Incidence 1990 Number ('000s)	Rate (per 100 000)	Prevalence 1990 Number ('000s)	Rate (per 100 000)	Avg. age at onset (years)	Average duration (years)	Deaths 1990 Number ('000s)	Rate (per 100 000)	Deaths 2000 (Projected) Number ('000s)	Rate (per 100 000)
Males										
0-4	10	24.1	43	105	0.0	61.5	0	0.9	1	1.1
5-14	0	0.0	68	105	-	-	0	0.0	0	0.0
15-44	0	0.0	119	105	-	-	0	0.0	0	0.0
45-59	0	0.0	23	105	-	-	0	0.0	0	0.0
60+	0	0.0	14	105	-	-	0	0.0	0	0.0
All ages	10	3.9	268	105	0.0	61.5	0	0.2	1	0.2
Females										
0-4	7	18.0	31	78	0.0	64.1	0	0.7	0	0.8
5-14	0	0.0	48	78	-	-	0	0.0	0	0.0
15-44	0	0.0	83	78	-	-	0	0.0	0	0.0
45-59	0	0.0	17	78	-	-	0	0.0	0	0.0
60+	0	0.0	12	78	-	-	0	0.0	0	0.0
All ages	7	2.9	192	78	0.0	64.1	0	0.1	0	0.1
Total	17	3.4	460	91	0.0	62.6	1	0.1	1	0.1

Table 200i **World - Mundo - Monde** Cleft lip - Cases

Age group (years)	Incidence 1990 Number ('000s)	Rate (per 100 000)	Prevalence 1990 Number ('000s)	Rate (per 100 000)	Avg. age at onset (years)	Average duration (years)	Deaths 1990 Number ('000s)	Rate (per 100 000)	Deaths 2000 (Projected) Number ('000s)	Rate (per 100 000)
Males										
0-4	85	26.5	376	117	0.0	60.6	3	0.9	4	1.1
5-14	0	0.0	642	117	-	-	0	0.0	0	0.0
15-44	0	0.0	1 498	120	-	-	0	0.0	0	0.0
45-59	0	0.0	371	119	-	-	0	0.0	0	0.0
60+	0	0.0	259	118	-	-	0	0.0	0	0.0
All ages	85	3.2	3 147	119	0.0	61.7	3	0.1	4	0.1
Females										
0-4	67	21.6	292	94	0.0	63.7	2	0.7	2	0.7
5-14	0	0.0	489	93	-	-	0	0.0	0	0.0
15-44	0	0.0	1 174	98	-	-	0	0.0	0	0.0
45-59	0	0.0	296	95	-	-	0	0.0	0	0.0
60+	0	0.0	252	93	-	-	0	0.0	0	0.0
All ages	67	2.6	2 502	96	0.0	65.3	2	0.1	2	0.1
Total	152	2.9	5 649	107	0.0	63.3	5	0.1	6	0.1

For epidemiological sources see Shibuya and Murray 1996c. For the methods used to estimate and project incidence, prevalence, and deaths see Murray and Lopez 1996a. See explanatory notes for definitions and caveats.

Table 201
Cleft palate

Cuadro 201
Paladar hendido

Tableau 201
Fissure du palais

Cases

Casos

Cas

Table 201a EME - PEMC - EMBE — Cleft palate - Cases

Age group (years)	Incidence 1990 Number ('000s)	Rate (per 100 000)	Prevalence 1990 Number ('000s)	Rate (per 100 000)	Avg. age at onset (years)	Average duration (years)	Deaths 1990 Number ('000s)	Rate (per 100 000)	Deaths 2000 (Projected) Number ('000s)	Rate (per 100 000)
Males										
0-4	3	11.2	14	51	0.0	68.1	0	0.6	0	0.7
5-14	0	0.0	27	51	-	-	0	0.0	0	0.0
15-44	0	0.0	94	51	-	-	0	0.0	0	0.0
45-59	0	0.0	34	51	-	-	0	0.0	0	0.0
60+	0	0.0	31	51	-	-	0	0.0	0	0.0
All ages	3	0.8	199	51	0.0	68.1	0	0.0	0	0.1
Females										
0-4	3	13.3	15	61	0.0	73.8	0	1.0	0	1.1
5-14	0	0.0	31	60	-	-	0	0.0	0	0.0
15-44	0	0.0	108	60	-	-	0	0.0	0	0.0
45-59	0	0.0	41	60	-	-	0	0.0	0	0.0
60+	0	0.0	51	60	-	-	0	0.0	0	0.0
All ages	3	0.8	246	60	0.0	73.8	0	0.1	0	0.1
Total	6	0.8	444	56	0.0	71.1	0	0.1	1	0.1

Table 201b FSE - PEAS - AESE — Cleft palate - Cases

Age group (years)	Incidence 1990 Number ('000s)	Rate (per 100 000)	Prevalence 1990 Number ('000s)	Rate (per 100 000)	Avg. age at onset (years)	Average duration (years)	Deaths 1990 Number ('000s)	Rate (per 100 000)	Deaths 2000 (Projected) Number ('000s)	Rate (per 100 000)
Males										
0-4	1	8.2	5	37	0.0	62.8	0	1.0	0	1.6
5-14	0	0.0	10	37	-	-	0	0.0	0	0.0
15-44	0	0.0	28	37	-	-	0	0.0	0	0.0
45-59	0	0.0	10	37	-	-	0	0.0	0	0.0
60+	0	0.0	8	37	-	-	0	0.0	0	0.0
All ages	1	0.7	61	37	0.0	62.8	0	0.1	0	0.1
Females										
0-4	1	9.7	6	44	0.0	70.7	0	1.0	0	1.4
5-14	0	0.0	12	44	-	-	0	0.0	0	0.0
15-44	0	0.0	33	44	-	-	0	0.0	0	0.0
45-59	0	0.0	13	44	-	-	0	0.0	0	0.0
60+	0	0.0	16	44	-	-	0	0.0	0	0.0
All ages	1	0.7	80	44	0.0	70.7	0	0.1	0	0.1
Total	2	0.7	141	41	0.0	67.0	0	0.1	0	0.1

Table 201c India - India - Inde — Cleft palate - Cases

Age group (years)	Incidence 1990 Number ('000s)	Rate (per 100 000)	Prevalence 1990 Number ('000s)	Rate (per 100 000)	Avg. age at onset (years)	Average duration (years)	Deaths 1990 Number ('000s)	Rate (per 100 000)	Deaths 2000 (Projected) Number ('000s)	Rate (per 100 000)
Males										
0-4	6	9.2	24	40	0.0	58.8	0	0.8	1	1.0
5-14	0	0.0	40	39	-	-	0	0.0	0	0.0
15-44	0	0.0	79	39	-	-	0	0.0	0	0.0
45-59	0	0.0	19	39	-	-	0	0.0	0	0.0
60+	0	0.0	12	39	-	-	0	0.0	0	0.0
All ages	6	1.3	174	40	0.0	58.8	0	0.1	1	0.1
Females										
0-4	6	11.0	27	47	0.0	59.7	0	0.8	1	0.9
5-14	0	0.0	45	47	-	-	0	0.0	0	0.0
15-44	0	0.0	86	47	-	-	0	0.0	0	0.0
45-59	0	0.0	22	47	-	-	0	0.0	0	0.0
60+	0	0.0	14	47	-	-	0	0.0	0	0.0
All ages	6	1.5	193	47	0.0	59.7	0	0.1	1	0.1
Total	12	1.4	366	43	0.0	59.3	1	0.1	1	0.1

For epidemiological sources see Shibuya and Murray 1996c. For the methods used to estimate and project incidence, prevalence, and deaths see Murray and Lopez 1996a. See explanatory notes for definitions and caveats.

Table 201
Cleft palate

Cuadro 201
Paladar hendido

Tableau 201
Fissure du palais

Cases   Casos   Cas

Table 201d   China - China - Chine   Cleft palate - Cases

Age group (years)	Incidence 1990 Number ('000s)	Rate (per 100 000)	Prevalence 1990 Number ('000s)	Rate (per 100 000)	Avg. age at onset (years)	Average duration (years)	Deaths 1990 Number ('000s)	Rate (per 100 000)	Deaths 2000 (Projected) Number ('000s)	Rate (per 100 000)
Males										
0-4	1	2.2	5	8.8	0.0	64.1	0	0.5	0	0.6
5-14	0	0.0	9	8.8	-	-	0	0.0	0	0.0
15-44	0	0.0	27	8.8	-	-	0	0.0	0	0.0
45-59	0	0.0	6	8.8	-	-	0	0.0	0	0.0
60+	0	0.0	4	8.8	-	-	0	0.0	0	0.0
All ages	1	0.2	51	8.8	0.0	64.1	0	0.1	0	0.1
Females										
0-4	2	2.6	6	10.7	0.0	66.9	0	0.5	0	0.5
5-14	0	0.0	10	10.7	-	-	0	0.0	0	0.0
15-44	0	0.0	30	10.7	-	-	0	0.0	0	0.0
45-59	0	0.0	7	10.7	-	-	0	0.0	0	0.0
60+	0	0.0	6	10.7	-	-	0	0.0	0	0.0
All ages	2	0.3	58	10.7	0.0	66.9	0	0.1	0	0.0
Total	3	0.2	110	9.7	0.0	65.6	1	0.1	1	0.0

Table 201e   OAI - OPAI - APAI   Cleft palate - Cases

Age group (years)	Incidence 1990 Number ('000s)	Rate (per 100 000)	Prevalence 1990 Number ('000s)	Rate (per 100 000)	Avg. age at onset (years)	Average duration (years)	Deaths 1990 Number ('000s)	Rate (per 100 000)	Deaths 2000 (Projected) Number ('000s)	Rate (per 100 000)
Males										
0-4	4	8.9	18	40	0.0	60.6	0	0.8	0	0.8
5-14	0	0.0	33	40	-	-	0	0.0	0	0.0
15-44	0	0.0	64	40	-	-	0	0.0	0	0.0
45-59	0	0.0	14	40	-	-	0	0.0	0	0.0
60+	0	0.0	8	40	-	-	0	0.0	0	0.0
All ages	4	1.1	137	40	0.0	60.6	0	0.1	0	0.1
Females										
0-4	4	10.7	20	48	0.0	64.5	0	0.6	0	0.6
5-14	0	0.0	38	48	-	-	0	0.0	0	0.0
15-44	0	0.0	76	48	-	-	0	0.0	0	0.0
45-59	0	0.0	17	48	-	-	0	0.0	0	0.0
60+	0	0.0	11	48	-	-	0	0.0	0	0.0
All ages	4	1.3	163	48	0.0	64.5	0	0.1	0	0.1
Total	8	1.2	300	44	0.0	62.7	1	0.1	1	0.1

Table 201f   SSA - ASS - ASS   Cleft palate - Cases

Age group (years)	Incidence 1990 Number ('000s)	Rate (per 100 000)	Prevalence 1990 Number ('000s)	Rate (per 100 000)	Avg. age at onset (years)	Average duration (years)	Deaths 1990 Number ('000s)	Rate (per 100 000)	Deaths 2000 (Projected) Number ('000s)	Rate (per 100 000)
Males										
0-4	5	9.7	19	39	0.0	51.1	0	0.3	0	0.3
5-14	0	0.0	28	39	-	-	0	0.0	0	0.0
15-44	0	0.0	41	39	-	-	0	0.0	0	0.0
45-59	0	0.0	8	39	-	-	0	0.0	0	0.0
60+	0	0.0	4	39	-	-	0	0.0	0	0.0
All ages	5	1.8	99	39	0.0	51.1	0	0.1	0	0.1
Females										
0-4	6	11.9	23	49	0.0	54.1	0	0.3	0	0.4
5-14	0	0.0	34	49	-	-	0	0.0	0	0.0
15-44	0	0.0	52	49	-	-	0	0.0	0	0.0
45-59	0	0.0	11	49	-	-	0	0.0	0	0.0
60+	0	0.0	6	49	-	-	0	0.0	0	0.0
All ages	6	2.2	126	49	0.0	54.1	0	0.1	0	0.1
Total	10	2.0	225	44	0.0	52.8	0	0.1	0	0.1

For epidemiological sources see Shibuya and Murray 1996c. For the methods used to estimate and project incidence, prevalence, and deaths see Murray and Lopez 1996a. See explanatory notes for definitions and caveats.

Table 201   **Cuadro 201**   **Tableau 201**
Cleft palate   **Paladar hendido**   **Fissure du palais**

Cases   Casos   Cas

Table 201g   LAC - ALC - ALC   Cleft palate - Cases

Age group (years)	Incidence 1990 Number ('000s)	Rate (per 100 000)	Prevalence 1990 Number ('000s)	Rate (per 100 000)	Avg. age at onset (years)	Average duration (years)	Deaths 1990 Number ('000s)	Rate (per 100 000)	Deaths 2000 (Projected) Number ('000s)	Rate (per 100 000)
Males										
0-4	2	8.7	11	38	0.0	63.4	0	0.8	0	0.9
5-14	0	0.0	20	38	-	-	0	0.0	0	0.0
15-44	0	0.0	39	38	-	-	0	0.0	0	0.0
45-59	0	0.0	8	38	-	-	0	0.0	0	0.0
60+	0	0.0	5	38	-	-	0	0.0	0	0.0
All ages	2	1.1	84	38	0.0	63.4	0	0.1	0	0.1
Females										
0-4	3	10.4	13	46	0.0	67.3	0	1.0	0	1.0
5-14	0	0.0	23	45	-	-	0	0.0	0	0.0
15-44	0	0.0	47	45	-	-	0	0.0	0	0.0
45-59	0	0.0	11	45	-	-	0	0.0	0	0.0
60+	0	0.0	8	45	-	-	0	0.0	0	0.0
All ages	3	1.3	101	45	0.0	67.3	0	0.1	0	0.1
Total	5	1.2	185	42	0.0	65.5	1	0.1	1	0.1

Table 201h   MEC - AOM - CMO   Cleft palate - Cases

Age group (years)	Incidence 1990 Number ('000s)	Rate (per 100 000)	Prevalence 1990 Number ('000s)	Rate (per 100 000)	Avg. age at onset (years)	Average duration (years)	Deaths 1990 Number ('000s)	Rate (per 100 000)	Deaths 2000 (Projected) Number ('000s)	Rate (per 100 000)
Males										
0-4	4	9.5	16	40	0.0	61.5	0	0.6	0	0.7
5-14	0	0.0	26	40	-	-	0	0.0	0	0.0
15-44	0	0.0	45	40	-	-	0	0.0	0	0.0
45-59	0	0.0	9	40	-	-	0	0.0	0	0.0
60+	0	0.0	5	40	-	-	0	0.0	0	0.0
All ages	4	1.5	102	40	0.0	61.5	0	0.1	0	0.1
Females										
0-4	5	11.5	19	48	0.0	64.1	0	0.7	0	0.8
5-14	0	0.0	30	48	-	-	0	0.0	0	0.0
15-44	0	0.0	52	48	-	-	0	0.0	0	0.0
45-59	0	0.0	11	48	-	-	0	0.0	0	0.0
60+	0	0.0	7	48	-	-	0	0.0	0	0.0
All ages	5	1.9	119	48	0.0	64.1	0	0.1	0	0.1
Total	8	1.7	221	44	0.0	62.9	1	0.1	1	0.1

Table 201i   World - Mundo - Monde   Cleft palate - Cases

Age group (years)	Incidence 1990 Number ('000s)	Rate (per 100 000)	Prevalence 1990 Number ('000s)	Rate (per 100 000)	Avg. age at onset (years)	Average duration (years)	Deaths 1990 Number ('000s)	Rate (per 100 000)	Deaths 2000 (Projected) Number ('000s)	Rate (per 100 000)
Males										
0-4	26	8.0	111	35	0.0	60.6	2	0.6	3	0.7
5-14	0	0.0	193	35	-	-	0	0.0	0	0.0
15-44	0	0.0	418	33	-	-	0	0.0	0	0.0
45-59	0	0.0	108	34	-	-	0	0.0	0	0.0
60+	0	0.0	78	35	-	-	0	0.0	0	0.0
All ages	26	1.0	907	34	0.0	61.7	2	0.1	3	0.1
Females										
0-4	30	9.7	129	42	0.0	63.7	2	0.7	2	0.7
5-14	0	0.0	222	42	-	-	0	0.0	0	0.0
15-44	0	0.0	485	40	-	-	0	0.0	0	0.0
45-59	0	0.0	131	42	-	-	0	0.0	0	0.0
60+	0	0.0	118	44	-	-	0	0.0	0	0.0
All ages	30	1.1	1 085	42	0.0	65.3	2	0.1	2	0.1
Total	56	1.1	1 992	38	0.0	63.7	4	0.1	5	0.1

For epidemiological sources see Shibuya and Murray 1996c. For the methods used to estimate and project incidence, prevalence, and deaths see Murray and Lopez 1996a. See explanatory notes for definitions and caveats.

Table 202
Oesophageal atresia

Cuadro 202
Atresia esofágica

Tableau 202
Atrésie de l'oesophage

Cases

Casos

Cas

Table 202a   EME - PEMC - EMBE   Oesophageal atresia - Cases

Age group (years)	Incidence 1990 Number ('000s)	Rate (per 100 000)	Prevalence 1990 Number ('000s)	Rate (per 100 000)	Avg. age at onset (years)	Average duration (years)	Deaths 1990 Number ('000s)	Rate (per 100 000)	Deaths 2000 (Projected) Number ('000s)	Rate (per 100 000)
Males										
0-4	1	1.9	0	0	0.0	0.01	0	0.4	0	0.5
5-14	0	0.0	0	0	-	-	0	0.0	0	0.0
15-44	0	0.0	0	0	-	-	0	0.0	0	0.0
45-59	0	0.0	0	0	-	-	0	0.0	0	0.0
60+	0	0.0	0	0	-	-	0	0.0	0	0.0
All ages	1	0.1	0	0	0.0	0.01	0	0.0	0	0.0
Females										
0-4	1	2.7	0	0	0.0	0.01	0	0.5	0	0.6
5-14	0	0.0	0	0	-	-	0	0.0	0	0.0
15-44	0	0.0	0	0	-	-	0	0.0	0	0.0
45-59	0	0.0	0	0	-	-	0	0.0	0	0.0
60+	0	0.0	0	0	-	-	0	0.0	0	0.0
All ages	1	0.2	0	0	0.0	0.01	0	0.0	0	0.0
Total	1	0.1	0	0	0.0	0.01	0	0.0	0	0.0

Table 202b   FSE - PEAS - AESE   Oesophageal atresia - Cases

Age group (years)	Incidence 1990 Number ('000s)	Rate (per 100 000)	Prevalence 1990 Number ('000s)	Rate (per 100 000)	Avg. age at onset (years)	Average duration (years)	Deaths 1990 Number ('000s)	Rate (per 100 000)	Deaths 2000 (Projected) Number ('000s)	Rate (per 100 000)
Males										
0-4	0	2.5	0	0	0.0	0.01	0	0.5	0	0.8
5-14	0	0.0	0	0	-	-	0	0.0	0	0.0
15-44	0	0.0	0	0	-	-	0	0.0	0	0.0
45-59	0	0.0	0	0	-	-	0	0.0	0	0.0
60+	0	0.0	0	0	-	-	0	0.0	0	0.0
All ages	0	0.2	0	0	0.0	0.01	0	0.0	0	0.1
Females										
0-4	0	2.2	0	0	0.0	0.01	0	0.4	0	0.6
5-14	0	0.0	0	0	-	-	0	0.0	0	0.0
15-44	0	0.0	0	0	-	-	0	0.0	0	0.0
45-59	0	0.0	0	0	-	-	0	0.0	0	0.0
60+	0	0.0	0	0	-	-	0	0.0	0	0.0
All ages	0	0.2	0	0	0.0	0.01	0	0.0	0	0.0
Total	1	0.2	0	0	0.0	0.01	0	0.0	0	0.0

Table 202c   India - India - Inde   Oesophageal atresia - Cases

Age group (years)	Incidence 1990 Number ('000s)	Rate (per 100 000)	Prevalence 1990 Number ('000s)	Rate (per 100 000)	Avg. age at onset (years)	Average duration (years)	Deaths 1990 Number ('000s)	Rate (per 100 000)	Deaths 2000 (Projected) Number ('000s)	Rate (per 100 000)
Males										
0-4	1	1.1	0	0.0	0.0	0.01	0	0.8	1	1.0
5-14	0	0.0	0	0.0	-	-	0	0.0	0	0.0
15-44	0	0.0	0	0.0	-	-	0	0.0	0	0.0
45-59	0	0.0	0	0.0	-	-	0	0.0	0	0.0
60+	0	0.0	0	0.0	-	-	0	0.0	0	0.0
All ages	1	0.2	0	0.0	0.0	0.01	0	0.1	1	0.1
Females										
0-4	1	1.0	0	0.0	0.0	0.01	0	0.7	0	0.9
5-14	0	0.0	0	0.0	-	-	0	0.0	0	0.0
15-44	0	0.0	0	0.0	-	-	0	0.0	0	0.0
45-59	0	0.0	0	0.0	-	-	0	0.0	0	0.0
60+	0	0.0	0	0.0	-	-	0	0.0	0	0.0
All ages	1	0.1	0	0.0	0.0	0.01	0	0.1	0	0.1
Total	1	0.1	0	0.0	0.0	0.01	1	0.1	1	0.1

For epidemiological sources see Shibuya and Murray 1996c. For the methods used to estimate and project incidence, prevalence, and deaths see Murray and Lopez 1996a. See explanatory notes for definitions and caveats.

Table 202
Oesophageal atresia

Cuadro 202
Atresia esofágica

Tableau 202
Atrésie de l'oesophage

Cases

Casos

Cas

Table 202d — China - China - Chine — Oesophageal atresia - Cases

Age group (years)	Incidence 1990 Number ('000s)	Rate (per 100 000)	Prevalence 1990 Number ('000s)	Rate (per 100 000)	Avg. age at onset (years)	Average duration (years)	Deaths 1990 Number ('000s)	Rate (per 100 000)	Deaths 2000 (Projected) Number ('000s)	Rate (per 100 000)
Males										
0-4	0	0.3	0	0	0.0	0.01	0	0.1	0	0.1
5-14	0	0.0	0	0	-	-	0	0.0	0	0.0
15-44	0	0.0	0	0	-	-	0	0.0	0	0.0
45-59	0	0.0	0	0	-	-	0	0.0	0	0.0
60+	0	0.0	0	0	-	-	0	0.0	0	0.0
All ages	0	0.0	0	0	0.0	0.01	0	0.0	0	0.0
Females										
0-4	0	0.3	0	0	0.0	0.01	0	0.1	0	0.1
5-14	0	0.0	0	0	-	-	0	0.0	0	0.0
15-44	0	0.0	0	0	-	-	0	0.0	0	0.0
45-59	0	0.0	0	0	-	-	0	0.0	0	0.0
60+	0	0.0	0	0	-	-	0	0.0	0	0.0
All ages	0	0.0	0	0	0.0	0.01	0	0.0	0	0.0
Total	0	0.0	0	0	0.0	0.01	0	0.0	0	0.0

Table 202e — OAI - OPAI - APAI — Oesophageal atresia - Cases

Age group (years)	Incidence 1990 Number ('000s)	Rate (per 100 000)	Prevalence 1990 Number ('000s)	Rate (per 100 000)	Avg. age at onset (years)	Average duration (years)	Deaths 1990 Number ('000s)	Rate (per 100 000)	Deaths 2000 (Projected) Number ('000s)	Rate (per 100 000)
Males										
0-4	1	1.2	0	0	0.0	0.01	0	0.7	0	0.7
5-14	0	0.0	0	0	-	-	0	0.0	0	0.0
15-44	0	0.0	0	0	-	-	0	0.0	0	0.0
45-59	0	0.0	0	0	-	-	0	0.0	0	0.0
60+	0	0.0	0	0	-	-	0	0.0	0	0.0
All ages	1	0.2	0	0	0.0	0.01	0	0.1	0	0.1
Females										
0-4	0	0.8	0	0	0.0	0.01	0	0.5	0	0.5
5-14	0	0.0	0	0	-	-	0	0.0	0	0.0
15-44	0	0.0	0	0	-	-	0	0.0	0	0.0
45-59	0	0.0	0	0	-	-	0	0.0	0	0.0
60+	0	0.0	0	0	-	-	0	0.0	0	0.0
All ages	0	0.1	0	0	0.0	0.01	0	0.1	0	0.1
Total	1	0.1	0	0	0.0	0.01	0	0.1	1	0.1

Table 202f — SSA - ASS - ASS — Oesophageal atresia - Cases

Age group (years)	Incidence 1990 Number ('000s)	Rate (per 100 000)	Prevalence 1990 Number ('000s)	Rate (per 100 000)	Avg. age at onset (years)	Average duration (years)	Deaths 1990 Number ('000s)	Rate (per 100 000)	Deaths 2000 (Projected) Number ('000s)	Rate (per 100 000)
Males										
0-4	0	0.4	0	0.0	0.0	0.01	0	0.3	0	0.3
5-14	0	0.0	0	0.0	-	-	0	0.0	0	0.0
15-44	0	0.0	0	0.0	-	-	0	0.0	0	0.0
45-59	0	0.0	0	0.0	-	-	0	0.0	0	0.0
60+	0	0.0	0	0.0	-	-	0	0.0	0	0.0
All ages	0	0.1	0	0.0	0.0	0.01	0	0.1	0	0.1
Females										
0-4	0	0.4	0	0.0	0.0	0.01	0	0.3	0	0.3
5-14	0	0.0	0	0.0	-	-	0	0.0	0	0.0
15-44	0	0.0	0	0.0	-	-	0	0.0	0	0.0
45-59	0	0.0	0	0.0	-	-	0	0.0	0	0.0
60+	0	0.0	0	0.0	-	-	0	0.0	0	0.0
All ages	0	0.1	0	0.0	0.0	0.01	0	0.1	0	0.1
Total	0	0.1	0	0.0	0.0	0.01	0	0.1	0	0.1

For epidemiological sources see Shibuya and Murray 1996c. For the methods used to estimate and project incidence, prevalence, and deaths see Murray and Lopez 1996a. See explanatory notes for definitions and caveats.

Table 202 — **Cuadro 202** — **Tableau 202**
Oesophageal atresia — **Atresia esofágica** — **Atrésie de l'oesophage**

Cases — Casos — Cas

Table 202g   LAC - ALC - ALC — Oesophageal atresia - Cases

Age group (years)	Incidence 1990 Number ('000s)	Rate (per 100 000)	Prevalence 1990 Number ('000s)	Rate (per 100 000)	Avg. age at onset (years)	Average duration (years)	Deaths 1990 Number ('000s)	Rate (per 100 000)	Deaths 2000 (Projected) Number ('000s)	Rate (per 100 000)
Males										
0-4	0	1.1	0	0.0	0.0	0.01	0	0.6	0	0.6
5-14	0	0.0	0	0.0	-	-	0	0.0	0	0.0
15-44	0	0.0	0	0.0	-	-	0	0.0	0	0.0
45-59	0	0.0	0	0.0	-	-	0	0.0	0	0.0
60+	0	0.0	0	0.0	-	-	0	0.0	0	0.0
All ages	0	0.1	0	0.0	0.0	0.01	0	0.1	0	0.1
Females										
0-4	0	1.1	0	0.0	0.0	0.01	0	0.6	0	0.7
5-14	0	0.0	0	0.0	-	-	0	0.0	0	0.0
15-44	0	0.0	0	0.0	-	-	0	0.0	0	0.0
45-59	0	0.0	0	0.0	-	-	0	0.0	0	0.0
60+	0	0.0	0	0.0	-	-	0	0.0	0	0.0
All ages	0	0.1	0	0.0	0.0	0.01	0	0.1	0	0.1
Total	1	0.1	0	0.0	0.0	0.01	0	0.1	0	0.1

Table 202h   MEC - AOM - CMO — Oesophageal atresia - Cases

Age group (years)	Incidence 1990 Number ('000s)	Rate (per 100 000)	Prevalence 1990 Number ('000s)	Rate (per 100 000)	Avg. age at onset (years)	Average duration (years)	Deaths 1990 Number ('000s)	Rate (per 100 000)	Deaths 2000 (Projected) Number ('000s)	Rate (per 100 000)
Males										
0-4	1	1.7	0	0.0	0.0	0.01	0	1.0	1	1.1
5-14	0	0.0	0	0.0	-	-	0	0.0	0	0.0
15-44	0	0.0	0	0.0	-	-	0	0.0	0	0.0
45-59	0	0.0	0	0.0	-	-	0	0.0	0	0.0
60+	0	0.0	0	0.0	-	-	0	0.0	0	0.0
All ages	1	0.3	0	0.0	0.0	0.01	0	0.2	1	0.2
Females										
0-4	0	1.0	0	0.0	0.0	0.01	0	0.5	0	0.6
5-14	0	0.0	0	0.0	-	-	0	0.0	0	0.0
15-44	0	0.0	0	0.0	-	-	0	0.0	0	0.0
45-59	0	0.0	0	0.0	-	-	0	0.0	0	0.0
60+	0	0.0	0	0.0	-	-	0	0.0	0	0.0
All ages	0	0.2	0	0.0	0.0	0.01	0	0.1	0	0.1
Total	1	0.2	0	0.0	0.0	0.01	1	0.1	1	0.1

Table 202i   World - Mundo - Monde — Oesophageal atresia - Cases

Age group (years)	Incidence 1990 Number ('000s)	Rate (per 100 000)	Prevalence 1990 Number ('000s)	Rate (per 100 000)	Avg. age at onset (years)	Average duration (years)	Deaths 1990 Number ('000s)	Rate (per 100 000)	Deaths 2000 (Projected) Number ('000s)	Rate (per 100 000)
Males										
0-4	3	1.1	0	0.0	0.0	0.01	2	0.5	2	0.6
5-14	0	0.0	0	0.0	-	-	0	0.0	0	0.0
15-44	0	0.0	0	0.0	-	-	0	0.0	0	0.0
45-59	0	0.0	0	0.0	-	-	0	0.0	0	0.0
60+	0	0.0	0	0.0	-	-	0	0.0	0	0.0
All ages	3	0.1	0	0.0	0.0	0.01	2	0.1	2	0.1
Females										
0-4	3	0.9	0	0.0	0.0	0.01	1	0.4	2	0.5
5-14	0	0.0	0	0.0	-	-	0	0.0	0	0.0
15-44	0	0.0	0	0.0	-	-	0	0.0	0	0.0
45-59	0	0.0	0	0.0	-	-	0	0.0	0	0.0
60+	0	0.0	0	0.0	-	-	0	0.0	0	0.0
All ages	3	0.1	0	0.0	0.0	0.01	1	0.1	2	0.1
Total	6	0.1	0	0.0	0.0	0.01	3	0.1	4	0.1

For epidemiological sources see Shibuya and Murray 1996c. For the methods used to estimate and project incidence, prevalence, and deaths see Murray and Lopez 1996a. See explanatory notes for definitions and caveats.

Table 203
Renal agenesis

Cuadro 203
Agenesia renal

Tableau 203
Agénésie rénale

Cases

Casos

Cas

Table 203a   EME - PEMC - EMBE   Renal agenesis - Cases

Age group (years)	Incidence 1990 Number ('000s)	Rate (per 100 000)	Prevalence 1990 Number ('000s)	Rate (per 100 000)	Avg. age at onset (years)	Average duration (years)	Deaths 1990 Number ('000s)	Rate (per 100 000)	Deaths 2000 (Projected) Number ('000s)	Rate (per 100 000)
Males										
0-4	1	3.6	0	0	0.0	0.01	1	3.6	1	4.3
5-14	0	0.0	0	0	-	-	0	0.0	0	0.0
15-44	0	0.0	0	0	-	-	0	0.0	0	0.0
45-59	0	0.0	0	0	-	-	0	0.0	0	0.0
60+	0	0.0	0	0	-	-	0	0.0	0	0.0
All ages	1	0.2	0	0	0.0	0.01	1	0.2	1	0.3
Females										
0-4	1	3.6	0	0	0.0	0.01	1	3.6	1	3.7
5-14	0	0.0	0	0	-	-	0	0.0	0	0.0
15-44	0	0.0	0	0	-	-	0	0.0	0	0.0
45-59	0	0.0	0	0	-	-	0	0.0	0	0.0
60+	0	0.0	0	0	-	-	0	0.0	0	0.0
All ages	1	0.2	0	0	0.0	0.01	1	0.2	1	0.2
Total	2	0.2	0	0	0.0	0.01	2	0.2	2	0.3

Table 203b   FSE - PEAS - AESE   Renal agenesis - Cases

Age group (years)	Incidence 1990 Number ('000s)	Rate (per 100 000)	Prevalence 1990 Number ('000s)	Rate (per 100 000)	Avg. age at onset (years)	Average duration (years)	Deaths 1990 Number ('000s)	Rate (per 100 000)	Deaths 2000 (Projected) Number ('000s)	Rate (per 100 000)
Males										
0-4	0	1.6	0	0	0.0	0.01	0	1.6	0	2.6
5-14	0	0.0	0	0	-	-	0	0.0	0	0.0
15-44	0	0.0	0	0	-	-	0	0.0	0	0.0
45-59	0	0.0	0	0	-	-	0	0.0	0	0.0
60+	0	0.0	0	0	-	-	0	0.0	0	0.0
All ages	0	0.1	0	0	0.0	0.01	0	0.1	0	0.2
Females										
0-4	0	1.7	0	0	0.0	0.01	0	1.7	0	2.4
5-14	0	0.0	0	0	-	-	0	0.0	0	0.0
15-44	0	0.0	0	0	-	-	0	0.0	0	0.0
45-59	0	0.0	0	0	-	-	0	0.0	0	0.0
60+	0	0.0	0	0	-	-	0	0.0	0	0.0
All ages	0	0.1	0	0	0.0	0.01	0	0.1	0	0.2
Total	0	0.1	0	0	0.0	0.01	0	0.1	1	0.2

Table 203c   India - India - Inde   Renal agenesis - Cases

Age group (years)	Incidence 1990 Number ('000s)	Rate (per 100 000)	Prevalence 1990 Number ('000s)	Rate (per 100 000)	Avg. age at onset (years)	Average duration (years)	Deaths 1990 Number ('000s)	Rate (per 100 000)	Deaths 2000 (Projected) Number ('000s)	Rate (per 100 000)
Males										
0-4	1	2.1	0	0	0.0	0.01	1	2.1	1	2.6
5-14	0	0.0	0	0	-	-	0	0.0	0	0.0
15-44	0	0.0	0	0	-	-	0	0.0	0	0.0
45-59	0	0.0	0	0	-	-	0	0.0	0	0.0
60+	0	0.0	0	0	-	-	0	0.0	0	0.0
All ages	1	0.3	0	0	0.0	0.01	1	0.3	1	0.3
Females										
0-4	1	2.1	0	0	0.0	0.01	1	2.1	1	2.6
5-14	0	0.0	0	0	-	-	0	0.0	0	0.0
15-44	0	0.0	0	0	-	-	0	0.0	0	0.0
45-59	0	0.0	0	0	-	-	0	0.0	0	0.0
60+	0	0.0	0	0	-	-	0	0.0	0	0.0
All ages	1	0.3	0	0	0.0	0.01	1	0.3	1	0.3
Total	2	0.3	0	0	0.0	0.01	2	0.3	3	0.3

For epidemiological sources see Shibuya and Murray 1996c. For the methods used to estimate and project incidence, prevalence, and deaths see Murray and Lopez 1996a. See explanatory notes for definitions and caveats.

Table 203
Renal agenesis

Cuadro 203
Agenesia renal

Tableau 203
Agénésie rénale

Cases

Casos

Cas

Table 203d — China - China - Chine — Renal agenesis - Cases

Age group (years)	Incidence 1990 Number ('000s)	Rate (per 100 000)	Prevalence 1990 Number ('000s)	Rate (per 100 000)	Avg. age at onset (years)	Average duration (years)	Deaths 1990 Number ('000s)	Rate (per 100 000)	Deaths 2000 (Projected) Number ('000s)	Rate (per 100 000)
Males										
0-4	0	0.4	0	0	0.0	0.01	0	0.4	0	0.5
5-14	0	0.0	0	0	-	-	0	0.0	0	0.0
15-44	0	0.0	0	0	-	-	0	0.0	0	0.0
45-59	0	0.0	0	0	-	-	0	0.0	0	0.0
60+	0	0.0	0	0	-	-	0	0.0	0	0.0
All ages	0	0.0	0	0	0.0	0.01	0	0.0	0	0.0
Females										
0-4	0	0.4	0	0	0.0	0.01	0	0.4	0	0.5
5-14	0	0.0	0	0	-	-	0	0.0	0	0.0
15-44	0	0.0	0	0	-	-	0	0.0	0	0.0
45-59	0	0.0	0	0	-	-	0	0.0	0	0.0
60+	0	0.0	0	0	-	-	0	0.0	0	0.0
All ages	0	0.0	0	0	0.0	0.01	0	0.0	0	0.0
Total	1	0.0	0	0	0.0	0.01	1	0.0	1	0.0

Table 203e — OAI - OPAI - APAI — Renal agenesis - Cases

Age group (years)	Incidence 1990 Number ('000s)	Rate (per 100 000)	Prevalence 1990 Number ('000s)	Rate (per 100 000)	Avg. age at onset (years)	Average duration (years)	Deaths 1990 Number ('000s)	Rate (per 100 000)	Deaths 2000 (Projected) Number ('000s)	Rate (per 100 000)
Males										
0-4	1	2.0	0	0	0.0	0.01	1	2.0	1	2.2
5-14	0	0.0	0	0	-	-	0	0.0	0	0.0
15-44	0	0.0	0	0	-	-	0	0.0	0	0.0
45-59	0	0.0	0	0	-	-	0	0.0	0	0.0
60+	0	0.0	0	0	-	-	0	0.0	0	0.0
All ages	1	0.3	0	0	0.0	0.01	1	0.3	1	0.2
Females										
0-4	1	2.0	0	0	0.0	0.01	1	2.0	1	2.2
5-14	0	0.0	0	0	-	-	0	0.0	0	0.0
15-44	0	0.0	0	0	-	-	0	0.0	0	0.0
45-59	0	0.0	0	0	-	-	0	0.0	0	0.0
60+	0	0.0	0	0	-	-	0	0.0	0	0.0
All ages	1	0.2	0	0	0.0	0.01	1	0.2	1	0.2
Total	2	0.3	0	0	0.0	0.01	2	0.3	2	0.2

Table 203f — SSA - ASS - ASS — Renal agenesis - Cases

Age group (years)	Incidence 1990 Number ('000s)	Rate (per 100 000)	Prevalence 1990 Number ('000s)	Rate (per 100 000)	Avg. age at onset (years)	Average duration (years)	Deaths 1990 Number ('000s)	Rate (per 100 000)	Deaths 2000 (Projected) Number ('000s)	Rate (per 100 000)
Males										
0-4	1	2.2	0	0	0.0	0.01	1	2.2	2	2.5
5-14	0	0.0	0	0	-	-	0	0.0	0	0.0
15-44	0	0.0	0	0	-	-	0	0.0	0	0.0
45-59	0	0.0	0	0	-	-	0	0.0	0	0.0
60+	0	0.0	0	0	-	-	0	0.0	0	0.0
All ages	1	0.4	0	0	0.0	0.01	1	0.4	2	0.5
Females										
0-4	1	2.2	0	0	0.0	0.01	1	2.2	2	2.5
5-14	0	0.0	0	0	-	-	0	0.0	0	0.0
15-44	0	0.0	0	0	-	-	0	0.0	0	0.0
45-59	0	0.0	0	0	-	-	0	0.0	0	0.0
60+	0	0.0	0	0	-	-	0	0.0	0	0.0
All ages	1	0.4	0	0	0.0	0.01	1	0.4	2	0.5
Total	2	0.4	0	0	0.0	0.01	2	0.4	3	0.5

For epidemiological sources see Shibuya and Murray 1996c. For the methods used to estimate and project incidence, prevalence, and deaths see Murray and Lopez 1996a. See explanatory notes for definitions and caveats.

Table 203	Cuadro 203	Tableau 203
Renal agenesis	Agenesia renal	Agénésie rénale
Cases	Casos	Cas

Table 203g — LAC - ALC - ALC — Renal agenesis - Cases

Age group (years)	Incidence 1990 Number ('000s)	Rate (per 100 000)	Prevalence 1990 Number ('000s)	Rate (per 100 000)	Avg. age at onset (years)	Average duration (years)	Deaths 1990 Number ('000s)	Rate (per 100 000)	Deaths 2000 (Projected) Number ('000s)	Rate (per 100 000)
Males										
0-4	0	1.6	0	0	0.0	0.01	0	1.6	1	1.8
5-14	0	0.0	0	0	-	-	0	0.0	0	0.0
15-44	0	0.0	0	0	-	-	0	0.0	0	0.0
45-59	0	0.0	0	0	-	-	0	0.0	0	0.0
60+	0	0.0	0	0	-	-	0	0.0	0	0.0
All ages	0	0.2	0	0	0.0	0.01	0	0.2	1	0.2
Females										
0-4	0	1.6	0	0	0.0	0.01	0	1.6	0	1.8
5-14	0	0.0	0	0	-	-	0	0.0	0	0.0
15-44	0	0.0	0	0	-	-	0	0.0	0	0.0
45-59	0	0.0	0	0	-	-	0	0.0	0	0.0
60+	0	0.0	0	0	-	-	0	0.0	0	0.0
All ages	0	0.2	0	0	0.0	0.01	0	0.2	0	0.2
Total	1	0.2	0	0	0.0	0.01	1	0.2	1	0.2

Table 203h — MEC - AOM - CMO — Renal agenesis - Cases

Age group (years)	Incidence 1990 Number ('000s)	Rate (per 100 000)	Prevalence 1990 Number ('000s)	Rate (per 100 000)	Avg. age at onset (years)	Average duration (years)	Deaths 1990 Number ('000s)	Rate (per 100 000)	Deaths 2000 (Projected) Number ('000s)	Rate (per 100 000)
Males										
0-4	1	2.1	0	0	0.0	0.01	1	2.1	1	2.4
5-14	0	0.0	0	0	-	-	0	0.0	0	0.0
15-44	0	0.0	0	0	-	-	0	0.0	0	0.0
45-59	0	0.0	0	0	-	-	0	0.0	0	0.0
60+	0	0.0	0	0	-	-	0	0.0	0	0.0
All ages	1	0.3	0	0	0.0	0.01	1	0.3	1	0.4
Females										
0-4	1	2.1	0	0	0.0	0.01	1	2.1	1	2.4
5-14	0	0.0	0	0	-	-	0	0.0	0	0.0
15-44	0	0.0	0	0	-	-	0	0.0	0	0.0
45-59	0	0.0	0	0	-	-	0	0.0	0	0.0
60+	0	0.0	0	0	-	-	0	0.0	0	0.0
All ages	1	0.3	0	0	0.0	0.01	1	0.3	1	0.4
Total	2	0.3	0	0	0.0	0.01	2	0.3	2	0.4

Table 203i — World - Mundo - Monde — Renal agenesis - Cases

Age group (years)	Incidence 1990 Number ('000s)	Rate (per 100 000)	Prevalence 1990 Number ('000s)	Rate (per 100 000)	Avg. age at onset (years)	Average duration (years)	Deaths 1990 Number ('000s)	Rate (per 100 000)	Deaths 2000 (Projected) Number ('000s)	Rate (per 100 000)
Males										
0-4	6	1.8	0	0	0.0	0.01	6	1.8	7	2.1
5-14	0	0.0	0	0	-	-	0	0.0	0	0.0
15-44	0	0.0	0	0	-	-	0	0.0	0	0.0
45-59	0	0.0	0	0	-	-	0	0.0	0	0.0
60+	0	0.0	0	0	-	-	0	0.0	0	0.0
All ages	6	0.2	0	0	0.0	0.01	6	0.2	7	0.2
Females										
0-4	6	1.9	0	0	0.0	0.01	6	1.9	7	2.1
5-14	0	0.0	0	0	-	-	0	0.0	0	0.0
15-44	0	0.0	0	0	-	-	0	0.0	0	0.0
45-59	0	0.0	0	0	-	-	0	0.0	0	0.0
60+	0	0.0	0	0	-	-	0	0.0	0	0.0
All ages	6	0.2	0	0	0.0	0.01	6	0.2	7	0.2
Total	12	0.2	0	0	0.0	0.01	12	0.2	14	0.2

For epidemiological sources see Shibuya and Murray 1996c. For the methods used to estimate and project incidence, prevalence, and deaths see Murray and Lopez 1996a. See explanatory notes for definitions and caveats.

Table 204
Down syndrome

Cuadro 204
Sindrome de Down

Tableau 204
Syndrome de Down

Cases | Casos | Cas

Table 204a   EME - PEMC - EMBE   Down syndrome - Cases

Age group (years)	Incidence 1990 Number ('000s)	Rate (per 100 000)	Prevalence 1990 Number ('000s)	Rate (per 100 000)	Avg. age at onset (years)	Average duration (years)	Deaths 1990 Number ('000s)	Rate (per 100 000)	Deaths 2000 (Projected) Number ('000s)	Rate (per 100 000)
Males										
0-4	6	23.7	25	94	0.0	68.1	1	2.9	1	3.6
5-14	0	0.0	52	98	-	-	0	0.1	0	0.2
15-44	0	0.0	178	97	-	-	0	0.0	0	0.1
45-59	0	0.0	61	92	-	-	0	0.5	0	0.5
60+	0	0.0	50	82	-	-	0	0.7	1	0.9
All ages	6	1.6	366	94	0.0	68.1	2	0.4	2	0.5
Females										
0-4	5	18.8	19	75	0.0	73.8	1	2.3	1	2.4
5-14	0	0.0	39	78	-	-	0	0.1	0	0.1
15-44	0	0.0	137	76	-	-	0	0.0	0	0.0
45-59	0	0.0	49	72	-	-	0	0.5	0	0.4
60+	0	0.0	53	63	-	-	0	0.4	1	0.6
All ages	5	1.2	297	73	0.0	73.8	1	0.3	2	0.4
Total	11	1.4	663	83	0.0	70.5	3	0.4	4	0.5

Table 204b   FSE - PEAS - AESE   Down syndrome - Cases

Age group (years)	Incidence 1990 Number ('000s)	Rate (per 100 000)	Prevalence 1990 Number ('000s)	Rate (per 100 000)	Avg. age at onset (years)	Average duration (years)	Deaths 1990 Number ('000s)	Rate (per 100 000)	Deaths 2000 (Projected) Number ('000s)	Rate (per 100 000)
Males										
0-4	2	16.4	9	65	0.0	62.8	0	2.6	1	4.2
5-14	0	0.0	18	67	-	-	0	0.3	0	0.4
15-44	0	0.0	49	64	-	-	0	0.1	0	0.1
45-59	0	0.0	16	60	-	-	0	0.6	0	0.6
60+	0	0.0	11	54	-	-	0	0.2	0	0.2
All ages	2	1.4	104	63	0.0	62.8	1	0.4	1	0.5
Females										
0-4	2	12.9	7	51	0.0	70.7	0	2.0	0	2.9
5-14	0	0.0	14	53	-	-	0	0.1	0	0.1
15-44	0	0.0	39	52	-	-	0	0.0	0	0.1
45-59	0	0.0	14	48	-	-	0	0.6	0	0.5
60+	0	0.0	15	41	-	-	0	0.1	0	0.1
All ages	2	0.9	89	49	0.0	70.7	1	0.3	1	0.3
Total	4	1.1	193	56	0.0	66.2	1	0.4	2	0.4

Table 204c   India - India - Inde   Down syndrome - Cases

Age group (years)	Incidence 1990 Number ('000s)	Rate (per 100 000)	Prevalence 1990 Number ('000s)	Rate (per 100 000)	Avg. age at onset (years)	Average duration (years)	Deaths 1990 Number ('000s)	Rate (per 100 000)	Deaths 2000 (Projected) Number ('000s)	Rate (per 100 000)
Males										
0-4	23	38.3	77	146	0.0	58.8	5	8.3	6	10.5
5-14	0	0.0	133	131	-	-	2	1.5	1	1.2
15-44	0	0.0	211	105	-	-	3	1.3	3	1.1
45-59	0	0.0	42	88	-	-	0	0.0	0	0.0
60+	0	0.0	26	88	-	-	0	0.0	0	0.0
All ages	23	5.2	489	113	0.0	58.8	9	2.1	10	1.9
Females										
0-4	17	30.6	60	107	0.0	59.7	3	5.7	4	7.1
5-14	0	0.0	102	107	-	-	1	1.5	1	1.2
15-44	0	0.0	152	83	-	-	2	1.1	2	0.8
45-59	0	0.0	31	67	-	-	0	0.0	0	0.0
60+	0	0.0	19	67	-	-	0	0.0	0	0.0
All ages	17	4.2	365	89	0.0	59.7	7	1.7	7	1.5
Total	40	4.7	854	101	0.0	59.2	16	1.9	17	1.7

For epidemiological sources see Shibuya and Murray 1996c. For the methods used to estimate and project incidence, prevalence, and deaths see Murray and Lopez 1996a. See explanatory notes for definitions and caveats.

Table 204
Down syndrome

Cuadro 204
Sindrome de Down

Tableau 204
Syndrome de Down

Cases

Casos

Cas

Table 204d — China - China - Chine — Down syndrome - Cases

Age group (years)	Incidence 1990 Number ('000s)	Rate (per 100 000)	Prevalence 1990 Number ('000s)	Rate (per 100 000)	Avg. age at onset (years)	Average duration (years)	Deaths 1990 Number ('000s)	Rate (per 100 000)	Deaths 2000 (Projected) Number ('000s)	Rate (per 100 000)
Males										
0-4	21	35.3	75	124	0.0	64.1	3	4.6	3	5.3
5-14	0	0.0	124	128	-	-	1	1.0	1	0.7
15-44	0	0.0	350	114	-	-	2	0.6	1	0.4
45-59	0	0.0	76	104	-	-	0	0.2	0	0.2
60+	0	0.0	50	102	-	-	0	0.0	0	0.0
All ages	21	3.6	675	115	0.0	64.1	6	1.0	6	0.9
Females										
0-4	17	29.1	57	99	0.0	66.9	3	4.7	3	5.4
5-14	0	0.0	89	98	-	-	1	1.3	1	0.9
15-44	0	0.0	222	78	-	-	3	0.9	2	0.6
45-59	0	0.0	41	64	-	-	0	0.3	0	0.3
60+	0	0.0	32	62	-	-	0	0.0	0	0.0
All ages	17	3.1	441	80	0.0	66.9	7	1.2	6	1.0
Total	38	3.4	1 116	98	0.0	65.4	12	1.1	12	0.9

Table 204e — OAI - OPAI - APAI — Down syndrome - Cases

Age group (years)	Incidence 1990 Number ('000s)	Rate (per 100 000)	Prevalence 1990 Number ('000s)	Rate (per 100 000)	Avg. age at onset (years)	Average duration (years)	Deaths 1990 Number ('000s)	Rate (per 100 000)	Deaths 2000 (Projected) Number ('000s)	Rate (per 100 000)
Males										
0-4	14	32.1	53	122	0.0	60.6	3	5.8	3	6.5
5-14	0	0.0	104	124	-	-	1	0.7	0	0.6
15-44	0	0.0	180	112	-	-	1	0.5	1	0.5
45-59	0	0.0	35	103	-	-	0	0.0	0	0.0
60+	0	0.0	21	103	-	-	0	0.0	0	0.0
All ages	14	4.1	393	115	0.0	60.6	4	1.2	4	1.1
Females										
0-4	11	25.8	42	99	0.0	64.5	1	3.1	1	3.4
5-14	0	0.0	82	102	-	-	0	0.5	0	0.5
15-44	0	0.0	149	93	-	-	1	0.3	0	0.2
45-59	0	0.0	31	88	-	-	0	0.0	0	0.0
60+	0	0.0	20	88	-	-	0	0.0	0	0.0
All ages	11	3.2	324	95	0.0	64.5	2	0.7	2	0.6
Total	25	3.6	717	105	0.0	62.3	6	0.9	7	0.8

Table 204f — SSA - ASS - ASS — Down syndrome - Cases

Age group (years)	Incidence 1990 Number ('000s)	Rate (per 100 000)	Prevalence 1990 Number ('000s)	Rate (per 100 000)	Avg. age at onset (years)	Average duration (years)	Deaths 1990 Number ('000s)	Rate (per 100 000)	Deaths 2000 (Projected) Number ('000s)	Rate (per 100 000)
Males										
0-4	19	40.2	70	147	0.0	51.1	1	3.1	2	3.6
5-14	0	0.0	110	157	-	-	1	1.1	1	0.9
15-44	0	0.0	137	132	-	-	1	1.1	1	1.0
45-59	0	0.0	23	114	-	-	0	0.0	0	0.0
60+	0	0.0	12	114	-	-	0	0.0	0	0.0
All ages	19	7.6	352	140	0.0	51.1	3	1.4	5	1.4
Females										
0-4	16	33.2	58	123	0.0	54.1	1	2.5	2	2.9
5-14	0	0.0	91	130	-	-	1	1.1	1	0.9
15-44	0	0.0	123	116	-	-	1	0.6	1	0.4
45-59	0	0.0	24	107	-	-	0	0.1	0	0.0
60+	0	0.0	14	107	-	-	0	0.0	0	0.0
All ages	16	6.1	309	120	0.0	54.1	3	1.0	3	0.9
Total	35	6.8	661	130	0.0	52.5	6	1.2	8	1.1

For epidemiological sources see Shibuya and Murray 1996c. For the methods used to estimate and project incidence, prevalence, and deaths see Murray and Lopez 1996a. See explanatory notes for definitions and caveats.

Table 204	Cuadro 204	Tableau 204
Down syndrome	Sindrome de Down	Syndrome de Down
Cases	Casos	Cas

Table 204g LAC - ALC - ALC — Down syndrome - Cases

Age group (years)	Incidence 1990 Number ('000s)	Rate (per 100 000)	Prevalence 1990 Number ('000s)	Rate (per 100 000)	Avg. age at onset (years)	Average duration (years)	Deaths 1990 Number ('000s)	Rate (per 100 000)	Deaths 2000 (Projected) Number ('000s)	Rate (per 100 000)
Males										
0-4	9	32.9	35	123	0.0	63.4	1	5.0	2	5.4
5-14	0	0.0	66	126	-	-	0	0.7	0	0.6
15-44	0	0.0	124	119	-	-	0	0.2	0	0.2
45-59	0	0.0	25	111	-	-	0	0.6	0	0.5
60+	0	0.0	15	106	-	-	0	0.1	0	0.1
All ages	9	4.3	265	120	0.0	63.4	2	1.0	2	0.9
Females										
0-4	7	26.3	27	99	0.0	67.3	1	4.1	1	4.5
5-14	0	0.0	51	101	-	-	0	0.6	0	0.5
15-44	0	0.0	97	93	-	-	0	0.3	0	0.2
45-59	0	0.0	19	82	-	-	0	0.7	0	0.6
60+	0	0.0	13	77	-	-	0	0.0	0	0.0
All ages	7	3.3	207	93	0.0	67.3	2	0.9	2	0.8
Total	17	3.8	473	106	0.0	65.1	4	0.9	4	0.8

Table 204h MEC - AOM - CMO — Down syndrome - Cases

Age group (years)	Incidence 1990 Number ('000s)	Rate (per 100 000)	Prevalence 1990 Number ('000s)	Rate (per 100 000)	Avg. age at onset (years)	Average duration (years)	Deaths 1990 Number ('000s)	Rate (per 100 000)	Deaths 2000 (Projected) Number ('000s)	Rate (per 100 000)
Males										
0-4	14	34.3	49	120	0.0	61.5	3	6.3	4	7.1
5-14	0	0.0	78	120	-	-	1	1.0	1	0.9
15-44	0	0.0	116	102	-	-	1	0.9	1	0.8
45-59	0	0.0	20	89	-	-	0	0.0	0	0.0
60+	0	0.0	12	89	-	-	0	0.0	0	0.0
All ages	14	5.5	276	107	0.0	61.5	4	1.7	5	1.6
Females										
0-4	14	34.4	39	98	0.0	64.1	2	4.6	2	5.1
5-14	0	0.0	60	97	-	-	1	1.3	1	1.1
15-44	0	0.0	84	78	-	-	1	0.8	1	0.6
45-59	0	0.0	15	67	-	-	0	0.0	0	0.0
60+	0	0.0	10	67	-	-	0	0.0	0	0.0
All ages	14	5.5	208	84	0.0	64.1	4	1.4	4	1.3
Total	28	5.5	484	96	0.0	62.8	8	1.6	10	1.5

Table 204i World - Mundo - Monde — Down syndrome - Cases

Age group (years)	Incidence 1990 Number ('000s)	Rate (per 100 000)	Prevalence 1990 Number ('000s)	Rate (per 100 000)	Avg. age at onset (years)	Average duration (years)	Deaths 1990 Number ('000s)	Rate (per 100 000)	Deaths 2000 (Projected) Number ('000s)	Rate (per 100 000)
Males										
0-4	109	34.1	394	123	0.0	60.1	17	5.3	21	6.1
5-14	0	0.0	686	125	-	-	5	0.9	5	0.8
15-44	0	0.0	1 345	108	-	-	8	0.6	8	0.6
45-59	0	0.0	298	95	-	-	1	0.3	1	0.2
60+	0	0.0	197	90	-	-	1	0.2	1	0.2
All ages	109	4.1	2 921	110	0.0	60.1	31	1.2	36	1.1
Females										
0-4	88	28.5	309	100	0.0	63.0	12	4.0	15	4.5
5-14	0	0.0	528	100	-	-	5	1.0	5	0.8
15-44	0	0.0	1 003	84	-	-	7	0.6	6	0.4
45-59	0	0.0	224	72	-	-	1	0.3	1	0.2
60+	0	0.0	176	66	-	-	0	0.1	1	0.2
All ages	88	3.4	2 240	86	0.0	63.0	26	1.0	27	0.9
Total	197	3.7	5 161	98	0.0	61.4	57	1.1	63	1.0

For epidemiological sources see Shibuya and Murray 1996c. For the methods used to estimate and project incidence, prevalence, and deaths see Murray and Lopez 1996a. See explanatory notes for definitions and caveats.

Table 205
Congenital heart anomalies
Cases

Cuadro 205
Anomalías congénitas del corazón
Casos

Tableau 205
Anomalies congénitales du coeur
Cas

Table 205a — EME - PEMC - EMBE — Congenital heart anomalies - Cases

Age group (years)	Incidence 1990 Number ('000s)	Rate (per 100 000)	Prevalence 1990 Number ('000s)	Rate (per 100 000)	Avg. age at onset (years)	Average duration (years)	Deaths 1990 Number ('000s)	Rate (per 100 000)	Deaths 2000 (Projected) Number ('000s)	Rate (per 100 000)
Males										
0-4	32	119.9	114	434	0.0	68.1	6	21.4	7	25.7
5-14	0	0.0	246	462	-	-	0	0.8	0	0.9
15-44	0	0.0	824	448	-	-	1	0.7	2	0.9
45-59	0	0.0	284	430	-	-	0	0.7	0	0.6
60+	0	0.0	249	411	-	-	1	1.2	1	1.5
All ages	32	8.1	1 718	440	0.0	68.1	9	2.2	11	2.7
Females										
0-4	30	119.9	113	452	0.0	73.8	4	17.9	5	18.6
5-14	0	0.0	245	484	-	-	0	0.7	0	0.9
15-44	0	0.0	851	475	-	-	1	0.5	1	0.6
45-59	0	0.0	315	464	-	-	0	0.6	0	0.4
60+	0	0.0	382	452	-	-	1	1.1	2	1.5
All ages	30	7.4	1 907	468	0.0	73.8	7	1.7	8	2.0
Total	62	7.7	3 625	454	0.0	70.9	16	2.0	19	2.3

Table 205b — FSE - PEAS - AESE — Congenital heart anomalies - Cases

Age group (years)	Incidence 1990 Number ('000s)	Rate (per 100 000)	Prevalence 1990 Number ('000s)	Rate (per 100 000)	Avg. age at onset (years)	Average duration (years)	Deaths 1990 Number ('000s)	Rate (per 100 000)	Deaths 2000 (Projected) Number ('000s)	Rate (per 100 000)
Males										
0-4	17	120.1	53	387	0.0	62.8	5	34.8	7	55.9
5-14	0	0.0	111	407	-	-	0	1.0	0	1.2
15-44	0	0.0	302	396	-	-	1	0.9	1	1.0
45-59	0	0.0	103	382	-	-	0	0.4	0	0.4
60+	0	0.0	78	371	-	-	0	0.4	0	0.4
All ages	17	10.0	647	392	0.0	62.8	6	3.6	8	4.9
Females										
0-4	16	119.3	54	412	0.0	70.7	4	29.7	5	41.9
5-14	0	0.0	115	436	-	-	0	0.9	0	1.4
15-44	0	0.0	320	427	-	-	0	0.5	0	0.6
45-59	0	0.0	125	415	-	-	0	0.3	0	0.3
60+	0	0.0	149	409	-	-	0	0.4	0	0.3
All ages	16	8.7	763	422	0.0	70.7	5	2.6	6	3.3
Total	32	9.3	1 410	407	0.0	66.6	11	3.1	15	4.1

Table 205c — India - India - Inde — Congenital heart anomalies - Cases

Age group (years)	Incidence 1990 Number ('000s)	Rate (per 100 000)	Prevalence 1990 Number ('000s)	Rate (per 100 000)	Avg. age at onset (years)	Average duration (years)	Deaths 1990 Number ('000s)	Rate (per 100 000)	Deaths 2000 (Projected) Number ('000s)	Rate (per 100 000)
Males										
0-4	74	125	171	286	0.0	58.8	24	39.8	28	50.2
5-14	0	0	282	277	-	-	3	2.5	2	2.0
15-44	0	0	524	261	-	-	2	0.9	2	0.8
45-59	0	0	114	239	-	-	1	2.4	1	2.0
60+	0	0	63	211	-	-	1	3.3	1	3.0
All ages	74	17	1 153	262	0.0	58.8	30	6.9	35	6.8
Females										
0-4	71	125	160	282	0.0	59.7	19	34.4	23	43.1
5-14	0	0	258	271	-	-	3	3.3	3	2.6
15-44	0	0	464	253	-	-	2	1.1	2	0.8
45-59	0	0	108	235	-	-	1	3.1	1	2.6
60+	0	0	61	212	-	-	1	4.1	2	3.9
All ages	71	17	1 051	256	0.0	59.7	27	6.6	31	6.4
Total	145	17	2 205	260	0.0	59.2	57	6.8	66	6.6

For epidemiological sources see Shibuya and Murray 1996c. For the methods used to estimate and project incidence, prevalence, and deaths see Murray and Lopez 1996a. See explanatory notes for definitions and caveats.

Table 205
Congenital heart anomalies

Cases

Cuadro 205
Anomalías congénitas del corazón

Casos

Tableau 205
Anomalies congénitales du coeur

Cas

Table 205d   China - China - Chine   Congenital heart anomalies - Cases

Age group (years)	Incidence 1990 Number ('000s)	Rate (per 100 000)	Prevalence 1990 Number ('000s)	Rate (per 100 000)	Avg. age at onset (years)	Average duration (years)	Deaths 1990 Number ('000s)	Rate (per 100 000)	Deaths 2000 (Projected) Number ('000s)	Rate (per 100 000)
Males										
0-4	79	132	251	417	0.0	64.1	11	18.6	13	21.6
5-14	0	0	429	443	-	-	2	2.1	2	1.5
15-44	0	0	1 314	429	-	-	3	1.0	2	0.8
45-59	0	0	300	413	-	-	0	0.2	0	0.2
60+	0	0	196	400	-	-	0	0.0	0	0.0
All ages	79	14	2 490	426	0.0	64.1	16	2.8	17	2.6
Females										
0-4	77	133	251	433	0.0	66.9	7	11.7	8	13.5
5-14	0	0	420	464	-	-	2	1.9	2	1.4
15-44	0	0	1 284	452	-	-	4	1.5	3	1.0
45-59	0	0	282	438	-	-	0	0.2	0	0.2
60+	0	0	222	429	-	-	0	0.0	0	0.0
All ages	77	14	2 459	448	0.0	66.9	13	2.4	12	1.9
Total	157	14	4 949	437	0.0	65.5	29	2.6	29	2.3

Table 205e   OAI - OPAI - APAI   Congenital heart anomalies - Cases

Age group (years)	Incidence 1990 Number ('000s)	Rate (per 100 000)	Prevalence 1990 Number ('000s)	Rate (per 100 000)	Avg. age at onset (years)	Average duration (years)	Deaths 1990 Number ('000s)	Rate (per 100 000)	Deaths 2000 (Projected) Number ('000s)	Rate (per 100 000)
Males										
0-4	52	120	144	330	0.0	60.6	14	31.1	15	34.5
5-14	0	0	273	325	-	-	1	1.7	1	1.5
15-44	0	0	492	306	-	-	1	0.8	1	0.7
45-59	0	0	95	279	-	-	1	1.8	1	1.6
60+	0	0	52	258	-	-	1	2.6	1	2.3
All ages	52	15	1 056	308	0.0	60.6	17	5.1	19	4.8
Females										
0-4	50	120	142	339	0.0	64.5	8	19.8	9	21.4
5-14	0	0	274	341	-	-	1	1.6	1	1.3
15-44	0	0	516	323	-	-	1	0.6	1	0.5
45-59	0	0	104	298	-	-	1	1.8	1	1.5
60+	0	0	63	277	-	-	1	2.3	1	2.2
All ages	50	15	1 099	324	0.0	64.5	12	3.4	12	3.1
Total	103	15	2 155	316	0.0	62.5	29	4.3	32	3.9

Table 205f   SSA - ASS - ASS   Congenital heart anomalies - Cases

Age group (years)	Incidence 1990 Number ('000s)	Rate (per 100 000)	Prevalence 1990 Number ('000s)	Rate (per 100 000)	Avg. age at onset (years)	Average duration (years)	Deaths 1990 Number ('000s)	Rate (per 100 000)	Deaths 2000 (Projected) Number ('000s)	Rate (per 100 000)
Males										
0-4	62	131	127	268	0.0	51.1	7	15.0	11	17.2
5-14	0	0	177	253	-	-	1	1.9	2	1.6
15-44	0	0	236	228	-	-	1	0.8	1	0.7
45-59	0	0	37	183	-	-	1	2.8	1	2.5
60+	0	0	10	99	-	-	1	5.0	1	4.4
All ages	62	25	588	233	0.0	51.1	10	4.1	15	4.4
Females										
0-4	61	130	131	278	0.0	54.1	7	14.7	11	16.8
5-14	0	0	186	267	-	-	2	2.3	2	1.9
15-44	0	0	259	244	-	-	1	0.6	0	0.3
45-59	0	0	45	204	-	-	1	3.4	1	2.8
60+	0	0	15	118	-	-	1	4.2	1	4.3
All ages	61	24	636	247	0.0	54.1	10	4.0	15	4.2
Total	123	24	1 224	240	0.0	52.6	21	4.1	30	4.3

For epidemiological sources see Shibuya and Murray 1996c. For the methods used to estimate and project incidence, prevalence, and deaths see Murray and Lopez 1996a. See explanatory notes for definitions and caveats.

Table 205 Congenital heart anomalies Cases	Cuadro 205 Anomalías congénitas del corazón Casos	Tableau 205 Anomalies congénitales du coeur Cas

Table 205g LAC - ALC - ALC — Congenital heart anomalies - Cases

Age group (years)	Incidence 1990 Number ('000s)	Rate (per 100 000)	Prevalence 1990 Number ('000s)	Rate (per 100 000)	Avg. age at onset (years)	Average duration (years)	Deaths 1990 Number ('000s)	Rate (per 100 000)	Deaths 2000 (Projected) Number ('000s)	Rate (per 100 000)
Males										
0-4	35	123	118	409	0.0	63.4	6	21.8	7	23.7
5-14	0	0	225	431	-	-	1	1.7	1	1.5
15-44	0	0	431	413	-	-	0	0.4	1	0.4
45-59	0	0	86	387	-	-	0	0.4	0	0.3
60+	0	0	53	369	-	-	0	2.1	0	2.0
All ages	35	16	912	411	0.0	63.4	8	3.6	9	3.3
Females										
0-4	34	123	120	432	0.0	67.3	5	18.6	6	20.1
5-14	0	0	234	461	-	-	1	1.4	1	1.2
15-44	0	0	462	444	-	-	1	0.8	1	0.6
45-59	0	0	98	421	-	-	0	0.6	0	0.5
60+	0	0	69	408	-	-	0	1.7	0	1.7
All ages	34	15	982	441	0.0	67.3	7	3.2	8	2.9
Total	69	16	1 894	426	0.0	65.3	15	3.4	17	3.1

Table 205h MEC - AOM - CMO — Congenital heart anomalies - Cases

Age group (years)	Incidence 1990 Number ('000s)	Rate (per 100 000)	Prevalence 1990 Number ('000s)	Rate (per 100 000)	Avg. age at onset (years)	Average duration (years)	Deaths 1990 Number ('000s)	Rate (per 100 000)	Deaths 2000 (Projected) Number ('000s)	Rate (per 100 000)
Males										
0-4	53	128	138	334	0.0	61.5	13	31.6	18	35.6
5-14	0	0	221	338	-	-	1	2.1	2	1.8
15-44	0	0	363	319	-	-	1	0.9	1	0.8
45-59	0	0	65	292	-	-	1	2.5	1	2.3
60+	0	0	37	271	-	-	0	3.6	1	3.2
All ages	53	21	824	321	0.0	61.5	16	6.4	22	6.5
Females										
0-4	51	128	133	335	0.0	64.1	9	22.9	12	25.5
5-14	0	0	210	339	-	-	1	2.4	2	2.0
15-44	0	0	344	321	-	-	1	0.8	1	0.6
45-59	0	0	66	297	-	-	1	3.2	1	2.7
60+	0	0	43	277	-	-	1	3.9	1	3.4
All ages	51	21	796	323	0.0	64.1	13	5.2	16	5.0
Total	104	21	1 620	322	0.0	62.8	29	5.8	38	5.8

Table 205i World - Mundo - Monde — Congenital heart anomalies - Cases

Age group (years)	Incidence 1990 Number ('000s)	Rate (per 100 000)	Prevalence 1990 Number ('000s)	Rate (per 100 000)	Avg. age at onset (years)	Average duration (years)	Deaths 1990 Number ('000s)	Rate (per 100 000)	Deaths 2000 (Projected) Number ('000s)	Rate (per 100 000)
Males										
0-4	404	126	1 116	347	0.0	60.5	85	26.6	107	30.9
5-14	0	0	1 964	356	-	-	10	1.9	10	1.6
15-44	0	0	4 486	359	-	-	11	0.8	11	0.8
45-59	0	0	1 085	347	-	-	4	1.1	4	1.0
60+	0	0	737	337	-	-	4	1.7	5	1.7
All ages	404	15	9 389	354	0.0	60.5	113	4.3	137	4.4
Females										
0-4	391	126	1 104	357	0.0	63.6	64	20.8	78	23.7
5-14	0	0	1 943	370	-	-	10	2.0	10	1.7
15-44	0	0	4 500	375	-	-	11	0.9	9	0.7
45-59	0	0	1 144	368	-	-	4	1.4	5	1.1
60+	0	0	1 003	373	-	-	4	1.6	6	1.7
All ages	391	15	9 694	371	0.0	63.6	94	3.6	108	3.5
Total	795	15	19 083	362	0.0	62.1	207	3.9	245	4.0

For epidemiological sources see Shibuya and Murray 1996c. For the methods used to estimate and project incidence, prevalence, and deaths see Murray and Lopez 1996a. See explanatory notes for definitions and caveats.

Table 206 | **Cuadro 206** | **Tableau 206**
Spina bifida | **Espina bífida** | **Spina bifida**

Cases | Casos | Cas

Table 206a   EME - PEMC - EMBE   Spina bifida - Cases

Age group (years)	Incidence 1990 Number ('000s)	Rate (per 100 000)	Prevalence 1990 Number ('000s)	Rate (per 100 000)	Avg. age at onset (years)	Average duration (years)	Deaths 1990 Number ('000s)	Rate (per 100 000)	Deaths 2000 (Projected) Number ('000s)	Rate (per 100 000)
Males										
0-4	2	6.8	6	23	0.0	68.1	1	2.4	1	2.9
5-14	0	0.0	11	21	-	-	0	0.2	0	0.2
15-44	0	0.0	35	19	-	-	0	0.1	0	0.1
45-59	0	0.0	12	18	-	-	0	0.0	0	0.0
60+	0	0.0	11	18	-	-	0	0.0	0	0.0
All ages	2	0.5	75	19	0.0	68.1	1	0.2	1	0.3
Females										
0-4	3	10.7	10	39	0.0	73.8	1	3.0	1	3.2
5-14	0	0.0	19	37	-	-	0	0.1	0	0.2
15-44	0	0.0	63	35	-	-	0	0.1	0	0.1
45-59	0	0.0	23	34	-	-	0	0.1	0	0.1
60+	0	0.0	29	34	-	-	0	0.0	0	0.1
All ages	3	0.7	143	35	0.0	73.8	1	0.3	1	0.3
Total	4	0.6	218	27	0.0	71.5	2	0.2	2	0.3

Table 206b   FSE - PEAS - AESE   Spina bifida - Cases

Age group (years)	Incidence 1990 Number ('000s)	Rate (per 100 000)	Prevalence 1990 Number ('000s)	Rate (per 100 000)	Avg. age at onset (years)	Average duration (years)	Deaths 1990 Number ('000s)	Rate (per 100 000)	Deaths 2000 (Projected) Number ('000s)	Rate (per 100 000)
Males										
0-4	1	8.6	3	18.9	0.0	62.8	1	6.9	1	11.0
5-14	0	0.0	2	8.8	-	-	0	0.3	0	0.4
15-44	0	0.0	6	7.9	-	-	0	0.1	0	0.1
45-59	0	0.0	2	7.5	-	-	0	0.0	0	0.0
60+	0	0.0	2	7.4	-	-	0	0.0	0	0.0
All ages	1	0.7	15	8.8	0.0	62.8	1	0.7	2	0.9
Females										
0-4	2	13.5	5	38.0	0.0	70.7	1	8.0	1	11.2
5-14	0	0.0	7	26.8	-	-	0	0.3	0	0.5
15-44	0	0.0	18	23.9	-	-	0	0.1	0	0.1
45-59	0	0.0	7	22.5	-	-	0	0.0	0	0.0
60+	0	0.0	8	22.1	-	-	0	0.0	0	0.0
All ages	2	1.0	45	24.7	0.0	70.7	1	0.7	2	0.8
Total	3	0.9	59	17.1	0.0	67.5	2	0.7	3	0.9

Table 206c   India - India - Inde   Spina bifida - Cases

Age group (years)	Incidence 1990 Number ('000s)	Rate (per 100 000)	Prevalence 1990 Number ('000s)	Rate (per 100 000)	Avg. age at onset (years)	Average duration (years)	Deaths 1990 Number ('000s)	Rate (per 100 000)	Deaths 2000 (Projected) Number ('000s)	Rate (per 100 000)
Males										
0-4	18	30.3	43	72	0.0	58.8	11	18.0	13	22.8
5-14	0	0.0	58	57	-	-	0	0.5	0	0.4
15-44	0	0.0	109	54	-	-	0	0.0	0	0.0
45-59	0	0.0	26	54	-	-	0	0.0	0	0.0
60+	0	0.0	16	53	-	-	0	0.1	0	0.0
All ages	18	4.1	252	57	0.0	58.8	11	2.6	13	2.6
Females										
0-4	27	48.2	87	154	0.0	59.7	9	15.2	10	19.1
5-14	0	0.0	136	143	-	-	1	0.6	1	0.5
15-44	0	0.0	247	135	-	-	0	0.2	0	0.2
45-59	0	0.0	59	129	-	-	0	0.3	0	0.2
60+	0	0.0	36	125	-	-	0	0.3	0	0.3
All ages	27	6.7	565	138	0.0	59.7	10	2.4	11	2.4
Total	45	5.3	817	96	0.0	59.3	21	2.5	25	2.5

For epidemiological sources see Shibuya and Murray 1996c. For the methods used to estimate and project incidence, prevalence, and deaths see Murray and Lopez 1996a. See explanatory notes for definitions and caveats.

Table 206 **Cuadro 206** **Tableau 206**
Spina bifida **Espina bífida** **Spina bifida**

Cases Casos Cas

Table 206d China - China - Chine Spina bifida - Cases

Age group (years)	Incidence 1990 Number ('000s)	Rate (per 100 000)	Prevalence 1990 Number ('000s)	Rate (per 100 000)	Avg. age at onset (years)	Average duration (years)	Deaths 1990 Number ('000s)	Rate (per 100 000)	Deaths 2000 (Projected) Number ('000s)	Rate (per 100 000)
Males										
0-4	12	20.2	32	52	0.0	64.1	6	9.7	7	11.3
5-14	0	0.0	38	39	-	-	1	0.9	1	0.7
15-44	0	0.0	109	36	-	-	0	0.0	0	0.0
45-59	0	0.0	26	35	-	-	0	0.0	0	0.0
60+	0	0.0	17	35	-	-	0	0.0	0	0.0
All ages	12	2.1	222	38	0.0	64.1	7	1.2	8	1.5
Females										
0-4	19	33.1	64	110	0.0	66.9	4	7.4	5	8.5
5-14	0	0.0	93	103	-	-	1	1.2	1	0.8
15-44	0	0.0	275	97	-	-	0	0.0	0	0.0
45-59	0	0.0	62	96	-	-	0	0.0	0	0.0
60+	0	0.0	50	96	-	-	0	0.0	0	0.0
All ages	19	3.5	544	99	0.0	66.9	5	1.0	6	1.2
Total	31	2.8	766	68	0.0	65.8	12	1.1	13	1.3

Table 206e OAI - OPAI - APAI Spina bifida - Cases

Age group (years)	Incidence 1990 Number ('000s)	Rate (per 100 000)	Prevalence 1990 Number ('000s)	Rate (per 100 000)	Avg. age at onset (years)	Average duration (years)	Deaths 1990 Number ('000s)	Rate (per 100 000)	Deaths 2000 (Projected) Number ('000s)	Rate (per 100 000)
Males										
0-4	4	9.4	9	21.1	0.0	60.6	3	6.1	3	6.7
5-14	0	0.0	10	12.4	-	-	0	0.5	0	0.4
15-44	0	0.0	16	9.8	-	-	0	0.0	0	0.0
45-59	0	0.0	3	9.5	-	-	0	0.0	0	0.0
60+	0	0.0	2	9.2	-	-	0	0.0	0	0.0
All ages	4	1.2	40	11.8	0.0	60.6	3	0.9	3	0.8
Females										
0-4	6	15.4	23	53.7	0.0	64.5	2	4.5	2	4.8
5-14	0	0.0	39	48.4	-	-	1	0.7	1	0.6
15-44	0	0.0	70	43.6	-	-	0	0.1	0	0.1
45-59	0	0.0	14	40.8	-	-	0	0.1	0	0.1
60+	0	0.0	9	39.1	-	-	0	0.1	0	0.1
All ages	6	1.9	154	45.4	0.0	64.5	3	0.8	3	0.7
Total	11	1.5	195	28.5	0.0	63.0	6	0.9	6	0.8

Table 206f SSA - ASS - ASS Spina bifida - Cases

Age group (years)	Incidence 1990 Number ('000s)	Rate (per 100 000)	Prevalence 1990 Number ('000s)	Rate (per 100 000)	Avg. age at onset (years)	Average duration (years)	Deaths 1990 Number ('000s)	Rate (per 100 000)	Deaths 2000 (Projected) Number ('000s)	Rate (per 100 000)
Males										
0-4	10	20.9	33	69	0.0	51.1	2	4.5	3	5.1
5-14	0	0.0	47	66	-	-	0	0.2	0	0.2
15-44	0	0.0	67	65	-	-	0	0.0	0	0.0
45-59	0	0.0	13	64	-	-	0	0.0	0	0.0
60+	0	0.0	7	63	-	-	0	0.1	0	0.1
All ages	10	3.9	166	66	0.0	51.1	2	0.9	4	1.1
Females										
0-4	16	34.3	62	131	0.0	54.1	2	4.4	3	5.0
5-14	0	0.0	90	129	-	-	0	0.3	0	0.2
15-44	0	0.0	136	128	-	-	0	0.1	0	0.1
45-59	0	0.0	28	125	-	-	0	0.3	0	0.2
60+	0	0.0	15	122	-	-	0	0.4	0	0.4
All ages	16	6.3	331	128	0.0	54.1	2	1.0	4	1.0
Total	26	5.1	497	97	0.0	53.0	5	0.9	7	1.0

For epidemiological sources see Shibuya and Murray 1996c. For the methods used to estimate and project incidence, prevalence, and deaths see Murray and Lopez 1996a. See explanatory notes for definitions and caveats.

Table 206   **Cuadro 206**   **Tableau 206**
Spina bifida   **Espina bífida**   **Spina bifida**

Cases   Casos   Cas

Table 206g   LAC - ALC - ALC   Spina bifida - Cases

Age group (years)	Incidence 1990 Number ('000s)	Rate (per 100 000)	Prevalence 1990 Number ('000s)	Rate (per 100 000)	Avg. age at onset (years)	Average duration (years)	Deaths 1990 Number ('000s)	Rate (per 100 000)	Deaths 2000 (Projected) Number ('000s)	Rate (per 100 000)
Males										
0-4	5	17.2	13	45	0.0	63.4	3	9.4	3	10.3
5-14	0	0.0	16	31	-	-	0	0.6	0	0.5
15-44	0	0.0	27	26	-	-	0	0.1	0	0.1
45-59	0	0.0	6	25	-	-	0	0.0	0	0.0
60+	0	0.0	4	25	-	-	0	0.0	0	0.0
All ages	5	2.2	66	30	0.0	63.4	3	1.4	3	1.3
Females										
0-4	8	27.3	24	87	0.0	67.3	3	9.7	3	10.5
5-14	0	0.0	39	77	-	-	0	0.6	0	0.6
15-44	0	0.0	73	70	-	-	0	0.1	0	0.1
45-59	0	0.0	16	67	-	-	0	0.1	0	0.0
60+	0	0.0	11	66	-	-	0	0.1	0	0.1
All ages	8	3.4	162	73	0.0	67.3	3	1.4	3	1.3
Total	13	2.8	228	51	0.0	65.8	6	1.4	7	1.3

Table 206h   MEC - AOM - CMO   Spina bifida - Cases

Age group (years)	Incidence 1990 Number ('000s)	Rate (per 100 000)	Prevalence 1990 Number ('000s)	Rate (per 100 000)	Avg. age at onset (years)	Average duration (years)	Deaths 1990 Number ('000s)	Rate (per 100 000)	Deaths 2000 (Projected) Number ('000s)	Rate (per 100 000)
Males										
0-4	4	10.0	9	21	0.0	61.5	2	5.7	3	6.4
5-14	0	0.0	11	17	-	-	0	0.2	0	0.2
15-44	0	0.0	18	16	-	-	0	0.0	0	0.0
45-59	0	0.0	3	15	-	-	0	0.0	0	0.0
60+	0	0.0	2	15	-	-	0	0.1	0	0.1
All ages	4	1.6	43	17	0.0	61.5	3	1.0	3	1.0
Females										
0-4	7	16.5	21	54	0.0	64.1	2	4.1	2	4.6
5-14	0	0.0	32	51	-	-	0	0.3	0	0.3
15-44	0	0.0	51	48	-	-	0	0.1	0	0.1
45-59	0	0.0	10	45	-	-	0	0.2	0	0.2
60+	0	0.0	7	44	-	-	0	0.1	0	0.1
All ages	7	2.7	121	49	0.0	64.1	2	0.8	3	0.8
Total	11	2.1	164	33	0.0	63.1	5	0.9	6	0.9

Table 206i   World - Mundo - Monde   Spina bifida - Cases

Age group (years)	Incidence 1990 Number ('000s)	Rate (per 100 000)	Prevalence 1990 Number ('000s)	Rate (per 100 000)	Avg. age at onset (years)	Average duration (years)	Deaths 1990 Number ('000s)	Rate (per 100 000)	Deaths 2000 (Projected) Number ('000s)	Rate (per 100 000)
Males										
0-4	56	17.5	147	46	0.0	60.6	28	8.7	35	10.0
5-14	0	0.0	194	35	-	-	3	0.5	3	0.4
15-44	0	0.0	387	31	-	-	0	0.0	0	0.0
45-59	0	0.0	90	29	-	-	0	0.0	0	0.0
60+	0	0.0	59	27	-	-	0	0.0	0	0.0
All ages	56	2.1	878	33	0.0	61.7	31	1.2	38	1.2
Females										
0-4	88	28.4	296	96	0.0	63.7	23	7.4	28	8.4
5-14	0	0.0	455	87	-	-	3	0.6	3	0.5
15-44	0	0.0	932	78	-	-	1	0.1	1	0.1
45-59	0	0.0	219	70	-	-	0	0.1	0	0.1
60+	0	0.0	165	61	-	-	0	0.1	0	0.1
All ages	88	3.4	2 066	79	0.0	65.3	28	1.1	33	1.1
Total	144	2.7	2 944	56	0.0	63.9	59	1.1	70	1.1

For epidemiological sources see Shibuya and Murray 1996c. For the methods used to estimate and project incidence, prevalence, and deaths see Murray and Lopez 1996a. See explanatory notes for definitions and caveats.

Table 207
Dental caries

Cuadro 207
Caries dentales

Tableau 207
Caries dentaires

Episodes

Episodios

Episodes

Table 207a EME - PEMC - EMBE Dental caries - Episodes

Age group (years)	Incidence 1990 Number ('000s)	Rate (per 100 000)	Prevalence 1990 Number ('000s)	Rate (per 100 000)	Avg. age at onset (years)	Average duration (years)	Deaths 1990 Number ('000s)	Rate (per 100 000)	Deaths 2000 (Projected) Number ('000s)	Rate (per 100 000)
Males										
0-4	18 469	70 000	354	1 342	3.0	0.02	0	0	0	0
5-14	40 011	75 000	767	1 438	10.0	0.02	0	0	0	0
15-44	36 813	20 000	706	384	25.0	0.02	0	0	0	0
45-59	9 921	15 000	190	288	55.0	0.02	0	0	0	0
60+	15 137	25 000	290	479	70.0	0.02	0	0	0	0
All ages	120 350	30 821	2 308	591	24.8	0.02	0	0	0	0
Females										
0-4	17 546	70 000	336	1 342	3.0	0.02	0	0	0	0
5-14	38 010	75 000	729	1 438	10.0	0.02	0	0	0	0
15-44	35 840	20 000	687	384	25.0	0.02	0	0	0	0
45-59	10 170	15 000	195	288	55.0	0.02	0	0	0	0
60+	21 141	25 000	405	479	70.0	0.02	0	0	0	0
All ages	122 707	30 126	2 353	578	27.4	0.02	0	0	0	0
Total	243 057	30 466	4 661	584	26.1	0.02	0	0	0	0

Table 207b FSE - PEAS - AESE Dental caries - Episodes

Age group (years)	Incidence 1990 Number ('000s)	Rate (per 100 000)	Prevalence 1990 Number ('000s)	Rate (per 100 000)	Avg. age at onset (years)	Average duration (years)	Deaths 1990 Number ('000s)	Rate (per 100 000)	Deaths 2000 (Projected) Number ('000s)	Rate (per 100 000)
Males										
0-4	23 390	170 000	449	3 260	3.0	0.02	0	0	0	0
5-14	12 307	45 000	236	863	10.0	0.02	0	0	0	0
15-44	19 070	25 000	366	479	25.0	0.02	0	0	0	0
45-59	12 138	45 000	233	863	55.0	0.02	0	0	0	0
60+	9 433	45 000	181	863	70.0	0.02	0	0	0	0
All ages	76 338	46 175	1 464	886	26.2	0.02	0	0	0	0
Females										
0-4	22 330	170 000	428	3 260	3.0	0.02	0	0	0	0
5-14	17 889	67 709	343	1 299	10.0	0.02	0	0	0	0
15-44	18 740	25 000	359	479	25.0	0.02	0	0	0	0
45-59	13 503	45 000	259	863	55.0	0.02	0	0	0	0
60+	16 377	45 000	314	863	70.0	0.02	0	0	0	0
All ages	88 839	49 105	1 704	942	29.3	0.02	0	0	0	0
Total	165 177	47 706	3 168	915	27.9	0.02	0	0	0	0

Table 207c India - India - Inde Dental caries - Episodes

Age group (years)	Incidence 1990 Number ('000s)	Rate (per 100 000)	Prevalence 1990 Number ('000s)	Rate (per 100 000)	Avg. age at onset (years)	Average duration (years)	Deaths 1990 Number ('000s)	Rate (per 100 000)	Deaths 2000 (Projected) Number ('000s)	Rate (per 100 000)
Males										
0-4	29 895	50 000	1 147	1 918	3.0	0.04	0	0	0	0
5-14	20 350	20 000	781	767	10.0	0.04	0	0	0	0
15-44	30 079	15 000	1 154	575	25.0	0.04	0	0	0	0
45-59	16 649	35 000	639	1 342	55.0	0.04	0	0	0	0
60+	17 861	60 000	685	2 301	70.0	0.04	0	0	0	0
All ages	114 833	26 134	4 405	1 002	28.0	0.04	0	0	0	0
Females										
0-4	28 340	50 000	1 087	1 918	3.0	0.04	0	0	0	0
5-14	19 053	20 000	731	767	10.0	0.04	0	0	0	0
15-44	27 486	15 000	1 054	575	25.0	0.04	0	0	0	0
45-59	16 102	35 000	618	1 342	55.0	0.04	0	0	0	0
60+	17 354	60 000	666	2 301	70.0	0.04	0	0	0	0
All ages	108 335	26 416	4 155	1 013	28.3	0.04	0	0	0	0
Total	223 168	26 270	8 560	1 008	28.1	0.04	0	0	0	0

For epidemiological sources see Barmes 1996. See explanatory notes for definitions and caveats.

Table 207
Dental caries

Cuadro 207
Caries dentales

Tableau 207
Caries dentaires

Episodes

Episodios

Episodes

Table 207d China - China - Chine — Dental caries - Episodes

Age group (years)	Incidence 1990 Number ('000s)	Rate (per 100 000)	Prevalence 1990 Number ('000s)	Rate (per 100 000)	Avg. age at onset (years)	Average duration (years)	Deaths 1990 Number ('000s)	Rate (per 100 000)	Deaths 2000 (Projected) Number ('000s)	Rate (per 100 000)
Males										
0-4	135 547	225 000	5 199	8 630	3.0	0.04	0	0	0	0
5-14	9 700	10 000	372	384	10.0	0.04	0	0	0	0
15-44	9 189	3 000	352	115	25.0	0.04	0	0	0	0
45-59	7 267	10 000	279	384	55.0	0.04	0	0	0	0
60+	4 898	10 000	188	384	70.0	0.04	0	0	0	0
All ages	166 601	28 469	6 390	1 092	8.9	0.04	0	0	0	0
Females										
0-4	130 379	225 000	5 001	8 630	3.0	0.04	0	0	0	0
5-14	9 040	10 000	347	384	10.0	0.04	0	0	0	0
15-44	8 522	3 000	327	115	25.0	0.04	0	0	0	0
45-59	6 440	10 000	247	384	55.0	0.04	0	0	0	0
60+	5 167	10 000	198	384	70.0	0.04	0	0	0	0
All ages	159 548	29 088	6 120	1 116	8.8	0.04	0	0	0	0
Total	326 149	28 769	12 510	1 103	8.8	0.04	0	0	0	0

Table 207e OAI - OPAI - APAI — Dental caries - Episodes

Age group (years)	Incidence 1990 Number ('000s)	Rate (per 100 000)	Prevalence 1990 Number ('000s)	Rate (per 100 000)	Avg. age at onset (years)	Average duration (years)	Deaths 1990 Number ('000s)	Rate (per 100 000)	Deaths 2000 (Projected) Number ('000s)	Rate (per 100 000)
Males										
0-4	21 882	50 000	839	1 918	3.0	0.04	0	0	0	0
5-14	12 605	15 000	483	575	10.0	0.04	0	0	0	0
15-44	24 124	15 000	925	575	25.0	0.04	0	0	0	0
45-59	17 069	50 000	655	1 918	55.0	0.04	0	0	0	0
60+	10 104	50 000	388	1 918	70.0	0.04	0	0	0	0
All ages	85 783	25 012	3 290	959	28.5	0.04	0	0	0	0
Females										
0-4	20 994	50 000	805	1 918	3.0	0.04	0	0	0	0
5-14	12 033	15 000	462	575	10.0	0.04	0	0	0	0
15-44	23 942	15 000	918	575	25.0	0.04	0	0	0	0
45-59	17 545	50 000	673	1 918	55.0	0.04	0	0	0	0
60+	11 331	50 000	435	1 918	70.0	0.04	0	0	0	0
All ages	85 844	25 280	3 293	970	29.6	0.04	0	0	0	0
Total	171 627	25 146	6 583	964	29.0	0.04	0	0	0	0

Table 207f SSA - ASS - ASS — Dental caries - Episodes

Age group (years)	Incidence 1990 Number ('000s)	Rate (per 100 000)	Prevalence 1990 Number ('000s)	Rate (per 100 000)	Avg. age at onset (years)	Average duration (years)	Deaths 1990 Number ('000s)	Rate (per 100 000)	Deaths 2000 (Projected) Number ('000s)	Rate (per 100 000)
Males										
0-4	33 239	70 000	1 275	2 685	3.0	0.04	0	0	0	0
5-14	14 052	20 000	539	767	10.0	0.04	0	0	0	0
15-44	7 263	7 000	279	268	25.0	0.04	0	0	0	0
45-59	3 046	15 000	117	575	55.0	0.04	0	0	0	0
60+	1 576	15 000	60	575	70.0	0.04	0	0	0	0
All ages	59 176	23 453	2 270	900	11.8	0.04	0	0	0	0
Females										
0-4	32 921	70 000	1 263	2 685	3.0	0.04	0	0	0	0
5-14	13 964	20 000	536	767	10.0	0.04	0	0	0	0
15-44	7 438	7 000	285	268	25.0	0.04	0	0	0	0
45-59	3 318	15 000	127	575	55.0	0.04	0	0	0	0
60+	1 910	15 000	73	575	70.0	0.04	0	0	0	0
All ages	59 550	23 086	2 284	885	12.4	0.04	0	0	0	0
Total	118 726	23 267	4 554	892	12.1	0.04	0	0	0	0

For epidemiological sources see Barmes 1996. See explanatory notes for definitions and caveats.

**Table 207
Dental caries**

**Cuadro 207
Caries dentales**

**Tableau 207
Caries dentaires**

Episodes

Episodios

Episodes

Table 207g   LAC - ALC - ALC   Dental caries - Episodes

Age group (years)	Incidence 1990 Number ('000s)	Rate (per 100 000)	Prevalence 1990 Number ('000s)	Rate (per 100 000)	Avg. age at onset (years)	Average duration (years)	Deaths 1990 Number ('000s)	Rate (per 100 000)	Deaths 2000 (Projected) Number ('000s)	Rate (per 100 000)
Males										
0-4	25 849	90 000	991	3 452	3.0	0.04	0	0	0	0
5-14	67 761	130 000	2 599	4 986	10.0	0.04	0	0	0	0
15-44	36 500	35 000	1 400	1 342	25.0	0.04	0	0	0	0
45-59	2 225	10 000	85	384	55.0	0.04	0	0	0	0
60+	1 423	10 000	55	384	70.0	0.04	0	0	0	0
All ages	133 758	60 357	5 130	2 315	14.1	0.04	0	0	0	0
Females										
0-4	24 908	90 000	955	3 452	3.0	0.04	0	0	0	0
5-14	65 967	130 000	2 530	4 986	10.0	0.04	0	0	0	0
15-44	36 430	35 000	1 397	1 342	25.0	0.04	0	0	0	0
45-59	2 336	10 000	90	384	55.0	0.04	0	0	0	0
60+	1 682	10 000	65	384	70.0	0.04	0	0	0	0
All ages	131 323	58 973	5 037	2 262	14.4	0.04	0	0	0	0
Total	265 081	59 663	10 168	2 288	14.3	0.04	0	0	0	0

Table 207h   MEC - AOM - CMO   Dental caries - Episodes

Age group (years)	Incidence 1990 Number ('000s)	Rate (per 100 000)	Prevalence 1990 Number ('000s)	Rate (per 100 000)	Avg. age at onset (years)	Average duration (years)	Deaths 1990 Number ('000s)	Rate (per 100 000)	Deaths 2000 (Projected) Number ('000s)	Rate (per 100 000)
Males										
0-4	61 742	150 000	2 368	5 753	3.0	0.04	0	0	0	0
5-14	29 405	45 000	1 128	1 726	10.0	0.04	0	0	0	0
15-44	22 779	20 000	874	767	25.0	0.04	0	0	0	0
45-59	11 169	50 000	428	1 918	55.0	0.04	0	0	0	0
60+	9 556	70 000	367	2 685	70.0	0.04	0	0	0	0
All ages	134 650	52 518	5 165	2 014	17.3	0.04	0	0	0	0
Females										
0-4	59 601	150 000	2 286	5 753	3.0	0.04	0	0	0	0
5-14	27 900	45 000	1 070	1 726	10.0	0.04	0	0	0	0
15-44	21 442	20 000	822	767	25.0	0.04	0	0	0	0
45-59	11 146	50 000	428	1 918	55.0	0.04	0	0	0	0
60+	10 815	70 000	415	2 685	70.0	0.04	0	0	0	0
All ages	130 904	53 065	5 021	2 035	18.1	0.04	0	0	0	0
Total	265 554	52 786	10 186	2 025	17.7	0.04	0	0	0	0

Table 207i   World - Mundo - Monde   Dental caries - Episodes

Age group (years)	Incidence 1990 Number ('000s)	Rate (per 100 000)	Prevalence 1990 Number ('000s)	Rate (per 100 000)	Avg. age at onset (years)	Average duration (years)	Deaths 1990 Number ('000s)	Rate (per 100 000)	Deaths 2000 (Projected) Number ('000s)	Rate (per 100 000)
Males										
0-4	350 011	108 936	12 622	3 929	3.0	0.04	0	0	0	0
5-14	206 191	37 408	6 905	1 253	10.0	0.03	0	0	0	0
15-44	185 816	14 866	6 055	484	25.0	0.03	0	0	0	0
45-59	79 483	25 445	2 626	841	55.0	0.03	0	0	0	0
60+	69 988	31 979	2 213	1 011	70.0	0.03	0	0	0	0
All ages	891 490	33 595	30 422	1 146	19.1	0.03	0	0	0	0
Females										
0-4	337 017	108 979	12 162	3 933	3.0	0.04	0	0	0	0
5-14	203 855	38 790	6 747	1 284	10.0	0.03	0	0	0	0
15-44	179 840	15 004	5 851	488	25.0	0.03	0	0	0	0
45-59	80 559	25 899	2 636	847	55.0	0.03	0	0	0	0
60+	85 778	31 862	2 571	955	70.0	0.03	0	0	0	0
All ages	887 048	33 939	29 967	1 147	20.3	0.03	0	0	0	0
Total	1 778 538	33 766	60 389	1 146	19.7	0.03	0	0	0	0

For epidemiological sources see Barmes 1996. See explanatory notes for definitions and caveats.

Table 208
Periodontal disease

Cuadro 208
Enfermedad periodontal

Tableau 208
Maladie périodontale

Episodes

Episodios

Episodes

Table 208a   EME - PEMC - EMBE   Periodontal disease - Episodes

Age group (years)	Incidence 1990 Number ('000s)	Rate (per 100 000)	Prevalence 1990 Number ('000s)	Rate (per 100 000)	Avg. age at onset (years)	Average duration (years)	Deaths 1990 Number ('000s)	Rate (per 100 000)	Deaths 2000 (Projected) Number ('000s)	Rate (per 100 000)
Males										
0-4	0	0	0	0	-	-	0	0	0	0
5-14	0	0	0	0	-	-	0	0	0	0
15-44	9 204	5 000	17 207	9 348	29.8	2.1	0	0	0	0
45-59	662	1 000	3 003	4 540	52.4	3.1	0	0	0	0
60+	606	1 000	2 187	3 612	71.1	3.0	0	0	0	0
All ages	10 471	2 682	22 397	5 736	33.6	2.2	0	0	0	0
Females										
0-4	0	0	0	0	-	-	0	0	0	0
5-14	0	0	0	0	-	-	0	0	0	0
15-44	8 960	5 000	16 764	9 355	29.9	2.1	0	0	0	0
45-59	678	1 001	3 065	4 521	52.5	3.2	0	0	0	0
60+	846	1 000	3 065	3 624	72.4	3.1	0	0	0	0
All ages	10 484	2 574	22 894	5 621	34.8	2.2	0	0	0	0
Total	20 955	2 627	45 291	5 677	34.2	2.2	0	0	0	0

Table 208b   FSE - PEAS - AESE   Periodontal disease - Episodes

Age group (years)	Incidence 1990 Number ('000s)	Rate (per 100 000)	Prevalence 1990 Number ('000s)	Rate (per 100 000)	Avg. age at onset (years)	Average duration (years)	Deaths 1990 Number ('000s)	Rate (per 100 000)	Deaths 2000 (Projected) Number ('000s)	Rate (per 100 000)
Males										
0-4	0	0	0	0	-	-	0	0	0	0
5-14	0	0	0	0	-	-	0	0	0	0
15-44	4 577	6 000	8 548	11 206	29.8	2.0	0	0	0	0
45-59	540	2 000	1 963	7 277	52.2	3.0	0	0	0	0
60+	419	2 000	1 542	7 357	70.0	3.0	0	0	0	0
All ages	5 536	3 348	12 053	7 291	35.0	2.2	0	0	0	0
Females										
0-4	0	0	0	0	-	-	0	0	0	0
5-14	0	0	0	0	-	-	0	0	0	0
15-44	4 498	6 000	8 415	11 226	29.8	2.1	0	0	0	0
45-59	600	2 000	2 169	7 228	52.5	3.1	0	0	0	0
60+	728	2 001	2 698	7 412	71.5	3.2	0	0	0	0
All ages	5 826	3 220	13 281	7 341	37.3	2.3	0	0	0	0
Total	11 362	3 281	25 334	7 317	36.2	2.3	0	0	0	0

Table 208c   India - India - Inde   Periodontal disease - Episodes

Age group (years)	Incidence 1990 Number ('000s)	Rate (per 100 000)	Prevalence 1990 Number ('000s)	Rate (per 100 000)	Avg. age at onset (years)	Average duration (years)	Deaths 1990 Number ('000s)	Rate (per 100 000)	Deaths 2000 (Projected) Number ('000s)	Rate (per 100 000)
Males										
0-4	0	0	0	0	-	-	0	0	0	0
5-14	0	0	0	0	-	-	0	0	0	0
15-44	18 048	9 000	33 100	16 507	29.6	2.0	0	0	0	0
45-59	2 854	6 000	8 577	18 032	52.3	3.0	0	0	0	0
60+	1 786	6 000	6 542	21 978	69.6	3.0	0	0	0	0
All ages	22 688	5 163	48 220	10 974	35.6	2.2	0	0	0	0
Females										
0-4	0	0	0	0	-	-	0	0	0	0
5-14	0	0	0	0	-	-	0	0	0	0
15-44	16 492	9 000	30 246	16 506	29.6	2.0	0	0	0	0
45-59	2 760	6 000	8 296	18 033	52.3	3.1	0	0	0	0
60+	1 735	6 000	6 373	22 035	70.0	3.1	0	0	0	0
All ages	20 988	5 118	44 916	10 952	35.9	2.2	0	0	0	0
Total	43 675	5 141	93 136	10 963	35.8	2.2	0	0	0	0

For epidemiological sources see Barmes 1996. See explanatory notes for definitions and caveats.

Table 208
Periodontal disease

Cuadro 208
Enfermedad periodontal

Tableau 208
Maladie périodontale

Episodes

Episodios

Episodes

Table 208d   China - China - Chine | Periodontal disease - Episodes

Age group (years)	Incidence 1990 Number ('000s)	Rate (per 100 000)	Prevalence 1990 Number ('000s)	Rate (per 100 000)	Avg. age at onset (years)	Average duration (years)	Deaths 1990 Number ('000s)	Rate (per 100 000)	Deaths 2000 (Projected) Number ('000s)	Rate (per 100 000)
Males										
0-4	0	0	0	0	-	-	0	0	0	0
5-14	0	0	0	0	-	-	0	0	0	0
15-44	9 189	3 000	16 860	5 504	29.8	2.0	0	0	0	0
45-59	727	1 000	2 557	3 519	52.4	3.0	0	0	0	0
60+	490	1 000	1 843	3 762	69.8	3.1	0	0	0	0
All ages	10 406	1 778	21 260	3 633	33.3	2.1	0	0	0	0
Females										
0-4	0	0	0	0	-	-	0	0	0	0
5-14	0	0	0	0	-	-	0	0	0	0
15-44	8 522	3 000	15 643	5 507	29.9	2.0	0	0	0	0
45-59	644	1 000	2 262	3 512	52.4	3.0	0	0	0	0
60+	517	1 000	1 954	3 782	70.6	3.2	0	0	0	0
All ages	9 683	1 765	19 859	3 621	33.6	2.1	0	0	0	0
Total	20 089	1 772	41 119	3 627	33.4	2.1	0	0	0	0

Table 208e   OAI - OPAI - APAI | Periodontal disease - Episodes

Age group (years)	Incidence 1990 Number ('000s)	Rate (per 100 000)	Prevalence 1990 Number ('000s)	Rate (per 100 000)	Avg. age at onset (years)	Average duration (years)	Deaths 1990 Number ('000s)	Rate (per 100 000)	Deaths 2000 (Projected) Number ('000s)	Rate (per 100 000)
Males										
0-4	0	0	0	0	-	-	0	0	0	0
5-14	0	0	0	0	-	-	0	0	0	0
15-44	8 042	5 000	14 736	9 163	29.6	2.0	0	0	0	0
45-59	1 366	4 000	3 972	11 635	52.2	3.0	0	0	0	0
60+	808	4 000	2 955	14 622	69.6	3.0	0	0	0	0
All ages	10 215	2 979	21 663	6 316	35.8	2.2	0	0	0	0
Females										
0-4	0	0	0	0	-	-	0	0	0	0
5-14	0	0	0	0	-	-	0	0	0	0
15-44	7 980	5 000	14 631	9 167	29.7	2.0	0	0	0	0
45-59	1 404	4 000	4 085	11 641	52.3	3.0	0	0	0	0
60+	906	4 000	3 327	14 683	70.3	3.1	0	0	0	0
All ages	10 290	3 030	22 044	6 492	36.4	2.2	0	0	0	0
Total	20 506	3 004	43 706	6 404	36.1	2.2	0	0	0	0

Table 208f   SSA - ASS - ASS | Periodontal disease - Episodes

Age group (years)	Incidence 1990 Number ('000s)	Rate (per 100 000)	Prevalence 1990 Number ('000s)	Rate (per 100 000)	Avg. age at onset (years)	Average duration (years)	Deaths 1990 Number ('000s)	Rate (per 100 000)	Deaths 2000 (Projected) Number ('000s)	Rate (per 100 000)
Males										
0-4	0	0	0	0	-	-	0	0	0	0
5-14	0	0	0	0	-	-	0	0	0	0
15-44	7 264	7 000	13 261	12 780	29.3	2.0	0	0	0	0
45-59	609	3 000	2 038	10 033	52.2	3.0	0	0	0	0
60+	105	1 000	553	5 264	69.3	3.0	0	0	0	0
All ages	7 978	3 162	15 851	6 282	31.6	2.1	0	0	0	0
Females										
0-4	0	0	0	0	-	-	0	0	0	0
5-14	0	0	0	0	-	-	0	0	0	0
15-44	7 438	7 000	13 594	12 793	29.4	2.0	0	0	0	0
45-59	664	3 000	2 216	10 019	52.3	3.0	0	0	0	0
60+	127	1 000	662	5 200	69.8	3.1	0	0	0	0
All ages	8 229	3 190	16 472	6 386	31.9	2.1	0	0	0	0
Total	16 206	3 176	32 323	6 334	31.7	2.1	0	0	0	0

For epidemiological sources see Barmes 1996. See explanatory notes for definitions and caveats.

Table 208 | **Cuadro 208** | **Tableau 208**
Periodontal disease | **Enfermedad periodontal** | **Maladie périodontale**

Episodes | Episodios | Episodes

Table 208g — LAC - ALC - ALC — Periodontal disease - Episodes

Age group (years)	Incidence 1990 Number ('000s)	Rate (per 100 000)	Prevalence 1990 Number ('000s)	Rate (per 100 000)	Avg. age at onset (years)	Average duration (years)	Deaths 1990 Number ('000s)	Rate (per 100 000)	Deaths 2000 (Projected) Number ('000s)	Rate (per 100 000)
Males										
0-4	0	0	0	0	-	-	0	0	0	0
5-14	0	0	0	0	-	-	0	0	0	0
15-44	2 086	2 000	3 823	3 666	29.8	2.0	0	0	0	0
45-59	2 225	10 000	5 596	25 151	52.1	3.0	0	0	0	0
60+	1 423	10 000	5 037	35 397	70.2	3.0	0	0	0	0
All ages	5 734	2 587	14 456	6 523	48.5	2.6	0	0	0	0
Females										
0-4	0	0	0	0	-	-	0	0	0	0
5-14	0	0	0	0	-	-	0	0	0	0
15-44	2 082	2 000	3 818	3 668	29.8	2.0	0	0	0	0
45-59	2 335	10 000	5 891	25 225	52.1	3.1	0	0	0	0
60+	1 682	10 000	5 981	35 549	71.0	3.1	0	0	0	0
All ages	6 100	2 739	15 690	7 046	49.7	2.7	0	0	0	0
Total	11 833	2 663	30 147	6 785	49.1	2.7	0	0	0	0

Table 208h — MEC - AOM - CMO — Periodontal disease - Episodes

Age group (years)	Incidence 1990 Number ('000s)	Rate (per 100 000)	Prevalence 1990 Number ('000s)	Rate (per 100 000)	Avg. age at onset (years)	Average duration (years)	Deaths 1990 Number ('000s)	Rate (per 100 000)	Deaths 2000 (Projected) Number ('000s)	Rate (per 100 000)
Males										
0-4	0	0	0	0	-	-	0	0	0	0
5-14	0	0	0	0	-	-	0	0	0	0
15-44	5 695	5 000	10 445	9 171	29.7	2.0	0	0	0	0
45-59	223	1 000	986	4 412	52.4	3.0	0	0	0	0
60+	137	1 000	502	3 679	69.7	3.0	0	0	0	0
All ages	6 055	2 362	11 933	4 654	31.4	2.1	0	0	0	0
Females										
0-4	0	0	0	0	-	-	0	0	0	0
5-14	0	0	0	0	-	-	0	0	0	0
15-44	5 360	5 000	9 835	9 174	29.8	2.0	0	0	0	0
45-59	223	1 000	980	4 395	52.4	3.1	0	0	0	0
60+	154	1 000	570	3 691	70.4	3.1	0	0	0	0
All ages	5 738	2 326	11 385	4 615	31.8	2.1	0	0	0	0
Total	11 793	2 344	23 318	4 635	31.6	2.1	0	0	0	0

Table 208i — World - Mundo - Monde — Periodontal disease - Episodes

Age group (years)	Incidence 1990 Number ('000s)	Rate (per 100 000)	Prevalence 1990 Number ('000s)	Rate (per 100 000)	Avg. age at onset (years)	Average duration (years)	Deaths 1990 Number ('000s)	Rate (per 100 000)	Deaths 2000 (Projected) Number ('000s)	Rate (per 100 000)
Males										
0-4	0	0	0	0	-	-	0	0	0	0
5-14	0	0	0	0	-	-	0	0	0	0
15-44	64 103	5 129	117 981	9 439	31.8	2.0	0	0	0	0
45-59	9 205	2 947	28 691	9 185	50.4	3.0	0	0	0	0
60+	5 774	2 638	21 161	9 669	66.3	3.0	0	0	0	0
All ages	79 082	2 980	167 833	6 325	36.5	2.2	0	0	0	0
Females										
0-4	0	0	0	0	-	-	0	0	0	0
5-14	0	0	0	0	-	-	0	0	0	0
15-44	61 332	5 117	112 946	9 423	29.7	2.0	0	0	0	0
45-59	9 308	2 993	28 964	9 312	52.3	3.1	0	0	0	0
60+	6 696	2 487	24 630	9 149	70.8	3.1	0	0	0	0
All ages	77 337	2 959	166 541	6 372	36.0	2.2	0	0	0	0
Total	156 419	2 970	334 374	6 348	36.2	2.2	0	0	0	0

For epidemiological sources see Barmes 1996. See explanatory notes for definitions and caveats.

Table 209	Cuadro 209	Tableau 209
Edentulism	Edentulismo	Edentation
Cases	Casos	Cas

Table 209a EME - PEMC - EMBE Edentulism - Cases

Age group (years)	Incidence 1990 Number ('000s)	Rate (per 100 000)	Prevalence 1990 Number ('000s)	Rate (per 100 000)	Avg. age at onset (years)	Average duration (years)	Deaths 1990 Number ('000s)	Rate (per 100 000)	Deaths 2000 (Projected) Number ('000s)	Rate (per 100 000)
Males										
0-4	0	0	0	0	-	-	0	0	0	0
5-14	0	0	0	0	-	-	0	0	0	0
15-44	369	200	5 552	3 016	29.7	44.9	0	0	0	0
45-59	595	900	8 488	12 833	52.2	24.6	0	0	0	0
60+	1 211	2 000	26 602	43 935	69.2	12.4	0	0	0	0
All ages	2 175	557	40 642	10 408	57.9	21.2	0	0	0	0
Females										
0-4	0	0	0	0	-	-	0	0	0	0
5-14	0	0	0	0	-	-	0	0	0	0
15-44	359	200	5 430	3 030	29.8	50.2	0	0	0	0
45-59	610	900	8 741	12 893	52.3	28.9	0	0	0	0
60+	1 691	2 000	40 223	47 565	70.1	14.3	0	0	0	0
All ages	2 660	653	54 395	13 355	60.6	22.5	0	0	0	0
Total	4 836	606	95 036	11 912	59.4	21.9	0	0	0	0

Table 209b FSE - PEAS - AESE Edentulism - Cases

Age group (years)	Incidence 1990 Number ('000s)	Rate (per 100 000)	Prevalence 1990 Number ('000s)	Rate (per 100 000)	Avg. age at onset (years)	Average duration (years)	Deaths 1990 Number ('000s)	Rate (per 100 000)	Deaths 2000 (Projected) Number ('000s)	Rate (per 100 000)
Males										
0-4	0	0	0	0	-	-	0	0	0	0
5-14	0	0	0	0	-	-	0	0	0	0
15-44	229	301	3 444	4 516	29.5	39.4	0	0	0	0
45-59	405	1 501	5 490	20 352	51.9	21.1	0	0	0	0
60+	314	1 500	9 949	47 461	68.7	10.8	0	0	0	0
All ages	949	574	18 883	11 422	52.0	22.1	0	0	0	0
Females										
0-4	0	0	0	0	-	-	0	0	0	0
5-14	0	0	0	0	-	-	0	0	0	0
15-44	225	301	3 423	4 566	29.7	47.0	0	0	0	0
45-59	450	1 500	6 199	20 660	52.0	26.4	0	0	0	0
60+	546	1 501	18 360	50 449	69.9	12.8	0	0	0	0
All ages	1 222	675	27 982	15 467	55.9	24.1	0	0	0	0
Total	2 170	627	46 866	13 536	54.2	23.2	0	0	0	0

Table 209c India - India - Inde Edentulism - Cases

Age group (years)	Incidence 1990 Number ('000s)	Rate (per 100 000)	Prevalence 1990 Number ('000s)	Rate (per 100 000)	Avg. age at onset (years)	Average duration (years)	Deaths 1990 Number ('000s)	Rate (per 100 000)	Deaths 2000 (Projected) Number ('000s)	Rate (per 100 000)
Males										
0-4	0	0	0	0	-	-	0	0	0	0
5-14	0	0	0	0	-	-	0	0	0	0
15-44	0	0	0	0	-	-	0	0	0	0
45-59	95	200	698	1 468	52.3	21.0	0	0	0	0
60+	298	1 000	3 851	12 936	69.1	10.0	0	0	0	0
All ages	393	89	4 549	1 035	65.0	12.7	0	0	0	0
Females										
0-4	0	0	0	0	-	-	0	0	0	0
5-14	0	0	0	0	-	-	0	0	0	0
15-44	0	0	0	0	-	-	0	0	0	0
45-59	92	200	682	1 482	52.3	22.5	0	0	0	0
60+	289	1 000	3 871	13 384	69.5	10.5	0	0	0	0
All ages	381	93	4 553	1 110	65.3	13.4	0	0	0	0
Total	774	91	9 102	1 071	65.2	13.0	0	0	0	0

For epidemiological sources see Barmes 1996. See explanatory notes for definitions and caveats.

Table 209	Cuadro 209	Tableau 209
Edentulism	Edentulismo	Edentation

Cases   Casos   Cas

Table 209d   China - China - Chine   Edentulism - Cases

Age group (years)	Incidence 1990 Number ('000s)	Rate (per 100 000)	Prevalence 1990 Number ('000s)	Rate (per 100 000)	Avg. age at onset (years)	Average duration (years)	Deaths 1990 Number ('000s)	Rate (per 100 000)	Deaths 2000 (Projected) Number ('000s)	Rate (per 100 000)
Males										
0-4	0	0	0	0	-	-	0	0	0	0
5-14	0	0	0	0	-	-	0	0	0	0
15-44	0	0	0	0	-	-	0	0	0	0
45-59	145	200	1 073	1 477	52.3	21.4	0	0	0	0
60+	490	1 000	6 400	13 067	69.2	10.1	0	0	0	0
All ages	635	109	7 474	1 277	65.3	12.7	0	0	0	0
Females										
0-4	0	0	0	0	-	-	0	0	0	0
5-14	0	0	0	0	-	-	0	0	0	0
15-44	0	0	0	0	-	-	0	0	0	0
45-59	129	200	958	1 488	52.4	23.8	0	0	0	0
60+	517	1 000	7 227	13 987	70.0	11.1	0	0	0	0
All ages	646	118	8 185	1 492	66.5	13.6	0	0	0	0
Total	1 281	113	15 659	1 381	65.9	13.2	0	0	0	0

Table 209e   OAI - OPAI - APAI   Edentulism - Cases

Age group (years)	Incidence 1990 Number ('000s)	Rate (per 100 000)	Prevalence 1990 Number ('000s)	Rate (per 100 000)	Avg. age at onset (years)	Average duration (years)	Deaths 1990 Number ('000s)	Rate (per 100 000)	Deaths 2000 (Projected) Number ('000s)	Rate (per 100 000)
Males										
0-4	0	0	0	0	-	-	0	0	0	0
5-14	0	0	0	0	-	-	0	0	0	0
15-44	113	70	1 667	1 036	29.7	38.8	0	0	0	0
45-59	171	500	1 976	5 789	52.2	20.4	0	0	0	0
60+	404	2 000	6 076	30 066	68.3	10.3	0	0	0	0
All ages	688	200	9 719	2 834	58.0	17.5	0	0	0	0
Females										
0-4	0	0	0	0	-	-	0	0	0	0
5-14	0	0	0	0	-	-	0	0	0	0
15-44	112	70	1 659	1 039	29.7	41.5	0	0	0	0
45-59	176	500	2 043	5 822	52.2	22.5	0	0	0	0
60+	453	2 000	7 209	31 811	68.9	11.2	0	0	0	0
All ages	741	218	10 911	3 213	59.0	18.5	0	0	0	0
Total	1 428	209	20 629	3 022	58.5	18.0	0	0	0	0

Table 209f   SSA - ASS - ASS   Edentulism - Cases

Age group (years)	Incidence 1990 Number ('000s)	Rate (per 100 000)	Prevalence 1990 Number ('000s)	Rate (per 100 000)	Avg. age at onset (years)	Average duration (years)	Deaths 1990 Number ('000s)	Rate (per 100 000)	Deaths 2000 (Projected) Number ('000s)	Rate (per 100 000)
Males										
0-4	0	0	0	0	-	-	0	0	0	0
5-14	0	0	0	0	-	-	0	0	0	0
15-44	0	0	0	0	-	-	0	0	0	0
45-59	41	200	298	1 468	52.2	19.1	0	0	0	0
60+	105	1 000	1 359	12 936	69.0	9.4	0	0	0	0
All ages	146	58	1 657	642	64.3	12.1	0	0	0	0
Females										
0-4	0	0	0	0	-	-	0	0	0	0
5-14	0	0	0	0	-	-	0	0	0	0
15-44	0	0	0	0	-	-	0	0	0	0
45-59	44	200	328	1 482	52.2	20.5	0	0	0	0
60+	127	1 000	1 704	13 384	69.5	9.9	0	0	0	0
All ages	172	68	2 031	788	65.0	12.7	0	0	0	0
Total	317	62	3 689	723	64.7	12.4	0	0	0	0

For epidemiological sources see Barmes 1996. See explanatory notes for definitions and caveats.

Table 209
Edentulism

Cuadro 209
Edentulismo

Tableau 209
Edentation

Cases

Casos

Cas

Table 209g   LAC - ALC - ALC   Edentulism - Cases

Age group (years)	Incidence 1990 Number ('000s)	Rate (per 100 000)	Prevalence 1990 Number ('000s)	Rate (per 100 000)	Avg. age at onset (years)	Average duration (years)	Deaths 1990 Number ('000s)	Rate (per 100 000)	Deaths 2000 (Projected) Number ('000s)	Rate (per 100 000)
Males										
0-4	0	0	0	0	-	-	0	0	0	0
5-14	0	0	0	0	-	-	0	0	0	0
15-44	0	0	0	0	-	-	0	0	0	0
45-59	22	100	164	738	52.3	22.4	0	0	0	0
60+	142	1 000	1 728	12 143	69.7	10.8	0	0	0	0
All ages	165	74	1 892	854	67.3	12.3	0	0	0	0
Females										
0-4	0	0	0	0	-	-	0	0	0	0
5-14	0	0	0	0	-	-	0	0	0	0
15-44	0	0	0	0	-	-	0	0	0	0
45-59	23	100	174	744	52.4	24.8	0	0	0	0
60+	168	1 000	2 184	12 983	70.5	11.6	0	0	0	0
All ages	192	86	2 358	1 059	68.3	13.3	0	0	0	0
Total	356	80	4 250	957	67.9	12.8	0	0	0	0

Table 209h   MEC - AOM - CMO   Edentulism - Cases

Age group (years)	Incidence 1990 Number ('000s)	Rate (per 100 000)	Prevalence 1990 Number ('000s)	Rate (per 100 000)	Avg. age at onset (years)	Average duration (years)	Deaths 1990 Number ('000s)	Rate (per 100 000)	Deaths 2000 (Projected) Number ('000s)	Rate (per 100 000)
Males										
0-4	0	0	0	0	-	-	0	0	0	0
5-14	0	0	0	0	-	-	0	0	0	0
15-44	171	150	2 553	2 242	29.7	40.1	0	0	0	0
45-59	201	900	2 509	11 234	52.1	21.0	0	0	0	0
60+	205	1 500	4 557	33 385	68.7	10.3	0	0	0	0
All ages	577	225	9 620	3 752	51.4	22.9	0	0	0	0
Females										
0-4	0	0	0	0	-	-	0	0	0	0
5-14	0	0	0	0	-	-	0	0	0	0
15-44	161	150	2 407	2 245	29.7	42.7	0	0	0	0
45-59	201	900	2 516	11 288	52.2	23.1	0	0	0	0
60+	232	1 500	5 346	34 600	69.3	11.2	0	0	0	0
All ages	593	240	10 269	4 163	52.8	23.7	0	0	0	0
Total	1 170	233	19 889	3 953	52.1	23.3	0	0	0	0

Table 209i   World - Mundo - Monde   Edentulism - Cases

Age group (years)	Incidence 1990 Number ('000s)	Rate (per 100 000)	Prevalence 1990 Number ('000s)	Rate (per 100 000)	Avg. age at onset (years)	Average duration (years)	Deaths 1990 Number ('000s)	Rate (per 100 000)	Deaths 2000 (Projected) Number ('000s)	Rate (per 100 000)
Males										
0-4	0	0	0	0	-	-	0	0	0	0
5-14	0	0	0	0	-	-	0	0	0	0
15-44	882	71	13 216	1 057	29.6	41.8	0	0	0	0
45-59	1 675	536	20 696	6 626	52.1	22.3	0	0	0	0
60+	3 169	1 448	60 523	27 654	69.0	11.1	0	0	0	0
All ages	5 726	216	94 436	3 559	58.0	19.2	0	0	0	0
Females										
0-4	0	0	0	0	-	-	0	0	0	0
5-14	0	0	0	0	-	-	0	0	0	0
15-44	857	71	12 919	1 078	29.7	46.8	0	0	0	0
45-59	1 725	555	21 641	6 957	52.2	26.1	0	0	0	0
60+	4 024	1 495	86 124	31 991	69.8	12.7	0	0	0	0
All ages	6 605	253	120 684	4 617	60.0	20.7	0	0	0	0
Total	12 332	234	215 120	4 084	59.0	20.0	0	0	0	0

For epidemiological sources see Barmes 1996. See explanatory notes for definitions and caveats.

Table 210
Road traffic accidents

Cuadro 210
Accidentes de tráfico

Tableau 210
Accidents de la voie publique

Episodes

Episodios

Episodes

Table 210a EME - PEMC - EMBE Road traffic accidents - Episodes

Age group (years)	Incidence 1990 Number ('000s)	Rate (per 100 000)	Prevalence 1990 Number ('000s)	Rate (per 100 000)	Avg. age at onset (years)	Average duration (years)	Deaths 1990 Number ('000s)	Rate (per 100 000)	Deaths 2000 (Projected) Number ('000s)	Rate (per 100 000)
Males										
0-4	21	78	-	-	2.5	-	1	5.2	2	5.2
5-14	162	304	-	-	10.0	-	3	6.3	3	5.4
15-44	934	507	-	-	29.9	-	57	31.2	51	29.0
45-59	212	321	-	-	52.4	-	13	19.9	13	15.9
60+	206	340	-	-	71.1	-	19	30.7	18	24.6
All ages	1 535	393	-	-	36.1	-	94	24.1	86	20.9
Females										
0-4	15	61	-	-	2.5	-	1	4.1	1	4.1
5-14	94	185	-	-	10.0	-	2	3.8	2	3.6
15-44	411	229	-	-	30.0	-	17	9.5	17	10.1
45-59	82	121	-	-	52.4	-	5	7.5	6	7.8
60+	135	160	-	-	72.4	-	12	14.5	13	13.6
All ages	738	181	-	-	37.2	-	37	9.2	40	9.3
Total	2 272	285	-	-	36.4	-	131	16.5	126	15.0

Table 210b FSE - PEAS - AESE Road traffic accidents - Episodes

Age group (years)	Incidence 1990 Number ('000s)	Rate (per 100 000)	Prevalence 1990 Number ('000s)	Rate (per 100 000)	Avg. age at onset (years)	Average duration (years)	Deaths 1990 Number ('000s)	Rate (per 100 000)	Deaths 2000 (Projected) Number ('000s)	Rate (per 100 000)
Males										
0-4	12	88	-	-	2.5	-	1	7.4	1	7.4
5-14	113	413	-	-	10.0	-	3	10.6	3	9.9
15-44	567	743	-	-	29.8	-	44	57.1	44	57.7
45-59	185	685	-	-	52.2	-	14	53.0	17	55.5
60+	81	388	-	-	70.0	-	9	43.9	12	47.1
All ages	958	579	-	-	34.9	-	71	42.9	76	44.7
Females										
0-4	7	55	-	-	2.5	-	1	4.6	1	4.6
5-14	57	215	-	-	10.0	-	1	5.6	1	5.5
15-44	94	126	-	-	29.9	-	7	9.7	8	10.5
45-59	49	164	-	-	52.4	-	4	12.7	5	13.5
60+	60	166	-	-	71.5	-	7	18.7	9	21.0
All ages	268	148	-	-	38.4	-	20	11.0	23	12.3
Total	1 226	354	-	-	35.6	-	91	26.3	99	27.8

Table 210c India - India - Inde Road traffic accidents - Episodes

Age group (years)	Incidence 1990 Number ('000s)	Rate (per 100 000)	Prevalence 1990 Number ('000s)	Rate (per 100 000)	Avg. age at onset (years)	Average duration (years)	Deaths 1990 Number ('000s)	Rate (per 100 000)	Deaths 2000 (Projected) Number ('000s)	Rate (per 100 000)
Males										
0-4	161	270	-	-	2.5	-	17	27.8	16	27.8
5-14	594	584	-	-	10.0	-	19	18.6	26	23.2
15-44	632	315	-	-	29.8	-	59	29.5	95	38.4
45-59	184	388	-	-	52.3	-	17	36.4	32	54.4
60+	89	298	-	-	69.7	-	12	41.7	24	64.5
All ages	1 661	378	-	-	24.7	-	124	28.3	193	37.7
Females										
0-4	47	82	-	-	2.5	-	5	8.5	5	8.5
5-14	428	449	-	-	10.0	-	14	14.3	19	18.0
15-44	144	79	-	-	29.8	-	14	7.4	22	9.5
45-59	102	222	-	-	52.4	-	10	20.9	16	27.3
60+	61	210	-	-	70.1	-	8	28.9	17	43.2
All ages	781	191	-	-	23.4	-	50	12.2	78	16.1
Total	2 443	288	-	-	24.3	-	174	20.5	271	27.2

For epidemiological sources see Lozano et al. 1996. For the methods used to estimate and project incidence, prevalence, and deaths see Murray and Lopez 1996a. See explanatory notes for definitions and caveats.

Table 210
Road traffic accidents

Cuadro 210
Accidentes de tráfico

Tableau 210
Accidents de la voie publique

Episodes

Episodios

Episodes

Table 210d China - China - Chine — Road traffic accidents - Episodes

Age group (years)	Incidence 1990 Number ('000s)	Rate (per 100 000)	Prevalence 1990 Number ('000s)	Rate (per 100 000)	Avg. age at onset (years)	Average duration (years)	Deaths 1990 Number ('000s)	Rate (per 100 000)	Deaths 2000 (Projected) Number ('000s)	Rate (per 100 000)
Males										
0-4	47	77	-	-	2.5	-	4	6.5	4	6.5
5-14	227	234	-	-	10.0	-	6	6.0	11	9.3
15-44	714	233	-	-	29.9	-	55	17.9	95	29.9
45-59	213	293	-	-	52.3	-	17	22.7	41	41.8
60+	139	283	-	-	69.8	-	16	32.0	44	73.4
All ages	1 340	229	-	-	33.3	-	97	16.5	196	29.8
Females										
0-4	34	59	-	-	2.5	-	3	4.9	3	4.9
5-14	212	235	-	-	10.0	-	5	6.1	11	9.3
15-44	201	71	-	-	29.9	-	15	5.4	25	8.3
45-59	98	152	-	-	52.4	-	8	11.8	17	18.1
60+	61	119	-	-	70.6	-	7	13.4	16	25.4
All ages	606	111	-	-	29.1	-	38	7.0	71	11.4
Total	1 946	172	-	-	32.0	-	135	11.9	267	20.8

Table 210e OAI - OPAI - APAI — Road traffic accidents - Episodes

Age group (years)	Incidence 1990 Number ('000s)	Rate (per 100 000)	Prevalence 1990 Number ('000s)	Rate (per 100 000)	Avg. age at onset (years)	Average duration (years)	Deaths 1990 Number ('000s)	Rate (per 100 000)	Deaths 2000 (Projected) Number ('000s)	Rate (per 100 000)
Males										
0-4	127	289	-	-	2.5	-	13	29.0	13	29
5-14	414	493	-	-	10.0	-	14	16.2	15	18
15-44	541	336	-	-	29.7	-	50	31.0	73	36
45-59	113	331	-	-	52.3	-	11	30.8	17	36
60+	53	265	-	-	69.6	-	7	35.9	13	45
All ages	1 248	364	-	-	24.2	-	94	27.4	130	32
Females										
0-4	115	274	-	-	2.5	-	12	27.5	12	27
5-14	220	274	-	-	10.0	-	7	8.5	8	10
15-44	134	84	-	-	29.8	-	12	7.7	20	10
45-59	43	124	-	-	52.3	-	4	11.5	6	14
60+	32	143	-	-	70.3	-	4	19.4	8	24
All ages	545	160	-	-	20.2	-	39	11.5	53	13
Total	1 793	263	-	-	23.0	-	133	19.5	183	23

Table 210f SSA - ASS - ASS — Road traffic accidents - Episodes

Age group (years)	Incidence 1990 Number ('000s)	Rate (per 100 000)	Prevalence 1990 Number ('000s)	Rate (per 100 000)	Avg. age at onset (years)	Average duration (years)	Deaths 1990 Number ('000s)	Rate (per 100 000)	Deaths 2000 (Projected) Number ('000s)	Rate (per 100 000)
Males										
0-4	72	151	-	-	2.4	-	10	20	13	20
5-14	690	982	-	-	10.0	-	30	43	38	41
15-44	467	450	-	-	29.4	-	57	55	79	55
45-59	87	428	-	-	52.2	-	11	54	14	54
60+	35	336	-	-	69.2	-	6	61	9	61
All ages	1 351	535	-	-	20.6	-	114	45	153	45
Females										
0-4	50	105	-	-	2.4	-	7	14	9	14
5-14	333	477	-	-	10.0	-	14	20	19	20
15-44	122	115	-	-	29.5	-	15	14	23	16
45-59	26	115	-	-	52.2	-	3	14	4	15
60+	10	77	-	-	69.7	-	2	14	3	15
All ages	540	209	-	-	16.8	-	41	16	58	17
Total	1 891	371	-	-	19.5	-	155	30	211	31

For epidemiological sources see Lozano et al. 1996. For the methods used to estimate and project incidence, prevalence, and deaths see Murray and Lopez 1996a. See explanatory notes for definitions and caveats.

Table 210
Road traffic accidents

Cuadro 210
Accidentes de tráfico

Tableau 210
Accidents de la voie publique

Episodes

Episodios

Episodes

Table 210g   LAC - ALC - ALC   Road traffic accidents - Episodes

Age group (years)	Incidence 1990 Number ('000s)	Rate (per 100 000)	Prevalence 1990 Number ('000s)	Rate (per 100 000)	Avg. age at onset (years)	Average duration (years)	Deaths 1990 Number ('000s)	Rate (per 100 000)	Deaths 2000 (Projected) Number ('000s)	Rate (per 100 000)
Males										
0-4	40	139	-	-	2.5	-	3	11.6	3	11.6
5-14	475	911	-	-	10.0	-	12	23.5	13	23.0
15-44	591	567	-	-	29.8	-	45	43.6	59	45.7
45-59	143	641	-	-	52.3	-	11	49.6	16	52.1
60+	73	511	-	-	70.3	-	8	57.8	12	62.1
All ages	1 321	596	-	-	26.5	-	80	36.2	104	39.0
Females										
0-4	30	108	-	-	2.5	-	2	9.0	3	9.0
5-14	238	470	-	-	10.0	-	6	12.1	7	12.6
15-44	178	171	-	-	29.9	-	14	13.2	20	15.3
45-59	42	179	-	-	52.4	-	3	13.8	5	15.3
60+	30	177	-	-	71.1	-	3	20.0	5	22.3
All ages	518	233	-	-	23.3	-	29	13.0	39	14.7
Total	1 839	414	-	-	25.6	-	109	24.6	143	26.8

Table 210h   MEC - AOM - CMO   Road traffic accidents - Episodes

Age group (years)	Incidence 1990 Number ('000s)	Rate (per 100 000)	Prevalence 1990 Number ('000s)	Rate (per 100 000)	Avg. age at onset (years)	Average duration (years)	Deaths 1990 Number ('000s)	Rate (per 100 000)	Deaths 2000 (Projected) Number ('000s)	Rate (per 100 000)
Males										
0-4	27	66	-	-	2.5	-	3	6.6	3	6.6
5-14	263	403	-	-	10.0	-	8	12.6	10	11.5
15-44	382	335	-	-	29.8	-	35	30.9	45	30.1
45-59	65	291	-	-	52.3	-	6	27.1	8	26.5
60+	24	176	-	-	69.7	-	3	23.9	4	23.3
All ages	761	297	-	-	25.2	-	55	21.6	71	21.2
Females										
0-4	24	59	-	-	2.5	-	2	6.0	3	6.0
5-14	123	198	-	-	10.0	-	4	6.2	5	6.1
15-44	59	55	-	-	29.8	-	5	5.0	8	5.6
45-59	17	76	-	-	52.3	-	2	7.1	2	7.4
60+	12	79	-	-	70.4	-	2	10.7	2	11.2
All ages	234	95	-	-	20.4	-	15	6.0	20	6.3
Total	995	198	-	-	24.0	-	70	14.0	91	13.9

Table 210i   World - Mundo - Monde   Road traffic accidents - Episodes

Age group (years)	Incidence 1990 Number ('000s)	Rate (per 100 000)	Prevalence 1990 Number ('000s)	Rate (per 100 000)	Avg. age at onset (years)	Average duration (years)	Deaths 1990 Number ('000s)	Rate (per 100 000)	Deaths 2000 (Projected) Number ('000s)	Rate (per 100 000)
Males										
0-4	506	158	-	-	2.5	-	51	16.0	55	16
5-14	2 938	533	-	-	10.0	-	95	17.3	118	19
15-44	4 827	386	-	-	29.8	-	403	32.2	541	37
45-59	1 203	385	-	-	52.3	-	100	32.0	159	39
60+	700	320	-	-	70.1	-	81	37.0	136	49
All ages	10 174	383	-	-	28.6	-	730	27.5	1 008	33
Females										
0-4	321	104	-	-	2.5	-	32	10.4	35	11
5-14	1 705	324	-	-	10.0	-	53	10.1	71	12
15-44	1 343	112	-	-	29.8	-	100	8.3	142	10
45-59	459	148	-	-	52.4	-	38	12.3	61	15
60+	402	149	-	-	71.2	-	46	16.9	73	22
All ages	4 231	162	-	-	26.4	-	269	10.3	382	12
Total	14 405	273	-	-	28.0	-	999	19.0	1 391	23

For epidemiological sources see Lozano et al. 1996. For the methods used to estimate and project incidence, prevalence, and deaths see Murray and Lopez 1996a. See explanatory notes for definitions and caveats.

Table 211
Road traffic accidents

Cuadro 211
Accidentes de tráfico

Tableau 211
Accidents de la voie publique

Fractured skull - long term   Fractura de cráneo - larga duración   Fracture du crâne - long terme

Table 211a   EME - PEMC - EMBE   Road traffic accidents - Fractured skull - long term

Age group (years)	Incidence 1990 Number ('000s)	Rate (per 100 000)	Prevalence 1990 Number ('000s)	Rate (per 100 000)	Avg. age at onset (years)	Average duration (years)	Deaths 1990 Number ('000s)	Rate (per 100 000)	Deaths 2000 (Projected) Number ('000s)	Rate (per 100 000)
Males										
0-4	0	0.3	0	0.8	2.5	70.2	-	-	-	-
5-14	1	1.2	4	7.5	10.0	63.6	-	-	-	-
15-44	2	1.3	60	32.4	29.9	44.8	-	-	-	-
45-59	1	0.8	38	57.7	52.4	24.5	-	-	-	-
60+	1	0.9	45	74.1	71.1	11.3	-	-	-	-
All ages	4	1.1	147	37.6	34.8	41.0	-	-	-	-
Females										
0-4	0	0.2	0	0.6	2.5	76.1	-	-	-	-
5-14	0	0.7	2	4.8	10.0	69.5	-	-	-	-
15-44	1	0.6	31	17.1	30.0	50.0	-	-	-	-
45-59	0	0.3	19	28.0	52.4	28.8	-	-	-	-
60+	0	0.4	30	35.8	72.4	12.7	-	-	-	-
All ages	2	0.5	82	20.2	35.6	45.3	-	-	-	-
Total	6	0.8	229	28.7	35.1	42.4	-	-	-	-

Table 211b   FSE - PEAS - AESE   Road traffic accidents - Fractured skull - long term

Age group (years)	Incidence 1990 Number ('000s)	Rate (per 100 000)	Prevalence 1990 Number ('000s)	Rate (per 100 000)	Avg. age at onset (years)	Average duration (years)	Deaths 1990 Number ('000s)	Rate (per 100 000)	Deaths 2000 (Projected) Number ('000s)	Rate (per 100 000)
Males										
0-4	0	0.3	0	0.9	2.5	63.5	-	-	-	-
5-14	0	1.6	3	9.8	10.0	57.3	-	-	-	-
15-44	1	1.9	35	45.4	29.8	39.2	-	-	-	-
45-59	0	1.7	23	86.4	52.2	20.8	-	-	-	-
60+	0	1.1	23	110.4	70.0	10.1	-	-	-	-
All ages	3	1.6	84	50.8	33.4	36.9	-	-	-	-
Females										
0-4	0	0.2	0	0.5	2.5	72.4	-	-	-	-
5-14	0	0.8	1	5.3	10.0	66.0	-	-	-	-
15-44	0	0.3	11	14.2	29.9	46.8	-	-	-	-
45-59	0	0.4	7	22.0	52.4	26.1	-	-	-	-
60+	0	0.5	11	30.4	71.5	11.8	-	-	-	-
All ages	1	0.4	30	16.5	35.7	42.4	-	-	-	-
Total	3	1.0	114	32.8	33.9	38.2	-	-	-	-

Table 211c   India - India - Inde   Road traffic accidents - Fractured skull - long term

Age group (years)	Incidence 1990 Number ('000s)	Rate (per 100 000)	Prevalence 1990 Number ('000s)	Rate (per 100 000)	Avg. age at onset (years)	Average duration (years)	Deaths 1990 Number ('000s)	Rate (per 100 000)	Deaths 2000 (Projected) Number ('000s)	Rate (per 100 000)
Males										
0-4	1	1.1	2	2.7	2.5	59.9	-	-	-	-
5-14	2	2.3	17	17.2	10.0	57.4	-	-	-	-
15-44	2	0.8	81	40.6	29.8	39.9	-	-	-	-
45-59	0	1.0	29	60.1	52.3	21.0	-	-	-	-
60+	0	0.8	23	75.9	69.7	9.7	-	-	-	-
All ages	5	1.2	152	34.5	21.6	47.0	-	-	-	-
Females										
0-4	0	0.3	0	0.8	2.5	60.8	-	-	-	-
5-14	2	1.8	10	10.7	10.0	59.1	-	-	-	-
15-44	0	0.2	41	22.6	29.8	41.7	-	-	-	-
45-59	0	0.6	14	29.9	52.4	22.5	-	-	-	-
60+	0	0.6	12	40.1	70.1	10.2	-	-	-	-
All ages	3	0.7	77	18.9	20.1	50.2	-	-	-	-
Total	8	0.9	229	27.0	21.1	48.1	-	-	-	-

For epidemiological sources see Lozano et al. 1996. For the methods used to estimate and project incidence, prevalence, and deaths see Lozano et al. 1996 and Murray and Lopez 1996a. See explanatory notes for definitions and caveats.

Table 211	Cuadro 211	Tableau 211
Road traffic accidents	**Accidentes de tráfico**	**Accidents de la voie publique**

Fractured skull - long term   Fractura de cráneo - larga duración   Fracture du crâne - long terme

Table 211d   China - China - Chine   Road traffic accidents - Fractured skull - long term

Age group (years)	Incidence 1990 Number ('000s)	Rate (per 100 000)	Prevalence 1990 Number ('000s)	Rate (per 100 000)	Avg. age at onset (years)	Average duration (years)	Deaths 1990 Number ('000s)	Rate (per 100 000)	Deaths 2000 (Projected) Number ('000s)	Rate (per 100 000)
Males										
0-4	0	0.3	0	0.7	2.5	65.5	-	-	-	-
5-14	1	0.9	6	6.1	10.0	59.9	-	-	-	-
15-44	2	0.6	59	19.4	29.9	41.2	-	-	-	-
45-59	1	0.7	24	33.7	52.3	21.4	-	-	-	-
60+	0	0.8	23	46.9	69.8	9.9	-	-	-	-
All ages	4	0.6	113	19.3	31.1	40.8	-	-	-	-
Females										
0-4	0	0.2	0	0.6	2.5	68.5	-	-	-	-
5-14	1	0.9	5	5.7	10.0	63.2	-	-	-	-
15-44	1	0.2	37	12.9	29.9	44.2	-	-	-	-
45-59	0	0.4	12	18.5	52.4	23.8	-	-	-	-
60+	0	0.3	13	24.8	70.6	10.8	-	-	-	-
All ages	2	0.3	67	12.2	25.8	48.6	-	-	-	-
Total	6	0.5	180	15.9	29.4	43.4	-	-	-	-

Table 211e   OAI - OPAI - APAI   Road traffic accidents - Fractured skull - long term

Age group (years)	Incidence 1990 Number ('000s)	Rate (per 100 000)	Prevalence 1990 Number ('000s)	Rate (per 100 000)	Avg. age at onset (years)	Average duration (years)	Deaths 1990 Number ('000s)	Rate (per 100 000)	Deaths 2000 (Projected) Number ('000s)	Rate (per 100 000)
Males										
0-4	0	1.1	1	2.8	2.5	59.8	-	-	-	-
5-14	2	1.9	13	15.2	10.0	56.2	-	-	-	-
15-44	1	0.8	60	37.3	29.7	38.8	-	-	-	-
45-59	0	0.8	19	56.3	52.3	20.3	-	-	-	-
60+	0	0.7	14	69.7	69.6	9.7	-	-	-	-
All ages	4	1.1	107	31.3	21.3	46.2	-	-	-	-
Females										
0-4	0	1.1	1	2.6	2.5	63.2	-	-	-	-
5-14	1	1.1	9	10.7	10.0	59.2	-	-	-	-
15-44	0	0.2	31	19.1	29.8	41.4	-	-	-	-
45-59	0	0.3	9	24.6	52.3	22.4	-	-	-	-
60+	0	0.4	7	31.1	70.3	10.5	-	-	-	-
All ages	2	0.5	56	16.4	17.2	52.3	-	-	-	-
Total	6	0.8	163	23.9	20.0	48.2	-	-	-	-

Table 211f   SSA - ASS - ASS   Road traffic accidents - Fractured skull - long term

Age group (years)	Incidence 1990 Number ('000s)	Rate (per 100 000)	Prevalence 1990 Number ('000s)	Rate (per 100 000)	Avg. age at onset (years)	Average duration (years)	Deaths 1990 Number ('000s)	Rate (per 100 000)	Deaths 2000 (Projected) Number ('000s)	Rate (per 100 000)
Males										
0-4	0	0.6	1	1.4	2.4	48.7	-	-	-	-
5-14	3	3.8	15	22.0	10.0	49.2	-	-	-	-
15-44	1	1.1	60	57.5	29.4	35.0	-	-	-	-
45-59	0	1.1	17	82.9	52.2	19.1	-	-	-	-
60+	0	0.9	10	99.9	69.2	9.3	-	-	-	-
All ages	4	1.8	103	40.9	18.0	43.1	-	-	-	-
Females										
0-4	0	0.4	0	1.0	2.4	51.9	-	-	-	-
5-14	1	1.8	8	11.2	10.0	51.9	-	-	-	-
15-44	0	0.3	26	24.7	29.5	37.2	-	-	-	-
45-59	0	0.3	7	31.3	52.2	20.5	-	-	-	-
60+	0	0.2	5	35.6	69.7	9.8	-	-	-	-
All ages	2	0.7	46	17.8	14.7	47.8	-	-	-	-
Total	6	1.2	149	29.2	17.0	44.5	-	-	-	-

For epidemiological sources see Lozano et al. 1996. For the methods used to estimate and project incidence, prevalence, and deaths see Lozano et al. 1996 and Murray and Lopez 1996a. See explanatory notes for definitions and caveats.

Table 211
Road traffic accidents

Cuadro 211
Accidentes de tráfico

Tableau 211
Accidents de la voie publique

Fractured skull - long term | Fractura de cráneo - larga duración | Fracture du crâne - long terme

Table 211g   LAC - ALC - ALC — Road traffic accidents - Fractured skull - long term

Age group (years)	Incidence 1990 Number ('000s)	Rate (per 100 000)	Prevalence 1990 Number ('000s)	Rate (per 100 000)	Avg. age at onset (years)	Average duration (years)	Deaths 1990 Number ('000s)	Rate (per 100 000)	Deaths 2000 (Projected) Number ('000s)	Rate (per 100 000)
Males										
0-4	0	0.5	0	1.3	2.5	63.9	-	-	-	-
5-14	2	3.5	11	20.5	10.0	59.3	-	-	-	-
15-44	1	1.4	62	59.3	29.8	41.4	-	-	-	-
45-59	0	1.6	21	92.8	52.3	22.3	-	-	-	-
60+	0	1.4	17	119.6	70.3	10.4	-	-	-	-
All ages	4	1.8	111	49.9	23.7	47.3	-	-	-	-
Females										
0-4	0	0.4	0	1.0	2.5	67.9	-	-	-	-
5-14	1	1.8	6	11.3	10.0	63.0	-	-	-	-
15-44	0	0.4	28	26.8	29.9	44.6	-	-	-	-
45-59	0	0.5	9	36.6	52.4	24.8	-	-	-	-
60+	0	0.5	8	45.5	71.1	11.3	-	-	-	-
All ages	2	0.8	50	22.5	20.4	53.5	-	-	-	-
Total	6	1.3	161	36.2	22.7	49.1	-	-	-	-

Table 211h   MEC - AOM - CMO — Road traffic accidents - Fractured skull - long term

Age group (years)	Incidence 1990 Number ('000s)	Rate (per 100 000)	Prevalence 1990 Number ('000s)	Rate (per 100 000)	Avg. age at onset (years)	Average duration (years)	Deaths 1990 Number ('000s)	Rate (per 100 000)	Deaths 2000 (Projected) Number ('000s)	Rate (per 100 000)
Males										
0-4	0	0.3	0	0.6	2.5	61.1	-	-	-	-
5-14	1	1.6	6	9.1	10.0	58.1	-	-	-	-
15-44	1	0.8	34	29.5	29.8	40.0	-	-	-	-
45-59	0	0.7	11	47.6	52.3	20.8	-	-	-	-
60+	0	0.5	8	58.0	69.7	9.8	-	-	-	-
All ages	2	0.9	58	22.8	22.5	46.7	-	-	-	-
Females										
0-4	0	0.2	0	0.6	2.5	63.7	-	-	-	-
5-14	0	0.8	3	5.0	10.0	60.9	-	-	-	-
15-44	0	0.1	12	10.9	29.8	42.6	-	-	-	-
45-59	0	0.2	3	14.4	52.3	22.9	-	-	-	-
60+	0	0.2	3	18.2	70.4	10.6	-	-	-	-
All ages	1	0.3	21	8.5	17.6	53.6	-	-	-	-
Total	3	0.6	79	15.8	21.3	48.5	-	-	-	-

Table 211i   World - Mundo - Monde — Road traffic accidents - Fractured skull - long term

Age group (years)	Incidence 1990 Number ('000s)	Rate (per 100 000)	Prevalence 1990 Number ('000s)	Rate (per 100 000)	Avg. age at onset (years)	Average duration (years)	Deaths 1990 Number ('000s)	Rate (per 100 000)	Deaths 2000 (Projected) Number ('000s)	Rate (per 100 000)
Males										
0-4	2	0.6	5	1.5	2.5	59.7	-	-	-	-
5-14	12	2.1	75	13.6	10.0	56.2	-	-	-	-
15-44	12	1.0	450	36.0	29.8	40.5	-	-	-	-
45-59	3	1.0	182	58.2	52.3	21.6	-	-	-	-
60+	2	0.9	163	74.5	70.2	10.3	-	-	-	-
All ages	31	1.2	875	33.0	25.4	43.9	-	-	-	-
Females										
0-4	1	0.4	3	1.0	2.5	63.0	-	-	-	-
5-14	7	1.3	44	8.5	10.0	59.7	-	-	-	-
15-44	3	0.3	216	18.0	29.9	45.0	-	-	-	-
45-59	1	0.4	79	25.3	52.4	24.4	-	-	-	-
60+	1	0.4	88	32.6	71.2	11.5	-	-	-	-
All ages	14	0.5	430	16.4	22.9	49.4	-	-	-	-
Total	44	0.8	1 304	24.8	24.6	45.6	-	-	-	-

For epidemiological sources see Lozano et al. 1996. For the methods used to estimate and project incidence, prevalence, and deaths see Lozano et al. 1996 and Murray and Lopez 1996a. See explanatory notes for definitions and caveats.

Table 212
Road traffic accidents

Cuadro 212
Accidentes de tráfico

Tableau 212
Accidents de la voie publique

Injured spinal cord   Lesión de la medula espinal   Lésion de la moelle épinière

Table 212a   EME - PEMC - EMBE   Road traffic accidents - Injured spinal cord

Age group (years)	Incidence 1990 Number ('000s)	Rate (per 100 000)	Prevalence 1990 Number ('000s)	Rate (per 100 000)	Avg. age at onset (years)	Average duration (years)	Deaths 1990 Number ('000s)	Rate (per 100 000)	Deaths 2000 (Projected) Number ('000s)	Rate (per 100 000)
Males										
0-4	0	0.3	0	0.7	2.5	57.1	-	-	-	-
5-14	1	1.0	3	6.4	10.0	51.1	-	-	-	-
15-44	26	13.9	390	211.7	29.9	33.6	-	-	-	-
45-59	6	8.8	286	432.1	52.4	15.6	-	-	-	-
60+	3	5.1	175	288.8	71.1	6.1	-	-	-	-
All ages	35	9.0	854	218.7	36.9	28.5	-	-	-	-
Females										
0-4	0	0.2	0	0.5	2.5	65.1	-	-	-	-
5-14	0	0.6	2	4.2	10.0	59.0	-	-	-	-
15-44	11	6.3	179	99.9	30.0	40.2	-	-	-	-
45-59	2	3.3	140	206.1	52.4	20.5	-	-	-	-
60+	2	2.4	139	164.8	72.4	7.8	-	-	-	-
All ages	16	3.9	460	113.0	38.1	33.7	-	-	-	-
Total	51	6.4	1 314	164.7	37.3	30.1	-	-	-	-

Table 212b   FSE - PEAS - AESE   Road traffic accidents - Injured spinal cord

Age group (years)	Incidence 1990 Number ('000s)	Rate (per 100 000)	Prevalence 1990 Number ('000s)	Rate (per 100 000)	Avg. age at onset (years)	Average duration (years)	Deaths 1990 Number ('000s)	Rate (per 100 000)	Deaths 2000 (Projected) Number ('000s)	Rate (per 100 000)
Males										
0-4	0	0.3	0	0.7	2.5	48.3	-	-	-	-
5-14	0	1.4	2	8.4	10.0	43.1	-	-	-	-
15-44	15	20.3	226	296.2	29.8	26.8	-	-	-	-
45-59	5	18.6	156	577.8	52.2	11.9	-	-	-	-
60+	1	5.8	70	333.3	70.0	5.2	-	-	-	-
All ages	22	13.4	454	274.7	36.7	22.5	-	-	-	-
Females										
0-4	0	0.2	0	0.5	2.5	59.8	-	-	-	-
5-14	0	0.7	1	4.5	10.0	54.5	-	-	-	-
15-44	3	3.4	44	58.5	29.9	36.2	-	-	-	-
45-59	1	4.5	39	131.1	52.4	17.4	-	-	-	-
60+	1	2.5	40	110.6	71.5	6.7	-	-	-	-
All ages	5	2.8	125	68.9	42.5	26.7	-	-	-	-
Total	27	7.9	579	167.2	37.8	23.3	-	-	-	-

Table 212c   India - India - Inde   Road traffic accidents - Injured spinal cord

Age group (years)	Incidence 1990 Number ('000s)	Rate (per 100 000)	Prevalence 1990 Number ('000s)	Rate (per 100 000)	Avg. age at onset (years)	Average duration (years)	Deaths 1990 Number ('000s)	Rate (per 100 000)	Deaths 2000 (Projected) Number ('000s)	Rate (per 100 000)
Males										
0-4	1	0.9	1	2.1	2.5	40.0	-	-	-	-
5-14	2	2.0	14	14.1	10.0	43.1	-	-	-	-
15-44	18	8.7	288	143.7	29.8	28.1	-	-	-	-
45-59	5	10.7	138	290.4	52.3	12.7	-	-	-	-
60+	1	4.7	57	192.2	69.7	4.9	-	-	-	-
All ages	27	6.1	499	113.6	34.1	25.3	-	-	-	-
Females										
0-4	0	0.3	0	0.6	2.5	40.1	-	-	-	-
5-14	1	1.6	9	8.9	10.0	44.5	-	-	-	-
15-44	4	2.2	84	45.7	29.8	30.0	-	-	-	-
45-59	3	6.2	49	107.4	52.4	14.3	-	-	-	-
60+	1	3.2	27	95.0	70.1	5.3	-	-	-	-
All ages	9	2.3	169	41.3	37.0	25.3	-	-	-	-
Total	36	4.2	668	78.7	34.8	25.3	-	-	-	-

For epidemiological sources see Lozano et al. 1996. For the methods used to estimate and project incidence, prevalence, and deaths see Lozano et al. 1996 and Murray and Lopez 1996a. See explanatory notes for definitions and caveats.

Table 212
Road traffic accidents

Cuadro 212
Accidentes de tráfico

Tableau 212
Accidents de la voie publique

Injured spinal cord

Lesión de la medula espinal

Lésion de la moelle épinière

Table 212d   China - China - Chine   Road traffic accidents - Injured spinal cord

Age group (years)	Incidence 1990 Number ('000s)	Rate (per 100 000)	Prevalence 1990 Number ('000s)	Rate (per 100 000)	Avg. age at onset (years)	Average duration (years)	Deaths 1990 Number ('000s)	Rate (per 100 000)	Deaths 2000 (Projected) Number ('000s)	Rate (per 100 000)
Males										
0-4	0	0.3	0	0.6	2.5	51.2	-	-	-	-
5-14	1	0.8	5	5.2	10.0	47.6	-	-	-	-
15-44	20	6.4	307	100.2	29.9	30.4	-	-	-	-
45-59	6	8.0	160	219.9	52.3	13.1	-	-	-	-
60+	2	4.3	74	151.9	69.8	5.0	-	-	-	-
All ages	28	4.9	547	93.4	36.8	25.6	-	-	-	-
Females										
0-4	0	0.2	0	0.5	2.5	54.2	-	-	-	-
5-14	1	0.8	4	4.9	10.0	51.4	-	-	-	-
15-44	6	1.9	104	36.7	29.9	33.6	-	-	-	-
45-59	3	4.2	56	87.0	52.4	15.4	-	-	-	-
60+	1	1.8	38	72.7	70.6	5.7	-	-	-	-
All ages	10	1.8	203	36.9	38.0	27.6	-	-	-	-
Total	38	3.4	749	66.1	37.1	26.1	-	-	-	-

Table 212e   OAI - OPAI - APAI   Road traffic accidents - Injured spinal cord

Age group (years)	Incidence 1990 Number ('000s)	Rate (per 100 000)	Prevalence 1990 Number ('000s)	Rate (per 100 000)	Avg. age at onset (years)	Average duration (years)	Deaths 1990 Number ('000s)	Rate (per 100 000)	Deaths 2000 (Projected) Number ('000s)	Rate (per 100 000)
Males										
0-4	0	1.0	1	2.3	2.5	41.2	-	-	-	-
5-14	1	1.7	11	12.6	10.0	41.5	-	-	-	-
15-44	15	9.2	233	145.2	29.7	26.7	-	-	-	-
45-59	3	9.0	95	277.7	52.3	11.8	-	-	-	-
60+	1	4.0	33	165.2	69.6	4.7	-	-	-	-
All ages	21	6.0	373	108.8	32.8	24.9	-	-	-	-
Females										
0-4	0	0.9	1	2.2	2.5	45.0	-	-	-	-
5-14	1	0.9	7	8.8	10.0	44.6	-	-	-	-
15-44	4	2.3	71	44.3	29.8	29.4	-	-	-	-
45-59	1	3.4	31	87.0	52.3	13.7	-	-	-	-
60+	0	2.2	15	65.4	70.3	5.4	-	-	-	-
All ages	6	1.9	124	36.5	33.1	27.4	-	-	-	-
Total	27	4.0	497	72.8	32.8	25.5	-	-	-	-

Table 212f   SSA - ASS - ASS   Road traffic accidents - Injured spinal cord

Age group (years)	Incidence 1990 Number ('000s)	Rate (per 100 000)	Prevalence 1990 Number ('000s)	Rate (per 100 000)	Avg. age at onset (years)	Average duration (years)	Deaths 1990 Number ('000s)	Rate (per 100 000)	Deaths 2000 (Projected) Number ('000s)	Rate (per 100 000)
Males										
0-4	0	0.5	1	1.1	2.4	25.2	-	-	-	-
5-14	2	3.3	12	17.7	10.0	31.1	-	-	-	-
15-44	13	12.3	186	179.1	29.4	21.3	-	-	-	-
45-59	2	11.7	63	311.8	52.2	10.6	-	-	-	-
60+	1	5.1	19	177.9	69.2	4.5	-	-	-	-
All ages	18	7.2	281	111.3	30.7	20.7	-	-	-	-
Females										
0-4	0	0.4	0	0.8	2.4	28.3	-	-	-	-
5-14	1	1.6	6	9.0	10.0	33.9	-	-	-	-
15-44	3	3.1	57	53.9	29.5	23.5	-	-	-	-
45-59	1	3.2	20	91.3	52.2	11.9	-	-	-	-
60+	0	1.2	7	54.9	69.7	4.9	-	-	-	-
All ages	5	2.1	91	35.3	28.7	23.8	-	-	-	-
Total	24	4.6	372	72.9	30.2	21.4	-	-	-	-

For epidemiological sources see Lozano et al. 1996. For the methods used to estimate and project incidence, prevalence, and deaths see Lozano et al. 1996 and Murray and Lopez 1996a. See explanatory notes for definitions and caveats.

Table 212	Cuadro 212	Tableau 212
Road traffic accidents	Accidentes de tráfico	Accidents de la voie publique

| Injured spinal cord | Lesión de la medula espinal | Lésion de la moelle épinière |

Table 212g LAC - ALC - ALC

Road traffic accidents - Injured spinal cord

Age group (years)	Incidence 1990 Number ('000s)	Rate (per 100 000)	Prevalence 1990 Number ('000s)	Rate (per 100 000)	Avg. age at onset (years)	Average duration (years)	Deaths 1990 Number ('000s)	Rate (per 100 000)	Deaths 2000 (Projected) Number ('000s)	Rate (per 100 000)
Males										
0-4	0	0.5	0	1.1	2.5	46.5	-	-	-	-
5-14	2	3.1	9	17.4	10.0	45.1	-	-	-	-
15-44	16	15.5	258	247.3	29.8	29.4	-	-	-	-
45-59	4	17.5	113	510.1	52.3	13.6	-	-	-	-
60+	1	7.7	49	346.4	70.3	5.4	-	-	-	-
All ages	23	10.3	430	194.1	34.0	26.8	-	-	-	-
Females										
0-4	0	0.4	0	0.9	2.5	51.7	-	-	-	-
5-14	1	1.6	5	9.6	10.0	49.5	-	-	-	-
15-44	5	4.7	87	83.3	29.8	33.0	-	-	-	-
45-59	1	4.9	39	166.6	52.4	16.2	-	-	-	-
60+	0	2.7	21	126.2	71.1	6.2	-	-	-	-
All ages	7	3.3	152	68.2	33.3	30.8	-	-	-	-
Total	30	6.8	582	131.0	33.8	27.8	-	-	-	-

Table 212h MEC - AOM - CMO

Road traffic accidents - Injured spinal cord

Age group (years)	Incidence 1990 Number ('000s)	Rate (per 100 000)	Prevalence 1990 Number ('000s)	Rate (per 100 000)	Avg. age at onset (years)	Average duration (years)	Deaths 1990 Number ('000s)	Rate (per 100 000)	Deaths 2000 (Projected) Number ('000s)	Rate (per 100 000)
Males										
0-4	0	0.2	0	0.5	2.5	42.6	-	-	-	-
5-14	1	1.4	5	7.7	10.0	44.6	-	-	-	-
15-44	10	9.2	163	142.9	29.8	28.5	-	-	-	-
45-59	2	8.0	62	279.0	52.3	12.3	-	-	-	-
60+	0	2.7	22	161.0	69.7	4.9	-	-	-	-
All ages	14	5.3	252	98.4	32.3	26.9	-	-	-	-
Females										
0-4	0	0.2	0	0.5	2.5	45.1	-	-	-	-
5-14	0	0.7	3	4.2	10.0	47.5	-	-	-	-
15-44	2	1.5	30	28.4	29.8	31.1	-	-	-	-
45-59	0	2.1	13	57.1	52.3	14.3	-	-	-	-
60+	0	1.2	7	42.7	70.4	5.5	-	-	-	-
All ages	3	1.1	53	21.3	32.6	29.4	-	-	-	-
Total	16	3.2	305	60.6	32.4	27.3	-	-	-	-

Table 212i World - Mundo - Monde

Road traffic accidents - Injured spinal cord

Age group (years)	Incidence 1990 Number ('000s)	Rate (per 100 000)	Prevalence 1990 Number ('000s)	Rate (per 100 000)	Avg. age at onset (years)	Average duration (years)	Deaths 1990 Number ('000s)	Rate (per 100 000)	Deaths 2000 (Projected) Number ('000s)	Rate (per 100 000)
Males										
0-4	2	0.5	4	1.2	2.5	40.8	-	-	-	-
5-14	10	1.8	62	11.3	10.0	41.3	-	-	-	-
15-44	132	10.6	2 050	164.1	29.8	28.7	-	-	-	-
45-59	33	10.5	1 073	343.7	52.3	13.0	-	-	-	-
60+	11	4.9	500	228.4	70.2	5.3	-	-	-	-
All ages	187	7.1	3 690	139.1	34.7	25.4	-	-	-	-
Females										
0-4	1	0.4	3	0.8	2.5	44.6	-	-	-	-
5-14	6	1.1	37	7.1	10.0	45.3	-	-	-	-
15-44	37	3.1	656	54.7	29.9	33.9	-	-	-	-
45-59	13	4.1	387	124.4	52.4	15.9	-	-	-	-
60+	6	2.3	294	109.3	71.2	6.5	-	-	-	-
All ages	62	2.4	1 377	52.7	36.1	28.8	-	-	-	-
Total	250	4.7	5 067	96.2	35.1	26.3	-	-	-	-

For epidemiological sources see Lozano et al. 1996. For the methods used to estimate and project incidence, prevalence, and deaths see Lozano et al. 1996 and Murray and Lopez 1996a. See explanatory notes for definitions and caveats.

Table 213
Road traffic accidents

Cuadro 213
Accidentes de tráfico

Tableau 213
Accidents de la voie publique

Fractured femur - long term

Fractura de femur - larga duración

Fracture du fémur - long terme

Table 213a **EME - PEMC - EMBE** Road traffic accidents - Fractured femur - long term

Age group (years)	Incidence 1990 Number ('000s)	Rate (per 100 000)	Prevalence 1990 Number ('000s)	Rate (per 100 000)	Avg. age at onset (years)	Average duration (years)	Deaths 1990 Number ('000s)	Rate (per 100 000)	Deaths 2000 (Projected) Number ('000s)	Rate (per 100 000)
Males										
0-4	0	0.4	0	0.9	2.5	70.2	-	-	-	-
5-14	1	1.4	5	8.8	10.0	63.6	-	-	-	-
15-44	4	2.1	87	47.0	29.9	44.8	-	-	-	-
45-59	1	1.3	58	88.3	52.4	24.5	-	-	-	-
60+	2	3.5	83	137.5	71.1	11.3	-	-	-	-
All ages	8	2.0	233	59.7	41.6	35.3	-	-	-	-
Females										
0-4	0	0.3	0	0.7	2.5	76.1	-	-	-	-
5-14	0	0.9	3	5.7	10.0	69.5	-	-	-	-
15-44	2	0.9	43	24.1	30.0	50.0	-	-	-	-
45-59	0	0.5	29	42.0	52.4	28.8	-	-	-	-
60+	1	1.7	56	66.4	72.4	12.7	-	-	-	-
All ages	4	1.0	131	32.1	44.3	37.5	-	-	-	-
Total	12	1.5	364	45.6	42.5	36.1	-	-	-	-

Table 213b **FSE - PEAS - AESE** Road traffic accidents - Fractured femur - long term

Age group (years)	Incidence 1990 Number ('000s)	Rate (per 100 000)	Prevalence 1990 Number ('000s)	Rate (per 100 000)	Avg. age at onset (years)	Average duration (years)	Deaths 1990 Number ('000s)	Rate (per 100 000)	Deaths 2000 (Projected) Number ('000s)	Rate (per 100 000)
Males										
0-4	0	0.4	0	1.0	2.5	63.5	-	-	-	-
5-14	1	1.9	3	11.6	10.0	57.3	-	-	-	-
15-44	2	3.1	51	66.3	29.8	39.2	-	-	-	-
45-59	1	2.8	36	133.3	52.2	20.8	-	-	-	-
60+	1	4.0	41	195.5	70.0	10.1	-	-	-	-
All ages	5	2.7	131	79.2	38.5	33.0	-	-	-	-
Females										
0-4	0	0.3	0	0.6	2.5	72.4	-	-	-	-
5-14	0	1.0	2	6.3	10.0	66.0	-	-	-	-
15-44	0	0.5	14	19.0	29.9	46.8	-	-	-	-
45-59	0	0.7	10	31.8	52.4	26.1	-	-	-	-
60+	1	1.7	21	56.8	71.5	11.8	-	-	-	-
All ages	2	0.8	46	25.5	46.1	33.4	-	-	-	-
Total	6	1.7	177	51.1	40.4	33.1	-	-	-	-

Table 213c **India - India - Inde** Road traffic accidents - Fractured femur - long term

Age group (years)	Incidence 1990 Number ('000s)	Rate (per 100 000)	Prevalence 1990 Number ('000s)	Rate (per 100 000)	Avg. age at onset (years)	Average duration (years)	Deaths 1990 Number ('000s)	Rate (per 100 000)	Deaths 2000 (Projected) Number ('000s)	Rate (per 100 000)
Males										
0-4	2	3.3	5	8.0	2.5	59.9	-	-	-	-
5-14	7	7.1	53	51.9	10.0	57.4	-	-	-	-
15-44	7	3.4	274	136.5	29.8	39.9	-	-	-	-
45-59	2	4.1	104	217.9	52.3	21.0	-	-	-	-
60+	2	8.1	98	328.3	69.7	9.7	-	-	-	-
All ages	20	4.6	533	121.2	27.1	42.6	-	-	-	-
Females										
0-4	1	1.0	1	2.4	2.5	60.8	-	-	-	-
5-14	5	5.4	31	32.4	10.0	59.1	-	-	-	-
15-44	2	0.8	131	71.7	29.8	41.7	-	-	-	-
45-59	1	2.4	47	102.1	52.4	22.5	-	-	-	-
60+	9	30.4	124	428.2	70.1	10.2	-	-	-	-
All ages	17	4.2	334	81.5	45.0	30.2	-	-	-	-
Total	37	4.4	867	102.1	35.3	36.9	-	-	-	-

For epidemiological sources see Lozano et al. 1996. For the methods used to estimate and project incidence, prevalence, and deaths see Lozano et al. 1996 and Murray and Lopez 1996a. See explanatory notes for definitions and caveats.

Table 213
Road traffic accidents

Cuadro 213
Accidentes de tráfico

Tableau 213
Accidents de la voie publique

Fractured femur - long term   Fractura de femur - larga duración   Fracture du fémur - long terme

| Table 213d | China - China - Chine | | | | | | Road traffic accidents - Fractured femur - long term | | | |

Age group (years)	Incidence 1990 Number ('000s)	Rate (per 100 000)	Prevalence 1990 Number ('000s)	Rate (per 100 000)	Avg. age at onset (years)	Average duration (years)	Deaths 1990 Number ('000s)	Rate (per 100 000)	Deaths 2000 (Projected) Number ('000s)	Rate (per 100 000)
Males										
0-4	0	0.5	1	1.2	2.5	65.5	-	-	-	-
5-14	1	1.4	9	9.4	10.0	59.9	-	-	-	-
15-44	4	1.3	108	35.2	29.9	41.2	-	-	-	-
45-59	1	1.6	48	65.9	52.3	21.4	-	-	-	-
60+	2	3.9	57	115.8	69.8	9.9	-	-	-	-
All ages	9	1.5	222	38.0	37.6	35.4	-	-	-	-
Females										
0-4	0	0.4	1	0.9	2.5	68.5	-	-	-	-
5-14	1	1.4	8	8.9	10.0	63.2	-	-	-	-
15-44	1	0.4	62	21.7	29.9	44.2	-	-	-	-
45-59	1	0.8	22	33.5	52.4	23.8	-	-	-	-
60+	1	1.6	29	56.9	70.6	10.8	-	-	-	-
All ages	4	0.7	121	22.1	33.6	41.8	-	-	-	-
Total	12	1.1	343	30.3	36.4	37.5	-	-	-	-

| Table 213e | OAI - OPAI - APAI | | | | | | Road traffic accidents - Fractured femur - long term | | | |

Age group (years)	Incidence 1990 Number ('000s)	Rate (per 100 000)	Prevalence 1990 Number ('000s)	Rate (per 100 000)	Avg. age at onset (years)	Average duration (years)	Deaths 1990 Number ('000s)	Rate (per 100 000)	Deaths 2000 (Projected) Number ('000s)	Rate (per 100 000)
Males										
0-4	1	2.2	2	5.3	2.5	59.8	-	-	-	-
5-14	3	3.7	25	29.2	10.0	56.2	-	-	-	-
15-44	4	2.2	130	80.7	29.7	38.8	-	-	-	-
45-59	1	2.2	45	131.1	52.3	20.3	-	-	-	-
60+	1	4.4	39	190.9	69.6	9.7	-	-	-	-
All ages	9	2.7	240	70.0	26.1	42.4	-	-	-	-
Females										
0-4	1	2.0	2	5.1	2.5	63.2	-	-	-	-
5-14	2	2.1	16	20.5	10.0	59.2	-	-	-	-
15-44	1	0.6	62	39.0	29.8	41.5	-	-	-	-
45-59	0	0.8	19	53.6	52.3	22.4	-	-	-	-
60+	1	2.4	19	84.8	70.3	10.5	-	-	-	-
All ages	4	1.2	119	35.0	23.3	47.4	-	-	-	-
Total	14	2.0	359	52.6	25.2	44.0	-	-	-	-

| Table 213f | SSA - ASS - ASS | | | | | | Road traffic accidents - Fractured femur - long term | | | |

Age group (years)	Incidence 1990 Number ('000s)	Rate (per 100 000)	Prevalence 1990 Number ('000s)	Rate (per 100 000)	Avg. age at onset (years)	Average duration (years)	Deaths 1990 Number ('000s)	Rate (per 100 000)	Deaths 2000 (Projected) Number ('000s)	Rate (per 100 000)
Males										
0-4	1	2.2	3	5.3	2.4	48.7	-	-	-	-
5-14	10	14.4	58	82.5	10.0	49.2	-	-	-	-
15-44	6	5.9	248	239.3	29.4	35.0	-	-	-	-
45-59	1	5.6	75	371.1	52.2	19.1	-	-	-	-
60+	1	11.0	54	516.7	69.2	9.3	-	-	-	-
All ages	20	7.7	438	173.8	21.6	40.7	-	-	-	-
Females										
0-4	1	1.5	2	3.7	2.4	51.9	-	-	-	-
5-14	5	6.9	29	42.2	10.0	51.9	-	-	-	-
15-44	2	1.5	105	98.8	29.5	37.2	-	-	-	-
45-59	0	1.5	29	133.1	52.2	20.5	-	-	-	-
60+	0	2.5	22	169.4	69.7	9.8	-	-	-	-
All ages	8	3.0	187	72.6	17.5	45.8	-	-	-	-
Total	27	5.4	626	122.6	20.4	42.1	-	-	-	-

For epidemiological sources see Lozano et al. 1996. For the methods used to estimate and project incidence, prevalence, and deaths see Lozano et al. 1996 and Murray and Lopez 1996a. See explanatory notes for definitions and caveats.

Table 213	Cuadro 213	Tableau 213
Road traffic accidents	**Accidentes de tráfico**	**Accidents de la voie publique**
Fractured femur - long term	Fractura de femur - larga duración	Fracture du fémur - long terme

Table 213g LAC - ALC - ALC

Road traffic accidents - Fractured femur - long term

Age group (years)	Incidence 1990 Number ('000s)	Rate (per 100 000)	Prevalence 1990 Number ('000s)	Rate (per 100 000)	Avg. age at onset (years)	Average duration (years)	Deaths 1990 Number ('000s)	Rate (per 100 000)	Deaths 2000 (Projected) Number ('000s)	Rate (per 100 000)
Males										
0-4	0	1.2	1	3.1	2.5	63.9	-	-	-	-
5-14	5	8.8	26	50.4	10.0	59.3	-	-	-	-
15-44	5	4.5	168	161.1	29.8	41.4	-	-	-	-
45-59	1	5.1	59	266.9	52.3	22.3	-	-	-	-
60+	1	10.2	59	411.4	70.3	10.5	-	-	-	-
All ages	12	5.5	313	141.2	28.5	43.4	-	-	-	-
Females										
0-4	0	1.0	1	2.4	2.5	67.9	-	-	-	-
5-14	2	4.2	13	25.8	10.0	63.0	-	-	-	-
15-44	1	1.4	70	66.9	29.9	44.6	-	-	-	-
45-59	0	1.4	23	98.0	52.4	24.8	-	-	-	-
60+	1	3.5	25	148.2	71.1	11.3	-	-	-	-
All ages	5	2.1	131	58.9	26.2	48.6	-	-	-	-
Total	17	3.8	444	100.0	27.8	44.8	-	-	-	-

Table 213h MEC - AOM - CMO

Road traffic accidents - Fractured femur - long term

Age group (years)	Incidence 1990 Number ('000s)	Rate (per 100 000)	Prevalence 1990 Number ('000s)	Rate (per 100 000)	Avg. age at onset (years)	Average duration (years)	Deaths 1990 Number ('000s)	Rate (per 100 000)	Deaths 2000 (Projected) Number ('000s)	Rate (per 100 000)
Males										
0-4	0	0.6	1	1.4	2.5	61.1	-	-	-	-
5-14	2	3.6	14	20.9	10.0	58.1	-	-	-	-
15-44	3	2.7	89	78.4	29.8	40.0	-	-	-	-
45-59	1	2.3	30	135.7	52.3	20.8	-	-	-	-
60+	0	3.5	26	187.9	69.7	9.8	-	-	-	-
All ages	7	2.6	160	62.2	26.4	43.5	-	-	-	-
Females										
0-4	0	0.5	1	1.3	2.5	63.7	-	-	-	-
5-14	1	1.8	7	11.5	10.0	60.9	-	-	-	-
15-44	0	0.4	29	26.8	29.8	42.6	-	-	-	-
45-59	0	0.6	8	37.8	52.3	22.9	-	-	-	-
60+	0	1.6	9	59.0	70.4	10.6	-	-	-	-
All ages	2	0.9	54	21.8	23.1	49.1	-	-	-	-
Total	9	1.7	213	42.4	25.6	44.9	-	-	-	-

Table 213i World - Mundo - Monde

Road traffic accidents - Fractured femur - long term

Age group (years)	Incidence 1990 Number ('000s)	Rate (per 100 000)	Prevalence 1990 Number ('000s)	Rate (per 100 000)	Avg. age at onset (years)	Average duration (years)	Deaths 1990 Number ('000s)	Rate (per 100 000)	Deaths 2000 (Projected) Number ('000s)	Rate (per 100 000)
Males										
0-4	5	1.6	12	3.8	2.5	58.4	-	-	-	-
5-14	30	5.4	192	34.9	10.0	55.2	-	-	-	-
15-44	34	2.7	1 154	92.3	29.7	39.8	-	-	-	-
45-59	8	2.7	456	145.9	52.3	21.2	-	-	-	-
60+	11	5.1	456	208.2	70.0	10.1	-	-	-	-
All ages	89	3.3	2 270	85.5	28.8	40.5	-	-	-	-
Females										
0-4	3	0.9	7	2.3	2.5	61.2	-	-	-	-
5-14	17	3.2	110	20.8	10.0	58.3	-	-	-	-
15-44	9	0.8	516	43.0	29.8	43.4	-	-	-	-
45-59	3	1.0	186	59.8	52.4	23.6	-	-	-	-
60+	13	5.0	305	113.3	70.5	10.6	-	-	-	-
All ages	46	1.7	1 124	43.0	34.3	39.0	-	-	-	-
Total	134	2.5	3 394	64.4	30.6	40.0	-	-	-	-

For epidemiological sources see Lozano et al. 1996. For the methods used to estimate and project incidence, prevalence, and deaths see Lozano et al. 1996 and Murray and Lopez 1996a. See explanatory notes for definitions and caveats.

Table 214
Road traffic accidents

Cuadro 214
Accidentes de tráfico

Tableau 214
Accidents de la voie publique

Intracranial injury - short term   Lesión intracraneal - corta duración   Lésions intra-crâniennes - court terme

Table 214a   EME - PEMC - EMBE   Road traffic accidents - Intracranial injury - short term

Age group (years)	Incidence 1990 Number ('000s)	Rate (per 100 000)	Prevalence 1990 Number ('000s)	Rate (per 100 000)	Avg. age at onset (years)	Average duration (years)	Deaths 1990 Number ('000s)	Rate (per 100 000)	Deaths 2000 (Projected) Number ('000s)	Rate (per 100 000)
Males										
0-4	10	38	1	2.5	2.5	0.07	-	-	-	-
5-14	78	146	5	9.8	10.0	0.07	-	-	-	-
15-44	314	171	21	11.4	29.9	0.07	-	-	-	-
45-59	71	108	5	7.2	52.4	0.07	-	-	-	-
60+	51	85	3	5.7	71.1	0.07	-	-	-	-
All ages	525	134	35	9.0	33.5	0.07	-	-	-	-
Females										
0-4	7	29	0	2.0	2.5	0.07	-	-	-	-
5-14	45	89	3	6.0	10.0	0.07	-	-	-	-
15-44	138	77	9	5.2	30.0	0.07	-	-	-	-
45-59	28	41	2	2.7	52.4	0.07	-	-	-	-
60+	34	40	2	2.7	72.4	0.07	-	-	-	-
All ages	252	62	17	4.2	33.8	0.07	-	-	-	-
Total	777	97	52	6.5	33.6	0.07	-	-	-	-

Table 214b   FSE - PEAS - AESE   Road traffic accidents - Intracranial injury - short term

Age group (years)	Incidence 1990 Number ('000s)	Rate (per 100 000)	Prevalence 1990 Number ('000s)	Rate (per 100 000)	Avg. age at onset (years)	Average duration (years)	Deaths 1990 Number ('000s)	Rate (per 100 000)	Deaths 2000 (Projected) Number ('000s)	Rate (per 100 000)
Males										
0-4	6	42	0	2.8	2.5	0.07	-	-	-	-
5-14	54	199	4	13.3	10.0	0.07	-	-	-	-
15-44	191	250	13	16.7	29.8	0.07	-	-	-	-
45-59	62	230	4	15.4	52.2	0.07	-	-	-	-
60+	20	97	1	6.5	70.0	0.07	-	-	-	-
All ages	333	202	22	13.5	32.7	0.07	-	-	-	-
Females										
0-4	3	26	0	1.8	2.5	0.07	-	-	-	-
5-14	27	104	2	6.9	10.0	0.07	-	-	-	-
15-44	32	42	2	2.8	29.9	0.07	-	-	-	-
45-59	17	55	1	3.7	52.4	0.07	-	-	-	-
60+	15	41	1	2.8	71.5	0.07	-	-	-	-
All ages	94	52	6	3.5	33.7	0.07	-	-	-	-
Total	427	123	29	8.3	32.9	0.07	-	-	-	-

Table 214c   India - India - Inde   Road traffic accidents - Intracranial injury - short term

Age group (years)	Incidence 1990 Number ('000s)	Rate (per 100 000)	Prevalence 1990 Number ('000s)	Rate (per 100 000)	Avg. age at onset (years)	Average duration (years)	Deaths 1990 Number ('000s)	Rate (per 100 000)	Deaths 2000 (Projected) Number ('000s)	Rate (per 100 000)
Males										
0-4	80	134	5	8.9	2.5	0.07	-	-	-	-
5-14	294	289	20	19.3	10.0	0.07	-	-	-	-
15-44	216	107	14	7.2	29.8	0.07	-	-	-	-
45-59	63	132	4	8.8	52.3	0.07	-	-	-	-
60+	23	77	2	5.1	69.7	0.07	-	-	-	-
All ages	675	154	45	10.3	21.4	0.07	-	-	-	-
Females										
0-4	23	41	2	2.7	2.5	0.07	-	-	-	-
5-14	211	222	14	14.9	10.0	0.07	-	-	-	-
15-44	49	27	3	1.8	29.8	0.07	-	-	-	-
45-59	35	76	2	5.1	52.4	0.07	-	-	-	-
60+	15	53	1	3.6	70.1	0.07	-	-	-	-
All ages	334	81	22	5.5	19.6	0.07	-	-	-	-
Total	1 009	119	68	8.0	20.8	0.07	-	-	-	-

For epidemiological sources see Lozano et al. 1996. For the methods used to estimate and project incidence, prevalence, and deaths see Lozano et al. 1996 and Murray and Lopez 1996a. See explanatory notes for definitions and caveats.

Table 214	Cuadro 214	Tableau 214
Road traffic accidents	Accidentes de tráfico	Accidents de la voie publique

Intracranial injury - short term   Lesión intracraneal - corta duración   Lésions intra-crâniennes - court terme

Table 214d China - China - Chine   Road traffic accidents - Intracranial injury - short term

Age group (years)	Incidence 1990 Number ('000s)	Rate (per 100 000)	Prevalence 1990 Number ('000s)	Rate (per 100 000)	Avg. age at onset (years)	Average duration (years)	Deaths 1990 Number ('000s)	Rate (per 100 000)	Deaths 2000 (Projected) Number ('000s)	Rate (per 100 000)
Males										
0-4	22	37	2	2.5	2.5	0.07	-	-	-	-
5-14	109	113	7	7.5	10.0	0.07	-	-	-	-
15-44	240	78	16	5.3	29.9	0.07	-	-	-	-
45-59	72	99	5	6.6	52.3	0.07	-	-	-	-
60+	35	71	2	4.8	69.8	0.07	-	-	-	-
All ages	478	82	32	5.5	30.3	0.07	-	-	-	-
Females										
0-4	16	28	1	1.9	2.5	0.07	-	-	-	-
5-14	102	113	7	7.6	10.0	0.07	-	-	-	-
15-44	68	24	5	1.6	29.9	0.07	-	-	-	-
45-59	33	51	2	3.4	52.4	0.07	-	-	-	-
60+	15	30	1	2.0	70.6	0.07	-	-	-	-
All ages	234	43	16	2.9	25.1	0.07	-	-	-	-
Total	713	63	48	4.2	28.6	0.07	-	-	-	-

Table 214e OAI - OPAI - APAI   Road traffic accidents - Intracranial injury - short term

Age group (years)	Incidence 1990 Number ('000s)	Rate (per 100 000)	Prevalence 1990 Number ('000s)	Rate (per 100 000)	Avg. age at onset (years)	Average duration (years)	Deaths 1990 Number ('000s)	Rate (per 100 000)	Deaths 2000 (Projected) Number ('000s)	Rate (per 100 000)
Males										
0-4	61	139	4	9.3	2.5	0.07	-	-	-	-
5-14	199	237	13	15.9	10.0	0.07	-	-	-	-
15-44	182	113	12	7.6	29.7	0.07	-	-	-	-
45-59	38	111	3	7.5	52.3	0.07	-	-	-	-
60+	13	66	1	4.4	69.6	0.07	-	-	-	-
All ages	493	144	33	9.6	21.2	0.07	-	-	-	-
Females										
0-4	55	132	4	8.8	2.5	0.07	-	-	-	-
5-14	106	132	7	8.8	10.0	0.07	-	-	-	-
15-44	45	28	3	1.9	29.8	0.07	-	-	-	-
45-59	15	42	1	2.8	52.3	0.07	-	-	-	-
60+	8	36	1	2.4	70.3	0.07	-	-	-	-
All ages	229	67	15	4.5	16.9	0.07	-	-	-	-
Total	722	106	48	7.1	19.9	0.07	-	-	-	-

Table 214f SSA - ASS - ASS   Road traffic accidents - Intracranial injury - short term

Age group (years)	Incidence 1990 Number ('000s)	Rate (per 100 000)	Prevalence 1990 Number ('000s)	Rate (per 100 000)	Avg. age at onset (years)	Average duration (years)	Deaths 1990 Number ('000s)	Rate (per 100 000)	Deaths 2000 (Projected) Number ('000s)	Rate (per 100 000)
Males										
0-4	35	73	2	4.9	2.4	0.07	-	-	-	-
5-14	332	472	22	31.6	10.0	0.07	-	-	-	-
15-44	157	151	11	10.1	29.4	0.07	-	-	-	-
45-59	29	144	2	9.7	52.2	0.07	-	-	-	-
60+	9	84	1	5.6	69.2	0.07	-	-	-	-
All ages	562	223	38	14.9	18.1	0.07	-	-	-	-
Females										
0-4	24	51	2	3.4	2.4	0.07	-	-	-	-
5-14	159	228	11	15.3	10.0	0.07	-	-	-	-
15-44	41	39	3	2.6	29.5	0.07	-	-	-	-
45-59	9	39	1	2.6	52.2	0.07	-	-	-	-
60+	2	19	0	1.3	69.7	0.07	-	-	-	-
All ages	235	91	16	6.1	14.8	0.07	-	-	-	-
Total	797	156	53	10.5	17.1	0.07	-	-	-	-

For epidemiological sources see Lozano et al. 1996. For the methods used to estimate and project incidence, prevalence, and deaths see Lozano et al. 1996 and Murray and Lopez 1996a. See explanatory notes for definitions and caveats.

Table 214	Cuadro 214	Tableau 214
Road traffic accidents	Accidentes de tráfico	Accidents de la voie publique

Intracranial injury - short term   Lesión intracraneal - corta duración   Lésions intra-crâniennes - court terme

Table 214g   LAC - ALC - ALC   Road traffic accidents - Intracranial injury - short term

Age group (years)	Incidence 1990 Number ('000s)	Rate (per 100 000)	Prevalence 1990 Number ('000s)	Rate (per 100 000)	Avg. age at onset (years)	Average duration (years)	Deaths 1990 Number ('000s)	Rate (per 100 000)	Deaths 2000 (Projected) Number ('000s)	Rate (per 100 000)
Males										
0-4	19	67	1	4.5	2.5	0.07	-	-	-	-
5-14	228	438	15	29.3	10.0	0.07	-	-	-	-
15-44	199	191	13	12.8	29.8	0.07	-	-	-	-
45-59	48	216	3	14.4	52.3	0.07	-	-	-	-
60+	18	128	1	8.6	70.3	0.07	-	-	-	-
All ages	513	231	34	15.5	23.5	0.07	-	-	-	-
Females										
0-4	14	52	1	3.5	2.5	0.07	-	-	-	-
5-14	115	226	8	15.1	10.0	0.07	-	-	-	-
15-44	60	58	4	3.9	29.9	0.07	-	-	-	-
45-59	14	60	1	4.0	52.4	0.07	-	-	-	-
60+	7	44	1	3.0	71.1	0.07	-	-	-	-
All ages	210	95	14	6.3	20.1	0.07	-	-	-	-
Total	723	163	48	10.9	22.5	0.07	-	-	-	-

Table 214h   MEC - AOM - CMO   Road traffic accidents - Intracranial injury - short term

Age group (years)	Incidence 1990 Number ('000s)	Rate (per 100 000)	Prevalence 1990 Number ('000s)	Rate (per 100 000)	Avg. age at onset (years)	Average duration (years)	Deaths 1990 Number ('000s)	Rate (per 100 000)	Deaths 2000 (Projected) Number ('000s)	Rate (per 100 000)
Males										
0-4	13	32	1	2.1	2.5	0.07	-	-	-	-
5-14	127	194	8	13.0	10.0	0.07	-	-	-	-
15-44	128	113	9	7.5	29.8	0.07	-	-	-	-
45-59	22	98	1	6.6	52.3	0.07	-	-	-	-
60+	6	44	0	2.9	69.7	0.07	-	-	-	-
All ages	296	115	20	7.7	22.6	0.07	-	-	-	-
Females										
0-4	11	29	1	1.9	2.5	0.07	-	-	-	-
5-14	59	95	4	6.4	10.0	0.07	-	-	-	-
15-44	20	18	1	1.2	29.8	0.07	-	-	-	-
45-59	6	26	0	1.7	52.3	0.07	-	-	-	-
60+	3	20	0	1.3	70.4	0.07	-	-	-	-
All ages	99	40	7	2.7	17.4	0.07	-	-	-	-
Total	395	78	26	5.3	21.3	0.07	-	-	-	-

Table 214i   World - Mundo - Monde   Road traffic accidents - Intracranial injury - short term

Age group (years)	Incidence 1990 Number ('000s)	Rate (per 100 000)	Prevalence 1990 Number ('000s)	Rate (per 100 000)	Avg. age at onset (years)	Average duration (years)	Deaths 1990 Number ('000s)	Rate (per 100 000)	Deaths 2000 (Projected) Number ('000s)	Rate (per 100 000)
Males										
0-4	246	76	16	5.1	2.5	0.07	-	-	-	-
5-14	1 421	258	95	17.3	10.0	0.07	-	-	-	-
15-44	1 626	130	109	8.7	29.8	0.07	-	-	-	-
45-59	405	130	27	8.7	52.3	0.07	-	-	-	-
60+	176	80	12	5.4	70.2	0.07	-	-	-	-
All ages	3 874	146	260	9.8	25.0	0.07	-	-	-	-
Females										
0-4	155	50	10	3.4	2.5	0.07	-	-	-	-
5-14	825	157	55	10.5	10.0	0.07	-	-	-	-
15-44	453	38	30	2.5	29.9	0.07	-	-	-	-
45-59	155	50	10	3.3	52.4	0.07	-	-	-	-
60+	101	37	7	2.5	71.2	0.07	-	-	-	-
All ages	1 688	65	113	4.3	22.2	0.07	-	-	-	-
Total	5 563	106	373	7.1	24.1	0.07	-	-	-	-

For epidemiological sources see Lozano et al. 1996. For the methods used to estimate and project incidence, prevalence, and deaths see Lozano et al. 1996 and Murray and Lopez 1996a. See explanatory notes for definitions and caveats.

Table 215
Road traffic accidents

Cuadro 215
Accidentes de tráfico

Tableau 215
Accidents de la voie publique

Intracranial injury - long term   Lesión intracraneal - larga duración   Lésions intra-crâniennes - long terme

Table 215a   EME - PEMC - EMBE   Road traffic accidents - Intracranial injury - long term

Age group (years)	Incidence 1990 Number ('000s)	Rate (per 100 000)	Prevalence 1990 Number ('000s)	Rate (per 100 000)	Avg. age at onset (years)	Average duration (years)	Deaths 1990 Number ('000s)	Rate (per 100 000)	Deaths 2000 (Projected) Number ('000s)	Rate (per 100 000)
Males										
0-4	0	1.9	1	4.7	2.5	70.2	-	-	-	-
5-14	4	7.3	2	4.6	10.0	63.6	-	-	-	-
15-44	16	8.5	385	209.4	29.9	44.8	-	-	-	-
45-59	4	5.4	250	377.6	52.4	24.5	-	-	-	-
60+	3	4.2	282	465.6	71.1	11.3	-	-	-	-
All ages	26	6.7	921	235.8	33.5	42.0	-	-	-	-
Females										
0-4	0	1.5	1	3.7	2.5	76.1	-	-	-	-
5-14	2	4.5	15	29.7	10.0	69.5	-	-	-	-
15-44	7	3.9	196	109.6	30.0	50.0	-	-	-	-
45-59	1	2.0	124	182.6	52.4	28.8	-	-	-	-
60+	2	2.0	188	222.8	72.4	12.7	-	-	-	-
All ages	13	3.1	525	128.8	33.8	46.9	-	-	-	-
Total	39	4.9	1 445	181.2	33.6	43.6	-	-	-	-

Table 215b   FSE - PEAS - AESE   Road traffic accidents - Intracranial injury - long term

Age group (years)	Incidence 1990 Number ('000s)	Rate (per 100 000)	Prevalence 1990 Number ('000s)	Rate (per 100 000)	Avg. age at onset (years)	Average duration (years)	Deaths 1990 Number ('000s)	Rate (per 100 000)	Deaths 2000 (Projected) Number ('000s)	Rate (per 100 000)
Males										
0-4	0	2.1	1	5.3	2.5	63.5	-	-	-	-
5-14	3	9.9	17	60.4	10.0	57.0	-	-	-	-
15-44	9	12.5	224	294.1	29.8	39.2	-	-	-	-
45-59	3	11.5	153	566.4	52.2	20.8	-	-	-	-
60+	1	4.8	148	703.7	70.0	10.1	-	-	-	-
All ages	17	10.0	542	327.7	32.7	37.3	-	-	-	-
Females										
0-4	0	1.3	0	3.3	2.5	72.4	-	-	-	-
5-14	1	5.2	9	32.6	10.0	66.0	-	-	-	-
15-44	2	2.1	67	90.0	29.9	46.8	-	-	-	-
45-59	1	2.8	43	142.2	52.4	26.1	-	-	-	-
60+	1	2.1	68	187.0	71.5	11.8	-	-	-	-
All ages	5	2.6	187	103.5	33.7	44.1	-	-	-	-
Total	21	6.2	729	210.6	32.9	38.8	-	-	-	-

Table 215c   India - India - Inde   Road traffic accidents - Intracranial injury - long term

Age group (years)	Incidence 1990 Number ('000s)	Rate (per 100 000)	Prevalence 1990 Number ('000s)	Rate (per 100 000)	Avg. age at onset (years)	Average duration (years)	Deaths 1990 Number ('000s)	Rate (per 100 000)	Deaths 2000 (Projected) Number ('000s)	Rate (per 100 000)
Males										
0-4	4	6.7	10	16.4	2.5	59.9	-	-	-	-
5-14	15	14.4	108	105.9	10.0	57.4	-	-	-	-
15-44	11	5.4	514	256.6	29.8	39.9	-	-	-	-
45-59	3	6.6	184	386.3	52.3	21.0	-	-	-	-
60+	1	3.8	141	473.8	69.7	9.7	-	-	-	-
All ages	34	7.7	957	217.8	21.4	47.1	-	-	-	-
Females										
0-4	1	2.0	3	5.0	2.5	60.8	-	-	-	-
5-14	11	11.1	63	66.2	10.0	59.1	-	-	-	-
15-44	2	1.3	258	140.9	29.8	41.7	-	-	-	-
45-59	2	3.8	87	189.4	52.4	22.5	-	-	-	-
60+	1	2.7	71	245.0	70.1	10.2	-	-	-	-
All ages	17	4.1	482	117.5	19.6	50.6	-	-	-	-
Total	50	5.9	1 439	169.4	20.8	48.3	-	-	-	-

For epidemiological sources see Lozano et al. 1996. For the methods used to estimate and project incidence, prevalence, and deaths see Lozano et al. 1996 and Murray and Lopez 1996a. See explanatory notes for definitions and caveats.

Table 215
Road traffic accidents

Intracranial injury - long term

Cuadro 215
Accidentes de tráfico

Lesión intracraneal - larga duración

Tableau 215
Accidents de la voie publique

Lésions intra-crâniennes - long terme

Table 215d China - China - Chine — Road traffic accidents - Intracranial injury - long term

Age group (years)	Incidence 1990 Number ('000s)	Rate (per 100 000)	Prevalence 1990 Number ('000s)	Rate (per 100 000)	Avg. age at onset (years)	Average duration (years)	Deaths 1990 Number ('000s)	Rate (per 100 000)	Deaths 2000 (Projected) Number ('000s)	Rate (per 100 000)
Males										
0-4	1	1.9	3	4.6	2.5	65.5	-	-	-	-
5-14	5	5.6	36	37.5	10.0	59.9	-	-	-	-
15-44	12	3.9	379	123.9	29.9	41.2	-	-	-	-
45-59	4	4.9	159	219.2	52.3	21.4	-	-	-	-
60+	2	3.5	143	291.6	69.8	9.9	-	-	-	-
All ages	24	4.1	721	123.2	30.3	41.4	-	-	-	-
Females										
0-4	1	1.4	2	3.5	2.5	68.5	-	-	-	-
5-14	5	5.6	32	35.3	10.0	63.2	-	-	-	-
15-44	3	1.2	231	81.2	29.9	44.2	-	-	-	-
45-59	2	2.5	76	118.0	52.4	23.8	-	-	-	-
60+	1	1.5	79	153.2	70.6	10.8	-	-	-	-
All ages	12	2.1	420	76.5	25.1	49.1	-	-	-	-
Total	36	3.1	1 140	100.6	28.6	43.9	-	-	-	-

Table 215e OAI - OPAI - APAI — Road traffic accidents - Intracranial injury - long term

Age group (years)	Incidence 1990 Number ('000s)	Rate (per 100 000)	Prevalence 1990 Number ('000s)	Rate (per 100 000)	Avg. age at onset (years)	Average duration (years)	Deaths 1990 Number ('000s)	Rate (per 100 000)	Deaths 2000 (Projected) Number ('000s)	Rate (per 100 000)
Males										
0-4	3	7.0	7	17	2.5	59.8	-	-	-	-
5-14	10	11.8	79	94	10.0	56.2	-	-	-	-
15-44	9	5.6	380	236	29.7	38.8	-	-	-	-
45-59	2	5.6	124	363	52.3	20.3	-	-	-	-
60+	1	3.3	88	437	69.6	9.7	-	-	-	-
All ages	25	7.2	678	198	21.2	46.2	-	-	-	-
Females										
0-4	3	6.6	7	16	2.5	63.2	-	-	-	-
5-14	5	6.6	53	66	10.0	59.2	-	-	-	-
15-44	2	1.4	191	120	29.8	41.5	-	-	-	-
45-59	1	2.1	55	156	52.3	22.4	-	-	-	-
60+	0	1.8	43	191	70.3	10.5	-	-	-	-
All ages	11	3.4	348	103	16.9	52.6	-	-	-	-
Total	36	5.3	1 027	150	19.8	48.2	-	-	-	-

Table 215f SSA - ASS - ASS — Road traffic accidents - Intracranial injury - long term

Age group (years)	Incidence 1990 Number ('000s)	Rate (per 100 000)	Prevalence 1990 Number ('000s)	Rate (per 100 000)	Avg. age at onset (years)	Average duration (years)	Deaths 1990 Number ('000s)	Rate (per 100 000)	Deaths 2000 (Projected) Number ('000s)	Rate (per 100 000)
Males										
0-4	2	3.6	4	8.7	2.4	48.7	-	-	-	-
5-14	17	23.6	95	135.6	10.0	49.2	-	-	-	-
15-44	8	7.5	376	362.7	29.4	35.0	-	-	-	-
45-59	1	7.2	108	531.8	52.2	19.1	-	-	-	-
60+	0	4.2	66	626.5	69.2	9.3	-	-	-	-
All ages	28	11.1	650	257.4	18.1	43.0	-	-	-	-
Females										
0-4	1	2.5	3	6.1	2.4	51.9	-	-	-	-
5-14	8	11.4	48	69.4	10.0	51.9	-	-	-	-
15-44	2	1.9	164	154.5	29.5	37.2	-	-	-	-
45-59	0	1.9	44	198.5	52.2	20.5	-	-	-	-
60+	0	1.0	28	222.9	69.7	9.8	-	-	-	-
All ages	12	4.6	288	111.6	14.8	47.8	-	-	-	-
Total	40	7.8	937	183.7	17.1	44.4	-	-	-	-

For epidemiological sources see Lozano et al. 1996. For the methods used to estimate and project incidence, prevalence, and deaths see Lozano et al. 1996 and Murray and Lopez 1996a. See explanatory notes for definitions and caveats.

Table 215 | **Cuadro 215** | **Tableau 215**
Road traffic accidents | **Accidentes de tráfico** | **Accidents de la voie publique**

Intracranial injury - long term | Lesión intracraneal - larga duración | Lésions intra-crâniennes - long terme

Table 215g   LAC - ALC - ALC — Road traffic accidents - Intracranial injury - long term

Age group (years)	Incidence 1990 Number ('000s)	Rate (per 100 000)	Prevalence 1990 Number ('000s)	Rate (per 100 000)	Avg. age at onset (years)	Average duration (years)	Deaths 1990 Number ('000s)	Rate (per 100 000)	Deaths 2000 (Projected) Number ('000s)	Rate (per 100 000)
Males										
0-4	1	3.4	2	8.3	2.5	63.9	-	-	-	-
5-14	11	21.9	66	126.5	10.0	59.3	-	-	-	-
15-44	10	9.5	392	376.2	29.8	41.4	-	-	-	-
45-59	2	10.7	133	599.1	52.3	22.3	-	-	-	-
60+	1	6.4	106	746.8	70.3	10.4	-	-	-	-
All ages	26	11.5	700	315.9	23.5	47.4	-	-	-	-
Females										
0-4	1	2.6	2	6.4	2.5	67.9	-	-	-	-
5-14	6	11.3	35	69.6	10.0	63.0	-	-	-	-
15-44	3	2.9	175	168.6	29.8	44.6	-	-	-	-
45-59	1	3.0	55	234.2	52.4	24.8	-	-	-	-
60+	0	2.2	47	281.6	71.1	11.3	-	-	-	-
All ages	11	4.7	315	141.3	20.1	53.7	-	-	-	-
Total	36	8.1	1 015	228.4	22.5	49.2	-	-	-	-

Table 215h   MEC - AOM - CMO — Road traffic accidents - Intracranial injury - long term

Age group (years)	Incidence 1990 Number ('000s)	Rate (per 100 000)	Prevalence 1990 Number ('000s)	Rate (per 100 000)	Avg. age at onset (years)	Average duration (years)	Deaths 1990 Number ('000s)	Rate (per 100 000)	Deaths 2000 (Projected) Number ('000s)	Rate (per 100 000)
Males										
0-4	1	1.6	2	3.9	2.5	61.1	-	-	-	-
5-14	6	9.7	37	56.5	10.0	58.1	-	-	-	-
15-44	6	5.6	214	188.2	29.8	40.0	-	-	-	-
45-59	1	4.9	69	309.1	52.3	20.8	-	-	-	-
60+	0	2.2	50	368.2	69.7	9.8	-	-	-	-
All ages	15	5.8	372	145.2	22.6	46.7	-	-	-	-
Females										
0-4	1	1.4	1	3.5	2.5	63.7	-	-	-	-
5-14	3	4.8	19	31.0	10.0	60.9	-	-	-	-
15-44	1	0.9	73	68.4	29.8	42.6	-	-	-	-
45-59	0	1.3	20	91.8	52.3	22.9	-	-	-	-
60+	0	1.0	17	111.9	70.4	10.6	-	-	-	-
All ages	5	2.0	132	53.4	17.4	53.8	-	-	-	-
Total	20	3.9	504	100.2	21.3	48.5	-	-	-	-

Table 215i   World - Mundo - Monde — Road traffic accidents - Intracranial injury - long term

Age group (years)	Incidence 1990 Number ('000s)	Rate (per 100 000)	Prevalence 1990 Number ('000s)	Rate (per 100 000)	Avg. age at onset (years)	Average duration (years)	Deaths 1990 Number ('000s)	Rate (per 100 000)	Deaths 2000 (Projected) Number ('000s)	Rate (per 100 000)
Males										
0-4	12	3.8	30	9.4	2.5	59.7	-	-	-	-
5-14	71	12.9	440	79.9	10.0	56.2	-	-	-	-
15-44	81	6.5	2 866	229.3	29.8	40.5	-	-	-	-
45-59	20	6.5	1 180	377.7	52.3	21.6	-	-	-	-
60+	9	4.0	1 024	467.9	70.2	10.3	-	-	-	-
All ages	193	7.3	5 540	208.8	25.0	44.2	-	-	-	-
Females										
0-4	8	2.5	19	6.2	2.5	63.0	-	-	-	-
5-14	41	7.8	274	52.2	10.0	59.7	-	-	-	-
15-44	23	1.9	1 356	113.2	29.9	45.0	-	-	-	-
45-59	8	2.5	504	161.9	52.4	24.4	-	-	-	-
60+	5	1.9	543	201.6	71.2	11.5	-	-	-	-
All ages	84	3.2	2 696	103.2	22.2	49.9	-	-	-	-
Total	278	5.3	8 237	156.4	24.1	45.9	-	-	-	-

For epidemiological sources see Lozano et al. 1996. For the methods used to estimate and project incidence, prevalence, and deaths see Lozano et al. 1996 and Murray and Lopez 1996a. See explanatory notes for definitions and caveats.

Table 216
Poisonings

Cuadro 216
Envenenamientos

Tableau 216
Empoisonnements

Episodes   Episodios   Episodes

Table 216a   EME - PEMC - EMBE   Poisonings - Episodes

Age group (years)	Incidence 1990 Number ('000s)	Rate (per 100 000)	Prevalence 1990 Number ('000s)	Rate (per 100 000)	Avg. age at onset (years)	Average duration (years)	Deaths 1990 Number ('000s)	Rate (per 100 000)	Deaths 2000 (Projected) Number ('000s)	Rate (per 100 000)
Males										
0-4	1 147	4 347	9	35.6	2.5	0.01	0	0.3	0	0.2
5-14	149	278	1	2.3	10.0	0.01	0	0.1	0	0.1
15-44	508	276	4	2.3	29.9	0.01	6	3.2	5	2.9
45-59	39	59	0	0.5	52.4	0.01	1	2.2	2	2.0
60+	28	47	0	0.4	71.1	0.01	1	2.2	2	2.1
All ages	1 871	479	15	3.9	12.6	0.01	9	2.3	8	2.0
Females										
0-4	794	3 168	7	26.0	2.5	0.01	0	0.3	0	0.2
5-14	98	193	1	1.6	10.0	0.01	0	0.1	0	0.1
15-44	143	80	1	0.7	30.0	0.01	2	0.9	2	1.0
45-59	18	26	0	0.2	52.4	0.01	1	1.0	1	1.0
60+	29	35	0	0.3	72.4	0.01	1	1.7	1	1.5
All ages	1 082	266	9	2.2	9.5	0.01	4	0.9	4	0.9
Total	2 953	370	24	3.0	11.5	0.01	13	1.6	12	1.5

Table 216b   FSE - PEAS - AESE   Poisonings - Episodes

Age group (years)	Incidence 1990 Number ('000s)	Rate (per 100 000)	Prevalence 1990 Number ('000s)	Rate (per 100 000)	Avg. age at onset (years)	Average duration (years)	Deaths 1990 Number ('000s)	Rate (per 100 000)	Deaths 2000 (Projected) Number ('000s)	Rate (per 100 000)
Males										
0-4	7 964	57 882	65	474.6	2.5	0.01	1	6.9	1	6.0
5-14	498	1 821	4	14.9	10.0	0.01	0	1.4	0	1.1
15-44	841	1 102	7	9.0	29.8	0.01	15	19.4	14	18.4
45-59	236	876	2	7.2	52.2	0.01	13	48.8	16	50.5
60+	66	313	1	2.6	70.0	0.01	5	22.6	6	22.2
All ages	9 605	5 810	79	47.6	7.0	0.01	34	20.6	36	21.3
Females										
0-4	5 829	44 380	48	363.9	2.5	0.01	1	5.3	1	4.7
5-14	367	1 390	3	11.4	10.0	0.01	0	1.0	0	0.9
15-44	162	216	1	1.8	29.9	0.01	3	3.8	3	3.9
45-59	61	205	1	1.7	52.4	0.01	3	11.4	4	11.4
60+	46	125	0	1.0	71.5	0.01	3	9.0	4	8.9
All ages	6 465	3 574	53	29.3	4.6	0.01	11	5.8	11	6.0
Total	16 070	4 641	132	38.1	6.0	0.01	45	12.9	48	13.3

Table 216c   India - India - Inde   Poisonings - Episodes

Age group (years)	Incidence 1990 Number ('000s)	Rate (per 100 000)	Prevalence 1990 Number ('000s)	Rate (per 100 000)	Avg. age at onset (years)	Average duration (years)	Deaths 1990 Number ('000s)	Rate (per 100 000)	Deaths 2000 (Projected) Number ('000s)	Rate (per 100 000)
Males										
0-4	6 547	10 950	54	89.8	2.5	0.01	5	7.9	5	7.9
5-14	1 193	1 172	10	9.6	10.0	0.01	3	2.6	2	1.9
15-44	108	54	1	0.4	29.8	0.01	6	2.8	6	2.6
45-59	10	20	0	0.2	52.3	0.01	2	3.3	2	3.3
60+	4	13	0	0.1	69.7	0.01	1	2.9	1	3.0
All ages	7 861	1 789	64	14.7	4.1	0.01	16	3.5	16	3.1
Females										
0-4	4 515	7 966	37	65.3	2.5	0.01	3	5.7	3	5.7
5-14	894	938	7	7.7	10.0	0.01	2	2.1	1	1.4
15-44	133	73	1	0.6	29.8	0.01	7	3.8	7	3.2
45-59	9 031	19 630	74	161.0	52.4	0.01	2	3.9	2	3.9
60+	894	3 090	7	25.3	70.1	0.01	0	1.0	0	1.2
All ages	15 467	3 771	127	30.9	36.2	0.01	14	3.5	14	3.0
Total	23 327	2 746	191	22.5	25.4	0.01	30	3.5	31	3.1

For epidemiological sources see Pronczuk and Hong 1996. For the methods used to estimate and project incidence, prevalence, and deaths see Murray and Lopez 1996a. See explanatory notes for definitions and caveats.

Table 216 — **Cuadro 216** — **Tableau 216**
Poisonings — Envenenamientos — Empoisonnements

Episodes — Episodios — Episodes

Table 216d China - China - Chine — Poisonings - Episodes

Age group (years)	Incidence 1990 Number ('000s)	Rate (per 100 000)	Prevalence 1990 Number ('000s)	Rate (per 100 000)	Avg. age at onset (years)	Average duration (years)	Deaths 1990 Number ('000s)	Rate (per 100 000)	Deaths 2000 (Projected) Number ('000s)	Rate (per 100 000)
Males										
0-4	31 171	51 742	256	424.3	2.5	0.01	5	8.3	4	7.5
5-14	1 558	1 606	13	13.2	10.0	0.01	2	1.6	1	1.0
15-44	571	186	5	1.5	29.9	0.01	13	4.4	12	3.7
45-59	121	166	1	1.4	52.3	0.01	9	12.4	11	10.8
60+	93	190	1	1.6	69.8	0.01	9	18.3	12	19.5
All ages	33 514	5 727	275	47.0	3.7	0.01	38	6.5	40	6.1
Females										
0-4	9 629	16 617	79	136.3	2.5	0.01	2	2.7	1	2.3
5-14	2 157	2 386	18	19.6	10.0	0.01	2	2.4	2	1.4
15-44	617	217	5	1.8	29.9	0.01	15	5.1	10	3.5
45-59	31	48	0	0.4	52.4	0.01	2	3.6	3	3.6
60+	70	136	1	1.1	70.6	0.01	7	13.1	11	16.6
All ages	12 504	2 280	103	18.7	5.7	0.01	27	5.0	27	4.4
Total	46 018	1 059	377	33.3	4.2	0.01	65	5.7	67	5.2

Table 216e OAI - OPAI - APAI — Poisonings - Episodes

Age group (years)	Incidence 1990 Number ('000s)	Rate (per 100 000)	Prevalence 1990 Number ('000s)	Rate (per 100 000)	Avg. age at onset (years)	Average duration (years)	Deaths 1990 Number ('000s)	Rate (per 100 000)	Deaths 2000 (Projected) Number ('000s)	Rate (per 100 000)
Males										
0-4	8 217	18 776	67	154.0	2.5	0.01	2	4.5	2	4.0
5-14	1 594	1 897	13	15.6	10.0	0.01	3	3.0	2	2.2
15-44	276	172	2	1.4	29.7	0.01	10	6.1	11	5.3
45-59	26	77	0	0.6	52.3	0.01	3	8.6	4	8.2
60+	14	71	0	0.6	69.6	0.01	2	10.2	3	10.2
All ages	10 128	2 953	83	24.2	4.6	0.01	19	5.6	21	5.2
Females										
0-4	7 447	17 736	61	145.4	2.5	0.01	2	4.3	2	3.8
5-14	1 754	2 187	14	17.9	10.0	0.01	3	3.3	2	2.3
15-44	252	158	2	1.3	29.8	0.01	9	5.6	10	4.8
45-59	13	37	0	0.3	52.3	0.01	1	4.1	2	4.1
60+	12	53	0	0.4	70.3	0.01	2	7.7	3	8.2
All ages	9 478	2 791	78	22.9	4.8	0.01	16	4.9	18	4.4
Total	19 606	2 873	161	23.6	4.7	0.01	36	5.2	39	4.8

Table 216f SSA - ASS - ASS — Poisonings - Episodes

Age group (years)	Incidence 1990 Number ('000s)	Rate (per 100 000)	Prevalence 1990 Number ('000s)	Rate (per 100 000)	Avg. age at onset (years)	Average duration (years)	Deaths 1990 Number ('000s)	Rate (per 100 000)	Deaths 2000 (Projected) Number ('000s)	Rate (per 100 000)
Males										
0-4	5 538	11 663.8	45	95.6	2.4	0.01	14	29.2	19	29.0
5-14	753	1 072.4	6	8.8	10.0	0.01	4	5.7	4	4.4
15-44	46	44.4	0	0.4	29.4	0.01	2	2.3	3	2.2
45-59	5	26.6	0	0.2	52.2	0.01	1	4.5	1	4.6
60+	4	34.9	0	0.3	69.2	0.01	1	7.6	1	8.0
All ages	6 347	2 515.5	52	20.6	3.6	0.01	22	8.7	29	8.4
Females										
0-4	4 077	8 669.7	33	71.1	2.4	0.01	10	21.7	14	21.9
5-14	391	560.6	3	4.6	10.0	0.01	2	2.9	2	2.2
15-44	39	36.8	0	0.3	29.5	0.01	2	1.9	3	1.9
45-59	1	6.2	0	0.1	52.2	0.01	0	1.0	0	1.0
60+	2	13.7	0	0.1	69.7	0.01	0	3.0	1	3.2
All ages	4 511	1 748.8	37	14.3	3.3	0.01	15	5.8	20	5.6
Total	10 858	2 127.9	89	17.4	3.5	0.01	37	7.2	48	7.0

For epidemiological sources see Pronczuk and Hong 1996. For the methods used to estimate and project incidence, prevalence, and deaths see Murray and Lopez 1996a. See explanatory notes for definitions and caveats.

Table 216 — Cuadro 216 — Tableau 216
Poisonings — Envenenamientos — Empoisonnements

Episodes — Episodios — Episodes

Table 216g LAC - ALC - ALC — Poisonings - Episodes

Age group (years)	Incidence 1990 Number ('000s)	Rate (per 100 000)	Prevalence 1990 Number ('000s)	Rate (per 100 000)	Avg. age at onset (years)	Average duration (years)	Deaths 1990 Number ('000s)	Rate (per 100 000)	Deaths 2000 (Projected) Number ('000s)	Rate (per 100 000)
Males										
0-4	3 975	13 838.9	33	113.5	2.5	0.01	1	2.2	1	2.0
5-14	396	760.0	3	6.2	10.0	0.01	0	0.8	0	0.6
15-44	50	47.6	0	0.4	29.8	0.01	1	1.1	1	1.0
45-59	4	19.8	0	0.2	52.3	0.01	0	1.5	0	1.5
60+	4	24.8	0	0.2	70.3	0.01	0	2.4	0	2.5
All ages	4 428	1 998.3	36	16.4	3.6	0.01	3	1.3	3	1.2
Females										
0-4	2 850	10 296.8	23	84.4	2.5	0.01	0	1.6	0	1.5
5-14	339	668.0	3	5.5	10.0	0.01	0	0.7	0	0.5
15-44	33	31.4	0	0.3	29.9	0.01	1	0.7	1	0.7
45-59	2	7.6	0	0.1	52.4	0.01	0	0.6	0	0.6
60+	2	14.1	0	0.1	71.1	0.01	0	1.4	0	1.4
All ages	3 226	1 448.5	26	11.9	3.6	0.01	2	0.9	2	0.8
Total	7 654	1 722.7	63	14.1	3.6	0.01	5	1.1	5	1.0

Table 216h MEC - AOM - CMO — Poisonings - Episodes

Age group (years)	Incidence 1990 Number ('000s)	Rate (per 100 000)	Prevalence 1990 Number ('000s)	Rate (per 100 000)	Avg. age at onset (years)	Average duration (years)	Deaths 1990 Number ('000s)	Rate (per 100 000)	Deaths 2000 (Projected) Number ('000s)	Rate (per 100 000)
Males										
0-4	6 130	14 893	50	122.1	2.5	0.01	1	3.6	2	3.5
5-14	368	564	3	4.6	10.0	0.01	1	0.9	1	0.7
15-44	107	94	1	0.8	29.8	0.01	4	3.3	5	3.2
45-59	13	60	0	0.5	52.3	0.01	1	6.6	2	6.9
60+	4	32	0	0.3	69.7	0.01	1	4.6	1	4.7
All ages	6 623	2 583	54	21.2	3.5	0.01	8	3.1	10	3.0
Females										
0-4	5 659	14 242	46	116.8	2.5	0.01	1	3.4	2	3.4
5-14	290	468	2	3.8	10.0	0.01	0	0.7	0	0.6
15-44	41	38	0	0.3	29.8	0.01	1	1.3	2	1.4
45-59	5	22	0	0.2	52.3	0.01	1	2.4	1	2.4
60+	3	22	0	0.2	70.4	0.01	0	3.1	1	3.2
All ages	5 999	2 432	49	19.9	3.1	0.01	4	1.7	5	1.7
Total	12 622	2 509	103	20.6	3.3	0.01	12	2.4	16	2.4

Table 216i World - Mundo - Monde — Poisonings - Episodes

Age group (years)	Incidence 1990 Number ('000s)	Rate (per 100 000)	Prevalence 1990 Number ('000s)	Rate (per 100 000)	Avg. age at onset (years)	Average duration (years)	Deaths 1990 Number ('000s)	Rate (per 100 000)	Deaths 2000 (Projected) Number ('000s)	Rate (per 100 000)
Males										
0-4	70 689	22 001	580	180.4	2.5	0.01	29	8.9	33	9.5
5-14	6 508	1 181	53	9.7	10.0	0.01	12	2.2	10	1.7
15-44	2 507	201	21	1.6	29.8	0.01	57	4.6	57	4.0
45-59	455	146	4	1.2	52.3	0.01	31	9.9	37	9.3
60+	217	99	2	0.8	70.0	0.01	20	9.0	25	9.2
All ages	80 377	3 029	659	24.8	4.4	0.01	148	5.6	164	5.3
Females										
0-4	40 801	13 193	335	108.2	2.5	0.01	19	6.3	23	6.8
5-14	6 291	1 197	52	9.8	10.0	0.01	10	1.9	8	1.3
15-44	1 420	118	12	1.0	29.9	0.01	39	3.3	38	2.7
45-59	9 162	2 945	75	24.2	52.4	0.01	10	3.4	13	3.3
60+	1 058	393	9	3.2	70.3	0.01	15	5.4	21	6.1
All ages	58 731	2 247	482	18.4	13.0	0.01	94	3.6	102	3.3
Total	139 108	2 641	1 141	21.7	8.0	0.01	242	4.6	265	4.3

For epidemiological sources see Pronczuk and Hong 1996. For the methods used to estimate and project incidence, prevalence, and deaths see Murray and Lopez 1996a. See explanatory notes for definitions and caveats.

Table 217   **Cuadro 217**   **Tableau 217**
Falls   **Caídas**   **Chutes**

Episodes   Episodios   Episodes

Table 217a   EME - PEMC - EMBE   Falls - Episodes

Age group (years)	Incidence 1990 Number ('000s)	Rate (per 100 000)	Prevalence 1990 Number ('000s)	Rate (per 100 000)	Avg. age at onset (years)	Average duration (years)	Deaths 1990 Number ('000s)	Rate (per 100 000)	Deaths 2000 (Projected) Number ('000s)	Rate (per 100 000)
Males										
0-4	187	709	-	-	2.5	-	0	0.8	0	0.6
5-14	261	489	-	-	10.0	-	0	0.4	0	0.3
15-44	787	428	-	-	29.9	-	4	2.4	4	2.1
45-59	374	566	-	-	52.4	-	4	6.5	5	5.9
60+	513	847	-	-	71.1	-	21	35.3	26	35.8
All ages	2 122	543	-	-	39.0	-	30	7.8	35	8.4
Females										
0-4	116	461	-	-	2.5	-	0	0.5	0	0.4
5-14	104	206	-	-	10.0	-	0	0.1	0	0.1
15-44	355	198	-	-	30.0	-	1	0.4	1	0.5
45-59	483	712	-	-	52.4	-	1	1.6	1	1.6
60+	1 560	1 844	-	-	72.4	-	37	44.2	40	41.4
All ages	2 617	643	-	-	57.4	-	39	9.7	43	9.9
Total	4 739	594	-	-	49.1	-	70	8.8	77	9.2

Table 217b   FSE - PEAS - AESE   Falls - Episodes

Age group (years)	Incidence 1990 Number ('000s)	Rate (per 100 000)	Prevalence 1990 Number ('000s)	Rate (per 100 000)	Avg. age at onset (years)	Average duration (years)	Deaths 1990 Number ('000s)	Rate (per 100 000)	Deaths 2000 (Projected) Number ('000s)	Rate (per 100 000)
Males										
0-4	260	1 891	-	-	2.5	-	0	2.1	0	1.9
5-14	507	1 852	-	-	10.0	-	0	1.3	0	1.1
15-44	920	1 207	-	-	29.8	-	5	6.7	5	6.5
45-59	324	1 202	-	-	52.2	-	4	13.8	4	14.3
60+	154	736	-	-	70.0	-	6	30.7	9	37.2
All ages	2 166	1 310	-	-	28.1	-	16	9.6	19	11.3
Females										
0-4	179	1 366	-	-	2.5	-	0	1.6	0	1.4
5-14	178	672	-	-	10.0	-	0	0.5	0	0.4
15-44	338	451	-	-	29.9	-	1	1.0	1	1.0
45-59	343	1 145	-	-	52.4	-	1	2.5	1	2.5
60+	462	1 270	-	-	71.5	-	11	30.4	14	34.3
All ages	1 501	830	-	-	42.2	-	13	7.1	16	8.6
Total	3 667	1 059	-	-	33.9	-	29	8.3	35	9.9

Table 217c   India - India - Inde   Falls - Episodes

Age group (years)	Incidence 1990 Number ('000s)	Rate (per 100 000)	Prevalence 1990 Number ('000s)	Rate (per 100 000)	Avg. age at onset (years)	Average duration (years)	Deaths 1990 Number ('000s)	Rate (per 100 000)	Deaths 2000 (Projected) Number ('000s)	Rate (per 100 000)
Males										
0-4	3 093	5 173	-	-	2.5	-	4	5.9	3	5.9
5-14	11 234	11 041	-	-	10.0	-	8	8.0	6	5.7
15-44	1 318	657	-	-	29.8	-	7	3.7	8	3.3
45-59	429	902	-	-	52.3	-	5	10.4	6	10.2
60+	151	506	-	-	69.7	-	6	21.1	9	23.4
All ages	16 224	3 692	-	-	11.9	-	30	6.9	33	6.4
Females										
0-4	3 287	5 800	-	-	2.5	-	4	6.6	4	6.5
5-14	4 863	5 105	-	-	10.0	-	4	3.7	3	2.4
15-44	1 248	681	-	-	29.8	-	3	1.5	3	1.3
45-59	887	1 927	-	-	52.4	-	2	4.3	2	4.3
60+	179	621	-	-	70.1	-	4	14.9	7	18.1
All ages	10 465	2 552	-	-	14.6	-	16	4.0	18	3.8
Total	26 689	3 142	-	-	12.9	-	46	5.5	51	5.1

For epidemiological sources see Fullerton et al. 1996. For the methods used to estimate and project incidence, prevalence, and deaths see Murray and Lopez 1996a. See explanatory notes for definitions and caveats.

Table 217   **Cuadro 217**   **Tableau 217**
Falls   **Caídas**   **Chutes**

Episodes   Episodios   Episodes

Table 217d   China - China - Chine   Falls - Episodes

Age group (years)	Incidence 1990 Number ('000s)	Rate (per 100 000)	Prevalence 1990 Number ('000s)	Rate (per 100 000)	Avg. age at onset (years)	Average duration (years)	Deaths 1990 Number ('000s)	Rate (per 100 000)	Deaths 2000 (Projected) Number ('000s)	Rate (per 100 000)
Males										
0-4	2 105	3 494	-	-	2.5	-	2	4.0	2	3.6
5-14	1 280	1 319	-	-	10.0	-	1	0.9	1	0.6
15-44	1 775	580	-	-	29.9	-	10	3.2	8	2.5
45-59	393	541	-	-	52.3	-	4	6.2	5	5.4
60+	353	721	-	-	69.8	-	15	30.1	19	32.3
All ages	5 906	1 009	-	-	19.7	-	32	5.5	36	5.4
Females										
0-4	3 170	5 470	-	-	2.5	-	4	6.2	3	5.3
5-14	1 048	1 159	-	-	10.0	-	1	0.8	1	0.5
15-44	912	321	-	-	29.9	-	2	0.7	2	0.5
45-59	1 462	2 269	-	-	52.4	-	3	5.1	5	5.1
60+	956	1 850	-	-	70.6	-	23	44.6	39	60.6
All ages	7 547	1 376	-	-	25.1	-	33	6.0	49	7.8
Total	13 453	1 187	-	-	22.8	-	65	5.7	84	6.6

Table 217e   OAI - OPAI - APAI   Falls - Episodes

Age group (years)	Incidence 1990 Number ('000s)	Rate (per 100 000)	Prevalence 1990 Number ('000s)	Rate (per 100 000)	Avg. age at onset (years)	Average duration (years)	Deaths 1990 Number ('000s)	Rate (per 100 000)	Deaths 2000 (Projected) Number ('000s)	Rate (per 100 000)
Males										
0-4	3 506	8 011	-	-	2.5	-	4	9.1	4	8.1
5-14	3 242	3 858	-	-	10.0	-	2	3.0	2	2.1
15-44	2 077	1 291	-	-	29.7	-	12	7.2	13	6.4
45-59	348	1 019	-	-	52.3	-	4	11.7	5	11.2
60+	67	332	-	-	69.6	-	3	13.8	4	14.2
All ages	9 239	2 694	-	-	13.6	-	25	7.2	27	6.8
Females										
0-4	2 661	6 338	-	-	2.5	-	3	7.2	3	6.4
5-14	1 506	1 878	-	-	10.0	-	1	1.4	1	1.0
15-44	1 059	664	-	-	29.8	-	2	1.5	3	1.3
45-59	469	1 337	-	-	52.3	-	1	3.0	1	3.0
60+	68	302	-	-	70.3	-	2	7.2	3	8.0
All ages	5 764	1 697	-	-	14.3	-	9	2.7	10	2.5
Total	15 003	2 198	-	-	13.9	-	34	5.0	38	4.7

Table 217f   SSA - ASS - ASS   Falls - Episodes

Age group (years)	Incidence 1990 Number ('000s)	Rate (per 100 000)	Prevalence 1990 Number ('000s)	Rate (per 100 000)	Avg. age at onset (years)	Average duration (years)	Deaths 1990 Number ('000s)	Rate (per 100 000)	Deaths 2000 (Projected) Number ('000s)	Rate (per 100 000)
Males										
0-4	788	1 660	-	-	2.4	-	1	1.9	1	1.9
5-14	2 303	3 278	-	-	10.0	-	2	2.5	2	1.9
15-44	926	892	-	-	29.4	-	5	5.0	6	4.5
45-59	127	626	-	-	52.2	-	1	7.3	2	7.5
60+	48	452	-	-	69.2	-	2	18.9	3	20.2
All ages	4 192	1 661	-	-	14.8	-	11	4.5	14	4.2
Females										
0-4	846	1 800	-	-	2.4	-	1	2.0	1	2.1
5-14	1 417	2 030	-	-	10.0	-	1	1.5	1	1.1
15-44	482	454	-	-	29.5	-	1	1.0	1	1.0
45-59	158	712	-	-	52.2	-	0	1.6	0	1.6
60+	124	975	-	-	69.7	-	3	23.3	4	25.6
All ages	3 027	1 174	-	-	15.6	-	6	2.5	9	2.5
Total	7 219	1 415	-	-	15.1	-	18	3.5	23	3.4

For epidemiological sources see Fullerton et al. 1996. For the methods used to estimate and project incidence, prevalence, and deaths see Murray and Lopez 1996a. See explanatory notes for definitions and caveats.

Table 217	Cuadro 217	Tableau 217
Falls	Caídas	Chutes

Episodes | Episodios | Episodes

Table 217g   LAC - ALC - ALC   Falls - Episodes

Age group (years)	Incidence 1990 Number ('000s)	Rate (per 100 000)	Prevalence 1990 Number ('000s)	Rate (per 100 000)	Avg. age at onset (years)	Average duration (years)	Deaths 1990 Number ('000s)	Rate (per 100 000)	Deaths 2000 (Projected) Number ('000s)	Rate (per 100 000)
Males										
0-4	578	2 013	-	-	2.5	-	1	2.2	1	2.0
5-14	1 517	2 910	-	-	10.0	-	1	2.1	1	1.6
15-44	790	757	-	-	29.8	-	4	4.2	5	3.9
45-59	152	684	-	-	52.3	-	2	7.8	2	7.8
60+	105	736	-	-	70.3	-	4	28.6	6	31.4
All ages	3 142	1 418	-	-	17.7	-	12	5.4	15	5.7
Females										
0-4	373	1 346	-	-	2.5	-	0	1.5	0	1.4
5-14	719	1 417	-	-	10.0	-	1	1.0	0	0.8
15-44	332	319	-	-	29.9	-	1	0.7	1	0.7
45-59	164	704	-	-	52.4	-	0	1.6	1	1.6
60+	189	1 126	-	-	71.1	-	5	27.0	7	30.1
All ages	1 777	798	-	-	22.6	-	7	3.0	9	3.5
Total	4 919	1 107	-	-	19.4	-	18	4.2	24	4.6

Table 217h   MEC - AOM - CMO   Falls - Episodes

Age group (years)	Incidence 1990 Number ('000s)	Rate (per 100 000)	Prevalence 1990 Number ('000s)	Rate (per 100 000)	Avg. age at onset (years)	Average duration (years)	Deaths 1990 Number ('000s)	Rate (per 100 000)	Deaths 2000 (Projected) Number ('000s)	Rate (per 100 000)
Males										
0-4	1 305	3 170	-	-	2.5	-	1	3.6	2	3.5
5-14	2 029	3 105	-	-	10.0	-	1	2.3	1	1.8
15-44	571	502	-	-	29.8	-	3	2.8	4	2.6
45-59	83	370	-	-	52.3	-	1	4.3	1	4.4
60+	22	162	-	-	69.7	-	1	6.8	1	7.5
All ages	4 010	1 564	-	-	11.6	-	8	3.1	10	3.0
Females										
0-4	1 107	2 787	-	-	2.5	-	1	3.2	2	3.2
5-14	845	1 364	-	-	10.0	-	1	1.0	1	0.8
15-44	257	240	-	-	29.8	-	1	0.5	1	0.5
45-59	97	437	-	-	52.3	-	0	1.0	0	1.0
60+	31	199	-	-	70.4	-	1	4.8	1	5.2
All ages	2 338	948	-	-	11.2	-	3	1.4	4	1.3
Total	6 348	1 262	-	-	11.4	-	11	2.3	14	2.2

Table 217i   World - Mundo - Monde   Falls - Episodes

Age group (years)	Incidence 1990 Number ('000s)	Rate (per 100 000)	Prevalence 1990 Number ('000s)	Rate (per 100 000)	Avg. age at onset (years)	Average duration (years)	Deaths 1990 Number ('000s)	Rate (per 100 000)	Deaths 2000 (Projected) Number ('000s)	Rate (per 100 000)
Males										
0-4	11 822	3 679	-	-	2.5	-	13	4.2	13	3.8
5-14	22 372	4 059	-	-	10.0	-	16	3.0	13	2.1
15-44	9 164	733	-	-	29.8	-	51	4.1	53	3.7
45-59	2 231	714	-	-	52.3	-	26	8.2	31	7.8
60+	1 412	645	-	-	70.1	-	59	26.8	78	28.3
All ages	47 001	1 771	-	-	19.5	-	165	6.2	189	6.1
Females										
0-4	11 740	3 796	-	-	2.5	-	13	4.3	13	3.8
5-14	10 680	2 032	-	-	10.0	-	8	1.5	6	1.0
15-44	4 983	416	-	-	29.8	-	11	0.9	12	0.8
45-59	4 063	1 306	-	-	52.4	-	9	2.9	12	3.0
60+	3 570	1 326	-	-	71.2	-	86	31.8	116	34.4
All ages	35 035	1 340	-	-	25.8	-	127	4.9	158	5.2
Total	82 036	1 557	-	-	22.2	-	292	5.5	347	5.6

For epidemiological sources see Fullerton et al. 1996. For the methods used to estimate and project incidence, prevalence, and deaths see Murray and Lopez 1996a. See explanatory notes for definitions and caveats.

Global Health Statistics

Table 218	Cuadro 218	Tableau 218
Falls	Caídas	Chutes

Fractured skull - long term   Fractura de cráneo - larga duración   Fracture du crâne - long terme

Table 218a　　EME - PEMC - EMBE

Falls - Fractured skull - long term

Age group (years)	Incidence 1990 Number ('000s)	Rate (per 100 000)	Prevalence 1990 Number ('000s)	Rate (per 100 000)	Avg. age at onset (years)	Average duration (years)	Deaths 1990 Number ('000s)	Rate (per 100 000)	Deaths 2000 (Projected) Number ('000s)	Rate (per 100 000)
Males										
0-4	0	1.7	1	4.2	2.5	70.2	-	-	-	-
5-14	1	1.1	7	14.0	10.0	63.6	-	-	-	-
15-44	1	0.5	49	26.8	29.9	44.7	-	-	-	-
45-59	0	0.6	26	38.7	52.4	24.5	-	-	-	-
60+	0	0.3	28	47.0	71.1	11.3	-	-	-	-
All ages	3	0.6	112	28.7	27.2	47.9	-	-	-	-
Females										
0-4	0	1.1	1	2.7	2.5	76.1	-	-	-	-
5-14	0	0.5	4	7.8	10.0	69.5	-	-	-	-
15-44	0	0.2	24	13.5	30.0	50.0	-	-	-	-
45-59	1	0.8	15	22.7	52.4	28.8	-	-	-	-
60+	1	0.7	31	37.2	72.4	12.7	-	-	-	-
All ages	2	0.5	76	18.6	42.0	39.5	-	-	-	-
Total	5	0.6	188	23.5	33.8	44.1	-	-	-	-

Table 218b　　FSE - PEAS - AESE

Falls - Fractured skull - long term

Age group (years)	Incidence 1990 Number ('000s)	Rate (per 100 000)	Prevalence 1990 Number ('000s)	Rate (per 100 000)	Avg. age at onset (years)	Average duration (years)	Deaths 1990 Number ('000s)	Rate (per 100 000)	Deaths 2000 (Projected) Number ('000s)	Rate (per 100 000)
Males										
0-4	1	4.4	2	11.1	2.5	63.5	-	-	-	-
5-14	1	4.3	12	43.9	10.0	57.3	-	-	-	-
15-44	1	1.3	65	85.4	29.8	39.2	-	-	-	-
45-59	0	1.3	31	115.4	52.2	20.8	-	-	-	-
60+	0	0.3	27	128.5	70.0	10.1	-	-	-	-
All ages	3	2.0	137	82.7	20.6	47.9	-	-	-	-
Females										
0-4	0	3.2	1	8.0	2.5	72.4	-	-	-	-
5-14	0	1.6	6	23.9	10.0	66.0	-	-	-	-
15-44	0	0.5	29	39.2	29.9	46.8	-	-	-	-
45-59	0	1.3	17	56.2	52.4	26.1	-	-	-	-
60+	0	0.5	26	71.3	71.5	11.8	-	-	-	-
All ages	2	1.0	80	44.0	27.6	49.5	-	-	-	-
Total	5	1.4	216	62.5	23.1	48.4	-	-	-	-

Table 218c　　India - India - Inde

Falls - Fractured skull - long term

Age group (years)	Incidence 1990 Number ('000s)	Rate (per 100 000)	Prevalence 1990 Number ('000s)	Rate (per 100 000)	Avg. age at onset (years)	Average duration (years)	Deaths 1990 Number ('000s)	Rate (per 100 000)	Deaths 2000 (Projected) Number ('000s)	Rate (per 100 000)
Males										
0-4	1	1.2	2	3.0	2.5	59.9	-	-	-	-
5-14	26	25.6	138	135.8	10.0	57.4	-	-	-	-
15-44	1	0.7	553	275.6	29.8	39.9	-	-	-	-
45-59	0	1.0	140	294.0	52.3	21.0	-	-	-	-
60+	0	0.2	90	303.5	69.7	9.7	-	-	-	-
All ages	29	6.5	923	210.0	11.6	55.9	-	-	-	-
Females										
0-4	8	13.6	19	33.3	2.5	60.8	-	-	-	-
5-14	11	12.0	122	127.7	10.0	59.1	-	-	-	-
15-44	1	0.8	363	198.0	29.8	41.7	-	-	-	-
45-59	1	2.1	104	225.3	52.4	22.5	-	-	-	-
60+	0	0.2	71	243.9	70.1	10.2	-	-	-	-
All ages	22	5.3	678	165.2	10.7	56.8	-	-	-	-
Total	50	5.9	1 600	188.4	11.2	56.3	-	-	-	-

For epidemiological sources see Fullerton et al. 1996. For the methods used to estimate and project incidence, prevalence, and deaths see Lozano et al. 1996 and Murray and Lopez 1996a. See explanatory notes for definitions and caveats.

Table 218	Cuadro 218	Tableau 218
Falls	Caídas	Chutes

Fractured skull - long term   Fractura de cráneo - larga duración   Fracture du crâne - long terme

Table 218d   China - China - Chine   Falls - Fractured skull - long term

Age group (years)	Incidence 1990 Number ('000s)	Rate (per 100 000)	Prevalence 1990 Number ('000s)	Rate (per 100 000)	Avg. age at onset (years)	Average duration (years)	Deaths 1990 Number ('000s)	Rate (per 100 000)	Deaths 2000 (Projected) Number ('000s)	Rate (per 100 000)
Males										
0-4	5	8.2	12	20	2.5	65.5	-	-	-	-
5-14	3	3.1	55	56	10.0	59.9	-	-	-	-
15-44	2	0.6	248	81	29.9	41.2	-	-	-	-
45-59	0	0.6	69	95	52.3	21.4	-	-	-	-
60+	0	0.3	50	102	69.8	9.9	-	-	-	-
All ages	10	1.8	434	74	12.7	56.8	-	-	-	-
Females										
0-4	7	12.8	18	32	2.5	68.5	-	-	-	-
5-14	2	2.7	70	77	10.0	63.2	-	-	-	-
15-44	1	0.4	273	96	29.9	44.2	-	-	-	-
45-59	2	2.5	78	120	52.4	23.8	-	-	-	-
60+	0	0.7	76	147	70.6	10.8	-	-	-	-
All ages	13	2.3	515	94	14.3	58.3	-	-	-	-
Total	23	2.1	949	84	13.6	57.7	-	-	-	-

Table 218e   OAI - OPAI - APAI   Falls - Fractured skull - long term

Age group (years)	Incidence 1990 Number ('000s)	Rate (per 100 000)	Prevalence 1990 Number ('000s)	Rate (per 100 000)	Avg. age at onset (years)	Average duration (years)	Deaths 1990 Number ('000s)	Rate (per 100 000)	Deaths 2000 (Projected) Number ('000s)	Rate (per 100 000)
Males										
0-4	8	18.8	20	46	2.5	59.8	-	-	-	-
5-14	8	9.0	117	139	10.0	56.2	-	-	-	-
15-44	2	1.4	330	205	29.7	38.8	-	-	-	-
45-59	0	1.1	80	235	52.3	20.3	-	-	-	-
60+	0	0.1	50	245	69.6	9.7	-	-	-	-
All ages	19	5.4	597	174	10.1	54.8	-	-	-	-
Females										
0-4	6	14.9	15	37	2.5	63.2	-	-	-	-
5-14	4	4.4	77	96	10.0	59.2	-	-	-	-
15-44	1	0.7	206	129	29.8	41.4	-	-	-	-
45-59	1	1.5	53	151	52.3	22.4	-	-	-	-
60+	0	0.1	37	164	70.3	10.5	-	-	-	-
All ages	12	3.4	388	114	10.0	57.8	-	-	-	-
Total	30	4.4	985	144	10.1	56.0	-	-	-	-

Table 218f   SSA - ASS - ASS   Falls - Fractured skull - long term

Age group (years)	Incidence 1990 Number ('000s)	Rate (per 100 000)	Prevalence 1990 Number ('000s)	Rate (per 100 000)	Avg. age at onset (years)	Average duration (years)	Deaths 1990 Number ('000s)	Rate (per 100 000)	Deaths 2000 (Projected) Number ('000s)	Rate (per 100 000)
Males										
0-4	2	3.9	4	9.4	2.4	48.7	-	-	-	-
5-14	5	7.7	41	57.7	10.0	49.2	-	-	-	-
15-44	1	1.0	115	110.7	29.4	35.0	-	-	-	-
45-59	0	0.7	27	131.3	52.2	19.1	-	-	-	-
60+	0	0.2	15	138.3	69.2	9.3	-	-	-	-
All ages	8	3.3	201	79.7	11.5	46.8	-	-	-	-
Females										
0-4	2	4.2	5	10.2	2.4	51.9	-	-	-	-
5-14	3	4.8	31	44.8	10.0	51.9	-	-	-	-
15-44	1	0.5	81	76.0	29.5	37.2	-	-	-	-
45-59	0	0.8	20	89.5	52.2	20.5	-	-	-	-
60+	0	0.4	13	99.2	69.7	9.8	-	-	-	-
All ages	6	2.4	149	57.8	10.9	49.4	-	-	-	-
Total	15	2.8	350	68.6	11.3	47.9	-	-	-	-

For epidemiological sources see Fullerton et al. 1996. For the methods used to estimate and project incidence, prevalence, and deaths see Lozano et al. 1996 and Murray and Lopez 1996a. See explanatory notes for definitions and caveats.

Table 218   **Cuadro 218**   **Tableau 218**
Falls   **Caídas**   **Chutes**

Fractured skull - long term   Fractura de cráneo - larga duración   Fracture du crâne - long terme

Table 218g   LAC - ALC - ALC   Falls - Fractured skull - long term

Age group (years)	Incidence 1990 Number ('000s)	Rate (per 100 000)	Prevalence 1990 Number ('000s)	Rate (per 100 000)	Avg. age at onset (years)	Average duration (years)	Deaths 1990 Number ('000s)	Rate (per 100 000)	Deaths 2000 (Projected) Number ('000s)	Rate (per 100 000)
Males										
0-4	1	4.6	3	11.5	2.5	63.9	-	-	-	-
5-14	3	6.7	30	56.8	10.0	59.3	-	-	-	-
15-44	1	0.8	107	102.5	29.8	41.4	-	-	-	-
45-59	0	0.8	27	120.7	52.3	22.3	-	-	-	-
60+	0	0.3	18	129.2	70.3	10.4	-	-	-	-
All ages	6	2.7	185	83.5	12.8	56.4	-	-	-	-
Females										
0-4	1	3.2	2	7.8	2.5	67.9	-	-	-	-
5-14	2	3.3	16	32.4	10.0	63.0	-	-	-	-
15-44	0	0.4	56	54.2	29.9	44.6	-	-	-	-
45-59	0	0.8	15	65.4	52.4	24.8	-	-	-	-
60+	0	0.4	13	76.0	71.1	11.3	-	-	-	-
All ages	3	1.4	103	46.3	14.0	58.9	-	-	-	-
Total	9	2.0	288	64.9	13.2	57.2	-	-	-	-

Table 218h   MEC - AOM - CMO   Falls - Fractured skull - long term

Age group (years)	Incidence 1990 Number ('000s)	Rate (per 100 000)	Prevalence 1990 Number ('000s)	Rate (per 100 000)	Avg. age at onset (years)	Average duration (years)	Deaths 1990 Number ('000s)	Rate (per 100 000)	Deaths 2000 (Projected) Number ('000s)	Rate (per 100 000)
Males										
0-4	3	7.4	8	18	2.5	61.1	-	-	-	-
5-14	5	7.3	48	74	10.0	58.1	-	-	-	-
15-44	1	0.6	135	118	29.8	40.0	-	-	-	-
45-59	0	0.4	29	130	52.3	20.8	-	-	-	-
60+	0	0.1	18	133	69.7	9.8	-	-	-	-
All ages	9	3.3	237	93	9.3	57.4	-	-	-	-
Females										
0-4	3	6.5	6	16	2.5	63.7	-	-	-	-
5-14	2	3.2	30	49	10.0	60.9	-	-	-	-
15-44	0	0.3	73	68	29.8	42.6	-	-	-	-
45-59	0	0.5	17	76	52.3	22.9	-	-	-	-
60+	0	0.1	12	81	70.4	10.6	-	-	-	-
All ages	5	2.0	139	56	8.3	60.3	-	-	-	-
Total	14	2.7	377	75	8.9	58.5	-	-	-	-

Table 218i   World - Mundo - Monde   Falls - Fractured skull - long term

Age group (years)	Incidence 1990 Number ('000s)	Rate (per 100 000)	Prevalence 1990 Number ('000s)	Rate (per 100 000)	Avg. age at onset (years)	Average duration (years)	Deaths 1990 Number ('000s)	Rate (per 100 000)	Deaths 2000 (Projected) Number ('000s)	Rate (per 100 000)
Males										
0-4	21	6.6	52	16	2.5	60.9	-	-	-	-
5-14	52	9.5	447	81	10.0	56.8	-	-	-	-
15-44	10	0.8	1 601	128	29.8	39.9	-	-	-	-
45-59	2	0.8	428	137	52.3	21.5	-	-	-	-
60+	1	0.2	296	135	70.3	10.4	-	-	-	-
All ages	86	3.3	2 825	106	12.1	54.5	-	-	-	-
Females										
0-4	28	8.9	68	22	2.5	63.6	-	-	-	-
5-14	25	4.8	357	68	10.0	59.2	-	-	-	-
15-44	6	0.5	1 106	92	29.8	42.8	-	-	-	-
45-59	5	1.5	318	102	52.4	24.0	-	-	-	-
60+	1	0.5	279	104	71.5	11.7	-	-	-	-
All ages	64	2.4	2 128	81	12.8	56.2	-	-	-	-
Total	150	2.9	4 954	94	12.4	55.2	-	-	-	-

For epidemiological sources see Fullerton et al. 1996. For the methods used to estimate and project incidence, prevalence, and deaths see Lozano et al. 1996 and Murray and Lopez 1996a. See explanatory notes for definitions and caveats.

Table 219 / **Cuadro 219** / **Tableau 219**
Falls / **Caídas** / **Chutes**

Injured spinal cord / Lesión de la medula espinal / Lésion de la moelle épinière

Table 219a EME - PEMC - EMBE — Falls - Injured spinal cord

Age group (years)	Incidence 1990 Number ('000s)	Rate (per 100 000)	Prevalence 1990 Number ('000s)	Rate (per 100 000)	Avg. age at onset (years)	Average duration (years)	Deaths 1990 Number ('000s)	Rate (per 100 000)	Deaths 2000 (Projected) Number ('000s)	Rate (per 100 000)
Males										
0-4	0	1.1	1	2.6	2.5	57.1	-	-	-	-
5-14	0	0.7	5	8.9	10.0	51.1	-	-	-	-
15-44	9	5.1	158	85.8	29.9	33.6	-	-	-	-
45-59	4	6.7	126	190.1	52.4	15.6	-	-	-	-
60+	3	5.1	95	156.1	71.1	6.1	-	-	-	-
All ages	18	4.5	384	98.3	41.9	25.0	-	-	-	-
Females										
0-4	0	0.7	0	1.7	2.5	65.1	-	-	-	-
5-14	0	0.3	3	5.0	10.0	59.0	-	-	-	-
15-44	4	2.4	74	41.3	30.0	40.2	-	-	-	-
45-59	6	8.5	90	133.2	52.4	20.5	-	-	-	-
60+	9	11.0	179	211.6	72.4	7.9	-	-	-	-
All ages	20	4.8	346	85.0	56.3	19.4	-	-	-	-
Total	37	4.7	730	91.5	49.5	22.1	-	-	-	-

Table 219b FSE - PEAS - AESE — Falls - Injured spinal cord

Age group (years)	Incidence 1990 Number ('000s)	Rate (per 100 000)	Prevalence 1990 Number ('000s)	Rate (per 100 000)	Avg. age at onset (years)	Average duration (years)	Deaths 1990 Number ('000s)	Rate (per 100 000)	Deaths 2000 (Projected) Number ('000s)	Rate (per 100 000)
Males										
0-4	0	2.9	1	7.0	2.5	48.3	-	-	-	-
5-14	1	2.3	8	27.8	10.0	43.1	-	-	-	-
15-44	11	14.4	182	238.3	29.8	26.8	-	-	-	-
45-59	4	14.3	118	436.8	52.2	11.9	-	-	-	-
60+	1	4.4	53	252.2	70.0	5.2	-	-	-	-
All ages	17	10.1	361	218.4	35.8	23.3	-	-	-	-
Females										
0-4	0	2.1	1	5.1	2.5	59.8	-	-	-	-
5-14	0	1.0	4	15.1	10.0	54.5	-	-	-	-
15-44	4	5.4	74	98.5	29.9	36.2	-	-	-	-
45-59	4	13.6	77	257.6	52.4	17.4	-	-	-	-
60+	3	7.6	94	257.2	71.5	6.7	-	-	-	-
All ages	11	6.3	249	137.9	46.9	23.3	-	-	-	-
Total	28	8.1	610	176.3	40.3	23.3	-	-	-	-

Table 219c India - India - Inde — Falls - Injured spinal cord

Age group (years)	Incidence 1990 Number ('000s)	Rate (per 100 000)	Prevalence 1990 Number ('000s)	Rate (per 100 000)	Avg. age at onset (years)	Average duration (years)	Deaths 1990 Number ('000s)	Rate (per 100 000)	Deaths 2000 (Projected) Number ('000s)	Rate (per 100 000)
Males										
0-4	5	7.8	10	18	2.5	40.3	-	-	-	-
5-14	17	16.6	118	115	10.0	43.1	-	-	-	-
15-44	16	7.8	581	290	29.8	28.1	-	-	-	-
45-59	5	10.7	186	391	52.3	12.7	-	-	-	-
60+	1	3.0	68	230	69.7	4.9	-	-	-	-
All ages	43	9.8	964	219	22.6	33.0	-	-	-	-
Females										
0-4	5	8.8	11	20	2.5	40.1	-	-	-	-
5-14	7	7.7	71	75	10.0	44.5	-	-	-	-
15-44	15	8.1	395	215	29.8	30.0	-	-	-	-
45-59	11	22.9	200	435	52.4	14.3	-	-	-	-
60+	1	3.7	95	328	70.1	5.3	-	-	-	-
All ages	39	9.5	772	188	29.8	29.1	-	-	-	-
Total	82	9.7	1 736	204	26.0	31.1	-	-	-	-

For epidemiological sources see Fullerton et al. 1996. For the methods used to estimate and project incidence, prevalence, and deaths see Lozano et al. 1996 and Murray and Lopez 1996a. See explanatory notes for definitions and caveats.

Table 219
Falls

Cuadro 219
Caídas

Tableau 219
Chutes

Injured spinal cord

Lesión de la medula espinal

Lésion de la moelle épinière

Table 219d   China - China - Chine   Falls - Injured spinal cord

Age group (years)	Incidence 1990 Number ('000s)	Rate (per 100 000)	Prevalence 1990 Number ('000s)	Rate (per 100 000)	Avg. age at onset (years)	Average duration (years)	Deaths 1990 Number ('000s)	Rate (per 100 000)	Deaths 2000 (Projected) Number ('000s)	Rate (per 100 000)
Males										
0-4	7	12.1	8	13	2.5	51.2	-	-	-	-
5-14	6	5.8	34	35	10.0	47.6	-	-	-	-
15-44	47	15.4	429	140	29.9	30.4	-	-	-	-
45-59	9	12.1	180	248	52.3	13.1	-	-	-	-
60+	1	2.0	78	158	69.8	5.0	-	-	-	-
All ages	70	11.9	728	124	28.8	31.4	-	-	-	-
Females										
0-4	6	9.6	12	20	2.5	54.2	-	-	-	-
5-14	3	2.8	43	48	10.0	51.4	-	-	-	-
15-44	22	7.9	310	109	29.9	33.6	-	-	-	-
45-59	4	6.1	216	335	52.4	15.4	-	-	-	-
60+	1	1.8	182	352	70.6	5.7	-	-	-	-
All ages	35	6.5	763	139	27.7	35.3	-	-	-	-
Total	**105**	**9.3**	**1 491**	**132**	**28.4**	**32.8**	-	-	-	-

Table 219e   OAI - OPAI - APAI   Falls - Injured spinal cord

Age group (years)	Incidence 1990 Number ('000s)	Rate (per 100 000)	Prevalence 1990 Number ('000s)	Rate (per 100 000)	Avg. age at onset (years)	Average duration (years)	Deaths 1990 Number ('000s)	Rate (per 100 000)	Deaths 2000 (Projected) Number ('000s)	Rate (per 100 000)
Males										
0-4	5	12.1	12	28	2.5	41.2	-	-	-	-
5-14	5	5.8	69	82	10.0	41.5	-	-	-	-
15-44	25	15.4	501	312	29.7	26.7	-	-	-	-
45-59	4	12.1	169	496	52.3	11.8	-	-	-	-
60+	0	2.0	52	256	69.6	4.7	-	-	-	-
All ages	39	11.5	804	234	26.4	28.7	-	-	-	-
Females										
0-4	4	9.6	9	22	2.5	45.0	-	-	-	-
5-14	2	2.8	46	57	10.0	44.6	-	-	-	-
15-44	13	7.9	280	175	29.8	29.4	-	-	-	-
45-59	2	6.1	122	347	52.3	13.7	-	-	-	-
60+	0	1.8	53	234	70.3	5.4	-	-	-	-
All ages	21	6.3	510	150	25.6	31.9	-	-	-	-
Total	**61**	**8.9**	**1 314**	**192**	**26.1**	**29.8**	-	-	-	-

Table 219f   SSA - ASS - ASS   Falls - Injured spinal cord

Age group (years)	Incidence 1990 Number ('000s)	Rate (per 100 000)	Prevalence 1990 Number ('000s)	Rate (per 100 000)	Avg. age at onset (years)	Average duration (years)	Deaths 1990 Number ('000s)	Rate (per 100 000)	Deaths 2000 (Projected) Number ('000s)	Rate (per 100 000)
Males										
0-4	1	2.5	2	5.2	2.4	25.2	-	-	-	-
5-14	3	4.9	23	32.9	10.0	31.1	-	-	-	-
15-44	2	1.8	185	178.1	29.4	21.3	-	-	-	-
45-59	2	7.5	54	268.2	52.2	10.6	-	-	-	-
60+	0	2.7	14	136.4	69.2	4.5	-	-	-	-
All ages	8	3.3	279	110.6	22.9	23.4	-	-	-	-
Females										
0-4	1	2.7	3	5.8	2.4	28.3	-	-	-	-
5-14	2	3.1	18	25.1	10.0	33.9	-	-	-	-
15-44	6	5.4	108	101.6	29.5	23.5	-	-	-	-
45-59	2	8.5	40	182.2	52.2	11.9	-	-	-	-
60+	1	5.8	17	134.7	69.7	4.9	-	-	-	-
All ages	12	4.6	186	72.0	29.2	22.9	-	-	-	-
Total	**20**	**3.9**	**465**	**91.1**	**26.6**	**23.1**	-	-	-	-

For epidemiological sources see Fullerton et al. 1996. For the methods used to estimate and project incidence, prevalence, and deaths see Lozano et al. 1996 and Murray and Lopez 1996a. See explanatory notes for definitions and caveats.

Table 219   **Cuadro 219**   **Tableau 219**
Falls   **Caídas**   **Chutes**

Injured spinal cord   Lesión de la medula espinal   Lésion de la moelle épinière

Table 219g   LAC - ALC - ALC   Falls - Injured spinal cord

Age group (years)	Incidence 1990 Number ('000s)	Rate (per 100 000)	Prevalence 1990 Number ('000s)	Rate (per 100 000)	Avg. age at onset (years)	Average duration (years)	Deaths 1990 Number ('000s)	Rate (per 100 000)	Deaths 2000 (Projected) Number ('000s)	Rate (per 100 000)
Males										
0-4	1	3.0	2	7.1	2.5	46.5	-	-	-	-
5-14	2	4.3	18	35.1	10.0	45.1	-	-	-	-
15-44	9	8.9	185	177.6	29.8	29.4	-	-	-	-
45-59	2	8.1	69	308.6	52.3	13.6	-	-	-	-
60+	1	4.1	28	196.5	70.3	5.4	-	-	-	-
All ages	15	6.7	302	136.4	29.5	29.9	-	-	-	-
Females										
0-4	1	2.0	1	4.9	2.5	51.7	-	-	-	-
5-14	1	2.1	10	20.1	10.0	49.5	-	-	-	-
15-44	4	3.8	87	83.2	29.8	33.0	-	-	-	-
45-59	2	8.4	42	179.0	52.4	16.2	-	-	-	-
60+	1	6.7	29	172.9	71.1	6.2	-	-	-	-
All ages	9	3.9	169	75.9	36.0	29.0	-	-	-	-
Total	24	5.3	471	106.1	32.0	29.6	-	-	-	-

Table 219h   MEC - AOM - CMO   Falls - Injured spinal cord

Age group (years)	Incidence 1990 Number ('000s)	Rate (per 100 000)	Prevalence 1990 Number ('000s)	Rate (per 100 000)	Avg. age at onset (years)	Average duration (years)	Deaths 1990 Number ('000s)	Rate (per 100 000)	Deaths 2000 (Projected) Number ('000s)	Rate (per 100 000)
Males										
0-4	2	4.8	4	11	2.5	42.6	-	-	-	-
5-14	3	4.7	29	44	10.0	44.6	-	-	-	-
15-44	7	6.0	168	147	29.8	28.5	-	-	-	-
45-59	1	4.4	49	219	52.3	12.3	-	-	-	-
60+	0	1.0	16	114	69.7	4.9	-	-	-	-
All ages	13	5.1	265	104	23.1	33.0	-	-	-	-
Females										
0-4	2	4.0	4	10	2.5	45.1	-	-	-	-
5-14	1	2.1	18	29	10.0	47.5	-	-	-	-
15-44	3	2.9	83	77	29.8	31.1	-	-	-	-
45-59	1	5.2	30	136	52.3	14.3	-	-	-	-
60+	0	1.2	14	94	70.4	5.5	-	-	-	-
All ages	7	3.0	149	60	25.0	33.7	-	-	-	-
Total	20	4.0	414	82	23.8	33.2	-	-	-	-

Table 219i   World - Mundo - Monde   Falls - Injured spinal cord

Age group (years)	Incidence 1990 Number ('000s)	Rate (per 100 000)	Prevalence 1990 Number ('000s)	Rate (per 100 000)	Avg. age at onset (years)	Average duration (years)	Deaths 1990 Number ('000s)	Rate (per 100 000)	Deaths 2000 (Projected) Number ('000s)	Rate (per 100 000)
Males										
0-4	22	6.8	41	13	2.5	44.1	-	-	-	-
5-14	37	6.8	303	55	10.0	42.8	-	-	-	-
15-44	126	10.1	2 389	191	29.8	29.0	-	-	-	-
45-59	31	9.8	951	304	52.3	12.9	-	-	-	-
60+	7	3.3	403	184	70.4	5.5	-	-	-	-
All ages	223	8.4	4 087	154	28.2	29.8	-	-	-	-
Females										
0-4	18	5.9	41	13	2.5	45.9	-	-	-	-
5-14	17	3.2	212	40	10.0	45.0	-	-	-	-
15-44	71	5.9	1 410	118	29.8	31.7	-	-	-	-
45-59	31	10.1	818	263	52.4	15.9	-	-	-	-
60+	17	6.2	663	246	71.7	7.0	-	-	-	-
All ages	154	5.9	3 145	120	33.5	29.0	-	-	-	-
Total	377	7.2	7 232	137	30.4	29.5	-	-	-	-

For epidemiological sources see Fullerton et al. 1996. For the methods used to estimate and project incidence, prevalence, and deaths see Lozano et al. 1996 and Murray and Lopez 1996a. See explanatory notes for definitions and caveats.

Table 220 | **Cuadro 220** | **Tableau 220**
Falls | **Caídas** | **Chutes**

Fractured femur - short term | Fractura de femur - corta duración | Fracture du fémur - court terme

---

Table 220a EME - PEMC - EMBE

Falls - Fractured femur - short term

Age group (years)	Incidence 1990 Number ('000s)	Rate (per 100 000)	Prevalence 1990 Number ('000s)	Rate (per 100 000)	Avg. age at onset (years)	Average duration (years)	Deaths 1990 Number ('000s)	Rate (per 100 000)	Deaths 2000 (Projected) Number ('000s)	Rate (per 100 000)
Males										
0-4	24	90	3	12.4	2.5	0.14	-	-	-	-
5-14	33	62	5	8.6	10.0	0.14	-	-	-	-
15-44	49	27	7	3.7	29.9	0.14	-	-	-	-
45-59	23	35	3	4.9	52.4	0.14	-	-	-	-
60+	259	428	36	59.5	71.1	0.14	-	-	-	-
All ages	388	99	54	13.8	55.4	0.14	-	-	-	-
Females										
0-4	15	58	2	8.1	2.5	0.14	-	-	-	-
5-14	13	26	2	3.6	10.0	0.14	-	-	-	-
15-44	22	12	3	1.7	30.0	0.14	-	-	-	-
45-59	30	44	4	6.1	52.4	0.14	-	-	-	-
60+	788	932	110	129.5	72.4	0.14	-	-	-	-
All ages	868	213	121	29.6	68.5	0.14	-	-	-	-
Total	1 255	157	175	21.9	64.5	0.14	-	-	-	-

Table 220b FSE - PEAS - AESE

Falls - Fractured femur - short term

Age group (years)	Incidence 1990 Number ('000s)	Rate (per 100 000)	Prevalence 1990 Number ('000s)	Rate (per 100 000)	Avg. age at onset (years)	Average duration (years)	Deaths 1990 Number ('000s)	Rate (per 100 000)	Deaths 2000 (Projected) Number ('000s)	Rate (per 100 000)
Males										
0-4	33	239	5	33.2	2.5	0.14	-	-	-	-
5-14	64	234	9	32.5	10.0	0.14	-	-	-	-
15-44	57	75	8	10.4	29.8	0.14	-	-	-	-
45-59	20	75	3	10.4	52.2	0.14	-	-	-	-
60+	78	372	11	51.7	70.0	0.14	-	-	-	-
All ages	252	152	35	21.2	35.4	0.14	-	-	-	-
Females										
0-4	23	173	3	24.0	2.5	0.14	-	-	-	-
5-14	22	85	3	11.8	10.0	0.14	-	-	-	-
15-44	21	28	3	3.9	29.9	0.14	-	-	-	-
45-59	21	71	3	9.9	52.4	0.14	-	-	-	-
60+	234	642	32	89.2	71.5	0.14	-	-	-	-
All ages	321	177	45	24.7	58.3	0.14	-	-	-	-
Total	573	165	80	23.0	48.3	0.14	-	-	-	-

Table 220c India - India - Inde

Falls - Fractured femur - short term

Age group (years)	Incidence 1990 Number ('000s)	Rate (per 100 000)	Prevalence 1990 Number ('000s)	Rate (per 100 000)	Avg. age at onset (years)	Average duration (years)	Deaths 1990 Number ('000s)	Rate (per 100 000)	Deaths 2000 (Projected) Number ('000s)	Rate (per 100 000)
Males										
0-4	391	653	54	90.8	2.5	0.14	-	-	-	-
5-14	1 419	1 394	197	193.8	10.0	0.14	-	-	-	-
15-44	82	41	11	5.7	29.8	0.14	-	-	-	-
45-59	27	56	4	7.8	52.3	0.14	-	-	-	-
60+	76	256	11	35.5	69.7	0.14	-	-	-	-
All ages	1 994	454	277	63.1	12.2	0.14	-	-	-	-
Females										
0-4	415	732	58	101.8	2.5	0.14	-	-	-	-
5-14	614	645	85	89.6	10.0	0.14	-	-	-	-
15-44	77	42	11	5.9	29.8	0.14	-	-	-	-
45-59	55	120	8	16.6	52.4	0.14	-	-	-	-
60+	91	314	13	43.6	70.1	0.14	-	-	-	-
All ages	1 252	305	174	42.4	15.0	0.14	-	-	-	-
Total	3 246	382	451	53.1	13.3	0.14	-	-	-	-

For epidemiological sources see Fullerton et al. 1996. For the methods used to estimate and project incidence, prevalence, and deaths see Lozano et al. 1996 and Murray and Lopez 1996a. See explanatory notes for definitions and caveats.

Table 220	Cuadro 220	Tableau 220
Falls	Caídas	Chutes

Fractured femur - short term	Fractura de femur - corta duración	Fracture du fémur - court terme

Table 220d China - China - Chine — Falls - Fractured femur - short term

Age group (years)	Incidence 1990 Number ('000s)	Rate (per 100 000)	Prevalence 1990 Number ('000s)	Rate (per 100 000)	Avg. age at onset (years)	Average duration (years)	Deaths 1990 Number ('000s)	Rate (per 100 000)	Deaths 2000 (Projected) Number ('000s)	Rate (per 100 000)
Males										
0-4	265	440	37	61.2	2.5	0.14	-	-	-	-
5-14	161	166	22	23.1	10.0	0.14	-	-	-	-
15-44	109	35	15	4.9	29.9	0.14	-	-	-	-
45-59	24	33	3	4.6	52.3	0.14	-	-	-	-
60+	179	365	25	50.8	69.8	0.14	-	-	-	-
All ages	738	126	103	17.5	26.1	0.14	-	-	-	-
Females										
0-4	400	691	56	96.0	2.5	0.14	-	-	-	-
5-14	132	146	18	20.3	10.0	0.14	-	-	-	-
15-44	56	20	8	2.7	29.9	0.14	-	-	-	-
45-59	92	142	13	19.8	52.4	0.14	-	-	-	-
60+	485	939	67	130.6	70.6	0.14	-	-	-	-
All ages	1 165	212	162	29.5	37.0	0.14	-	-	-	-
Total	1 903	168	265	23.3	32.8	0.14	-	-	-	-

Table 220e OAI - OPAI - APAI — Falls - Fractured femur - short term

Age group (years)	Incidence 1990 Number ('000s)	Rate (per 100 000)	Prevalence 1990 Number ('000s)	Rate (per 100 000)	Avg. age at onset (years)	Average duration (years)	Deaths 1990 Number ('000s)	Rate (per 100 000)	Deaths 2000 (Projected) Number ('000s)	Rate (per 100 000)
Males										
0-4	443	1 012	62	140.6	2.5	0.14	-	-	-	-
5-14	409	487	57	67.7	10.0	0.14	-	-	-	-
15-44	129	80	18	11.1	29.7	0.14	-	-	-	-
45-59	22	63	3	8.8	52.3	0.14	-	-	-	-
60+	34	168	5	23.3	69.6	0.14	-	-	-	-
All ages	1 036	302	144	42.0	12.1	0.14	-	-	-	-
Females										
0-4	336	800	47	111.2	2.5	0.14	-	-	-	-
5-14	190	237	26	33.0	10.0	0.14	-	-	-	-
15-44	66	41	9	5.7	29.8	0.14	-	-	-	-
45-59	29	84	4	11.6	52.3	0.14	-	-	-	-
60+	35	152	5	21.2	70.3	0.14	-	-	-	-
All ages	656	193	91	26.8	13.2	0.14	-	-	-	-
Total	1 692	248	235	34.5	12.5	0.14	-	-	-	-

Table 220f SSA - ASS - ASS — Falls - Fractured femur - short term

Age group (years)	Incidence 1990 Number ('000s)	Rate (per 100 000)	Prevalence 1990 Number ('000s)	Rate (per 100 000)	Avg. age at onset (years)	Average duration (years)	Deaths 1990 Number ('000s)	Rate (per 100 000)	Deaths 2000 (Projected) Number ('000s)	Rate (per 100 000)
Males										
0-4	100	210	14	29.1	2.4	0.14	-	-	-	-
5-14	291	414	40	57.5	10.0	0.14	-	-	-	-
15-44	58	56	8	7.8	29.4	0.14	-	-	-	-
45-59	8	39	1	5.4	52.2	0.14	-	-	-	-
60+	24	229	3	31.8	69.2	0.14	-	-	-	-
All ages	480	190	67	26.5	14.4	0.14	-	-	-	-
Females										
0-4	107	227	15	31.6	2.4	0.14	-	-	-	-
5-14	179	256	25	35.6	10.0	0.14	-	-	-	-
15-44	30	28	4	3.9	29.5	0.14	-	-	-	-
45-59	10	44	1	6.1	52.2	0.14	-	-	-	-
60+	63	493	9	68.5	69.7	0.14	-	-	-	-
All ages	388	150	54	20.9	20.1	0.14	-	-	-	-
Total	869	170	121	23.7	17.0	0.14	-	-	-	-

For epidemiological sources see Fullerton et al. 1996. For the methods used to estimate and project incidence, prevalence, and deaths see Lozano et al. 1996 and Murray and Lopez 1996a. See explanatory notes for definitions and caveats.

Table 220   **Cuadro 220**   **Tableau 220**
Falls   **Caídas**   **Chutes**

Fractured femur - short term   Fractura de femur - corta duración   Fracture du fémur - court terme

Table 220g   LAC - ALC - ALC

Falls - Fractured femur - short term

Age group (years)	Incidence 1990 Number ('000s)	Rate (per 100 000)	Prevalence 1990 Number ('000s)	Rate (per 100 000)	Avg. age at onset (years)	Average duration (years)	Deaths 1990 Number ('000s)	Rate (per 100 000)	Deaths 2000 (Projected) Number ('000s)	Rate (per 100 000)
Males										
0-4	72	250	10	34.7	2.5	0.14	-	-	-	-
5-14	188	361	26	50.2	10.0	0.14	-	-	-	-
15-44	49	47	7	6.5	29.8	0.14	-	-	-	-
45-59	9	42	1	5.9	52.3	0.14	-	-	-	-
60+	49	347	7	48.3	70.3	0.14	-	-	-	-
All ages	367	166	51	23.0	20.4	0.14	-	-	-	-
Females										
0-4	47	170	7	23.6	2.5	0.14	-	-	-	-
5-14	91	179	13	24.9	10.0	0.14	-	-	-	-
15-44	21	20	3	2.7	29.9	0.14	-	-	-	-
45-59	10	44	1	6.1	52.4	0.14	-	-	-	-
60+	96	569	13	79.0	71.1	0.14	-	-	-	-
All ages	264	119	37	16.5	34.0	0.14	-	-	-	-
Total	632	142	88	19.8	26.0	0.14	-	-	-	-

Table 220h   MEC - AOM - CMO

Falls - Fractured femur - short term

Age group (years)	Incidence 1990 Number ('000s)	Rate (per 100 000)	Prevalence 1990 Number ('000s)	Rate (per 100 000)	Avg. age at onset (years)	Average duration (years)	Deaths 1990 Number ('000s)	Rate (per 100 000)	Deaths 2000 (Projected) Number ('000s)	Rate (per 100 000)
Males										
0-4	165	400	23	55.6	2.5	0.14	-	-	-	-
5-14	256	392	36	54.5	10.0	0.14	-	-	-	-
15-44	35	31	5	4.3	29.8	0.14	-	-	-	-
45-59	5	23	1	3.2	52.3	0.14	-	-	-	-
60+	11	82	2	11.4	69.7	0.14	-	-	-	-
All ages	473	184	66	25.6	10.7	0.14	-	-	-	-
Females										
0-4	140	352	19	48.9	2.5	0.14	-	-	-	-
5-14	107	172	15	23.9	10.0	0.14	-	-	-	-
15-44	16	15	2	2.1	29.8	0.14	-	-	-	-
45-59	6	27	1	3.8	52.3	0.14	-	-	-	-
60+	15	100	2	13.9	70.4	0.14	-	-	-	-
All ages	284	115	39	16.0	11.6	0.14	-	-	-	-
Total	757	150	105	20.9	11.1	0.14	-	-	-	-

Table 220i   World - Mundo - Monde

Falls - Fractured femur - short term

Age group (years)	Incidence 1990 Number ('000s)	Rate (per 100 000)	Prevalence 1990 Number ('000s)	Rate (per 100 000)	Avg. age at onset (years)	Average duration (years)	Deaths 1990 Number ('000s)	Rate (per 100 000)	Deaths 2000 (Projected) Number ('000s)	Rate (per 100 000)
Males										
0-4	1 491	464	207	64.5	2.5	0.14	-	-	-	-
5-14	2 821	512	392	71.1	10.0	0.14	-	-	-	-
15-44	568	45	79	6.3	29.8	0.14	-	-	-	-
45-59	138	44	19	6.1	52.3	0.14	-	-	-	-
60+	710	325	99	45.1	70.3	0.14	-	-	-	-
All ages	5 728	216	796	30.0	18.5	0.14	-	-	-	-
Females										
0-4	1 482	479	206	66.6	2.5	0.14	-	-	-	-
5-14	1 348	257	187	35.7	10.0	0.14	-	-	-	-
15-44	309	26	43	3.6	29.8	0.14	-	-	-	-
45-59	253	81	35	11.3	52.4	0.14	-	-	-	-
60+	1 806	671	251	93.2	71.5	0.14	-	-	-	-
All ages	5 199	199	723	27.6	32.5	0.14	-	-	-	-
Total	10 927	207	1 519	28.8	25.1	0.14	-	-	-	-

For epidemiological sources see Fullerton et al. 1996. For the methods used to estimate and project incidence, prevalence, and deaths see Lozano et al. 1996 and Murray and Lopez 1996a. See explanatory notes for definitions and caveats.

Table 221	Cuadro 221	Tableau 221
Falls	Caídas	Chutes

Fractured femur - long term	Fractura de femur - larga duración	Fracture du fémur - long terme

Table 221a   EME - PEMC - EMBE   Falls - Fractured femur - long term

Age group (years)	Incidence 1990 Number ('000s)	Rate (per 100 000)	Prevalence 1990 Number ('000s)	Rate (per 100 000)	Avg. age at onset (years)	Average duration (years)	Deaths 1990 Number ('000s)	Rate (per 100 000)	Deaths 2000 (Projected) Number ('000s)	Rate (per 100 000)
Males										
0-4	2	6.5	4	16	2.5	70.2	-	-	-	-
5-14	2	4.5	29	55	10.0	63.6	-	-	-	-
15-44	4	1.9	195	106	29.9	44.7	-	-	-	-
45-59	2	2.5	102	154	52.4	24.5	-	-	-	-
60+	19	30.9	312	516	71.1	11.3	-	-	-	-
All ages	28	7.2	642	164	55.4	24.4	-	-	-	-
Females										
0-4	1	4.2	3	11	2.5	76.1	-	-	-	-
5-14	1	1.9	15	30	10.0	69.5	-	-	-	-
15-44	2	0.9	95	53	30.0	50.0	-	-	-	-
45-59	2	3.2	61	90	52.4	28.8	-	-	-	-
60+	57	67.0	800	947	72.4	12.7	-	-	-	-
All ages	62	15.3	975	239	68.5	16.2	-	-	-	-
Total	90	11.3	1 617	203	64.4	18.7	-	-	-	-

Table 221b   FSE - PEAS - AESE   Falls - Fractured femur - long term

Age group (years)	Incidence 1990 Number ('000s)	Rate (per 100 000)	Prevalence 1990 Number ('000s)	Rate (per 100 000)	Avg. age at onset (years)	Average duration (years)	Deaths 1990 Number ('000s)	Rate (per 100 000)	Deaths 2000 (Projected) Number ('000s)	Rate (per 100 000)
Males										
0-4	2	17.3	6	43	2.5	63.5	-	-	-	-
5-14	5	16.9	47	171	10.0	57.3	-	-	-	-
15-44	4	5.4	256	335	29.8	39.2	-	-	-	-
45-59	1	5.4	123	457	52.2	20.8	-	-	-	-
60+	6	26.8	161	767	70.0	10.1	-	-	-	-
All ages	18	11.0	593	358	35.4	36.5	-	-	-	-
Females										
0-4	2	12.5	4	31	2.5	72.4	-	-	-	-
5-14	2	6.2	25	93	10.0	66.0	-	-	-	-
15-44	2	2.0	115	154	29.9	46.8	-	-	-	-
45-59	2	5.1	67	223	52.4	26.1	-	-	-	-
60+	17	46.2	290	796	71.5	11.8	-	-	-	-
All ages	23	12.8	501	277	58.3	23.1	-	-	-	-
Total	41	11.9	1 093	316	48.2	29.0	-	-	-	-

Table 221c   India - India - Inde   Falls - Fractured femur - long term

Age group (years)	Incidence 1990 Number ('000s)	Rate (per 100 000)	Prevalence 1990 Number ('000s)	Rate (per 100 000)	Avg. age at onset (years)	Average duration (years)	Deaths 1990 Number ('000s)	Rate (per 100 000)	Deaths 2000 (Projected) Number ('000s)	Rate (per 100 000)
Males										
0-4	72	120.5	177	295	2.5	59.9	-	-	-	-
5-14	258	253.1	1 906	1 873	10.0	57.4	-	-	-	-
15-44	15	7.3	6 494	3 239	29.8	39.9	-	-	-	-
45-59	5	10.0	1 628	3 423	52.3	21.0	-	-	-	-
60+	14	45.5	1 173	3 940	69.7	9.7	-	-	-	-
All ages	363	82.5	11 378	2 589	12.1	55.0	-	-	-	-
Females										
0-4	77	135.2	188	331	2.5	60.8	-	-	-	-
5-14	112	117.8	1 203	1 263	10.0	59.1	-	-	-	-
15-44	14	7.7	3 587	1 957	29.8	41.7	-	-	-	-
45-59	10	21.7	1 028	2 234	52.4	22.5	-	-	-	-
60+	16	56.4	859	2 970	70.1	10.2	-	-	-	-
All ages	229	55.9	6 864	1 674	14.8	53.5	-	-	-	-
Total	592	69.7	18 242	2 147	13.2	54.4	-	-	-	-

For epidemiological sources see Fullerton et al. 1996. For the methods used to estimate and project incidence, prevalence, and deaths see Lozano et al. 1996 and Murray and Lopez 1996a. See explanatory notes for definitions and caveats.

Table 221   **Cuadro 221**   **Tableau 221**
Falls   **Caídas**   **Chutes**

Fractured femur - long term   Fractura de femur - larga duración   Fracture du fémur - long terme

Table 221d   China - China - Chine   Falls - Fractured femur - long term

Age group (years)	Incidence 1990 Number ('000s)	Rate (per 100 000)	Prevalence 1990 Number ('000s)	Rate (per 100 000)	Avg. age at onset (years)	Average duration (years)	Deaths 1990 Number ('000s)	Rate (per 100 000)	Deaths 2000 (Projected) Number ('000s)	Rate (per 100 000)
Males										
0-4	25	41.8	63	104	2.5	65.5	-	-	-	-
5-14	15	15.7	278	287	10.0	59.9	-	-	-	-
15-44	10	3.4	1 271	415	29.9	41.2	-	-	-	-
45-59	2	3.1	355	489	52.3	21.4	-	-	-	-
60+	2	3.4	417	851	69.8	9.9	-	-	-	-
All ages	55	9.3	2 384	407	13.9	55.8	-	-	-	-
Females										
0-4	38	65.5	94	163	2.5	68.5	-	-	-	-
5-14	13	13.8	357	395	10.0	63.2	-	-	-	-
15-44	5	1.9	1 397	492	29.9	44.2	-	-	-	-
45-59	9	13.4	399	619	52.4	23.8	-	-	-	-
60+	45	87.8	857	1 658	70.6	10.8	-	-	-	-
All ages	110	20.0	3 104	566	36.8	39.3	-	-	-	-
Total	164	14.5	5 489	484	29.2	44.8	-	-	-	-

Table 221e   OAI - OPAI - APAI   Falls - Fractured femur - long term

Age group (years)	Incidence 1990 Number ('000s)	Rate (per 100 000)	Prevalence 1990 Number ('000s)	Rate (per 100 000)	Avg. age at onset (years)	Average duration (years)	Deaths 1990 Number ('000s)	Rate (per 100 000)	Deaths 2000 (Projected) Number ('000s)	Rate (per 100 000)
Males										
0-4	52	118.5	128	292	2.5	59.8	-	-	-	-
5-14	48	56.7	735	874	10.0	56.2	-	-	-	-
15-44	15	9.3	2 081	1 294	29.7	38.8	-	-	-	-
45-59	3	7.3	508	1 489	52.3	20.3	-	-	-	-
60+	4	19.4	350	1 732	69.6	9.7	-	-	-	-
All ages	121	35.3	3 802	1 109	12.0	53.4	-	-	-	-
Females										
0-4	39	93.8	97	232	2.5	63.2	-	-	-	-
5-14	22	27.7	486	606	10.0	59.2	-	-	-	-
15-44	8	4.8	1 300	815	29.8	41.4	-	-	-	-
45-59	3	9.7	337	959	52.3	22.4	-	-	-	-
60+	4	17.7	276	1 217	70.3	10.5	-	-	-	-
All ages	77	22.6	2 496	735	13.2	55.3	-	-	-	-
Total	198	29.0	6 298	923	12.5	54.1	-	-	-	-

Table 221f   SSA - ASS - ASS   Falls - Fractured femur - long term

Age group (years)	Incidence 1990 Number ('000s)	Rate (per 100 000)	Prevalence 1990 Number ('000s)	Rate (per 100 000)	Avg. age at onset (years)	Average duration (years)	Deaths 1990 Number ('000s)	Rate (per 100 000)	Deaths 2000 (Projected) Number ('000s)	Rate (per 100 000)
Males										
0-4	23	48.2	55	116	2.4	48.7	-	-	-	-
5-14	66	94.5	500	711	10.0	49.2	-	-	-	-
15-44	13	12.7	1 420	1 368	29.4	35.0	-	-	-	-
45-59	2	8.8	331	1 629	52.2	19.1	-	-	-	-
60+	5	51.5	229	2 175	69.2	9.3	-	-	-	-
All ages	110	43.5	2 534	1 004	14.4	45.0	-	-	-	-
Females										
0-4	25	52.2	59	126	2.4	51.9	-	-	-	-
5-14	41	58.6	386	552	10.0	51.9	-	-	-	-
15-44	7	6.4	998	939	29.5	37.2	-	-	-	-
45-59	2	10.1	246	1 112	52.2	20.5	-	-	-	-
60+	14	110.8	289	2 270	69.7	9.8	-	-	-	-
All ages	89	34.4	1 978	767	20.0	43.3	-	-	-	-
Total	198	38.9	4 512	884	16.9	44.2	-	-	-	-

For epidemiological sources see Fullerton et al. 1996. For the methods used to estimate and project incidence, prevalence, and deaths see Lozano et al. 1996 and Murray and Lopez 1996a. See explanatory notes for definitions and caveats.

Table 221   **Cuadro 221**   **Tableau 221**
Falls   **Caídas**   **Chutes**

Fractured femur - long term   Fractura de femur - larga duración   Fracture du fémur - long terme

Table 221g   LAC - ALC - ALC   Falls - Fractured femur - long term

Age group (years)	Incidence 1990 Number ('000s)	Rate (per 100 000)	Prevalence 1990 Number ('000s)	Rate (per 100 000)	Avg. age at onset (years)	Average duration (years)	Deaths 1990 Number ('000s)	Rate (per 100 000)	Deaths 2000 (Projected) Number ('000s)	Rate (per 100 000)
Males										
0-4	10	34.9	25	86	2.5	63.9	-	-	-	-
5-14	26	50.3	222	427	10.0	59.3	-	-	-	-
15-44	7	6.5	806	773	29.8	41.4	-	-	-	-
45-59	1	5.8	203	914	52.3	22.3	-	-	-	-
60+	7	48.0	207	1 456	70.3	10.4	-	-	-	-
All ages	51	23.1	1 464	661	20.3	50.4	-	-	-	-
Females										
0-4	7	23.8	16	59	2.5	67.9	-	-	-	-
5-14	13	25.0	124	244	10.0	63.0	-	-	-	-
15-44	3	2.8	426	409	29.9	44.6	-	-	-	-
45-59	1	6.1	116	496	52.4	24.8	-	-	-	-
60+	13	78.5	238	1 416	71.1	11.3	-	-	-	-
All ages	37	16.5	920	413	33.8	42.4	-	-	-	-
Total	88	19.8	2 384	537	25.9	47.0	-	-	-	-

Table 221h   MEC - AOM - CMO   Falls - Fractured femur - long term

Age group (years)	Incidence 1990 Number ('000s)	Rate (per 100 000)	Prevalence 1990 Number ('000s)	Rate (per 100 000)	Avg. age at onset (years)	Average duration (years)	Deaths 1990 Number ('000s)	Rate (per 100 000)	Deaths 2000 (Projected) Number ('000s)	Rate (per 100 000)
Males										
0-4	23	56.0	57	137	2.5	61.1	-	-	-	-
5-14	36	54.6	361	553	10.0	58.1	-	-	-	-
15-44	5	4.3	1 012	889	29.8	40.0	-	-	-	-
45-59	1	3.2	218	977	52.3	20.8	-	-	-	-
60+	2	11.4	152	1 113	69.7	9.8	-	-	-	-
All ages	66	25.7	1 800	702	10.7	56.3	-	-	-	-
Females										
0-4	20	49.2	48	121	2.5	63.7	-	-	-	-
5-14	15	24.0	227	365	10.0	60.9	-	-	-	-
15-44	2	2.1	553	516	29.8	42.6	-	-	-	-
45-59	1	3.8	128	575	52.3	22.9	-	-	-	-
60+	2	14.0	116	750	70.4	10.6	-	-	-	-
All ages	40	16.1	1 072	434	11.6	57.7	-	-	-	-
Total	106	21.0	2 871	571	11.0	56.8	-	-	-	-

Table 221i   World - Mundo - Monde   Falls - Fractured femur - long term

Age group (years)	Incidence 1990 Number ('000s)	Rate (per 100 000)	Prevalence 1990 Number ('000s)	Rate (per 100 000)	Avg. age at onset (years)	Average duration (years)	Deaths 1990 Number ('000s)	Rate (per 100 000)	Deaths 2000 (Projected) Number ('000s)	Rate (per 100 000)
Males										
0-4	209	65.1	514	160	2.5	59.8	-	-	-	-
5-14	456	82.7	4 078	740	10.0	56.4	-	-	-	-
15-44	72	5.8	13 535	1 083	29.7	39.3	-	-	-	-
45-59	16	5.3	3 469	1 111	52.3	21.2	-	-	-	-
60+	57	26.2	3 000	1 371	70.2	10.3	-	-	-	-
All ages	811	30.6	24 597	927	14.9	51.8	-	-	-	-
Females										
0-4	207	67.1	510	165	2.5	62.3	-	-	-	-
5-14	218	41.5	2 822	537	10.0	58.4	-	-	-	-
15-44	42	3.5	8 472	707	29.8	42.0	-	-	-	-
45-59	30	9.7	2 381	766	52.4	23.5	-	-	-	-
60+	169	62.6	3 725	1 384	71.2	11.4	-	-	-	-
All ages	666	25.5	17 910	685	26.3	45.1	-	-	-	-
Total	1 477	28.0	42 506	807	20.1	48.8	-	-	-	-

For epidemiological sources see Fullerton et al. 1996. For the methods used to estimate and project incidence, prevalence, and deaths see Lozano et al. 1996 and Murray and Lopez 1996a. See explanatory notes for definitions and caveats.

Table 222 **Cuadro 222** **Tableau 222**
Falls **Caídas** **Chutes**

Intracranial injury - long term   Lesión intracraneal - larga duración   Lésions intra-crâniennes - long terme

Table 222a   EME - PEMC - EMBE   Falls - Intracranial injury - long term

Age group (years)	Incidence 1990 Number ('000s)	Rate (per 100 000)	Prevalence 1990 Number ('000s)	Rate (per 100 000)	Avg. age at onset (years)	Average duration (years)	Deaths 1990 Number ('000s)	Rate (per 100 000)	Deaths 2000 (Projected) Number ('000s)	Rate (per 100 000)
Males										
0-4	3	10.3	7	26	2.5	70.2	-	-	-	-
5-14	4	7.1	46	87	10.0	63.6	-	-	-	-
15-44	7	4.0	336	182	29.9	44.7	-	-	-	-
45-59	4	5.3	187	282	52.4	24.5	-	-	-	-
60+	2	3.3	218	360	71.1	11.3	-	-	-	-
All ages	19	5.0	793	203	30.5	44.9	-	-	-	-
Females										
0-4	2	6.7	4	17	2.5	76.1	-	-	-	-
5-14	2	3.0	25	48	10.0	69.5	-	-	-	-
15-44	3	1.9	164	91	30.0	50.0	-	-	-	-
45-59	5	6.7	115	169	52.4	28.8	-	-	-	-
60+	6	7.1	263	311	72.4	12.7	-	-	-	-
All ages	17	4.2	570	140	46.4	35.5	-	-	-	-
Total	37	4.6	1 363	171	37.9	40.5	-	-	-	-

Table 222b   FSE - PEAS - AESE   Falls - Intracranial injury - long term

Age group (years)	Incidence 1990 Number ('000s)	Rate (per 100 000)	Prevalence 1990 Number ('000s)	Rate (per 100 000)	Avg. age at onset (years)	Average duration (years)	Deaths 1990 Number ('000s)	Rate (per 100 000)	Deaths 2000 (Projected) Number ('000s)	Rate (per 100 000)
Males										
0-4	2	17.9	6	45	2.5	63.5	-	-	-	-
5-14	2	7.2	34	125	10.0	57.3	-	-	-	-
15-44	7	9.6	231	302	29.8	39.2	-	-	-	-
45-59	3	12.1	144	535	52.2	20.8	-	-	-	-
60+	2	7.7	148	706	70.0	10.1	-	-	-	-
All ages	17	10.0	563	341	31.7	38.5	-	-	-	-
Females										
0-4	2	12.9	4	32	2.5	72.4	-	-	-	-
5-14	1	2.6	20	77	10.0	66.0	-	-	-	-
15-44	1	1.4	84	112	29.9	46.8	-	-	-	-
45-59	1	2.2	45	150	52.4	26.1	-	-	-	-
60+	3	7.5	93	255	71.5	11.8	-	-	-	-
All ages	7	3.8	246	136	40.0	39.0	-	-	-	-
Total	23	6.8	810	234	34.1	38.7	-	-	-	-

Table 222c   India - India - Inde   Falls - Intracranial injury - long term

Age group (years)	Incidence 1990 Number ('000s)	Rate (per 100 000)	Prevalence 1990 Number ('000s)	Rate (per 100 000)	Avg. age at onset (years)	Average duration (years)	Deaths 1990 Number ('000s)	Rate (per 100 000)	Deaths 2000 (Projected) Number ('000s)	Rate (per 100 000)
Males										
0-4	45	75.3	110	185	2.5	59.9	-	-	-	-
5-14	162	159.0	1 199	1 179	10.0	57.4	-	-	-	-
15-44	12	6.1	4 114	2 051	29.8	39.9	-	-	-	-
45-59	4	8.3	1 049	2 205	52.3	21.0	-	-	-	-
60+	1	2.0	681	2 287	69.7	9.7	-	-	-	-
All ages	224	50.9	7 153	1 628	10.5	56.2	-	-	-	-
Females										
0-4	48	84.5	117	207	2.4	60.8	-	-	-	-
5-14	70	73.8	753	790	10.0	59.1	-	-	-	-
15-44	12	6.3	2 287	1 248	29.8	41.7	-	-	-	-
45-59	8	17.9	680	1 477	52.4	22.5	-	-	-	-
60+	1	2.4	474	1 638	70.1	10.2	-	-	-	-
All ages	139	33.8	4 310	1 051	11.9	55.8	-	-	-	-
Total	362	42.6	11 463	1 349	11.0	56.1	-	-	-	-

For epidemiological sources see Fullerton et al. 1996. For the methods used to estimate and project incidence, prevalence, and deaths see Lozano et al. 1996 and Murray and Lopez 1996a. See explanatory notes for definitions and caveats.

Table 222   **Cuadro 222**   **Tableau 222**
Falls   **Caídas**   **Chutes**

Intracranial injury - long term   Lesión intracraneal - larga duración   Lésions intra-crâniennes - long terme

Table 222d   China - China - Chine   Falls - Intracranial injury - long term

Age group (years)	Incidence 1990 Number ('000s)	Rate (per 100 000)	Prevalence 1990 Number ('000s)	Rate (per 100 000)	Avg. age at onset (years)	Average duration (years)	Deaths 1990 Number ('000s)	Rate (per 100 000)	Deaths 2000 (Projected) Number ('000s)	Rate (per 100 000)
Males										
0-4	19	31.5	47	78	2.5	65.5	-	-	-	-
5-14	5	4.9	176	181	10.0	59.9	-	-	-	-
15-44	13	4.3	827	270	29.9	41.2	-	-	-	-
45-59	4	5.2	271	373	52.3	21.4	-	-	-	-
60+	4	7.2	237	484	69.8	9.9	-	-	-	-
All ages	44	7.6	1 558	266	21.1	49.5	-	-	-	-
Females										
0-4	29	49.4	71	123	2.5	68.5	-	-	-	-
5-14	4	4.3	242	267	10.0	63.2	-	-	-	-
15-44	3	1.0	860	303	29.9	44.2	-	-	-	-
45-59	3	4.3	225	349	52.4	23.8	-	-	-	-
60+	5	10.6	256	496	70.6	10.8	-	-	-	-
All ages	43	7.9	1 654	301	16.7	56.4	-	-	-	-
Total	88	7.7	3 212	283	18.9	52.9	-	-	-	-

Table 222e   OAI - OPAI - APAI   Falls - Intracranial injury - long term

Age group (years)	Incidence 1990 Number ('000s)	Rate (per 100 000)	Prevalence 1990 Number ('000s)	Rate (per 100 000)	Avg. age at onset (years)	Average duration (years)	Deaths 1990 Number ('000s)	Rate (per 100 000)	Deaths 2000 (Projected) Number ('000s)	Rate (per 100 000)
Males										
0-4	30	69.3	75	171	2.5	59.8	-	-	-	-
5-14	12	13.7	347	413	10.0	56.2	-	-	-	-
15-44	15	9.3	997	620	29.7	38.8	-	-	-	-
45-59	3	9.4	284	831	52.3	20.3	-	-	-	-
60+	1	3.2	189	934	69.6	9.7	-	-	-	-
All ages	61	17.7	1 891	551	14.0	51.3	-	-	-	-
Females										
0-4	23	54.8	57	135	2.5	63.2	-	-	-	-
5-14	5	6.7	246	306	10.0	59.2	-	-	-	-
15-44	3	1.9	587	368	29.8	41.4	-	-	-	-
45-59	1	2.4	146	415	52.3	22.4	-	-	-	-
60+	0	1.7	102	450	70.3	10.5	-	-	-	-
All ages	33	9.6	1 138	335	8.4	58.8	-	-	-	-
Total	93	13.7	3 029	444	12.0	54.0	-	-	-	-

Table 222f   SSA - ASS - ASS   Falls - Intracranial injury - long term

Age group (years)	Incidence 1990 Number ('000s)	Rate (per 100 000)	Prevalence 1990 Number ('000s)	Rate (per 100 000)	Avg. age at onset (years)	Average duration (years)	Deaths 1990 Number ('000s)	Rate (per 100 000)	Deaths 2000 (Projected) Number ('000s)	Rate (per 100 000)
Males										
0-4	5	11.5	13	28	2.4	48.7	-	-	-	-
5-14	7	9.4	73	104	10.0	49.2	-	-	-	-
15-44	5	5.2	235	226	29.4	35.0	-	-	-	-
45-59	1	4.6	69	341	52.2	19.1	-	-	-	-
60+	0	3.5	43	410	69.2	9.3	-	-	-	-
All ages	19	7.4	433	172	16.7	42.7	-	-	-	-
Females										
0-4	6	12.5	14	30	2.4	51.9	-	-	-	-
5-14	4	5.8	63	91	10.0	51.9	-	-	-	-
15-44	1	1.1	144	135	29.5	37.2	-	-	-	-
45-59	0	1.0	35	159	52.2	20.5	-	-	-	-
60+	1	4.3	27	209	69.7	9.8	-	-	-	-
All ages	12	4.6	283	110	11.6	48.0	-	-	-	-
Total	31	6.0	717	140	14.7	44.7	-	-	-	-

For epidemiological sources see Fullerton et al. 1996. For the methods used to estimate and project incidence, prevalence, and deaths see Lozano et al. 1996 and Murray and Lopez 1996a. See explanatory notes for definitions and caveats.

Table 222	Cuadro 222	Tableau 222
Falls	Caídas	Chutes

Intracranial injury - long term   Lesión intracraneal - larga duración   Lésions intra-crâniennes - long terme

Table 222g   LAC - ALC - ALC — Falls - Intracranial injury - long term

Age group (years)	Incidence 1990 Number ('000s)	Rate (per 100 000)	Prevalence 1990 Number ('000s)	Rate (per 100 000)	Avg. age at onset (years)	Average duration (years)	Deaths 1990 Number ('000s)	Rate (per 100 000)	Deaths 2000 (Projected) Number ('000s)	Rate (per 100 000)
Males										
0-4	5	17.9	13	44	2.5	63.9	-	-	-	-
5-14	6	10.6	74	142	10.0	59.3	-	-	-	-
15-44	6	5.7	292	280	29.8	41.4	-	-	-	-
45-59	1	6.5	92	414	52.3	22.3	-	-	-	-
60+	1	6.8	76	535	70.3	10.4	-	-	-	-
All ages	19	8.6	547	247	20.5	49.7	-	-	-	-
Females										
0-4	3	12.2	8	30	2.5	67.9	-	-	-	-
5-14	3	5.3	44	87	10.0	63.0	-	-	-	-
15-44	1	1.0	133	128	29.8	44.6	-	-	-	-
45-59	0	1.3	35	152	52.4	24.8	-	-	-	-
60+	1	6.4	39	234	71.1	11.3	-	-	-	-
All ages	8	3.8	260	117	18.7	54.8	-	-	-	-
Total	27	6.2	807	182	19.9	51.2	-	-	-	-

Table 222h   MEC - AOM - CMO — Falls - Intracranial injury - long term

Age group (years)	Incidence 1990 Number ('000s)	Rate (per 100 000)	Prevalence 1990 Number ('000s)	Rate (per 100 000)	Avg. age at onset (years)	Average duration (years)	Deaths 1990 Number ('000s)	Rate (per 100 000)	Deaths 2000 (Projected) Number ('000s)	Rate (per 100 000)
Males										
0-4	11	27.4	28	67	2.5	61.1	-	-	-	-
5-14	7	11.1	126	192	10.0	58.1	-	-	-	-
15-44	4	3.6	343	301	29.8	40.0	-	-	-	-
45-59	1	3.4	85	382	52.3	20.8	-	-	-	-
60+	0	1.6	58	423	69.7	9.8	-	-	-	-
All ages	24	9.2	639	249	11.8	54.7	-	-	-	-
Females										
0-4	10	24.1	24	59	2.5	63.7	-	-	-	-
5-14	3	4.9	90	144	10.0	60.9	-	-	-	-
15-44	1	0.7	192	179	29.8	42.6	-	-	-	-
45-59	0	0.8	44	195	52.3	22.9	-	-	-	-
60+	0	1.1	33	213	70.4	10.6	-	-	-	-
All ages	14	5.6	381	155	7.1	60.7	-	-	-	-
Total	37	7.4	1 021	203	10.1	56.9	-	-	-	-

Table 222i   World - Mundo - Monde — Falls - Intracranial injury - long term

Age group (years)	Incidence 1990 Number ('000s)	Rate (per 100 000)	Prevalence 1990 Number ('000s)	Rate (per 100 000)	Avg. age at onset (years)	Average duration (years)	Deaths 1990 Number ('000s)	Rate (per 100 000)	Deaths 2000 (Projected) Number ('000s)	Rate (per 100 000)
Males										
0-4	121	37.8	299	93	2.5	60.8	-	-	-	-
5-14	203	36.9	2 076	377	10.0	57.4	-	-	-	-
15-44	71	5.7	7 373	590	29.8	40.1	-	-	-	-
45-59	21	6.7	2 181	698	52.3	21.5	-	-	-	-
60+	10	4.5	1 650	754	70.1	10.2	-	-	-	-
All ages	426	16.1	13 579	512	14.6	52.6	-	-	-	-
Females										
0-4	122	39.4	300	97	2.5	63.4	-	-	-	-
5-14	92	17.4	1 482	282	10.0	59.3	-	-	-	-
15-44	25	2.1	4 451	371	29.8	43.2	-	-	-	-
45-59	18	5.7	1 324	426	52.4	24.4	-	-	-	-
60+	17	6.4	1 286	478	71.4	11.6	-	-	-	-
All ages	273	10.4	8 842	338	15.0	54.4	-	-	-	-
Total	699	13.3	22 421	426	14.8	53.3	-	-	-	-

For epidemiological sources see Fullerton et al. 1996. For the methods used to estimate and project incidence, prevalence, and deaths see Lozano et al. 1996 and Murray and Lopez 1996a. See explanatory notes for definitions and caveats.

Table 223	Cuadro 223	Tableau 223
Fires	Fuegos	Incendies
Episodes	Episodios	Episodes

Table 223a   EME - PEMC - EMBE   Fires - Episodes

Age group (years)	Incidence 1990 Number ('000s)	Rate (per 100 000)	Prevalence 1990 Number ('000s)	Rate (per 100 000)	Avg. age at onset (years)	Average duration (years)	Deaths 1990 Number ('000s)	Rate (per 100 000)	Deaths 2000 (Projected) Number ('000s)	Rate (per 100 000)
Males										
0-4	12	45.4	-	-	2.5	-	1	2.5	0	1.7
5-14	37	68.7	-	-	10.0	-	0	0.7	0	0.6
15-44	28	15.1	-	-	29.9	-	2	1.0	2	0.9
45-59	12	17.7	-	-	52.4	-	1	1.5	1	1.4
60+	7	12.2	-	-	71.1	-	2	3.7	3	3.6
All ages	95	24.5	-	-	24.8	-	6	1.6	6	1.5
Females										
0-4	9	36.6	-	-	2.5	-	0	2.0	0	1.4
5-14	29	57.8	-	-	10.0	-	0	0.6	0	0.5
15-44	12	6.4	-	-	30.0	-	1	0.4	1	0.5
45-59	5	8.0	-	-	52.4	-	0	0.7	1	0.7
60+	7	8.6	-	-	72.4	-	2	2.6	2	2.4
All ages	63	15.4	-	-	23.4	-	4	1.1	4	1.0
Total	158	19.8	-	24.2		-	11	1.3	10	1.3

Table 223b   FSE - PEAS - AESE   Fires - Episodes

Age group (years)	Incidence 1990 Number ('000s)	Rate (per 100 000)	Prevalence 1990 Number ('000s)	Rate (per 100 000)	Avg. age at onset (years)	Average duration (years)	Deaths 1990 Number ('000s)	Rate (per 100 000)	Deaths 2000 (Projected) Number ('000s)	Rate (per 100 000)
Males										
0-4	7	51.5	-	-	2.5	-	0	3.4	0	2.9
5-14	15	56.1	-	-	10.0	-	0	0.7	0	0.6
15-44	23	30.0	-	-	29.8	-	2	2.5	2	2.4
45-59	13	47.0	-	-	52.2	-	1	4.9	2	5.1
60+	3	15.0	-	-	70.0	-	1	5.5	2	6.3
All ages	61	37.0	-	-	28.4	-	5	3.0	6	3.2
Females										
0-4	6	44.0	-	-	2.5	-	0	2.9	0	2.6
5-14	10	38.9	-	-	10.0	-	0	0.5	0	0.4
15-44	5	6.9	-	-	29.9	-	0	0.6	0	0.6
45-59	4	12.0	-	-	52.4	-	0	1.3	0	1.3
60+	4	10.6	-	-	71.5	-	1	3.9	2	4.1
All ages	29	15.9	-	-	25.7	-	3	1.5	3	1.6
Total	90	25.9	-	-	27.5	-	8	2.2	9	2.4

Table 223c   India - India - Inde   Fires - Episodes

Age group (years)	Incidence 1990 Number ('000s)	Rate (per 100 000)	Prevalence 1990 Number ('000s)	Rate (per 100 000)	Avg. age at onset (years)	Average duration (years)	Deaths 1990 Number ('000s)	Rate (per 100 000)	Deaths 2000 (Projected) Number ('000s)	Rate (per 100 000)
Males										
0-4	111	185	-	-	2.5	-	9	15.1	9	15.2
5-14	250	245	-	-	10.0	-	4	3.9	3	2.8
15-44	149	74	-	-	29.8	-	16	7.7	17	6.9
45-59	44	92	-	-	52.3	-	6	12.0	7	11.8
60+	6	22	-	-	69.7	-	3	9.9	4	10.9
All ages	560	127	-	-	17.8	-	37	8.5	40	7.8
Females										
0-4	95	168	-	-	2.5	-	8	13.8	7	13.6
5-14	785	824	-	-	10.0	-	12	13.1	9	8.5
15-44	514	280	-	-	29.8	-	53	29.2	55	24.0
45-59	49	107	-	-	52.4	-	6	13.9	8	13.9
60+	15	53	-	-	70.1	-	7	24.4	11	28.5
All ages	1 458	356	-	-	18.5	-	87	21.2	90	18.7
Total	2 018	238	-	-	18.3	-	124	14.6	130	13.1

For epidemiological sources see Goodreau et al. 1996. For the methods used to estimate and project incidence, prevalence, and deaths see Murray and Lopez 1996a. See explanatory notes for definitions and caveats.

Table 223   **Cuadro 223**   **Tableau 223**
Fires   **Fuegos**   **Incendies**

Episodes   Episodios   Episodes

Table 223d   China - China - Chine   Fires - Episodes

Age group (years)	Incidence 1990 Number ('000s)	Rate (per 100 000)	Prevalence 1990 Number ('000s)	Rate (per 100 000)	Avg. age at onset (years)	Average duration (years)	Deaths 1990 Number ('000s)	Rate (per 100 000)	Deaths 2000 (Projected) Number ('000s)	Rate (per 100 000)
Males										
0-4	37	61.0	-	-	2.5	-	3	4.3	2	3.9
5-14	47	48.9	-	-	10.0	-	1	0.7	1	0.4
15-44	45	14.6	-	-	29.9	-	4	1.3	3	1.1
45-59	10	13.3	-	-	52.3	-	1	1.5	1	1.3
60+	13	27.0	-	-	69.8	-	5	10.7	7	12.2
All ages	152	25.9	-	-	21.9	-	14	2.3	15	2.3
Females										
0-4	26	44.1	-	-	2.5	-	2	3.1	1	2.7
5-14	68	75.5	-	-	10.0	-	1	1.0	1	0.6
15-44	17	5.9	-	-	29.9	-	2	0.5	1	0.4
45-59	9	14.2	-	-	52.4	-	1	1.6	1	1.6
60+	13	24.8	-	-	70.6	-	5	9.8	9	13.4
All ages	133	24.2	-	-	19.9	-	10	1.9	13	2.1
Total	284	25.1	-	-	21.0	-	24	2.1	28	2.2

Table 223e   OAI - OPAI - APAI   Fires - Episodes

Age group (years)	Incidence 1990 Number ('000s)	Rate (per 100 000)	Prevalence 1990 Number ('000s)	Rate (per 100 000)	Avg. age at onset (years)	Average duration (years)	Deaths 1990 Number ('000s)	Rate (per 100 000)	Deaths 2000 (Projected) Number ('000s)	Rate (per 100 000)
Males										
0-4	29	66.2	-	-	2.5	-	2	4.5	2	4.0
5-14	54	64.2	-	-	10.0	-	1	0.9	1	0.7
15-44	25	15.5	-	-	29.7	-	2	1.3	2	1.2
45-59	4	12.6	-	-	52.3	-	0	1.4	1	1.3
60+	1	5.8	-	-	69.6	-	0	2.2	1	2.3
All ages	113	33.1	-	-	14.6	-	6	1.7	6	1.5
Females										
0-4	30	71.5	-	-	2.5	-	2	4.9	2	4.3
5-14	61	75.7	-	-	10.0	-	1	1.0	1	0.7
15-44	12	7.6	-	-	29.8	-	1	0.7	1	0.6
45-59	2	5.2	-	-	52.3	-	0	0.6	0	0.6
60+	1	4.3	-	-	70.3	-	0	1.6	1	1.8
All ages	106	31.1	-	-	11.4	-	4	1.3	4	1.1
Total	219	32.1	-	-	13.1	-	10	1.5	10	1.3

Table 223f   SSA - ASS - ASS   Fires - Episodes

Age group (years)	Incidence 1990 Number ('000s)	Rate (per 100 000)	Prevalence 1990 Number ('000s)	Rate (per 100 000)	Avg. age at onset (years)	Average duration (years)	Deaths 1990 Number ('000s)	Rate (per 100 000)	Deaths 2000 (Projected) Number ('000s)	Rate (per 100 000)
Males										
0-4	145	305	-	-	2.4	-	13	28.2	18	28.0
5-14	331	471	-	-	10.0	-	6	8.9	6	6.9
15-44	90	86	-	-	29.4	-	11	10.2	13	9.3
45-59	14	68	-	-	52.2	-	2	10.1	3	10.4
60+	4	42	-	-	69.2	-	2	21.7	3	23.7
All ages	583	231	-	-	12.5	-	35	13.7	44	12.9
Females										
0-4	124	263	-	-	2.4	-	11	24.4	16	24.7
5-14	462	662	-	-	10.0	-	8	12.1	9	9.2
15-44	68	64	-	-	29.5	-	8	7.6	11	7.4
45-59	10	45	-	-	52.2	-	1	6.7	2	6.7
60+	5	39	-	-	69.7	-	3	20.3	4	21.6
All ages	669	259	-	-	11.7	-	32	12.4	41	11.7
Total	1 252	245	-	-	12.1	-	67	13.1	85	12.3

For epidemiological sources see Goodreau et al. 1996. For the methods used to estimate and project incidence, prevalence, and deaths see Murray and Lopez 1996a. See explanatory notes for definitions and caveats.

Table 223   **Cuadro 223**   **Tableau 223**
Fires   **Fuegos**   **Incendies**

Episodes   Episodios   Episodes

Table 223g   LAC - ALC - ALC   Fires - Episodes

Age group (years)	Incidence 1990 Number ('000s)	Rate (per 100 000)	Prevalence 1990 Number ('000s)	Rate (per 100 000)	Avg. age at onset (years)	Average duration (years)	Deaths 1990 Number ('000s)	Rate (per 100 000)	Deaths 2000 (Projected) Number ('000s)	Rate (per 100 000)
Males										
0-4	15	51.1	-	-	2.5	-	1	3.6	1	3.2
5-14	44	83.9	-	-	10.0	-	1	1.2	1	0.9
15-44	15	14.7	-	-	29.8	-	1	1.3	2	1.2
45-59	3	15.4	-	-	52.3	-	0	1.7	1	1.7
60+	1	10.0	-	-	70.3	-	1	4.0	1	4.2
All ages	79	35.5	-	-	15.4	-	4	1.8	4	1.7
Females										
0-4	13	47.8	-	-	2.5	-	1	3.4	1	3.1
5-14	43	84.1	-	-	10.0	-	1	1.2	0	0.9
15-44	9	8.2	-	-	29.9	-	1	0.7	1	0.7
45-59	2	8.5	-	-	52.4	-	0	1.0	0	1.0
60+	1	6.5	-	-	71.1	-	0	2.6	1	2.8
All ages	68	30.3	-	-	13.3	-	3	1.3	3	1.2
Total	146	32.9	-	-	14.4	-	7	1.6	8	1.4

Table 223h   MEC - AOM - CMO   Fires - Episodes

Age group (years)	Incidence 1990 Number ('000s)	Rate (per 100 000)	Prevalence 1990 Number ('000s)	Rate (per 100 000)	Avg. age at onset (years)	Average duration (years)	Deaths 1990 Number ('000s)	Rate (per 100 000)	Deaths 2000 (Projected) Number ('000s)	Rate (per 100 000)
Males										
0-4	30	72.9	-	-	2.5	-	2	5.4	3	5.2
5-14	74	114.0	-	-	10.0	-	1	1.6	1	1.3
15-44	26	22.8	-	-	29.8	-	2	2.1	3	2.0
45-59	4	19.4	-	-	52.3	-	1	2.3	1	2.4
60+	1	6.4	-	-	69.7	-	0	2.6	1	2.8
All ages	136	52.9	-	-	13.9	-	7	2.6	8	2.4
Females										
0-4	31	76.8	-	-	2.5	-	2	5.6	3	5.6
5-14	77	124.8	-	-	10.0	-	1	1.8	1	1.4
15-44	38	35.5	-	-	29.8	-	4	3.3	5	3.3
45-59	3	15.2	-	-	52.3	-	0	1.8	1	1.8
60+	2	9.8	-	-	70.4	-	1	4.0	1	4.3
All ages	151	61.1	-	-	15.0	-	8	3.2	10	3.1
Total	287	57.0	-	-	14.5	-	15	2.9	18	2.7

Table 223i   World - Mundo - Monde   Fires - Episodes

Age group (years)	Incidence 1990 Number ('000s)	Rate (per 100 000)	Prevalence 1990 Number ('000s)	Rate (per 100 000)	Avg. age at onset (years)	Average duration (years)	Deaths 1990 Number ('000s)	Rate (per 100 000)	Deaths 2000 (Projected) Number ('000s)	Rate (per 100 000)
Males										
0-4	385	120	-	-	2.5	-	31	9.8	36	10.3
5-14	852	155	-	-	10.0	-	14	2.5	13	2.0
15-44	401	32	-	-	29.8	-	40	3.2	44	3.1
45-59	103	33	-	-	52.3	-	13	4.0	16	3.9
60+	38	17	-	-	70.1	-	15	7.0	21	7.6
All ages	1 779	67	-	-	18.9	-	113	4.3	129	4.2
Females										
0-4	333	108	-	-	2.5	-	27	8.8	31	9.3
5-14	1 535	292	-	-	10.0	-	25	4.7	21	3.4
15-44	674	56	-	-	29.8	-	70	5.8	75	5.4
45-59	84	27	-	-	52.4	-	11	3.4	13	3.3
60+	48	18	-	-	71.2	-	20	7.3	30	8.8
All ages	2 675	102	-	-	17.7	-	152	5.8	169	5.5
Total	4 454	85	-	-	18.2	-	265	5.0	298	4.8

For epidemiological sources see Goodreau et al. 1996. For the methods used to estimate and project incidence, prevalence, and deaths see Murray and Lopez 1996a. See explanatory notes for definitions and caveats.

Table 224
Fires

Cuadro 224
Fuegos

Tableau 224
Incendies

Injured spinal cord   Lesión de la medula espinal   Lésion de la moelle épinière

Table 224a   EME - PEMC - EMBE   Fires - Injured spinal cord

Age group (years)	Incidence 1990 Number ('000s)	Rate (per 100 000)	Prevalence 1990 Number ('000s)	Rate (per 100 000)	Avg. age at onset (years)	Average duration (years)	Deaths 1990 Number ('000s)	Rate (per 100 000)	Deaths 2000 (Projected) Number ('000s)	Rate (per 100 000)
Males										
0-4	0	0	0	0.0	-	-	-	-	-	-
5-14	0	0	0	0.0	-	-	-	-	-	-
15-44	0	0	0	0.3	29.9	33.6	-	-	-	-
45-59	0	0	0	0.6	52.4	15.6	-	-	-	-
60+	0	0	0	0.4	-	-	-	-	-	-
All ages	0	0	1	0.3	36.5	28.3	-	-	-	-
Females										
0-4	0	0	0	0.0	-	-	-	-	-	-
5-14	0	0	0	0.0	-	-	-	-	-	-
15-44	0	0	0	0.1	30.0	40.2	-	-	-	-
45-59	0	0	0	0.3	52.4	20.5	-	-	-	-
60+	0	0	0	0.2	-	-	-	-	-	-
All ages	0	0	1	0.1	36.7	34.3	-	-	-	-
Total	0	0	2	0.2	36.6	30.1	-	-	-	-

Table 224b   FSE - PEAS - AESE   Fires - Injured spinal cord

Age group (years)	Incidence 1990 Number ('000s)	Rate (per 100 000)	Prevalence 1990 Number ('000s)	Rate (per 100 000)	Avg. age at onset (years)	Average duration (years)	Deaths 1990 Number ('000s)	Rate (per 100 000)	Deaths 2000 (Projected) Number ('000s)	Rate (per 100 000)
Males										
0-4	0	0.0	0	0.0	-	-	-	-	-	-
5-14	0	0.0	0	0.0	-	-	-	-	-	-
15-44	0	0.0	0	0.5	29.8	26.8	-	-	-	-
45-59	0	0.1	0	1.1	52.2	11.9	-	-	-	-
60+	0	0.0	0	0.7	-	-	-	-	-	-
All ages	0	0.0	1	0.5	37.8	21.4	-	-	-	-
Females										
0-4	0	0.0	0	0.0	-	-	-	-	-	-
5-14	0	0.0	0	0.0	-	-	-	-	-	-
15-44	0	0.0	0	0.1	29.9	36.2	-	-	-	-
45-59	0	0.0	0	0.3	52.4	17.4	-	-	-	-
60+	0	0.0	0	0.2	-	-	-	-	-	-
All ages	0	0.0	0	0.2	39.2	28.4	-	-	-	-
Total	0	0.0	1	0.3	38.1	22.8	-	-	-	-

Table 224c   India - India - Inde   Fires - Injured spinal cord

Age group (years)	Incidence 1990 Number ('000s)	Rate (per 100 000)	Prevalence 1990 Number ('000s)	Rate (per 100 000)	Avg. age at onset (years)	Average duration (years)	Deaths 1990 Number ('000s)	Rate (per 100 000)	Deaths 2000 (Projected) Number ('000s)	Rate (per 100 000)
Males										
0-4	0	0.0	0	0.0	-	-	-	-	-	-
5-14	0	0.0	0	0.0	-	-	-	-	-	-
15-44	0	0.1	2	1.2	29.8	28.1	-	-	-	-
45-59	0	0.0	1	2.1	52.3	12.7	-	-	-	-
60+	0	0.0	0	1.0	-	-	-	-	-	-
All ages	0	0.0	4	0.8	30.5	27.6	-	-	-	-
Females										
0-4	0	0.0	0	0.0	-	-	-	-	-	-
5-14	0	0.0	0	0.0	-	-	-	-	-	-
15-44	1	0.3	9	4.9	29.8	30.0	-	-	-	-
45-59	0	0.1	5	10.8	52.4	13.9	-	-	-	-
60+	0	0.0	3	11.7	-	-	-	-	-	-
All ages	1	0.2	17	4.2	31.8	28.6	-	-	-	-
Total	1	0.1	21	2.5	31.5	28.4	-	-	-	-

For epidemiological sources see Goodreau et al. 1996. For the methods used to estimate and project incidence, prevalence, and deaths see Lozano et al. 1996 and Murray and Lopez 1996a. See explanatory notes for definitions and caveats.

Table 224	Cuadro 224	Tableau 224
Fires	Fuegos	Incendies

Injured spinal cord	Lesión de la medula espinal	Lésion de la moelle épinière

Table 224d China - China - Chine — Fires - Injured spinal cord

Age group (years)	Incidence 1990 Number ('000s)	Rate (per 100 000)	Prevalence 1990 Number ('000s)	Rate (per 100 000)	Avg. age at onset (years)	Average duration (years)	Deaths 1990 Number ('000s)	Rate (per 100 000)	Deaths 2000 (Projected) Number ('000s)	Rate (per 100 000)
Males										
0-4	0	0	0	0.0	-	-	-	-	-	-
5-14	0	0	0	0.0	-	-	-	-	-	-
15-44	0	0	1	0.2	29.9	30.4	-	-	-	-
45-59	0	0	0	0.5	52.3	13.1	-	-	-	-
60+	0	0	0	0.3	-	-	-	-	-	-
All ages	0	0	1	0.2	34.0	27.3	-	-	-	-
Females										
0-4	0	0	0	0.0	-	-	-	-	-	-
5-14	0	0	0	0.0	-	-	-	-	-	-
15-44	0	0	0	0.1	29.9	33.6	-	-	-	-
45-59	0	0	0	0.3	52.4	15.4	-	-	-	-
60+	0	0	0	0.2	-	-	-	-	-	-
All ages	0	0	1	0.1	37.9	27.1	-	-	-	-
Total	0	0	2	0.2	35.3	27.2	-	-	-	-

Table 224e OAI - OPAI - APAI — Fires - Injured spinal cord

Age group (years)	Incidence 1990 Number ('000s)	Rate (per 100 000)	Prevalence 1990 Number ('000s)	Rate (per 100 000)	Avg. age at onset (years)	Average duration (years)	Deaths 1990 Number ('000s)	Rate (per 100 000)	Deaths 2000 (Projected) Number ('000s)	Rate (per 100 000)
Males										
0-4	0	0	0	0.0	-	-	-	-	-	-
5-14	0	0	0	0.0	-	-	-	-	-	-
15-44	0	0	0	0.3	29.7	26.7	-	-	-	-
45-59	0	0	0	0.5	52.3	11.8	-	-	-	-
60+	0	0	0	0.3	-	-	-	-	-	-
All ages	0	0	1	0.2	33.1	24.4	-	-	-	-
Females										
0-4	0	0	0	0.0	-	-	-	-	-	-
5-14	0	0	0	0.0	-	-	-	-	-	-
15-44	0	0	0	0.1	29.8	29.4	-	-	-	-
45-59	0	0	0	0.3	52.3	13.7	-	-	-	-
60+	0	0	0	0.1	-	-	-	-	-	-
All ages	0	0	0	0.1	32.7	27.4	-	-	-	-
Total	0	0	1	0.1	33.0	25.4	-	-	-	-

Table 224f SSA - ASS - ASS — Fires - Injured spinal cord

Age group (years)	Incidence 1990 Number ('000s)	Rate (per 100 000)	Prevalence 1990 Number ('000s)	Rate (per 100 000)	Avg. age at onset (years)	Average duration (years)	Deaths 1990 Number ('000s)	Hate (per 100 000)	Deaths 2000 (Projected) Number ('000s)	Rate (per 100 000)
Males										
0-4	0	0.0	0	0.0	-	-	-	-	-	-
5-14	0	0.0	0	0.0	-	-	-	-	-	-
15-44	0	0.1	1	1.3	29.4	21.3	-	-	-	-
45-59	0	0.1	0	2.3	52.2	10.6	-	-	-	-
60+	0	0.0	0	1.1	-	-	-	-	-	-
All ages	0	0.0	2	0.7	32.4	19.9	-	-	-	-
Females										
0-4	0	0.0	0	0.0	-	-	-	-	-	-
5-14	0	0.0	0	0.0	-	-	-	-	-	-
15-44	0	0.1	1	1.0	29.5	23.5	-	-	-	-
45-59	0	0.1	0	1.8	52.2	11.9	-	-	-	-
60+	0	0.0	0	0.9	-	-	-	-	-	-
All ages	0	0.0	2	0.6	32.4	22.0	-	-	-	-
Total	0	0.0	3	0.7	32.4	20.8	-	-	-	-

For epidemiological sources see Goodreau et al. 1996. For the methods used to estimate and project incidence, prevalence, and deaths see Lozano et al. 1996 and Murray and Lopez 1996a. See explanatory notes for definitions and caveats.

Table 224   **Cuadro 224**   **Tableau 224**
Fires   **Fuegos**   **Incendies**

Injured spinal cord   Lesión de la medula espinal   Lésion de la moelle épinière

Table 224g   LAC - ALC - ALC   Fires - Injured spinal cord

Age group (years)	Incidence 1990 Number ('000s)	Rate (per 100 000)	Prevalence 1990 Number ('000s)	Rate (per 100 000)	Avg. age at onset (years)	Average duration (years)	Deaths 1990 Number ('000s)	Rate (per 100 000)	Deaths 2000 (Projected) Number ('000s)	Rate (per 100 000)
Males										
0-4	0	0	0	0.0	-	-	-	-	-	-
5-14	0	0	0	0.0	-	-	-	-	-	-
15-44	0	0	0	0.2	29.8	29.4	-	-	-	-
45-59	0	0	0	0.5	52.3	13.6	-	-	-	-
60+	0	0	0	0.3	-	-	-	-	-	-
All ages	0	0	0	0.2	33.9	26.5	-	-	-	-
Females										
0-4	0	0	0	0.0	-	-	-	-	-	-
5-14	0	0	0	0.0	-	-	-	-	-	-
15-44	0	0	0	0.1	29.9	33.0	-	-	-	-
45-59	0	0	0	0.3	52.4	16.2	-	-	-	-
60+	0	0	0	0.2	-	-	-	-	-	-
All ages	0	0	0	0.1	34.0	29.9	-	-	-	-
Total	0	0	1	0.2	34.0	27.8	-	-	-	-

Table 224h   MEC - AOM - CMO   Fires - Injured spinal cord

Age group (years)	Incidence 1990 Number ('000s)	Rate (per 100 000)	Prevalence 1990 Number ('000s)	Rate (per 100 000)	Avg. age at onset (years)	Average duration (years)	Deaths 1990 Number ('000s)	Rate (per 100 000)	Deaths 2000 (Projected) Number ('000s)	Rate (per 100 000)
Males										
0-4	0	0	0	0.0	-	-	-	-	-	-
5-14	0	0	0	0.0	-	-	-	-	-	-
15-44	0	0	0	0.4	29.8	28.5	-	-	-	-
45-59	0	0	0	0.8	52.3	12.3	-	-	-	-
60+	0	0	0	0.4	-	-	-	-	-	-
All ages	0	0	1	0.3	33.0	26.2	-	-	-	-
Females										
0-4	0	0	0	0.0	-	-	-	-	-	-
5-14	0	0	0	0.0	-	-	-	-	-	-
15-44	0	0	1	0.6	29.8	31.1	-	-	-	-
45-59	0	0	0	1.2	52.3	14.3	-	-	-	-
60+	0	0	0	0.6	-	-	-	-	-	-
All ages	0	0	1	0.4	31.6	29.7	-	-	-	-
Total	0	0	2	0.3	32.2	28.2	-	-	-	-

Table 224i   World - Mundo - Monde   Fires - Injured spinal cord

Age group (years)	Incidence 1990 Number ('000s)	Rate (per 100 000)	Prevalence 1990 Number ('000s)	Rate (per 100 000)	Avg. age at onset (years)	Average duration (years)	Deaths 1990 Number ('000s)	Rate (per 100 000)	Deaths 2000 (Projected) Number ('000s)	Rate (per 100 000)
Males										
0-4	0	0.0	0	0.0	-	-	-	-	-	-
5-14	0	0.0	0	0.0	-	-	-	-	-	-
15-44	0	0.0	6	0.5	29.8	28.8	-	-	-	-
45-59	0	0.0	3	1.0	52.3	13.1	-	-	-	-
60+	0	0.0	1	0.5	-	-	-	-	-	-
All ages	1	0.0	11	0.4	33.7	25.9	-	-	-	-
Females										
0-4	0	0.0	0	0.0	-	-	-	-	-	-
5-14	0	0.0	0	0.0	-	-	-	-	-	-
15-44	1	0.1	12	1.0	29.8	32.5	-	-	-	-
45-59	0	0.0	6	2.0	52.4	14.4	-	-	-	-
60+	0	0.0	4	1.5	-	-	-	-	-	-
All ages	1	0.0	22	0.8	34.7	30.5	-	-	-	-
Total	1	0.0	32	0.6	34.3	28.7	-	-	-	-

For epidemiological sources see Goodreau et al. 1996. For the methods used to estimate and project incidence, prevalence, and deaths see Lozano et al. 1996 and Murray and Lopez 1996a. See explanatory notes for definitions and caveats.

Table 225	Cuadro 225	Tableau 225
Fires	Fuegos	Incendies

Burns <20% - short term   Quemaduras <20% - corta duración   Brûlures <20% - court terme

Table 225a   EME - PEMC - EMBE   Fires - Burns <20% - short term

Age group (years)	Incidence 1990 Number ('000s)	Rate (per 100 000)	Prevalence 1990 Number ('000s)	Rate (per 100 000)	Avg. age at onset (years)	Average duration (years)	Deaths 1990 Number ('000s)	Rate (per 100 000)	Deaths 2000 (Projected) Number ('000s)	Rate (per 100 000)
Males										
0-4	11	42.9	1	3.6	2.5	0.08	-	-	-	-
5-14	35	64.9	3	5.4	10.0	0.08	-	-	-	-
15-44	22	12.1	2	1.0	29.9	0.08	-	-	-	-
45-59	9	14.2	1	1.2	52.4	0.08	-	-	-	-
60+	6	9.6	0	0.8	71.1	0.08	-	-	-	-
All ages	84	21.4	7	1.8	23.3	0.08	-	-	-	-
Females										
0-4	9	34.6	1	2.9	2.5	0.08	-	-	-	-
5-14	28	54.7	2	4.5	10.0	0.08	-	-	-	-
15-44	9	5.2	1	0.4	30.0	0.08	-	-	-	-
45-59	4	6.4	0	0.5	52.4	0.08	-	-	-	-
60+	6	6.8	0	0.6	72.4	0.08	-	-	-	-
All ages	56	13.7	5	1.1	21.9	0.08	-	-	-	-
Total	139	17.5	12	1.4	22.7	0.08	-	-	-	-

Table 225b   FSE - PEAS - AESE   Fires - Burns <20% - short term

Age group (years)	Incidence 1990 Number ('000s)	Rate (per 100 000)	Prevalence 1990 Number ('000s)	Rate (per 100 000)	Avg. age at onset (years)	Average duration (years)	Deaths 1990 Number ('000s)	Rate (per 100 000)	Deaths 2000 (Projected) Number ('000s)	Rate (per 100 000)
Males										
0-4	7	48.7	1	4.0	2.5	0.08	-	-	-	-
5-14	15	53.1	1	4.4	10.0	0.08	-	-	-	-
15-44	18	24.1	2	2.0	29.8	0.08	-	-	-	-
45-59	10	37.7	1	3.1	52.2	0.08	-	-	-	-
60+	2	11.8	0	1.0	70.0	0.08	-	-	-	-
All ages	52	31.6	4	2.6	27.1	0.08	-	-	-	-
Females										
0-4	5	41.6	0	3.5	2.5	0.08	-	-	-	-
5-14	10	36.8	1	3.1	10.0	0.08	-	-	-	-
15-44	4	5.6	0	0.5	29.9	0.08	-	-	-	-
45-59	3	9.7	0	0.8	52.4	0.08	-	-	-	-
60+	3	8.3	0	0.7	71.5	0.08	-	-	-	-
All ages	25	14.0	2	1.2	23.9	0.08	-	-	-	-
Total	78	22.4	6	1.9	26.0	0.08	-	-	-	-

Table 225c   India - India - Inde   Fires - Burns <20% - short term

Age group (years)	Incidence 1990 Number ('000s)	Rate (per 100 000)	Prevalence 1990 Number ('000s)	Rato (per 100 000)	Avg. age at onset (years)	Average duration (years)	Deaths 1990 Number ('000s)	Hate (per 100 000)	Deaths 2000 (Projected) Number ('000s)	Rate (per 100 000)
Males										
0-4	105	175	9	14.5	2.5	0.08	-	-	-	-
5-14	236	232	20	19.3	10.0	0.08	-	-	-	-
15-44	120	60	10	5.0	29.8	0.08	-	-	-	-
45-59	35	74	3	6.1	52.3	0.08	-	-	-	-
60+	5	17	0	1.4	69.7	0.08	-	-	-	-
All ages	501	114	42	9.5	16.7	0.08	-	-	-	-
Females										
0-4	90	159	7	13.2	2.5	0.08	-	-	-	-
5-14	742	779	62	64.7	10.0	0.08	-	-	-	-
15-44	412	225	34	18.7	29.8	0.08	-	-	-	-
45-59	39	86	3	7.1	52.4	0.08	-	-	-	-
60+	12	42	1	3.5	70.1	0.08	-	-	-	-
All ages	1 297	316	108	26.2	17.6	0.08	-	-	-	-
Total	1 798	212	149	17.6	17.4	0.08	-	-	-	-

For epidemiological sources see Goodreau et al. 1996. For the methods used to estimate and project incidence, prevalence, and deaths see Lozano et al. 1996 and Murray and Lopez 1996a. See explanatory notes for definitions and caveats.

Table 225	Cuadro 225	Tableau 225
Fires	Fuegos	Incendies

Burns <20% - short term   Quemaduras <20% - corta duración   Brûlures <20% - court terme

Table 225d   China - China - Chine

Fires - Burns <20% - short term

Age group (years)	Incidence 1990 Number ('000s)	Rate (per 100 000)	Prevalence 1990 Number ('000s)	Rate (per 100 000)	Avg. age at onset (years)	Average duration (years)	Deaths 1990 Number ('000s)	Rate (per 100 000)	Deaths 2000 (Projected) Number ('000s)	Rate (per 100 000)
Males										
0-4	35	57.7	3	4.8	2.5	0.08	-	-	-	-
5-14	45	46.2	4	3.8	10.0	0.08	-	-	-	-
15-44	36	11.7	3	1.0	29.9	0.08	-	-	-	-
45-59	8	10.6	1	0.9	52.3	0.08	-	-	-	-
60+	10	21.4	1	1.8	69.8	0.08	-	-	-	-
All ages	134	22.8	11	1.9	20.5	0.08	-	-	-	-
Females										
0-4	24	41.7	2	3.5	2.5	0.08	-	-	-	-
5-14	65	71.4	5	5.9	10.0	0.08	-	-	-	-
15-44	13	4.8	1	0.4	29.9	0.08	-	-	-	-
45-59	7	11.4	1	0.9	52.4	0.08	-	-	-	-
60+	10	19.6	1	1.6	70.6	0.08	-	-	-	-
All ages	120	21.8	10	1.8	18.5	0.08	-	-	-	-
Total	253	22.3	21	1.9	19.5	0.08	-	-	-	-

Table 225e   OAI - OPAI - APAI

Fires - Burns <20% - short term

Age group (years)	Incidence 1990 Number ('000s)	Rate (per 100 000)	Prevalence 1990 Number ('000s)	Rate (per 100 000)	Avg. age at onset (years)	Average duration (years)	Deaths 1990 Number ('000s)	Rate (per 100 000)	Deaths 2000 (Projected) Number ('000s)	Rate (per 100 000)
Males										
0-4	27	62.6	2	5.2	2.5	0.08	-	-	-	-
5-14	51	60.7	4	5.0	10.0	0.08	-	-	-	-
15-44	20	12.5	2	1.0	29.7	0.08	-	-	-	-
45-59	3	10.1	0	0.8	52.3	0.08	-	-	-	-
60+	1	4.6	0	0.4	69.6	0.08	-	-	-	-
All ages	103	30.0	9	2.5	13.8	0.08	-	-	-	-
Females										
0-4	28	67.6	2	5.6	2.5	0.08	-	-	-	-
5-14	57	71.6	5	5.9	10.0	0.08	-	-	-	-
15-44	10	6.1	1	0.5	29.8	0.08	-	-	-	-
45-59	1	4.2	0	0.3	52.3	0.08	-	-	-	-
60+	1	3.4	0	0.3	70.3	0.08	-	-	-	-
All ages	98	28.8	8	2.4	10.9	0.08	-	-	-	-
Total	201	29.4	17	2.4	12.4	0.08	-	-	-	-

Table 225f   SSA - ASS - ASS

Fires - Burns <20% - short term

Age group (years)	Incidence 1990 Number ('000s)	Rate (per 100 000)	Prevalence 1990 Number ('000s)	Rate (per 100 000)	Avg. age at onset (years)	Average duration (years)	Deaths 1990 Number ('000s)	Rate (per 100 000)	Deaths 2000 (Projected) Number ('000s)	Rate (per 100 000)
Males										
0-4	137	288	11	23.9	2.4	0.08	-	-	-	-
5-14	313	445	26	37.0	10.0	0.08	-	-	-	-
15-44	72	69	6	5.8	29.4	0.08	-	-	-	-
45-59	11	54	1	4.5	52.2	0.08	-	-	-	-
60+	3	33	0	2.7	69.2	0.08	-	-	-	-
All ages	536	213	45	17.6	11.9	0.08	-	-	-	-
Females										
0-4	117	249	10	20.7	2.4	0.08	-	-	-	-
5-14	437	626	36	51.9	10.0	0.08	-	-	-	-
15-44	55	52	5	4.3	29.5	0.08	-	-	-	-
45-59	8	36	1	3.0	52.2	0.08	-	-	-	-
60+	4	31	0	2.6	69.7	0.08	-	-	-	-
All ages	621	241	52	20.0	11.2	0.08	-	-	-	-
Total	1 157	227	96	18.8	11.5	0.08	-	-	-	-

For epidemiological sources see Goodreau et al. 1996. For the methods used to estimate and project incidence, prevalence, and deaths see Lozano et al. 1996 and Murray and Lopez 1996a. See explanatory notes for definitions and caveats.

Table 225	Cuadro 225	Tableau 225
Fires	Fuegos	Incendies

Burns <20% - short term　　Quemaduras <20% - corta duración　　Brûlures <20% - court terme

Table 225g　　LAC - ALC - ALC　　Fires - Burns <20% - short term

Age group (years)	Incidence 1990 Number ('000s)	Rate (per 100 000)	Prevalence 1990 Number ('000s)	Rate (per 100 000)	Avg. age at onset (years)	Average duration (years)	Deaths 1990 Number ('000s)	Rate (per 100 000)	Deaths 2000 (Projected) Number ('000s)	Rate (per 100 000)
Males										
0-4	14	48.4	1	4.0	2.5	0.08	-	-	-	-
5-14	41	79.3	3	6.6	10.0	0.08	-	-	-	-
15-44	12	11.8	1	1.0	29.8	0.08	-	-	-	-
45-59	3	12.3	0	1.0	52.3	0.08	-	-	-	-
60+	1	7.9	0	0.7	70.3	0.08	-	-	-	-
All ages	71	32.2	6	2.7	14.5	0.08	-	-	-	-
Females										
0-4	13	45.2	1	3.7	2.5	0.08	-	-	-	-
5-14	40	79.5	3	6.6	10.0	0.08	-	-	-	-
15-44	7	6.6	1	0.5	29.9	0.08	-	-	-	-
45-59	2	6.9	0	0.6	52.4	0.08	-	-	-	-
60+	1	5.2	0	0.4	71.1	0.08	-	-	-	-
All ages	62	27.9	5	2.3	12.6	0.08	-	-	-	-
Total	134	30.1	11	2.5	13.7	0.08	-	-	-	-

Table 225h　　MEC - AOM - CMO　　Fires - Burns <20% - short term

Age group (years)	Incidence 1990 Number ('000s)	Rate (per 100 000)	Prevalence 1990 Number ('000s)	Rate (per 100 000)	Avg. age at onset (years)	Average duration (years)	Deaths 1990 Number ('000s)	Rate (per 100 000)	Deaths 2000 (Projected) Number ('000s)	Rate (per 100 000)
Males										
0-4	28	69.0	2	5.7	2.5	0.08	-	-	-	-
5-14	70	107.8	6	8.9	10.0	0.08	-	-	-	-
15-44	21	18.3	2	1.5	29.8	0.08	-	-	-	-
45-59	3	15.5	0	1.3	52.3	0.08	-	-	-	-
60+	1	5.1	0	0.4	69.7	0.08	-	-	-	-
All ages	124	48.3	10	4.0	13.1	0.08	-	-	-	-
Females										
0-4	29	72.6	2	6.0	2.5	0.08	-	-	-	-
5-14	73	118.0	6	9.8	10.0	0.08	-	-	-	-
15-44	31	28.5	3	2.4	29.8	0.08	-	-	-	-
45-59	3	12.2	0	1.0	52.3	0.08	-	-	-	-
60+	1	7.7	0	0.6	70.4	0.08	-	-	-	-
All ages	136	55.3	11	4.6	14.2	0.08	-	-	-	-
Total	260	51.8	22	4.3	13.7	0.08	-	-	-	-

Table 225i　　World - Mundo - Monde　　Fires - Burns <20% - short term

Age group (years)	Incidence 1990 Number ('000s)	Rate (per 100 000)	Prevalence 1990 Number ('000s)	Rate (per 100 000)	Avg. age at onset (years)	Average duration (years)	Deaths 1990 Number ('000s)	Rate (per 100 000)	Deaths 2000 (Projected) Number ('000s)	Rate (per 100 000)
Males										
0-4	364	113	30	9.4	2.5	0.08	-	-	-	-
5-14	806	146	67	12.1	10.0	0.08	-	-	-	-
15-44	322	26	27	2.1	29.8	0.08	-	-	-	-
45-59	83	27	7	2.2	52.3	0.08	-	-	-	-
60+	30	14	2	1.1	70.1	0.08	-	-	-	-
All ages	1 605	60	133	5.0	17.8	0.08	-	-	-	-
Females										
0-4	315	102	26	8.5	2.5	0.08	-	-	-	-
5-14	1 452	276	121	22.9	10.0	0.08	-	-	-	-
15-44	541	45	45	3.7	29.8	0.08	-	-	-	-
45-59	68	22	6	1.8	52.4	0.08	-	-	-	-
60+	38	14	3	1.2	71.2	0.08	-	-	-	-
All ages	2 415	92	200	7.7	16.6	0.08	-	-	-	-
Total	4 019	76	334	6.3	17.1	0.08	-	-	-	-

For epidemiological sources see Goodreau et al. 1996. For the methods used to estimate and project incidence, prevalence, and deaths see Lozano et al. 1996 and Murray and Lopez 1996a. See explanatory notes for definitions and caveats.

Table 226 Fires	Cuadro 226 Fuegos	Tableau 226 Incendies

Burns <20% - long term   Quemaduras <20% - larga duración   Brûlures <20% - long terme

Table 226a   EME - PEMC - EMBE

Fires - Burns <20% - long term

Age group (years)	Incidence 1990 Number ('000s)	Rate (per 100 000)	Prevalence 1990 Number ('000s)	Rate (per 100 000)	Avg. age at onset (years)	Average duration (years)	Deaths 1990 Number ('000s)	Rate (per 100 000)	Deaths 2000 (Projected) Number ('000s)	Rate (per 100 000)
Males										
0-4	11	42.8	28	107	2.5	70.2	-	-	-	-
5-14	34	64.6	287	538	10.0	63.6	-	-	-	-
15-44	22	12.0	1 911	1 038	29.9	44.7	-	-	-	-
45-59	9	14.0	875	1 323	52.4	24.5	-	-	-	-
60+	6	9.5	929	1 535	71.1	11.3	-	-	-	-
All ages	83	21.2	4 031	1 032	23.3	51.5	-	-	-	-
Females										
0-4	9	34.6	22	86	2.5	76.1	-	-	-	-
5-14	28	54.4	226	446	10.0	69.5	-	-	-	-
15-44	9	5.1	1 422	793	30.0	50.0	-	-	-	-
45-59	4	6.3	622	918	52.4	28.8	-	-	-	-
60+	6	6.7	887	1 048	72.4	12.7	-	-	-	-
All ages	55	13.6	3 178	780	21.8	58.3	-	-	-	-
Total	138	17.3	7 209	904	22.7	54.2	-	-	-	-

Table 226b   FSE - PEAS - AESE

Fires - Burns <20% - long term

Age group (years)	Incidence 1990 Number ('000s)	Rate (per 100 000)	Prevalence 1990 Number ('000s)	Rate (per 100 000)	Avg. age at onset (years)	Average duration (years)	Deaths 1990 Number ('000s)	Rate (per 100 000)	Deaths 2000 (Projected) Number ('000s)	Rate (per 100 000)
Males										
0-4	7	48.7	17	121	2.5	63.5	-	-	-	-
5-14	14	52.8	139	508	10.0	57.3	-	-	-	-
15-44	18	23.8	856	1 122	29.8	39.2	-	-	-	-
45-59	10	37.1	473	1 753	52.2	20.8	-	-	-	-
60+	2	11.6	452	2 156	70.0	10.1	-	-	-	-
All ages	52	31.3	1 936	1 171	27.0	42.5	-	-	-	-
Females										
0-4	5	41.6	14	104	2.5	72.4	-	-	-	-
5-14	10	36.7	103	391	10.0	66.0	-	-	-	-
15-44	4	5.5	492	656	29.9	46.8	-	-	-	-
45-59	3	9.6	243	810	52.4	26.1	-	-	-	-
60+	3	8.3	356	978	71.5	11.8	-	-	-	-
All ages	25	13.9	1 208	668	23.8	53.2	-	-	-	-
Total	77	22.2	3 144	908	25.9	46.0	-	-	-	-

Table 226c   India - India - Inde

Fires - Burns <20% - long term

Age group (years)	Incidence 1990 Number ('000s)	Rate (per 100 000)	Prevalence 1990 Number ('000s)	Rate (per 100 000)	Avg. age at onset (years)	Average duration (years)	Deaths 1990 Number ('000s)	Rate (per 100 000)	Deaths 2000 (Projected) Number ('000s)	Rate (per 100 000)
Males										
0-4	104	175	256	428	2.5	59.9	-	-	-	-
5-14	231	227	2 052	2 016	10.0	57.4	-	-	-	-
15-44	115	57	7 997	3 988	29.8	39.9	-	-	-	-
45-59	33	70	2 556	5 373	52.3	21.0	-	-	-	-
60+	5	16	1 805	6 062	69.7	9.7	-	-	-	-
All ages	489	111	14 666	3 338	16.5	50.9	-	-	-	-
Females										
0-4	90	159	220	389	2.5	60.8	-	-	-	-
5-14	709	744	4 380	4 598	10.0	59.1	-	-	-	-
15-44	366	200	20 563	11 222	29.8	41.7	-	-	-	-
45-59	34	73	6 791	14 761	52.4	22.5	-	-	-	-
60+	10	36	4 534	15 675	70.1	10.2	-	-	-	-
All ages	1 209	295	36 488	8 897	17.1	52.5	-	-	-	-
Total	1 698	200	51 154	6 022	17.0	52.0	-	-	-	-

For epidemiological sources see Goodreau et al. 1996. For the methods used to estimate and project incidence, prevalence, and deaths see Lozano et al. 1996 and Murray and Lopez 1996a. See explanatory notes for definitions and caveats.

Table 226 / **Cuadro 226** / **Tableau 226**
Fires / **Fuegos** / **Incendies**

Burns <20% - long term / Quemaduras <20% - larga duración / Brûlures <20% - long terme

Table 226d — China - China - Chine
Fires - Burns <20% - long term

Age group (years)	Incidence 1990 Number ('000s)	Rate (per 100 000)	Prevalence 1990 Number ('000s)	Rate (per 100 000)	Avg. age at onset (years)	Average duration (years)	Deaths 1990 Number ('000s)	Rate (per 100 000)	Deaths 2000 (Projected) Number ('000s)	Rate (per 100 000)
Males										
0-4	35	57.6	86	143	2.5	65.5	-	-	-	-
5-14	45	46.0	502	518	10.0	59.9	-	-	-	-
15-44	36	11.6	2 815	919	29.9	41.2	-	-	-	-
45-59	8	10.5	851	1 172	52.3	21.4	-	-	-	-
60+	10	21.1	714	1 459	69.8	9.9	-	-	-	-
All ages	133	22.7	4 969	849	20.4	50.3	-	-	-	-
Females										
0-4	24	41.7	60	103	2.5	68.5	-	-	-	-
5-14	64	71.0	510	564	10.0	63.2	-	-	-	-
15-44	13	4.7	2 804	987	29.9	44.2	-	-	-	-
45-59	7	11.3	735	1 141	52.4	23.8	-	-	-	-
60+	10	19.3	740	1 433	70.6	10.8	-	-	-	-
All ages	119	21.7	4 849	884	18.4	55.3	-	-	-	-
Total	252	22.2	9 819	866	19.5	52.7	-	-	-	-

Table 226e — OAI - OPAI - APAI
Fires - Burns <20% - long term

Age group (years)	Incidence 1990 Number ('000s)	Rate (per 100 000)	Prevalence 1990 Number ('000s)	Rate (per 100 000)	Avg. age at onset (years)	Average duration (years)	Deaths 1990 Number ('000s)	Rate (per 100 000)	Deaths 2000 (Projected) Number ('000s)	Rate (per 100 000)
Males										
0-4	3	6.3	67	154	2.5	59.8	-	-	-	-
5-14	51	60.4	516	614	10.0	56.2	-	-	-	-
15-44	20	12.3	1 764	1 097	29.7	38.8	-	-	-	-
45-59	3	10.0	463	1 357	52.3	20.3	-	-	-	-
60+	1	4.5	299	1 478	69.6	9.7	-	-	-	-
All ages	78	22.6	3 109	907	17.3	49.7	-	-	-	-
Females										
0-4	28	67.5	70	167	2.5	63.2	-	-	-	-
5-14	57	71.1	556	693	10.0	59.2	-	-	-	-
15-44	10	6.1	1 814	1 136	29.8	41.4	-	-	-	-
45-59	1	4.1	442	1 259	52.3	22.4	-	-	-	-
60+	1	3.3	300	1 325	70.3	10.5	-	-	-	-
All ages	97	28.6	3 182	937	10.9	57.6	-	-	-	-
Total	175	25.6	6 291	922	13.7	54.1	-	-	-	-

Table 226f — SSA - ASS - ASS
Fires - Burns <20% - long term

Age group (years)	Incidence 1990 Number ('000s)	Rate (per 100 000)	Prevalence 1990 Number ('000s)	Rate (per 100 000)	Avg. age at onset (years)	Average duration (years)	Deaths 1990 Number ('000s)	Rate (per 100 000)	Deaths 2000 (Projected) Number ('000s)	Rate (per 100 000)
Males										
0-4	136	286	328	690	2.4	48.7	-	-	-	-
5-14	302	430	2 514	3 578	10.0	49.2	-	-	-	-
15-44	67	65	6 907	6 657	29.4	35.0	-	-	-	-
45-59	10	50	1 629	8 023	52.2	19.1	-	-	-	-
60+	3	30	913	8 692	69.2	9.3	-	-	-	-
All ages	518	205	12 292	4 871	11.7	46.4	-	-	-	-
Females										
0-4	116	248	282	600	2.4	51.9	-	-	-	-
5-14	418	599	2 966	4 248	10.0	51.9	-	-	-	-
15-44	51	48	8 410	7 915	29.5	37.2	-	-	-	-
45-59	7	33	1 966	8 891	52.2	20.5	-	-	-	-
60+	4	28	1 199	9 419	69.7	9.8	-	-	-	-
All ages	596	231	14 824	5 747	11.0	50.0	-	-	-	-
Total	1 115	218	27 115	5 314	11.4	48.4	-	-	-	-

For epidemiological sources see Goodreau et al. 1996. For the methods used to estimate and project incidence, prevalence, and deaths see Lozano et al. 1996 and Murray and Lopez 1996a. See explanatory notes for definitions and caveats.

Table 226
Fires

Burns <20% - long term

Cuadro 226
Fuegos

Quemaduras <20% - larga duración

Tableau 226
Incendies

Brûlures <20% - long terme

Table 226g   LAC - ALC - ALC

Fires - Burns <20% - long term

Age group (years)	Incidence 1990 Number ('000s)	Rate (per 100 000)	Prevalence 1990 Number ('000s)	Rate (per 100 000)	Avg. age at onset (years)	Average duration (years)	Deaths 1990 Number ('000s)	Rate (per 100 000)	Deaths 2000 (Projected) Number ('000s)	Rate (per 100 000)
Males										
0-4	14	48.3	34	120	2.5	63.9	-	-	-	-
5-14	41	78.8	332	636	10.0	59.3	-	-	-	-
15-44	12	11.7	1 253	1 202	29.8	41.4	-	-	-	-
45-59	3	12.2	327	1 468	52.3	22.3	-	-	-	-
60+	1	7.8	234	1 642	70.3	10.4	-	-	-	-
All ages	71	32.0	2 179	983	14.5	55.0	-	-	-	-
Females										
0-4	12	45.1	31	112	2.5	67.9	-	-	-	-
5-14	40	79.0	316	622	10.0	63.0	-	-	-	-
15-44	7	6.5	1 158	1 112	29.9	44.6	-	-	-	-
45-59	2	6.8	295	1 262	52.4	24.8	-	-	-	-
60+	1	5.1	230	1 370	71.1	11.3	-	-	-	-
All ages	62	27.8	2 029	911	12.6	60.3	-	-	-	-
Total	133	29.9	4 209	947	13.6	57.4	-	-	-	-

Table 226h   MEC - AOM - CMO

Fires - Burns <20% - long term

Age group (years)	Incidence 1990 Number ('000s)	Rate (per 100 000)	Prevalence 1990 Number ('000s)	Rate (per 100 000)	Avg. age at onset (years)	Average duration (years)	Deaths 1990 Number ('000s)	Rate (per 100 000)	Deaths 2000 (Projected) Number ('000s)	Rate (per 100 000)
Males										
0-4	28	68.9	70	169	2.5	61.1	-	-	-	-
5-14	70	106.9	575	880	10.0	58.1	-	-	-	-
15-44	21	18.0	1 912	1 679	29.8	40.0	-	-	-	-
45-59	3	15.2	461	2 064	52.3	20.8	-	-	-	-
60+	1	4.9	304	2 229	69.7	9.8	-	-	-	-
All ages	123	47.9	3 322	1 296	13.1	54.5	-	-	-	-
Females										
0-4	29	72.5	71	178	2.5	63.7	-	-	-	-
5-14	72	116.9	588	948	10.0	60.9	-	-	-	-
15-44	30	27.9	2 086	1 945	29.8	42.6	-	-	-	-
45-59	3	11.9	547	2 455	52.3	22.9	-	-	-	-
60+	1	7.5	406	2 625	70.4	10.6	-	-	-	-
All ages	135	54.7	3 697	1 499	14.1	56.2	-	-	-	-
Total	258	51.3	7 019	1 395	13.6	55.4	-	-	-	-

Table 226i   World - Mundo - Monde

Fires - Burns <20% - long term

Age group (years)	Incidence 1990 Number ('000s)	Rate (per 100 000)	Prevalence 1990 Number ('000s)	Rate (per 100 000)	Avg. age at onset (years)	Average duration (years)	Deaths 1990 Number ('000s)	Rate (per 100 000)	Deaths 2000 (Projected) Number ('000s)	Rate (per 100 000)
Males										
0-4	338	105	886	276	2.5	60.8	-	-	-	-
5-14	788	143	6 916	1 255	10.0	57.5	-	-	-	-
15-44	311	25	25 416	2 033	29.8	40.5	-	-	-	-
45-59	80	26	7 635	2 444	52.3	21.7	-	-	-	-
60+	29	13	5 650	2 582	70.1	10.3	-	-	-	-
All ages	1 546	58	46 505	1 752	18.2	50.4	-	-	-	-
Females										
0-4	314	102	770	249	2.5	64.0	-	-	-	-
5-14	1 398	266	9 644	1 835	10.0	60.8	-	-	-	-
15-44	490	41	38 748	3 233	29.8	43.7	-	-	-	-
45-59	61	20	11 641	3 742	52.4	24.5	-	-	-	-
60+	35	13	8 652	3 214	71.2	11.4	-	-	-	-
All ages	2 299	88	69 455	2 657	16.5	55.5	-	-	-	-
Total	3 845	73	115 960	2 202	17.2	53.5	-	-	-	-

For epidemiological sources see Goodreau et al. 1996. For the methods used to estimate and project incidence, prevalence, and deaths see Lozano et al. 1996 and Murray and Lopez 1996a. See explanatory notes for definitions and caveats.

Table 227
Fires
Burns >20% and <60% -
short term

Cuadro 227
Fuegos
Quemaduras >20% y <60% -
corta duración

Tableau 227
Incendies
Brûlures >20% et <60%-
court terme

Table 227a   EME - PEMC - EMBE   Fires - Burns >20% and <60% - short term

Age group (years)	Incidence 1990 Number ('000s)	Rate (per 100 000)	Prevalence 1990 Number ('000s)	Rate (per 100 000)	Avg. age at onset (years)	Average duration (years)	Deaths 1990 Number ('000s)	Rate (per 100 000)	Deaths 2000 (Projected) Number ('000s)	Rate (per 100 000)
Males										
0-4	0	0.8	0	0.2	2.5	0.28	-	-	-	-
5-14	1	1.1	0	0.3	10.0	0.28	-	-	-	-
15-44	1	0.4	0	0.1	29.9	0.28	-	-	-	-
45-59	0	0.4	0	0.1	52.4	0.28	-	-	-	-
60+	0	0.5	0	0.1	71.1	0.28	-	-	-	-
All ages	2	0.5	1	0.1	30.2	0.28	-	-	-	-
Females										
0-4	0	0.6	0	0.2	2.5	0.28	-	-	-	-
5-14	0	1.0	0	0.3	10.0	0.28	-	-	-	-
15-44	0	0.2	0	0.0	30.0	0.28	-	-	-	-
45-59	0	0.2	0	0.1	52.4	0.28	-	-	-	-
60+	0	0.3	0	0.1	72.4	0.28	-	-	-	-
All ages	1	0.3	0	0.1	30.7	0.28	-	-	-	-
Total	3	0.4	1	0.1	30.4	0.28	-	-	-	-

Table 227b   FSE - PEAS - AESE   Fires - Burns >20% and <60% - short term

Age group (years)	Incidence 1990 Number ('000s)	Rate (per 100 000)	Prevalence 1990 Number ('000s)	Rate (per 100 000)	Avg. age at onset (years)	Average duration (years)	Deaths 1990 Number ('000s)	Rate (per 100 000)	Deaths 2000 (Projected) Number ('000s)	Rate (per 100 000)
Males										
0-4	0	0.9	0	0.2	2.5	0.28	-	-	-	-
5-14	0	0.9	0	0.3	10.0	0.28	-	-	-	-
15-44	1	0.7	0	0.2	29.8	0.28	-	-	-	-
45-59	0	1.1	0	0.3	52.2	0.28	-	-	-	-
60+	0	0.6	0	0.2	70.0	0.28	-	-	-	-
All ages	1	0.8	0	0.2	32.4	0.28	-	-	-	-
Females										
0-4	0	0.7	0	0.2	2.5	0.28	-	-	-	-
5-14	0	0.6	0	0.2	10.0	0.28	-	-	-	-
15-44	0	0.2	0	0.0	29.9	0.28	-	-	-	-
45-59	0	0.3	0	0.1	52.4	0.28	-	-	-	-
60+	0	0.4	0	0.1	71.5	0.28	-	-	-	-
All ages	1	0.3	0	0.1	33.3	0.28	-	-	-	-
Total	2	0.6	1	0.2	32.7	0.28	-	-	-	-

Table 227c   India - India - Inde   Fires - Burns >20% and <60% - short term

Age group (years)	Incidence 1990 Number ('000s)	Rate (per 100 000)	Prevalence 1990 Number ('000s)	Rate (per 100 000)	Avg. age at onset (years)	Average duration (years)	Deaths 1990 Number ('000s)	Rate (per 100 000)	Deaths 2000 (Projected) Number ('000s)	Rate (per 100 000)
Males										
0-4	2	3.1	1	0.9	2.5	0.28	-	-	-	-
5-14	4	4.1	1	1.1	10.0	0.28	-	-	-	-
15-44	4	1.8	1	0.5	29.8	0.28	-	-	-	-
45-59	1	2.2	0	0.6	52.3	0.28	-	-	-	-
60+	0	0.8	0	0.2	69.7	0.28	-	-	-	-
All ages	11	2.5	3	0.7	20.8	0.28	-	-	-	-
Females										
0-4	2	2.8	0	0.8	2.5	0.28	-	-	-	-
5-14	13	13.7	4	3.8	10.0	0.28	-	-	-	-
15-44	12	6.8	3	1.9	29.8	0.28	-	-	-	-
45-59	1	2.6	0	0.7	52.4	0.28	-	-	-	-
60+	1	2.1	0	0.6	70.1	0.28	-	-	-	-
All ages	29	7.0	8	2.0	21.1	0.28	-	-	-	-
Total	40	4.7	11	1.3	21.0	0.28	-	-	-	-

For epidemiological sources see Goodreau et al. 1996. For the methods used to estimate and project incidence, prevalence, and deaths see Lozano et al. 1996 and Murray and Lopez 1996a. See explanatory notes for definitions and caveats.

Table 227	Cuadro 227	Tableau 227
Fires	**Fuegos**	**Incendies**
Burns >20% and <60% - short term	Quemaduras >20% y <60% - corta duración	Brûlures >20% et <60%- court terme

Table 227d — China - China - Chine — Fires - Burns >20% and <60% - short term

Age group (years)	Incidence 1990 Number ('000s)	Rate (per 100 000)	Prevalence 1990 Number ('000s)	Rate (per 100 000)	Avg. age at onset (years)	Average duration (years)	Deaths 1990 Number ('000s)	Rate (per 100 000)	Deaths 2000 (Projected) Number ('000s)	Rate (per 100 000)
Males										
0-4	1	1.0	0	0.3	2.5	0.28	-	-	-	-
5-14	1	0.8	0	0.2	10.0	0.28	-	-	-	-
15-44	1	0.4	0	0.1	29.9	0.28	-	-	-	-
45-59	0	0.3	0	0.1	52.3	0.28	-	-	-	-
60+	1	1.1	0	0.3	69.8	0.28	-	-	-	-
All ages	3	0.6	1	0.2	27.9	0.28	-	-	-	-
Females										
0-4	0	0.7	0	0.2	2.5	0.28	-	-	-	-
5-14	1	1.3	0	0.3	10.0	0.28	-	-	-	-
15-44	0	0.1	0	0.0	29.9	0.28	-	-	-	-
45-59	0	0.3	0	0.1	52.4	0.28	-	-	-	-
60+	0	1.0	0	0.3	70.6	0.28	-	-	-	-
All ages	3	0.5	1	0.1	26.6	0.28	-	-	-	-
Total	6	0.5	2	0.1	27.3	0.28	-	-	-	-

Table 227e — OAI - OPAI - APAI — Fires - Burns >20% and <60% - short term

Age group (years)	Incidence 1990 Number ('000s)	Rate (per 100 000)	Prevalence 1990 Number ('000s)	Rate (per 100 000)	Avg. age at onset (years)	Average duration (years)	Deaths 1990 Number ('000s)	Rate (per 100 000)	Deaths 2000 (Projected) Number ('000s)	Rate (per 100 000)
Males										
0-4	0	1.1	0	0.3	2.5	0.28	-	-	-	-
5-14	1	1.1	0	0.3	10.0	0.28	-	-	-	-
15-44	1	0.4	0	0.1	29.7	0.28	-	-	-	-
45-59	0	0.3	0	0.1	52.3	0.28	-	-	-	-
60+	0	0.2	0	0.1	69.6	0.28	-	-	-	-
All ages	2	0.6	1	0.2	17.2	0.28	-	-	-	-
Females										
0-4	0	1.2	0	0.3	2.5	0.28	-	-	-	-
5-14	1	1.3	0	0.4	10.0	0.28	-	-	-	-
15-44	0	0.2	0	0.1	29.8	0.28	-	-	-	-
45-59	0	0.1	0	0.0	52.3	0.28	-	-	-	-
60+	0	0.2	0	0.0	70.3	0.28	-	-	-	-
All ages	2	0.6	1	0.2	13.3	0.28	-	-	-	-
Total	4	0.6	1	0.2	15.4	0.28	-	-	-	-

Table 227f — SSA - ASS - ASS — Fires - Burns >20% and <60% - short term

Age group (years)	Incidence 1990 Number ('000s)	Rate (per 100 000)	Prevalence 1990 Number ('000s)	Rate (per 100 000)	Avg. age at onset (years)	Average duration (years)	Deaths 1990 Number ('000s)	Rate (per 100 000)	Deaths 2000 (Projected) Number ('000s)	Rate (per 100 000)
Males										
0-4	2	5.1	1	1.4	2.4	0.28	-	-	-	-
5-14	5	7.8	2	2.2	10.0	0.28	-	-	-	-
15-44	2	2.1	1	0.6	29.4	0.28	-	-	-	-
45-59	0	1.6	0	0.5	52.2	0.28	-	-	-	-
60+	0	1.6	0	0.5	69.2	0.28	-	-	-	-
All ages	11	4.2	3	1.2	14.5	0.28	-	-	-	-
Females										
0-4	2	4.4	1	1.2	2.4	0.28	-	-	-	-
5-14	8	11.0	2	3.1	10.0	0.28	-	-	-	-
15-44	2	1.6	0	0.4	29.5	0.28	-	-	-	-
45-59	0	1.1	0	0.3	52.2	0.28	-	-	-	-
60+	0	1.5	0	0.4	69.7	0.28	-	-	-	-
All ages	12	4.6	3	1.3	13.3	0.28	-	-	-	-
Total	22	4.4	6	1.2	13.9	0.28	-	-	-	-

For epidemiological sources see Goodreau et al. 1996. For the methods used to estimate and project incidence, prevalence, and deaths see Lozano et al. 1996 and Murray and Lopez 1996a. See explanatory notes for definitions and caveats.

Table 227
Fires
Burns >20% and <60% -
short term

Cuadro 227
Fuegos
Quemaduras >20% y <60% -
corta duración

Tableau 227
Incendies
Brûlures >20% et <60%-
court terme

Table 227g LAC - ALC - ALC — Fires - Burns >20% and <60% - short term

Age group (years)	Incidence 1990 Number ('000s)	Rate (per 100 000)	Prevalence 1990 Number ('000s)	Rate (per 100 000)	Avg. age at onset (years)	Average duration (years)	Deaths 1990 Number ('000s)	Rate (per 100 000)	Deaths 2000 (Projected) Number ('000s)	Rate (per 100 000)
Males										
0-4	0	0.8	0	0.2	2.5	0.28	-	-	-	-
5-14	1	1.4	0	0.4	10.0	0.28	-	-	-	-
15-44	0	0.4	0	0.1	29.8	0.28	-	-	-	-
45-59	0	0.4	0	0.1	52.3	0.28	-	-	-	-
60+	0	0.4	0	0.1	70.3	0.28	-	-	-	-
All ages	1	0.7	0	0.2	18.4	0.28	-	-	-	-
Females										
0-4	0	0.8	0	0.2	2.5	0.28	-	-	-	-
5-14	1	1.4	0	0.4	10.0	0.28	-	-	-	-
15-44	0	0.2	0	0.1	29.9	0.28	-	-	-	-
45-59	0	0.2	0	0.1	52.4	0.28	-	-	-	-
60+	0	0.3	0	0.1	71.1	0.28	-	-	-	-
All ages	1	0.6	0	0.2	15.8	0.28	-	-	-	-
Total	3	0.6	1	0.2	17.2	0.28				

Table 227h MEC - AOM - CMO — Fires - Burns >20% and <60% - short term

Age group (years)	Incidence 1990 Number ('000s)	Rate (per 100 000)	Prevalence 1990 Number ('000s)	Rate (per 100 000)	Avg. age at onset (years)	Average duration (years)	Deaths 1990 Number ('000s)	Rate (per 100 000)	Deaths 2000 (Projected) Number ('000s)	Rate (per 100 000)
Males										
0-4	0	1.2	0	0.3	2.5	0.28	-	-	-	-
5-14	1	1.9	0	0.5	10.0	0.28	-	-	-	-
15-44	1	0.6	0	0.2	29.8	0.28	-	-	-	-
45-59	0	0.5	0	0.1	52.3	0.28	-	-	-	-
60+	0	0.2	0	0.1	69.7	0.28	-	-	-	-
All ages	3	1.0	1	0.3	16.1	0.28	-	-	-	-
Females										
0-4	1	1.3	0	0.4	2.5	0.28	-	-	-	-
5-14	1	2.1	0	0.6	10.0	0.28	-	-	-	-
15-44	1	0.9	0	0.2	29.8	0.28	-	-	-	-
45-59	0	0.4	0	0.1	52.3	0.28	-	-	-	-
60+	0	0.4	0	0.1	70.4	0.28	-	-	-	-
All ages	3	1.2	1	0.3	17.5	0.28	-	-	-	-
Total	5	1.1	1	0.3	16.8	0.28	-	-	-	-

Table 227i World - Mundo - Monde — Fires - Burns >20% and <60% - short term

Age group (years)	Incidence 1990 Number ('000s)	Rate (per 100 000)	Prevalence 1990 Number ('000s)	Rate (per 100 000)	Avg. age at onset (years)	Average duration (years)	Deaths 1990 Number ('000s)	Rate (per 100 000)	Deaths 2000 (Projected) Number ('000s)	Rate (per 100 000)
Males										
0-4	6	2.0	2	0.6	2.5	0.28	-	-	-	-
5-14	14	2.6	4	0.7	10.0	0.28	-	-	-	-
15-44	10	0.8	3	0.2	29.8	0.28	-	-	-	-
45-59	3	0.8	1	0.2	52.3	0.28	-	-	-	-
60+	1	0.7	0	0.2	70.1	0.28	-	-	-	-
All ages	34	1.3	10	0.4	22.7	0.28	-	-	-	-
Females										
0-4	6	1.8	2	0.5	2.5	0.28	-	-	-	-
5-14	25	4.9	7	1.4	10.0	0.28	-	-	-	-
15-44	16	1.4	5	0.4	29.8	0.28	-	-	-	-
45-59	2	0.7	1	0.2	52.4	0.28	-	-	-	-
60+	2	0.7	1	0.2	71.2	0.28	-	-	-	-
All ages	51	2.0	14	0.5	22.0	0.28	-	-	-	-
Total	85	1.6	24	0.5	22.3	0.28	-	-	-	-

For epidemiological sources see Goodreau et al. 1996. For the methods used to estimate and project incidence, prevalence, and deaths see Lozano et al. 1996 and Murray and Lopez 1996a. See explanatory notes for definitions and caveats.

Table 228 | **Cuadro 228** | **Tableau 228**
Fires | Fuegos | Incendies
Burns >20% and <60% - long term | Quemaduras >20% y <60% - larga duración | Brûlures >20% et <60% - long terme

Table 228a   EME - PEMC - EMBE   Fires - Burns >20% and <60% - long term

Age group (years)	Incidence 1990 Number ('000s)	Rate (per 100 000)	Prevalence 1990 Number ('000s)	Rate (per 100 000)	Avg. age at onset (years)	Average duration (years)	Deaths 1990 Number ('000s)	Rate (per 100 000)	Deaths 2000 (Projected) Number ('000s)	Rate (per 100 000)
Males										
0-4	0	0.8	0	1.3	2.5	3.9	-	-	-	-
5-14	1	1.1	2	3.7	10.0	3.6	-	-	-	-
15-44	1	0.4	3	1.4	29.9	2.7	-	-	-	-
45-59	0	0.4	0	0.8	52.4	1.6	-	-	-	-
60+	0	0.5	0	0.6	71.1	1.2	-	-	-	-
All ages	2	0.5	6	1.5	30.2	2.7	-	-	-	-
Females										
0-4	0	0.6	0	1.0	2.5	3.9	-	-	-	-
5-14	0	1.0	2	3.1	10.0	3.6	-	-	-	-
15-44	0	0.2	1	0.7	30.0	2.7	-	-	-	-
45-59	0	0.2	0	0.3	52.4	1.6	-	-	-	-
60+	0	0.3	0	0.4	72.4	1.2	-	-	-	-
All ages	1	0.3	4	0.9	30.7	2.7	-	-	-	-
Total	3	0.4	9	1.2	30.4	2.7	-	-	-	-

Table 228b   FSE - PEAS - AESE   Fires - Burns >20% and <60% - long term

Age group (years)	Incidence 1990 Number ('000s)	Rate (per 100 000)	Prevalence 1990 Number ('000s)	Rate (per 100 000)	Avg. age at onset (years)	Average duration (years)	Deaths 1990 Number ('000s)	Rate (per 100 000)	Deaths 2000 (Projected) Number ('000s)	Rate (per 100 000)
Males										
0-4	0	0.9	0	1.2	2.5	2.46	-	-	-	-
5-14	0	0.9	1	2.2	10.0	2.29	-	-	-	-
15-44	1	0.7	1	1.3	29.8	1.64	-	-	-	-
45-59	0	1.1	0	1.4	52.2	1.21	-	-	-	-
60+	0	0.6	0	0.6	70.0	0.94	-	-	-	-
All ages	1	0.8	2	1.4	32.4	1.67	-	-	-	-
Females										
0-4	0	0.7	0	1.0	2.5	2.47	-	-	-	-
5-14	0	0.6	1	1.6	10.0	2.29	-	-	-	-
15-44	0	0.2	0	0.4	29.9	1.64	-	-	-	-
45-59	0	0.3	0	0.4	52.4	1.22	-	-	-	-
60+	0	0.4	0	0.4	71.5	0.96	-	-	-	-
All ages	1	0.3	1	0.6	33.4	1.72	-	-	-	-
Total	2	0.6	3	1.0	32.7	1.69	-	-	-	-

Table 228c   India - India - Inde   Fires - Burns >20% and <60% - long term

Age group (years)	Incidence 1990 Number ('000s)	Rate (per 100 000)	Prevalence 1990 Number ('000s)	Rate (per 100 000)	Avg. age at onset (years)	Average duration (years)	Deaths 1990 Number ('000s)	Rate (per 100 000)	Deaths 2000 (Projected) Number ('000s)	Rate (per 100 000)
Males										
0-4	2	3.1	3	4.4	2.5	2.36	-	-	-	-
5-14	4	4.1	10	9.4	10.0	2.29	-	-	-	-
15-44	4	1.8	7	3.4	29.8	1.64	-	-	-	-
45-59	1	2.2	1	2.8	52.3	1.21	-	-	-	-
60+	0	0.8	0	0.9	69.7	0.94	-	-	-	-
All ages	11	2.5	21	4.7	20.8	1.95	-	-	-	-
Females										
0-4	2	2.8	4	6.4	2.5	2.35	-	-	-	-
5-14	13	13.7	27	28.5	10.0	2.29	-	-	-	-
15-44	12	6.8	20	11.1	29.8	1.64	-	-	-	-
45-59	1	2.6	1	3.1	52.4	1.22	-	-	-	-
60+	1	2.1	1	2.0	70.1	0.95	-	-	-	-
All ages	29	7.0	53	13.0	21.1	1.94	-	-	-	-
Total	40	4.7	74	8.7	21.0	1.94	-	-	-	-

For epidemiological sources see Goodreau et al. 1996. For the methods used to estimate and project incidence, prevalence, and deaths see Lozano et al. 1996 and Murray and Lopez 1996a. See explanatory notes for definitions and caveats.

Table 228
Fires
Burns >20% and <60% -
long term

Cuadro 228
Fuegos
Quemaduras >20% y <60% -
larga duración

Tableau 228
Incendies
Brûlures >20% et <60% -
long terme

Table 228d   China - China - Chine   Fires - Burns >20% and <60% - long term

Age group (years)	Incidence 1990 Number ('000s)	Rate (per 100 000)	Prevalence 1990 Number ('000s)	Rate (per 100 000)	Avg. age at onset (years)	Average duration (years)	Deaths 1990 Number ('000s)	Rate (per 100 000)	Deaths 2000 (Projected) Number ('000s)	Rate (per 100 000)
Males										
0-4	1	1.0	1	1.4	2.5	2.45	-	-	-	-
5-14	1	0.8	2	2.1	10.0	2.29	-	-	-	-
15-44	1	0.4	2	0.7	29.9	1.64	-	-	-	-
45-59	0	0.3	0	0.4	52.3	1.22	-	-	-	-
60+	1	1.1	0	1.0	69.8	0.94	-	-	-	-
All ages	3	0.6	6	1.0	27.9	1.81	-	-	-	-
Females										
0-4	0	0.7	1	1.0	2.5	2.45	-	-	-	-
5-14	1	1.3	2	2.8	10.0	2.29	-	-	-	-
15-44	0	0.1	1	0.4	29.9	1.64	-	-	-	-
45-59	0	0.3	0	0.4	52.4	1.22	-	-	-	-
60+	0	1.0	0	0.9	70.6	0.95	-	-	-	-
All ages	3	0.5	5	0.9	26.6	1.88	-	-	-	-
Total	6	0.5	11	0.9	27.3	1.84	-	-	-	-

Table 228e   OAI - OPAI - APAI   Fires - Burns >20% and <60% - long term

Age group (years)	Incidence 1990 Number ('000s)	Rate (per 100 000)	Prevalence 1990 Number ('000s)	Rate (per 100 000)	Avg. age at onset (years)	Average duration (years)	Deaths 1990 Number ('000s)	Rate (per 100 000)	Deaths 2000 (Projected) Number ('000s)	Rate (per 100 000)
Males										
0-4	0	1.1	1	1.6	2.5	2.41	-	-	-	-
5-14	1	1.1	2	2.6	10.0	2.29	-	-	-	-
15-44	1	0.4	1	0.7	29.7	1.63	-	-	-	-
45-59	0	0.3	0	0.4	52.3	1.21	-	-	-	-
60+	0	0.2	0	0.2	69.6	0.94	-	-	-	-
All ages	2	0.6	4	1.2	17.2	2.05	-	-	-	-
Females										
0-4	0	1.2	1	1.7	2.5	2.42	-	-	-	-
5-14	1	1.3	2	3.0	10.0	2.29	-	-	-	-
15-44	0	0.2	1	0.5	29.8	1.64	-	-	-	-
45-59	0	0.1	0	0.2	52.3	1.22	-	-	-	-
60+	0	0.2	0	0.2	70.3	0.95	-	-	-	-
All ages	2	0.6	4	1.2	13.3	2.17	-	-	-	-
Total	4	0.6	8	1.2	15.4	2.10	-	-	-	-

Table 228f   SSA - ASS - ASS   Fires - Burns >20% and <60% - long term

Age group (years)	Incidence 1990 Number ('000s)	Rate (per 100 000)	Prevalence 1990 Number ('000s)	Rate (per 100 000)	Avg. age at onset (years)	Average duration (years)	Deaths 1990 Number ('000s)	Rate (per 100 000)	Deaths 2000 (Projected) Number ('000s)	Rate (per 100 000)
Males										
0-4	2	5.1	3	7.0	2.4	2.30	-	-	-	-
5-14	5	7.8	12	17.5	10.0	2.27	-	-	-	-
15-44	2	2.1	5	4.4	29.4	1.62	-	-	-	-
45-59	0	1.6	0	2.2	52.2	1.20	-	-	-	-
60+	0	1.6	0	1.7	69.2	0.93	-	-	-	-
All ages	11	4.2	21	8.2	14.5	2.09	-	-	-	-
Females										
0-4	2	4.4	3	6.1	2.4	2.33	-	-	-	-
5-14	8	11.0	16	23.1	10.0	2.27	-	-	-	-
15-44	2	1.6	4	4.0	29.5	1.63	-	-	-	-
45-59	0	1.1	0	1.5	52.2	1.21	-	-	-	-
60+	0	1.5	0	1.5	69.7	0.94	-	-	-	-
All ages	12	4.6	24	9.2	13.2	2.15	-	-	-	-
Total	22	4.4	45	8.7	13.9	2.12	-	-	-	-

For epidemiological sources see Goodreau et al. 1996. For the methods used to estimate and project incidence, prevalence, and deaths see Lozano et al. 1996 and Murray and Lopez 1996a. See explanatory notes for definitions and caveats.

Table 228
Fires
Burns >20% and <60% -
long term

Cuadro 228
Fuegos
Quemaduras >20% y <60% -
larga duración

Tableau 228
Incendies
Brûlures >20% et <60% -
long terme

Table 228g   LAC - ALC - ALC   Fires - Burns >20% and <60% - long term

Age group (years)	Incidence 1990 Number ('000s)	Rate (per 100 000)	Prevalence 1990 Number ('000s)	Rate (per 100 000)	Avg. age at onset (years)	Average duration (years)	Deaths 1990 Number ('000s)	Rate (per 100 000)	Deaths 2000 (Projected) Number ('000s)	Rate (per 100 000)
Males										
0-4	0	0.8	0	1.2	2.5	2.43	-	-	-	-
5-14	1	1.4	2	3.1	10.0	2.29	-	-	-	-
15-44	0	0.4	1	0.8	29.8	1.64	-	-	-	-
45-59	0	0.4	0	0.5	52.3	1.22	-	-	-	-
60+	0	0.4	0	0.4	70.3	0.95	-	-	-	-
All ages	1	0.7	3	1.3	18.4	2.04	-	-	-	-
Females										
0-4	0	0.8	0	1.1	2.5	2.44	-	-	-	-
5-14	1	1.4	2	3.1	10.0	2.29	-	-	-	-
15-44	0	0.2	1	0.5	29.9	1.64	-	-	-	-
45-59	0	0.2	0	0.3	52.4	1.22	-	-	-	-
60+	0	0.3	0	0.3	71.1	0.95	-	-	-	-
All ages	1	0.6	2	1.1	15.8	2.12	-	-	-	-
Total	3	0.6	5	1.2	17.2	2.07	-	-	-	-

Table 228h   MEC - AOM - CMO   Fires - Burns >20% and <60% - long term

Age group (years)	Incidence 1990 Number ('000s)	Rate (per 100 000)	Prevalence 1990 Number ('000s)	Rate (per 100 000)	Avg. age at onset (years)	Average duration (years)	Deaths 1990 Number ('000s)	Rate (per 100 000)	Deaths 2000 (Projected) Number ('000s)	Rate (per 100 000)
Males										
0-4	0	1.2	1	1.7	2.5	2.39	-	-	-	-
5-14	1	1.9	3	4.2	10.0	2.29	-	-	-	-
15-44	1	0.6	1	1.1	29.8	1.64	-	-	-	-
45-59	0	0.5	0	0.6	52.3	1.21	-	-	-	-
60+	0	0.2	0	0.3	69.7	0.94	-	-	-	-
All ages	3	1.0	5	1.9	16.1	2.08	-	-	-	-
Females										
0-4	1	1.3	1	1.8	2.5	2.39	-	-	-	-
5-14	1	2.1	3	4.6	10.0	2.29	-	-	-	-
15-44	1	0.9	2	1.6	29.8	1.64	-	-	-	-
45-59	1	3.7	1	4.3	52.3	1.22	-	-	-	-
60+	0	0.4	0	0.6	70.4	0.95	-	-	-	-
All ages	4	1.5	6	2.6	24.7	1.87	-	-	-	-
Total	6	1.2	11	2.2	21.1	1.96	-	-	-	-

Table 228i   World - Mundo - Monde   Fires - Burns >20% and <60% - long term

Age group (years)	Incidence 1990 Number ('000s)	Rate (per 100 000)	Prevalence 1990 Number ('000s)	Rate (per 100 000)	Avg. age at onset (years)	Average duration (years)	Deaths 1990 Number ('000s)	Rate (per 100 000)	Deaths 2000 (Projected) Number ('000s)	Rate (per 100 000)
Males										
0-4	6	2.0	9	2.8	2.5	2.5	-	-	-	-
5-14	14	2.6	33	6.0	10.0	2.4	-	-	-	-
15-44	10	0.8	20	1.6	29.8	1.8	-	-	-	-
45-59	3	0.8	3	1.1	52.3	1.3	-	-	-	-
60+	1	0.7	2	0.7	70.1	1.0	-	-	-	-
All ages	34	1.3	67	2.5	22.7	2.1	-	-	-	-
Females										
0-4	6	1.8	9	3.0	2.5	2.5	-	-	-	-
5-14	25	4.8	55	10.4	10.0	2.4	-	-	-	-
15-44	16	1.4	30	2.5	29.8	1.8	-	-	-	-
45-59	3	0.9	3	1.1	52.4	1.3	-	-	-	-
60+	2	0.7	2	0.7	71.2	1.0	-	-	-	-
All ages	52	2.0	99	3.8	22.7	2.1	-	-	-	-
Total	86	1.6	167	3.2	22.7	2.1	-	-	-	-

For epidemiological sources see Goodreau et al. 1996. For the methods used to estimate and project incidence, prevalence, and deaths see Lozano et al. 1996 and Murray and Lopez 1996a. See explanatory notes for definitions and caveats.

Table 229
Drownings

Cuadro 229
Ahogamientos

Tableau 229
Noyades

Episodes

Episodios

Episodes

Table 229a   EME - PEMC - EMBE — Drownings - Episodes

Age group (years)	Incidence 1990 Number ('000s)	Rate (per 100 000)	Prevalence 1990 Number ('000s)	Rate (per 100 000)	Avg. age at onset (years)	Average duration (years)	Deaths 1990 Number ('000s)	Rate (per 100 000)	Deaths 2000 (Projected) Number ('000s)	Rate (per 100 000)
Males										
0-4	3	10.2	-	-	2.5	-	1	4.1	1	2.8
5-14	2	4.4	-	-	10.0	-	1	1.8	1	1.3
15-44	10	5.5	-	-	29.9	-	4	2.2	3	1.9
45-59	3	5.3	-	-	52.4	-	1	2.1	2	1.9
60+	6	9.3	-	-	71.1	-	2	3.7	3	3.5
All ages	24	6.2	-	-	37.7	-	10	2.5	9	2.2
Females										
0-4	1	5.4	-	-	2.5	-	1	2.2	0	1.5
5-14	1	1.1	-	-	10.0	-	0	0.4	0	0.4
15-44	1	0.8	-	-	30.0	-	1	0.3	1	0.3
45-59	1	1.2	-	-	52.5	-	0	0.5	0	0.5
60+	4	4.6	-	-	72.4	-	2	1.8	2	1.7
All ages	8	2.0	-	-	34.9	-	3	0.8	3	0.8
Total	32	4.0	-	-	37.2	-	13	1.6	12	1.4

Table 229b   FSE - PEAS - AESE — Drownings - Episodes

Age group (years)	Incidence 1990 Number ('000s)	Rate (per 100 000)	Prevalence 1990 Number ('000s)	Rate (per 100 000)	Avg. age at onset (years)	Average duration (years)	Deaths 1990 Number ('000s)	Rate (per 100 000)	Deaths 2000 (Projected) Number ('000s)	Rate (per 100 000)
Males										
0-4	3	19.3	-	-	2.5	-	1	7.7	1	6.7
5-14	6	22.8	-	-	10.0	-	2	9.1	2	7.4
15-44	27	35.4	-	-	29.8	-	11	14.2	10	13.8
45-59	9	34.2	-	-	52.2	-	4	13.7	4	14.1
60+	4	19.9	-	-	70.0	-	2	7.9	2	8.2
All ages	49	29.8	-	-	33.4	-	20	11.9	20	11.5
Females										
0-4	1	8.8	-	-	2.5	-	0	3.5	0	3.1
5-14	2	7.8	-	-	10.0	-	1	3.1	1	2.7
15-44	3	3.5	-	-	29.9	-	1	1.4	1	1.5
45-59	1	4.6	-	-	52.4	-	1	1.8	1	1.8
60+	2	6.3	-	-	71.5	-	1	2.5	1	2.6
All ages	9	5.2	-	-	35.5	-	4	2.1	4	2.1
Total	59	17.0	-	-	33.7	-	24	6.8	24	6.6

Table 229c   India - India - Inde — Drownings - Episodes

Age group (years)	Incidence 1990 Number ('000s)	Rate (per 100 000)	Prevalence 1990 Number ('000s)	Rate (per 100 000)	Avg. age at onset (years)	Average duration (years)	Deaths 1990 Number ('000s)	Rate (per 100 000)	Deaths 2000 (Projected) Number ('000s)	Rate (per 100 000)
Males										
0-4	27	45	-	-	2.5	-	11	18.0	10	18.1
5-14	41	40	-	-	10.0	-	16	16.1	13	11.4
15-44	35	18	-	-	29.8	-	14	7.1	15	6.2
45-59	8	17	-	-	52.3	-	3	6.9	4	6.8
60+	8	25	-	-	69.7	-	3	10.1	4	11.2
All ages	119	27	-	-	20.9	-	48	10.8	47	9.1
Females										
0-4	22	39	-	-	2.5	-	9	15.6	8	15.4
5-14	39	41	-	-	10.0	-	16	16.5	11	10.8
15-44	23	13	-	-	29.8	-	9	5.1	10	4.2
45-59	8	18	-	-	52.4	-	3	7.3	4	7.3
60+	9	32	-	-	70.1	-	4	12.7	6	15.4
All ages	102	25	-	-	18.5	-	41	10.0	39	8.2
Total	221	26	-	-	19.9	-	89	10.4	86	8.6

For the methods used to estimate and project incidence, prevalence, and deaths see Murray and Lopez 1996a. See explanatory notes for definitions and caveats.

Table 229	Cuadro 229	Tableau 229
Drownings	**Ahogamientos**	**Noyades**

Episodes   Episodios   Episodes

Table 229d   China - China - Chine   Drownings - Episodes

Age group (years)	Incidence 1990 Number ('000s)	Incidence 1990 Rate (per 100 000)	Prevalence 1990 Number ('000s)	Prevalence 1990 Rate (per 100 000)	Avg. age at onset (years)	Average duration (years)	Deaths 1990 Number ('000s)	Deaths 1990 Rate (per 100 000)	Deaths 2000 (Projected) Number ('000s)	Deaths 2000 (Projected) Rate (per 100 000)
Males										
0-4	76	125.9	-	-	2.5	-	30	50.4	27	45.4
5-14	55	56.5	-	-	10.0	-	22	22.5	17	14.3
15-44	66	21.7	-	-	29.9	-	27	8.7	20	6.2
45-59	11	15.3	-	-	52.3	-	4	6.1	5	5.4
60+	20	39.8	-	-	69.8	-	8	15.9	10	17.1
All ages	228	38.9	-	-	20.5	-	91	15.5	79	12.0
Females										
0-4	64	110.4	-	-	2.5	-	26	44.2	21	38.0
5-14	27	29.4	-	-	10.0	-	11	11.8	8	6.7
15-44	25	9.0	-	-	29.9	-	10	3.6	7	2.3
45-59	5	8.2	-	-	52.4	-	2	3.3	3	3.3
60+	17	33.8	-	-	70.6	-	7	13.6	11	17.8
All ages	139	25.3	-	-	19.4	-	56	10.1	50	8.0
Total	366	32.3	-	-	20.1	-	147	12.9	129	10.1

Table 229e   OAI - OPAI - APAI   Drownings - Episodes

Age group (years)	Incidence 1990 Number ('000s)	Incidence 1990 Rate (per 100 000)	Prevalence 1990 Number ('000s)	Prevalence 1990 Rate (per 100 000)	Avg. age at onset (years)	Average duration (years)	Deaths 1990 Number ('000s)	Deaths 1990 Rate (per 100 000)	Deaths 2000 (Projected) Number ('000s)	Deaths 2000 (Projected) Rate (per 100 000)
Males										
0-4	48	109.4	-	-	2.5	-	19	43.8	17	39.1
5-14	48	57.4	-	-	10.0	-	21	24.4	15	17.7
15-44	37	22.9	-	-	29.7	-	15	9.1	16	7.8
45-59	6	17.3	-	-	52.3	-	2	6.9	3	6.6
60+	5	25.4	-	-	69.6	-	2	10.2	3	10.5
All ages	144	42.0	-	-	16.4	-	59	17.1	54	13.3
Females										
0-4	30	70.7	-	-	2.5	-	12	28.3	11	25.2
5-14	20	24.9	-	-	10.0	-	8	10.0	6	7.1
15-44	11	6.8	-	-	29.8	-	4	2.7	5	2.4
45-59	2	5.6	-	-	52.3	-	1	2.2	1	2.2
60+	3	11.4	-	-	70.3	-	1	4.6	2	4.9
All ages	65	19.2	-	-	13.5	-	26	7.7	24	5.9
Total	209	30.6	-	-	15.5	-	85	12.4	77	9.6

Table 229f   SSA - ASS - ASS   Drownings - Episodes

Age group (years)	Incidence 1990 Number ('000s)	Incidence 1990 Rate (per 100 000)	Prevalence 1990 Number ('000s)	Prevalence 1990 Rate (per 100 000)	Avg. age at onset (years)	Average duration (years)	Deaths 1990 Number ('000s)	Deaths 1990 Rate (per 100 000)	Deaths 2000 (Projected) Number ('000s)	Deaths 2000 (Projected) Rate (per 100 000)
Males										
0-4	39	82.8	-	-	2.4	-	16	33.1	22	32.9
5-14	79	112.1	-	-	10.0	-	33	47.5	34	36.5
15-44	36	34.3	-	-	29.4	-	14	13.7	18	12.4
45-59	4	22.1	-	-	52.2	-	2	9.0	2	9.2
60+	3	31.1	-	-	69.2	-	1	12.5	2	13.3
All ages	161	64.0	-	-	14.8	-	66	26.3	78	22.8
Females										
0-4	20	42.5	-	-	2.4	-	8	17.0	11	17.2
5-14	33	46.7	-	-	10.0	-	13	19.1	13	14.4
15-44	6	5.9	-	-	29.5	-	3	2.4	3	2.3
45-59	1	4.8	-	-	52.2	-	0	1.9	1	1.9
60+	1	8.6	-	-	69.7	-	0	3.4	1	3.7
All ages	61	23.7	-	-	11.3	-	25	9.6	29	8.3
Total	222	43.6	-	-	13.8	-	91	17.9	107	15.5

For the methods used to estimate and project incidence, prevalence, and deaths see Murray and Lopez 1996a. See explanatory notes for definitions and caveats.

Table 229
Drownings

Cuadro 229
Ahogamientos

Tableau 229
Noyades

Episodes

Episodios

Episodes

Table 229g   LAC - ALC - ALC   Drownings - Episodes

Age group (years)	Incidence 1990 Number ('000s)	Rate (per 100 000)	Prevalence 1990 Number ('000s)	Rate (per 100 000)	Avg. age at onset (years)	Average duration (years)	Deaths 1990 Number ('000s)	Rate (per 100 000)	Deaths 2000 (Projected) Number ('000s)	Rate (per 100 000)
Males										
0-4	7	25.6	-	-	2.5	-	3	10.2	3	9.1
5-14	14	27.7	-	-	10.0	-	6	11.1	5	8.5
15-44	28	26.5	-	-	29.8	-	11	10.6	12	9.5
45-59	4	18.5	-	-	52.3	-	2	7.4	2	7.3
60+	2	16.4	-	-	70.3	-	1	6.6	1	6.8
All ages	56	25.2	-	-	24.4	-	22	10.1	23	8.8
Females										
0-4	5	16.8	-	-	2.5	-	2	6.7	2	6.1
5-14	5	10.0	-	-	10.0	-	2	4.0	2	3.1
15-44	4	4.3	-	-	29.9	-	2	1.7	2	1.6
45-59	1	2.5	-	-	52.4	-	0	1.0	0	1.0
60+	1	3.3	-	-	71.1	-	0	1.3	0	1.4
All ages	15	6.9	-	-	17.4	-	6	2.8	6	2.3
Total	71	16.0	-	-	22.9	-	28	6.4	29	5.5

Table 229h   MEC - AOM - CMO   Drownings - Episodes

Age group (years)	Incidence 1990 Number ('000s)	Rate (per 100 000)	Prevalence 1990 Number ('000s)	Rate (per 100 000)	Avg. age at onset (years)	Average duration (years)	Deaths 1990 Number ('000s)	Rate (per 100 000)	Deaths 2000 (Projected) Number ('000s)	Rate (per 100 000)
Males										
0-4	14	34.4	-	-	2.5	-	6	13.7	7	13.4
5-14	14	21.3	-	-	10.0	-	6	8.6	6	6.7
15-44	18	15.9	-	-	29.8	-	7	6.4	9	5.9
45-59	2	8.8	-	-	52.3	-	1	3.5	1	3.7
60+	1	8.8	-	-	69.7	-	0	3.5	1	3.7
All ages	49	19.2	-	-	18.3	-	20	7.7	23	6.9
Females										
0-4	12	30.4	-	-	2.5	-	5	12.2	6	12.2
5-14	4	6.2	-	-	10.0	-	2	2.5	2	2.0
15-44	3	2.7	-	-	29.8	-	1	1.1	2	1.1
45-59	0	1.9	-	-	52.3	-	0	0.8	0	0.8
60+	0	2.8	-	-	70.4	-	0	1.1	0	1.2
All ages	20	8.0	-	-	10.5	-	8	3.2	9	2.9
Total	69	13.7	-	-	16.0	-	28	5.5	32	4.9

Table 229i   World - Mundo - Monde   Drownings - Episodes

Age group (years)	Incidence 1990 Number ('000s)	Rate (per 100 000)	Prevalence 1990 Number ('000s)	Rate (per 100 000)	Avg. age at onset (years)	Average duration (years)	Deaths 1990 Number ('000s)	Rate (per 100 000)	Deaths 2000 (Projected) Number ('000s)	Rate (per 100 000)
Males										
0-4	217	67.5	-	-	2.5	-	87	27.0	87	25.1
5-14	260	47.1	-	-	10.0	-	107	19.4	92	14.6
15-44	257	20.6	-	-	29.8	-	103	8.2	103	7.2
45-59	49	15.5	-	-	52.3	-	19	6.2	24	6.0
60+	49	22.3	-	-	69.9	-	20	8.9	26	9.4
All ages	831	31.3	-	-	20.1	-	335	12.6	332	10.7
Females										
0-4	155	50.1	-	-	2.5	-	62	20.1	59	18.0
5-14	130	24.7	-	-	10.0	-	52	10.0	42	7.0
15-44	77	6.5	-	-	29.8	-	31	2.6	30	2.2
45-59	20	6.4	-	-	52.4	-	8	2.6	10	2.6
60+	37	13.9	-	-	70.7	-	15	5.6	23	6.8
All ages	420	16.1	-	-	17.3	-	168	6.4	165	5.4
Total	1 251	23.7	-	-	19.2	-	504	9.6	497	8.1

For the methods used to estimate and project incidence, prevalence, and deaths see Murray and Lopez 1996a. See explanatory notes for definitions and caveats.

Table 230	Cuadro 230	Tableau 230
Drownings	Ahogamientos	Noyades

Quadriplegia	Cuadriplejia	Quadriplégie

Table 230a — EME - PEMC - EMBE — Drownings - Quadriplegia

Age group (years)	Incidence 1990 Number ('000s)	Rate (per 100 000)	Prevalence 1990 Number ('000s)	Rate (per 100 000)	Avg. age at onset (years)	Average duration (years)	Deaths 1990 Number ('000s)	Rate (per 100 000)	Deaths 2000 (Projected) Number ('000s)	Rate (per 100 000)
Males										
0-4	0	0.3	0	0.8	2.5	62.1	-	-	-	-
5-14	0	0.1	1	2.4	10.0	55.9	-	-	-	-
15-44	0	0.2	11	5.8	29.9	37.7	-	-	-	-
45-59	0	0.2	6	9.2	52.4	18.7	-	-	-	-
60+	0	0.3	6	9.7	71.1	7.9	-	-	-	-
All ages	1	0.2	24	6.2	37.7	32.5	-	-	-	-
Females										
0-4	0	0.2	0	0.4	2.5	69.5	-	-	-	-
5-14	0	0.0	1	1.1	10.0	63.1	-	-	-	-
15-44	0	0.0	3	1.6	30.0	44.0	-	-	-	-
45-59	0	0.0	1	2.1	52.5	23.6	-	-	-	-
60+	0	0.1	2	2.3	72.4	9.7	-	-	-	-
All ages	0	0.0	7	1.7	34.9	41.0	-	-	-	-
Total	1	0.1	31	3.9	37.2	34.0	-	-	-	-

Table 230b — FSE - PEAS - AESE — Drownings - Quadriplegia

Age group (years)	Incidence 1990 Number ('000s)	Rate (per 100 000)	Prevalence 1990 Number ('000s)	Rate (per 100 000)	Avg. age at onset (years)	Average duration (years)	Deaths 1990 Number ('000s)	Rate (per 100 000)	Deaths 2000 (Projected) Number ('000s)	Rate (per 100 000)
Males										
0-4	0	0.6	0	1.6	2.5	54.1	-	-	-	-
5-14	0	0.8	2	7.0	10.0	48.4	-	-	-	-
15-44	1	1.2	21	27.3	29.8	31.3	-	-	-	-
45-59	0	1.1	13	46.9	52.2	14.9	-	-	-	-
60+	0	0.7	8	38.5	70.0	6.7	-	-	-	-
All ages	2	1.0	44	26.4	33.4	29.5	-	-	-	-
Females										
0-4	0	0.3	0	0.7	2.5	64.7	-	-	-	-
5-14	0	0.3	1	2.8	10.0	58.9	-	-	-	-
15-44	0	0.1	4	5.7	29.9	40.2	-	-	-	-
45-59	0	0.2	2	8.1	52.4	20.6	-	-	-	-
60+	0	0.2	3	8.5	71.5	8.5	-	-	-	-
All ages	0	0.2	11	5.9	35.5	36.8	-	-	-	-
Total	2	0.6	54	15.7	33.7	30.7	-	-	-	-

Table 230c — India - India - Inde — Drownings - Quadriplegia

Age group (years)	Incidence 1990 Number ('000s)	Rate (per 100 000)	Prevalence 1990 Number ('000s)	Rate (per 100 000)	Avg. age at onset (years)	Average duration (years)	Deaths 1990 Number ('000s)	Rate (per 100 000)	Deaths 2000 (Projected) Number ('000s)	Rate (per 100 000)
Males										
0-4	1	1.5	2	3.5	2.5	48.0	-	-	-	-
5-14	1	1.3	14	13.6	10.0	48.6	-	-	-	-
15-44	1	0.6	56	27.7	29.8	32.4	-	-	-	-
45-59	0	0.6	17	36.4	52.3	15.6	-	-	-	-
60+	0	0.8	9	31.3	69.7	6.4	-	-	-	-
All ages	4	0.9	98	22.3	20.9	38.7	-	-	-	-
Females										
0-4	1	2.3	3	5.4	2.5	48.5	-	-	-	-
5-14	0	0.5	13	13.2	10.0	50.1	-	-	-	-
15-44	1	0.3	36	19.4	29.8	34.4	-	-	-	-
45-59	0	0.3	11	23.6	52.4	17.1	-	-	-	-
60+	0	1.0	7	23.8	70.1	6.9	-	-	-	-
All ages	3	0.7	69	16.8	18.5	40.3	-	-	-	-
Total	7	0.8	167	19.7	19.9	39.3	-	-	-	-

For the methods used to estimate and project incidence, prevalence, and deaths see Murray and Lopez 1996a. See explanatory notes for definitions and caveats.

Table 230 — **Cuadro 230** — **Tableau 230**
Drownings — **Ahogamientos** — **Noyades**

Quadriplegia — Cuadriplejia — Quadriplégie

Table 230d   China - China - Chine   Drownings - Quadriplegia

Age group (years)	Incidence 1990 Number ('000s)	Rate (per 100 000)	Prevalence 1990 Number ('000s)	Rate (per 100 000)	Avg. age at onset (years)	Average duration (years)	Deaths 1990 Number ('000s)	Rate (per 100 000)	Deaths 2000 (Projected) Number ('000s)	Rate (per 100 000)
Males										
0-4	3	4.2	6	10.3	2.5	56.7	-	-	-	-
5-14	2	1.9	29	29.8	10.0	52.2	-	-	-	-
15-44	2	0.7	149	48.8	29.9	34.4	-	-	-	-
45-59	0	0.5	42	58.0	52.3	15.9	-	-	-	-
60+	1	1.3	24	48.2	69.8	6.5	-	-	-	-
All ages	8	1.3	250	42.8	20.5	42.8	-	-	-	-
Females										
0-4	2	3.7	5	9.0	2.5	59.8	-	-	-	-
5-14	1	1.0	21	22.7	10.0	55.8	-	-	-	-
15-44	1	0.3	90	31.5	29.9	37.5	-	-	-	-
45-59	0	0.3	23	35.6	52.4	18.3	-	-	-	-
60+	1	1.1	18	34.2	70.6	7.4	-	-	-	-
All ages	5	0.8	156	28.4	19.4	46.8	-	-	-	-
Total	12	1.1	406	35.8	20.1	44.3	-	-	-	-

Table 230e   OAI - OPAI - APAI   Drownings - Quadriplegia

Age group (years)	Incidence 1990 Number ('000s)	Rate (per 100 000)	Prevalence 1990 Number ('000s)	Rate (per 100 000)	Avg. age at onset (years)	Average duration (years)	Deaths 1990 Number ('000s)	Rate (per 100 000)	Deaths 2000 (Projected) Number ('000s)	Rate (per 100 000)
Males										
0-4	2	3.6	4	8.7	2.5	48.4	-	-	-	-
5-14	2	1.9	22	26.7	10.0	47.0	-	-	-	-
15-44	1	0.8	73	45.2	29.7	31.1	-	-	-	-
45-59	0	0.6	18	53.2	52.3	14.7	-	-	-	-
60+	0	0.8	8	40.1	69.6	6.3	-	-	-	-
All ages	5	1.4	125	36.5	16.4	40.6	-	-	-	-
Females										
0-4	1	2.4	2	5.7	2.5	52.2	-	-	-	-
5-14	1	0.8	12	15.3	10.0	50.2	-	-	-	-
15-44	0	0.2	35	21.9	29.8	33.8	-	-	-	-
45-59	0	0.2	8	23.9	52.3	16.7	-	-	-	-
60+	0	0.4	4	19.1	70.3	7.0	-	-	-	-
All ages	2	0.6	62	18.3	13.5	45.6	-	-	-	-
Total	7	1.0	187	27.5	15.5	42.2	-	-	-	-

Table 230f   SSA - ASS - ASS   Drownings - Quadriplegia

Age group (years)	Incidence 1990 Number ('000s)	Rate (per 100 000)	Prevalence 1990 Number ('000s)	Rate (per 100 000)	Avg. age at onset (years)	Average duration (years)	Deaths 1990 Number ('000s)	Rate (per 100 000)	Deaths 2000 (Projected) Number ('000s)	Rate (per 100 000)
Males										
0-4	1	2.8	3	6.2	2.4	33.8	-	-	-	-
5-14	3	3.7	21	30.1	10.0	37.8	-	-	-	-
15-44	1	1.1	61	58.5	29.4	26.2	-	-	-	-
45-59	0	0.7	13	64.7	52.2	13.4	-	-	-	-
60+	0	1.0	5	46.6	69.2	6.0	-	-	-	-
All ages	5	2.1	103	40.7	14.8	32.9	-	-	-	-
Females										
0-4	1	1.4	2	3.2	2.4	37.1	-	-	-	-
5-14	1	1.6	10	13.8	10.0	40.6	-	-	-	-
15-44	0	0.2	24	22.1	29.5	28.5	-	-	-	-
45-59	0	0.2	5	21.5	52.2	14.8	-	-	-	-
60+	0	0.3	2	15.6	69.7	6.4	-	-	-	-
All ages	2	0.8	41	16.0	11.3	37.2	-	-	-	-
Total	7	1.5	144	28.3	13.8	34.1	-	-	-	-

For the methods used to estimate and project incidence, prevalence, and deaths see Murray and Lopez 1996a. See explanatory notes for definitions and caveats.

Table 230
Drownings

Cuadro 230
Ahogamientos

Tableau 230
Noyades

Quadriplegia

Cuadriplejia

Quadriplégie

Table 230g LAC - ALC - ALC   Drownings - Quadriplegia

Age group (years)	Incidence 1990 Number ('000s)	Rate (per 100 000)	Prevalence 1990 Number ('000s)	Rate (per 100 000)	Avg. age at onset (years)	Average duration (years)	Deaths 1990 Number ('000s)	Rate (per 100 000)	Deaths 2000 (Projected) Number ('000s)	Rate (per 100 000)
Males										
0-4	0	0.9	1	2.1	2.5	53.3	-	-	-	-
5-14	0	0.9	5	8.7	10.0	50.5	-	-	-	-
15-44	1	0.9	27	25.5	29.8	33.8	-	-	-	-
45-59	0	0.6	9	39.3	52.3	16.6	-	-	-	-
60+	0	0.5	5	32.3	70.3	7.0	-	-	-	-
All ages	2	0.8	45	20.3	24.4	38.3	-	-	-	-
Females										
0-4	0	0.6	0	1.4	2.5	58.2	-	-	-	-
5-14	0	0.3	2	4.4	10.0	54.7	-	-	-	-
15-44	0	0.1	8	7.9	29.9	37.4	-	-	-	-
45-59	0	0.1	2	9.9	52.4	19.2	-	-	-	-
60+	0	0.1	1	8.2	71.1	7.9	-	-	-	-
All ages	1	0.2	15	6.5	17.4	47.7	-	-	-	-
Total	2	0.5	60	13.4	22.9	40.3	-	-	-	-

Table 230h MEC - AOM - CMO   Drownings - Quadriplegia

Age group (years)	Incidence 1990 Number ('000s)	Rate (per 100 000)	Prevalence 1990 Number ('000s)	Rate (per 100 000)	Avg. age at onset (years)	Average duration (years)	Deaths 1990 Number ('000s)	Rate (per 100 000)	Deaths 2000 (Projected) Number ('000s)	Rate (per 100 000)
Males										
0-4	0	1.1	1	2.7	2.5	49.9	-	-	-	-
5-14	0	0.7	6	8.9	10.0	49.7	-	-	-	-
15-44	1	0.5	22	19.6	29.8	32.6	-	-	-	-
45-59	0	0.3	6	26.7	52.3	15.2	-	-	-	-
60+	0	0.3	3	19.7	69.7	6.4	-	-	-	-
All ages	2	0.6	38	14.8	18.3	41.0	-	-	-	-
Females										
0-4	0	1.0	1	2.4	2.5	52.5	-	-	-	-
5-14	0	0.2	4	5.7	10.0	52.6	-	-	-	-
15-44	0	0.1	8	7.9	29.8	35.3	-	-	-	-
45-59	0	0.1	2	8.8	52.3	17.3	-	-	-	-
60+	0	0.1	1	6.8	70.4	7.2	-	-	-	-
All ages	1	0.3	16	6.5	10.5	48.2	-	-	-	-
Total	2	0.5	54	10.7	16.0	43.1	-	-	-	-

Table 230i World - Mundo - Monde   Drownings - Quadriplegia

Age group (years)	Incidence 1990 Number ('000s)	Rate (per 100 000)	Prevalence 1990 Number ('000s)	Rate (per 100 000)	Avg. age at onset (years)	Average duration (years)	Deaths 1990 Number ('000s)	Rate (per 100 000)	Deaths 2000 (Projected) Number ('000s)	Rate (per 100 000)
Males										
0-4	7	2.2	17	5.3	2.5	49.1	-	-	-	-
5-14	9	1.6	100	18.1	10.0	46.0	-	-	-	-
15-44	9	0.7	419	33.5	29.8	32.1	-	-	-	-
45-59	2	0.5	124	39.8	52.3	15.5	-	-	-	-
60+	2	0.7	67	30.7	69.9	6.6	-	-	-	-
All ages	28	1.0	727	27.4	20.1	38.4	-	-	-	-
Females										
0-4	6	1.9	14	4.4	2.5	52.8	-	-	-	-
5-14	4	0.7	62	11.8	10.0	49.2	-	-	-	-
15-44	2	0.2	207	17.3	29.8	35.5	-	-	-	-
45-59	0	0.2	55	17.7	52.4	18.0	-	-	-	-
60+	1	0.4	38	14.2	70.6	7.4	-	-	-	-
All ages	13	0.5	377	14.4	17.1	43.5	-	-	-	-
Total	41	0.8	1 104	21.0	19.2	40.1	-	-	-	-

For the methods used to estimate and project incidence, prevalence, and deaths see Murray and Lopez 1996a. See explanatory notes for definitions and caveats.

Table 231
Other unintentional injuries

Episodes

Cuadro 231
Otras lesiones no
intencionales

Episodios

Tableau 231
Autres traumatismes
non-intentionnels

Episodes

Table 231a — EME - PEMC - EMBE — Other unintentional injuries - Episodes

Age group (years)	Incidence 1990 Number ('000s)	Rate (per 100 000)	Prevalence 1990 Number ('000s)	Rate (per 100 000)	Avg. age at onset (years)	Average duration (years)	Deaths 1990 Number ('000s)	Rate (per 100 000)	Deaths 2000 (Projected) Number ('000s)	Rate (per 100 000)
Males										
0-4	154	583	-	-	2.5	-	2	7.5	2	5.2
5-14	107	201	-	-	10.0	-	1	2.6	1	2.0
15-44	1 315	714	-	-	29.9	-	16	8.9	14	7.8
45-59	711	1 076	-	-	52.4	-	9	13.4	10	12.1
60+	1 050	1 734	-	-	71.1	-	17	27.7	19	26.7
All ages	3 337	855	-	-	45.8	-	45	11.6	45	11.0
Females										
0-4	98	390	-	-	2.5	-	1	5.0	1	3.6
5-14	36	71	-	-	10.0	-	0	0.9	0	0.8
15-44	218	122	-	-	30.0	-	3	1.5	3	1.6
45-59	166	245	-	-	52.4	-	2	3.1	2	3.1
60+	830	981	-	-	72.4	-	13	15.7	14	14.5
All ages	1 348	331	-	-	56.3	-	20	4.8	21	4.8
Total	4 685	587	-	-	48.8	-	65	8.2	66	7.9

Table 231b — FSE - PEAS - AESE — Other unintentional injuries - Episodes

Age group (years)	Incidence 1990 Number ('000s)	Rate (per 100 000)	Prevalence 1990 Number ('000s)	Rate (per 100 000)	Avg. age at onset (years)	Average duration (years)	Deaths 1990 Number ('000s)	Rate (per 100 000)	Deaths 2000 (Projected) Number ('000s)	Rate (per 100 000)
Males										
0-4	197	1 430	-	-	2.5	-	3	18.3	2	15.9
5-14	137	502	-	-	10.0	-	2	6.4	1	5.2
15-44	1 614	2 116	-	-	29.8	-	20	26.3	19	25.5
45-59	903	3 347	-	-	52.2	-	11	41.6	13	43.1
60+	382	1 822	-	-	70.0	-	6	29.1	8	30.8
All ages	3 233	1 956	-	-	38.3	-	42	25.2	44	25.7
Females										
0-4	137	1 046	-	-	2.5	-	2	13.4	1	11.9
5-14	38	142	-	-	10.0	-	0	1.8	0	1.6
15-44	221	295	-	-	29.9	-	3	3.7	3	3.8
45-59	192	641	-	-	52.4	-	2	8.0	3	8.0
60+	279	768	-	-	71.5	-	4	12.3	5	12.7
All ages	868	480	-	-	43.1	-	12	6.5	13	6.8
Total	4 101	1 184	-	-	39.3	-	54	15.5	57	15.8

Table 231c — India - India - Inde — Other unintentional injuries - Episodes

Age group (years)	Incidence 1990 Number ('000s)	Rate (per 100 000)	Prevalence 1990 Number ('000s)	Rate (per 100 000)	Avg. age at onset (years)	Average duration (years)	Deaths 1990 Number ('000s)	Rate (per 100 000)	Deaths 2000 (Projected) Number ('000s)	Rate (per 100 000)
Males										
0-4	1 661	2 777	-	-	2.5	-	22	38	21	37.8
5-14	1 809	1 778	-	-	10.0	-	25	24	19	17.1
15-44	2 671	1 332	-	-	29.8	-	34	17	39	15.6
45-59	1 304	2 741	-	-	52.3	-	17	35	21	34.6
60+	782	2 628	-	-	69.7	-	14	46	18	49.9
All ages	8 227	1 872	-	-	27.3	-	112	25	118	23.0
Females										
0-4	1 399	2 467	-	-	2.5	-	19	33	18	33.1
5-14	1 282	1 346	-	-	10.0	-	17	18	12	11.9
15-44	1 408	768	-	-	29.8	-	18	10	19	8.3
45-59	655	1 424	-	-	52.4	-	8	18	10	18.2
60+	701	2 424	-	-	70.1	-	12	42	19	48.7
All ages	5 445	1 328	-	-	26.0	-	75	18	79	16.3
Total	13 672	1 609	-	-	26.8	-	187	22	197	19.7

For the methods used to estimate and project incidence, prevalence, and deaths see Murray and Lopez 1996a. See explanatory notes for definitions and caveats.

Table 231
Other unintentional injuries

Episodes

Cuadro 231
Otras lesiones no intencionales

Episodios

Tableau 231
Autres traumatismes non-intentionnels

Episodes

Table 231d — China - China - Chine — Other unintentional injuries - Episodes

Age group (years)	Incidence 1990 Number ('000s)	Rate (per 100 000)	Prevalence 1990 Number ('000s)	Rate (per 100 000)	Avg. age at onset (years)	Average duration (years)	Deaths 1990 Number ('000s)	Rate (per 100 000)	Deaths 2000 (Projected) Number ('000s)	Rate (per 100 000)
Males										
0-4	2 063	3 424	-	-	2.5	-	26	43.8	23	39.5
5-14	578	596	-	-	10.0	-	7	7.7	6	4.9
15-44	4 775	1 559	-	-	29.9	-	59	19.4	49	15.2
45-59	1 271	1 748	-	-	52.3	-	16	21.7	19	19.0
60+	1 201	2 452	-	-	69.8	-	19	39.1	25	40.7
All ages	9 887	1 690	-	-	30.7	-	128	21.9	121	18.4
Females										
0-4	2 079	3 589	-	-	2.5	-	27	45.9	22	39.4
5-14	288	318	-	-	10.0	-	4	4.1	3	2.3
15-44	1 145	403	-	-	29.9	-	14	4.8	10	3.4
45-59	484	751	-	-	52.4	-	6	9.3	9	9.3
60+	732	1 416	-	-	70.6	-	12	22.6	19	30.2
All ages	4 728	862	-	-	25.2	-	62	11.2	63	10.0
Total	14 615	1 289	-	-	29.0	-	190	16.7	184	14.3

Table 231e — OAI - OPAI - APAI — Other unintentional injuries - Episodes

Age group (years)	Incidence 1990 Number ('000s)	Rate (per 100 000)	Prevalence 1990 Number ('000s)	Rate (per 100 000)	Avg. age at onset (years)	Average duration (years)	Deaths 1990 Number ('000s)	Rate (per 100 000)	Deaths 2000 (Projected) Number ('000s)	Rate (per 100 000)
Males										
0-4	922	2 107	-	-	2.5	-	12	27.0	11	24.1
5-14	1 030	1 225	-	-	10.0	-	13	15.7	9	11.3
15-44	3 984	2 477	-	-	29.7	-	50	30.8	55	26.8
45-59	874	2 561	-	-	52.3	-	11	31.8	14	30.3
60+	375	1 856	-	-	69.6	-	6	29.8	8	30.1
All ages	7 185	2 095	-	-	28.2	-	91	26.6	97	23.9
Females										
0-4	915	2 179	-	-	2.5	-	12	27.9	11	24.9
5-14	477	595	-	-	10.0	-	6	7.6	4	5.4
15-44	979	613	-	-	29.8	-	12	7.6	14	6.8
45-59	252	718	-	-	52.3	-	3	8.9	4	8.9
60+	225	992	-	-	70.3	-	4	15.9	5	16.9
All ages	2 848	839	-	-	22.9	-	37	10.8	38	9.5
Total	10 033	1 470	-	-	26.7	-	128	18.8	135	16.7

Table 231f — SSA - ASS - ASS — Other unintentional injuries - Episodes

Age group (years)	Incidence 1990 Number ('000s)	Rate (per 100 000)	Prevalence 1990 Number ('000s)	Rate (per 100 000)	Avg. age at onset (years)	Average duration (years)	Deaths 1990 Number ('000s)	Rate (per 100 000)	Deaths 2000 (Projected) Number ('000s)	Rate (per 100 000)
Males										
0-4	1 061	2 234	-	-	2.4	-	14	29	19	28
5-14	1 381	1 966	-	-	10.0	-	18	25	18	19
15-44	6 381	6 150	-	-	29.4	-	79	76	99	69
45-59	821	4 042	-	-	52.2	-	10	50	14	52
60+	361	3 438	-	-	69.2	-	6	55	8	58
All ages	10 005	3 965	-	-	27.2	-	126	50	158	46
Females										
0-4	771	1 639	-	-	2.4	-	10	21	13	21
5-14	1 087	1 557	-	-	10.0	-	14	20	14	15
15-44	900	847	-	-	29.5	-	11	11	15	10
45-59	188	850	-	-	52.2	-	2	11	3	11
60+	152	1 191	-	-	69.7	-	2	19	4	20
All ages	3 098	1 201	-	-	19.3	-	40	15	49	14
Total	13 103	2 568	-	-	25.3	-	166	33	207	30

For the methods used to estimate and project incidence, prevalence, and deaths see Murray and Lopez 1996a. See explanatory notes for definitions and caveats.

Table 231
Other unintentional injuries

Episodes

Cuadro 231
**Otras lesiones no
intencionales**
Episodios

Tableau 231
**Autres traumatismes
non-intentionnels**
Episodes

Table 231g   LAC - ALC - ALC   Other unintentional injuries - Episodes

Age group (years)	Incidence 1990 Number ('000s)	Rate (per 100 000)	Prevalence 1990 Number ('000s)	Rate (per 100 000)	Avg. age at onset (years)	Average duration (years)	Deaths 1990 Number ('000s)	Rate (per 100 000)	Deaths 2000 (Projected) Number ('000s)	Rate (per 100 000)
Males										
0-4	571	1 988	-	-	2.5	-	7	25.4	7	22.7
5-14	568	1 089	-	-	10.0	-	7	13.9	6	10.7
15-44	2 181	2 091	-	-	29.8	-	27	26.0	31	24.1
45-59	620	2 787	-	-	52.3	-	8	34.7	11	34.4
60+	476	3 342	-	-	70.3	-	8	53.4	11	56.0
All ages	4 415	1 992	-	-	31.2	-	57	25.7	65	24.6
Females										
0-4	447	1 616	-	-	2.5	-	6	20.7	5	18.7
5-14	241	475	-	-	10.0	-	3	6.1	3	4.7
15-44	656	630	-	-	29.9	-	8	7.8	10	7.5
45-59	162	694	-	-	52.4	-	2	8.6	3	8.6
60+	262	1 555	-	-	71.1	-	4	24.8	6	26.6
All ages	1 768	794	-	-	28.4	-	23	10.4	27	9.9
Total	6 183	1 392	-	-	30.4	-	80	18.0	92	17.2

Table 231h   MEC - AOM - CMO   Other unintentional injuries - Episodes

Age group (years)	Incidence 1990 Number ('000s)	Rate (per 100 000)	Prevalence 1990 Number ('000s)	Rate (per 100 000)	Avg. age at onset (years)	Average duration (years)	Deaths 1990 Number ('000s)	Rate (per 100 000)	Deaths 2000 (Projected) Number ('000s)	Rate (per 100 000)
Males										
0-4	766	1 860	-	-	2.5	-	10	23.8	12	23.3
5-14	512	784	-	-	10.0	-	7	10.0	7	7.9
15-44	1 605	1 409	-	-	29.8	-	20	17.5	25	16.5
45-59	349	1 562	-	-	52.3	-	4	19.4	6	20.2
60+	203	1 488	-	-	69.7	-	3	23.8	5	25.5
All ages	3 435	1 340	-	-	25.4	-	44	17.1	54	16.2
Females										
0-4	627	1 579	-	-	2.5	-	8	20.2	10	20.2
5-14	214	345	-	-	10.0	-	3	4.4	3	3.5
15-44	339	316	-	-	29.8	-	4	3.9	6	4.0
45-59	103	461	-	-	52.3	-	1	5.7	2	5.7
60+	127	821	-	-	70.4	-	2	13.1	3	14.0
All ages	1 410	572	-	-	19.9	-	18	7.4	23	7.1
Total	4 845	963	-	-	23.8	-	62	12.4	77	11.7

Table 231i   World - Mundo - Monde   Other unintentional injuries - Episodes

Age group (years)	Incidence 1990 Number ('000s)	Rate (per 100 000)	Prevalence 1990 Number ('000s)	Rate (per 100 000)	Avg. age at onset (years)	Average duration (years)	Deaths 1990 Number ('000s)	Rate (per 100 000)	Deaths 2000 (Projected) Number ('000s)	Rate (per 100 000)
Males										
0-4	7 394	2 301	-	-	2.5	-	96	29.8	96	27.7
5-14	6 123	1 111	-	-	10.0	-	80	14.5	67	10.7
15-44	24 526	1 962	-	-	29.8	-	306	24.5	329	22.8
45-59	6 853	2 194	-	-	52.3	-	86	27.4	107	26.5
60+	4 830	2 207	-	-	70.1	-	78	35.8	103	37.3
All ages	49 725	1 874	-	-	31.7	-	645	24.3	702	22.7
Females										
0-4	6 473	2 093	-	-	2.5	-	84	27.1	81	24.5
5-14	3 663	697	-	-	10.0	-	48	9.1	40	6.6
15-44	5 866	489	-	-	29.8	-	73	6.1	78	5.6
45-59	2 202	708	-	-	52.4	-	28	8.9	36	8.9
60+	3 306	1 228	-	-	71.2	-	54	20.0	76	22.6
All ages	21 511	823	-	-	30.3	-	286	11.0	311	10.2
Total	71 236	1 352	-	-	31.3	-	932	17.7	1 013	16.4

For the methods used to estimate and project incidence, prevalence, and deaths see Murray and Lopez 1996a. See explanatory notes for definitions and caveats.

Table 232
Other unintentional injuries
Injured spinal cord

Cuadro 232
Otras lesiones no intencionales
Lesión de la medula espinal

Tableau 232
Autres traumatismes non-intentionnels
Lésion de la moelle épinière

Table 232a   **EME - PEMC - EMBE**   Other unintentional injuries - Injured spinal cord

Age group (years)	Incidence 1990 Number ('000s)	Rate (per 100 000)	Prevalence 1990 Number ('000s)	Rate (per 100 000)	Avg. age at onset (years)	Average duration (years)	Deaths 1990 Number ('000s)	Rate (per 100 000)	Deaths 2000 (Projected) Number ('000s)	Rate (per 100 000)
Males										
0-4	0	0.2	0	0.4	2.5	57.1	-	-	-	-
5-14	0	0.1	1	1.2	10.0	51.1	-	-	-	-
15-44	5	2.6	71	38.4	29.9	33.6	-	-	-	-
45-59	3	3.8	62	94.5	52.4	15.6	-	-	-	-
60+	7	11.8	82	136.0	71.1	6.1	-	-	-	-
All ages	14	3.7	216	55.4	54.1	17.0	-	-	-	-
Females										
0-4	0	0.1	0	0.3	2.5	65.1	-	-	-	-
5-14	0	0.0	0	0.7	10.0	59.0	-	-	-	-
15-44	1	0.4	13	7.2	30.0	40.2	-	-	-	-
45-59	1	0.9	13	19.2	52.4	20.5	-	-	-	-
60+	6	6.7	58	68.3	72.4	7.9	-	-	-	-
All ages	7	1.7	84	20.7	65.6	12.8	-	-	-	-
Total	22	2.7	300	37.7	57.9	15.6	-	-	-	-

Table 232b   **FSE - PEAS - AESE**   Other unintentional injuries - Injured spinal cord

Age group (years)	Incidence 1990 Number ('000s)	Rate (per 100 000)	Prevalence 1990 Number ('000s)	Rate (per 100 000)	Avg. age at onset (years)	Average duration (years)	Deaths 1990 Number ('000s)	Rate (per 100 000)	Deaths 2000 (Projected) Number ('000s)	Rate (per 100 000)
Males										
0-4	0	0.4	0	1.1	2.5	48.3	-	-	-	-
5-14	0	0.2	1	2.9	10.0	43.1	-	-	-	-
15-44	6	7.6	83	108.3	29.8	26.8	-	-	-	-
45-59	3	11.9	66	244.6	52.2	11.9	-	-	-	-
60+	3	12.4	43	206.7	70.0	5.2	-	-	-	-
All ages	12	7.1	193	116.6	44.7	18.0	-	-	-	-
Females										
0-4	0	0.3	0	0.8	2.5	59.8	-	-	-	-
5-14	0	0.0	0	1.8	10.0	54.5	-	-	-	-
15-44	1	1.1	13	17.4	29.9	36.2	-	-	-	-
45-59	1	2.3	14	46.1	52.4	17.4	-	-	-	-
60+	2	5.2	26	71.2	71.5	6.7	-	-	-	-
All ages	3	1.9	53	29.5	57.0	16.5	-	-	-	-
Total	15	4.4	246	71.1	47.5	17.7	-	-	-	-

Table 232c   **India - India - Inde**   Other unintentional injuries - Injured spinal cord

Age group (years)	Incidence 1990 Number ('000s)	Rate (per 100 000)	Prevalence 1990 Number ('000s)	Rate (per 100 000)	Avg. age at onset (years)	Average duration (years)	Deaths 1990 Number ('000s)	Rate (per 100 000)	Deaths 2000 (Projected) Number ('000s)	Rate (per 100 000)
Males										
0-4	1	0.9	1	2.0	2.5	40.0	-	-	-	-
5-14	1	0.6	7	6.7	10.0	43.1	-	-	-	-
15-44	1	4.9	16	77.2	29.8	28.1	-	-	-	-
45-59	5	10.0	89	187.0	52.3	12.7	-	-	-	-
60+	6	19.5	65	216.7	69.7	4.9	-	-	-	-
All ages	13	4.9	177	68.4	54.4	12.9	-	-	-	-
Females										
0-4	0	0.8	1	1.8	2.5	40.1	-	-	-	-
5-14	0	0.4	5	5.5	10.0	44.5	-	-	-	-
15-44	5	2.9	86	46.9	29.8	30.0	-	-	-	-
45-59	2	5.2	51	110.6	52.4	14.3	-	-	-	-
60+	5	18.0	49	171.0	70.1	5.3	-	-	-	-
All ages	14	3.3	193	47.0	47.5	18.7	-	-	-	-
Total	26	3.9	370	55.3	50.8	15.9	-	-	-	-

For the methods used to estimate and project incidence, prevalence, and deaths see Lozano et al. 1996 and Murray and Lopez 1996a. See explanatory notes for definitions and caveats.

Table 232
Other unintentional injuries

Injured spinal cord

Cuadro 232
Otras lesiones no
intencionales

Lesión de la medula espinal

Tableau 232
Autres traumatismes
non-intentionnels

Lésion de la moelle épinière

Table 232d   China - China - Chine   Other unintentional injuries - Injured spinal cord

Age group (years)	Incidence 1990 Number ('000s)	Rate (per 100 000)	Prevalence 1990 Number ('000s)	Rate (per 100 000)	Avg. age at onset (years)	Average duration (years)	Deaths 1990 Number ('000s)	Rate (per 100 000)	Deaths 2000 (Projected) Number ('000s)	Rate (per 100 000)
Males										
0-4	1	1.1	2	2.5	2.5	51.2	-	-	-	-
5-14	0	0.2	6	5.9	10.0	47.6	-	-	-	-
15-44	17	5.6	264	86.3	29.9	30.4	-	-	-	-
45-59	5	6.2	135	185.7	52.3	13.1	-	-	-	-
60+	8	16.7	93	190.8	69.8	5.0	-	-	-	-
All ages	31	5.2	500	85.4	43.2	21.6	-	-	-	-
Females										
0-4	1	1.1	2	2.7	2.5	54.2	-	-	-	-
5-14	0	0.1	5	5.7	10.0	51.4	-	-	-	-
15-44	4	1.4	74	26.0	29.9	33.6	-	-	-	-
45-59	2	2.7	39	59.8	52.4	15.4	-	-	-	-
60+	5	9.6	50	97.2	70.6	5.7	-	-	-	-
All ages	11	2.1	169	30.9	49.5	19.9	-	-	-	-
Total	42	3.7	669	59.0	44.9	21.1	-	-	-	-

Table 232e   OAI - OPAI - APAI   Other unintentional injuries - Injured spinal cord

Age group (years)	Incidence 1990 Number ('000s)	Rate (per 100 000)	Prevalence 1990 Number ('000s)	Rate (per 100 000)	Avg. age at onset (years)	Average duration (years)	Deaths 1990 Number ('000s)	Rate (per 100 000)	Deaths 2000 (Projected) Number ('000s)	Rate (per 100 000)
Males										
0-4	0	0.6	1	1.5	2.5	41.2	-	-	-	-
5-14	0	0.4	4	4.7	10.0	41.5	-	-	-	-
15-44	14	8.8	205	127.3	29.7	26.7	-	-	-	-
45-59	3	9.1	89	260.5	52.3	11.8	-	-	-	-
60+	0	12.7	4	199.5	69.6	4.7	-	-	-	-
All ages	18	5.6	302	93.1	33.4	24.3	-	-	-	-
Females										
0-4	0	0.7	1	1.6	2.5	45.0	-	-	-	-
5-14	0	0.2	3	3.9	10.0	44.6	-	-	-	-
15-44	3	2.2	56	34.9	29.8	29.4	-	-	-	-
45-59	1	2.6	26	72.7	52.3	13.7	-	-	-	-
60+	2	6.8	18	80.0	70.3	5.4	-	-	-	-
All ages	6	1.9	103	30.4	41.1	22.4	-	-	-	-
Total	25	3.7	406	61.0	35.4	23.8	-	-	-	-

Table 232f   SSA - ASS - ASS   Other unintentional injuries - Injured spinal cord

Age group (years)	Incidence 1990 Number ('000s)	Rate (per 100 000)	Prevalence 1990 Number ('000s)	Rate (per 100 000)	Avg. age at onset (years)	Average duration (years)	Deaths 1990 Number ('000s)	Rate (per 100 000)	Deaths 2000 (Projected) Number ('000s)	Rate (per 100 000)
Males										
0-4	0	0.7	1	1.4	2.4	25.2	-	-	-	-
5-14	0	0.6	4	5.4	10.0	31.1	-	-	-	-
15-44	23	21.9	287	276.8	29.4	21.3	-	-	-	-
45-59	3	14.4	100	491.1	52.2	10.6	-	-	-	-
60+	2	23.3	35	335.1	69.2	4.5	-	-	-	-
All ages	29	11.4	427	169.1	34.5	19.0	-	-	-	-
Females										
0-4	0	0.5	1	1.1	2.4	28.3	-	-	-	-
5-14	0	0.5	3	4.2	10.0	33.9	-	-	-	-
15-44	3	3.0	46	43.7	29.5	23.5	-	-	-	-
45-59	1	3.0	18	82.5	52.2	11.9	-	-	-	-
60+	1	8.1	11	84.4	69.7	4.9	-	-	-	-
All ages	5	2.1	79	30.6	37.5	19.4	-	-	-	-
Total	34	6.7	506	99.1	35.0	19.1	-	-	-	-

For the methods used to estimate and project incidence, prevalence, and deaths see Lozano et al. 1996 and Murray and Lopez 1996a. See explanatory notes for definitions and caveats.

Table 232
Other unintentional injuries

Cuadro 232
Otras lesiones no intencionales

Tableau 232
Autres traumatismes non-intentionnels

Injured spinal cord

Lesión de la medula espinal

Lésion de la moelle épinière

Table 232g   LAC - ALC - ALC   Other unintentional injuries - Injured spinal cord

Age group (years)	Incidence 1990 Number ('000s)	Rate (per 100 000)	Prevalence 1990 Number ('000s)	Rate (per 100 000)	Avg. age at onset (years)	Average duration (years)	Deaths 1990 Number ('000s)	Rate (per 100 000)	Deaths 2000 (Projected) Number ('000s)	Rate (per 100 000)
Males										
0-4	0	0.6	0	1.4	2.5	46.5	-	-	-	-
5-14	0	0.3	2	4.5	10.0	45.1	-	-	-	-
15-44	8	7.5	115	110.1	29.4	29.4	-	-	-	-
45-59	2	9.9	55	248.6	52.3	13.4	-	-	-	-
60+	3	22.7	39	275.3	70.3	5.4	-	-	-	-
All ages	14	6.1	212	95.7	42.5	21.5	-	-	-	-
Females										
0-4	0	0.5	0	1.2	2.5	51.7	-	-	-	-
5-14	0	0.1	2	3.0	10.0	49.5	-	-	-	-
15-44	2	2.3	37	35.6	29.8	33.0	-	-	-	-
45-59	1	2.5	18	77.2	52.4	16.2	-	-	-	-
60+	2	10.6	20	116.6	71.1	6.2	-	-	-	-
All ages	5	2.2	77	34.4	46.4	22.1	-	-	-	-
Total	18	4.2	289	65.0	43.5	21.7	-	-	-	-

Table 232h   MEC - AOM - CMO   Other unintentional injuries - Injured spinal cord

Age group (years)	Incidence 1990 Number ('000s)	Rate (per 100 000)	Prevalence 1990 Number ('000s)	Rate (per 100 000)	Avg. age at onset (years)	Average duration (years)	Deaths 1990 Number ('000s)	Rate (per 100 000)	Deaths 2000 (Projected) Number ('000s)	Rate (per 100 000)
Males										
0-4	0	0.6	1	1.3	2.5	42.6	-	-	-	-
5-14	0	0.2	2	3.7	10.0	44.6	-	-	-	-
15-44	6	5.0	86	75.5	29.8	28.5	-	-	-	-
45-59	1	5.6	35	158.6	52.3	12.3	-	-	-	-
60+	1	10.1	19	137.1	69.7	4.9	-	-	-	-
All ages	9	3.4	143	55.8	38.2	23.1	-	-	-	-
Females										
0-4	0	0.5	0	1.1	2.5	45.1	-	-	-	-
5-14	0	0.1	2	2.6	10.0	47.5	-	-	-	-
15-44	1	1.1	20	19.0	29.8	31.1	-	-	-	-
45-59	0	1.6	9	41.6	52.3	14.3	-	-	-	-
60+	1	5.6	9	57.5	70.4	5.5	-	-	-	-
All ages	3	1.1	41	16.5	43.4	22.0	-	-	-	-
Total	11	2.3	184	36.5	39.4	22.9	-	-	-	-

Table 232i   World - Mundo - Monde   Other unintentional injuries - Injured spinal cord

Age group (years)	Incidence 1990 Number ('000s)	Rate (per 100 000)	Prevalence 1990 Number ('000s)	Rate (per 100 000)	Avg. age at onset (years)	Average duration (years)	Deaths 1990 Number ('000s)	Rate (per 100 000)	Deaths 2000 (Projected) Number ('000s)	Rate (per 100 000)
Males										
0-4	2	0.7	5	1.6	2.5	42.5	-	-	-	-
5-14	2	0.3	27	4.8	10.0	41.0	-	-	-	-
15-44	79	6.3	1 126	90.1	29.7	26.8	-	-	-	-
45-59	25	7.9	632	202.3	52.3	12.6	-	-	-	-
60+	31	14.2	381	174.0	70.1	5.2	-	-	-	-
All ages	139	5.2	2 170	81.8	42.0	19.9	-	-	-	-
Females										
0-4	2	0.7	5	1.5	2.5	45.9	-	-	-	-
5-14	1	0.2	21	3.9	10.0	42.7	-	-	-	-
15-44	21	1.8	345	28.8	29.8	30.6	-	-	-	-
45-59	8	2.5	187	60.2	52.4	15.1	-	-	-	-
60+	23	8.5	241	89.4	71.0	6.2	-	-	-	-
All ages	55	2.1	799	30.6	48.8	19.0	-	-	-	-
Total	194	3.7	2 969	56.4	43.9	19.7	-	-	-	-

For the methods used to estimate and project incidence, prevalence, and deaths see Lozano et al. 1996 and Murray and Lopez 1996a. See explanatory notes for definitions and caveats.

Table 233
Other unintentional injuries

Intracranial injury - long term

Cuadro 233
Otras lesiones no intencionales

Lesión intracraneal - larga duración

Tableau 233
Autres traumatismes non-intentionnels

Lésions intra-crâniennes - long terme

Table 233a EME - PEMC - EMBE Other unintentional injuries - Intracranial injury - long term

Age group (years)	Incidence 1990 Number ('000s)	Rate (per 100 000)	Prevalence 1990 Number ('000s)	Rate (per 100 000)	Avg. age at onset (years)	Average duration (years)	Deaths 1990 Number ('000s)	Rate (per 100 000)	Deaths 2000 (Projected) Number ('000s)	Rate (per 100 000)
Males										
0-4	1	4.8	3	11.9	2.5	70.2	-	-	-	-
5-14	1	1.6	17	32.0	10.0	63.6	-	-	-	-
15-44	5	2.7	148	80.3	29.9	44.8	-	-	-	-
45-59	3	4.1	100	150.8	52.4	24.5	-	-	-	-
60+	4	7.1	158	260.6	71.1	11.3	-	-	-	-
All ages	14	3.6	426	109.0	43.1	34.1	-	-	-	-
Females										
0-4	1	3.2	2	8.0	2.5	76.1	-	-	-	-
5-14	0	0.6	10	18.7	10.0	69.5	-	-	-	-
15-44	1	0.5	51	28.5	30.0	50.0	-	-	-	-
45-59	1	0.9	29	42.2	52.4	28.8	-	-	-	-
60+	3	4.0	84	99.1	72.4	12.7	-	-	-	-
All ages	6	1.5	175	43.0	52.0	30.9	-	-	-	-
Total	20	2.5	601	75.3	45.7	33.1	-	-	-	-

Table 233b FSE - PEAS - AESE Other unintentional injuries - Intracranial injury - long term

Age group (years)	Incidence 1990 Number ('000s)	Rate (per 100 000)	Prevalence 1990 Number ('000s)	Rate (per 100 000)	Avg. age at onset (years)	Average duration (years)	Deaths 1990 Number ('000s)	Rate (per 100 000)	Deaths 2000 (Projected) Number ('000s)	Rate (per 100 000)
Males										
0-4	2	11.7	4	29	2.5	63.5	-	-	-	-
5-14	1	4.1	22	79	10.0	57.3	-	-	-	-
15-44	6	8.0	165	217	29.8	39.2	-	-	-	-
45-59	3	12.6	115	428	52.2	20.8	-	-	-	-
60+	2	7.5	126	600	70.0	10.1	-	-	-	-
All ages	14	8.3	432	261	35.1	35.7	-	-	-	-
Females										
0-4	1	8.5	3	21	2.5	72.4	-	-	-	-
5-14	0	1.2	13	48	10.0	66.0	-	-	-	-
15-44	1	1.1	53	71	29.9	46.8	-	-	-	-
45-59	1	2.4	32	105	52.4	26.1	-	-	-	-
60+	1	3.2	58	160	71.5	11.8	-	-	-	-
All ages	4	2.3	158	88	36.5	41.8	-	-	-	-
Total	18	5.2	590	170	35.4	37.1	-	-	-	-

Table 233c India - India - Inde Other unintentional injuries - Intracranial injury - long term

Age group (years)	Incidence 1990 Number ('000s)	Rate (per 100 000)	Prevalence 1990 Number ('000s)	Rate (per 100 000)	Avg. age at onset (years)	Average duration (years)	Deaths 1990 Number ('000s)	Rate (per 100 000)	Deaths 2000 (Projected) Number ('000s)	Rate (per 100 000)
Males										
0-4	14	24.0	35	59	2.5	59.9	-	-	-	-
5-14	16	15.4	199	196	10.0	57.4	-	-	-	-
15-44	10	5.2	698	348	29.8	39.9	-	-	-	-
45-59	5	10.6	240	504	52.3	21.0	-	-	-	-
60+	3	11.7	208	698	69.7	9.7	-	-	-	-
All ages	49	11.1	1 380	314	20.6	47.3	-	-	-	-
Females										
0-4	12	21.3	30	52	2.5	60.8	-	-	-	-
5-14	11	11.7	157	164	10.0	59.1	-	-	-	-
15-44	6	3.0	489	267	29.8	41.7	-	-	-	-
45-59	3	5.5	162	353	52.3	22.5	-	-	-	-
60+	3	10.9	146	504	70.1	10.2	-	-	-	-
All ages	34	8.4	983	240	19.1	49.8	-	-	-	-
Total	83	9.8	2 363	278	20.0	48.3	-	-	-	-

For the methods used to estimate and project incidence, prevalence, and deaths see Lozano et al. 1996 and Murray and Lopez 1996a. See explanatory notes for definitions and caveats.

Table 233
Other unintentional injuries

Intracranial injury - long term

Cuadro 233
Otras lesiones no intencionales

Lesión intracraneal - larga duración

Tableau 233
Autres traumatismes non-intentionnels

Lésions intra-crâniennes - long terme

Table 233d   China - China - Chine   Other unintentional injuries - Intracranial injury - long term

Age group (years)	Incidence 1990 Number ('000s)	Rate (per 100 000)	Prevalence 1990 Number ('000s)	Rate (per 100 000)	Avg. age at onset (years)	Average duration (years)	Deaths 1990 Number ('000s)	Rate (per 100 000)	Deaths 2000 (Projected) Number ('000s)	Rate (per 100 000)
Males										
0-4	17	28.0	42	69	2.5	65.5	-	-	-	-
5-14	5	4.9	159	163	10.0	59.9	-	-	-	-
15-44	18	5.9	841	275	29.9	41.2	-	-	-	-
45-59	5	6.6	299	411	52.3	21.4	-	-	-	-
60+	5	10.1	274	559	69.8	9.9	-	-	-	-
All ages	49	8.4	1 614	276	24.8	46.3	-	-	-	-
Females										
0-4	17	29.3	42	73	2.5	68.5	-	-	-	-
5-14	2	2.6	144	159	10.0	63.2	-	-	-	-
15-44	4	1.5	549	193	29.9	44.2	-	-	-	-
45-59	2	2.8	152	236	52.4	23.8	-	-	-	-
60+	3	5.8	165	319	70.6	10.8	-	-	-	-
All ages	28	5.2	1 052	192	17.6	55.5	-	-	-	-
Total	78	6.8	2 666	235	22.1	49.6	-	-	-	-

Table 233e   OAI - OPAI - APAI   Other unintentional injuries - Intracranial injury - long term

Age group (years)	Incidence 1990 Number ('000s)	Rate (per 100 000)	Prevalence 1990 Number ('000s)	Rate (per 100 000)	Avg. age at onset (years)	Average duration (years)	Deaths 1990 Number ('000s)	Rate (per 100 000)	Deaths 2000 (Projected) Number ('000s)	Rate (per 100 000)
Males										
0-4	8	17.2	19	42	2.5	59.8	-	-	-	-
5-14	8	10.0	114	136	10.0	56.2	-	-	-	-
15-44	15	9.3	519	323	29.7	38.8	-	-	-	-
45-59	3	9.6	182	534	52.3	20.3	-	-	-	-
60+	2	7.7	138	681	69.6	9.7	-	-	-	-
All ages	36	10.4	971	283	23.1	44.4	-	-	-	-
Females										
0-4	7	17.8	18	44	2.5	63.2	-	-	-	-
5-14	4	4.9	91	113	10.0	59.2	-	-	-	-
15-44	4	2.3	273	171	29.8	41.5	-	-	-	-
45-59	1	2.7	79	226	52.3	22.4	-	-	-	-
60+	1	4.1	65	289	70.3	10.5	-	-	-	-
All ages	17	5.0	527	155	16.7	52.4	-	-	-	-
Total	53	7.7	1 498	219	21.1	46.9	-	-	-	-

Table 233f   SSA - ASS - ASS   Other unintentional injuries - Intracranial injury - long term

Age group (years)	Incidence 1990 Number ('000s)	Rate (per 100 000)	Prevalence 1990 Number ('000s)	Rate (per 100 000)	Avg. age at onset (years)	Average duration (years)	Deaths 1990 Number ('000s)	Rate (per 100 000)	Deaths 2000 (Projected) Number ('000s)	Rate (per 100 000)
Males										
0-4	9	18.2	21	44	2.4	48.7	-	-	-	-
5-14	11	16.1	120	171	10.0	49.2	-	-	-	-
15-44	24	23.1	604	582	29.3	35.0	-	-	-	-
45-59	3	15.2	213	1 048	52.2	19.1	-	-	-	-
60+	1	14.1	136	1 297	69.2	9.3	-	-	-	-
All ages	48	19.2	1 094	434	22.7	39.0	-	-	-	-
Females										
0-4	6	13.4	15	32	2.4	51.9	-	-	-	-
5-14	9	12.7	91	130	10.0	51.9	-	-	-	-
15-44	3	3.2	255	240	29.5	37.2	-	-	-	-
45-59	1	3.2	69	312	52.2	20.5	-	-	-	-
60+	1	4.9	49	384	69.7	9.8	-	-	-	-
All ages	20	7.7	478	185	14.3	47.0	-	-	-	-
Total	68	13.4	1 572	308	20.2	41.3	-	-	-	-

For the methods used to estimate and project incidence, prevalence, and deaths see Lozano et al. 1996 and Murray and Lopez 1996a. See explanatory notes for definitions and caveats.

Table 233
Other unintentional injuries

Intracranial injury - long term

Cuadro 233
Otras lesiones no intencionales

Lesión intracraneal - larga duración

Tableau 233
Autres traumatismes non-intentionnels

Lésions intra-crâniennes - long terme

Table 233g　　LAC - ALC - ALC　　Other unintentional injuries - Intracranial injury - long term

Age group (years)	Incidence 1990 Number ('000s)	Rate (per 100 000)	Prevalence 1990 Number ('000s)	Rate (per 100 000)	Avg. age at onset (years)	Average duration (years)	Deaths 1990 Number ('000s)	Rate (per 100 000)	Deaths 2000 (Projected) Number ('000s)	Rate (per 100 000)
Males										
0-4	5	16.2	12	40	2.5	63.9	-	-	-	-
5-14	5	8.9	65	125	10.0	59.3	-	-	-	-
15-44	8	7.9	298	286	29.8	41.5	-	-	-	-
45-59	2	10.5	107	481	52.3	22.3	-	-	-	-
60+	2	13.7	100	702	70.3	10.4	-	-	-	-
All ages	22	9.8	582	263	25.8	45.2	-	-	-	-
Females										
0-4	4	13.2	9	33	2.5	67.9	-	-	-	-
5-14	2	3.9	43	85	10.0	63.0	-	-	-	-
15-44	2	2.4	145	140	29.8	44.6	-	-	-	-
45-59	1	2.6	45	195	52.4	24.8	-	-	-	-
60+	1	6.4	48	285	71.1	11.3	-	-	-	-
All ages	10	4.4	291	131	21.6	52.1	-	-	-	-
Total	32	7.1	873	196	24.5	47.4	-	-	-	-

Table 233h　　MEC - AOM - CMO　　Other unintentional injuries - Intracranial injury - long term

Age group (years)	Incidence 1990 Number ('000s)	Rate (per 100 000)	Prevalence 1990 Number ('000s)	Rate (per 100 000)	Avg. age at onset (years)	Average duration (years)	Deaths 1990 Number ('000s)	Rate (per 100 000)	Deaths 2000 (Projected) Number ('000s)	Rate (per 100 000)
Males										
0-4	6	15.2	15	37	2.5	61.1	-	-	-	-
5-14	4	6.4	70	108	10.0	58.1	-	-	-	-
15-44	6	5.3	248	218	29.8	40.0	-	-	-	-
45-59	1	5.9	76	341	52.3	20.8	-	-	-	-
60+	1	6.1	61	445	69.7	9.8	-	-	-	-
All ages	19	7.3	471	184	19.5	48.5	-	-	-	-
Females										
0-4	5	12.9	13	32	2.5	63.7	-	-	-	-
5-14	2	2.8	49	78	10.0	60.9	-	-	-	-
15-44	1	1.2	118	110	29.8	42.6	-	-	-	-
45-59	0	1.7	31	141	52.3	22.9	-	-	-	-
60+	1	3.4	29	189	70.4	10.6	-	-	-	-
All ages	9	3.7	240	97	13.8	55.4	-	-	-	-
Total	28	5.5	710	141	17.7	50.7	-	-	-	-

Table 233i　　World - Mundo - Monde　　Other unintentional injuries - Intracranial injury - long term

Age group (years)	Incidence 1990 Number ('000s)	Rate (per 100 000)	Prevalence 1990 Number ('000s)	Rate (per 100 000)	Avg. age at onset (years)	Average duration (years)	Deaths 1990 Number ('000s)	Rate (per 100 000)	Deaths 2000 (Projected) Number ('000s)	Rate (per 100 000)
Males										
0-4	61	19.0	150	47	2.5	60.6	-	-	-	-
5-14	51	9.2	766	139	10.0	56.0	-	-	-	-
15-44	93	7.4	3 522	282	29.7	39.1	-	-	-	-
45-59	26	8.3	1 332	426	52.3	21.2	-	-	-	-
60+	20	9.2	1 200	548	70.1	10.2	-	-	-	-
All ages	251	9.4	6 970	263	24.6	43.6	-	-	-	-
Females										
0-4	54	17.3	132	43	2.5	63.8	-	-	-	-
5-14	31	5.8	595	113	10.0	57.8	-	-	-	-
15-44	22	1.8	1 933	161	29.8	42.3	-	-	-	-
45-59	8	2.7	600	193	52.3	23.6	-	-	-	-
60+	14	5.1	644	239	71.0	11.2	-	-	-	-
All ages	128	4.9	3 903	149	19.6	50.4	-	-	-	-
Total	379	7.2	10 873	206	22.9	45.9	-	-	-	-

For the methods used to estimate and project incidence, prevalence, and deaths see Lozano et al. 1996 and Murray and Lopez 1996a. See explanatory notes for definitions and caveats.

Table 234
Other unintentional injuries

Amputated finger

Cuadro 234
Otras lesiones no
intencionales

Amputación de dedo de la mano

Tableau 234
Autres traumatismes
non-intentionnels

Amputation d'un doigt

Table 234a EME - PEMC - EMBE Other unintentional injuries - Amputated finger

Age group (years)	Incidence 1990 Number ('000s)	Rate (per 100 000)	Prevalence 1990 Number ('000s)	Rate (per 100 000)	Avg. age at onset (years)	Average duration (years)	Deaths 1990 Number ('000s)	Rate (per 100 000)	Deaths 2000 (Projected) Number ('000s)	Rate (per 100 000)
Males										
0-4	2	8.8	6	22	2.5	70.2	-	-	-	-
5-14	2	3.0	31	59	10.0	63.6	-	-	-	-
15-44	16	8.8	377	205	29.9	44.7	-	-	-	-
45-59	9	13.2	287	435	52.4	24.5	-	-	-	-
60+	14	23.7	482	796	71.1	11.3	-	-	-	-
All ages	43	11.1	1 183	303	45.9	31.6	-	-	-	-
Females										
0-4	1	5.8	4	15	2.5	76.1	-	-	-	-
5-14	1	1.1	17	34	10.0	69.5	-	-	-	-
15-44	3	1.5	111	62	30.0	50.0	-	-	-	-
45-59	2	3.0	73	107	52.5	28.8	-	-	-	-
60+	11	13.4	250	295	72.4	12.7	-	-	-	-
All ages	18	4.4	455	112	56.3	26.9	-	-	-	-
Total	61	7.7	1 638	205	49.0	30.2	-	-	-	-

Table 234b FSE - PEAS - AESE Other unintentional injuries - Amputated finger

Age group (years)	Incidence 1990 Number ('000s)	Rate (per 100 000)	Prevalence 1990 Number ('000s)	Rate (per 100 000)	Avg. age at onset (years)	Average duration (years)	Deaths 1990 Number ('000s)	Rate (per 100 000)	Deaths 2000 (Projected) Number ('000s)	Rate (per 100 000)
Males										
0-4	3	21.4	7	53	2.5	63.5	-	-	-	-
5-14	2	7.5	39	144	10.0	57.3	-	-	-	-
15-44	20	26.0	430	564	29.8	39.2	-	-	-	-
45-59	11	41.1	338	1 251	52.2	20.8	-	-	-	-
60+	5	24.9	380	1 811	70.0	10.1	-	-	-	-
All ages	41	24.9	1 194	722	38.0	33.2	-	-	-	-
Females										
0-4	2	15.7	5	39	2.5	72.4	-	-	-	-
5-14	1	2.1	23	89	10.0	66.0	-	-	-	-
15-44	3	3.6	115	153	30.0	46.8	-	-	-	-
45-59	2	7.9	80	266	52.4	26.1	-	-	-	-
60+	4	10.5	162	446	71.5	11.8	-	-	-	-
All ages	12	6.4	386	213	42.4	36.4	-	-	-	-
Total	53	15.2	1 580	456	39.0	33.9	-	-	-	-

Table 234c India - India - Inde Other unintentional injuries - Amputated finger

Age group (years)	Incidence 1990 Number ('000s)	Rate (per 100 000)	Prevalence 1990 Number ('000s)	Rate (per 100 000)	Avg. age at onset (years)	Average duration (years)	Deaths 1990 Number ('000s)	Rate (per 100 000)	Deaths 2000 (Projected) Number ('000s)	Rate (per 100 000)
Males										
0-4	26	44	64	108	2.5	59.9	-	-	-	-
5-14	29	28	365	359	10.0	57.4	-	-	-	-
15-44	34	17	1 497	747	29.8	39.9	-	-	-	-
45-59	16	35	596	1 253	52.3	21.0	-	-	-	-
60+	12	39	562	1 887	69.7	9.7	-	-	-	-
All ages	117	27	3 085	702	25.9	43.0	-	-	-	-
Females										
0-4	22	39	54	96	2.5	60.8	-	-	-	-
5-14	20	21	287	301	10.0	59.1	-	-	-	-
15-44	18	10	1 012	552	29.8	41.7	-	-	-	-
45-59	8	18	383	833	52.4	22.5	-	-	-	-
60+	10	36	384	1 329	70.1	10.2	-	-	-	-
All ages	79	19	2 120	517	24.7	45.4	-	-	-	-
Total	196	23	5 205	613	25.4	44.0	-	-	-	-

For the methods used to estimate and project incidence, prevalence, and deaths see Lozano et al. 1996 and Murray and Lopez 1996a. See explanatory notes for definitions and caveats.

Table 234
Other unintentional injuries
Amputated finger

Cuadro 234
Otras lesiones no intencionales
Amputación de dedo de la mano

Tableau 234
Autres traumatismes non-intentionnels
Amputation d'un doigt

Table 234d China - China - Chine — Other unintentional injuries - Amputated finger

Age group (years)	Incidence 1990 Number ('000s)	Rate (per 100 000)	Prevalence 1990 Number ('000s)	Rate (per 100 000)	Avg. age at onset (years)	Average duration (years)	Deaths 1990 Number ('000s)	Rate (per 100 000)	Deaths 2000 (Projected) Number ('000s)	Rate (per 100 000)
Males										
0-4	31	51.3	77	127	2.5	65.5	-	-	-	-
5-14	9	8.9	290	299	10.0	59.9	-	-	-	-
15-44	59	19.1	1 921	627	29.9	41.2	-	-	-	-
45-59	16	21.5	778	1 071	52.3	21.4	-	-	-	-
60+	16	33.4	762	1 556	69.8	9.9	-	-	-	-
All ages	130	22.2	3 828	654	29.8	41.9	-	-	-	-
Females										
0-4	31	53.7	77	133	2.5	68.5	-	-	-	-
5-14	4	4.8	263	291	10.0	63.2	-	-	-	-
15-44	13	4.7	1 094	385	29.9	44.2	-	-	-	-
45-59	6	9.2	338	524	52.4	23.8	-	-	-	-
60+	10	19.3	412	798	70.6	10.8	-	-	-	-
All ages	65	11.8	2 184	398	23.7	50.1	-	-	-	-
Total	195	17.2	6 012	530	27.8	44.6	-	-	-	-

Table 234e OAI - OPAI - APAI — Other unintentional injuries - Amputated finger

Age group (years)	Incidence 1990 Number ('000s)	Rate (per 100 000)	Prevalence 1990 Number ('000s)	Rate (per 100 000)	Avg. age at onset (years)	Average duration (years)	Deaths 1990 Number ('000s)	Rate (per 100 000)	Deaths 2000 (Projected) Number ('000s)	Rate (per 100 000)
Males										
0-4	14	31.6	34	78	2.5	59.8	-	-	-	-
5-14	15	18.4	209	249	10.0	56.2	-	-	-	-
15-44	49	30.4	1 264	786	29.7	38.8	-	-	-	-
45-59	11	31.5	502	1 471	52.3	20.3	-	-	-	-
60+	5	25.5	394	1 951	69.6	9.7	-	-	-	-
All ages	94	27.4	2 403	701	27.2	41.0	-	-	-	-
Females										
0-4	14	32.6	34	81	2.5	63.2	-	-	-	-
5-14	7	8.9	166	207	10.0	59.2	-	-	-	-
15-44	12	7.5	578	362	229.8	41.4	-	-	-	-
45-59	3	8.8	187	534	52.3	22.4	-	-	-	-
60+	3	13.5	169	747	70.3	10.5	-	-	-	-
All ages	39	11.5	1 135	334	83.2	48.4	-	-	-	-
Total	133	19.5	3 538	518	43.6	43.2	-	-	-	-

Table 234f SSA - ASS - ASS — Other unintentional injuries - Amputated finger

Age group (years)	Incidence 1990 Number ('000s)	Rate (per 100 000)	Prevalence 1990 Number ('000s)	Rate (per 100 000)	Avg. age at onset (years)	Average duration (years)	Deaths 1990 Number ('000s)	Rate (per 100 000)	Deaths 2000 (Projected) Number ('000s)	Rate (per 100 000)
Males										
0-4	16	33	38	80	2.4	48.7	-	-	-	-
5-14	21	29	219	312	10.0	49.2	-	-	-	-
15-44	78	75	1 592	1 534	29.4	35.0	-	-	-	-
45-59	10	50	616	3 035	52.2	19.1	-	-	-	-
60+	5	47	402	3 829	69.2	9.3	-	-	-	-
All ages	130	51	2 869	1 137	26.3	36.7	-	-	-	-
Females										
0-4	12	25	28	59	2.4	51.9	-	-	-	-
5-14	16	23	166	238	10.0	51.9	-	-	-	-
15-44	11	10	536	505	29.5	37.2	-	-	-	-
45-59	2	10	164	740	52.3	20.5	-	-	-	-
60+	2	16	124	977	69.7	9.8	-	-	-	-
All ages	43	17	1 018	395	18.1	44.5	-	-	-	-
Total	173	34	3 887	762	24.2	38.7	-	-	-	-

For the methods used to estimate and project incidence, prevalence, and deaths see Lozano et al. 1996 and Murray and Lopez 1996a. See explanatory notes for definitions and caveats.

Table 234
Other unintentional injuries

Amputated finger

Cuadro 234
Otras lesiones no
intencionales
Amputación de dedo de la mano

Tableau 234
Autres traumatismes
non-intentionnels
Amputation d'un doigt

Table 234g LAC - ALC - ALC Other unintentional injuries - Amputated finger

Age group (years)	Incidence 1990 Number ('000s)	Rate (per 100 000)	Prevalence 1990 Number ('000s)	Rate (per 100 000)	Avg. age at onset (years)	Average duration (years)	Deaths 1990 Number ('000s)	Rate (per 100 000)	Deaths 2000 (Projected) Number ('000s)	Rate (per 100 000)
Males										
0-4	9	29.8	21	74	2.5	63.9	-	-	-	-
5-14	9	16.3	120	230	10.0	59.3	-	-	-	-
15-44	27	25.7	719	689	29.8	41.4	-	-	-	-
45-59	8	34.2	295	1 324	52.3	22.3	-	-	-	-
60+	6	45.6	291	2 045	70.3	10.4	-	-	-	-
All ages	58	26.1	1 445	652	30.4	41.4	-	-	-	-
Females										
0-4	7	24.2	17	60	2.5	67.9	-	-	-	-
5-14	4	7.1	79	156	10.0	63.0	-	-	-	-
15-44	8	7.7	319	306	29.9	44.6	-	-	-	-
45-59	2	8.5	113	486	52.4	24.8	-	-	-	-
60+	4	21.2	132	784	71.1	11.3	-	-	-	-
All ages	24	10.7	660	296	27.2	47.3	-	-	-	-
Total	82	18.4	2 105	474	29.4	43.1	-	-	-	-

Table 234h MEC - AOM - CMO Other unintentional injuries - Amputated finger

Age group (years)	Incidence 1990 Number ('000s)	Rate (per 100 000)	Prevalence 1990 Number ('000s)	Rate (per 100 000)	Avg. age at onset (years)	Average duration (years)	Deaths 1990 Number ('000s)	Rate (per 100 000)	Deaths 2000 (Projected) Number ('000s)	Rate (per 100 000)
Males										
0-4	11	27.9	28	68	2.5	61.1	-	-	-	-
5-14	8	11.7	129	197	10.0	58.1	-	-	-	-
15-44	20	17.3	582	511	29.8	40.0	-	-	-	-
45-59	4	19.2	204	911	52.3	20.8	-	-	-	-
60+	3	20.3	171	1 254	69.7	9.8	-	-	-	-
All ages	46	17.9	1 114	435	24.2	44.7	-	-	-	-
Females										
0-4	9	23.6	23	58	2.5	63.7	-	-	-	-
5-14	3	5.2	89	143	10.0	60.9	-	-	-	-
15-44	4	3.9	243	227	29.9	42.6	-	-	-	-
45-59	1	5.7	73	327	52.4	22.9	-	-	-	-
60+	2	11.2	75	487	70.4	10.6	-	-	-	-
All ages	20	8.0	503	204	18.6	51.5	-	-	-	-
Total	66	13.1	1 617	321	22.5	46.7	-	-	-	-

Table 234i World - Mundo - Monde Other unintentional injuries - Amputated finger

Age group (years)	Incidence 1990 Number ('000s)	Rate (per 100 000)	Prevalence 1990 Number ('000s)	Rate (per 100 000)	Avg. age at onset (years)	Average duration (years)	Deaths 1990 Number ('000s)	Rate (per 100 000)	Deaths 2000 (Projected) Number ('000s)	Rate (per 100 000)
Males										
0-4	112	34.9	276	86	2.5	60.6	-	-	-	-
5-14	93	16.9	1 403	255	10.0	56.0	-	-	-	-
15-44	302	24.2	8 382	671	29.7	39.1	-	-	-	-
45-59	85	27.1	3 616	1 158	52.3	21.2	-	-	-	-
60+	67	30.6	3 445	1 574	70.1	10.2	-	-	-	-
All ages	659	24.8	17 122	645	29.3	39.9	-	-	-	-
Females										
0-4	98	31.7	242	78	2.5	63.8	-	-	-	-
5-14	56	10.7	1 090	207	10.0	57.8	-	-	-	-
15-44	72	6.0	4 007	334	63.1	42.3	-	-	-	-
45-59	27	8.8	1 410	453	52.4	23.6	-	-	-	-
60+	46	17.1	1 710	635	71.0	11.2	-	-	-	-
All ages	300	11.5	8 459	324	33.5	45.8	-	-	-	-
Total	959	18.2	25 581	486	30.6	41.7	-	-	-	-

For the methods used to estimate and project incidence, prevalence, and deaths see Lozano et al. 1996 and Murray and Lopez 1996a. See explanatory notes for definitions and caveats.

Table 235
Other unintentional injuries

Burns <20% - long term

Cuadro 235
Otras lesiones no intencionales

Quemaduras <20% - larga duración

Tableau 235
Autres traumatismes non-intentionnels

Brûlures <20% - long terme

Table 235a   EME - PEMC - EMBE   Other unintentional injuries - Burns <20% - long term

Age group (years)	Incidence 1990 Number ('000s)	Rate (per 100 000)	Prevalence 1990 Number ('000s)	Rate (per 100 000)	Avg. age at onset (years)	Average duration (years)	Deaths 1990 Number ('000s)	Rate (per 100 000)	Deaths 2000 (Projected) Number ('000s)	Rate (per 100 000)
Males										
0-4	45	169	111	422	2.5	70.2	-	-	-	-
5-14	31	59	600	1 124	10.0	63.6	-	-	-	-
15-44	194	105	5 424	2 947	29.9	44.8	-	-	-	-
45-59	105	159	3 701	5 597	52.4	24.5	-	-	-	-
60+	49	81	4 577	7 560	71.1	11.3	-	-	-	-
All ages	424	109	14 414	3 691	35.9	39.9	-	-	-	-
Females										
0-4	28	113	71	282	2.5	76.2	-	-	-	-
5-14	10	20	333	658	10.0	69.5	-	-	-	-
15-44	32	18	1 837	1 025	30.0	50.0	-	-	-	-
45-59	24	36	1 056	1 558	52.4	28.8	-	-	-	-
60+	39	46	2 013	2 381	72.4	12.7	-	-	-	-
All ages	134	33	5 310	1 304	39.0	42.4	-	-	-	-
Total	558	70	19 724	2 472	36.6	40.5	-	-	-	-

Table 235b   FSE - PEAS - AESE   Other unintentional injuries - Burns <20% - long term

Age group (years)	Incidence 1990 Number ('000s)	Rate (per 100 000)	Prevalence 1990 Number ('000s)	Rate (per 100 000)	Avg. age at onset (years)	Average duration (years)	Deaths 1990 Number ('000s)	Rate (per 100 000)	Deaths 2000 (Projected) Number ('000s)	Rate (per 100 000)
Males										
0-4	57	415	141	1 027	2.5	63.5	-	-	-	-
5-14	40	146	750	2 741	10.0	57.3	-	-	-	-
15-44	238	311	5 924	7 766	29.8	39.2	-	-	-	-
45-59	133	493	4 084	15 139	52.2	20.8	-	-	-	-
60+	18	85	3 987	19 019	70.0	10.1	-	-	-	-
All ages	485	293	14 885	9 004	32.6	37.4	-	-	-	-
Females										
0-4	40	303	99	752	2.5	72.4	-	-	-	-
5-14	11	41	446	1 687	10.0	66.0	-	-	-	-
15-44	33	43	1 891	2 523	29.9	46.8	-	-	-	-
45-59	28	94	1 151	3 836	52.4	26.1	-	-	-	-
60+	13	36	1 788	4 913	71.5	11.8	-	-	-	-
All ages	125	69	5 375	2 971	28.9	48.3	-	-	-	-
Total	610	176	20 260	5 851	31.8	39.7	-	-	-	-

Table 235c   India - India - Inde   Other unintentional injuries - Burns <20% - long term

Age group (years)	Incidence 1990 Number ('000s)	Rate (per 100 000)	Prevalence 1990 Number ('000s)	Rate (per 100 000)	Avg. age at onset (years)	Average duration (years)	Deaths 1990 Number ('000s)	Rate (per 100 000)	Deaths 2000 (Projected) Number ('000s)	Rate (per 100 000)
Males										
0-4	508	850	1 229	2 056	2.5	59.9	-	-	-	-
5-14	556	546	6 826	6 709	10.0	57.5	-	-	-	-
15-44	407	203	23 819	11 878	29.8	39.9	-	-	-	-
45-59	197	414	8 143	17 119	52.3	21.0	-	-	-	-
60+	40	133	6 175	20 745	69.7	9.7	-	-	-	-
All ages	1 707	388	46 192	10 513	18.8	48.7	-	-	-	-
Females										
0-4	429	757	1 038	1 831	2.5	60.8	-	-	-	-
5-14	395	415	5 393	5 662	10.0	59.1	-	-	-	-
15-44	216	118	16 827	9 183	29.8	41.9	-	-	-	-
45-59	99	215	5 617	12 210	52.4	22.5	-	-	-	-
60+	36	123	4 252	14 702	70.1	10.2	-	-	-	-
All ages	1 175	287	33 129	8 078	16.3	52.0	-	-	-	-
Total	2 882	339	79 321	9 337	17.8	50.0	-	-	-	-

For the methods used to estimate and project incidence, prevalence, and deaths see Lozano et al. 1996 and Murray and Lopez 1996a. See explanatory notes for definitions and caveats.

Table 235
Other unintentional injuries

Burns <20% - long term

Cuadro 235
Otras lesiones no intencionales

Quemaduras <20% - larga duración

Tableau 235
Autres traumatismes non-intentionnels

Brûlures <20% - long terme

Table 235d   China - China - Chine   Other unintentional injuries - Burns <20% - long term

Age group (years)	Incidence 1990 Number ('000s)	Rate (per 100 000)	Prevalence 1990 Number ('000s)	Rate (per 100 000)	Avg. age at onset (years)	Average duration (years)	Deaths 1990 Number ('000s)	Rate (per 100 000)	Deaths 2000 (Projected) Number ('000s)	Rate (per 100 000)
Males										
0-4	598	992	1 463	2 428	2.5	65.5	-	-	-	-
5-14	168	173	5 430	5 598	10.0	59.9	-	-	-	-
15-44	702	229	31 810	10 385	29.9	41.3	-	-	-	-
45-59	187	257	11 554	15 899	52.3	21.4	-	-	-	-
60+	56	114	9 039	18 454	69.8	9.9	-	-	-	-
All ages	1 711	292	59 296	10 133	22.1	48.4	-	-	-	-
Females										
0-4	603	1 040	1 472	2 541	2.5	68.5	-	-	-	-
5-14	83	92	4 914	5 435	10.0	63.2	-	-	-	-
15-44	161	57	18 922	6 661	29.9	44.2	-	-	-	-
45-59	71	110	5 290	8 214	52.4	23.8	-	-	-	-
60+	34	66	4 968	9 616	70.6	10.8	-	-	-	-
All ages	953	174	35 566	6 484	14.0	58.5	-	-	-	-
Total	2 664	235	94 862	8 368	19.2	52.0	-	-	-	-

Table 235e   OAI - OPAI - APAI   Other unintentional injuries - Burns <20% - long term

Age group (years)	Incidence 1990 Number ('000s)	Rate (per 100 000)	Prevalence 1990 Number ('000s)	Rate (per 100 000)	Avg. age at onset (years)	Average duration (years)	Deaths 1990 Number ('000s)	Rate (per 100 000)	Deaths 2000 (Projected) Number ('000s)	Rate (per 100 000)
Males										
0-4	267	611	653	1 491	2.5	59.8	-	-	-	-
5-14	299	355	3 942	4 691	10.0	56.2	-	-	-	-
15-44	586	364	18 058	11 228	29.7	38.8	-	-	-	-
45-59	129	377	6 259	18 335	52.3	20.3	-	-	-	-
60+	18	87	4 312	21 338	69.6	9.7	-	-	-	-
All ages	1 298	379	33 224	9 687	22.3	44.9	-	-	-	-
Females										
0-4	265	632	649	1 545	2.5	63.2	-	-	-	-
5-14	138	172	3 133	3 906	10.0	59.2	-	-	-	-
15-44	144	90	9 554	5 986	29.8	41.5	-	-	-	-
45-59	37	106	2 803	7 988	52.3	22.4	-	-	-	-
60+	10	46	2 077	9 164	70.3	10.5	-	-	-	-
All ages	595	175	18 216	5 364	15.1	53.5	-	-	-	-
Total	1 893	277	51 439	7 537	20.1	47.6	-	-	-	-

Table 235f   SSA - ASS - ASS   Other unintentional injuries - Burns <20% - long term

Age group (years)	Incidence 1990 Number ('000s)	Rate (per 100 000)	Prevalence 1990 Number ('000s)	Rate (per 100 000)	Avg. age at onset (years)	Average duration (years)	Deaths 1990 Number ('000s)	Rate (per 100 000)	Deaths 2000 (Projected) Number ('000s)	Rate (per 100 000)
Males										
0-4	307	647	734	1 546	2.4	48.7	-	-	-	-
5-14	400	569	4 125	5 871	10.0	49.3	-	-	-	-
15-44	938	904	20 223	19 489	29.4	35.1	-	-	-	-
45-59	121	594	6 740	33 189	52.2	19.1	-	-	-	-
60+	17	160	3 906	37 170	69.2	9.3	-	-	-	-
All ages	1 783	707	35 728	14 160	22.3	39.3	-	-	-	-
Females										
0-4	223	475	538	1 143	2.4	51.9	-	-	-	-
5-14	315	451	3 144	4 503	10.0	52.0	-	-	-	-
15-44	132	125	8 819	8 299	29.5	37.2	-	-	-	-
45-59	28	125	2 404	10 872	52.2	20.5	-	-	-	-
60+	7	55	1 554	12 204	69.7	9.8	-	-	-	-
All ages	705	273	16 459	6 380	13.5	47.5	-	-	-	-
Total	2 489	488	52 186	10 227	19.8	41.6	-	-	-	-

For the methods used to estimate and project incidence, prevalence, and deaths see Lozano et al. 1996 and Murray and Lopez 1996a. See explanatory notes for definitions and caveats.

Table 235	Cuadro 235	Tableau 235
Other unintentional injuries	Otras lesiones no intencionales	Autres traumatismes non-intentionnels
Burns <20% - long term	Quemaduras <20% - larga duración	Brûlures <20% - long terme

Table 235g LAC - ALC - ALC Other unintentional injuries - Burns <20% - long term

Age group (years)	Incidence 1990 Number ('000s)	Rate (per 100 000)	Prevalence 1990 Number ('000s)	Rate (per 100 000)	Avg. age at onset (years)	Average duration (years)	Deaths 1990 Number ('000s)	Rate (per 100 000)	Deaths 2000 (Projected) Number ('000s)	Rate (per 100 000)
Males										
0-4	166	576	406	1 413	2.5	63.9	-	-	-	-
5-14	165	316	2 262	4 339	10.0	59.3	-	-	-	-
15-44	321	308	10 429	10 000	29.8	41.5	-	-	-	-
45-59	91	410	3 712	16 682	52.3	22.3	-	-	-	-
60+	22	156	2 924	20 547	70.3	10.5	-	-	-	-
All ages	764	345	19 732	8 904	23.5	47.0	-	-	-	-
Females										
0-4	130	468	319	1 153	2.5	67.9	-	-	-	-
5-14	70	138	1 502	2 959	10.0	63.0	-	-	-	-
15-44	96	93	5 139	4 937	29.9	44.6	-	-	-	-
45-59	24	102	1 628	6 970	52.4	24.8	-	-	-	-
60+	12	72	1 418	8 427	71.1	11.3	-	-	-	-
All ages	332	149	10 005	4 493	18.1	54.9	-	-	-	-
Total	1 096	247	29 737	6 693	21.9	49.4	-	-	-	-

Table 235h MEC - AOM - CMO Other unintentional injuries - Burns <20% - long term

Age group (years)	Incidence 1990 Number ('000s)	Rate (per 100 000)	Prevalence 1990 Number ('000s)	Rate (per 100 000)	Avg. age at onset (years)	Average duration (years)	Deaths 1990 Number ('000s)	Rate (per 100 000)	Deaths 2000 (Projected) Number ('000s)	Rate (per 100 000)
Males										
0-4	222	539	541	1 314	2.5	61.1	-	-	-	-
5-14	148	227	2 441	3 736	10.0	58.1	-	-	-	-
15-44	236	207	8 758	7 689	29.8	40.0	-	-	-	-
45-59	51	230	2 691	12 049	52.3	20.8	-	-	-	-
60+	9	69	1 935	14 173	69.7	9.8	-	-	-	-
All ages	667	260	16 366	6 383	18.6	49.1	-	-	-	-
Females										
0-4	182	458	444	1 117	2.5	63.7	-	-	-	-
5-14	62	100	1 689	2 724	10.0	60.9	-	-	-	-
15-44	50	47	4 151	3 872	29.8	42.6	-	-	-	-
45-59	15	68	1 120	5 024	52.3	22.9	-	-	-	-
60+	6	38	910	5 890	70.4	10.6	-	-	-	-
All ages	315	128	8 313	3 370	12.0	56.8	-	-	-	-
Total	982	195	24 679	4 906	16.5	51.6	-	-	-	-

Table 235i World - Mundo - Monde Other unintentional injuries - Burns <20% - long term

Age group (years)	Incidence 1990 Number ('000s)	Rate (per 100 000)	Prevalence 1990 Number ('000s)	Rate (per 100 000)	Avg. age at onset (years)	Average duration (years)	Deaths 1990 Number ('000s)	Rate (per 100 000)	Deaths 2000 (Projected) Number ('000s)	Rate (per 100 000)
Males										
0-4	2 170	675	5 278	1 643	2.5	60.6	-	-	-	-
5-14	1 806	328	26 376	4 785	10.0	56.0	-	-	-	-
15-44	3 622	290	124 444	9 956	29.7	39.1	-	-	-	-
45-59	1 014	325	46 884	15 009	52.3	21.2	-	-	-	-
60+	228	104	36 855	16 840	70.1	10.2	-	-	-	-
All ages	8 840	333	239 837	9 038	22.6	45.0	-	-	-	-
Females										
0-4	1 900	614	4 629	1 497	2.5	63.8	-	-	-	-
5-14	1 085	207	20 554	3 911	10.0	57.9	-	-	-	-
15-44	865	72	67 139	5 601	29.8	42.4	-	-	-	-
45-59	327	105	21 070	6 774	52.4	23.6	-	-	-	-
60+	157	58	18 980	7 050	71.0	11.2	-	-	-	-
All ages	4 334	166	132 372	5 065	16.1	53.1	-	-	-	-
Total	13 174	250	372 209	7 066	20.5	47.7	-	-	-	-

For the methods used to estimate and project incidence, prevalence, and deaths see Lozano et al. 1996 and Murray and Lopez 1996a. See explanatory notes for definitions and caveats.

Table 236	Cuadro 236	Tableau 236
Other unintentional injuries	**Otras lesiones no intencionales**	**Autres traumatismes non-intentionnels**
Injured nerves	Traumatismo de nervios	Lésions des nerfs

Table 236a   EME - PEMC - EMBE   Other unintentional injuries - Injured nerves

Age group (years)	Incidence 1990 Number ('000s)	Rate (per 100 000)	Prevalence 1990 Number ('000s)	Rate (per 100 000)	Avg. age at onset (years)	Average duration (years)	Deaths 1990 Number ('000s)	Rate (per 100 000)	Deaths 2000 (Projected) Number ('000s)	Rate (per 100 000)
Males										
0-4	1	4.7	3	11.7	2.5	70.2	-	-	-	-
5-14	1	1.6	17	31.4	10.0	63.6	-	-	-	-
15-44	49	26.6	801	435.0	29.9	44.7	-	-	-	-
45-59	27	40.1	746	1 127.8	52.4	24.5	-	-	-	-
60+	10	16.3	973	1 607.4	71.1	11.3	-	-	-	-
All ages	87	22.4	2 540	650.4	40.8	35.4	-	-	-	-
Females										
0-4	1	3.1	2	7.8	2.5	76.1	-	-	-	-
5-14	0	0.6	9	18.4	10.0	69.5	-	-	-	-
15-44	8	4.5	159	89.0	30.0	50.0	-	-	-	-
45-59	6	9.1	153	225.0	52.5	28.8	-	-	-	-
60+	8	9.2	345	407.6	72.4	12.7	-	-	-	-
All ages	23	5.7	668	164.0	49.1	32.9	-	-	-	-
Total	111	13.9	3 208	402.1	42.5	34.8	-	-	-	-

Table 236b   FSE - PEAS - AESE   Other unintentional injuries - Injured nerves

Age group (years)	Incidence 1990 Number ('000s)	Rate (per 100 000)	Prevalence 1990 Number ('000s)	Rate (per 100 000)	Avg. age at onset (years)	Average duration (years)	Deaths 1990 Number ('000s)	Rate (per 100 000)	Deaths 2000 (Projected) Number ('000s)	Rate (per 100 000)
Males										
0-4	2	11.5	4	29	2.5	63.5	-	-	-	-
5-14	1	4.0	21	77	10.0	57.3	-	-	-	-
15-44	60	78.7	954	1 250	29.8	39.2	-	-	-	-
45-59	34	124.5	890	3 301	52.2	20.8	-	-	-	-
60+	4	17.1	922	4 397	70.0	10.1	-	-	-	-
All ages	100	60.4	2 791	1 688	38.1	32.5	-	-	-	-
Females										
0-4	1	8.4	3	21	2.5	72.4	-	-	-	-
5-14	0	1.1	13	47	10.0	66.0	-	-	-	-
15-44	8	11.0	162	217	29.9	46.8	-	-	-	-
45-59	7	23.8	167	557	52.4	26.1	-	-	-	-
60+	3	7.2	298	820	71.5	11.8	-	-	-	-
All ages	19	10.7	643	356	42.0	36.2	-	-	-	-
Total	119	34.4	3 434	992	38.8	33.1	-	-	-	-

Table 236c   India - India - Inde   Other unintentional injuries - Injured nerves

Age group (years)	Incidence 1990 Number ('000s)	Rate (per 100 000)	Prevalence 1990 Number ('000s)	Rate (per 100 000)	Avg. age at onset (years)	Average duration (years)	Deaths 1990 Number ('000s)	Rate (per 100 000)	Deaths 2000 (Projected) Number ('000s)	Rate (per 100 000)
Males										
0-4	14	23	34	58	2.5	59.9	-	-	-	-
5-14	15	15	195	192	10.0	57.4	-	-	-	-
15-44	103	51	2 046	1 021	29.8	39.9	-	-	-	-
45-59	50	105	1 209	2 542	52.3	21.0	-	-	-	-
60+	8	27	1 063	3 572	69.7	9.7	-	-	-	-
All ages	190	43	4 549	1 035	33.8	36.6	-	-	-	-
Females										
0-4	12	21	29	51	2.5	60.8	-	-	-	-
5-14	11	11	153	161	10.0	59.1	-	-	-	-
15-44	55	30	1 206	658	29.8	41.7	-	-	-	-
45-59	25	54	692	1 505	52.4	22.5	-	-	-	-
60+	7	25	624	2 157	70.1	10.2	-	-	-	-
All ages	110	27	2 704	659	32.7	39.1	-	-	-	-
Total	300	35	7 253	854	33.4	37.5	-	-	-	-

For the methods used to estimate and project incidence, prevalence, and deaths see Lozano et al. 1996 and Murray and Lopez 1996a. See explanatory notes for definitions and caveats.

Table 236
Other unintentional injuries

Injured nerves

Cuadro 236
Otras lesiones no intencionales

Traumatismo de nervios

Tableau 236
Autres traumatismes non-intentionnels

Lésions des nerfs

Table 236d   China - China - Chine   Other unintentional injuries - Injured nerves

Age group (years)	Incidence 1990 Number ('000s)	Rate (per 100 000)	Prevalence 1990 Number ('000s)	Rate (per 100 000)	Avg. age at onset (years)	Average duration (years)	Deaths 1990 Number ('000s)	Rate (per 100 000)	Deaths 2000 (Projected) Number ('000s)	Rate (per 100 000)
Males										
0-4	17	27.4	41	68	2.5	65.5	-	-	-	-
5-14	5	4.8	155	160	10.0	59.9	-	-	-	-
15-44	177	57.9	3 185	1 040	29.9	41.2	-	-	-	-
45-59	47	65.0	1 723	2 371	52.3	21.4	-	-	-	-
60+	11	23.1	1 506	3 075	69.8	9.9	-	-	-	-
All ages	257	43.9	6 611	1 130	33.6	38.1	-	-	-	-
Females										
0-4	17	28.7	41	71	2.5	68.5	-	-	-	-
5-14	2	2.6	141	156	10.0	63.2	-	-	-	-
15-44	41	14.3	1 085	382	29.9	44.2	-	-	-	-
45-59	18	27.9	517	802	52.4	23.8	-	-	-	-
60+	7	13.3	596	1 153	70.6	10.8	-	-	-	-
All ages	85	15.4	2 379	434	32.1	42.4	-	-	-	-
Total	342	30.1	8 990	793	33.3	30.2	-	-	-	-

Table 236e   OAI - OPAI - APAI   Other unintentional injuries - Injured nerves

Age group (years)	Incidence 1990 Number ('000s)	Rate (per 100 000)	Prevalence 1990 Number ('000s)	Rate (per 100 000)	Avg. age at onset (years)	Average duration (years)	Deaths 1990 Number ('000s)	Rate (per 100 000)	Deaths 2000 (Projected) Number ('000s)	Rate (per 100 000)
Males										
0-4	7	16.9	18	42	2.5	59.8	-	-	-	-
5-14	8	9.8	112	133	10.0	56.2	-	-	-	-
15-44	148	92.1	2 453	1 525	29.7	38.8	-	-	-	-
45-59	33	95.2	1 219	3 572	52.3	20.3	-	-	-	-
60+	4	17.6	897	4 441	69.6	9.7	-	-	-	-
All ages	200	58.2	4 700	1 370	32.3	36.7	-	-	-	-
Females										
0-4	7	17.5	18	43	2.5	63.2	-	-	-	-
5-14	4	4.8	89	111	10.0	59.2	-	-	-	-
15-44	36	22.8	751	470	29.8	41.4	-	-	-	-
45-59	9	26.7	354	1 010	52.3	22.4	-	-	-	-
60+	2	9.3	296	1 307	70.3	10.5	-	-	-	-
All ages	59	17.4	1 508	444	30.2	41.2	-	-	-	-
Total	259	37.9	6 208	910	31.8	37.8	-	-	-	-

Table 236f   SSA - ASS - ASS   Other unintentional injuries - Injured nerves

Age group (years)	Incidence 1990 Number ('000s)	Rate (per 100 000)	Prevalence 1990 Number ('000s)	Rate (per 100 000)	Avg. age at onset (years)	Average duration (years)	Deaths 1990 Number ('000s)	Rate (per 100 000)	Deaths 2000 (Projected) Number ('000s)	Rate (per 100 000)
Males										
0-4	8	18	20	43	2.4	48.7	-	-	-	-
5-14	11	16	117	167	10.0	49.2	-	-	-	-
15-44	237	228	3 588	3 458	29.4	35.0	-	-	-	-
45-59	31	150	1 595	7 854	52.2	19.1	-	-	-	-
60+	3	32	967	9 204	69.2	9.3	-	-	-	-
All ages	291	115	6 288	2 492	30.7	34.0	-	-	-	-
Females										
0-4	6	13	15	32	2.4	51.9	-	-	-	-
5-14	9	12	89	127	10.0	51.9	-	-	-	-
15-44	33	31	684	644	29.5	37.2	-	-	-	-
45-59	7	32	300	1 354	52.3	20.5	-	-	-	-
60+	1	11	217	1 703	69.7	9.8	-	-	-	-
All ages	57	22	1 304	506	27.4	38.3	-	-	-	-
Total	347	68	7 592	1 488	30.2	34.7	-	-	-	-

For the methods used to estimate and project incidence, prevalence, and deaths see Lozano et al. 1996 and Murray and Lopez 1996a. See explanatory notes for definitions and caveats.

Table 236	Cuadro 236	Tableau 236
Other unintentional injuries	**Otras lesiones no intencionales**	**Autres traumatismes non-intentionnels**
Injured nerves	Traumatismo de nervios	Lésions des nerfs

Table 236g LAC - ALC - ALC — Other unintentional injuries - Injured nerves

Age group (years)	Incidence 1990 Number ('000s)	Rate (per 100 000)	Prevalence 1990 Number ('000s)	Rate (per 100 000)	Avg. age at onset (years)	Average duration (years)	Deaths 1990 Number ('000s)	Rate (per 100 000)	Deaths 2000 (Projected) Number ('000s)	Rate (per 100 000)
Males										
0-4	5	15.9	11	39	2.5	63.9	-	-	-	-
5-14	5	8.7	64	123	10.0	59.3	-	-	-	-
15-44	81	77.7	1 363	1 307	29.8	41.4	-	-	-	-
45-59	23	103.6	713	3 206	52.3	22.3	-	-	-	-
60+	4	31.4	610	4 284	70.3	10.4	-	-	-	-
All ages	118	53.1	2 761	1 246	33.9	38.1	-	-	-	-
Females										
0-4	4	12.9	9	32	2.5	67.9	-	-	-	-
5-14	2	3.8	42	83	10.0	63.0	-	-	-	-
15-44	24	23.4	468	449	29.9	44.6	-	-	-	-
45-59	6	25.8	231	991	52.4	24.8	-	-	-	-
60+	2	14.6	226	1 345	71.1	11.3	-	-	-	-
All ages	38	17.2	977	439	32.5	42.5	-	-	-	-
Total	156	35.1	3 738	841	33.6	39.2	-	-	-	-

Table 236h MEC - AOM - CMO — Other unintentional injuries - Injured nerves

Age group (years)	Incidence 1990 Number ('000s)	Rate (per 100 000)	Prevalence 1990 Number ('000s)	Rate (per 100 000)	Avg. age at onset (years)	Average duration (years)	Deaths 1990 Number ('000s)	Rate (per 100 000)	Deaths 2000 (Projected) Number ('000s)	Rate (per 100 000)
Males										
0-4	6	14.9	15	37	2.5	61.1	-	-	-	-
5-14	4	6.3	69	106	10.0	58.1	-	-	-	-
15-44	60	52.4	1 035	909	29.8	40.0	-	-	-	-
45-59	13	58.1	471	2 110	52.3	20.8	-	-	-	-
60+	2	14.0	366	2 680	69.7	9.8	-	-	-	-
All ages	85	33.1	1 956	763	31.2	38.8	-	-	-	-
Females										
0-4	5	12.6	12	31	2.5	63.7	-	-	-	-
5-14	2	2.8	48	77	10.0	60.9	-	-	-	-
15-44	13	11.8	284	265	29.9	42.6	-	-	-	-
45-59	4	17.1	127	568	52.4	22.9	-	-	-	-
60+	1	7.7	120	778	70.4	10.6	-	-	-	-
All ages	24	9.9	591	239	28.4	43.6	-	-	-	-
Total	109	21.7	2 547	506	30.6	39.8	-	-	-	-

Table 236i World - Mundo - Monde — Other unintentional injuries - Injured nerves

Age group (years)	Incidence 1990 Number ('000s)	Rate (per 100 000)	Prevalence 1990 Number ('000s)	Rate (per 100 000)	Avg. age at onset (years)	Average duration (years)	Deaths 1990 Number ('000s)	Rate (per 100 000)	Deaths 2000 (Projected) Number ('000s)	Rate (per 100 000)
Males										
0-4	60	18.7	147	46	2.5	60.6	-	-	-	-
5-14	50	9.1	751	136	10.0	56.0	-	-	-	-
15-44	915	73.2	15 426	1 234	29.7	39.1	-	-	-	-
45-59	256	82.0	8 568	2 743	52.3	21.2	-	-	-	-
60+	46	21.1	7 305	3 338	70.1	10.2	-	-	-	-
All ages	1 327	50.0	32 196	1 213	33.5	36.2	-	-	-	-
Females										
0-4	52	17.0	129	42	2.5	63.8	-	-	-	-
5-14	30	5.7	583	111	10.0	57.8	-	-	-	-
15-44	219	18.2	4 799	400	29.8	42.3	-	-	-	-
45-59	83	26.5	2 541	817	52.4	23.6	-	-	-	-
60+	32	11.8	2 722	1 011	71.0	11.2	-	-	-	-
All ages	415	15.9	10 774	412	32.5	40.0	-	-	-	-
Total	1 742	33.1	42 971	816	33.3	37.1	-	-	-	-

For the methods used to estimate and project incidence, prevalence, and deaths see Lozano et al. 1996 and Murray and Lopez 1996a. See explanatory notes for definitions and caveats.

Table 237
Self-inflicted injuries

Cuadro 237
Lesiones autoinfligidas

Tableau 237
Traumatismes auto-infligés

Episodes

Episodios

Episodes

Table 237a   EME - PEMC - EMBE   Self-inflicted injuries - Episodes

Age group (years)	Incidence 1990 Number ('000s)	Rate (per 100 000)	Prevalence 1990 Number ('000s)	Rate (per 100 000)	Avg. age at onset (years)	Average duration (years)	Deaths 1990 Number ('000s)	Rate (per 100 000)	Deaths 2000 (Projected) Number ('000s)	Rate (per 100 000)
Males										
0-4	0	0.0	-	-	-	-	0	0.0	0	0.0
5-14	1	2.4	-	-	10.0	-	0	0.7	0	0.7
15-44	140	76.2	-	-	29.9	-	39	20.9	37	21.2
45-59	48	72.0	-	-	52.4	-	18	27.7	22	27.7
60+	45	74.8	-	-	71.1	-	23	38.7	29	40.1
All ages	235	60.1	-	-	42.3	-	81	20.7	89	21.6
Females										
0-4	0	0.0	-	-	-	-	0	0.0	0	0.0
5-14	1	2.7	-	-	10.0	-	0	0.2	0	0.2
15-44	139	77.8	-	-	30.0	-	11	6.3	11	6.4
45-59	51	74.5	-	-	52.4	-	8	11.1	9	11.1
60+	48	56.3	-	-	72.4	-	13	14.8	15	15.1
All ages	239	58.7	-	-	43.1	-	31	7.7	35	8.1
Total	474	59.4	-	-	42.7	-	112	14.0	123	14.7

Table 237b   FSE - PEAS - AESE   Self-inflicted injuries - Episodes

Age group (years)	Incidence 1990 Number ('000s)	Rate (per 100 000)	Prevalence 1990 Number ('000s)	Rate (per 100 000)	Avg. age at onset (years)	Average duration (years)	Deaths 1990 Number ('000s)	Rate (per 100 000)	Deaths 2000 (Projected) Number ('000s)	Rate (per 100 000)
Males										
0-4	0	0.0	-	-	-	-	0	0.0	0	0.0
5-14	2	6.8	-	-	10.0	-	1	1.9	0	1.9
15-44	111	145.0	-	-	29.8	-	30	39.8	29	38.9
45-59	47	175.3	-	-	52.2	-	18	67.5	21	67.5
60+	25	117.7	-	-	70.0	-	13	61.0	17	65.2
All ages	184	111.5	-	-	40.7	-	62	37.4	68	39.5
Females										
0-4	0	0.0	-	-	-	-	0	0.0	0	0.0
5-14	1	4.9	-	-	10.0	-	0	0.4	0	0.4
15-44	67	90.0	-	-	29.9	-	5	7.2	5	7.1
45-59	32	107.5	-	-	52.4	-	5	16.0	5	16.0
60+	32	87.2	-	-	71.5	-	8	22.9	10	24.1
All ages	133	73.4	-	-	45.1	-	19	10.3	21	11.1
Total	317	91.6	-	-	42.6	-	81	23.3	88	24.7

Table 237c   India - India - Inde   Self-inflicted injuries - Episodes

Age group (years)	Incidence 1990 Number ('000s)	Rate (per 100 000)	Prevalence 1990 Number ('000s)	Rate (per 100 000)	Avg. age at onset (years)	Average duration (years)	Deaths 1990 Number ('000s)	Rate (per 100 000)	Deaths 2000 (Projected) Number ('000s)	Rate (per 100 000)
Males										
0-4	0	0.0	-	-	-	-	0	0.0	0	0.0
5-14	10	10.0	-	-	10.0	-	3	2.8	3	2.8
15-44	123	61.4	-	-	29.8	-	34	16.8	42	16.9
45-59	32	67.1	-	-	52.3	-	12	25.8	15	25.8
60+	9	30.7	-	-	69.7	-	5	15.9	6	16.4
All ages	174	39.7	-	-	34.9	-	54	12.2	66	13.0
Females										
0-4	0	0.0	-	-	-	-	0	0.0	0	0.0
5-14	34	36.0	-	-	10.0	-	3	2.9	3	2.9
15-44	446	243.5	-	-	29.8	-	36	19.6	44	19.4
45-59	36	77.5	-	-	52.4	-	5	11.5	7	11.5
60+	5	18.5	-	-	70.1	-	1	5.0	2	5.1
All ages	522	127.2	-	-	30.5	-	45	11.1	56	11.6
Total	696	81.9	-	-	31.6	-	99	11.7	122	12.3

For epidemiological sources see Ruzika and Gakidou 1996. For the methods used to estimate and project incidence, prevalence, and deaths see Murray and Lopez 1996a. See explanatory notes for definitions and caveats.

Table 237
Self-inflicted injuries

Cuadro 237
Lesiones autoinfligidas

Tableau 237
Traumatismes auto-infligés

Episodes

Episodios

Episodes

Table 237d China - China - Chine · Self-inflicted injuries - Episodes

Age group (years)	Incidence 1990 Number ('000s)	Rate (per 100 000)	Prevalence 1990 Number ('000s)	Rate (per 100 000)	Avg. age at onset (years)	Average duration (years)	Deaths 1990 Number ('000s)	Rate (per 100 000)	Deaths 2000 (Projected) Number ('000s)	Rate (per 100 000)
Males										
0-4	0	0.0	-	-	-	-	0	0.0	0	0.0
5-14	9	8.8	-	-	10.0	-	2	2.5	3	2.5
15-44	286	93.4	-	-	29.9	-	79	25.7	84	26.4
45-59	71	97.5	-	-	52.3	-	27	37.6	37	37.6
60+	98	200.7	-	-	69.8	-	51	103.9	64	106.5
All ages	464	79.3	-	-	41.4	-	159	27.2	188	28.7
Females										
0-4	0	0.0	-	-	-	-	0	0.0	0	0.0
5-14	21	23.3	-	-	10.0	-	2	1.9	2	1.9
15-44	1 349	475.0	-	-	29.9	-	108	38.2	109	36.6
45-59	175	271.3	-	-	52.4	-	26	40.3	37	40.3
60+	182	351.5	-	-	70.6	-	48	92.5	61	94.7
All ages	1 727	314.8	-	-	36.2	-	184	33.5	209	33.5
Total	2 191	193.2	-	-	37.3	-	343	30.3	397	31.0

Table 237e OAI - OPAI - APAI · Self-inflicted injuries - Episodes

Age group (years)	Incidence 1990 Number ('000s)	Rate (per 100 000)	Prevalence 1990 Number ('000s)	Rate (per 100 000)	Avg. age at onset (years)	Average duration (years)	Deaths 1990 Number ('000s)	Rate (per 100 000)	Deaths 2000 (Projected) Number ('000s)	Rate (per 100 000)
Males										
0-4	0	0.0	-	-	-	-	0	0.0	0	0.0
5-14	7	8.2	-	-	10.0	-	2	2.3	2	2.3
15-44	97	60.1	-	-	29.7	-	27	16.5	34	16.5
45-59	16	46.3	-	-	52.3	-	6	17.8	8	17.8
60+	11	54.9	-	-	69.6	-	6	28.4	8	29.0
All ages	130	38.0	-	-	34.8	-	40	11.7	52	12.8
Females										
0-4	0	0.0	-	-	-	-	0	0.0	0	0.0
5-14	14	17.7	-	-	10.0	-	1	1.4	1	1.4
15-44	253	158.3	-	-	29.8	-	20	12.7	25	12.5
45-59	17	47.7	-	-	52.3	-	2	7.1	3	7.1
60+	11	46.8	-	-	70.3	-	3	12.3	4	12.6
All ages	294	86.6	-	-	31.6	-	27	7.9	34	8.4
Total	425	62.2	-	-	32.6	-	67	9.8	85	10.6

Table 237f SSA - ASS - ASS · Self-inflicted injuries - Episodes

Age group (years)	Incidence 1990 Number ('000s)	Rate (per 100 000)	Prevalence 1990 Number ('000s)	Rate (per 100 000)	Avg. age at onset (years)	Average duration (years)	Deaths 1990 Number ('000s)	Rate (per 100 000)	Deaths 2000 (Projected) Number ('000s)	Rate (per 100 000)
Males										
0-4	0	0.0	-	-	-	-	0	0.0	0	0.0
5-14	5	7.1	-	-	10.0	-	1	2.0	2	2.0
15-44	34	32.6	-	-	29.4	-	9	9.0	13	9.0
45-59	4	17.5	-	-	52.2	-	1	6.7	2	6.7
60+	2	15.8	-	-	69.2	-	1	8.2	1	8.2
All ages	44	17.5	-	-	30.5	-	13	5.1	18	5.1
Females										
0-4	0	0.0	-	-	-	-	0	0.0	0	0.0
5-14	0	0.0	-	-	-	-	0	0.0	0	0.0
15-44	28	26.2	-	-	29.5	-	2	2.1	3	2.1
45-59	3	12.8	-	-	52.2	-	0	1.9	1	1.9
60+	0	3.6	-	-	69.7	-	0	0.9	0	0.9
All ages	31	12.1	-	-	32.2	-	3	1.1	4	1.1
Total	75	14.7	-	-	31.2	-	16	3.1	21	3.1

For epidemiological sources see Ruzika and Gakidou 1996. For the methods used to estimate and project incidence, prevalence, and deaths see Murray and Lopez 1996a. See explanatory notes for definitions and caveats.

Table 237
Self-inflicted injuries

Cuadro 237
Lesiones autoinfligidas

Tableau 237
Traumatismes auto-infligés

Episodes

Episodios

Episodes

Table 237g   LAC - ALC - ALC

Self-inflicted injuries - Episodes

Age group (years)	Incidence 1990 Number ('000s)	Rate (per 100 000)	Prevalence 1990 Number ('000s)	Rate (per 100 000)	Avg. age at onset (years)	Average duration (years)	Deaths 1990 Number ('000s)	Rate (per 100 000)	Deaths 2000 (Projected) Number ('000s)	Rate (per 100 000)
Males										
0-4	0	0.0	-	-	-	-	0	0.0	0	0.0
5-14	2	3.1	-	-	10.0	-	0	0.9	0	0.9
15-44	36	34.1	-	-	29.8	-	10	9.4	12	9.4
45-59	7	32.7	-	-	52.3	-	3	12.6	4	12.6
60+	5	36.9	-	-	70.3	-	3	19.1	4	19.4
All ages	50	22.4	-	-	36.7	-	16	7.1	20	7.6
Females										
0-4	0	0.0	-	-	-	-	0	0.0	0	0.0
5-14	4	8.5	-	-	10.0	-	0	0.7	0	0.7
15-44	59	56.5	-	-	29.9	-	5	4.5	6	4.5
45-59	6	25.9	-	-	52.4	-	1	3.8	1	3.8
60+	3	17.6	-	-	71.1	-	1	4.6	1	4.6
All ages	72	32.4	-	-	32.3	-	7	3.0	8	3.2
Total	122	27.4	-	-	34.1	-	22	5.1	29	5.4

Table 237h   MEC - AOM - CMO

Self-inflicted injuries - Episodes

Age group (years)	Incidence 1990 Number ('000s)	Rate (per 100 000)	Prevalence 1990 Number ('000s)	Rate (per 100 000)	Avg. age at onset (years)	Average duration (years)	Deaths 1990 Number ('000s)	Rate (per 100 000)	Deaths 2000 (Projected) Number ('000s)	Rate (per 100 000)
Males										
0-4	0	0.0	-	-	-	-	0	0.0	0	0.0
5-14	30	45.2	-	-	10.0	-	8	12.5	10	12.5
15-44	59	51.6	-	-	29.8	-	16	14.2	21	14.2
45-59	11	50.5	-	-	52.3	-	4	19.5	6	19.5
60+	7	47.9	-	-	69.7	-	3	24.8	5	25.6
All ages	106	41.4	-	-	29.1	-	32	12.5	43	12.8
Females										
0-4	0	0.0	-	-	-	-	0	0.0	0	0.0
5-14	45	73.2	-	-	10.0	-	4	5.9	5	5.9
15-44	82	76.4	-	-	29.8	-	7	6.1	9	6.1
45-59	11	48.0	-	-	52.3	-	2	7.1	2	7.1
60+	9	60.4	-	-	70.4	-	2	15.9	4	16.4
All ages	147	59.8	-	-	27.9	-	14	5.8	19	6.0
Total	254	50.4	-	-	28.4	-	46	9.2	62	9.4

Table 237i   World - Mundo - Monde

Self-inflicted injuries - Episodes

Age group (years)	Incidence 1990 Number ('000s)	Rate (per 100 000)	Prevalence 1990 Number ('000s)	Rate (per 100 000)	Avg. age at onset (years)	Average duration (years)	Deaths 1990 Number ('000s)	Rate (per 100 000)	Deaths 2000 (Projected) Number ('000s)	Rate (per 100 000)
Males										
0-4	0	0.0	-	-	-	-	0	0.0	0	0.0
5-14	65	11.8	-	-	10.0	-	18	3.3	22	3.4
15-44	885	70.8	-	-	29.8	-	243	19.4	273	18.9
45-59	236	75.4	-	-	52.3	-	91	29.1	115	28.6
60+	202	92.3	-	-	70.1	-	105	47.8	134	48.5
All ages	1 387	52.3	-	-	37.0	-	456	17.2	543	17.5
Females										
0-4	0	0.0	-	-	-	-	0	0.0	0	0.0
5-14	122	23.2	-	-	10.0	-	10	1.9	12	1.9
15-44	2 424	202.2	-	-	29.8	-	195	16.3	212	15.3
45-59	329	105.9	-	-	52.4	-	49	15.7	65	16.2
60+	290	107.6	-	-	71.2	-	76	28.3	96	28.6
All ages	3 165	121.1	-	-	34.9	-	330	12.6	386	12.6
Total	4 552	86.4	-	-	35.5	-	786	14.9	929	15.1

For epidemiological sources see Ruzika and Gakidou 1996. For the methods used to estimate and project incidence, prevalence, and deaths see Murray and Lopez 1996a. See explanatory notes for definitions and caveats.

Table 238
Violence

Cuadro 238
Violencias

Tableau 238
Violence

Episodes

Episodios

Episodes

Table 238a EME - PEMC - EMBE

Violence - Episodes

Age group (years)	Incidence 1990 Number ('000s)	Rate (per 100 000)	Prevalence 1990 Number ('000s)	Rate (per 100 000)	Avg. age at onset (years)	Average duration (years)	Deaths 1990 Number ('000s)	Rate (per 100 000)	Deaths 2000 (Projected) Number ('000s)	Rate (per 100 000)
Males										
0-4	12	46	-	-	2.5	-	1	2.1	1	2.1
5-14	12	23	-	-	10.0	-	0	0.8	0	0.8
15-44	403	219	-	-	29.9	-	17	9.3	16	9.3
45-59	40	61	-	-	52.4	-	3	4.4	4	4.4
60+	16	26	-	-	71.1	-	2	2.8	2	2.7
All ages	483	124	-	-	31.9	-	23	5.8	23	5.6
Females										
0-4	12	46	-	-	2.5	-	1	2.1	1	2.1
5-14	9	18	-	-	10.0	-	0	0.6	0	0.6
15-44	108	60	-	-	30.0	-	5	2.6	4	2.6
45-59	13	19	-	-	52.4	-	1	1.4	1	1.4
60+	11	13	-	-	72.4	-	1	1.3	1	1.3
All ages	153	38	-	-	31.6	-	8	1.9	8	1.8
Total	636	80	-	-	31.8	-	30	3.8	31	3.6

Table 238b FSE - PEAS - AESE

Violence - Episodes

Age group (years)	Incidence 1990 Number ('000s)	Rate (per 100 000)	Prevalence 1990 Number ('000s)	Rate (per 100 000)	Avg. age at onset (years)	Average duration (years)	Deaths 1990 Number ('000s)	Rate (per 100 000)	Deaths 2000 (Projected) Number ('000s)	Rate (per 100 000)
Males										
0-4	3	25	-	-	2.5	-	0	1.4	0	1.4
5-14	5	18	-	-	10.0	-	0	0.8	0	0.8
15-44	289	379	-	-	29.8	-	15	20.2	15	20.0
45-59	48	179	-	-	52.2	-	4	16.4	5	16.4
60+	14	67	-	-	70.0	-	2	8.7	2	8.7
All ages	359	217	-	-	33.9	-	22	13.4	23	13.3
Females										
0-4	3	26	-	-	2.5	-	0	1.5	0	1.5
5-14	4	16	-	-	10.0	-	0	0.7	0	0.7
15-44	73	98	-	-	29.9	-	4	5.2	4	5.1
45-59	20	66	-	-	52.4	-	2	6.1	2	6.1
60+	14	38	-	-	71.5	-	2	5.0	2	5.2
All ages	115	63	-	-	37.3	-	8	4.4	8	4.5
Total	474	137	-	-	34.7	-	30	8.7	31	8.7

Table 238c India - India - Inde

Violence - Episodes

Age group (years)	Incidence 1990 Number ('000s)	Rate (per 100 000)	Prevalence 1990 Number ('000s)	Rate (per 100 000)	Avg. age at onset (years)	Average duration (years)	Deaths 1990 Number ('000s)	Rate (per 100 000)	Deaths 2000 (Projected) Number ('000s)	Rate (per 100 000)
Males										
0-4	81	135	-	-	2.5	-	6	9.6	5	9.6
5-14	30	30	-	-	10.0	-	2	1.6	2	1.6
15-44	203	101	-	-	29.8	-	14	7.0	18	7.1
45-59	56	117	-	-	52.3	-	7	14.3	9	14.3
60+	31	104	-	-	69.7	-	5	16.4	6	16.7
All ages	400	91	-	-	29.0	-	33	7.5	40	7.7
Females										
0-4	100	176	-	-	2.5	-	7	12.6	7	12.6
5-14	26	27	-	-	10.0	-	1	1.5	2	1.5
15-44	58	31	-	-	29.8	-	4	2.2	5	2.2
45-59	49	107	-	-	52.4	-	6	13.2	8	13.2
60+	25	88	-	-	70.1	-	4	13.9	5	13.8
All ages	258	63	-	-	25.5	-	23	5.5	26	5.4
Total	658	77	-	-	27.6	-	56	6.6	66	6.6

For epidemiological sources see Sandiford 1996. For the methods used to estimate and project incidence, prevalence, and deaths see Murray and Lopez 1996a. See explanatory notes for definitions and caveats.

Table 238 / **Cuadro 238** / **Tableau 238**
Violence / **Violencias** / **Violence**

Episodes / Episodios / Episodes

Table 238d   China - China - Chine — Violence - Episodes

Age group (years)	Incidence 1990 Number ('000s)	Rate (per 100 000)	Prevalence 1990 Number ('000s)	Rate (per 100 000)	Avg. age at onset (years)	Average duration (years)	Deaths 1990 Number ('000s)	Rate (per 100 000)	Deaths 2000 (Projected) Number ('000s)	Rate (per 100 000)
Males										
0-4	83	137	-	-	2.5	-	5	7.9	5	7.9
5-14	22	23	-	-	10.0	-	1	1.0	1	1.0
15-44	338	110	-	-	29.9	-	20	6.5	20	6.4
45-59	26	36	-	-	52.3	-	3	3.7	4	3.7
60+	16	33	-	-	69.8	-	2	4.3	3	4.2
All ages	485	83	-	-	26.9	-	30	5.2	32	4.9
Females										
0-4	153	263	-	-	2.5	-	9	15.2	8	15.2
5-14	30	33	-	-	10.0	-	1	1.5	2	1.5
15-44	102	36	-	-	29.9	-	6	2.1	7	2.3
45-59	16	25	-	-	52.4	-	2	2.5	2	2.5
60+	19	37	-	-	70.6	-	3	4.9	3	4.9
All ages	320	58	-	-	18.6	-	20	3.7	23	3.6
Total	806	71	-	-	23.6	-	51	4.5	55	4.3

Table 238e   OAI - OPAI - APAI — Violence - Episodes

Age group (years)	Incidence 1990 Number ('000s)	Rate (per 100 000)	Prevalence 1990 Number ('000s)	Rate (per 100 000)	Avg. age at onset (years)	Average duration (years)	Deaths 1990 Number ('000s)	Rate (per 100 000)	Deaths 2000 (Projected) Number ('000s)	Rate (per 100 000)
Males										
0-4	17	38	-	-	2.5	-	1	2.6	1	2.6
5-14	37	44	-	-	10.0	-	2	2.5	2	2.5
15-44	404	251	-	-	29.7	-	28	17.7	36	17.9
45-59	53	154	-	-	52.3	-	6	18.6	9	18.6
60+	18	88	-	-	69.6	-	3	13.8	4	14.2
All ages	528	154	-	-	31.1	-	41	11.9	52	12.9
Females										
0-4	19	45	-	-	2.5	-	1	3.1	1	3.1
5-14	24	30	-	-	10.0	-	1	1.6	1	1.6
15-44	87	54	-	-	29.8	-	6	3.8	8	3.9
45-59	9	25	-	-	52.3	-	1	3.0	1	3.0
60+	4	19	-	-	70.3	-	1	2.9	1	2.9
All ages	143	42	-	-	25.5	-	10	3.1	13	3.2
Total	670	98	-	-	29.9	-	51	7.5	65	8.0

Table 238f   SSA - ASS - ASS — Violence - Episodes

Age group (years)	Incidence 1990 Number ('000s)	Rate (per 100 000)	Prevalence 1990 Number ('000s)	Rate (per 100 000)	Avg. age at onset (years)	Average duration (years)	Deaths 1990 Number ('000s)	Rate (per 100 000)	Deaths 2000 (Projected) Number ('000s)	Rate (per 100 000)
Males										
0-4	44	93	-	-	2.4	-	4	8.6	6	8.6
5-14	104	148	-	-	10.0	-	8	11.0	10	11.0
15-44	1 540	1 484	-	-	29.4	-	145	139.5	198	139.5
45-59	86	423	-	-	52.2	-	14	69.0	18	69.0
60+	25	243	-	-	69.2	-	5	50.8	7	50.7
All ages	1 799	713	-	-	29.3	-	176	69.7	240	70.0
Females										
0-4	22	47	-	-	2.4	-	2	4.4	3	4.4
5-14	44	64	-	-	10.0	-	3	4.6	4	4.6
15-44	200	189	-	-	29.5	-	19	17.7	26	17.7
45-59	18	81	-	-	52.2	-	3	13.1	4	13.1
60+	9	69	-	-	69.7	-	2	14.4	3	14.5
All ages	294	114	-	-	27.1	-	29	11.2	39	11.2
Total	2 093	410	-	-	29.0	-	205	40.1	279	40.3

For epidemiological sources see Sandiford 1996. For the methods used to estimate and project incidence, prevalence, and deaths see Murray and Lopez 1996a. See explanatory notes for definitions and caveats.

Table 238
Violence

Cuadro 238
Violencias

Tableau 238
Violence

Episodes

Episodios

Episodes

Table 238g LAC - ALC - ALC   Violence - Episodes

Age group (years)	Incidence 1990 Number ('000s)	Rate (per 100 000)	Prevalence 1990 Number ('000s)	Rate (per 100 000)	Avg. age at onset (years)	Average duration (years)	Deaths 1990 Number ('000s)	Rate (per 100 000)	Deaths 2000 (Projected) Number ('000s)	Rate (per 100 000)
Males										
0-4	19	66	-	-	2.5	-	1	3.8	1	3.8
5-14	67	128	-	-	10.0	-	3	5.6	3	5.6
15-44	1 309	1 255	-	-	29.8	-	71	68.5	88	68.4
45-59	103	463	-	-	52.3	-	10	43.2	13	43.2
60+	28	199	-	-	70.3	-	4	25.9	5	25.8
All ages	1 526	688	-	-	30.9	-	89	40.0	111	41.7
Females										
0-4	14	51	-	-	2.5	-	1	2.9	1	2.9
5-14	27	53	-	-	10.0	-	1	2.3	1	2.3
15-44	166	160	-	-	29.9	-	9	8.7	11	8.6
45-59	12	49	-	-	52.4	-	1	4.6	1	4.6
60+	6	34	-	-	71.1	-	1	4.4	1	4.5
All ages	225	101	-	-	28.0	-	13	5.8	16	5.9
Total	1 750	394	-	-	30.5	-	102	22.9	126	23.7

Table 238h MEC - AOM - CMO   Violence - Episodes

Age group (years)	Incidence 1990 Number ('000s)	Rate (per 100 000)	Prevalence 1990 Number ('000s)	Rate (per 100 000)	Avg. age at onset (years)	Average duration (years)	Deaths 1990 Number ('000s)	Rate (per 100 000)	Deaths 2000 (Projected) Number ('000s)	Rate (per 100 000)
Males										
0-4	5	11.4	-	-	2.5	-	6	14.1	7	14.1
5-14	4	6.2	-	-	10.0	-	2	3.1	3	3.1
15-44	154	135.3	-	-	29.8	-	14	12.1	18	12.1
45-59	14	61.8	-	-	52.3	-	2	9.2	3	9.2
60+	4	32.4	-	-	69.7	-	1	9.1	2	9.2
All ages	181	70.6	-	-	31.3	-	25	9.7	32	9.7
Females										
0-4	4	9.8	-	-	2.5	-	6	15.9	8	15.9
5-14	3	5.1	-	-	10.0	-	2	3.4	3	3.4
15-44	30	27.9	-	-	29.8	-	4	3.4	5	3.4
45-59	5	20.8	-	-	52.3	-	1	3.8	1	3.8
60+	2	15.6	-	-	70.4	-	1	4.4	1	4.6
All ages	44	17.9	-	-	30.6	-	14	5.5	17	5.4
Total	225	44.8	-	-	31.2	-	39	7.7	50	7.6

Table 238i World - Mundo - Monde   Violence - Episodes

Age group (years)	Incidence 1990 Number ('000s)	Rate (per 100 000)	Prevalence 1990 Number ('000s)	Rate (per 100 000)	Avg. age at onset (years)	Average duration (years)	Deaths 1990 Number ('000s)	Rate (per 100 000)	Deaths 2000 (Projected) Number ('000s)	Rate (per 100 000)
Males										
0-4	264	82	-	-	2.5	-	23	7.3	26	7.5
5-14	281	51	-	-	10.0	-	18	3.3	22	3.5
15-44	4 638	371	-	-	29.8	-	325	26.0	410	28.4
45-59	426	136	-	-	52.3	-	49	15.6	64	15.8
60+	153	70	-	-	70.1	-	24	10.7	31	11.2
All ages	5 762	217	-	-	29.9	-	439	16.5	553	17.9
Females										
0-4	327	106	-	-	2.5	-	27	8.8	29	8.6
5-14	168	32	-	-	10.0	-	11	2.1	13	2.2
15-44	825	69	-	-	29.8	-	56	4.7	69	5.0
45-59	141	45	-	-	52.4	-	16	5.3	21	5.2
60+	90	34	-	-	71.2	-	13	5.0	18	5.2
All ages	1 551	59	-	-	26.6	-	124	4.7	150	4.9
Total	7 313	139	-	-	29.2	-	563	10.7	702	11.4

For epidemiological sources see Sandiford 1996. For the methods used to estimate and project incidence, prevalence, and deaths see Murray and Lopez 1996a. See explanatory notes for definitions and caveats.

Table 239
Violence

Cuadro 239
Violencias

Tableau 239
Violence

Fractured skull - long term | Fractura de cráneo - larga duración | Fracture du crâne - long terme

Table 239a — EME - PEMC - EMBE — Violence - Fractured skull - long term

Age group (years)	Incidence 1990 Number ('000s)	Rate (per 100 000)	Prevalence 1990 Number ('000s)	Rate (per 100 000)	Avg. age at onset (years)	Average duration (years)	Deaths 1990 Number ('000s)	Rate (per 100 000)	Deaths 2000 (Projected) Number ('000s)	Rate (per 100 000)
Males										
0-4	0	0.3	0	0.6	2.5	70.2	-	-	-	-
5-14	0	0.1	1	1.9	10.0	63.6	-	-	-	-
15-44	1	0.4	16	8.7	29.9	44.8	-	-	-	-
45-59	0	0.1	10	15.7	52.4	24.5	-	-	-	-
60+	0	0.1	11	17.4	71.1	11.3	-	-	-	-
All ages	1	0.3	38	9.8	30.3	44.7	-	-	-	-
Females										
0-4	0	0.3	0	0.6	2.5	76.1	-	-	-	-
5-14	0	0.1	1	1.8	10.0	69.5	-	-	-	-
15-44	0	0.1	7	4.0	30.0	50.0	-	-	-	-
45-59	0	0.0	4	6.0	52.4	28.8	-	-	-	-
60+	0	0.0	6	6.7	72.4	12.7	-	-	-	-
All ages	0	0.1	18	4.4	27.5	52.7	-	-	-	-
Total	1	0.2	56	7.0	29.6	46.8	-	-	-	-

Table 239b — FSE - PEAS - AESE — Violence - Fractured skull - long term

Age group (years)	Incidence 1990 Number ('000s)	Rate (per 100 000)	Prevalence 1990 Number ('000s)	Rate (per 100 000)	Avg. age at onset (years)	Average duration (years)	Deaths 1990 Number ('000s)	Rate (per 100 000)	Deaths 2000 (Projected) Number ('000s)	Rate (per 100 000)
Males										
0-4	0	1.4	0	0.3	2.5	63.5	-	-	-	-
5-14	0	0.1	0	1.2	10.0	57.3	-	-	-	-
15-44	1	0.7	9	12.2	29.8	39.2	-	-	-	-
45-59	0	0.3	7	25.4	52.2	20.8	-	-	-	-
60+	0	0.2	6	30.0	70.0	10.1	-	-	-	-
All ages	1	0.5	23	13.8	27.5	41.7	-	-	-	-
Females										
0-4	0	0.1	0	0.4	2.5	72.4	-	-	-	-
5-14	0	0.1	0	1.2	10.0	66.0	-	-	-	-
15-44	0	0.2	3	4.3	29.9	46.8	-	-	-	-
45-59	0	0.1	2	8.0	52.4	26.1	-	-	-	-
60+	0	0.1	4	10.3	71.5	11.8	-	-	-	-
All ages	0	0.1	10	5.4	35.9	41.9	-	-	-	-
Total	1	0.3	33	9.4	29.4	41.7	-	-	-	-

Table 239c — India - India - Inde — Violence - Fractured skull - long term

Age group (years)	Incidence 1990 Number ('000s)	Rate (per 100 000)	Prevalence 1990 Number ('000s)	Rate (per 100 000)	Avg. age at onset (years)	Average duration (years)	Deaths 1990 Number ('000s)	Rate (per 100 000)	Deaths 2000 (Projected) Number ('000s)	Rate (per 100 000)
Males										
0-4	0	0.8	1	1.9	2.5	59.9	-	-	-	-
5-14	0	0.2	5	4.6	10.0	57.4	-	-	-	-
15-44	1	0.4	22	10.9	29.8	39.9	-	-	-	-
45-59	0	0.4	9	19.6	52.3	21.0	-	-	-	-
60+	0	0.3	8	25.9	69.7	9.7	-	-	-	-
All ages	2	0.4	45	10.2	25.2	43.2	-	-	-	-
Females										
0-4	1	1.0	1	2.5	2.5	60.8	-	-	-	-
5-14	0	0.2	5	5.8	10.0	59.1	-	-	-	-
15-44	0	0.1	15	8.2	29.8	41.7	-	-	-	-
45-59	0	0.4	6	12.9	52.4	22.5	-	-	-	-
60+	0	0.3	5	18.6	70.1	10.2	-	-	-	-
All ages	1	0.3	33	8.1	20.3	48.1	-	-	-	-
Total	3	0.3	78	9.2	23.1	45.3	-	-	-	-

For epidemiological sources see Sandiford 1996. For the methods used to estimate and project incidence, prevalence, and deaths see Lozano et al. 1996 and Murray and Lopez 1996a. See explanatory notes for definitions and caveats.

Table 239 **Cuadro 239** **Tableau 239**
Violence Violencias Violence

Fractured skull - long term Fractura de cráneo - larga duración Fracture du crâne - long terme

---

Table 239d	China - China - Chine						Violence - Fractured skull - long term			
Age group (years)	Incidence 1990		Prevalence 1990		Avg. age at onset (years)	Average duration (years)	Deaths 1990		Deaths 2000 (Projected)	
	Number ('000s)	Rate (per 100 000)	Number ('000s)	Rate (per 100 000)			Number ('000s)	Rate (per 100 000)	Number ('000s)	Rate (per 100 000)
Males										
0-4	0	0.8	1	1.9	2.5	65.5	-	-	-	-
5-14	0	0.1	4	4.4	10.0	59.9	-	-	-	-
15-44	1	0.4	34	11.1	29.9	41.2	-	-	-	-
45-59	0	0.1	13	18.2	52.3	21.4	-	-	-	-
60+	0	0.1	10	20.2	69.8	9.9	-	-	-	-
All ages	2	0.3	62	10.7	24.3	46.3	-	-	-	-
Females										
0-4	1	1.5	2	3.6	2.5	68.5	-	-	-	-
5-14	0	0.2	7	8.2	10.0	63.2	-	-	-	-
15-44	0	0.1	31	11.0	29.9	44.2	-	-	-	-
45-59	0	0.1	9	13.7	52.4	23.8	-	-	-	-
60+	0	0.1	8	15.6	70.6	10.8	-	-	-	-
All ages	2	0.3	58	10.5	14.7	57.9	-	-	-	-
Total	3	0.3	120	10.6	20.2	51.3	-	-	-	-

Table 239e	OAI - OPAI - APAI						Violence - Fractured skull - long term			
Age group (years)	Incidence 1990		Prevalence 1990		Avg. age at onset (years)	Average duration (years)	Deaths 1990		Deaths 2000 (Projected)	
	Number ('000s)	Rate (per 100 000)	Number ('000s)	Rate (per 100 000)			Number ('000s)	Rate (per 100 000)	Number ('000s)	Rate (per 100 000)
Males										
0-4	0	0.2	0	0.5	2.5	59.8	-	-	-	-
5-14	0	0.2	2	2.3	10.0	56.2	-	-	-	-
15-44	1	0.9	27	17.1	29.7	38.8	-	-	-	-
45-59	0	0.6	12	35.3	52.3	20.3	-	-	-	-
60+	0	0.3	9	42.1	69.6	9.7	-	-	-	-
All ages	2	0.6	50	14.6	29.7	39.0	-	-	-	-
Females										
0-4	0	0.3	0	0.6	2.5	63.2	-	-	-	-
5-14	0	0.2	2	2.1	10.0	59.2	-	-	-	-
15-44	0	0.2	9	5.9	29.8	41.5	-	-	-	-
45-59	0	0.1	3	9.6	52.3	22.4	-	-	-	-
60+	0	0.1	2	10.8	70.3	10.5	-	-	-	-
All ages	1	0.2	17	5.0	22.7	47.5	-	-	-	-
Total	3	0.4	67	9.9	28.1	40.9	-	-	-	-

Table 239f	SSA - ASS - ASS						Violence - Fractured skull - long term			
Age group (years)	Incidence 1990		Prevalence 1990		Avg. age at onset (years)	Average duration (years)	Deaths 1990		Deaths 2000 (Projected)	
	Number ('000s)	Rate (per 100 000)	Number ('000s)	Rate (per 100 000)			Number ('000s)	Rate (per 100 000)	Number ('000s)	Rate (per 100 000)
Males										
0-4	0	0.5	1	1.2	2.4	48.7	-	-	-	-
5-14	1	0.8	5	6.6	10.0	49.2	-	-	-	-
15-44	6	5.4	93	89.3	29.4	35.0	-	-	-	-
45-59	0	1.6	38	185.4	52.2	19.1	-	-	-	-
60+	0	0.7	21	204.1	69.2	9.3	-	-	-	-
All ages	7	2.7	157	62.2	28.3	35.7	-	-	-	-
Females										
0-4	0	0.3	0	0.6	2.4	51.9	-	-	-	-
5-14	0	0.4	2	3.1	10.0	51.9	-	-	-	-
15-44	1	0.7	16	14.9	29.5	37.2	-	-	-	-
45-59	0	0.3	6	27.8	52.2	20.5	-	-	-	-
60+	0	0.2	4	32.1	69.7	9.8	-	-	-	-
All ages	1	0.5	28	11.0	24.8	40.2	-	-	-	-
Total	8	1.6	185	36.3	27.8	36.4	-	-	-	-

For epidemiological sources see Sandiford 1996. For the methods used to estimate and project incidence, prevalence, and deaths see Lozano et al. 1996 and Murray and Lopez 1996a. See explanatory notes for definitions and caveats.

Table 239
Violence

Cuadro 239
Violencias

Tableau 239
Violence

Fractured skull - long term Fractura de cráneo - larga duración Fracture du crâne - long terme

Table 239g — LAC - ALC - ALC — Violence - Fractured skull - long term

Age group (years)	Incidence 1990 Number ('000s)	Rate (per 100 000)	Prevalence 1990 Number ('000s)	Rate (per 100 000)	Avg. age at onset (years)	Average duration (years)	Deaths 1990 Number ('000s)	Rate (per 100 000)	Deaths 2000 (Projected) Number ('000s)	Rate (per 100 000)
Males										
0-4	0	0.4	0	0.9	2.5	63.9	-	-	-	-
5-14	0	0.7	3	5.4	10.0	59.3	-	-	-	-
15-44	1	1.4	31	29.7	29.8	41.4	-	-	-	-
45-59	0	0.5	12	54.7	52.3	22.3	-	-	-	-
60+	0	0.6	9	64.7	70.3	10.4	-	-	-	-
All ages	2	1.0	55	25.0	27.8	43.4	-	-	-	-
Females										
0-4	0	0.3	0	0.7	2.5	67.9	-	-	-	-
5-14	0	0.3	1	2.9	10.0	63.0	-	-	-	-
15-44	0	0.2	7	7.0	29.9	44.6	-	-	-	-
45-59	0	0.1	2	10.1	52.4	24.8	-	-	-	-
60+	0	0.1	2	11.6	71.1	11.3	-	-	-	-
All ages	0	0.2	13	5.9	20.6	53.1	-	-	-	-
Total	3	0.6	69	15.4	26.6	45.1	-	-	-	-

Table 239h — MEC - AOM - CMO — Violence - Fractured skull - long term

Age group (years)	Incidence 1990 Number ('000s)	Rate (per 100 000)	Prevalence 1990 Number ('000s)	Rate (per 100 000)	Avg. age at onset (years)	Average duration (years)	Deaths 1990 Number ('000s)	Rate (per 100 000)	Deaths 2000 (Projected) Number ('000s)	Rate (per 100 000)
Males										
0-4	0	0.1	0	0.2	2.5	61.1	-	-	-	-
5-14	0	0.0	0	0.5	10.0	58.1	-	-	-	-
15-44	2	1.5	3	2.9	29.8	40.0	-	-	-	-
45-59	0	0.1	1	5.7	52.3	20.8	-	-	-	-
60+	0	0.1	1	7.1	69.7	9.8	-	-	-	-
All ages	2	0.7	6	2.3	29.6	40.1	-	-	-	-
Females										
0-4	0	0.1	0	0.1	2.5	63.7	-	-	-	-
5-14	0	0.0	0	0.4	10.0	60.9	-	-	-	-
15-44	0	0.0	1	1.0	29.8	42.6	-	-	-	-
45-59	0	0.0	0	1.7	52.3	22.9	-	-	-	-
60+	0	0.0	0	2.3	70.4	10.6	-	-	-	-
All ages	0	0.0	2	0.9	23.6	47.8	-	-	-	-
Total	2	0.4	8	1.6	29.4	40.5	-	-	-	-

Table 239i — World - Mundo - Monde — Violence - Fractured skull - long term

Age group (years)	Incidence 1990 Number ('000s)	Rate (per 100 000)	Prevalence 1990 Number ('000s)	Rate (per 100 000)	Avg. age at onset (years)	Average duration (years)	Deaths 1990 Number ('000s)	Rate (per 100 000)	Deaths 2000 (Projected) Number ('000s)	Rate (per 100 000)
Males										
0-4	2	0.5	4	1.1	2.5	60.9	-	-	-	-
5-14	2	0.3	20	3.6	10.0	55.2	-	-	-	-
15-44	14	1.1	235	18.8	29.6	38.3	-	-	-	-
45-59	1	0.4	103	33.0	52.3	20.7	-	-	-	-
60+	0	0.2	75	34.1	69.9	10.0	-	-	-	-
All ages	18	0.7	437	16.5	27.9	40.0	-	-	-	-
Females										
0-4	2	0.6	5	1.5	2.5	64.9	-	-	-	-
5-14	1	0.2	20	3.7	10.0	59.3	-	-	-	-
15-44	2	0.2	90	7.5	29.7	41.9	-	-	-	-
45-59	0	0.1	33	10.8	52.4	23.1	-	-	-	-
60+	0	0.1	32	11.8	70.7	10.9	-	-	-	-
All ages	6	0.2	180	6.9	21.3	49.4	-	-	-	-
Total	24	0.5	616	11.7	26.3	42.2	-	-	-	-

For epidemiological sources see Sandiford 1996. For the methods used to estimate and project incidence, prevalence, and deaths see Lozano et al. 1996 and Murray and Lopez 1996a. See explanatory notes for definitions and caveats.

Table 240 | **Cuadro 240** | **Tableau 240**
Violence | **Violencias** | **Violence**

Injured spinal cord | Lesión de la medula espinal | Lésion de la moelle épinière

Table 240a   EME - PEMC - EMBE   Violence - Injured spinal cord

Age group (years)	Incidence 1990 Number ('000s)	Rate (per 100 000)	Prevalence 1990 Number ('000s)	Rate (per 100 000)	Avg. age at onset (years)	Average duration (years)	Deaths 1990 Number ('000s)	Rate (per 100 000)	Deaths 2000 (Projected) Number ('000s)	Rate (per 100 000)
Males										
0-4	0	0.0	0	0.0	-	-	-	-	-	-
5-14	0	0.0	0	0.0	-	-	-	-	-	-
15-44	2	1.0	26	14.0	29.9	33.6	-	-	-	-
45-59	0	0.3	18	27.2	52.4	15.6	-	-	-	-
60+	0	0.2	10	15.9	71.1	6.1	-	-	-	-
All ages	2	0.5	53	13.7	33.7	30.8	-	-	-	-
Females										
0-4	0	0.0	0	0.0	-	-	-	-	-	-
5-14	0	0.0	0	0.0	-	-	-	-	-	-
15-44	0	0.3	7	4.0	30.0	40.2	-	-	-	-
45-59	0	0.1	6	8.1	52.4	20.5	-	-	-	-
60+	0	0.1	5	6.1	72.4	7.8	-	-	-	-
All ages	1	0.1	18	4.4	36.4	35.0	-	-	-	-
Total	3	0.3	71	8.9	34.3	31.8	-	-	-	-

Table 240b   FSE - PEAS - AESE   Violence - Injured spinal cord

Age group (years)	Incidence 1990 Number ('000s)	Rate (per 100 000)	Prevalence 1990 Number ('000s)	Rate (per 100 000)	Avg. age at onset (years)	Average duration (years)	Deaths 1990 Number ('000s)	Rate (per 100 000)	Deaths 2000 (Projected) Number ('000s)	Rate (per 100 000)
Males										
0-4	0	0.0	0	0.0	-	-	-	-	-	-
5-14	0	0.0	0	0.0	-	-	-	-	-	-
15-44	1	1.7	18	23.3	29.8	26.8	-	-	-	-
45-59	0	0.8	11	42.2	52.2	11.9	-	-	-	-
60+	0	0.4	5	21.9	70.0	5.2	-	-	-	-
All ages	2	1.0	34	20.4	34.9	23.7	-	-	-	-
Females										
0-4	0	0.0	0	0.0	-	-	-	-	-	-
5-14	0	0.0	0	0.0	-	-	-	-	-	-
15-44	0	0.4	5	6.4	29.9	36.2	-	-	-	-
45-59	0	0.3	4	13.7	52.4	17.4	-	-	-	-
60+	0	0.2	4	10.5	71.5	6.7	-	-	-	-
All ages	0	0.3	13	7.0	40.7	28.0	-	-	-	-
Total	2	0.6	46	13.4	36.3	24.7	-	-	-	-

Table 240c   India - India - Inde   Violence - Injured spinal cord

Age group (years)	Incidence 1990 Number ('000s)	Rate (per 100 000)	Prevalence 1990 Number ('000s)	Rate (per 100 000)	Avg. age at onset (years)	Average duration (years)	Deaths 1990 Number ('000s)	Rate (per 100 000)	Deaths 2000 (Projected) Number ('000s)	Rate (per 100 000)
Males										
0-4	0	0.0	0	0.0	-	-	-	-	-	-
5-14	0	0.0	0	0.0	-	-	-	-	-	-
15-44	0	0.0	0	0.0	-	-	-	-	-	-
45-59	0	0.0	0	0.0	-	-	-	-	-	-
60+	0	0.6	1	2.9	69.7	4.9	-	-	-	-
All ages	0	0.0	1	0.2	69.7	4.9	-	-	-	-
Females										
0-4	0	0.0	0	0.0	-	-	-	-	-	-
5-14	0	0.0	0	0.0	-	-	-	-	-	-
15-44	0	0.0	0	0.0	-	-	-	-	-	-
45-59	0	0.0	0	0.0	-	-	-	-	-	-
60+	0	0.5	1	2.7	70.1	5.3	-	-	-	-
All ages	0	0.0	1	0.2	70.1	5.3	-	-	-	-
Total	0	0.0	2	0.2	69.9	5.1	-	-	-	-

For epidemiological sources see Sandiford 1996. For the methods used to estimate and project incidence, prevalence, and deaths see Lozano et al. 1996 and Murray and Lopez 1996a. See explanatory notes for definitions and caveats.

Table 240	Cuadro 240	Tableau 240
Violence	Violencias	Violence
Injured spinal cord	Lesión de la medula espinal	Lésion de la moelle épinière

Table 240d   China - China - Chine   Violence - Injured spinal cord

Age group (years)	Incidence 1990 Number ('000s)	Rate (per 100 000)	Prevalence 1990 Number ('000s)	Rate (per 100 000)	Avg. age at onset (years)	Average duration (years)	Deaths 1990 Number ('000s)	Rate (per 100 000)	Deaths 2000 (Projected) Number ('000s)	Rate (per 100 000)
Males										
0-4	0	0.0	0	0.0	-	-	-	-	-	-
5-14	0	0.0	0	0.0	-	-	-	-	-	-
15-44	0	0.0	0	0.0	-	-	-	-	-	-
45-59	0	0.0	0	0.0	-	-	-	-	-	-
60+	0	0.2	0	0.9	69.8	5.0	-	-	-	-
All ages	0	0.0	0	0.1	69.8	5.0	-	-	-	-
Females										
0-4	0	0.0	0	0.0	-	-	-	-	-	-
5-14	0	0.0	0	0.0	-	-	-	-	-	-
15-44	0	0.0	0	0.0	-	-	-	-	-	-
45-59	0	0.0	0	0.0	-	-	-	-	-	-
60+	0	0.2	1	1.2	70.6	5.7	-	-	-	-
All ages	0	0.0	1	0.1	70.6	5.7	-	-	-	-
Total	0	0.0	1	0.1	70.2	5.4	-	-	-	-

Table 240e   OAI - OPAI - APAI   Violence - Injured spinal cord

Age group (years)	Incidence 1990 Number ('000s)	Rate (per 100 000)	Prevalence 1990 Number ('000s)	Rate (per 100 000)	Avg. age at onset (years)	Average duration (years)	Deaths 1990 Number ('000s)	Rate (per 100 000)	Deaths 2000 (Projected) Number ('000s)	Rate (per 100 000)
Males										
0-4	0	0.0	0	0.0	-	-	-	-	-	-
5-14	0	0.0	0	0.0	-	-	-	-	-	-
15-44	0	0.0	0	0.0	-	-	-	-	-	-
45-59	0	0.0	0	0.0	-	-	-	-	-	-
60+	0	0.5	0	2.4	69.6	4.7	-	-	-	-
All ages	0	0.0	0	0.1	69.6	4.7	-	-	-	-
Females										
0-4	0	0.0	0	0.0	-	-	-	-	-	-
5-14	0	0.0	0	0.0	-	-	-	-	-	-
15-44	0	0.0	0	0.0	-	-	-	-	-	-
45-59	0	0.0	0	0.0	-	-	-	-	-	-
60+	0	0.1	0	0.6	70.3	5.4	-	-	-	-
All ages	0	0.0	0	0.0	70.3	5.4	-	-	-	-
Total	0	0.0	1	0.1	69.7	4.9	-	-	-	-

Table 240f   SSA - ASS - ASS   Violence - Injured spinal cord

Age group (years)	Incidence 1990 Number ('000s)	Rate (per 100 000)	Prevalence 1990 Number ('000s)	Rate (per 100 000)	Avg. age at onset (years)	Average duration (years)	Deaths 1990 Number ('000s)	Rate (per 100 000)	Deaths 2000 (Projected) Number ('000s)	Rate (per 100 000)
Males										
0-4	0	0.0	0	0.0	-	-	-	-	-	-
5-14	0	0.0	0	0.0	-	-	-	-	-	-
15-44	0	0.0	0	0.0	-	-	-	-	-	-
45-59	0	0.0	0	0.0	-	-	-	-	-	-
60+	0	1.4	1	6.2	69.2	4.5	-	-	-	-
All ages	0	0.1	1	0.3	69.2	4.5	-	-	-	-
Females										
0-4	0	0.0	0	0.0	-	-	-	-	-	-
5-14	0	0.0	0	0.0	-	-	-	-	-	-
15-44	0	0.0	0	0.0	-	-	-	-	-	-
45-59	0	0.0	0	0.0	-	-	-	-	-	-
60+	0	0.4	0	1.9	69.7	4.9	-	-	-	-
All ages	0	0.0	0	0.1	69.7	4.9	-	-	-	-
Total	0	0.0	1	0.2	69.3	4.6	-	-	-	-

For epidemiological sources see Sandiford 1996. For the methods used to estimate and project incidence, prevalence, and deaths see Lozano et al. 1996 and Murray and Lopez 1996a. See explanatory notes for definitions and caveats.

Table 240
Violence

Cuadro 240
Violencias

Tableau 240
Violence

Injured spinal cord

Lesión de la medula espinal

Lésion de la moelle épinière

Table 240g   LAC - ALC - ALC   Violence - Injured spinal cord

Age group (years)	Incidence 1990 Number ('000s)	Rate (per 100 000)	Prevalence 1990 Number ('000s)	Rate (per 100 000)	Avg. age at onset (years)	Average duration (years)	Deaths 1990 Number ('000s)	Rate (per 100 000)	Deaths 2000 (Projected) Number ('000s)	Rate (per 100 000)
Males										
0-4	0	0.0	0	0.0	-	-	-	-	-	-
5-14	0	0.0	0	0.0	-	-	-	-	-	-
15-44	4	4.1	60	57.6	29.8	29.4	-	-	-	-
45-59	0	1.5	24	108.1	52.3	13.6	-	-	-	-
60+	0	1.1	9	61.9	70.3	5.4	-	-	-	-
All ages	5	2.2	93	41.9	32.8	27.5	-	-	-	-
Females										
0-4	0	0.0	0	0.0	-	-	-	-	-	-
5-14	0	0.0	0	0.0	-	-	-	-	-	-
15-44	1	0.5	8	7.5	29.9	33.0	-	-	-	-
45-59	0	0.2	3	14.4	52.4	16.2	-	-	-	-
60+	0	0.2	2	9.5	71.1	6.2	-	-	-	-
All ages	1	0.3	13	5.7	33.5	30.6	-	-	-	-
Total	5	1.2	106	23.8	32.8	27.9	-	-	-	-

Table 240h   MEC - AOM - CMO   Violence - Injured spinal cord

Age group (years)	Incidence 1990 Number ('000s)	Rate (per 100 000)	Prevalence 1990 Number ('000s)	Rate (per 100 000)	Avg. age at onset (years)	Average duration (years)	Deaths 1990 Number ('000s)	Rate (per 100 000)	Deaths 2000 (Projected) Number ('000s)	Rate (per 100 000)
Males										
0-4	0	0.0	0	0.0	-	-	-	-	-	-
5-14	0	0.0	0	0.0	-	-	-	-	-	-
15-44	1	0.4	7	6.3	29.8	28.5	-	-	-	-
45-59	0	0.2	3	11.8	52.3	12.3	-	-	-	-
60+	0	0.2	1	6.7	69.7	4.9	-	-	-	-
All ages	1	0.2	11	4.2	33.3	26.2	-	-	-	-
Females										
0-4	0	0.0	0	0.0	-	-	-	-	-	-
5-14	0	0.0	0	0.0	-	-	-	-	-	-
15-44	0	0.1	1	1.3	29.8	31.1	-	-	-	-
45-59	0	0.1	1	2.7	52.3	14.3	-	-	-	-
60+	0	0.1	0	2.1	70.4	5.5	-	-	-	-
All ages	0	0.1	2	0.9	36.9	26.3	-	-	-	-
Total	1	0.1	13	2.6	34.0	26.2	-	-	-	-

Table 240i   World - Mundo - Monde   Violence - Injured spinal cord

Age group (years)	Incidence 1990 Number ('000s)	Rate (per 100 000)	Prevalence 1990 Number ('000s)	Rate (per 100 000)	Avg. age at onset (years)	Average duration (years)	Deaths 1990 Number ('000s)	Rate (per 100 000)	Deaths 2000 (Projected) Number ('000s)	Rate (per 100 000)
Males										
0-4	0	0.0	0	0.0	-	-	-	-	-	-
5-14	0	0.0	0	0.0	-	-	-	-	-	-
15-44	8	0.6	111	8.9	29.8	29.9	-	-	-	-
45-59	1	0.2	56	17.9	52.3	13.5	-	-	-	-
60+	1	0.4	26	12.1	69.9	5.1	-	-	-	-
All ages	10	0.4	193	7.3	35.3	26.3	-	-	-	-
Females										
0-4	0	0.0	0	0.0	-	-	-	-	-	-
5-14	0	0.0	0	0.0	-	-	-	-	-	-
15-44	1	0.1	21	1.8	29.9	36.0	-	-	-	-
45-59	0	0.1	14	4.4	52.4	17.8	-	-	-	-
60+	1	0.2	13	4.7	70.7	5.9	-	-	-	-
All ages	2	0.1	47	1.8	41.7	27.1	-	-	-	-
Total	12	0.2	241	4.6	36.5	26.4	-	-	-	-

For epidemiological sources see Sandiford 1996. For the methods used to estimate and project incidence, prevalence, and deaths see Lozano et al. 1996 and Murray and Lopez 1996a. See explanatory notes for definitions and caveats.

Table 241
Violence

Cuadro 241
Violencias

Tableau 241
Violence

Intracranial injury - short term   Lesión intracraneal - corta duración   Lésions intra-crâniennes - court terme

Table 241a   EME - PEMC - EMBE   Violence - Intracranial injury - short term

Age group (years)	Incidence 1990 Number ('000s)	Rate (per 100 000)	Prevalence 1990 Number ('000s)	Rate (per 100 000)	Avg. age at onset (years)	Average duration (years)	Deaths 1990 Number ('000s)	Rate (per 100 000)	Deaths 2000 (Projected) Number ('000s)	Rate (per 100 000)
Males										
0-4	5	17.2	0	1.2	2.5	0.07	-	-	-	-
5-14	5	8.6	0	0.6	10.0	0.07	-	-	-	-
15-44	164	88.9	11	6.2	29.9	0.07	-	-	-	-
45-59	16	24.6	1	1.7	52.4	0.07	-	-	-	-
60+	5	8.3	0	0.6	71.1	0.07	-	-	-	-
All ages	194	49.7	14	3.5	31.7	0.07	-	-	-	-
Females										
0-4	4	17.3	0	1.2	2.5	0.07	-	-	-	-
5-14	3	6.9	0	0.5	10.0	0.07	-	-	-	-
15-44	44	24.5	3	1.7	30.0	0.07	-	-	-	-
45-59	5	7.9	0	0.6	52.4	0.07	-	-	-	-
60+	3	3.9	0	0.3	72.4	0.07	-	-	-	-
All ages	60	14.8	4	1.0	31.2	0.07	-	-	-	-
Total	254	31.9	18	2.2	31.6	0.07	-	-	-	-

Table 241b   FSE - PEAS - AESE   Violence - Intracranial injury - short term

Age group (years)	Incidence 1990 Number ('000s)	Rate (per 100 000)	Prevalence 1990 Number ('000s)	Rate (per 100 000)	Avg. age at onset (years)	Average duration (years)	Deaths 1990 Number ('000s)	Rate (per 100 000)	Deaths 2000 (Projected) Number ('000s)	Rate (per 100 000)
Males										
0-4	1	9.3	0	0.6	2.5	0.07	-	-	-	-
5-14	2	6.5	0	0.5	10.0	0.07	-	-	-	-
15-44	117	153.8	8	10.8	29.8	0.07	-	-	-	-
45-59	20	72.9	1	5.1	52.2	0.07	-	-	-	-
60+	4	20.9	0	1.5	70.0	0.07	-	-	-	-
All ages	144	87.3	10	6.1	33.6	0.07	-	-	-	-
Females										
0-4	1	9.6	0	0.7	2.5	0.07	-	-	-	-
5-14	2	6.0	0	0.4	10.0	0.07	-	-	-	-
15-44	30	39.7	2	2.8	29.9	0.07	-	-	-	-
45-59	8	26.9	1	1.9	52.4	0.07	-	-	-	-
60+	4	12.1	0	0.8	71.5	0.07	-	-	-	-
All ages	45	24.9	3	1.7	36.5	0.07	-	-	-	-
Total	189	54.7	13	3.8	34.3	0.07	-	-	-	-

Table 241c   India - India - Inde   Violence - Intracranial injury - short term

Age group (years)	Incidence 1990 Number ('000s)	Rate (per 100 000)	Prevalence 1990 Number ('000s)	Rate (per 100 000)	Avg. age at onset (years)	Average duration (years)	Deaths 1990 Number ('000s)	Rate (per 100 000)	Deaths 2000 (Projected) Number ('000s)	Rate (per 100 000)
Males										
0-4	31	52	2	3.6	2.5	0.07	-	-	-	-
5-14	11	11	1	0.8	10.0	0.07	-	-	-	-
15-44	70	35	5	2.4	29.8	0.07	-	-	-	-
45-59	20	41	1	2.9	52.3	0.07	-	-	-	-
60+	10	33	1	2.3	69.7	0.07	-	-	-	-
All ages	142	32	10	2.3	28.1	0.07	-	-	-	-
Females										
0-4	39	68	3	4.8	2.5	0.07	-	-	-	-
5-14	10	10	1	0.7	10.0	0.07	-	-	-	-
15-44	20	11	1	0.8	29.8	0.07	-	-	-	-
45-59	18	38	1	2.7	52.4	0.07	-	-	-	-
60+	8	28	1	1.9	70.1	0.07	-	-	-	-
All ages	94	23	7	1.6	24.2	0.07	-	-	-	-
Total	236	28	17	1.9	26.6	0.07	-	-	-	-

For epidemiological sources see Sandiford 1996. For the methods used to estimate and project incidence, prevalence, and deaths see Lozano et al. 1996 and Murray and Lopez 1996a. See explanatory notes for definitions and caveats.

Table 241   **Cuadro 241**   **Tableau 241**
Violence   **Violencias**   **Violence**

Intracranial injury - short term   Lesión intracraneal - corta duración   Lésions intra-crâniennes - court terme

Table 241d   China - China - Chine   Violence - Intracranial injury - short term

Age group (years)	Incidence 1990 Number ('000s)	Rate (per 100 000)	Prevalence 1990 Number ('000s)	Rate (per 100 000)	Avg. age at onset (years)	Average duration (years)	Deaths 1990 Number ('000s)	Rate (per 100 000)	Deaths 2000 (Projected) Number ('000s)	Rate (per 100 000)
Males										
0-4	31	51.1	2	3.6	2.5	0.07	-	-	-	-
5-14	8	8.6	1	0.6	10.0	0.07	-	-	-	-
15-44	118	38.7	8	2.7	29.9	0.07	-	-	-	-
45-59	9	12.8	1	0.9	52.3	0.07	-	-	-	-
60+	5	10.3	0	0.7	69.8	0.07	-	-	-	-
All ages	172	29.4	12	2.1	26.4	0.07	-	-	-	-
Females										
0-4	57	98.0	4	6.9	2.5	0.07	-	-	-	-
5-14	11	12.3	1	0.9	10.0	0.07	-	-	-	-
15-44	36	12.6	3	0.9	29.9	0.07	-	-	-	-
45-59	6	8.8	0	0.6	52.4	0.07	-	-	-	-
60+	6	11.7	0	0.8	70.6	0.07	-	-	-	-
All ages	116	21.1	8	1.5	17.7	0.07	-	-	-	-
Total	287	25.4	20	1.8	22.9	0.07	-	-	-	-

Table 241e   OAI - OPAI - APAI   Violence - Intracranial injury - short term

Age group (years)	Incidence 1990 Number ('000s)	Rate (per 100 000)	Prevalence 1990 Number ('000s)	Rate (per 100 000)	Avg. age at onset (years)	Average duration (years)	Deaths 1990 Number ('000s)	Rate (per 100 000)	Deaths 2000 (Projected) Number ('000s)	Rate (per 100 000)
Males										
0-4	6	14.1	0	1.0	2.5	0.07	-	-	-	-
5-14	14	16.4	1	1.1	10.0	0.07	-	-	-	-
15-44	142	88.0	10	6.2	29.7	0.07	-	-	-	-
45-59	18	54.0	1	3.8	52.3	0.07	-	-	-	-
60+	6	27.6	0	1.9	69.6	0.07	-	-	-	-
All ages	186	54.1	13	3.8	30.8	0.07	-	-	-	-
Females										
0-4	7	16.9	0	1.2	2.5	0.07	-	-	-	-
5-14	9	11.0	1	0.8	10.0	0.07	-	-	-	-
15-44	30	19.1	2	1.3	29.8	0.07	-	-	-	-
45-59	3	8.8	0	0.6	52.3	0.07	-	-	-	-
60+	1	5.8	0	0.4	70.3	0.07	-	-	-	-
All ages	51	15.0	4	1.0	24.9	0.07	-	-	-	-
Total	236	34.6	17	2.4	29.5	0.07	-	-	-	-

Table 241f   SSA - ASS - ASS   Violence - Intracranial injury - short term

Age group (years)	Incidence 1990 Number ('000s)	Rate (per 100 000)	Prevalence 1990 Number ('000s)	Rate (per 100 000)	Avg. age at onset (years)	Average duration (years)	Deaths 1990 Number ('000s)	Rate (per 100 000)	Deaths 2000 (Projected) Number ('000s)	Rate (per 100 000)
Males										
0-4	17	35	1	2.4	2.4	0.07	-	-	-	-
5-14	39	55	3	3.9	10.0	0.07	-	-	-	-
15-44	540	520	38	36.4	29.4	0.07	-	-	-	-
45-59	30	148	2	10.4	52.2	0.07	-	-	-	-
60+	8	76	1	5.3	69.2	0.07	-	-	-	-
All ages	633	251	44	17.6	29.1	0.07	-	-	-	-
Females										
0-4	8	18	1	1.2	2.4	0.07	-	-	-	-
5-14	17	24	1	1.7	10.0	0.07	-	-	-	-
15-44	70	66	5	4.6	29.5	0.07	-	-	-	-
45-59	6	28	0	2.0	52.2	0.07	-	-	-	-
60+	3	22	0	1.5	69.7	0.07	-	-	-	-
All ages	104	40	7	2.8	26.7	0.07	-	-	-	-
Total	737	144	52	10.1	28.8	0.07	-	-	-	-

For epidemiological sources see Sandiford 1996. For the methods used to estimate and project incidence, prevalence, and deaths see Lozano et al. 1996 and Murray and Lopez 1996a. See explanatory notes for definitions and caveats.

Table 241
Violence

Cuadro 241
Violencias

Tableau 241
Violence

Intracranial injury - short term   Lesión intracraneal - corta duración   Lésions intra-crâniennes - court terme

Table 241g LAC - ALC - ALC   Violence - Intracranial injury - short term

Age group (years)	Incidence 1990 Number ('000s)	Rate (per 100 000)	Prevalence 1990 Number ('000s)	Rate (per 100 000)	Avg. age at onset (years)	Average duration (years)	Deaths 1990 Number ('000s)	Rate (per 100 000)	Deaths 2000 (Projected) Number ('000s)	Rate (per 100 000)
Males										
0-4	7	24.7	0	1.7	2.5	0.07	-	-	-	-
5-14	25	47.6	2	3.3	10.0	0.07	-	-	-	-
15-44	196	187.8	14	13.1	29.8	0.07	-	-	-	-
45-59	15	69.2	1	4.8	52.3	0.07	-	-	-	-
60+	9	62.4	1	4.4	70.3	0.07	-	-	-	-
All ages	252	113.7	18	8.0	29.9	0.07	-	-	-	-
Females										
0-4	5	18.9	0	1.3	2.5	0.07	-	-	-	-
5-14	10	19.8	1	1.4	10.0	0.07	-	-	-	-
15-44	25	23.9	2	1.7	29.9	0.07	-	-	-	-
45-59	2	7.4	0	0.5	52.4	0.07	-	-	-	-
60+	2	10.7	0	0.7	71.1	0.07	-	-	-	-
All ages	44	19.6	3	1.4	24.6	0.07	-	-	-	-
Total	296	66.5	21	4.7	29.1	0.07	-	-	-	-

Table 241h MEC - AOM - CMO   Violence - Intracranial injury - short term

Age group (years)	Incidence 1990 Number ('000s)	Rate (per 100 000)	Prevalence 1990 Number ('000s)	Rate (per 100 000)	Avg. age at onset (years)	Average duration (years)	Deaths 1990 Number ('000s)	Rate (per 100 000)	Deaths 2000 (Projected) Number ('000s)	Rate (per 100 000)
Males										
0-4	2	4.2	0	0.3	2.5	0.07	-	-	-	-
5-14	2	2.3	0	0.2	10.0	0.07	-	-	-	-
15-44	23	20.2	2	1.4	29.8	0.07	-	-	-	-
45-59	2	9.2	0	0.6	52.3	0.07	-	-	-	-
60+	1	10.2	0	0.7	69.7	0.07	-	-	-	-
All ages	30	11.6	2	0.8	30.6	0.07	-	-	-	-
Females										
0-4	1	3.7	0	0.3	2.5	0.07	-	-	-	-
5-14	1	1.9	0	0.1	10.0	0.07	-	-	-	-
15-44	4	4.2	0	0.3	29.8	0.07	-	-	-	-
45-59	1	3.1	0	0.2	52.3	0.07	-	-	-	-
60+	1	4.9	0	0.3	70.4	0.07	-	-	-	-
All ages	9	3.5	1	0.2	27.9	0.07	-	-	-	-
Total	38	7.6	3	0.5	30.0	0.07	-	-	-	-

Table 241i World - Mundo - Monde   Violence - Intracranial injury - short term

Age group (years)	Incidence 1990 Number ('000s)	Rate (per 100 000)	Prevalence 1990 Number ('000s)	Rate (per 100 000)	Avg. age at onset (years)	Average duration (years)	Deaths 1990 Number ('000s)	Rate (per 100 000)	Deaths 2000 (Projected) Number ('000s)	Rate (per 100 000)
Males										
0-4	99	31	7	2.2	2.5	0.07	-	-	-	-
5-14	105	19	7	1.3	10.0	0.07	-	-	-	-
15-44	1 369	110	96	7.7	29.7	0.07	-	-	-	-
45-59	131	42	9	2.9	52.3	0.07	-	-	-	-
60+	48	22	3	1.5	69.9	0.07	-	-	-	-
All ages	1 752	66	123	4.6	29.7	0.07	-	-	-	-
Females										
0-4	123	40	9	2.8	2.5	0.07	-	-	-	-
5-14	63	12	4	0.8	10.0	0.07	-	-	-	-
15-44	260	22	18	1.5	29.8	0.07	-	-	-	-
45-59	49	16	3	1.1	52.4	0.07	-	-	-	-
60+	28	11	2	0.7	70.7	0.07	-	-	-	-
All ages	522	20	37	1.4	25.3	0.07	-	-	-	-
Total	2 275	43	159	3.0	28.7	0.07	-	-	-	-

For epidemiological sources see Sandiford 1996. For the methods used to estimate and project incidence, prevalence, and deaths see Lozano et al. 1996 and Murray and Lopez 1996a. See explanatory notes for definitions and caveats.

Table 242
Violence

Cuadro 242
Violencias

Tableau 242
Violence

Intracranial injury - long term   Lesión intracraneal - larga duración   Lésions intra-crâniennes - long terme

Table 242a   EME - PEMC - EMBE   Violence - Intracranial injury - long term

Age group (years)	Incidence 1990 Number ('000s)	Rate (per 100 000)	Prevalence 1990 Number ('000s)	Rate (per 100 000)	Avg. age at onset (years)	Average duration (years)	Deaths 1990 Number ('000s)	Rate (per 100 000)	Deaths 2000 (Projected) Number ('000s)	Rate (per 100 000)
Males										
0-4	0	0.9	1	2.1	2.5	70.2	-	-	-	-
5-14	0	0.4	3	6.4	10.0	63.6	-	-	-	-
15-44	8	4.4	138	74.8	29.9	44.8	-	-	-	-
45-59	1	1.2	100	150.8	52.4	24.5	-	-	-	-
60+	0	0.4	100	164.8	71.1	11.3	-	-	-	-
All ages	10	2.5	341	87.4	31.7	43.2	-	-	-	-
Females										
0-4	0	0.9	1	2.2	2.5	76.1	-	-	-	-
5-14	0	0.3	3	6.0	10.0	69.5	-	-	-	-
15-44	2	1.2	47	26.1	30.0	50.0	-	-	-	-
45-59	0	0.4	32	47.4	52.4	28.8	-	-	-	-
60+	0	0.2	45	52.8	72.4	12.7	-	-	-	-
All ages	3	0.7	127	31.2	31.2	49.1	-	-	-	-
Total	13	1.6	468	58.7	31.6	44.6	-	-	-	-

Table 242b   FSE - PEAS - AESE   Violence - Intracranial injury - long term

Age group (years)	Incidence 1990 Number ('000s)	Rate (per 100 000)	Prevalence 1990 Number ('000s)	Rate (per 100 000)	Avg. age at onset (years)	Average duration (years)	Deaths 1990 Number ('000s)	Rate (per 100 000)	Deaths 2000 (Projected) Number ('000s)	Rate (per 100 000)
Males										
0-4	0	0.5	0	1.2	2.5	63.5	-	-	-	-
5-14	0	0.3	1	3.9	10.0	57.3	-	-	-	-
15-44	6	7.7	91	119.2	29.8	39.2	-	-	-	-
45-59	1	3.6	71	262.3	52.2	20.8	-	-	-	-
60+	0	1.0	63	300.9	70.0	10.1	-	-	-	-
All ages	7	4.4	226	136.7	33.6	36.2	-	-	-	-
Females										
0-4	0	0.5	0	1.2	2.5	72.4	-	-	-	-
5-14	0	0.3	1	3.9	10.0	66.0	-	-	-	-
15-44	1	2.0	26	35.1	29.9	46.8	-	-	-	-
45-59	0	1.3	22	74.9	52.4	26.1	-	-	-	-
60+	0	0.6	34	92.1	71.5	11.8	-	-	-	-
All ages	2	1.2	83	46.1	36.5	41.1	-	-	-	-
Total	9	2.7	309	89.4	34.3	37.4	-	-	-	-

Table 242c   India - India - Inde   Violence - Intracranial injury - long term

Age group (years)	Incidence 1990 Number ('000s)	Rate (per 100 000)	Prevalence 1990 Number ('000s)	Rate (per 100 000)	Avg. age at onset (years)	Average duration (years)	Deaths 1990 Number ('000s)	Rate (per 100 000)	Deaths 2000 (Projected) Number ('000s)	Rate (per 100 000)
Males										
0-4	2	2.6	4	6.4	2.5	59.9	-	-	-	-
5-14	1	0.6	16	15.6	10.0	57.4	-	-	-	-
15-44	3	1.7	89	44.2	29.8	39.9	-	-	-	-
45-59	1	2.1	41	85.9	52.3	21.0	-	-	-	-
60+	0	1.6	35	117.7	69.7	9.7	-	-	-	-
All ages	7	1.6	184	41.9	28.1	41.0	-	-	-	-
Females										
0-4	2	3.4	5	8.3	2.5	60.8	-	-	-	-
5-14	0	0.5	18	19.4	10.0	59.1	-	-	-	-
15-44	1	0.5	55	30.0	29.8	41.7	-	-	-	-
45-59	1	1.9	24	52.4	52.3	22.5	-	-	-	-
60+	0	1.4	23	81.1	70.1	10.2	-	-	-	-
All ages	5	1.1	126	30.6	24.2	45.1	-	-	-	-
Total	12	1.4	310	36.5	26.6	42.6	-	-	-	-

For epidemiological sources see Sandiford 1996. For the methods used to estimate and project incidence, prevalence, and deaths see Lozano et al. 1996 and Murray and Lopez 1996a. See explanatory notes for definitions and caveats.

Table 242 / **Cuadro 242** / **Tableau 242**
Violence / Violencias / Violence

Intracranial injury - long term / Lesión intracraneal - larga duración / Lésions intra-crâniennes - long terme

Table 242d China - China - Chine — Violence - Intracranial injury - long term

Age group (years)	Incidence 1990 Number ('000s)	Rate (per 100 000)	Prevalence 1990 Number ('000s)	Rate (per 100 000)	Avg. age at onset (years)	Average duration (years)	Deaths 1990 Number ('000s)	Rate (per 100 000)	Deaths 2000 (Projected) Number ('000s)	Rate (per 100 000)
Males										
0-4	2	2.6	4	6.4	2.5	65.5	-	-	-	-
5-14	0	0.4	14	14.9	10.0	59.9	-	-	-	-
15-44	6	1.9	140	45.8	29.9	41.2	-	-	-	-
45-59	0	0.6	58	79.7	52.3	21.4	-	-	-	-
60+	0	0.5	44	89.6	69.8	9.9	-	-	-	-
All ages	9	1.5	260	44.5	26.4	44.5	-	-	-	-
Females										
0-4	3	4.9	7	12.2	2.5	68.5	-	-	-	-
5-14	1	0.6	25	27.5	10.0	63.2	-	-	-	-
15-44	2	0.6	113	40.0	29.9	44.2	-	-	-	-
45-59	0	0.4	34	52.7	52.4	23.8	-	-	-	-
60+	0	0.6	32	62.3	70.6	10.8	-	-	-	-
All ages	6	1.1	212	38.6	17.7	55.2	-	-	-	-
Total	14	1.3	472	41.6	22.9	48.8	-	-	-	-

Table 242e OAI - OPAI - APAI — Violence - Intracranial injury - long term

Age group (years)	Incidence 1990 Number ('000s)	Rate (per 100 000)	Prevalence 1990 Number ('000s)	Rate (per 100 000)	Avg. age at onset (years)	Average duration (years)	Deaths 1990 Number ('000s)	Rate (per 100 000)	Deaths 2000 (Projected) Number ('000s)	Rate (per 100 000)
Males										
0-4	0	0.7	1	1.7	2.5	59.8	-	-	-	-
5-14	1	0.8	6	7.6	10.0	56.2	-	-	-	-
15-44	7	4.4	123	76.6	29.7	38.8	-	-	-	-
45-59	1	2.7	56	163.3	52.3	20.3	-	-	-	-
60+	0	1.4	40	197.4	69.6	9.7	-	-	-	-
All ages	9	2.7	226	65.9	30.8	38.1	-	-	-	-
Females										
0-4	0	0.8	1	2.1	2.5	63.2	-	-	-	-
5-14	0	0.6	6	7.0	10.0	59.2	-	-	-	-
15-44	2	1.0	38	23.8	29.8	41.5	-	-	-	-
45-59	0	0.4	15	41.6	52.3	22.4	-	-	-	-
60+	0	0.3	11	47.9	70.3	10.5	-	-	-	-
All ages	3	0.7	70	20.6	24.9	45.6	-	-	-	-
Total	12	1.7	296	43.4	29.5	39.7	-	-	-	-

Table 242f SSA - ASS - ASS — Violence - Intracranial injury - long term

Age group (years)	Incidence 1990 Number ('000s)	Rate (per 100 000)	Prevalence 1990 Number ('000s)	Rate (per 100 000)	Avg. age at onset (years)	Average duration (years)	Deaths 1990 Number ('000s)	Rate (per 100 000)	Deaths 2000 (Projected) Number ('000s)	Rate (per 100 000)
Males										
0-4	1	1.7	2	4.2	2.4	48.7	-	-	-	-
5-14	2	2.8	16	22.4	10.0	49.2	-	-	-	-
15-44	27	25.9	425	409.9	29.3	35.0	-	-	-	-
45-59	1	7.4	176	866.3	52.2	19.1	-	-	-	-
60+	0	3.8	101	958.7	69.2	9.3	-	-	-	-
All ages	32	12.5	720	285.2	29.0	35.2	-	-	-	-
Females										
0-4	0	0.9	1	2.1	2.4	51.9	-	-	-	-
5-14	1	1.2	7	10.3	10.0	51.9	-	-	-	-
15-44	4	3.3	68	64.2	29.5	37.2	-	-	-	-
45-59	0	1.4	28	125.7	52.2	20.5	-	-	-	-
60+	0	1.1	19	147.2	69.7	9.8	-	-	-	-
All ages	5	2.0	123	47.6	26.7	39.0	-	-	-	-
Total	37	7.2	843	165.1	28.7	35.7	-	-	-	-

For epidemiological sources see Sandiford 1996. For the methods used to estimate and project incidence, prevalence, and deaths see Lozano et al. 1996 and Murray and Lopez 1996a. See explanatory notes for definitions and caveats.

Table 242
Violence

Cuadro 242
Violencias

Tableau 242
Violence

Intracranial injury - long term   Lesión intracraneal - larga duración   Lésions intra-crâniennes - long terme

Table 242g   LAC - ALC - ALC   Violence - Intracranial injury - long term

Age group (years)	Incidence 1990 Number ('000s)	Rate (per 100 000)	Prevalence 1990 Number ('000s)	Rate (per 100 000)	Avg. age at onset (years)	Average duration (years)	Deaths 1990 Number ('000s)	Rate (per 100 000)	Deaths 2000 (Projected) Number ('000s)	Rate (per 100 000)
Males										
0-4	0	1.2	1	3.1	2.5	63.9	-	-	-	-
5-14	1	2.4	9	18.1	10.0	59.3	-	-	-	-
15-44	10	9.4	176	168.8	29.8	41.5	-	-	-	-
45-59	1	3.5	75	336.4	52.3	22.3	-	-	-	-
60+	0	3.1	56	395.0	70.3	10.4	-	-	-	-
All ages	13	5.7	317	143.2	29.9	41.6	-	-	-	-
Females										
0-4	0	0.9	1	2.3	2.5	67.9	-	-	-	-
5-14	1	1.0	5	9.7	10.0	63.0	-	-	-	-
15-44	1	1.2	34	32.4	29.8	44.6	-	-	-	-
45-59	0	0.4	12	53.2	52.4	24.8	-	-	-	-
60+	0	0.5	10	61.9	71.1	11.3	-	-	-	-
All ages	2	1.0	62	27.9	24.6	49.5	-	-	-	-
Total	15	3.3	379	85.4	29.1	42.8	-	-	-	-

Table 242h   MEC - AOM - CMO   Violence - Intracranial injury - long term

Age group (years)	Incidence 1990 Number ('000s)	Rate (per 100 000)	Prevalence 1990 Number ('000s)	Rate (per 100 000)	Avg. age at onset (years)	Average duration (years)	Deaths 1990 Number ('000s)	Rate (per 100 000)	Deaths 2000 (Projected) Number ('000s)	Rate (per 100 000)
Males										
0-4	0	0.2	0	0.5	2.5	61.1	-	-	-	-
5-14	0	0.1	1	1.6	10.0	58.1	-	-	-	-
15-44	1	1.0	20	17.2	29.8	40.0	-	-	-	-
45-59	0	0.5	8	36.0	52.3	20.8	-	-	-	-
60+	0	0.5	6	44.5	69.7	9.8	-	-	-	-
All ages	1	0.6	35	13.7	30.6	39.4	-	-	-	-
Females										
0-4	0	0.2	0	0.4	2.5	63.7	-	-	-	-
5-14	0	0.1	1	1.4	10.0	60.9	-	-	-	-
15-44	0	0.2	5	5.0	29.8	42.6	-	-	-	-
45-59	0	0.2	2	9.3	52.3	22.9	-	-	-	-
60+	0	0.2	2	13.0	70.4	10.6	-	-	-	-
All ages	0	0.2	10	4.2	27.9	44.2	-	-	-	-
Total	2	0.4	45	9.0	30.0	40.5	-	-	-	-

Table 242i   World - Mundo - Monde   Violence - Intracranial injury - long term

Age group (years)	Incidence 1990 Number ('000s)	Rate (per 100 000)	Prevalence 1990 Number ('000s)	Rate (per 100 000)	Avg. age at onset (years)	Average duration (years)	Deaths 1990 Number ('000s)	Rate (per 100 000)	Deaths 2000 (Projected) Number ('000s)	Rate (per 100 000)
Males										
0-4	5	1.5	12	3.8	2.5	60.6	-	-	-	-
5-14	5	1.0	67	12.2	10.0	55.2	-	-	-	-
15-44	68	5.5	1 202	96.1	29.6	38.7	-	-	-	-
45-59	7	2.1	584	186.9	52.3	21.0	-	-	-	-
60+	2	1.1	445	203.2	69.9	10.0	-	-	-	-
All ages	87	3.3	2 310	87.0	29.7	38.9	-	-	-	-
Females										
0-4	6	2.0	15	4.9	2.5	64.9	-	-	-	-
5-14	3	0.6	66	12.5	10.0	59.3	-	-	-	-
15-44	13	1.1	387	32.3	29.8	43.1	-	-	-	-
45-59	2	0.8	170	54.5	52.3	23.8	-	-	-	-
60+	1	0.5	176	65.3	70.7	10.9	-	-	-	-
All ages	26	1.0	813	31.1	25.3	46.6	-	-	-	-
Total	114	2.2	3 123	59.3	28.7	40.6	-	-	-	-

For epidemiological sources see Sandiford 1996. For the methods used to estimate and project incidence, prevalence, and deaths see Lozano et al. 1996 and Murray and Lopez 1996a. See explanatory notes for definitions and caveats.

Table 243	Cuadro 243	Tableau 243
Violence	Violencias	Violence

Injured nerves	Traumatismo de nervios	Lésions des nerfs

Table 243a EME - PEMC - EMBE — Violence - Injured nerves

Age group (years)	Incidence 1990 Number ('000s)	Rate (per 100 000)	Prevalence 1990 Number ('000s)	Rate (per 100 000)	Avg. age at onset (years)	Average duration (years)	Deaths 1990 Number ('000s)	Rate (per 100 000)	Deaths 2000 (Projected) Number ('000s)	Rate (per 100 000)
Males										
0-4	0	0.2	0	0.4	2.5	70.2	-	-	-	-
5-14	0	0.1	1	1.1	10.0	63.6	-	-	-	-
15-44	2	1.0	30	16.5	29.9	44.7	-	-	-	-
45-59	0	0.3	22	33.6	52.4	24.5	-	-	-	-
60+	0	0.2	23	37.4	71.1	11.3	-	-	-	-
All ages	2	0.6	76	19.4	32.6	42.5	-	-	-	-
Females										
0-4	0	0.2	0	0.4	2.5	76.1	-	-	-	-
5-14	0	0.1	1	1.1	10.0	69.5	-	-	-	-
15-44	0	0.3	10	5.5	30.0	50.0	-	-	-	-
45-59	0	0.1	7	10.3	52.5	28.8	-	-	-	-
60+	0	0.1	10	11.9	72.4	12.7	-	-	-	-
All ages	1	0.2	28	6.8	33.2	47.2	-	-	-	-
Total	3	0.4	104	13.0	32.8	43.6	-	-	-	-

Table 243b FSE - PEAS - AESE — Violence - Injured nerves

Age group (years)	Incidence 1990 Number ('000s)	Rate (per 100 000)	Prevalence 1990 Number ('000s)	Rate (per 100 000)	Avg. age at onset (years)	Average duration (years)	Deaths 1990 Number ('000s)	Rate (per 100 000)	Deaths 2000 (Projected) Number ('000s)	Rate (per 100 000)
Males										
0-4	0	0.1	0	0.2	2.5	63.5	-	-	-	-
5-14	0	0.1	0	0.7	10.0	57.3	-	-	-	-
15-44	1	1.7	20	26.6	29.8	39.2	-	-	-	-
45-59	0	0.8	16	59.0	52.2	20.8	-	-	-	-
60+	0	0.4	14	69.2	70.0	10.1	-	-	-	-
All ages	2	1.0	51	30.8	34.4	35.6	-	-	-	-
Females										
0-4	0	0.1	0	0.2	2.5	72.4	-	-	-	-
5-14	0	0.1	0	0.7	10.0	66.0	-	-	-	-
15-44	0	0.4	6	7.7	29.9	46.8	-	-	-	-
45-59	0	0.3	5	16.7	52.4	26.1	-	-	-	-
60+	0	0.2	8	21.5	71.5	11.8	-	-	-	-
All ages	1	0.3	19	10.4	38.9	39.0	-	-	-	-
Total	2	0.6	70	20.1	35.5	36.5	-	-	-	-

Table 243c India - India - Inde — Violence - Injured nerves

Age group (years)	Incidence 1990 Number ('000s)	Rate (per 100 000)	Prevalence 1990 Number ('000s)	Rate (por 100 000)	Avg. age at onset (years)	Average duration (years)	Deaths 1990 Number ('000s)	Rate (per 100 000)	Deaths 2000 (Projected) Number ('000s)	Rate (per 100 000)
Males										
0-4	0	0.5	1	1.1	2.5	59.9	-	-	-	-
5-14	0	0.1	3	2.8	10.0	57.4	-	-	-	-
15-44	2	0.9	33	16.3	29.8	39.9	-	-	-	-
45-59	0	1.0	18	37.3	52.3	21.0	-	-	-	-
60+	0	0.6	15	51.0	69.7	9.7	-	-	-	-
All ages	3	0.6	69	15.7	32.9	37.2	-	-	-	-
Females										
0-4	0	0.6	1	1.5	2.5	60.8	-	-	-	-
5-14	0	0.1	3	3.4	10.0	59.1	-	-	-	-
15-44	1	0.3	15	7.9	29.8	41.7	-	-	-	-
45-59	0	1.0	9	19.2	52.4	22.5	-	-	-	-
60+	0	0.5	9	31.7	70.1	10.2	-	-	-	-
All ages	2	0.4	37	8.9	33.0	38.4	-	-	-	-
Total	4	0.5	106	12.4	32.9	37.6	-	-	-	-

For epidemiological sources see Sandiford 1996. For the methods used to estimate and project incidence, prevalence, and deaths see Lozano et al. 1996 and Murray and Lopez 1996a. See explanatory notes for definitions and caveats.

Table 243 | **Cuadro 243** | **Tableau 243**
Violence | Violencias | Violence

Table 243
Violence

Injured nerves

Cuadro 243
Violencias

Traumatismo de nervios

Tableau 243
Violence

Lésions des nerfs

Table 243d China - China - Chine — Violence - Injured nerves

Age group (years)	Incidence 1990 Number ('000s)	Rate (per 100 000)	Prevalence 1990 Number ('000s)	Rate (per 100 000)	Avg. age at onset (years)	Average duration (years)	Deaths 1990 Number ('000s)	Rate (per 100 000)	Deaths 2000 (Projected) Number ('000s)	Rate (per 100 000)
Males										
0-4	0	0.5	1	1.1	2.5	65.5	-	-	-	-
5-14	0	0.1	3	2.6	10.0	59.9	-	-	-	-
15-44	3	1.0	54	17.5	29.9	41.2	-	-	-	-
45-59	0	0.3	25	34.6	52.3	21.4	-	-	-	-
60+	0	0.2	19	38.9	69.8	9.9	-	-	-	-
All ages	4	0.6	101	17.3	29.9	41.4	-	-	-	-
Females										
0-4	1	0.9	1	2.2	2.5	68.5	-	-	-	-
5-14	0	0.1	4	4.9	10.0	63.2	-	-	-	-
15-44	1	0.3	29	10.2	29.9	44.2	-	-	-	-
45-59	0	0.2	11	16.6	52.4	23.8	-	-	-	-
60+	0	0.2	11	20.6	70.6	10.8	-	-	-	-
All ages	2	0.3	56	10.2	25.3	48.5	-	-	-	-
Total	5	0.5	157	13.8	28.4	43.7	-	-	-	-

Table 243e OAI - OPAI - APAI — Violence - Injured nerves

Age group (years)	Incidence 1990 Number ('000s)	Rate (per 100 000)	Prevalence 1990 Number ('000s)	Rate (per 100 000)	Avg. age at onset (years)	Average duration (years)	Deaths 1990 Number ('000s)	Rate (per 100 000)	Deaths 2000 (Projected) Number ('000s)	Rate (per 100 000)
Males										
0-4	0	0.1	0	0.3	2.5	59.8	-	-	-	-
5-14	0	0.1	1	1.4	10.0	56.2	-	-	-	-
15-44	4	2.2	56	34.7	29.7	38.8	-	-	-	-
45-59	0	1.4	27	78.4	52.3	20.3	-	-	-	-
60+	0	0.5	19	93.7	69.6	9.7	-	-	-	-
All ages	4	1.3	103	30.0	32.2	36.9	-	-	-	-
Females										
0-4	0	0.2	0	0.4	2.5	63.2	-	-	-	-
5-14	0	0.1	1	1.2	10.0	59.2	-	-	-	-
15-44	1	0.5	14	8.8	29.8	41.4	-	-	-	-
45-59	0	0.2	6	17.8	52.3	22.4	-	-	-	-
60+	0	0.1	5	20.5	70.3	10.5	-	-	-	-
All ages	1	0.3	26	7.7	29.2	42.0	-	-	-	-
Total	5	0.8	129	18.9	31.6	37.8	-	-	-	-

Table 243f SSA - ASS - ASS — Violence - Injured nerves

Age group (years)	Incidence 1990 Number ('000s)	Rate (per 100 000)	Prevalence 1990 Number ('000s)	Rate (per 100 000)	Avg. age at onset (years)	Average duration (years)	Deaths 1990 Number ('000s)	Rate (per 100 000)	Deaths 2000 (Projected) Number ('000s)	Rate (per 100 000)
Males										
0-4	0	0.3	0	0.7	2.4	48.7	-	-	-	-
5-14	0	0.5	3	4.0	10.0	49.2	-	-	-	-
15-44	14	13.1	202	194.7	29.4	35.0	-	-	-	-
45-59	1	3.7	86	425.1	52.2	19.1	-	-	-	-
60+	0	1.4	49	466.9	69.2	9.3	-	-	-	-
All ages	15	5.9	341	135.0	30.2	34.4	-	-	-	-
Females										
0-4	0	0.2	0	0.4	2.4	51.9	-	-	-	-
5-14	0	0.2	1	1.8	10.0	51.9	-	-	-	-
15-44	2	1.7	29	27.0	29.5	37.2	-	-	-	-
45-59	0	0.7	13	58.0	52.3	20.5	-	-	-	-
60+	0	0.4	9	67.3	69.7	9.8	-	-	-	-
All ages	2	0.9	52	20.0	29.8	36.8	-	-	-	-
Total	17	3.4	392	76.9	30.2	34.7	-	-	-	-

For epidemiological sources see Sandiford 1996. For the methods used to estimate and project incidence, prevalence, and deaths see Lozano et al. 1996 and Murray and Lopez 1996a. See explanatory notes for definitions and caveats.

Table 243	Cuadro 243	Tableau 243
Violence	Violencias	Violence
Injured nerves	Traumatismo de nervios	Lésions des nerfs

Table 243g LAC - ALC - ALC — Violence - Injured nerves

Age group (years)	Incidence 1990 Number ('000s)	Rate (per 100 000)	Prevalence 1990 Number ('000s)	Rate (per 100 000)	Avg. age at onset (years)	Average duration (years)	Deaths 1990 Number ('000s)	Rate (per 100 000)	Deaths 2000 (Projected) Number ('000s)	Rate (per 100 000)
Males										
0-4	0	0.2	0	0.5	2.5	63.9	-	-	-	-
5-14	0	0.4	2	3.2	10.0	59.3	-	-	-	-
15-44	8	7.2	117	112.6	29.8	41.4	-	-	-	-
45-59	1	2.7	54	242.2	52.3	22.3	-	-	-	-
60+	0	1.1	39	274.4	70.3	10.4	-	-	-	-
All ages	9	3.9	212	95.8	31.4	40.2	-	-	-	-
Females										
0-4	0	0.2	0	0.4	2.5	67.9	-	-	-	-
5-14	0	0.2	1	1.7	10.0	63.0	-	-	-	-
15-44	1	0.9	17	16.3	29.9	44.6	-	-	-	-
45-59	0	0.3	8	32.4	52.4	24.8	-	-	-	-
60+	0	0.2	6	36.7	71.1	11.3	-	-	-	-
All ages	1	0.5	32	14.2	29.7	44.9	-	-	-	-
Total	10	2.2	244	54.9	31.2	40.7	-	-	-	-

Table 243h MEC - AOM - CMO — Violence - Injured nerves

Age group (years)	Incidence 1990 Number ('000s)	Rate (per 100 000)	Prevalence 1990 Number ('000s)	Rate (per 100 000)	Avg. age at onset (years)	Average duration (years)	Deaths 1990 Number ('000s)	Rate (per 100 000)	Deaths 2000 (Projected) Number ('000s)	Rate (per 100 000)
Males										
0-4	0	0.0	0	0.1	2.5	61.1	-	-	-	-
5-14	0	0.0	0	0.3	10.0	58.1	-	-	-	-
15-44	1	0.8	14	12.0	29.8	40.0	-	-	-	-
45-59	0	0.4	6	26.5	52.3	20.8	-	-	-	-
60+	0	0.2	4	31.0	69.7	9.8	-	-	-	-
All ages	1	0.4	24	9.4	31.9	38.3	-	-	-	-
Females										
0-4	0	0.0	0	0.1	2.5	63.7	-	-	-	-
5-14	0	0.0	0	0.2	10.0	60.9	-	-	-	-
15-44	0	0.2	3	2.7	29.9	42.6	-	-	-	-
45-59	0	0.1	1	6.1	52.4	22.9	-	-	-	-
60+	0	0.1	1	7.9	70.4	10.6	-	-	-	-
All ages	0	0.1	6	2.3	32.4	40.5	-	-	-	-
Total	1	0.3	30	5.9	32.0	38.7	-	-	-	-

Table 243i World - Mundo - Monde — Violence - Injured nerves

Age group (years)	Incidence 1990 Number ('000s)	Rate (per 100 000)	Prevalence 1990 Number ('000s)	Rate (per 100 000)	Avg. age at onset (years)	Average duration (years)	Deaths 1990 Number ('000s)	Rate (per 100 000)	Deaths 2000 (Projected) Number ('000s)	Rate (per 100 000)
Males										
0-4	1	0.3	2	0.7	2.5	60.6	-	-	-	-
5-14	1	0.2	12	2.2	10.0	55.2	-	-	-	-
15-44	33	2.7	526	42.1	29.6	38.5	-	-	-	-
45-59	3	1.0	254	81.3	52.3	20.9	-	-	-	-
60+	1	0.4	183	83.5	69.9	10.0	-	-	-	-
All ages	39	1.5	977	36.8	31.2	37.4	-	-	-	-
Females										
0-4	1	0.4	3	0.9	2.5	64.9	-	-	-	-
5-14	1	0.1	12	2.2	10.0	59.3	-	-	-	-
15-44	6	0.5	122	10.2	29.8	42.2	-	-	-	-
45-59	1	0.3	60	19.1	52.4	23.2	-	-	-	-
60+	1	0.2	58	21.7	70.7	10.9	-	-	-	-
All ages	9	0.3	254	9.7	30.3	42.0	-	-	-	-
Total	48	0.9	1 231	23.4	31.0	38.3	-	-	-	-

For epidemiological sources see Sandiford 1996. For the methods used to estimate and project incidence, prevalence, and deaths see Lozano et al. 1996 and Murray and Lopez 1996a. See explanatory notes for definitions and caveats.

Table 244   **Cuadro 244**   **Tableau 244**
War   **Guerra**   **Guerre**

Episodes   Episodios   Episodes

Table 244a   EME - PEMC - EMBE   War - Episodes

Age group (years)	Incidence 1990 Number ('000s)	Rate (per 100 000)	Prevalence 1990 Number ('000s)	Rate (per 100 000)	Avg. age at onset (years)	Average duration (years)	Deaths 1990 Number ('000s)	Rate (per 100 000)	Deaths 2000 (Projected) Number ('000s)	Rate (per 100 000)
Males										
0-4	0	0.0	-	-	2.5	-	0	0.0	0	0.0
5-14	0	0.0	-	-	10.0	-	0	0.0	0	0.0
15-44	0	0.1	-	-	29.9	-	0	0.0	0	0.0
45-59	0	0.2	-	-	52.4	-	0	0.0	0	0.0
60+	0	0.4	-	-	71.1	-	0	0.1	0	0.1
All ages	1	0.2	-	-	51.5	-	0	0.0	0	0.0
Females										
0-4	0	0.0	-	-	-	-	0	0.0	0	0.0
5-14	0	0.0	-	-	10.0	-	0	0.0	0	0.0
15-44	0	0.0	-	-	30.0	-	0	0.0	0	0.0
45-59	0	0.0	-	-	52.4	-	0	0.0	0	0.0
60+	0	0.1	-	-	72.4	-	0	0.0	0	0.0
All ages	0	0.0	-	-	50.1	-	0	0.0	0	0.0
Total	1	0.1	-	-	51.2	-	0	0.0	0	0.0

Table 244b   FSE - PEAS - AESE   War - Episodes

Age group (years)	Incidence 1990 Number ('000s)	Rate (per 100 000)	Prevalence 1990 Number ('000s)	Rate (per 100 000)	Avg. age at onset (years)	Average duration (years)	Deaths 1990 Number ('000s)	Rate (per 100 000)	Deaths 2000 (Projected) Number ('000s)	Rate (per 100 000)
Males										
0-4	9	65.8	-	-	2.5	-	3	21.4	3	21.4
5-14	5	19.8	-	-	10.0	-	2	6.4	2	6.4
15-44	98	128.1	-	-	29.8	-	11	13.9	11	14.4
45-59	8	30.2	-	-	52.2	-	1	3.3	1	3.3
60+	3	12.9	-	-	70.0	-	1	2.8	1	2.7
All ages	123	74.4	-	-	29.3	-	17	10.1	17	9.9
Females										
0-4	9	68.9	-	-	2.5	-	3	22.4	3	22.4
5-14	7	27.4	-	-	10.0	-	1	4.5	1	4.5
15-44	65	86.9	-	-	29.9	-	7	9.4	7	9.8
45-59	5	18.1	-	-	52.4	-	1	2.0	1	2.0
60+	3	7.5	-	-	71.5	-	1	1.6	1	1.5
All ages	90	49.5	-	-	28.1	-	12	6.8	12	6.6
Total	213	61.4	-	-	28.8	-	29	8.4	29	8.2

Table 244c   India - India - Inde   War - Episodes

Age group (years)	Incidence 1990 Number ('000s)	Rate (per 100 000)	Prevalence 1990 Number ('000s)	Rate (per 100 000)	Avg. age at onset (years)	Average duration (years)	Deaths 1990 Number ('000s)	Rate (per 100 000)	Deaths 2000 (Projected) Number ('000s)	Rate (per 100 000)
Males										
0-4	0	0.0	-	-	-	-	0	0.0	0	0.0
5-14	0	0.0	-	-	-	-	0	0.0	0	0.0
15-44	29	14.4	-	-	29.8	-	3	1.5	4	1.5
45-59	0	0.0	-	-	-	-	0	0.0	0	0.0
60+	0	0.0	-	-	-	-	0	0.0	0	0.0
All ages	29	6.6	-	-	29.8	-	3	0.7	4	0.7
Females										
0-4	0	0.0	-	-	-	-	0	0.0	0	0.0
5-14	0	0.0	-	-	-	-	0	0.0	0	0.0
15-44	0	0.0	-	-	-	-	0	0.0	0	0.0
45-59	0	0.0	-	-	-	-	0	0.0	0	0.0
60+	0	0.0	-	-	-	-	0	0.0	0	0.0
All ages	0	0.0	-	-	-	-	0	0.0	0	0.0
Total	29	3.4	-	-	29.8	-	3	0.4	4	0.4

For epidemiological sources see Zwi 1996. For the methods used to estimate and project incidence, prevalence, and deaths see Murray and Lopez 1996a. See explanatory notes for definitions and caveats.

Table 244	Cuadro 244	Tableau 244
War	Guerra	Guerre
Episodes	Episodios	Episodes

Table 244d — China - China - Chine — War - Episodes

Age group (years)	Incidence 1990 Number ('000s)	Rate (per 100 000)	Prevalence 1990 Number ('000s)	Rate (per 100 000)	Avg. age at onset (years)	Average duration (years)	Deaths 1990 Number ('000s)	Rate (per 100 000)	Deaths 2000 (Projected) Number ('000s)	Rate (per 100 000)
Males										
0-4	0	0.0	-	-	-	-	0	0.0	0	0.0
5-14	0	0.0	-	-	-	-	0	0.0	0	0.0
15-44	6	1.8	-	-	29.9	-	1	0.2	1	0.2
45-59	0	0.0	-	-	-	-	0	0.0	0	0.0
60+	0	0.0	-	-	-	-	0	0.0	0	0.0
All ages	6	0.9	-	-	29.9	-	1	0.1	1	0.1
Females										
0-4	0	0.0	-	-	-	-	0	0.0	0	0.0
5-14	0	0.0	-	-	-	-	0	0.0	0	0.0
15-44	0	0.0	-	-	-	-	0	0.0	0	0.0
45-59	0	0.0	-	-	-	-	0	0.0	0	0.0
60+	0	0.0	-	-	-	-	0	0.0	0	0.0
All ages	0	0.0	-	-	-	-	0	0.0	0	0.0
Total	6	0.5	-	-	29.9	-	1	0.1	1	0.0

Table 244e — OAI - OPAI - APAI — War - Episodes

Age group (years)	Incidence 1990 Number ('000s)	Rate (per 100 000)	Prevalence 1990 Number ('000s)	Rate (per 100 000)	Avg. age at onset (years)	Average duration (years)	Deaths 1990 Number ('000s)	Rate (per 100 000)	Deaths 2000 (Projected) Number ('000s)	Rate (per 100 000)
Males										
0-4	5	10.6	-	-	2.5	-	2	3.4	2	3.4
5-14	3	3.3	-	-	10.0	-	1	1.1	1	1.1
15-44	50	31.1	-	-	29.7	-	5	3.4	7	3.3
45-59	4	12.2	-	-	52.3	-	0	1.3	1	1.3
60+	1	6.9	-	-	69.6	-	0	1.5	0	1.5
All ages	63	18.4	-	-	29.2	-	9	2.5	10	2.5
Females										
0-4	5	11.0	-	-	2.5	-	2	3.6	2	3.6
5-14	4	4.6	-	-	10.0	-	1	0.8	1	0.8
15-44	33	20.9	-	-	29.8	-	4	2.3	4	2.2
45-59	3	7.9	-	-	52.3	-	0	0.9	0	0.9
60+	1	6.1	-	-	70.3	-	0	1.3	0	1.3
All ages	46	13.5	-	-	28.0	-	6	1.9	7	1.8
Total	109	16.0	-	-	28.7	-	15	2.2	18	2.2

Table 244f — SSA - ASS - ASS — War - Episodes

Age group (years)	Incidence 1990 Number ('000s)	Rate (per 100 000)	Prevalence 1990 Number ('000s)	Rate (per 100 000)	Avg. age at onset (years)	Average duration (years)	Deaths 1990 Number ('000s)	Rate (per 100 000)	Deaths 2000 (Projected) Number ('000s)	Rate (per 100 000)
Males										
0-4	83	175	-	-	2.4	-	27	57	37	57
5-14	50	71	-	-	10.0	-	16	23	22	23
15-44	898	866	-	-	29.4	-	97	94	133	94
45-59	75	369	-	-	52.2	-	8	40	11	40
60+	25	237	-	-	69.2	-	5	51	7	51
All ages	1 131	448	-	-	28.9	-	154	61	210	61
Females										
0-4	83	177	-	-	2.4	-	27	57	37	57
5-14	67	95	-	-	10.0	-	11	15	14	15
15-44	599	564	-	-	29.5	-	65	61	88	61
45-59	50	226	-	-	52.2	-	5	24	7	24
60+	25	196	-	-	69.7	-	5	42	7	42
All ages	824	319	-	-	27.8	-	114	44	154	44
Total	1 955	383	-	-	28.5	-	268	52	364	53

For epidemiological sources see Zwi 1996. For the methods used to estimate and project incidence, prevalence, and deaths see Murray and Lopez 1996a. See explanatory notes for definitions and caveats.

Table 244 | **Cuadro 244** | **Tableau 244**
War | Guerra | Guerre

Episodes | Episodios | Episodes

Table 244g   LAC - ALC - ALC   War - Episodes

Age group (years)	Incidence 1990 Number ('000s)	Rate (per 100 000)	Prevalence 1990 Number ('000s)	Rate (per 100 000)	Avg. age at onset (years)	Average duration (years)	Deaths 1990 Number ('000s)	Rate (per 100 000)	Deaths 2000 (Projected) Number ('000s)	Rate (per 100 000)
Males										
0-4	5	18.8	-	-	2.5	-	2	6.1	2	6.1
5-14	3	6.2	-	-	10.0	-	1	2.0	1	2.0
15-44	58	55.8	-	-	29.8	-	6	6.0	8	6.0
45-59	5	21.8	-	-	52.3	-	1	2.4	1	2.4
60+	2	11.4	-	-	70.3	-	0	2.5	0	2.4
All ages	73	33.1	-	-	29.3	-	10	4.5	12	4.5
Females										
0-4	5	19.5	-	-	2.5	-	2	6.3	2	6.3
5-14	4	8.5	-	-	10.0	-	1	1.4	1	1.4
15-44	39	37.3	-	-	29.9	-	4	4.0	5	4.0
45-59	3	13.8	-	-	52.4	-	0	1.5	0	1.5
60+	2	9.6	-	-	71.1	-	0	2.1	0	2.0
All ages	53	23.9	-	-	28.1	-	7	3.3	9	3.2
Total	127	28.5	-	-	28.8	-	17	3.9	20	3.8

Table 244h   MEC - AOM - CMO   War - Episodes

Age group (years)	Incidence 1990 Number ('000s)	Rate (per 100 000)	Prevalence 1990 Number ('000s)	Rate (per 100 000)	Avg. age at onset (years)	Average duration (years)	Deaths 1990 Number ('000s)	Rate (per 100 000)	Deaths 2000 (Projected) Number ('000s)	Rate (per 100 000)
Males										
0-4	53	128	-	-	2.5	-	17	42	21	42
5-14	32	48	-	-	10.0	-	10	16	13	16
15-44	568	499	-	-	29.8	-	62	54	81	54
45-59	47	212	-	-	30.8	-	5	23	7	23
60+	16	116	-	-	69.7	-	3	25	5	25
All ages	716	279	-	-	27.9	-	97	38	126	38
Females										
0-4	53	132	-	-	2.5	-	17	43	20	43
5-14	42	68	-	-	10.0	-	7	11	9	11
15-44	379	353	-	-	29.8	-	41	38	54	38
45-59	32	142	-	-	52.3	-	3	15	5	15
60+	16	102	-	-	70.4	-	3	22	5	22
All ages	521	211	-	-	28.0	-	72	29	93	29
Total	1 237	246	-	-	27.9	-	169	34	219	33

Table 244i   World - Mundo - Monde   War - Episodes

Age group (years)	Incidence 1990 Number ('000s)	Rate (per 100 000)	Prevalence 1990 Number ('000s)	Rate (per 100 000)	Avg. age at onset (years)	Average duration (years)	Deaths 1990 Number ('000s)	Rate (per 100 000)	Deaths 2000 (Projected) Number ('000s)	Rate (per 100 000)
Males										
0-4	155	48	-	-	2.5	-	50	15.7	64	18.6
5-14	93	17	-	-	10.0	-	30	5.5	39	6.1
15-44	1 707	137	-	-	29.8	-	185	14.8	244	16.9
45-59	140	45	-	-	50.8	-	15	4.8	20	5.0
60+	47	21	-	-	70.1	-	10	4.6	14	4.9
All ages	2 141	81	-	-	32.6	-	291	11.0	380	12.3
Females										
0-4	155	50	-	-	2.5	-	50	16.3	63	19.1
5-14	124	24	-	-	10.0	-	20	3.8	26	4.3
15-44	1 115	93	-	-	29.8	-	121	10.1	160	11.5
45-59	93	30	-	-	52.4	-	10	3.2	13	3.3
60+	47	17	-	-	71.2	-	10	3.7	14	4.0
All ages	1 533	59	-	-	28.1	-	211	8.1	275	9.0
Total	3 675	70	-	-	30.7	-	502	9.5	656	10.6

For epidemiological sources see Zwi 1996. For the methods used to estimate and project incidence, prevalence, and deaths see Murray and Lopez 1996a. See explanatory notes for definitions and caveats.

Table 245   **Cuadro 245**   **Tableau 245**
War   **Guerra**   **Guerre**

Intracranial injury - long term   Lesión intracraneal - larga duración   Lésions intra-crâniennes - long terme

Table 245a   EME - PEMC - EMBE   War - Intracranial injury - long term

Age group (years)	Incidence 1990 Number ('000s)	Rate (per 100 000)	Prevalence 1990 Number ('000s)	Rate (per 100 000)	Avg. age at onset (years)	Average duration (years)	Deaths 1990 Number ('000s)	Rate (per 100 000)	Deaths 2000 (Projected) Number ('000s)	Rate (per 100 000)
Males										
0-4	0	0	0	0.0	2.5	70.2	-	-	-	-
5-14	0	0	0	0.0	10.0	63.6	-	-	-	-
15-44	0	0	0	0.1	29.9	44.7	-	-	-	-
45-59	0	0	0	0.3	52.4	24.5	-	-	-	-
60+	0	0	0	0.6	71.1	11.3	-	-	-	-
All ages	0	0	1	0.2	51.4	26.8	-	-	-	-
Females										
0-4	0	0	0	0.0	-	-	-	-	-	-
5-14	0	0	0	0.0	10.0	69.5	-	-	-	-
15-44	0	0	0	0.0	30.0	50.0	-	-	-	-
45-59	0	0	0	0.1	52.4	28.8	-	-	-	-
60+	0	0	0	0.2	72.4	12.7	-	-	-	-
All ages	0	0	0	0.1	50.0	32.3	-	-	-	-
Total	0	0	1	0.1	51.1	28.1	-	-	-	-

Table 245b   FSE - PEAS - AESE   War - Intracranial injury - long term

Age group (years)	Incidence 1990 Number ('000s)	Rate (per 100 000)	Prevalence 1990 Number ('000s)	Rate (per 100 000)	Avg. age at onset (years)	Average duration (years)	Deaths 1990 Number ('000s)	Rate (per 100 000)	Deaths 2000 (Projected) Number ('000s)	Rate (per 100 000)
Males										
0-4	0	3.6	1	8.9	2.5	63.5	-	-	-	-
5-14	0	1.1	6	23.1	10.0	57.3	-	-	-	-
15-44	5	6.9	100	130.9	29.8	39.2	-	-	-	-
45-59	0	1.6	67	248.1	52.2	20.8	-	-	-	-
60+	0	0.7	56	267.8	70.0	10.1	-	-	-	-
All ages	7	4.0	230	139.4	29.3	39.9	-	-	-	-
Females										
0-4	0	3.7	1	9.3	2.5	72.4	-	-	-	-
5-14	0	1.5	7	26.0	10.0	66.0	-	-	-	-
15-44	4	4.7	78	103.7	29.9	46.8	-	-	-	-
45-59	0	1.0	55	181.7	52.4	26.1	-	-	-	-
60+	0	0.4	71	193.8	71.5	11.8	-	-	-	-
All ages	5	2.7	211	116.6	28.1	48.6	-	-	-	-
Total	12	3.3	441	127.5	28.8	43.6	-	-	-	-

Table 245c   India - India - Inde   War - Intracranial injury - long term

Age group (years)	Incidence 1990 Number ('000s)	Rate (per 100 000)	Prevalence 1990 Number ('000s)	Rate (per 100 000)	Avg. age at onset (years)	Average duration (years)	Deaths 1990 Number ('000s)	Rate (per 100 000)	Deaths 2000 (Projected) Number ('000s)	Rate (per 100 000)
Males										
0-4	0	0.0	0	0.0	-	-	-	-	-	-
5-14	0	0.0	0	0.0	-	-	-	-	-	-
15-44	0	0.1	2	0.8	29.8	39.9	-	-	-	-
45-59	0	0.0	1	1.6	-	-	-	-	-	-
60+	0	0.0	0	1.6	-	-	-	-	-	-
All ages	0	0.0	3	0.6	29.8	39.9	-	-	-	-
Females										
0-4	0	0.0	0	0.0	-	-	-	-	-	-
5-14	0	0.0	0	0.0	-	-	-	-	-	-
15-44	0	0.0	0	0.0	-	-	-	-	-	-
45-59	0	0.0	0	0.0	-	-	-	-	-	-
60+	0	0.0	0	0.0	-	-	-	-	-	-
All ages	0	0.0	0	0.0	-	-	-	-	-	-
Total	0	0.0	3	0.3	29.8	39.9	-	-	-	-

For epidemiological sources see Zwi 1996. For the methods used to estimate and project incidence, prevalence, and deaths see Lozano et al. 1996 and Murray and Lopez 1996a. See explanatory notes for definitions and caveats.

Table 245 | **Cuadro 245** | **Tableau 245**
War | **Guerra** | **Guerre**

Intracranial injury - long term | Lesión intracraneal - larga duración | Lésions intra-crâniennes - long terme

Table 245d China - China - Chine — War - Intracranial injury - long term

Age group (years)	Incidence 1990 Number ('000s)	Rate (per 100 000)	Prevalence 1990 Number ('000s)	Rate (per 100 000)	Avg. age at onset (years)	Average duration (years)	Deaths 1990 Number ('000s)	Rate (per 100 000)	Deaths 2000 (Projected) Number ('000s)	Rate (per 100 000)
Males										
0-4	0	0.0	0	0.0	-	-	-	-	-	-
5-14	0	0.0	0	0.0	-	-	-	-	-	-
15-44	0	0.1	4	1.5	29.9	41.2	-	-	-	-
45-59	0	0.0	2	2.9	-	-	-	-	-	-
60+	0	0.0	1	2.9	-	-	-	-	-	-
All ages	0	0.1	8	1.4	29.9	41.2	-	-	-	-
Females										
0-4	0	0.0	0	0.0	-	-	-	-	-	-
5-14	0	0.0	0	0.0	-	-	-	-	-	-
15-44	0	0.0	0	0.0	-	-	-	-	-	-
45-59	0	0.0	0	0.0	-	-	-	-	-	-
60+	0	0.0	0	0.0	-	-	-	-	-	-
All ages	0	0.0	0	0.0	-	-	-	-	-	-
Total	0	0.0	8	0.7	29.9	41.2	-	-	-	-

Table 245e OAI - OPAI - APAI — War - Intracranial injury - long term

Age group (years)	Incidence 1990 Number ('000s)	Rate (per 100 000)	Prevalence 1990 Number ('000s)	Rate (per 100 000)	Avg. age at onset (years)	Average duration (years)	Deaths 1990 Number ('000s)	Rate (per 100 000)	Deaths 2000 (Projected) Number ('000s)	Rate (per 100 000)
Males										
0-4	0	0.6	1	1.4	2.5	59.8	-	-	-	-
5-14	0	0.2	3	3.8	10.0	56.2	-	-	-	-
15-44	3	1.7	47	29.5	29.7	38.8	-	-	-	-
45-59	0	0.7	20	60.0	52.3	20.3	-	-	-	-
60+	0	0.4	14	68.7	69.6	9.7	-	-	-	-
All ages	3	1.0	86	25.0	29.2	39.2	-	-	-	-
Females										
0-4	0	0.6	1	1.5	2.5	63.2	-	-	-	-
5-14	0	0.3	3	4.2	10.0	59.2	-	-	-	-
15-44	2	1.1	35	22.2	29.8	41.4	-	-	-	-
45-59	0	0.4	15	42.6	52.3	22.4	-	-	-	-
60+	0	0.3	11	49.3	70.3	10.5	-	-	-	-
All ages	2	0.7	66	19.3	28.0	43.0	-	-	-	-
Total	6	0.9	151	22.2	28.7	40.8	-	-	-	-

Table 245f SSA - ASS - ASS — War - Intracranial injury - long term

Age group (years)	Incidence 1990 Number ('000s)	Rate (per 100 000)	Prevalence 1990 Number ('000s)	Rate (per 100 000)	Avg. age at onset (years)	Average duration (years)	Deaths 1990 Number ('000s)	Rate (per 100 000)	Deaths 2000 (Projected) Number ('000s)	Rate (per 100 000)
Males										
0-4	5	9.5	11	23	2.4	48.7	-	-	-	-
5-14	3	3.8	47	66	10.0	49.2	-	-	-	-
15-44	49	46.9	786	757	29.4	35.0	-	-	-	-
45-59	4	20.0	330	1 623	52.2	19.1	-	-	-	-
60+	1	12.9	199	1 893	69.2	9.3	-	-	-	-
All ages	61	24.3	1 372	544	28.9	35.0	-	-	-	-
Females										
0-4	5	9.6	11	23	2.4	51.9	-	-	-	-
5-14	4	5.2	51	73	10.0	51.9	-	-	-	-
15-44	32	30.5	574	540	29.5	37.2	-	-	-	-
45-59	3	12.2	243	1 098	52.2	20.5	-	-	-	-
60+	1	10.6	165	1 293	69.7	9.8	-	-	-	-
All ages	45	17.3	1 044	405	27.8	38.0	-	-	-	-
Total	106	20.7	2 415	473	28.5	36.3	-	-	-	-

For epidemiological sources see Zwi 1996. For the methods used to estimate and project incidence, prevalence, and deaths see Lozano et al. 1996 and Murray and Lopez 1996a. See explanatory notes for definitions and caveats.

Table 245
War

Cuadro 245
Guerra

Tableau 245
Guerre

Intracranial injury - long term   Lesión intracraneal - larga duración   Lésions intra-crâniennes - long terme

Table 245g   LAC - ALC - ALC

War - Intracranial injury - long term

Age group (years)	Incidence 1990 Number ('000s)	Rate (per 100 000)	Prevalence 1990 Number ('000s)	Rate (per 100 000)	Avg. age at onset (years)	Average duration (years)	Deaths 1990 Number ('000s)	Rate (per 100 000)	Deaths 2000 (Projected) Number ('000s)	Rate (per 100 000)
Males										
0-4	0	1.0	1	2.5	2.5	63.9	-	-	-	-
5-14	0	0.3	4	6.7	10.0	59.3	-	-	-	-
15-44	3	3.0	55	53.1	29.8	41.4	-	-	-	-
45-59	0	1.2	24	107.6	52.3	22.3	-	-	-	-
60+	0	0.6	18	123.0	70.3	10.4	-	-	-	-
All ages	4	1.8	101	45.6	29.3	41.9	-	-	-	-
Females										
0-4	0	1.1	1	2.6	2.5	67.9	-	-	-	-
5-14	0	0.5	4	7.6	10.0	63.0	-	-	-	-
15-44	2	2.0	41	39.8	29.9	44.6	-	-	-	-
45-59	0	0.7	18	75.9	52.4	24.8	-	-	-	-
60+	0	0.5	15	87.4	71.1	11.3	-	-	-	-
All ages	3	1.3	78	35.2	28.1	46.2	-	-	-	-
Total	7	1.5	180	40.4	28.8	43.7	-	-	-	-

Table 245h   MEC - AOM - CMO

War - Intracranial injury - long term

Age group (years)	Incidence 1990 Number ('000s)	Rate (per 100 000)	Prevalence 1990 Number ('000s)	Rate (per 100 000)	Avg. age at onset (years)	Average duration (years)	Deaths 1990 Number ('000s)	Rate (per 100 000)	Deaths 2000 (Projected) Number ('000s)	Rate (per 100 000)
Males										
0-4	3	6.9	7	17	2.5	61.1	-	-	-	-
5-14	2	2.6	31	48	10.0	58.1	-	-	-	-
15-44	31	27.0	524	460	29.8	40.0	-	-	-	-
45-59	3	11.5	212	951	52.3	20.8	-	-	-	-
60+	1	6.3	150	1 099	69.7	9.8	-	-	-	-
All ages	39	15.1	925	361	29.3	40.4	-	-	-	-
Females										
0-4	3	7.2	7	18	2.5	63.7	-	-	-	-
5-14	2	3.7	34	54	10.0	60.9	-	-	-	-
15-44	21	19.1	382	356	29.8	42.6	-	-	-	-
45-59	2	7.7	156	701	52.3	22.9	-	-	-	-
60+	1	5.5	126	816	70.4	10.6	-	-	-	-
All ages	28	11.4	705	286	28.0	44.0	-	-	-	-
Total	67	13.3	1 629	324	28.8	41.9	-	-	-	-

Table 245i   World - Mundo - Monde

War - Intracranial injury - long term

Age group (years)	Incidence 1990 Number ('000s)	Rate (per 100 000)	Prevalence 1990 Number ('000s)	Rate (per 100 000)	Avg. age at onset (years)	Average duration (years)	Deaths 1990 Number ('000s)	Rate (per 100 000)	Deaths 2000 (Projected) Number ('000s)	Rate (per 100 000)
Males										
0-4	8	2.6	20	6.4	2.4	54.6	-	-	-	-
5-14	5	0.9	91	16.5	10.0	53.3	-	-	-	-
15-44	91	7.3	1 519	121.5	29.6	37.3	-	-	-	-
45-59	8	2.4	656	210.1	52.2	19.9	-	-	-	-
60+	3	1.2	439	200.5	69.5	9.6	-	-	-	-
All ages	115	4.3	2 726	102.7	29.1	37.5	-	-	-	-
Females										
0-4	8	2.7	20	6.6	2.4	58.0	-	-	-	-
5-14	7	1.3	99	18.8	10.0	56.4	-	-	-	-
15-44	60	5.0	1 111	92.6	29.6	40.0	-	-	-	-
45-59	5	1.6	486	156.3	52.3	21.9	-	-	-	-
60+	3	0.9	387	143.9	70.1	10.3	-	-	-	-
All ages	83	3.2	2 103	80.5	27.9	41.1	-	-	-	-
Total	198	3.8	4 829	91.7	28.5	38.9	-	-	-	-

For epidemiological sources see Zwi 1996. For the methods used to estimate and project incidence, prevalence, and deaths see Lozano et al. 1996 and Murray and Lopez 1996a. See explanatory notes for definitions and caveats.

Table 246	Cuadro 246	Tableau 246
War	Guerra	Guerre

Amputated arm	Amputación de brazo	Amputation d'un bras

Table 246a   EME - PEMC - EMBE   War - Amputated arm

Age group (years)	Incidence 1990 Number ('000s)	Rate (per 100 000)	Prevalence 1990 Number ('000s)	Rate (per 100 000)	Avg. age at onset (years)	Average duration (years)	Deaths 1990 Number ('000s)	Rate (per 100 000)	Deaths 2000 (Projected) Number ('000s)	Rate (per 100 000)
Males										
0-4	0	0	0	0.0	2.5	70.2	-	-	-	-
5-14	0	0	0	0.0	10.0	63.6	-	-	-	-
15-44	0	0	0	0.0	29.9	44.7	-	-	-	-
45-59	0	0	0	0.1	52.4	24.5	-	-	-	-
60+	0	0	0	0.3	71.1	11.3	-	-	-	-
All ages	0	0	0	0.1	51.4	26.8	-	-	-	-
Females										
0-4	0	0	0	0.0	-	-	-	-	-	-
5-14	0	0	0	0.0	10.0	69.5	-	-	-	-
15-44	0	0	0	0.0	30.0	50.0	-	-	-	-
45-59	0	0	0	0.0	52.5	28.8	-	-	-	-
60+	0	0	0	0.1	72.4	12.7	-	-	-	-
All ages	0	0	0	0.0	50.0	32.3	-	-	-	-
Total	0	0	0	0.1	51.1	28.1	-	-	-	-

Table 246b   FSE - PEAS - AESE   War - Amputated arm

Age group (years)	Incidence 1990 Number ('000s)	Rate (per 100 000)	Prevalence 1990 Number ('000s)	Rate (per 100 000)	Avg. age at onset (years)	Average duration (years)	Deaths 1990 Number ('000s)	Rate (per 100 000)	Deaths 2000 (Projected) Number ('000s)	Rate (per 100 000)
Males										
0-4	0	2.1	1	5.3	2.5	63.5	-	-	-	-
5-14	0	0.6	4	13.9	10.0	57.3	-	-	-	-
15-44	3	4.2	60	78.5	29.8	39.2	-	-	-	-
45-59	0	1.0	40	148.8	52.2	20.8	-	-	-	-
60+	0	0.4	34	160.6	70.0	10.1	-	-	-	-
All ages	4	2.4	138	83.6	29.3	39.9	-	-	-	-
Females										
0-4	0	2.2	1	5.6	2.5	72.4	-	-	-	-
5-14	0	0.9	4	15.6	10.0	66.0	-	-	-	-
15-44	2	2.8	47	62.2	30.0	46.8	-	-	-	-
45-59	0	0.6	33	109.0	52.4	26.1	-	-	-	-
60+	0	0.2	42	116.2	71.5	11.8	-	-	-	-
All ages	3	1.6	126	69.9	28.2	48.6	-	-	-	-
Total	7	2.0	265	76.4	28.8	43.6	-	-	-	-

Table 246c   India - India - Inde   War - Amputated arm

Age group (years)	Incidence 1990 Number ('000s)	Rate (per 100 000)	Prevalence 1990 Number ('000s)	Rate (per 100 000)	Avg. age at onset (years)	Average duration (years)	Deaths 1990 Number ('000s)	Rate (per 100 000)	Deaths 2000 (Projected) Number ('000s)	Rate (per 100 000)
Males										
0-4	0	0.0	0	0.0	-	-	-	-	-	-
5-14	0	0.0	0	0.0	-	-	-	-	-	-
15-44	1	0.5	14	6.9	29.8	39.9	-	-	-	-
45-59	0	0.0	7	14.1	-	-	-	-	-	-
60+	0	0.0	4	14.1	-	-	-	-	-	-
All ages	1	0.2	25	5.7	29.8	39.9	-	-	-	-
Females										
0-4	0	0.0	0	0.0	-	-	-	-	-	-
5-14	0	0.0	0	0.0	-	-	-	-	-	-
15-44	0	0.0	0	0.0	-	-	-	-	-	-
45-59	0	0.0	0	0.0	-	-	-	-	-	-
60+	0	0.0	0	0.0	-	-	-	-	-	-
All ages	0	0.0	0	0.0	-	-	-	-	-	-
Total	1	0.1	25	2.9	29.8	39.9	-	-	-	-

For epidemiological sources see Zwi 1996. For the methods used to estimate and project incidence, prevalence, and deaths see Lozano et al. 1996 and Murray and Lopez 1996a. See explanatory notes for definitions and caveats.

Table 246	Cuadro 246	Tableau 246
War	Guerra	Guerre

Amputated arm	Amputación de brazo	Amputation d'un bras

Table 246d China - China - Chine — War - Amputated arm

Age group (years)	Incidence 1990 Number ('000s)	Rate (per 100 000)	Prevalence 1990 Number ('000s)	Rate (per 100 000)	Avg. age at onset (years)	Average duration (years)	Deaths 1990 Number ('000s)	Rate (per 100 000)	Deaths 2000 (Projected) Number ('000s)	Rate (per 100 000)
Males										
0-4	0	0.0	0	0.0	-	-	-	-	-	-
5-14	0	0.0	0	0.0	-	-	-	-	-	-
15-44	0	0.1	3	0.9	29.9	41.2	-	-	-	-
45-59	0	0.0	1	1.8	-	-	-	-	-	-
60+	0	0.0	1	1.8	-	-	-	-	-	-
All ages	0	0.0	5	0.8	29.9	41.2	-	-	-	-
Females										
0-4	0	0.0	0	0.0	-	-	-	-	-	-
5-14	0	0.0	0	0.0	-	-	-	-	-	-
15-44	0	0.0	0	0.0	-	-	-	-	-	-
45-59	0	0.0	0	0.0	-	-	-	-	-	-
60+	0	0.0	0	0.0	-	-	-	-	-	-
All ages	0	0.0	0	0.0	-	-	-	-	-	-
Total	0	0.0	5	0.4	29.9	41.2	-	-	-	-

Table 246e OAI - OPAI - APAI — War - Amputated arm

Age group (years)	Incidence 1990 Number ('000s)	Rate (per 100 000)	Prevalence 1990 Number ('000s)	Rate (per 100 000)	Avg. age at onset (years)	Average duration (years)	Deaths 1990 Number ('000s)	Rate (per 100 000)	Deaths 2000 (Projected) Number ('000s)	Rate (per 100 000)
Males										
0-4	0	0.3	0	0.8	2.5	59.8	-	-	-	-
5-14	0	0.1	2	2.2	10.0	56.2	-	-	-	-
15-44	2	1.0	28	17.7	29.7	38.8	-	-	-	-
45-59	0	0.4	12	36.0	52.3	20.3	-	-	-	-
60+	0	0.2	8	41.2	69.6	9.7	-	-	-	-
All ages	2	0.6	51	15.0	29.2	39.2	-	-	-	-
Females										
0-4	0	0.4	0	0.9	2.5	63.2	-	-	-	-
5-14	0	0.2	2	2.5	10.0	59.2	-	-	-	-
15-44	1	0.7	21	13.4	29.8	41.4	-	-	-	-
45-59	0	0.3	9	25.6	52.3	22.4	-	-	-	-
60+	0	0.2	7	29.7	70.3	10.5	-	-	-	-
All ages	1	0.4	39	11.6	28.0	43.0	-	-	-	-
Total	4	0.5	91	13.3	28.7	40.8	-	-	-	-

Table 246f SSA - ASS - ASS — War - Amputated arm

Age group (years)	Incidence 1990 Number ('000s)	Rate (per 100 000)	Prevalence 1990 Number ('000s)	Rate (per 100 000)	Avg. age at onset (years)	Average duration (years)	Deaths 1990 Number ('000s)	Rate (per 100 000)	Deaths 2000 (Projected) Number ('000s)	Rate (per 100 000)
Males										
0-4	3	5.7	7	14	2.4	48.7	-	-	-	-
5-14	2	2.3	28	40	10.0	49.2	-	-	-	-
15-44	29	28.1	472	455	29.4	35.0	-	-	-	-
45-59	2	12.0	198	977	52.2	19.1	-	-	-	-
60+	1	7.7	120	1 140	69.2	9.3	-	-	-	-
All ages	37	14.6	825	327	28.9	35.0	-	-	-	-
Females										
0-4	3	5.7	7	14	2.4	51.9	-	-	-	-
5-14	2	3.1	31	44	10.0	51.9	-	-	-	-
15-44	19	18.3	345	324	29.5	37.2	-	-	-	-
45-59	2	7.3	146	660	52.3	20.5	-	-	-	-
60+	1	6.4	99	778	69.7	9.8	-	-	-	-
All ages	27	10.4	627	243	27.8	38.0	-	-	-	-
Total	64	12.4	1 452	285	28.5	36.3	-	-	-	-

For epidemiological sources see Zwi 1996. For the methods used to estimate and project incidence, prevalence, and deaths see Lozano et al. 1996 and Murray and Lopez 1996a. See explanatory notes for definitions and caveats.

Table 246   **Cuadro 246**   **Tableau 246**
War   **Guerra**   **Guerre**

Amputated arm   Amputación de brazo   Amputation d'un bras

Table 246g   LAC - ALC - ALC   War - Amputated arm

Age group (years)	Incidence 1990 Number ('000s)	Rate (per 100 000)	Prevalence 1990 Number ('000s)	Rate (per 100 000)	Avg. age at onset (years)	Average duration (years)	Deaths 1990 Number ('000s)	Rate (per 100 000)	Deaths 2000 (Projected) Number ('000s)	Rate (per 100 000)
Males										
0-4	0	0.6	0	1.5	2.5	63.9	-	-	-	-
5-14	0	0.2	2	4.0	10.0	59.3	-	-	-	-
15-44	2	1.8	33	31.8	29.8	41.4	-	-	-	-
45-59	0	0.7	14	64.5	52.3	22.3	-	-	-	-
60+	0	0.4	11	73.8	70.3	10.4	-	-	-	-
All ages	2	1.1	61	27.3	29.3	41.9	-	-	-	-
Females										
0-4	0	0.6	0	1.6	2.5	67.9	-	-	-	-
5-14	0	0.3	2	4.5	10.0	63.0	-	-	-	-
15-44	1	1.2	25	23.9	29.9	44.6	-	-	-	-
45-59	0	0.4	11	45.6	52.4	24.8	-	-	-	-
60+	0	0.3	9	52.4	71.1	11.3	-	-	-	-
All ages	2	0.8	47	21.1	28.1	46.2	-	-	-	-
Total	4	0.9	108	24.2	28.8	43.7	-	-	-	-

Table 246h   MEC - AOM - CMO   War - Amputated arm

Age group (years)	Incidence 1990 Number ('000s)	Rate (per 100 000)	Prevalence 1990 Number ('000s)	Rate (per 100 000)	Avg. age at onset (years)	Average duration (years)	Deaths 1990 Number ('000s)	Rate (per 100 000)	Deaths 2000 (Projected) Number ('000s)	Rate (per 100 000)
Males										
0-4	2	4.2	4	10	2.5	61.1	-	-	-	-
5-14	1	1.6	19	29	10.0	58.1	-	-	-	-
15-44	18	16.2	315	277	29.8	40.0	-	-	-	-
45-59	2	6.9	128	572	52.3	20.8	-	-	-	-
60+	1	3.8	90	661	69.7	9.8	-	-	-	-
All ages	23	9.1	556	217	29.3	40.4	-	-	-	-
Females										
0-4	2	4.3	4	11	2.5	63.7	-	-	-	-
5-14	1	2.2	20	32	10.0	60.9	-	-	-	-
15-44	12	11.5	229	214	29.9	42.6	-	-	-	-
45-59	1	4.6	94	421	52.4	22.9	-	-	-	-
60+	1	3.3	76	490	70.4	10.6	-	-	-	-
All ages	17	6.9	423	172	28.1	44.0	-	-	-	-
Total	40	8.0	979	195	28.8	41.9	-	-	-	-

Table 246i   World - Mundo - Monde   War - Amputated arm

Age group (years)	Incidence 1990 Number ('000s)	Rate (per 100 000)	Prevalence 1990 Number ('000s)	Rate (per 100 000)	Avg. age at onset (years)	Average duration (years)	Deaths 1990 Number ('000s)	Rate (per 100 000)	Deaths 2000 (Projected) Number ('000s)	Rate (per 100 000)
Males										
0-4	5	1.6	12	3.8	2.4	54.6	-	-	-	-
5-14	3	0.5	54	9.9	10.0	53.3	-	-	-	-
15-44	55	4.4	926	74.1	29.6	37.3	-	-	-	-
45-59	5	1.5	401	128.4	52.2	19.9	-	-	-	-
60+	2	0.7	268	122.4	69.5	9.6	-	-	-	-
All ages	70	2.6	1 661	62.6	29.1	37.5	-	-	-	-
Females										
0-4	5	1.6	12	4.0	2.4	58.0	-	-	-	-
5-14	4	0.8	59	11.3	10.0	56.4	-	-	-	-
15-44	36	3.0	667	55.6	35.7	40.0	-	-	-	-
45-59	3	1.0	292	93.9	52.3	21.9	-	-	-	-
60+	2	0.6	233	86.4	70.1	10.3	-	-	-	-
All ages	50	1.9	1 263	48.3	27.9	41.1	-	-	-	-
Total	119	2.3	2 924	55.5	28.6	38.7	-	-	-	-

For epidemiological sources see Zwi 1996. For the methods used to estimate and project incidence, prevalence, and deaths see Lozano et al. 1996 and Murray and Lopez 1996a. See explanatory notes for definitions and caveats.

Table 247	Cuadro 247	Tableau 247
War	Guerra	Guerre

Amputated foot	Amputación del pie	Amputation d'un pied

Table 247a — EME - PEMC - EMBE — War - Amputated foot

Age group (years)	Incidence 1990 Number ('000s)	Incidence 1990 Rate (per 100 000)	Prevalence 1990 Number ('000s)	Prevalence 1990 Rate (per 100 000)	Avg. age at onset (years)	Average duration (years)	Deaths 1990 Number ('000s)	Deaths 1990 Rate (per 100 000)	Deaths 2000 (Projected) Number ('000s)	Deaths 2000 (Projected) Rate (per 100 000)
Males										
0-4	0	0	0	0.0	2.5	70.2	-	-	-	-
5-14	0	0	0	0.0	-	-	-	-	-	-
15-44	0	0	0	0.1	29.9	44.7	-	-	-	-
45-59	0	0	0	0.2	52.4	24.5	-	-	-	-
60+	0	0	0	0.5	71.1	11.3	-	-	-	-
All ages	0	0	1	0.2	53.3	25.3	-	-	-	-
Females										
0-4	0	0	0	0.0	-	-	-	-	-	-
5-14	0	0	0	0.0	-	-	-	-	-	-
15-44	0	0	0	0.0	30.0	50.0	-	-	-	-
45-59	0	0	0	0.0	52.4	28.8	-	-	-	-
60+	0	0	0	0.1	72.4	12.7	-	-	-	-
All ages	0	0	0	0.0	56.4	26.5	-	-	-	-
Total	0	0	1	0.1	53.8	25.4	-	-	-	-

Table 247b — FSE - PEAS - AESE — War - Amputated foot

Age group (years)	Incidence 1990 Number ('000s)	Incidence 1990 Rate (per 100 000)	Prevalence 1990 Number ('000s)	Prevalence 1990 Rate (per 100 000)	Avg. age at onset (years)	Average duration (years)	Deaths 1990 Number ('000s)	Deaths 1990 Rate (per 100 000)	Deaths 2000 (Projected) Number ('000s)	Deaths 2000 (Projected) Rate (per 100 000)
Males										
0-4	0	2.8	1	7.1	2.5	63.5	-	-	-	-
5-14	0	0.9	5	18.5	10.0	57.3	-	-	-	-
15-44	4	5.6	80	104.8	29.8	39.2	-	-	-	-
45-59	0	1.3	54	198.8	52.2	20.8	-	-	-	-
60+	0	0.6	45	214.6	70.0	10.1	-	-	-	-
All ages	5	3.2	185	111.7	29.3	39.9	-	-	-	-
Females										
0-4	0	3.0	1	7.4	2.5	72.4	-	-	-	-
5-14	0	1.2	5	20.8	10.0	66.0	-	-	-	-
15-44	3	3.8	62	83.1	29.9	46.8	-	-	-	-
45-59	0	0.8	4	14.6	52.4	26.1	-	-	-	-
60+	0	0.3	56	155.2	71.5	11.8	-	-	-	-
All ages	4	2.1	130	71.6	28.1	48.6	-	-	-	-
Total	9	2.7	314	90.7	28.8	43.6	-	-	-	-

Table 247c — India - India - Inde — War - Amputated foot

Age group (years)	Incidence 1990 Number ('000s)	Incidence 1990 Rate (per 100 000)	Prevalence 1990 Number ('000s)	Prevalence 1990 Rate (per 100 000)	Avg. age at onset (years)	Average duration (years)	Deaths 1990 Number ('000s)	Deaths 1990 Rate (per 100 000)	Deaths 2000 (Projected) Number ('000s)	Deaths 2000 (Projected) Rate (per 100 000)
Males										
0-4	0	0.0	0	0.0	-	-	-	-	-	-
5-14	0	0.0	0	0.0	-	-	-	-	-	-
15-44	1	0.6	19	9.2	29.8	39.9	-	-	-	-
45-59	0	0.0	9	18.7	-	-	-	-	-	-
60+	0	0.0	6	18.7	-	-	-	-	-	-
All ages	1	0.3	33	7.5	29.8	39.9	-	-	-	-
Females										
0-4	0	0.0	0	0.0	-	-	-	-	-	-
5-14	0	0.0	0	0.0	-	-	-	-	-	-
15-44	0	0.0	0	0.0	-	-	-	-	-	-
45-59	0	0.0	0	0.0	-	-	-	-	-	-
60+	0	0.0	0	0.0	-	-	-	-	-	-
All ages	0	0.0	0	0.0	-	-	-	-	-	-
Total	1	0.1	33	3.9	29.8	39.9	-	-	-	-

For epidemiological sources see Zwi 1996. For the methods used to estimate and project incidence, prevalence, and deaths see Lozano et al. 1996 and Murray and Lopez 1996a. See explanatory notes for definitions and caveats.

Table 247   **Cuadro 247**   **Tableau 247**
War   **Guerra**   **Guerre**

Amputated foot   Amputación del pie   Amputation d'un pied

Table 247d   China - China - Chine   War - Amputated foot

Age group (years)	Incidence 1990 Number ('000s)	Rate (per 100 000)	Prevalence 1990 Number ('000s)	Rate (per 100 000)	Avg. age at onset (years)	Average duration (years)	Deaths 1990 Number ('000s)	Rate (per 100 000)	Deaths 2000 (Projected) Number ('000s)	Rate (per 100 000)
Males										
0-4	0	0.0	0	0.0	-	-	-	-	-	-
5-14	0	0.0	0	0.0	-	-	-	-	-	-
15-44	0	0.1	4	1.2	29.9	41.2	-	-	-	-
45-59	0	0.0	2	2.3	-	-	-	-	-	-
60+	0	0.0	1	2.3	-	-	-	-	-	-
All ages	0	0.0	6	1.1	29.9	41.2	-	-	-	-
Females										
0-4	0	0.0	0	0.0	-	-	-	-	-	-
5-14	0	0.0	0	0.0	-	-	-	-	-	-
15-44	0	0.0	0	0.0	-	-	-	-	-	-
45-59	0	0.0	0	0.0	-	-	-	-	-	-
60+	0	0.0	0	0.0	-	-	-	-	-	-
All ages	0	0.0	0	0.0	-	-	-	-	-	-
Total	0	0.0	6	0.6	29.9	41.2	-	-	-	-

Table 247e   OAI - OPAI - APAI   War - Amputated foot

Age group (years)	Incidence 1990 Number ('000s)	Rate (per 100 000)	Prevalence 1990 Number ('000s)	Rate (per 100 000)	Avg. age at onset (years)	Average duration (years)	Deaths 1990 Number ('000s)	Rate (per 100 000)	Deaths 2000 (Projected) Number ('000s)	Rate (per 100 000)
Males										
0-4	0	0.5	0	1.1	2.5	59.8	-	-	-	-
5-14	0	0.1	3	3.0	10.0	56.2	-	-	-	-
15-44	2	1.3	38	23.6	29.7	38.8	-	-	-	-
45-59	0	0.5	16	48.1	52.3	20.3	-	-	-	-
60+	0	0.3	11	55.0	69.6	9.7	-	-	-	-
All ages	3	0.8	68	20.0	29.2	39.2	-	-	-	-
Females										
0-4	0	0.5	1	1.2	2.5	63.2	-	-	-	-
5-14	0	0.2	3	3.4	10.0	59.2	-	-	-	-
15-44	1	0.9	29	17.9	29.8	41.4	-	-	-	-
45-59	0	0.3	12	34.2	52.3	22.4	-	-	-	-
60+	0	0.3	9	39.6	70.3	10.5	-	-	-	-
All ages	2	0.6	53	15.5	28.0	43.0	-	-	-	-
Total	5	0.7	121	17.8	28.7	40.8	-	-	-	-

Table 247f   SSA - ASS - ASS   War - Amputated foot

Age group (years)	Incidence 1990 Number ('000s)	Rate (per 100 000)	Prevalence 1990 Number ('000s)	Rate (per 100 000)	Avg. age at onset (years)	Average duration (years)	Deaths 1990 Number ('000s)	Rate (per 100 000)	Deaths 2000 (Projected) Number ('000s)	Rate (per 100 000)
Males										
0-4	4	7.6	9	18	2.4	48.7	-	-	-	-
5-14	2	3.1	37	53	10.0	49.2	-	-	-	-
15-44	39	37.5	632	609	29.4	35.0	-	-	-	-
45-59	3	16.0	266	1 309	52.2	19.1	-	-	-	-
60+	1	10.3	161	1 529	69.2	9.3	-	-	-	-
All ages	49	19.4	1 104	438	28.9	35.0	-	-	-	-
Females										
0-4	4	7.7	9	19	2.4	51.9	-	-	-	-
5-14	3	4.1	41	59	10.0	51.9	-	-	-	-
15-44	26	24.4	461	434	29.5	37.2	-	-	-	-
45-59	2	9.8	195	883	52.3	20.5	-	-	-	-
60+	1	8.5	133	1 042	69.7	9.8	-	-	-	-
All ages	36	13.8	838	325	27.8	38.0	-	-	-	-
Total	85	16.6	1 943	381	28.5	36.3	-	-	-	-

For epidemiological sources see Zwi 1996. For the methods used to estimate and project incidence, prevalence, and deaths see Lozano et al. 1996 and Murray and Lopez 1996a. See explanatory notes for definitions and caveats.

Table 247	Cuadro 247	Tableau 247
War	Guerra	Guerre

Amputated foot	Amputación del pie	Amputation d'un pied

Table 247g — LAC - ALC - ALC — War - Amputated foot

Age group (years)	Incidence 1990 Number ('000s)	Rate (per 100 000)	Prevalence 1990 Number ('000s)	Rate (per 100 000)	Avg. age at onset (years)	Average duration (years)	Deaths 1990 Number ('000s)	Rate (per 100 000)	Deaths 2000 (Projected) Number ('000s)	Rate (per 100 000)
Males										
0-4	0	0.8	1	2.0	2.5	63.9	-	-	-	-
5-14	0	0.3	3	5.4	10.0	59.3	-	-	-	-
15-44	3	2.4	44	42.6	29.8	41.4	-	-	-	-
45-59	0	0.9	19	86.2	52.3	22.3	-	-	-	-
60+	0	0.5	14	98.5	70.3	10.4	-	-	-	-
All ages	3	1.4	81	36.6	29.3	41.9	-	-	-	-
Females										
0-4	0	0.8	1	2.1	2.5	67.9	-	-	-	-
5-14	0	0.4	3	6.0	10.0	63.0	-	-	-	-
15-44	2	1.6	33	31.8	29.9	44.6	-	-	-	-
45-59	0	0.6	14	60.6	52.4	24.8	-	-	-	-
60+	0	0.4	12	69.8	71.1	11.3	-	-	-	-
All ages	2	1.0	63	28.1	28.1	46.2	-	-	-	-
Total	5	1.2	144	32.3	28.8	43.7	-	-	-	-

Table 247h — MEC - AOM - CMO — War - Amputated foot

Age group (years)	Incidence 1990 Number ('000s)	Rate (per 100 000)	Prevalence 1990 Number ('000s)	Rate (per 100 000)	Avg. age at onset (years)	Average duration (years)	Deaths 1990 Number ('000s)	Rate (per 100 000)	Deaths 2000 (Projected) Number ('000s)	Rate (per 100 000)
Males										
0-4	2	5.5	6	14	2.5	61.1	-	-	-	-
5-14	1	2.1	25	38	10.0	58.1	-	-	-	-
15-44	25	21.6	421	369	29.8	40.0	-	-	-	-
45-59	2	9.2	171	764	52.3	20.8	-	-	-	-
60+	1	5.0	121	884	69.7	9.8	-	-	-	-
All ages	31	12.1	742	290	29.3	40.4	-	-	-	-
Females										
0-4	2	5.7	6	14	2.5	63.7	-	-	-	-
5-14	2	2.9	27	43	10.0	60.9	-	-	-	-
15-44	16	15.3	306	286	29.9	42.6	-	-	-	-
45-59	1	6.1	125	563	52.4	22.9	-	-	-	-
60+	1	4.4	101	656	70.4	10.6	-	-	-	-
All ages	23	9.2	565	229	28.1	44.0	-	-	-	-
Total	54	10.7	1 308	260	28.8	41.9	-	-	-	-

Table 247i — World - Mundo - Monde — War - Amputated foot

Age group (years)	Incidence 1990 Number ('000s)	Rate (per 100 000)	Prevalence 1990 Number ('000s)	Rate (per 100 000)	Avg. age at onset (years)	Average duration (years)	Deaths 1990 Number ('000s)	Rate (per 100 000)	Deaths 2000 (Projected) Number ('000s)	Rate (per 100 000)
Males										
0-4	7	2.1	16	5.1	2.5	60.8	-	-	-	-
5-14	4	0.7	73	13.2	10.0	57.5	-	-	-	-
15-44	74	5.9	1 237	99.0	29.8	40.5	-	-	-	-
45-59	6	1.9	536	171.7	52.3	21.7	-	-	-	-
60+	2	0.9	358	163.8	70.1	10.3	-	-	-	-
All ages	93	3.5	2 221	83.7	33.0	37.7	-	-	-	-
Females										
0-4	7	2.2	16	5.3	2.5	64.0	-	-	-	-
5-14	5	1.0	79	15.1	10.0	60.8	-	-	-	-
15-44	48	4.0	891	74.3	29.9	43.7	-	-	-	-
45-59	4	1.3	351	112.9	52.4	24.5	-	-	-	-
60+	2	0.7	311	115.6	71.2	11.4	-	-	-	-
All ages	66	2.5	1 649	63.1	23.1	48.8	-	-	-	-
Total	159	3.0	3 869	73.5	28.9	42.4	-	-	-	-

For epidemiological sources see Zwi 1996. For the methods used to estimate and project incidence, prevalence, and deaths see Lozano et al. 1996 and Murray and Lopez 1996a. See explanatory notes for definitions and caveats.

Table 248 War	Cuadro 248 Guerra	Tableau 248 Guerre
Burns <20% - long term	Quemaduras <20% - larga duración	Brûlures <20% - long terme

Table 248a   EME - PEMC - EMBE   War - Burns <20% - long term

Age group (years)	Incidence 1990 Number ('000s)	Rate (per 100 000)	Prevalence 1990 Number ('000s)	Rate (per 100 000)	Avg. age at onset (years)	Average duration (years)	Deaths 1990 Number ('000s)	Rate (per 100 000)	Deaths 2000 (Projected) Number ('000s)	Rate (per 100 000)
Males										
0-4	0	0	0	0.0	2.5	70.2	-	-	-	-
5-14	0	0	0	0.0	10.0	63.6	-	-	-	-
15-44	0	0	0	0.1	29.9	44.7	-	-	-	-
45-59	0	0	0	0.3	52.4	24.5	-	-	-	-
60+	0	0	0	0.6	71.1	11.3	-	-	-	-
All ages	0	0	1	0.2	51.4	26.8	-	-	-	-
Females										
0-4	0	0	0	0.0	-	-	-	-	-	-
5-14	0	0	0	0.0	10.0	69.5	-	-	-	-
15-44	0	0	0	0.0	30.0	50.0	-	-	-	-
45-59	0	0	0	0.1	52.4	28.8	-	-	-	-
60+	0	0	0	0.2	72.4	12.7	-	-	-	-
All ages	0	0	0	0.1	50.0	32.3	-	-	-	-
Total	0	0	1	0.1	51.1	28.1	-	-	-	-

Table 248b   FSE - PEAS - AESE   War - Burns <20% - long term

Age group (years)	Incidence 1990 Number ('000s)	Rate (per 100 000)	Prevalence 1990 Number ('000s)	Rate (per 100 000)	Avg. age at onset (years)	Average duration (years)	Deaths 1990 Number ('000s)	Rate (per 100 000)	Deaths 2000 (Projected) Number ('000s)	Rate (per 100 000)
Males										
0-4	0	3.6	1	8.9	2.5	63.5	-	-	-	-
5-14	0	1.1	6	23.1	10.0	57.3	-	-	-	-
15-44	5	6.9	100	130.9	29.8	39.2	-	-	-	-
45-59	0	1.6	67	248.1	52.2	20.8	-	-	-	-
60+	0	0.7	56	267.8	70.0	10.1	-	-	-	-
All ages	7	4.0	230	139.4	29.3	39.9	-	-	-	-
Females										
0-4	0	3.7	1	9.3	2.5	72.4	-	-	-	-
5-14	0	1.5	7	26.0	10.0	66.0	-	-	-	-
15-44	4	4.7	78	103.7	29.9	46.8	-	-	-	-
45-59	0	1.0	55	181.7	52.4	26.1	-	-	-	-
60+	0	0.4	71	193.8	71.5	11.8	-	-	-	-
All ages	5	2.7	211	116.6	28.1	48.6	-	-	-	-
Total	12	3.3	441	127.5	28.8	43.6	-	-	-	-

Table 248c   India - India - Inde   War - Burns <20% - long term

Age group (years)	Incidence 1990 Number ('000s)	Rate (per 100 000)	Prevalence 1990 Number ('000s)	Rate (per 100 000)	Avg. age at onset (years)	Average duration (years)	Deaths 1990 Number ('000s)	Rate (per 100 000)	Deaths 2000 (Projected) Number ('000s)	Rate (per 100 000)
Males										
0-4	0	0.0	0	0.0	-	-	-	-	-	-
5-14	0	0.0	0	0.0	-	-	-	-	-	-
15-44	2	0.8	23	11.5	29.8	39.9	-	-	-	-
45-59	0	0.0	11	23.3	-	-	-	-	-	-
60+	0	0.0	7	23.3	-	-	-	-	-	-
All ages	2	0.4	41	9.4	29.8	39.9	-	-	-	-
Females										
0-4	0	0.0	0	0.0	-	-	-	-	-	-
5-14	0	0.0	0	0.0	-	-	-	-	-	-
15-44	0	0.0	0	0.0	-	-	-	-	-	-
45-59	0	0.0	0	0.0	-	-	-	-	-	-
60+	0	0.0	0	0.0	-	-	-	-	-	-
All ages	0	0.0	0	0.0	-	-	-	-	-	-
Total	2	0.2	41	4.8	29.8	39.9	-	-	-	-

For epidemiological sources see Zwi 1996. For the methods used to estimate and project incidence, prevalence, and deaths see Lozano et al. 1996 and Murray and Lopez 1996a. See explanatory notes for definitions and caveats.

Table 248
War

Cuadro 248
Guerra

Tableau 248
Guerre

Burns <20% - long term   Quemaduras <20% - larga duración   Brûlures <20% - long terme

Table 248d   China - China - Chine   War - Burns <20% - long term

Age group (years)	Incidence 1990 Number ('000s)	Rate (per 100 000)	Prevalence 1990 Number ('000s)	Rate (per 100 000)	Avg. age at onset (years)	Average duration (years)	Deaths 1990 Number ('000s)	Rate (per 100 000)	Deaths 2000 (Projected) Number ('000s)	Rate (per 100 000)
Males										
0-4	0	0.0	0	0.0	-	-	-	-	-	-
5-14	0	0.0	0	0.0	-	-	-	-	-	-
15-44	0	0.1	4	1.5	29.9	41.2	-	-	-	-
45-59	0	0.0	2	2.9	-	-	-	-	-	-
60+	0	0.0	1	2.9	-	-	-	-	-	-
All ages	0	0.1	8	1.4	29.9	41.2	-	-	-	-
Females										
0-4	0	0.0	0	0.0	-	-	-	-	-	-
5-14	0	0.0	0	0.0	-	-	-	-	-	-
15-44	0	0.0	0	0.0	-	-	-	-	-	-
45-59	0	0.0	0	0.0	-	-	-	-	-	-
60+	0	0.0	0	0.0	-	-	-	-	-	-
All ages	0	0.0	0	0.0	-	-	-	-	-	-
Total	0	0.0	8	0.7	29.9	41.2	-	-	-	-

Table 248e   OAI - OPAI - APAI   War - Burns <20% - long term

Age group (years)	Incidence 1990 Number ('000s)	Rate (per 100 000)	Prevalence 1990 Number ('000s)	Rate (per 100 000)	Avg. age at onset (years)	Average duration (years)	Deaths 1990 Number ('000s)	Rate (per 100 000)	Deaths 2000 (Projected) Number ('000s)	Rate (per 100 000)
Males										
0-4	0	0.6	1	1.4	2.5	59.8	-	-	-	-
5-14	0	0.2	3	3.8	10.0	56.2	-	-	-	-
15-44	3	1.7	47	29.5	29.7	38.8	-	-	-	-
45-59	0	0.7	20	60.0	52.3	20.3	-	-	-	-
60+	0	0.4	14	68.7	69.6	9.7	-	-	-	-
All ages	3	1.0	86	25.0	29.2	39.2	-	-	-	-
Females										
0-4	0	0.6	1	1.5	2.5	63.2	-	-	-	-
5-14	0	0.3	3	4.2	10.0	59.2	-	-	-	-
15-44	2	1.1	35	22.2	29.8	41.4	-	-	-	-
45-59	0	0.4	15	42.6	52.3	22.4	-	-	-	-
60+	0	0.3	11	49.3	70.3	10.5	-	-	-	-
All ages	2	0.7	66	19.3	28.0	43.0	-	-	-	-
Total	6	0.9	151	22.2	28.7	40.8	-	-	-	-

Table 248f   SSA - ASS - ASS   War - Burns <20% - long term

Age group (years)	Incidence 1990 Number ('000s)	Rate (per 100 000)	Prevalence 1990 Number ('000s)	Rate (per 100 000)	Avg. age at onset (years)	Average duration (years)	Deaths 1990 Number ('000s)	Rate (per 100 000)	Deaths 2000 (Projected) Number ('000s)	Rate (per 100 000)
Males										
0-4	5	9.5	11	23	2.4	48.7	-	-	-	-
5-14	3	3.8	47	66	10.0	49.2	-	-	-	-
15-44	49	46.9	786	757	29.4	35.0	-	-	-	-
45-59	4	20.0	330	1 623	52.2	19.1	-	-	-	-
60+	1	12.9	199	1 893	69.2	9.3	-	-	-	-
All ages	61	24.3	1 372	544	28.9	35.0	-	-	-	-
Females										
0-4	5	9.6	11	23	2.4	51.9	-	-	-	-
5-14	4	5.2	51	73	10.0	51.9	-	-	-	-
15-44	32	30.5	574	540	29.5	37.2	-	-	-	-
45-59	3	12.2	243	1 098	52.2	20.5	-	-	-	-
60+	1	10.6	165	1 293	69.7	9.8	-	-	-	-
All ages	45	17.3	1 044	405	27.8	38.0	-	-	-	-
Total	106	20.7	2 415	473	28.5	36.3	-	-	-	-

For epidemiological sources see Zwi 1996. For the methods used to estimate and project incidence, prevalence, and deaths see Lozano et al. 1996 and Murray and Lopez 1996a. See explanatory notes for definitions and caveats.

Table 248	Cuadro 248	Tableau 248
War	Guerra	Guerre

Burns <20% - long term   Quemaduras <20% - larga duración   Brûlures <20% - long terme

Table 248g   LAC - ALC - ALC   War - Burns <20% - long term

Age group (years)	Incidence 1990 Number ('000s)	Rate (per 100 000)	Prevalence 1990 Number ('000s)	Rate (per 100 000)	Avg. age at onset (years)	Average duration (years)	Deaths 1990 Number ('000s)	Rate (per 100 000)	Deaths 2000 (Projected) Number ('000s)	Rate (per 100 000)
Males										
0-4	0	1.0	1	2.5	2.5	63.9	-	-	-	-
5-14	0	0.3	4	6.7	10.0	59.3	-	-	-	-
15-44	3	3.0	55	53.1	29.8	41.4	-	-	-	-
45-59	0	1.2	24	107.6	52.3	22.3	-	-	-	-
60+	0	0.6	18	123.0	70.3	10.4	-	-	-	-
All ages	4	1.8	101	45.6	29.3	41.9	-	-	-	-
Females										
0-4	0	1.1	1	2.6	2.5	67.9	-	-	-	-
5-14	0	0.5	4	7.6	10.0	63.0	-	-	-	-
15-44	2	2.0	41	39.8	29.9	44.6	-	-	-	-
45-59	0	0.7	18	75.9	52.4	24.8	-	-	-	-
60+	0	0.5	15	87.4	71.1	11.3	-	-	-	-
All ages	3	1.3	78	35.2	28.1	46.2	-	-	-	-
Total	7	1.5	180	40.4	28.8	43.7	-	-	-	-

Table 248h   MEC - AOM - CMO   War - Burns <20% - long term

Age group (years)	Incidence 1990 Number ('000s)	Rate (per 100 000)	Prevalence 1990 Number ('000s)	Rate (per 100 000)	Avg. age at onset (years)	Average duration (years)	Deaths 1990 Number ('000s)	Rate (per 100 000)	Deaths 2000 (Projected) Number ('000s)	Rate (per 100 000)
Males										
0-4	3	6.9	7	17	2.5	61.1	-	-	-	-
5-14	2	2.6	31	48	10.0	58.1	-	-	-	-
15-44	31	27.0	524	460	29.8	40.0	-	-	-	-
45-59	3	11.5	212	951	52.3	20.8	-	-	-	-
60+	1	6.3	150	1 099	69.7	9.8	-	-	-	-
All ages	39	15.1	925	361	29.3	40.4	-	-	-	-
Females										
0-4	3	7.2	7	18	2.5	63.7	-	-	-	-
5-14	2	3.7	34	54	10.0	60.9	-	-	-	-
15-44	21	19.1	382	356	29.8	42.6	-	-	-	-
45-59	2	7.7	156	701	52.3	22.9	-	-	-	-
60+	1	5.5	126	816	70.4	10.6	-	-	-	-
All ages	28	11.4	705	286	28.0	44.0	-	-	-	-
Total	67	13.3	1 629	324	28.8	41.9	-	-	-	-

Table 248i   World - Mundo - Monde   War - Burns <20% - long term

Age group (years)	Incidence 1990 Number ('000s)	Rate (per 100 000)	Prevalence 1990 Number ('000s)	Rate (per 100 000)	Avg. age at onset (years)	Average duration (years)	Deaths 1990 Number ('000s)	Rate (per 100 000)	Deaths 2000 (Projected) Number ('000s)	Rate (per 100 000)
Males										
0-4	8	2.6	20	6.4	2.4	54.6	-	-	-	-
5-14	5	0.9	91	16.5	10.0	53.3	-	-	-	-
15-44	92	7.4	1 541	123.3	29.6	37.3	-	-	-	-
45-59	8	2.4	667	213.4	52.2	19.9	-	-	-	-
60+	3	1.2	445	203.4	69.5	9.6	-	-	-	-
All ages	116	4.4	2 764	104.2	29.1	37.5	-	-	-	-
Females										
0-4	8	2.7	20	6.6	2.4	58.0	-	-	-	-
5-14	7	1.3	99	18.8	10.0	56.4	-	-	-	-
15-44	60	5.0	1 111	92.6	29.6	40.0	-	-	-	-
45-59	5	1.6	486	156.3	52.3	21.9	-	-	-	-
60+	3	0.9	387	143.9	70.1	10.3	-	-	-	-
All ages	83	3.2	2 103	80.5	27.9	41.1	-	-	-	-
Total	199	3.8	4 867	92.4	28.6	39.0	-	-	-	-

For epidemiological sources see Zwi 1996. For the methods used to estimate and project incidence, prevalence, and deaths see Lozano et al. 1996 and Murray and Lopez 1996a. See explanatory notes for definitions and caveats.

Table 249 War	Cuadro 249 Guerra	Tableau 249 Guerre

Injured nerves	Traumatismo de nervios	Lésions des nerfs

Table 249a   EME - PEMC - EMBE   War - Injured nerves

Age group (years)	Incidence 1990 Number ('000s)	Rate (per 100 000)	Prevalence 1990 Number ('000s)	Rate (per 100 000)	Avg. age at onset (years)	Average duration (years)	Deaths 1990 Number ('000s)	Rate (per 100 000)	Deaths 2000 (Projected) Number ('000s)	Rate (per 100 000)
Males										
0-4	0	0	0	0.0	2.5	70.2	-	-	-	-
5-14	0	0	0	0.0	10.0	63.6	-	-	-	-
15-44	0	0	0	0.2	29.9	44.7	-	-	-	-
45-59	0	0	0	0.6	52.4	24.5	-	-	-	-
60+	0	0	1	1.3	71.1	11.3	-	-	-	-
All ages	0	0	2	0.4	51.4	26.8	-	-	-	-
Females										
0-4	0	0	0	0.0	-	-	-	-	-	-
5-14	0	0	0	0.0	10.0	69.5	-	-	-	-
15-44	0	0	0	0.1	30.0	50.0	-	-	-	-
45-59	0	0	0	0.2	52.5	28.8	-	-	-	-
60+	0	0	0	0.3	72.4	12.7	-	-	-	-
All ages	0	0	1	0.1	50.0	32.3	-	-	-	-
Total	0	0	2	0.3	51.1	28.1	-	-	-	-

Table 249b   FSE - PEAS - AESE   War - Injured nerves

Age group (years)	Incidence 1990 Number ('000s)	Rate (per 100 000)	Prevalence 1990 Number ('000s)	Rate (per 100 000)	Avg. age at onset (years)	Average duration (years)	Deaths 1990 Number ('000s)	Rate (per 100 000)	Deaths 2000 (Projected) Number ('000s)	Rate (per 100 000)
Males										
0-4	1	7.1	2	18	2.5	63.5	-	-	-	-
5-14	1	2.1	13	46	10.0	57.3	-	-	-	-
15-44	11	13.9	200	262	29.8	39.2	-	-	-	-
45-59	1	3.3	134	496	52.2	20.8	-	-	-	-
60+	0	1.4	112	535	70.0	10.1	-	-	-	-
All ages	13	8.1	461	279	29.3	39.9	-	-	-	-
Females										
0-4	1	7.5	2	19	2.5	72.4	-	-	-	-
5-14	1	3.0	14	52	10.0	66.0	-	-	-	-
15-44	7	9.4	155	207	30.0	46.8	-	-	-	-
45-59	1	2.0	109	363	52.4	26.1	-	-	-	-
60+	0	0.8	141	387	71.5	11.8	-	-	-	-
All ages	10	5.4	421	233	28.2	48.6	-	-	-	-
Total	23	6.7	882	255	28.8	43.6	-	-	-	-

Table 249c   India - India - Inde   War - Injured nerves

Age group (years)	Incidence 1990 Number ('000s)	Rate (per 100 000)	Prevalence 1990 Number ('000s)	Rate (per 100 000)	Avg. age at onset (years)	Average duration (years)	Deaths 1990 Number ('000s)	Rate (per 100 000)	Deaths 2000 (Projected) Number ('000s)	Rate (per 100 000)
Males										
0-4	0	0.0	0	0	-	-	-	-	-	-
5-14	0	0.0	0	0	-	-	-	-	-	-
15-44	3	1.6	46	23	29.8	39.9	-	-	-	-
45-59	0	0.0	22	47	-	-	-	-	-	-
60+	0	0.0	14	47	-	-	-	-	-	-
All ages	3	0.7	82	19	29.8	39.9	-	-	-	-
Females										
0-4	0	0.0	0	0	-	-	-	-	-	-
5-14	0	0.0	0	0	-	-	-	-	-	-
15-44	0	0.0	0	0	-	-	-	-	-	-
45-59	0	0.0	0	0	-	-	-	-	-	-
60+	0	0.0	0	0	-	-	-	-	-	-
All ages	0	0.0	0	0	-	-	-	-	-	-
Total	3	0.4	82	10	29.8	39.9	-	-	-	-

For epidemiological sources see Zwi 1996. For the methods used to estimate and project incidence, prevalence, and deaths see Lozano et al. 1996 and Murray and Lopez 1996a. See explanatory notes for definitions and caveats.

Table 249	Cuadro 249	Tableau 249
War	Guerra	Guerre

| Injured nerves | Traumatismo de nervios | Lésions des nerfs |

Table 249d   China - China - Chine   War - Injured nerves

Age group (years)	Incidence 1990 Number ('000s)	Rate (per 100 000)	Prevalence 1990 Number ('000s)	Rate (per 100 000)	Avg. age at onset (years)	Average duration (years)	Deaths 1990 Number ('000s)	Rate (per 100 000)	Deaths 2000 (Projected) Number ('000s)	Rate (per 100 000)
Males										
0-4	0	0.0	0	0.0	-	-	-	-	-	-
5-14	0	0.0	0	0.0	-	-	-	-	-	-
15-44	1	0.2	9	2.9	29.9	41.2	-	-	-	-
45-59	0	0.0	4	5.9	-	-	-	-	-	-
60+	0	0.0	3	5.9	-	-	-	-	-	-
All ages	1	0.1	16	2.7	29.9	41.2	-	-	-	-
Females										
0-4	0	0.0	0	0.0	-	-	-	-	-	-
5-14	0	0.0	0	0.0	-	-	-	-	-	-
15-44	0	0.0	0	0.0	-	-	-	-	-	-
45-59	0	0.0	0	0.0	-	-	-	-	-	-
60+	0	0.0	0	0.0	-	-	-	-	-	-
All ages	0	0.0	0	0.0	-	-	-	-	-	-
Total	1	0.1	16	1.4	29.9	41.2	-	-	-	-

Table 249e   OAI - OPAI - APAI   War - Injured nerves

Age group (years)	Incidence 1990 Number ('000s)	Rate (per 100 000)	Prevalence 1990 Number ('000s)	Rate (per 100 000)	Avg. age at onset (years)	Average duration (years)	Deaths 1990 Number ('000s)	Rate (per 100 000)	Deaths 2000 (Projected) Number ('000s)	Rate (per 100 000)
Males										
0-4	1	1.1	1	2.8	2.5	59.8	-	-	-	-
5-14	0	0.4	6	7.5	10.0	56.2	-	-	-	-
15-44	5	3.4	95	59.0	29.7	38.8	-	-	-	-
45-59	0	1.3	41	120.0	52.3	20.3	-	-	-	-
60+	0	0.7	28	137.4	69.6	9.7	-	-	-	-
All ages	7	2.0	171	49.9	29.2	39.2	-	-	-	-
Females										
0-4	1	1.2	1	3.0	2.5	63.2	-	-	-	-
5-14	0	0.5	7	8.5	10.0	59.2	-	-	-	-
15-44	4	2.3	71	44.4	29.8	41.4	-	-	-	-
45-59	0	0.9	30	85.2	52.3	22.4	-	-	-	-
60+	0	0.7	22	98.6	70.3	10.5	-	-	-	-
All ages	5	1.5	131	38.6	28.0	43.0	-	-	-	-
Total	12	1.7	302	44.3	28.7	40.8	-	-	-	-

Table 249f   SSA - ASS - ASS   War - Injured nerves

Age group (years)	Incidence 1990 Number ('000s)	Rate (per 100 000)	Prevalence 1990 Number ('000s)	Rate (per 100 000)	Avg. age at onset (years)	Average duration (years)	Deaths 1990 Number ('000s)	Rate (per 100 000)	Deaths 2000 (Projected) Number ('000s)	Rate (per 100 000)
Males										
0-4	9	19.0	22	46	2.4	48.7	-	-	-	-
5-14	5	7.7	93	133	10.0	49.2	-	-	-	-
15-44	97	93.8	1 564	1 508	29.4	35.0	-	-	-	-
45-59	8	39.9	654	3 219	52.2	19.1	-	-	-	-
60+	3	25.7	394	3 751	69.2	9.3	-	-	-	-
All ages	123	48.6	2 727	1 081	28.9	35.0	-	-	-	-
Females										
0-4	9	19.2	22	46	2.4	51.9	-	-	-	-
5-14	7	10.3	102	147	10.0	51.9	-	-	-	-
15-44	65	61.0	1 144	1 077	29.5	37.2	-	-	-	-
45-59	5	24.4	483	2 184	52.3	20.5	-	-	-	-
60+	3	21.2	327	2 570	69.7	9.8	-	-	-	-
All ages	89	34.6	2 078	806	27.8	38.0	-	-	-	-
Total	212	41.5	4 805	942	28.5	36.3	-	-	-	-

For epidemiological sources see Zwi 1996. For the methods used to estimate and project incidence, prevalence, and deaths see Lozano et al. 1996 and Murray and Lopez 1996a. See explanatory notes for definitions and caveats.

Table 249	Cuadro 249	Tableau 249
War	Guerra	Guerre

Injured nerves	Traumatismo de nervios	Lésions des nerfs

Table 249g LAC - ALC - ALC

War - Injured nerves

Age group (years)	Incidence 1990 Number ('000s)	Rate (per 100 000)	Prevalence 1990 Number ('000s)	Rate (per 100 000)	Avg. age at onset (years)	Average duration (years)	Deaths 1990 Number ('000s)	Rate (per 100 000)	Deaths 2000 (Projected) Number ('000s)	Rate (per 100 000)
Males										
0-4	1	2.0	1	5.0	2.5	63.9	-	-	-	-
5-14	0	0.7	7	13.5	10.0	59.3	-	-	-	-
15-44	6	6.0	111	106.2	29.8	41.4	-	-	-	-
45-59	1	2.4	48	215.2	52.3	22.3	-	-	-	-
60+	0	1.2	35	245.9	70.3	10.4	-	-	-	-
All ages	8	3.6	202	91.2	29.3	41.9	-	-	-	-
Females										
0-4	1	2.1	1	5.2	2.5	67.9	-	-	-	-
5-14	0	0.9	8	15.1	10.0	63.0	-	-	-	-
15-44	4	4.0	83	79.6	29.9	44.6	-	-	-	-
45-59	0	1.5	35	151.7	52.4	24.8	-	-	-	-
60+	0	1.0	29	174.6	71.1	11.3	-	-	-	-
All ages	6	2.6	157	70.4	28.1	46.2	-	-	-	-
Total	14	3.1	359	80.8	28.8	43.7	-	-	-	-

Table 249h MEC - AOM - CMO

War - Injured nerves

Age group (years)	Incidence 1990 Number ('000s)	Rate (per 100 000)	Prevalence 1990 Number ('000s)	Rate (per 100 000)	Avg. age at onset (years)	Average duration (years)	Deaths 1990 Number ('000s)	Rate (per 100 000)	Deaths 2000 (Projected) Number ('000s)	Rate (per 100 000)
Males										
0-4	6	13.8	14	34	2.5	61.1	-	-	-	-
5-14	3	5.2	62	95	10.0	58.1	-	-	-	-
15-44	62	54.1	1 045	918	29.8	40.0	-	-	-	-
45-59	5	23.0	423	1 893	52.3	20.8	-	-	-	-
60+	2	12.5	298	2 186	69.7	9.8	-	-	-	-
All ages	78	30.2	1 843	719	29.3	40.4	-	-	-	-
Females										
0-4	6	14.3	14	35	2.5	63.7	-	-	-	-
5-14	5	7.4	67	108	10.0	60.9	-	-	-	-
15-44	41	38.3	762	711	29.9	42.6	-	-	-	-
45-59	3	15.3	311	1 397	52.4	22.9	-	-	-	-
60+	2	11.1	251	1 626	70.4	10.6	-	-	-	-
All ages	56	22.9	1 406	570	28.1	44.0	-	-	-	-
Total	134	26.6	3 248	646	28.8	41.9	-	-	-	-

Table 249i World - Mundo - Monde

War - Injured nerves

Age group (years)	Incidence 1990 Number ('000s)	Rate (per 100 000)	Prevalence 1990 Number ('000s)	Rate (per 100 000)	Avg. age at onset (years)	Average duration (years)	Deaths 1990 Number ('000s)	Rate (per 100 000)	Deaths 2000 (Projected) Number ('000s)	Rate (per 100 000)
Males										
0-4	17	5.2	41	13	2.4	54.6	-	-	-	-
5-14	10	1.8	181	33	10.0	53.3	-	-	-	-
15-44	185	14.8	3 070	246	29.6	37.3	-	-	-	-
45-59	15	4.8	1 326	424	52.2	19.9	-	-	-	-
60+	5	2.3	885	404	69.5	9.6	-	-	-	-
All ages	232	8.7	5 503	207	29.1	37.5	-	-	-	-
Females										
0-4	17	5.4	41	13	2.4	58.0	-	-	-	-
5-14	13	2.6	198	38	10.0	56.4	-	-	-	-
15-44	121	10.1	2 215	185	29.7	40.0	-	-	-	-
45-59	10	3.2	969	311	52.3	21.9	-	-	-	-
60+	5	1.9	771	287	70.1	10.3	-	-	-	-
All ages	166	6.4	4 194	160	27.9	41.1	-	-	-	-
Total	398	7.6	9 697	184	28.6	39.0	-	-	-	-

For epidemiological sources see Zwi 1996. For the methods used to estimate and project incidence, prevalence, and deaths see Lozano et al. 1996 and Murray and Lopez 1996a. See explanatory notes for definitions and caveats.

EXPLANATORY NOTES

Symbols—In the mortality columns, a 0 indicates that we estimate that zero deaths are caused by the condition whereas a '–' indicates that we are unable to provide a meaningful estimate of mortality due to that sequela. The '–' is used when estimates of mortality from all sequelae of a disease or injury have been made but this mortality has not been disaggregated by specific sequelae.

IA1 Tuberculosis—Cases refer to individuals with clinical tuberculosis, normally pulmonary sputum culture positives and extra-pulmonary cases. We have distinguished incidence and death from clinical tuberculosis in HIV negative individuals (IA1-1) and incidence and death from clinical tuberculosis in HIV positives (IA1-2). The HIV/TB estimates have been generated by using information on the prevalence of tuberculosis infection by age, sex and region and the age-specific prevalence of HIV infection combined with estimates of the co-infection breakdown rate. Deaths in the primary mortality tabulations (Murray and Lopez 1996b) show deaths due to tuberculosis in HIV negative individuals while deaths from tuberculosis in HIV positives are included in the HIV-related mortality estimates.

IA2a Syphilis—Congenital syphilis rates are expressed as a rate for the population aged 0 to 4 years. To avoid double counting, the effects of low birth weight on mortality and development due to syphilis are included in the low birth weight tables under *Conditions arising during the perinatal period— low birth weight* (ID1-1) and low birth weight infants that continue to be wasted or stunted are included in IE1: *Protein energy malnutrition*. Mortality due to syphilis is included in the tables for congenital syphilis and tertiary syphilis but not primary or secondary syphilis. This division is somewhat arbitrary but reflects the types of syphilis that account for the majority of deaths.

IA2b Chlamydia—To avoid double counting, the effects of low birth weight on mortality and development due to chlamydia are included in the low birth weight tables under *Conditions arising during the perinatal period—low birth weight* (ID1-1) and low birth weight infants that continue to be wasted or stunted are included in IE1: *Protein energy malnutrition*. Chlamydia neonatal pneumonia (IA2b-6) does not include pneumonia due to chlamydia contracted through respiratory transmission. *PID* (IA2b-7) includes both acute and recurrent PID due to chlamydia. *Infertility* (IA2b-11) is the total of infertility due to chlamydia-related PID and ectopic pregancy in women and epididymitis in men. Mortality from chlamydia has been estimated for ectopic pregnancy (IA2b-8) and for tubo-ovarian abscess (IA2b-9). In the primary cause-of-death tabulations in the Global Burden of Disease Study, deaths from ectopic pregnancy are included under *Abortion* (IC5).

IA2c Gonorrhoea—To avoid double counting, the effects of low birth weight on mortality and development due to gonorrhoea are included in the low birth weight tables under *Conditions arising during the perinatal period—low birth weight* (ID1-1) and low birth weight infants that continue to be wasted or stunted are included in IE1: *Protein-energy malnutrition. PID* (IA2c-6) includes both acute and recurrent PID due to gonorrhoea. *Infertility* (IA2c-10) is the total of infertility due to gonorrhoea-related PID and ectopic pregnancy in women and epididymitis in men.

IA3 HIV — As an arbitrary convention, we have listed all HIV-related deaths under the sequela *AIDS* (IA3-2) as most causes of HIV-related death are themselves AIDS-defining conditions. IA3-1 provides information on the incidence of new HIV infection in 1990 and the prevalence of HIV infection in 1990. IA3-2 provides estimates of AIDS incidence and prevalence in 1990. The projections of AIDS deaths for 2000 are based on projections developed by the former WHO Global Programme on AIDS as described in the chapter by Low-Beer et al. 1996, slightly modified by Murray and Lopez (1996a) for years after 2000.

IA4 Diarrhoeal diseases—Following the convention for this study, deaths of children with both measles and diarrhoea or both LRI and diarrhoea are not included in the estimates of diarrhoea mortality shown in the table. The estimates of incidence and prevalence are for episodes of diarrhoea including acute watery diarrhoea, persistent diarrhoea and dysentery.

IA5a Pertussis—All deaths related to pertussis are presented in Table IA5a-1. The prevalence of mental retardation from pertussis does not decline with age, implying that the relative risk of death of those with this condition compared to the general population is 1.0. This assumption is probably unrealistic for some developing regions, but there are virtually no follow-up studies in any region to provide a relative risk of death for this patient group.

IA5b Poliomyelitis— *Lameness* (IA5b-2) includes both upper and lower limb involvement.

IA5c Diphtheria—Deaths due to diphtheria are all shown under *Myocarditis* (IA5c-3) based on the simplifying assumption that all individuals who die from diphtheria must have some form of myocardial involvement; clearly, there may be exceptions to this assumption but for convenience all deaths are shown in this table and consequently no deaths are listed for acute episodes of diphtheria (IA5c-1). IA5c-2: *Neurological complications* are most often cranial and peripheral nerve palsies.

IA5d Measles—Late effects of measles on child mortality, months or years after the episode, are not included in the estimates of mortality shown in the table.

IA5e Tetanus—This category includes both neonatal tetanus and adult tetanus.

IA6 Bacterial meningitis and meningococcaemia—For reasons of space, the name was abbreviated to "Bacterial meningitis" in tables 57–65. This category includes bacterial meningitis due to Streptococcus pneumonia, Hemophilus influenzae and Neisseria meningitidis and meningococcaemia without meningitis. Based on the data sources and methods used for estimation, meningitis from other bacteria (e.g. Listeria, gram negative organisms, etc.) are included in the estimates of mortality in EME, FSE and LAC but not in other regions. The estimates of all forms of incidence in all regions, however, are based only on estimates of the S. pneumococcus, H. influenzae and N. meningitidis. As other forms of meningitis are less common, this inconsistency should not substantially affect the results.

IA7 Hepatitis B and hepatitis C—Because of the limitations of the ICD-9 Basic Tabulation List codes for viral hepatitis, estimates of mortality from hepatitis B and C in EME, FSE and LAC include a limited number of deaths due to hepatitis A. Symptomatic cirrhosis (IA7-2) and hepatoma (IA7-3) attributed to hepatitis B are based on estimates of the attributable fraction of symptomatic cirrhosis (II.I2-1) and hepatoma (IIA5-1) thought to be caused by hepatitis B.

IA8 Malaria—Anaemia (IA8-2) is defined using WHO criteria for mild to very severe anaemia. Neurological sequelae from cerebral malaria (IA8-3) include hemiplegia, aphasia, ataxia and cortical blindness.

IA9b Chagas disease—All deaths related to Chagas are shown with the table for the prevalence of infection (IA9b-1). With available information, we have been unable to distinguish deaths due to acute infection, heart failure or megaviscera. To indicate this gap in information, the columns of death numbers for cardiomyopathy without congestive heart failure (IA9b-2), cardiomyopathy with congestive heart failure (IA9b-3) and megaviscera (IA9b-4) show a '–' for mortality.

IA9c Schistosomiasis—Estimates have been made only for the prevalence of infection and associated direct mortality from schistosomiasis. We have not included estimates of mortality from bladder cancer, cirrhosis or colon cancer that may be related to schistosomiasis.

IA9d Leishmaniasis—All deaths related to leishmaniasis are shown for convenience in the table for visceral leishmaniasis (IA9d-1).

IA9e Lymphatic filariasis—Based on the chapter analyzing lymphatic filariasis, we have assumed that there are few if any deaths directly caused by filariasis. This may be an underestimate of the effects of acute filarial infection.

IA10 Leprosy—Leprosy cases (IA10-1) provide the incidence and prevalence of case numbers following the WHO case definition. Prevalence is the prevalence of individuals meeting the WHO case definition and is not the same as the prevalence of individuals with clinical leprosy. The prevalence rates shown for disabling leprosy (IA10-2) are estimates of the true prevalence of disability from leprosy.

IA11 Dengue—Dengue was not included in Version 3 or Version 4 of the Global Burden of Disease Study. Estimates have been made only for dengue haemorrhagic fever (IA11-1) and global and regional estimates of all forms of dengue have not been undertaken.

IA12 Japanese encephalitis—All deaths due to Japanese encephalitis are shown under episodes (IA12-1).

IA14a Ascariasis—The table on high intensity infection (IA14a-1) provides estimates of the prevalence of infections with more than 10 worms in children aged 0–4 years, more than 15 worms at ages 5–9, and more than 20 worms in those over age 20. Incidence estimates have not been developed for high intensity infection. Deaths directly attributable to ascaris infection are shown with the incidence and prevalence of intestinal obstruction (IA14a-4) as this is considered the primary mechanism of directly attributable mortality. "Cotemporaneous cognitive deficit" (IA14a-2) is a term used by Bundy et al. (1996) to refer to cognitive deficits that are a function of current worm burden and are not due to developmental delays caused by prior high worm burdens. "Cognitive impairment" (IA14a-3) refers to permanent changes caused by high worm burdens during childhood and adolescent years.

IA14b Trichuriasis—The table on the high intensity infection (IA14b-1) provides estimates of the prevalence of infections with more than 90 worms in children aged 0–4 years, more than 130 worms at ages 5–9, and more than 180 worms in those over age 20. Incidence estimates have not been developed for high intensity infection. Deaths directly attributable to trichuris infection are shown with the incidence and prevalence of massive dysentery syndrome as this is considered the primary mechanism of directly attributable mortality. "Cotemporaneous cognitive deficit" (IA14b-2) is a term used by Bundy et al. (1996) to refer to cognitive deficits that are a function of current worm burden and are not due to developmental delays caused by prior high worm burdens. "Cognitive impairment" (IA14b-4) refers to permanent changes caused by high worm burdens during childhood and adolescent years.

IA14c Ancylostomiasis and necatoriasis—The table on the high intensity infection (IA14c-1) provides estimates of the prevalence of infections with more than 20 worms in children aged 0–4 years, more than 30 worms at ages 5–9, and more than 40 worms in those over age 20. Incidence estimates have not been developed for high intensity infection. Deaths directly attributable to ancylostomiasis and necatoriasis are shown in IA14c-1.

IB2 Lower respiratory infections—Chronic sequelae (IB2-2) include bronchiectasis and impaired lung function as measured by a decrease in FEV_1. While these chronic sequelae can certainly cause mortality, the magnitude of this mortality has not been estimated. In the primary mortality tabulations, they would appear along with other chronic respiratory conditions (IIH).

IB3 Otitis media—*Episodes* (IB3-1) refers to episodes of acute otitis media.

IC1 Maternal haemorrhage—For convenience, all deaths directly attributable to maternal haemorrhage are shown with the incidence of maternal haemorrhage (IC1-1).

IC3 Hypertensive disorders of pregnancy—This category includes pre-eclampsia and eclampsia. Mortality shown in the table with incidence and prevalence (IC3-1) of episodes is total mortality due to hypertensive disorders of pregnancy including eclampsia.

ID Conditions arising during the perinatal period—Care must be taken not to confuse conditions arising during the perinatal period, which is a particular cluster of causes of death that are peculiar to the first weeks of a newborn's life, with the perinatal mortality rate which is the death rate from 28 weeks gestation to 4 weeks after birth.

ID1 Low birth weight—This category includes small-for-gestational-age infants and premature infants. Unlike many of the other diseases in this study, all the developmental sequelae due to low birth weight have been clustered into one outcome which includes cerebral palsy, mental retardation, epilepsy, hearing loss and visual loss (ID1-1). Shibuya and Murray (1996a) explain in detail why this approach has been taken, based largely on the nature of the cohort studies that have been undertaken. In this study, "perinatal" is used to refer to conditions arising during the perinatal period. Incident cases do not include those that die soon after birth.

ID2 Birth asphyxia and birth trauma—Unlike many of the other diseases in this study, all the developmental sequelae due to birth asphyxia and birth trauma have been clustered into one outcome which includes cerebral palsy, mental retardation, epilepsy, hearing loss and visual loss (ID2-1). Shibuya and Murray (1996b) explain in detail why this approach has been taken, based largely on the nature of the cohort studies that have been undertaken. Incident cases do not include those that die soon after birth.

IE1 Protein-energy malnutrition—Wasting (IE1-1) is the prevalence of children who have a weight for height more than 2 standard deviations below the NCHS reference population mean. Stunting (IE1-2) is the prevalence of children who have a height for age more than 2 standard deviations below the NCHS reference population mean. Many children who are wasted may also be stunted and vice-versa. The same child may appear in the tables for wasting and stunting. For convenience, we have arbitrarily chosen to present mortality directly attributable to protein energy malnutrition in the table for wasting (IE1-1). Malnutrition is likely to be a risk factor for mortality from many other causes such as diarrhoea and respiratory infections. See Mason et al. (1996) for an analysis of mortality associated with malnutrition in children under age 5 years. Wasting and stunting in adults has not been estimated in this study.

IE2 Iodine deficiency—For convenience, we have arbitrarily chosen to present mortality directly attributable to iodine deficiency in the table for cretinism (IE2-6); Grade 2 goitre and cretinoidism may also contribute to the total estimated mortality from iodine deficiency. Cretinoids (IE2-5) are defined as having bilateral perceptive auditory loss, psychomotor delay and impaired intellectual development. Grade 0 goitre (IE2-1) is not palpable or visible in a normal position, Grade 1 goitre (IE2-2) is palpable but not visible in a normal position, and Grade 2 goitre (IE2-3) is visible in a normal position.

IE3 Vitamin A deficiency—Xerophthalmia (IE3-1) includes all ocular manifestations of vitamin A deficiency: night blindness, Bitot's spots, corneal xerosis, corneal ulceration and corneal scarring. Corneal scarring (IE3-2) is not synonymous with blindness. Direct deaths due to vitamin A deficiency have not been disaggregated into those due to corneal scar and those due to other forms of vitamin A deficiency. Vitamin A deficiency is likely to be a risk factor for mortality from many other causes such as diarrhoea and respiratory infections. See Murray and Lopez (1996b) for estimates of mortality associated with vitamin A deficiency.

IE4 Iron-deficiency anaemia—Mortality directly attributable to iron deficiency is shown with the prevalence of all forms of iron-deficiency anaemia (IE4-1); mortality has not been disaggregated into deaths attributable to mild, moderate, severe and very severe anaemia. Mild anaemia (IE4-2) is defined by a haemoglobin of 100–109 g/l in pregnant women, 110–119 g/l in children and adult women and 120–129 g/l in adult men. Moderate anaemia (IE4-3) is defined by a haemoglobin of 70–99 g/l in pregnant women, 80–109 g/l in children and adult women and 90–119 g/l in adult men. Severe anaemia(IE4-4) is defined by a haemoglobin of 40–69 g/l in pregnant women, 50–79 g/l in children and adult women and 60–89 g/l in adult men. Very severe anaemia (IE4-5) is defined by a haemoglobin of <40 g/l in pregnant women, <50 g/l in children and adult women and <60 g/l in adult men.

IIA Malignant neoplasms—For all malignant neoplasms, a case of cancer has by convention been assumed to remain a case until surviving five years from the time of onset. Any case surviving after five years has been assumed to be cured for the purpose of defining prevalence.

IIC Diabetes mellitus—For convenience, we have arbitrarily chosen to present mortality directly attributable to diabetes mellitus in the table for the incidence and prevalence of diabetes mellitus itself (IIC-1). Cases of diabetes mellitus (IIC-1) include insulin dependent diabetes mellitus (IDDM) and non-insulin dependent diabetes mellitus (NIDDM). Individuals suffering from diabetes mellitus have an elevated relative risk of death due to cardiovascular disease and other causes—see McKeigue and King (1996) for a review of these studies and Murray and Lopez (1996a) for estimates of mortality indirectly attributable to diabetes mellitus.

IIE1 Unipolar major depression—Unipolar major depression could be analyzed as an episodic disease or as a lifetime chronic condition with intermittent symptoms. Based on a consensus of the psychiatrists reviewing this study, we have chosen to present incidence and prevalence estimates for episodes of major depression.

IIE5 Alcohol use—Deaths include deaths directly attributed to alcohol dependence, non-dependent use of alcohol and alcoholic psychosis.

IIE6 Dementia and other degenerative and hereditary CNS disorders—For reasons of space, the name was abbreviated to Dementia in table 168. The vast majority of cases included in this category are due to Alzheimer's but some of the deaths at younger ages are due to other conditions such as Huntington's chorea, etc.

IIE9 Drug use—Deaths include deaths directly attributed to drug use. The prevalence estimates are for dysfunctional and harmful drug use (IIE9-1). Only prevalence numbers and rates are shown. No information was available on the average duration or incidence of dysfunctional and harmful drug use. For the calculation of YLDs, we have assumed that duration is one year and incidence equals prevalence.

IIF1 Glaucoma—Glaucoma related blindness (IIF1-1) includes primary angle-closure glaucoma and primary open angle glaucoma. There is no chapter on glaucoma in the *Global Burden of Disease and Injury Series*; the data shown here that were used to calculate YLDs from glaucoma were based on a review of published and unpublished sources of information provided by the World Health Organization. In all regions other than China, no deaths are directly attributed to glaucoma, although the literature suggests that the relative risk of death of the blind compared with the sighted of the same age is greater than 1. In China, the Disease Surveillance Points system assigns a small number of deaths to glaucoma. We have chosen to include those deaths in these tabulations.

IIF2 Cataracts—In all regions other than China, no deaths are directly attributed to cataracts although the literature suggests that the relative risk of death of the blind compared with the sighted of the same age is greater than 1. In China, the Disease Surveillance Points system assigns a small number of deaths to cataract. We have chosen to include those deaths in these tabulations.

IIG1 Rheumatic heart disease—Only the major sequela of rheumatic heart disease, i.e. congestive heart failure (IIG1-1), has been evaluated. Estimates of the incidence of acute rheumatic fever have not been undertaken.

IIG2 Ischaemic heart disease—For convenience, we have arbitrarily chosen to present mortality directly attributable to ischaemic heart disease in the table for acute myocardial infarction (IIG2-1). Acute MI rates are based on MONICA definitions (Beaglehole et al. 1996) and show rates for first MI, not including subsequent MIs. In the table for angina pectoris (IIG2-2), zeros are shown for mortality; we assume that all individuals dying from ischaemic heart disease die from acute myocardial infarction or congestive heart failure. *Congestive heart failure* (IIG2-3) shows '–'s for deaths because all deaths due to ischaemic heart disease are arbitrarily shown with acute myocardial infarction.

IIG3 Cerebrovascular diseases—The incidence figures are for first-ever stroke (IIG3-1) and do not include recurrent stroke rates. The prevalence estimates measure the prevalence of ever having had a stroke; they include the approximately one-third of stroke victims who do not suffer any residual disability. Incidence estimates for ages under 15 do not include non-fatal stroke.

IIG4 Inflammatory heart diseases—This category includes myocarditis (IIG4-1), pericarditis (IIG4-2), endocarditis (IIG4-3) and cardiomyopathies (IIG4-4). For each of these conditions, we have estimated the incidence and prevalence of symptomatic cases. For myocarditis (IIG4-1) and cardiomyopathies (IIG4-4), the main symptomatic outcome is congestive heart failure.

IIH1 Chronic obstructive pulmonary disease—For the purposes of this study, symptomatic COPD (IIH1-1) has been defined as an FEV_1 of less than 1 liter, which is consistently associated with significant symptoms. For the tabulations in this book, we have excluded the small number of incident cases and deaths that occur under age 15.

IIH2 Asthma—The estimates of incidence and prevalence refer to individuals with asthma, not to episodes of acute asthma.

II.I1 Peptic ulcer —Estimates of incidence and prevalence refer to individuals with peptic ulcers, most of whom have recurrent intermittent symptoms.

II.I2 Cirrhosis of the liver—Incidence and prevalence estimates are for individuals with symptomatic cirrhosis (II.I2-1).

IIJ1 Nephritis and nephrosis—The analysis of this large cluster of conditions has been undertaken for two aggregates, acute glomerulonephritis/nephrosis (IIJ1-1) and end-stage renal disease (IIJ1-2).

IIJ2 Benign prostatic hypertrophy—Estimates are presented for individuals with some albeit intermittent symptoms from benign prostatic hypertrophy (IIJ2-1). The prevalence of hypertrophy of the prostate is much higher but many of these individuals have not yet had symptoms. Prevalence rates are generally higher in developing regions because access to treatment that ameliorates symptoms such as transurethral prostatectomy is much lower.

IIL1 Rheumatoid arthritis—The table for rheumatoid arthritis cases (IIL1-1) includes deaths directly attributed to rheumatoid arthritis. In addition, there is evidence that individuals who have rheumatoid arthritis have an elevated relative risk of death from other causes (Symmons 1996); see Murray and Lopez (1996b) for estimates of indirect mortality.

IIL2 Osteoarthritis—Fewer than 500 deaths globally are directly attributed to osteoarthritis. Because of the small number of deaths and the difficulty of assigning these deaths to osteoarthritis of the hip or knee, the tables for hip osteoarthritis (IIL2-1) and for knee osteoarthritis (IIL2-2) show no deaths due to osteoarthritis.

IIM Congenital anomalies—The incidence rates shown for all of the congenital anomalies are in reality the number of live-born infants born with a congenital anomaly divided by the mid-year population aged 0–4 years. Readers interested in the birth prevalences of these congenital anomalies should divide the incident numbers by the number of live births in each region in 1990.

IIM4 Cleft lip—The prevalence estimates shown include individuals who have had surgical correction. In the calculation of YLDs, a different disability weight has been used for those individuals who have had surgical correction as compared with those who have not had surgical correction.

IIM5 Cleft palate—The prevalence estimates shown include individuals who have had surgical correction. In the calculation of YLDs, a different disability weight has been used for those individuals who have had surgical correction as compared to those who have not had surgical correction.

IIN1 Dental caries—The incidence rates and prevalence rates are per person, not per tooth, quadrant or sextant.

III Injuries—Because the datasets used to estimate the incidence and prevalence rates for injury events are based on health care provision data, for each injury our definition of incidence is an injury severe enough to warrant medical attention or that leads immediately to death. In other words, injuries that are severe enough that if an individual had access to a medical facility he or she would seek attention. For each cause of injury in the Global Burden of Disease Study, we have estimated the incidence and prevalence of 40 types of specific injuries, including distinguishing short-term and long-term consequences for a number of conditions such as fracture of the femur. In the tables of this book, we provide incidence and prevalence estimates of the 5 sequelae that contribute the most to the burden of disability from each cause of injury. Poisonings have only one sequela and drownings only two. Based on available datasets, we have evaluated all 40 possible types of injuries for suicide but the number of suicide attempts leading to each specific outcome is low enough that we have chosen to present only the incidence of suicide attempts warranting medical attention. For each injury the table labelled "episodes" shows only incidence rates and numbers as there is no meaning to the prevalence of events such as motor vehicle accidents or fires. The tables for each sequela, however, provide estimates of incidence and prevalence.

IIIA1 Road traffic accidents—*Episodes* (IIIA1-1) includes crashes and pedestrian injuries due to motor vehicles.

IIIA2 Poisonings—Only one outcome is included for poisonings.

IIIA4 Fires—Most of the sequelae of fires are due to burns. Some individuals, however, jump from buildings or are otherwise injured due to fires.

IIIA5 Drownings—Other than the drowning and near-drowning rates (IIIA5-1), the only major disabling sequelae from near-drowning included in this study is quadriplegia (IIIA5-2).

IIIA6 Other unintentional injuries—Unlike other residual categories in the GBD study, for other unintentional injuries there are data on the distribution of different types of sequelae which form the basis of the estimates shown here (Lozano et al. 1996).

IIIB1 Self-inflicted injuries—Incidence rates (IIIB1-1) are for suicide attempts.

IIIB3 War—Incidence of injuries and mortality from war include deaths directly attributable to war in non-combatants. For example, the estimates of mortality include deaths to children and adults from landmines.

Notas Explicativas

Símbolos—En las columnas de mortalidad, un 0 indica que esas 0 muertes que estimamos están causadas por la condición considerada. Por otra parte, el símbolo '–' que indica que no somos capaces de proveer una estimación de mortalidad con algún significado debido a esa secuela. El '–' se usa cuando ha estimado la mortalidad de todas las secuelas de una enfermedad o lesión pero para esa mortalidad no ha sido desagregada para ninguna secuela en específico.

IA1 Tuberculosis—Los casos se refieren a individuos con tuberculosis clínica, normalmente con de cultivos positivos esputo pulmonar, y tuberculosis extra-pulmonar. Hemos distinguido incidencia y muerte por tuberculosis de la tuberculosis clínica en individuos VIH negativos (IA1-1) e incidencia y muerte de tuberculosis clínica en VIH positivos (IA1-2). Las estimaciones de VIH/TB han sido generadas usando información de prevelencia de la infección por tuberculosis por edad, sexo y región y la prevalencia específica por edad de la infección por VIH combinada con estimaciones de la tasa de coinfección. Las muertes en las tabulaciones primarias de mortalidad (Murray y Lopez 1996b) muestran defunciones debidas a tuberculosis en individuos VIH negativos mientras que las muertes por tuberculosis en individuos VIH positivos se incluyen en las estimaciones de mortalidad relacionadas con VIH.

IA2a Sífilis—La tasa de sífilis congénita se expresa solo en la población de 0 a 4 años de edad. Para evitar doble conteo, los efectos en la mortalidad del bajo peso al nacer desarrollados por la sífilis se incluyen en las tablas en la definición de *Condiciones surgidas durante el período perinatal*—*bajo peso al nacer* (ID1-1) y los niños con peso bajo para su edad o por debajo de su talla se incluyen en IE1: *Desnutrición proteínico-calórica*. La mortalidad debida a sífilis se incluye en los cuadros en sífilis congénita y sífilis terciaria pero no en sífilis primaria o secundaria. Esta división es algo arbitraria pero refleja los tipos de sífilis que explican la mayoría de muertes.

IA2b Clamidia—Para evitar el doble conteo, los efectos del bajo peso al nacer en la mortalidad y en el desarrollo de los niños se incluyen en las tablas en el rubro de *Condiciones surgidas en el período perinatal*—*bajo peso al nacer*

(ID1-1) y los niños con peso bajo para su edad o por debajo de su talla se incluyen en IE1: *Desnutrición proteínico-calórica*. La neumonía neonatal por Clamidia (IA2b-6) no incluye los casos de neumonía contraídos por transmisión respiratoria. *La enfermedad inflamatoria pélvica* (EIP) (IA2b-7) incluye casos agudos y recurrentes debidos a clamidia. *Infertilidad* (IA2b-11) se refiere a la infertilidad total causada por clamidia debida a enfermedad infecciosa pélvica o embar-azo ectópico en las mujeres o por epididimitis en los hombres. La mortalidad por clamidia ha sido estimada por embarazo ectópico (IA2b-8) y por absceso tuboovárico (IA2b-9). En las tabulaciones primarias de defunciones del Estudio de la Carga Global de la Enfermedad, las muertes por embarazo ectópico aparecen en el rubro de *Aborto* (IC5).

IA2c Gonorrea—Para evitar el doble conteo, los efectos del bajo peso al nacer en la mortalidad y en el desarrollo de los niños se incluyen en los cuadros en el rubro de *Condiciones surgidas en el período perinatal—bajo peso al nacer* (ID1-1) y los niños con peso bajo para su edad o por debajo de su talla se incluyen en IE1: *Desnutrición proteínico-calórica*. *La enfermedad inflamatoria pélvica* (EIP) (IA2c-6) incluye casos agudos y recurrentes debidos a gonorrea. *Infertilidad* (IA2c-10) se refiere a la infertilidad total causada por gonorrea debida a enfermedad inflamatoria pélvica o embarazo ectópico en las mujeres o por epididimitis en los hombres.

IA3 VIH—Como una convención arbitraria, hemos listado todas las muertes relacionadas con VIH con la secuela del *SIDA* (IA3-2) puesto que la mayoría de causas de muerte relacionadas con VIH eran por si mismas condiciones definidas de SIDA. IA3-1 provee información en la incidencia de nuevos casos de infección por VIH en 1990 y de prevalencia por infección de VIH en 1990. IA3-2 provee estimaciones de incidencia y prevalencia del SIDA en 1990. Las proyecciones de muertes por SIDA para el año 2000 se basan en proyecciones desarrolladas por el Programa Mundial SIDA detallado en el capítulo por Low-Beer et al. 1996, ligeramente modificado por Murray y Lopez (1996a) para años después del 2000.

IA4 Enfermedades diarreicas—Siguiendo la convención para este estudio, las muertes en niños con sarampión y diarrea o infecciones de las vías respiratorias inferiores y diarrea no se incluyen en las estimaciones de mortalidad por diarrea que se muestran en la tabla. Las estimaciones de incidencia y prevalencia son por episodios de diarrea incluyendo diarrea aguda, diarrea persistente y disentería.

IA5a Tosferina—Todas las muertes relacionadas con tosferina se presentan en el Cuadro IA5a-1. La prevalencia de retraso mental por tosferina no disminuye con la edad edad. Esto implica que el riesgo relativo de morir de los casos con esa condición es de 1.0 con respecto a la población general. Esta supuesto probablemente no es realista para algunas regiones en desarrollo, pero virtualmente no hay ningún estudio de seguimiento en ninguna región que proporcione un riesgo relativo de morir para este grupo de pacientes.

IA5b Poliomielitis—*Paralítica* incluye complicaciones del miembro superior e inferior.

IA5c Difteria—Las muertes debidas a difteria se aparecen en *Miocarditis* (IA5c-3) basados bajo en el supuesto simplificado de que todos los individuos que mueren por difteria debieron tener alguna forma de complicación del miocardio; aunque puede haber excepciones, por conveniencia se muestran en esta tabla todas muertes y por consiguiente, no hay ninguna muerte asignada a los episodios agudos de difteria (IA5c-1). IA5c-2: *Las complicaciones neurológicas* son más a menudo de nervios craneales y paralisis periféricas.

IA5d Sarampión—Los efectos tardios del sarampión en la mortalidad durante la infancia, meses o años después del episodio, no se incluyen en las estimaciones de mortalidad que se muestran en la tabla.

IA5e Tétanos—Esta categoría incluye tétanos neonatal y tétanos del adulto.

IA6 Meningitis bacteriana y meningococcemia—Por razones de espacio, el nombre fue abreviado a «Meningitis bacteriana» en los cuadros 57–65. Esta categoría incluye meningitis bacteriana debida a Streptoccus pneumonia, Haemophilus influenzae, Neisseria meningitidis y meningococcemia sin meningitis. Basados en las fuentes de datos y métodos empleados para la estimación, las meningitis por otras bacterias (e.g. Listeria, organismos gram negativos, etc) se incluyen en las estimaciones de mortalidad en PEMC, PEAS y ALC pero no en otras regiones. Sin embargo, las estimaciones de todas las formas de incidencia en el total de regiones, estan basadas sólo en estimaciones de S. pneumococcus, H. influenzae y N. meningitidis. Puesto que otras formas de meningitis son menos comunes, esta inconsistencia no debe confundir substancialmente los resultados.

IA7 Hepatitis B y hepatitis C—A causa de las limitaciones de la CIE 9a revisión sobre la lista de códigos para hepatitis viral, se estimó la mortalidad por hepatitis B y C en las regiones de PEMC, PEAS y ALC incluyendo un número limitado de muertes debido a hepatitis A. La cirrosis sintomática (IA7-2) y el hepatoma (IA7-3) atribuidas a hepatitis B se basaron en estimaciones de la fracción atribuíble de cirrosis sintomática (II.I2-1) y hepatoma (IIA5-1) de las cuales se cree que estan causadan por hepatitis B.

IA8 Paludismo—La anemia (IA8-2) se definió usando los criterios de la OMS para anemia media y muy severa. La secuela neurológica por paludismo cerebral (IA8-3) incluye hemiplegia, afasia, ataxia y ceguera cortical.

IA9b Enfermedad de Chagas—Todas las muertes relacionadas con la enfermedad de Chagas se muestran en la tabla con la prevalencia de la infección (IA9b-1). Con la información disponible no hemos sido capaces de distinguir muertes debidas a infección aguda, deficiencia cardíaca o megaviscera. Las columnas de numero de muertes por cardiomiopatía sin insuficiencia cardíaca congestiva (IA9b-2), cardiomiopatía con insuficiencia cardíaca congestiva (IA9b-3) y megaviscera (IA9b-4) muestra el símbolo '–' en la mortalidad.

IA9c Esquistosomiasis—Las estimaciones han sido hechas sólo para la prevalencia de infección asociada directamente a la mortalidad por esquistosomiasis. No hemos incluido estimaciones de mortalidad por cáncer de vejiga, cirrosis o cáncer del colon que puede relacionarse con esquistosomiasis.

IA9d Leishmaniasis—Por conveniencia todas las muertes relacionadas con leishmaniasis que se muestran en la tabla corresponden a leishmaniasis visceral (IA9d-1).

IA9e Filariasis linfática—Basados en el capítulo donde se analiza la filariasis linfática hemos asumido que hay pocas muertes directamente causadas por la filariasis. Esto podría introducir una subestimación de los efectos de la infección aguda por filaria.

IA10 Lepra—Los casos de lepra (IA10-1) provienen de la incidencia y prevalencia que se obtiene al seguir la definición de casos de la OMS. Prevalencia esta no es la misma prevalencia de los individuos con lepra clínica. La tasa de prevalencia de lepra discapacitante (IA10-2) se estima a partir de la verdadera prevalencia de discapacidad por lepra.

IA11 Dengue—No se incluyó en la versión 3 o 4 del Estudio de la Carga Global de la Enfermedad. Las estimaciones han sido preparadas sólo para dengue hemorrágico (IA11-1). y aún no se han generado las estimaciones mundiales y regionales de todas las formas de dengue.

IA12 Encefalitis japonesa—Todas las muertes debidas a Encefalitis japonesa se muestran como episodios (IA12-1).

IA14a Ascaridiasis—El cuadro IA14a-1 proviene estimaciones de la prevalencia de infecciones con más de 10 gusanos en niños de 0–4, más de 15 en niños de 5–9, y más de 20 en la población mayor de 20 años de edad. Las estimaciones de la incidencia de elevada concentración de gusanos no han sido desarrolladas. Las muertes directamente atribuíbles a infestación del ascaris se muestran con la incidencia y prevalencia de obstrucción intestinal (IA14a-4), dado que éste se considera el mecanismo primario directamente atribuíble a la mortalidad. «El déficit contemporáneo cognocitivo» (IA14a-2) es un término usado por Bundy et al. (1996) y se refiere a los défits cognocitivos que estan una función de la concentración de gusanos presentes y no debido a retrasos del desarrollo causados por cargas elevadas del gusano en edades previas. «La deficienca cognocitiva» (IA14a-4) se refiere a los cambios permanentes causados por las elevadas concentraciones del gusano durante la niñez y en los años juveniles.

IA14b Tricocefalosis—El cuadro IA14b-1 proviene estimaciones de la prevalencia de infecciones con más de 90 gusanos en niños de 0–4, más de 130 en niños de 5–9, y más de 180 en población mayor de 20 años de edad. Las estimaciones de la incidencia de elevada concentración de gusanos no han sido desarrolladas. Las muertes directamente atribuíbles a infestación por tricocéfalos se muestran con la incidencia y prevalencia del síndrome de disentería masiva dado que éste se considera el mecanismo primario directamente atribuíble a la mortalidad. «El déficit contemporáneo cognocitivo» (IA14b-2) es un término usado por Bundy et al. (1996) y se refiere a los défits cognocitivos que estan una función de la concentración de gusanos presentes y no debido a retrasos del desarrollo causados por cargas elevadas del gusano en edad es previas. «La deficiencia cognocitiva» (IA14b-4) se refiere a los cambios permanentes causados por las elevadas concentraciones del gusano durante la niñez y en los años juveniles.

IA14c Anquilostomiasis y necatoriasis—El cuadro IA14c-1 proviene estimaciones de la prevalencia de infecciones con más de 20 gusanos en niños de 0–4, más de 30 en niños de 5–9, y más de 40 en población mayor de 20 años de edad. Las estimaciones de la incidencia de elevada concentración de gusanos no han sido desarrolladas. Las muertes directamente atribuíbles a infestación por uncinarias se muestran en el Cuadro IA14c-1.

IB2 Infecciones de las vías respiratorias inferiores—Las secuelas crónicas (IB2-2) incluyen bronquiectasias y daños de la función pulmonar medidas por una disminución en la FEV_1. Aún cuando estas secuelas crónicas pueden causar la muerte, no se ha estimado la magnitud de esta mortalidad. En las tabulaciones primarias de la mortalidad, estas secuelas aparecerían en otros condiciones respiratorias crónicas (IIH).

IB3 Otitis media—*Episodios* (IB3-1) se refiere a episodios de otitis media aguda.

IC1 Hemorragia materna—Por conveniencia, todas las muertes directamente atribuíbles a hemorragia materna se muestra con la incidencia de hemorragia materna (IC1-1).

IC3 Trastornos hipertensivos del embarazo—Esta categoría incluye pre-eclampsia y eclampsia. La mortalidad mostrada en la tabla con la incidencia y prevalencia (IC3-1) de episodios es el total de alteraciones hipertensivas debidas al embarazo, incluyendo eclampsia.

ID Condiciones que aparecen durante el período perinatal—Una equivocación común es confundir las condiciones que surgen durante el período perinatal, las cuales son un conjunto de causas de muerte que son peculiares de las primeras semanas de vida del recién nacido, con la mortalidad perinatal que representa las muertes que suceden entre la semana 28 gestación y las 4 semanas después del nacimiento.

ID1 Peso bajo al nacer—Esta categoría incluye a los niños pequeños para su edad gestational y a los prematuros. Diferentes enfermedades en este estudio y todas las secuelas realacionadas con bajo peso al nacer han sido agrupadas en un solo resultado el cual incluye parálisis cerebral, retraso mental, epilepsia, pérdida del oído y pérdida visual (ID1-1). Shibuya y Murray (1996a) explica en detalle porqué esta decisión ha sido tomada basándose principalmente en la naturaleza de los estudios de cohorte considerados. En este estudio el término «condiciones perinatales» es usado para referirse a las condiciones que surgen durante el período perinatal. La incidencia aquí considerada no incluye casos de muertes tempranas ocurridas después del nacimiento.

ID2 Asfixia y trauma al nacer—Diferentes enfermedades en este estudio y todas las secuelas realacionadas con asfixia al nacer y traumatismos al nacer han sido agrupadas en un solo resultado el cual incluye parálisis cerebral, retraso mental, epilepsia, pérdida del oído y pérdida visual (ID2-1). Shibuya y Murray (1996b) explica en detalle porqué esta decisión ha sido tomada, basándose principalmente en el naturaleza de los estudios de cohorte considerados. La incidencia aquí considerada no incluye casos de muertes tempranas ocurridas después del nacimiento.

IE1 Desnutrición proteínico-calórica—La emaciación (IE1-1) es la prevalencia de niños que presentan un bajo peso para su estatura y ésta se encuentra 2 desviaciones estándar por abajo de la media de la población de referencia del NCHS. El retraso de crecimiento (IE1-2) es la prevalencia de niños que tienen una estatura baja para su edad y ésta se encuentra 2 desviaciones estándar por abajo de la media de la población de refrencia del NCHS. Muchos niños que han presentado emanciación pueden haber tenido retraso en el crecimiento y viceversa. El mismo niño puede aparrarecer en la tablas con retraso en el crecimiento y con emaciación. Por conveniencia, arbitrariamente hemos escogido presentar la mortalidad directamente atribuíble a desnutrición proteínico-calórica en la tabla como emaciación (IE1-1). Es probable que la desnutrición sea un factor del riesgo de morir por muchas otras causas como diarrea o infecciones respiratorias. Ver a Mason et al. (1996) para el análisis de mortalidad asociado con desnutrición en niños menores de 5 años. Arbitrariamente hemos elegido no estimar emaciación o retraso en el crecimiento en adultos.

IE2 Deficiencia de yodo—Por conveniencia, arbitrariamente hemos escogido presentar la mortalidad directamente atribuíble a deficiencia de yodo el cuadro bajo el rubro de cretinismo (IE2-6); el bocio grado 2 y el cretinoidismo también contribuyen al total de defunciones estimadas por deficiencia de yodo. El cretinoidismo (IE2-5) se define como la pérdida de la percepción auditiva bilateral, retraso del desarrollo psicomotor y daño intelectual. En el bocio grado 0 (IE2-1) la tiroides no está palpable o visible en una posición normal, en el bocio grado 1 (IE2-2) la tiroides está palpable pero no visible en un posición normal y en el bocio grado 2 (IE2-3) está visible en un posición normal.

IE3 Deficiencia de vitamina A—La xeroftalmia (IE3-1) incluye todas las manifestaciones oculares de la deficiencia de vitamina A: ceguera nocturna, las manchas de Bitot, xerosis corneal, ulceración de la cornea y cicatriz corneal. La cicatriz de la córnea (IE3-2) no es sinónimo de ceguera. Las muertes directas debidas a deficiencia de vitamina A no han sido desagregadas en aquellas debidas a cicatriz de la córnea y a otras formas de deficiencia de vitamina A. La deficiencia de Vitamina A es probablemente un factor del riesgo de morir de muchos otras causas como diarrea e infecciones respiratorias. Ver Murray y Lopez (1996) para las estimaciones de mortalidad asociada con deficiencia de vitamina A.

IE4 Anemia por deficiencia de hierro—La mortalidad directamente atribuíble a la deficiencia de hierro se muestra con la prevalencia de todas las formas de anemia (IE4-1). Las estimaciones de esta mortalidad no han sido desagregadas por muertes atribuíbles a anemia leve, moderada, severa y muy severa. La anemia leve (IE4-2) en mujeres embarazadas corresponde a niveles de hemoglobina de 100–109 g/l, 110–119 g/l para niños y mujeres adultas y 120–129 g/l para hombres adultos; la anemia moderada (IE4-3) en mujeres embarazadas corresponde a una hemoglobina de 70–99 g/l, 80–109 g/l en niños y mujeres adultas y 90–119 g/l para hombres adultos; la anemia severa (IE4-4) en mujeres embarazadas corresponde a una hemoglobina de 40–69 g/l, 50–79 g/l en niños y mujeres adultas y 60–89 g/l en hombres adultos; y anemia muy severa (IE4-5) en mujeres embarazadas corresponde a una hemoglobina <40 g/l,<50 g/l en niños y mujeres adultas y <60 g/l en hombres adultos.

IIA Neoplasias malignas—Para todas las neoplasias malignas, se asume por conveniencia que un caso de cáncer es aquel que sobrevive hasta cinco años despues de la edad de inicio. Cualquier caso que sobreviva después de cinco años para los propósitos de definir prevalencia se considera como un caso curado.

IIC Diabetes mellitus—Por conveniencia, arbitrariamente hemos escogido presentar en la tabla la mortalidad directamente atribuíble a diabetes mellitus para la incidencia y prevalencia de misma enfermedad (IIC-1). Los casos de diabetes mellitus (IIC-1) incluyen diabetes insulino dependientes (IDDM) y no insulino dependientes (NIDDM). Los individuos que padecen diabetes mellitus presentan un riesgo relativo elevado de muerte debido a enfermedades cardiovasculares y otras causas—ver McKeigue y King (1996) para una revisión de estos estudios y Murray y Lopez (1996) para estimar la mortalidad indirectamente atribuíble a diabetes mellitus.

IIE1 Depresión mayor unipolar—La depresión mayor unipolar puede ser analizada como un episodio de una enfermedad o como condición crónica con síntomas intermitentes de por vida. Basado en un acuerdo general de las psiquiatras que revisaron este estudio, hemos escogido presentar la incidencia y prevalencia estimadas para episodios de depresión mayor.

IIE5 Uso de alcohol—Definiciones del síndrome de dependencia del alcohol. Las muertes incluyen aquellas directamente atribuíbles a dependencia del alcohol, comsumo de alcohol no dependiente y psícosis alcohólica.

IIE6 Dementia y otros trastornos degenerativos y hereditarios del sistema nervioso central—Por razones de espacio, el nombre fue abreviado a «Dementia» en el cuadro 168. La mayoría de los casos incluídos en esta categoría son debidos a Alzheimer pero algunas de las muertes a edades más jóvenes son debidas a otras condiciones como la corea de Huntington.

IIE9 Uso de drogas—Las muertes incluyen defunciones directamente atribuíbles a uso de narcóticos y las estimaciones de la prevalencia son por uso disfuncional y dañino de drogas (IIE9-1). Solo se muestran números de prevalencia. No hubo información disponible sobre la duración media o de la incidencia del uso disfuncional y dañino de drogas. Para los calculos de los AVD, hemos asumido que la duración es de un año y la incidencia es igual a la prevalencia.

IIF1 Glaucoma—La ceguera relacionada con glaucoma (IIF1-1) incluye glaucoma del ángulo-cerrado primario y glaucoma de ángulo abierto. No hay ningún capítulo de glaucoma en la *Serie de la Carga Global de Enfermedad y Lesión*. Los datos mostrados usados para los cálculos de los AVD para glaucoma se basaron en la revisión de datos publicados y en datos inéditos de la Organización Mundial de la Salud. En todas las regiones menos en China, no hay muertes que se atribuyan directamente a glaucoma sin embarge se ha reportado en la literatura un riesgo relativo mayor de 1 de morir ciego comparado con el vidente de la misma edad. En China, el sistema de Vigilancia de la Enfermadad le asigna un número pequeño de muertes a glaucoma. Hemos escogido incluir esas muertes en estas tabulaciones.

IIF2 Cataratas—En todas las regiones menos en China, no hay muertes que se atribuyan directamente a catarata sin embarge se ha reportado en la literatura un riesgo relativo mayor de 1 de morir ciego comparado con el vidente de la misma edad. En China, el sistema de Vigilancia de la Enfermedad le asigna un número pequeño de muertes a catarata. Hemos escogido incluir esas muertes en estas tabulaciones.

IIG1 Cardiopatía reumática—Sólo la secuela mayor de la cardiopatía reumática, insuficiencia cardíaca congestiva (IIG1-1) se han evaluado. No se incoporaron estimaciones de la incidencia de fiebre reumática aguda.

IIG2 Cardiopatía isquémica—Por conveniencia, arbitrariamente hemos escogido presentar en la tabla la mortalidad directamente atribuida a enfermedad isquémica del corazón por infarto agudo del miocardio (IIG2-1). El infarto agudo se basa en las definiciones del estudio de MONICA (Beaglehole et al. 1996). En la tabla se muestra la mortalidad por angina de pecho (IIG2-2), en ceros pues asumimos que todos los individuos que mueren de enfermedad isquémica del corazónes por infarto agudo del miocardio o de insuficiencia cardiaca congestiva. La insuficiencia cardíaca congestiva (IIG2-3) muestra el símbolo '–' para muertes ya que todas las defunciones debidas a enfermedad isquémica del corazón se muestran arbitrariamente en infarto agudo del miocardio.

IIG3 Enfermedad cerebrovascular—La incidencia de estas enfermedades fué calculada solo para el primer accidente vascular cerebral experimentado por persona (IIG3-1) sin incluir accidentes recurrentes. Las estimaciones de la prevalencia son de las personas que alguna vez hayan tenido un AVC; incluyen aproximadamente un tercio de las víctimas del AVC sin ninguna discapacidad residual. Las estimaciones de incidencia para las edades menores que 15 años no incluyen casos de accidente vascular cerebral no fatales.

IIG4 Enfermedades inflamatorias del corazón—Esta categoría incluye miocarditis (IIG4-1), pericarditis (IIG4-2), endocarditis (IIG4-3) y cardiomiopatias (IIG4-4). Para cada una de estas condiciones hemos estimado la incidencia y prevalencia de casos sintomáticos. Para miocarditis (IIG4-1) y cardiomiopatias (IIG4-4), el resultado principal es insuficiencia cardíaca congestiva.

IIH1 Enfermedad pulmonar obstructiva crónica—Para los propósitos de este estudio, se ha definido como un EPOC sintomático (IIH1-1) a una condición con un FEV_1 de menos de 1 litro, la cual indica sintomas significativos de una manera consistente. En las tabulaciones de este libro, hemos excluído el número reducido de casos y muertes que occurren antes de la edad de 15 años.

IIH2 Asma—Las estimaciones de incidencia y prevalencia se refieren a individuos con asma y no a los episodios de asma aguda.

II.I1 Ulcera péptica—Las estimaciones de incidencia y prevalencia se refieren a individuos con úlcera péptica que tienen síntomas recurrentes e intermitentes.

II.I2 Cirrosis hepática—Las estimaciones de incidencia y prevalencia son para individuos con cirrosis sintomática (II.I2-1).

IIJ1 Nefritis y nefrosis—El análisis de este grupo amplio de condiciones se llevó a cabo para los siguientes subgrupos: glomerulonefritis aguda/nefrosis (IIJ1-1) y estado terminal de la enfermedad renal (IIJ1-2).

IIJ2 Hipertrofia prostática benigna—Se presentan estimaciones para individuos con algunos síntomas intermitentes de hipertrofia prostática benigna (IIJ2-1). En realidad, la prevalencia de hipertrofia prostática benigna es mucho más alta para muchos de estos individuos que no han tenido todavía síntomas. La tasas de prevalencia generalmente son más altas en regiones desarrolladas porque el acceso al tratamiento que mejora síntomas, como la prostatectomía trasureteral es mucho más bajo.

IIL1 Artritis reumatoide—El cuadro para casos de artritis reumatoide (IIL1-1) incluye muertes directamente atribuíbles a esta condición. Además, hay evidencia que los individuos que ha tenido artritis reumatoide presentan un elevado riesgo de muerte por otro causas (Symmons 1996); ver Murray y Lopez (1996) para estimaciones indirectas de la mortalidad.

IIL2 Osteoartritis—Menos de 500 muertes a nivel mundial se atribuyen directamente a osteoartritis. A causa del número pequeño de muertes y la dificultad de asignarles a estas muertes, las tablas de osteoartritis de cadera OA (IIL2-1) y rodilla OA (IIL2-2) no muestran ninguna muerte debido a osteoartritis.

IIM Anomalías congénitas—La tasa de incidencia que se muestra para todas las anomalías congénitas es en realidad el número de recien nacidos con una anomalía congénita dividido por la población de 0 a 4 años de edad. Los lectores interesados en la prevalencia de estas anomalías congénitas al nacer debe dividir los números de casos incidentes entre el número de nacidos vivos en cada región en 1990.

IIM4 Labio leporino—La prevalencia estimada incluye individuos que han tenido corrección quirúrgica. En los cálculos de los AVD, se ha usado diferentes ponderaciones de la discapacidad para los individuos que han recibido corrección quirúrgica y los que no ha tenido corrección quirúrgica.

IIM5 Paladar hendido—La prevalencia estimada incluye individuos que han tenido corrección quirúrgica. En los cálculos de los AVD, se ha usado diferentes ponderaciones de la discapacidad para los individuos que han recibido corrección quirúrgica y los que no ha tenido corrección quirúrgica.

IIN1 Caries dentales—La tasa de incidencia y la tasa de prevalencia son por persona y no por diente, cuadrante o sextante.

III Lesiones—Dado que las bases de datos utilizadas para estimar las tasas de incidencia y prevalencia de las lesiones son basadas en oferta de servicios de salud, nuestra definición de incidencia es sobre una lesión bastante severa que requiere atención médica o si no llevaría inmediatamente a la muerte. En otras palabras, son lesiones bastan severas que si el individuo tiene acceso a servicios médicos seguramente recibirá atención. Para cada causa de lesión en el estudio de la Carga Global de la Enfermedad, hemos estimado la incidencia y pre-valencia de 40 tipos de lesiones específicas, incluyendo distinciones entre consecuencias de corto y largo plazo para varias condiciones como la fractura del fémur. En las tablas de este libro proveemos de estimaciones de incidencia y prevalencia para las 5 secuelas que más contribuyen a la carga de discapacidad de cada causa de lesión. Los envenenamientos solo tienen una secuela y los ahogamientos sólo dos. Basados en los datos disponibles, hemos evaluado 40 tipos posibles de lesiones para suicidio pero el número de intentos de suicidio es bastante raro por lo que hemos escogido sólo presentar la incidencia de intentos de suicidio que requiere atención médica. Para cada lesión en la tabla nombrada «episodios» solo se muestran tasas de incidencia, puesto que no tiene sentido calcular la prevalencia de ciertos accidentes como los de vehículo de motor y de quemaduras. Los cuadros en cada secuela, sin embargo, proveen estimaciones de incidencia y prevalencia.

IIIA1 Accidentes de tráfico—*Episodios* (IIIA1-1) incluyen choques y atropellados relacionados con vehículos de motor.

IIIA2 Envenenamientos—Solo se incluye un resultado por envenenamientos

IIIA4 Fuegos—La mayoría de las secuelas por accidente por fuego son las quemaduras. Sin embargo algunos individuos saltan de los edificios o se dañan de otra forma debido al fuego.

IIIA5 Ahogamientos—Se distingue entre los individuos que se ahogan y los que casi se ahogan. Sin embargo la unica secuela mayor considerada fue la quadriplegia en los casos cercanos a ahogarse (IIIA5-1,2).

IIIA6 Otras lesiones no intencionales—A diferencia de otras categorías residuales en el estudio de la CGE, para otras lesiones no intencionales existen datos acerca de la distribución de tipos diferentes de secuela. Estos datos forman la base de las estimaciones que aquí se muestran (Lozano et al. 1996).

IIIB1 Lesiónes autoinfligidas—La tasa de incidencia (IIIB1-1) es por intento de suicidio.

IIIB3 Guerra—La incidencia de las lesiones y la mortalidad por guerra incluyen muertes directamente atribuíbles a la guerra en no combatientes. Por ejemplo las estimaciones de mortalidad incluyen muertes en niños y adultos en campos minados.

Notes Explicatives

Symboles—Dans la colonne relative à la mortalité, un 0 indique que la condition cause 0 décès alors qu'un '−' indique que nous ne sommes pas en mesure de donner une estimation significative de la mortalité due à cette séquelle. Le '−' est utilisé lorsque les estimations de mortalité ont été faites pour l'ensemble des séquelles d'une maladie ou d'un traumatisme, mais que la mortalité due à chacune des séquelles spécifiques n'a pas été estimée.

IA1 Tuberculose—Les cas se réfèrent aux individus ayant une tuberculose clinique, en général pulmonaire avec des cultures de sputum positives, et aux cas de tuberculose extra-pulmonaire. Nous avons distingué entre l'incidence et les décès de tuberculose clinique chez les individus séro-négatifs pour le VIH (IA1-1), et l'incidence et les décès de tuberculose clinique chez les individus séro-positifs pour le VIH (IA1-2). Les estimations du VIH/TB ont été faites à partir de l'information sur la prévalence de l'infection tuberculeuse selon l'âge, le sexe, et la région et la prévalence de l'infection à VIH selon l'âge spécifique, combinée aux estimations du taux de coinfection. Les décès rapportés dans les tabulations primaires de mortalité (Murray et Lopez 1996b) sont les décès dûs à la tuberculose chez les individus séro-négatifs pour le VIH alors que les décès dûs à la tuberculose chez les individus séro-positifs pour le VIH sont inclus dans les estimations de mortalité en rapport avec le VIH.

IA2a Syphilis—Les taux de syphilis congénitale sont exprimés en tant que taux pour la population de 0–4 ans. Pour éviter de compter les décès à double, les effets d'un poids insuffisant à la naissance sur la mortalité et le développement dûs à la syphilis sont inclus dans les tableaux sur le poids insuffisant à la naissance sous *Poids insuffisant à la naissance — toutes les séquelles* (ID1-1) et les enfants ayant un poids insuffisant à la naissance qui continuent à avoir une insuffisance pondéral ou une insuffisance staturale sont inclus dans le tableau IE1: *Malnutrition protéino-calorique*. La mortalité due à la syphilis est incluse dans les tableaux sur la syphilis congénitale et la syphilis tertiaire, mais non dans celles sur la syphilis primaire et secondaire. Cette division est quelque peu arbitraire mais reflète les types de syphilis qui causent la majorité des décès.

IA2b Chlamydiose—Pour éviter de compter les décès à double, les effets d'un poids insuffisant à la naissance sur la mortalité et le développement dus à la chlamydiose sont inclus dans les tableaux sur le poids insuffisant à la naissance sous *Poids insuffisant à la naissance — toutes les séquelles* (ID1-1) et les enfants ayant un poids insuffisant à la naissance qui continuent à avoir une insuffisance pondéral ou une insuffisance staturale sont inclus dans le tableau IE1: *Malnutrition protéino-calorique*. La pneumonie néonatale à Chlamydia (IA2b-6) n'inclut pas les pneumonies à Chlamydia secondaires à une transmission aérienne. Le tableau *PID* (IA2b-6) inclut les inflammations aiguës et récidiventes à Chlamydia des organes pelviens. La *Stérilité* (IA2b-11) comprend toutes les formes de stérilité survenues à la suite d'inflamation des organes pelviens à Chlamydia, à la suite de grossesses ectopiques chez la femme, et à la suite d'épidymites chez l'homme. La mortalité due à la chlamydiose a été estimée pour les grossesses ectopiques (IA2b-8) et pour les abcès tubo-ovariens (IA2b-9). Dans les tabulations primaires des causes de décès de l'Etude de la Charge Globale des Maladies, les décès dus à une grossesse ectopique sont inclus dans les *Avortements* (IC5).

IA2c Gonorrhée—Pour éviter de compter les décès à double, les effets d'un poids léger pour l'âge gestationnel sur la mortalité et le développement dûs à la gonorrhée sont inclus dans les tableaux sur le poids léger pour l'âge gestationnel sous *Poids insuffisant à la naissance — toutes les séquelles* (ID1-1) et les enfants légers pour l'âge gestationnel qui continuent à avoir une insuffisance pondéral ou une insuffisance staturale sont inclus dans le tableau IE1: *Malnutrition protéino-calorique*. Les tableaux *PID* (IA2c-6) incluent les inflammations aiguës et récidiventes gonococciques des organes pelviens. La *Stérilité* (IA2c-10) comprend toutes les formes de stérilité survenues à la suite d'inflammation des organes pelviens à gonocoques, à la suite de grossesse ectopique chez la femme, et à la suite d'épididymite chez l'homme.

IA3 VIH—Suivant une convention arbitraire nous avons catalogué tous les décès en rapport avec le VIH comme séquelle du *SIDA* (IA3-2) du fait que la plupart des causes de décès en rapport avec le VIH sont elles-mêmes des conditions qui définissent le SIDA. Le Tableau IA3-1 indique l'incidence des nouvelles infections à VIH en 1990 et la prévalence des infections à VIH en 1990. Le tableau IA3-2 donne des estimations de l'incidence et de la prévalence du SIDA en 1990. Les projections des cas de décès dûs au SIDA d'ici à l'an 2000 sont basées sur les projections développées par le Programme Global sur le SIDA dont les détails sont donnés dans le chapitre par Low-Beer et al. 1996, légèrement modifiées par Murray et Lopez (1996a) pour les années au delà de l'an 2000.

IA4 Maladies diarrhéiques—Selon la convention adoptée pour cette étude, les décès survenus chez des enfants ayant la rougeole avec des diarrhées, et des infections respiratoires aiguës, avec des diarrhées, ne sont pas inclus dans les estimations de la mortalité due aux diarrhées rapportées dans ce tableau. Les estimations d'incidence et de prévalence se rapportent aux épisodes de diarrhée et comprennent les maladies diarrhéiques aqueuses aiguës, les diarrhées persistantes et les dysenteries.

IA5a Coqueluche—Tous les décès en rapport avec la coqueluche sont présentés dans le Tableau IA5a-1. La prévalence du retard mental secondaire à la coqueluche ne diminue pas avec l'âge, ce qui implique un risque relatif de décès chez ceux qui souffrent de cette condition, comparé à la population générale, égal à 1.0. Cette supposition n'est probablement pas réaliste pour certaines régions en voie de développement mais il n'existe virtuellement aucune étude longitudinale dans aucune région qui donne un risque relatif de décès pour ce groupe de patients.

IA5b Poliomyélite—Dans le tableau IA5b-2, la paralysie inclut l'atteinte des membres supérieur et inférieur.

IA5c Diphtérie—Les décès dûs à la diphtérie sont rapportés avec la *Myocardite* (IA5c-3), ceci à partir de la supposition simplificatrice que tous les individus qui décèdent de diphtérie doivent avoir un certain degré d'atteinte myocardique; il peut bien sûr y avoir des exceptions mais, par convenance, tous les décès sont inclus dans ce tableau et par conséquent aucun décès n'est attribué aux épisodes aigus de diphtérie (IA5c-1). IA5c-2: *Complications neurologiques* sont le plus souvent des paralysies des nerfs crâniens et des nerfs périphériques.

IA5d Rougeole—Les effets tardifs de la rougeole sur la mortalité infantile, survenant des mois ou années après l'épisode, ne sont pas inclus dans les estimations de mortalité présentées dans le tableau.

IA5e Tétanos—Cette catégorie inclut à la fois le tétanos néonatal et le tétanos adulte.

IA6 Méningite bactérienne et méningococcémie—A la suite de manque de place, le nom a été abrégé à «Méningite bactérienne» dans les tableaux 57–65. Cette catégorie inclut les méningites bactériennes à Streptococcus pneumonia, à Hemophilus influenzae, et à Neisseria meningitidis et les méningococcémies sans méningite. Du fait des sources de données et des méthodes utilisées pour les estimations, les méningites causées par d'autres bactéries (Listeria, organismes Gram négatifs, etc.) sont incluses dans les estimations de mortalité pour les EMBE, les AESE et l'ALC mais non dans celles des autres régions. Les estimations de l'incidence de toutes les formes de méningite dans toutes les régions sont néanmoins basées uniquement sur les estimations pour les méningites à S. Pneumonia, à H. influenza, et à N. meningitidis. Du fait que les autres formes de méningite sont moins communes, cette inconsistance ne devrait pas confondre les résultats de manière importante.

IA7 Hépatite B et hépatite C—A cause des limitations des tabulations de base de la CIM-9 pour l'hépatite virale, les estimations de la mortalité de l'hépatite B et C dans les EMBE, les AESE, et l'ALC incluent un nombre limité de décès dûs à l'hépatite A. Les cirrhoses symptomatiques (IA7-2) et les hépatomes (IA7-3) attribués à l'hépatite B sont basés sur l'estimation de la fraction attribuable des cirrhoses symptomatiques (II.I2-1) et des hépatomes (IIA5-1) que l'on pense être causés par l'hépatite B.

IA8 Paludisme—L'anémie (IA8-2) est définie selon les critères de l'OMS pour les anémies légères à très graves. Les séquelles neurologiques du paludisme cérébral (IA8-3) incluent l'hémiplégie, l'aphasie, l'ataxie, et la cécité corticale.

IA9b Maladie de Chagas—Tous les décès en rapport avec la maladie de Chagas sont donnés avec le tableau de la prévalence de l'infection (IA9b-1). L'information disponibles ne nous a pas permis de distinguer entre les décès dus à l'infection aiguë, à l'insuffisance cardiaque, et à la mégaviscerose. Afin d'indiquer cette lacune d'information, les colonnes des décès pour la cardiomyopathie sans insuffisance cardiaque congestive (IA9b-2), la cardiomyopathie avec insuffisance cardiaque congestive (IA9b-3), et la mégaviscérose (IA9b-4) indiquent un '–' pour la mortalité.

IA9c Schistosomiase—Les estimations ont été faites uniquement pour la prévalence de l'infection et la mortalité directement associée à la schistosomiase. Nous n'avons pas inclus les estimations de la mortalité dûs au cancer de la vessie, à la cirrhose du foie, ou au cancer du colon qui pourrait être en rapport avec la schistosomiase.

IA9d Leishmaniose—Par convenance tous les décès en rapport avec la leishmaniose sont rapportés dans le tableau de la leishmaniose viscérale (IA9d-1).

IA9e Filariose lymphatique—En accord avec le chapitre analysant la filariose lymphatique, nous avons estimé que peu ou pas de décès du tout étaient directement dûs à la filariose. Il se peut que cette approche sous-estime les effets de l'infection aiguë à filariose.

IA10 Lèpre—Le tableau (IA10-1) donne l'incidence et la prévalence des cas selon la définition de l'OMS. La prévalence est la prévalence d'individus qui remplissent les critères de définition des cas selon l'OMS qui n'est pas équivalente à la prévalence d'individus avec une lèpre clinique. Les taux de prévalence donnés pour la lèpre débilitante (IA10-2) sont des estimations de la prévalence réelle de l'invalidité causée par la lèpre.

IA11 Dengue—La dengue n'était pas incluse dans les Versions 3 et 4 de l'Etude de la Charge Globale des Maladies. Les estimations ont été faites uniquement pour la fièvre hémorragique de la dengue (IA11-1). Jusqu'à maintenant il n'existe pas d'estimations globales ou régionales de toutes les formes de la dengue.

IA12 Encéphalite japonaise—Tous les décès dûs à l'encéphalite japonaise sont rapportés avec les épisodes (IA12-1).

IA14a Ascaridose—Le tableau sur l'infection de forte intensité à ascaris (IA14a-1) donne des estimations de la prévalence d'infections dépassant 10 vers chez les enfants de 0–4 ans, 15 vers chez ceux de 5–9 ans et 20 vers au dessus de l'âge de 20 ans. Nous n'avons pas développé d'estimations de l'incidence de l'infection intense. Les décès directement attribuables à l'infection ascaridienne sont donnés avec l'incidence et la prévalence de l'obstruction intestinale (IA14a-4) du fait que celle-ci est considérée comme étant le mécanisme principal de mortalité directement attribuable. Le «déficit cognitif simultané» (IA14a-2) est un terme utilisé par Bundy et al. (1996) pour désigner les déficits cognitifs qui sont fonction de la charge actuelle de vers et qui ne sont pas dûs à des retards de développement causés par une charge élevée de vers préalable. Le terme «déficience cognitive» (IA14a-3) désigne des changements permanents causés par une charge élevée de vers pendant l'enfance et l'adolescence.

IA14b Tricocéphalose—Le tableau sur l'infection de forte intensité (IA14b-1) donne des estimations de la prévalence d'infections dépassant 90 vers chez les enfants de 0–4 ans, 130 vers chez ceux de 5–9 ans et 180 vers au dessus de l'âge de 20 ans. Nous n'avons pas développé d'estimations de l'incidence de l'infection de forte intensité. Les décès directement attribuables à l'infection à la tricocéphalose sont donnés avec l'incidence et la prévalence du syndrome dysentérique massif avec obstruction intestinale du fait que celui-ci est considéré comme étant le mécanisme principal de la mortalité directement attribuable. Le «déficit cognitif simultané» (IA14b-2) est un terme utilisé par Bundy et al. (1996) pour désigner les déficits cognitifs qui sont fonction de la charge actuelle de vers et qui ne sont pas dûs à des retards de développement causés par une charge élevée de vers préalable. Le terme «déficience cognitive» (IA14b-4) désigne les changements permanents causés par une charge élevée de vers pendant l'enfance et l'adolescence.

IA14c Ankylostomiase et néctariose—Le tableau sur l'infection de forte intensité (IA14c-1) donne des estimations de la prévalence d'infections dépassant 20 vers chez les enfants de 0–4 ans, 30 vers chez ceux de 5–9 ans et 40 vers au dessus de l'âge de 20 ans. Nous n'avons pas développé d'estimations de l'incidence de l'infection de forte intensité. Les décès directement attribuables à l'ankylostomiase et à la nectarisose sont rapportées l'incidence et la prévalence de l'infection.

IB2 Infections des voies respiratoires inférieures—Les séquelles chroniques (IB2-2) incluent les bronchectasies et les altérations de la fonction pulmonaire mesurées par une diminution du VEF_1. Bien que ces séquelles puissent sans doute causer la mort, la magnitude de cette mortalité n'a pas été estimée. Dans les tabulations primaires de mortalité de l'Etude de la Charge Globale des Maladies, elles étaient rapportées avec d'autres infections respiratoires chroniques (IIH).

IB3 Otite moyenne—Les *Episodes* (IB3-1) désignent les épisodes d'otite moyenne aiguë.

IC1 Hémorragie maternelle—Par convenance, tous les décès directement attribuables à une hémorragie maternelle sont rapportés avec l'incidence de l'hémorragie maternelle (IC1-1).

IC3 Troubles hypertensifs de la grossesse—Cette catégorie inclut la pré-éclampsie et l'éclampsie. La mortalité donnée dans le tableau de l'incidence et de la prévalence des épisodes (IC3-1) représente le total dû aux troubles hypertensifs de la grossesse, y compris l'éclampsie.

ID Affections de la période périnatale —Une erreur commune est de confondre les affections de la période périnatale qui comprennent une constellation particulière de causes de décès survenant au cours de la première semaine de vie d'un nouveau-né avec la mortalité périnatale qui est le taux de mortalité entre la 28ème semaine de gestation et la quatrième semaine après la naissance.

ID1 Poids insuffisant à la naissance—Cette catégorie comprends les nouveaux-nés de poids insuffisant à la naissance, et les prématurés. L'ensemble des séquelles au niveau du développement à la suite d'un poids insuffisant à la naissance a été regroupé en une seule issue qui inclut la paralysie infantile, l'épilepsie, et les déficits visuels et auditifs (ID1-1). Cette approche diffère de celle adoptée pour de nombreuses autres maladies dans cette étude. Shibuya et al. (1996) explique en détail les raisons de ce choix, largement basé sur la nature des études de cohorte qui ont été entreprises. Dans cette étude le terme «périnatal» désigne les affections de la période périnatale. Les cas incidents n'incluent pas ceux qui décèdent peu après la naissance.

ID2 Asphyxie néonatale et traumatismes de l'accouchement—L'ensemble des séquelles au niveau du développement dues à une asphyxie néonatale ou à un traumatisme de l'accouchement a été regroupé en une seule issue qui inclut la paralysie infantile, l'épilepsie, et les déficits visuels et auditifs (ID2-1). Cette approche diffère de celle adoptée pour de nombreuses autres maladies dans cette étude. Shibuya et al. (1996) explique en détail les raisons de ce choix, largement basé sur la nature des études de cohorte qui ont été entreprises. Les cas incidents n'incluent pas ceux qui décèdent peu après la naissance.

IE1 Malnutrition protéino-calorique—l'insuffisance pondéral (IE1-1) inclut la prévalence des enfants ayant un rapport poids/taille plus de 2 déviations standards au-dessous de la moyenne NCHS de la population de référence. Le retard de croissance (IE1-2) inclut la prévalence des enfants qui ont un rapport taille/âge plus de 2 déviations standards au-dessous de la moyenne pour la population de référence NCHS. De nombreux enfants ayant une insuffisance pondéral peuvent également avoir une insuffisance staturale, et vice-versa. Le même enfant peut ainsi apparaître dans les tableaux d'insuffisance pondéral et dans celles du d'insuffisance staturale. Par convenance, nous avons arbitrairement choisi de présenter la mortalité directement attribuable à la malnutrition protéino-calorique dans le tableau l'insuffisance pondéral (IE1-1). La malnutrition est vraisemblablement un facteur de risque pour la mortalité due à de nombreuses autres causes telles les affections diarrhéiques et respiratoires. Référez vous à Mason et al. (1996) pour l'analyse de la mortalité associée à la malnutrition chez les enfants en-dessous de 5 ans. Nous avons arbitrairement choisi de ne pas estimer l'insuffisance pondéral et l'insuffisance staturale chez les adultes.

IE2 Déficience en iode—Par convenance, nous avons arbitrairement choisi de présenter la mortalité directement attribuable à la déficience en iode dans la tableau sur le crétinisme (IE2-6); le goitre de Grade 2 et le crétinoidisme peuvent aussi contribuer à l'estimation totale de la mortalité due à la déficience en iode. Les crétinoïdes (IE2-5) sont définis par une perte bilatérale de la perception auditive, un retard psychomoteur, et un développement intellectuel déficitaire. Le goitre de Grade 0 (IE2-1) n'est ni palpable, ni visible en position normale, le goitre de Grade 1 (IE2-2) est palpable mais n'est pas visible en position normale, et le goitre de Grade 2 (IE2-3) est visible en position normale.

IE3 Avitaminose A—La xérophtalmie (IE3-1) inclut toutes les manifestations oculaires de l'avitaminose A: cécité nocturne, taches de Bitot, xérose de la cornée, ulcération de la cornée et cicatrices de la cornée. Les cicatrices de la cornée (IE3-2) ne sont pas synonymes de cécité. Les décès directement dûs à une avitaminose A n'ont pas été ventilés selon la cause—ceux dûs aux cicatrices de la cornée et ceux dûs à d'autres formes d'avitaminose A. L'avitaminose A est un facteur de risque probable pour la mortalité due à d'autres causes, telles les affections diarrhéiques et respiratoires. Veuillez vous référer à Murray et Lopez (1996b) pour les estimations de la mortalité associée à une avitaminose A.

IE4 Anémie ferriprive—la mortalité directement attribuable à l'anémie ferriprive est donnée avec la prévalence de toutes les formes d'anémie ferriprive

(IE4-1); la mortalité n'a pas été ventilée selon les décès attribuables à des anémies ferriprives légère, modérée, grave et très grave. Une anémie légère (IE4-2) chez la femme enceinte correspond à une hémoglobine de 100–109 g/l; de 110–119 g/l chez l'enfant et la femme adulte, et de 120–129 g/l chez l'homme adulte. Une anémie modérée (IE4-3) chez la femme enceinte correspond à une hémoglobine de 70–99 g/l; de 80–109 g/l chez l'enfant et la femme adulte, et de 90–119 g/l chez l'homme adulte. Une anémie grave (IE4-4) chez la femme enceinte correspond à une hémoglobine de 40–69 g/l; de 50–79 g/l chez l'enfant et la femme adulte, et de 60–89 g/l chez l'homme adulte. Une anémie très grave (IE4-5) chez la femme enceinte correspond à une hémoglobine de <40 g/l; de <50 g/l chez l'enfant et la femme adulte, et de <60 g/l chez l'homme adulte.

IIA Tumeurs malignes—Pour toutes les tumeurs malignes, un cas de cancer a par convention été considéré comme restant un cas jusqu'à ce qu'il ait survécu 5 ans à partir du début. Tout cas survivant au-delà de 5 ans a été considéré guéri lorsqu'il s'agissait de définir la prévalence.

IIC Diabète sucré—Par convenance nous avons arbitrairement choisi de présenter la mortalité directement attribuable au diabète sucré dans le tableau de l'incidence et de la prévalence du diabète même (IIC-1). Les cas de diabète sucré (IIC-1) comprennent le diabète insulino-dépendant (IDDM) et le diabète non insulino-dépendant (NIDDM). Les individus souffrant de diabète sucré ont un risque relatif élevé de décès à la suite de maladies cardio-vasculaires et d'autres causes—référez vous à McKeigue et King (1996) pour une revue de ces études et à Murray et Lopez (1996a) pour les estimations de la mortalité indirectement attribuable au diabète sucré.

IIE1 Dépression unipolaire majeure—La dépression unipolaire majeure peut être analysée comme une maladie épisodique ou comme une condition chronique qui dure toute la vie avec une symptomatologie intermittente. Suivant le consensus des psychiatres qui ont révisé cette étude, nous avons choisi de présenter les estimations de l'incidence et de la prévalence pour les épisodes dépressifs majeurs.

IIE5 Usage d'alcool—Les décès comprennent les décès directement liés à la dépendance alcoolique, l'usage d'alcool sans dépendance, et la psychose alcoolique.

IIE6 Démence et autres maladies dégénératives et héréditaires du SNC—A la suite de manque de place, le nom a été abrégé à Démence dans le tableau 168. La grande majorité des cas inclus dans cette catégorie sont dûs à la maladie d'Alzheimer mais certains décès survenant à des âges plus jeunes sont dûs à d'autres conditions telles la chorée de Huntington, etc.

IIE9 Usage de drogues—Les décès incluent les décès directement attribués à l'usage de drogues et les estimations d'incidence et de prévalence se rapportent aux usagers de drogues disfonctionnel et nocif (IIE9-1). Pour le calcul des années de vie perdues à la suite d'un décès prématuré (YLD), nous avons supposé que la durée était d'un an et que l'incidence était égale à la prévalence.

IIF1 Glaucome—La cécité liée au glaucome (IIF1-1) comprend le glaucome primaire à angle fermé et le glaucome primaire à angle ouvert. Il n'y a pas de chapitre sur le glaucome dans la *Série sur la Charge Globale des Maladies et Traumatismes*; les données rapportées ici et celles utilisées pour calculer YLD (années de vie perdues à la suite d'invalidité) pour le glaucome furent basées sur une revue de sources d'information publiées et non publiées mises à disposition par l'Organisation Mondiale de la Santé. Dans toutes les régions hormis la China, aucun décès n'est attribué directement au glaucome bien qu'il existe des articles dans la littérature montrant que le risque relatif de décès d'un aveugle comparativement à une personne du même âge ayant la vue est supérieur à 1. En Chine, le système des Points de Surveillance des Maladies assigne un petit nombre de décès au glaucome. Nous avons choisi d'inclure ces décès dans les tabulations.

IIF2 Cataractes—Dans toutes les régions hormis la Chine, aucun décès n'est attribué directement à la cataracte bien qu'il existe des articles dans la littérature montrant que le risque relatif de décès d'un aveugle comparativement à une personne du même âge ayant la vue est supérieur à 1. En Chine, le système des Points de Surveillance des Maladies assigne un petit nombre de décès à la cataracte. Nous avons choisi d'inclure ces décès dans les tabulations.

IIG1 Cardiopathie rhumatismale —Seule la séquelle majeure des cardiopathies rhumatismales, l'insuffisance cardiaque congestive, a été évaluée. Les estimations de l'incidence du rhumatisme articulaire aigu n'ont pas été faites et ne sont pas présentées.

IIG2 Cardiopathie ischémique—Par convenance, nous avons arbitrairement choisi de présenter la mortalité directement attribuable à la cardiopathie ischémique dans la tableau de l'infarctus aigu du myocarde (IIG2-1). Les taux relatifs à l'infarctus aigu du myocarde sont basés sur les définition de MONICA (Beaglehole et al. 1996). Dans le tableau pour l'angine de poitrine (IIG2-2), des '0' sont donnés pour la mortalité; nous supposons que tous les individus décédant de cardiopathie ischémique décèdent d'infarctus aigu du myocarde ou d'insuffisance cardiaque congestive. Le tableau sur l'insuffisance cardiaque congestive (IIG2-3) montre '–' pour les décès du fait que tous les décès dûs à une cardiopathie ischémique sont arbitrairement rapportés avec l'infarctus aigu du myocarde.

IIG3 Maladie cérébrovasculaire—Les données d'incidence se rapportent aux premiers accidents vasculaire cérébral (IIG3-1) et n'incluent pas le taux des accidents cérébrales récidivantes. Les estimations de prévalence sont la prévalence d'avoir eu une fois un accident cérébral; elles comprennent les victimes d'accidents cérébraux, dont approximativement le tiers ne cause aucune invalidité résiduelle. Les estimations de l'incidence pour les moins de 15 ans n'incluent pas les épisodes d'attaque cérébral dont l'issue n'est pas fatale.

IIG4 Maladies cardiaques inflammatoires—Cette catégorie inclut la myocardite (IIG4-1). La péricardite (IIG4-2), l'endocardite (IIG4-3) et les cardiomyopathies (IIG4-4). Pour chacune de ces conditions nous avons estimé l'incidence et la prévalence des cas symptomatiques. Pour les myocardites (IIG4-1) et les cardiomyopathies (IIG4-4), l'issue symptomatique principale est l'insuffisance cardiaque congestive.

IIH1 Maladie pulmonaire obstructive chronique—Pour cette étude, les cas symptomatiques (IIH1-1) ont été définis comme ayant un VEF$_1$ inférieur à 1 litre, ce qui concorde bien avec l'occurrence de symptômes significatifs. Les tabulations incluses dans ce volume ne comprennent pas le petit nombre de cas incidents et de décès survenant chez ceux de moins de 15 ans.

IIH2 Asthme—Les estimations de l'incidence et de la prévalence se réfèrent aux individus souffrant d'asthme et non aux épisodes d'asthme aigu.

II.I1 Ulcère peptique—Les estimations de l'incidence et de la prévalence se réfèrent aux individus ayant un ulcère peptique, dont la plupart souffre de symptômes intermittents et récurrents.

II.I2 Cirrhose de foie—Les estimations de l'incidence et de la prévalence se réfèrent aux individus ayant une cirrhose symptomatique (II.I2-1).

IIJ1 Néphrites et Néphroses—L'analyse de ce grand groupe de conditions a été entrepris pour deux agrégats, les glomerulonéphrites aiguës/néphrose (IIJ1-1) et les maladies rénales terminales (IIJ1-2).

IIJ2 Hypertrophie bénigne de la prostate—Les estimations sont données pour les individus ayant quelques symptômes dûs à l'hypertrophie bénigne de la prostate, bien que ceux-ci soient intermittents (IIJ2-1). La prévalence de l'hypertrophie de la prostate est beaucoup plus élevée mais de nombreux individus n'ont pas encore de symptômes. Les taux de prévalence sont en général plus élevés dans les régions en voie de développement du fait que les traitements qui améliorent les symptômes, tels que la prostatectomie transurétrale, sont beaucoup moins répandus.

IIL1 Arthrite rhumatoïde—Le tableau pour les cas d'arthrite rhumatoïde (IIL1-1) inclut les décès directement attribués à l'arthrite rhumatoïde. De plus, il existe une évidence que les individus souffrant d'arthrite rhumatoïde ont un risque relatif plus élevé de décès d'autres causes (Symmons 1996); voir Murray et Lopez (1996b) pour les estimations de mortalité indirecte.

IIL2 Ostéoarthrite—Moins de 500 décès globalement sont attribués directement à l'ostéoarthrite. Du fait du petit nombre de décès et de la difficulté d'attribuer ces décès à l'ostéoarthrite de la hanche ou du genou, les tableaux pour l'ostéoarthrite de la hanche (IIL2-1) et pour l'ostéoarthrite du genou (IIL2-2) n'indiquent pas de décès dûs à l'ostéoarthrite.

IIM Anomalies congénitales—Les taux d'incidence indiqués pour toutes les anomalies congénitales sont en réalité le nombre d'enfants vivants nés avec une anomalie congénitale divisé par la population à mi-année de 0–4 ans. Les lecteurs intéressés aux prévalences à la naissance de ces anomalies congénitales devraient diviser les nombres de cas incidents par le nombre de naissances vivantes dans chaque région en 1990.

IIM4 Bec de lièvre—Les estimations de prévalence données se rapportent aux individus qui ont subit une correction chirurgicale. Dans le calcul des années de vie perdues à la suite d'une invalidité (YLD), une pondération différente a été utilisée pour les individus qui ont eu une correction chirurgicale de celle utilisée pour ceux qui n'ont pas eu de correction chirurgicale.

IIM5 Fissure du palais—Les estimations de prévalence données se rapportent aux individus qui ont subit une correction chirurgicale. Dans le calcul des années de vie perdues à la suite d'une invalidité (YLD), une pondération différente a été utilisée pour les individus qui ont eu une correction chirurgicale de celle utilisée pour ceux qui n'ont pas eu de correction chirurgicale.

IIN1 Caries dentaires—Les taux d'incidence et de prévalence sont donnés par personne, et non par dent, quadrant ou sextant.

III Traumatismes—Du fait que les bases de données utilisées pour estimer les taux d'incidence et de prévalence des traumatismes ont été établies à partir de la provision de soins, notre définition d'incidence pour chaque traumatisme est un traumatisme qui soit suffisamment grave pour nécessiter une attention médicale ou qui entraîne immédiatement la mort. Autrement dit, les traumatismes suffisamment graves sont ceux pour lesquels tout individu ayant accès à un service médical demanderait de l'attention. Pour chaque cause de traumatisme dans l'Etude de la Charge Globale de Maladies, nous avons estimé l'incidence et la prévalence de 40 types de traumatismes spécifiques, y compris la distinction entre les conséquences à court et long terme pour un certain nombre de conditions telles la fracture du fémur. Dans les tableaux de ce livre, nous donnons des estimations des 5 séquelles qui contribuent le plus à la charge d'invalidité de chacune des causes de traumatisme. Les empoisonnements ont seulement une séquelle et les noyades deux. A partir des bases de données disponibles nous avons évalué les 40 types possibles de traumatismes pour les suicides mais pour les tentatives de suicide nous avons choisi de présenter seulement ceux qui demandent une attention médicale. Pour chaque traumatisme un tableau libellée épisodes donne seulement les taux d'incidence et les nombres, ceci du fait que la prévalence d'évènements tels que les accidents de la voie publique ou les incendies n'a pas de signification. Les tableaux se rapportant à chacune des séquelles donnent toutefois des estimations de l'incidence et de la prévalence.

IIIAI Accidents de la voie publique—Tous les accidents incluent des collisions, ou des traumatismes de piétons causés par des véhicules à moteur.

IIIA2 Empoisonnements—Seule une issue est incluse pour les empoisonnements.

IIIA4 Incendies—La plupart des séquelles d'incendies sont dues à des brûlures. Certains individus, toutefois, sautent d'immeubles en feu ou subissent d'autres traumatismes causés par des incendies.

IIIA5 Noyades—En plus des taux de noyades ou semi-noyades (IIIA5-1), la seule séquelle invalidante incluse dans cette étude est la quadriplégie. (IIIA5-2).

IIIA6 Autres traumatismes non-intentionnels—Contrairement aux autres catégories résiduelles incluses dans l'Etude de la Charge Globale des Maladies, pour les autres traumatismes non-intentionnels il existe des données relatives à la distribution des différents types de séquelles qui constituent la base des estimations rapportées ici (Lozano et al. 1996).

IIIB1 Auto-infligés—Les taux d'incidence (IIIB1) se rapportent aux tentatives de suicide.

IIIB3 Guerre—L'incidence des traumatismes et de la mortalité à la suite de guerres comprend les décès directement attribuables à la guerre chez les non-combattants. Par exemple, les estimations de la mortalité incluent les décès chez des enfants et des adultes dûs à des mines.

BIBLIOGRAPHY

Abou-Zahr C (1996a) Haemorrhage. In: Murray CJL, Lopez AD, eds. *Health dimensions of sex and reproduction: the global burden of sexually transmitted diseases, HIV, maternal conditions, perinatal disorders and congenital anomalies.* Cambridge, Harvard University Press.

Abou-Zahr C (1996b) Obstructed labour. In: Murray CJL, Lopez AD, eds. *Health dimensions of sex and reproduction: the global burden of sexually transmitted diseases, HIV, maternal conditions, perinatal disorders and congenital anomalies.* Cambridge, Harvard University Press.

Abou-Zahr C, Ähman E (1996) Abortion. In: Murray CJL, Lopez AD, eds. *Health dimensions of sex and reproduction: the global burden of sexually transmitted diseases, HIV, maternal conditions, perinatal disorders and congenital anomalies.* Cambridge, Harvard University Press.

Abou-Zahr C, Guidotti R (1996a) Maternal sepsis. In: Murray CJL, Lopez AD, eds. *Health dimensions of sex and reproduction: the global burden of sexually transmitted diseases, HIV, maternal conditions, perinatal disorders and congenital anomalies.* Cambridge, Harvard University Press.

Abou-Zahr C, Guidotti R (1996b) Hypertensive disorders of pregnancy. In: Murray CJL, Lopez AD, eds. *Health dimensions of sex and reproduction: the global burden of sexually transmitted diseases, HIV, maternal conditions, perinatal disorders and congenital anomalies.* Cambridge, Harvard University Press.

Andrews G (1996) Anxiety disorders. In: Murray CJL, Lopez AD, eds. *Neuropsychiatric disorders and global health: the epidemiology of schizophrenia, dementia, substance abuse, epilepsy and affective, neurotic and stress-related disorders.* Cambridge, Harvard University Press.

Ashley R et al. (1996) Appendicitis. In: Murray CJL, Lopez AD, eds. *Global perspectives on non-communicable diseases: the epidemiology of cancers, cardiovascular diseases, diabetes mellitus, respiratory disorders and other major conditions.* Cambridge, Harvard University Press.

Bailey K (1996) Iodine deficiency. In: Murray CJL, Lopez AD, eds. *Malnutrition and the burden of disease: the global epidemiology of protein-energy malnutrition, anaemias and vitamin deficiencies.* Cambridge, Harvard University Press.

Bailey K, Abou-Zahr C (1996) Anaemia. In: Murray CJL, Lopez AD, eds. *Malnutrition and the burden of disease: the global epidemiology of protein-energy malnutrition, anaemias and vitamin deficiencies.* Cambridge, Harvard University Press.

Bailey K, de Onis M, Bloessner M (1996) Protein energy malnutrition. In: Murray CJL, Lopez AD, eds. *Malnutrition and the burden of disease: the global epidemiology of protein-energy malnutrition, anaemias and vitamin deficiencies.* Cambridge, Harvard University Press.

Barmes D (1996) Oral health. In: Murray CJL, Lopez AD, eds. *Global perspectives on non-communicable diseases: the epidemiology of cancers, cardiovascular diseases, diabetes mellitus, respiratory disorders and other major conditions.* Cambridge, Harvard University Press.

Beaglehole R et al. (1996) Ischaemic heart disease. In: Murray CJL, Lopez AD, eds. *Global perspectives on non-communicable diseases: the epidemiology of cancers, cardiovascular diseases, diabetes mellitus, respiratory disorders and other major conditions.* Cambridge, Harvard University Press.

Bern C et al. (1996) Diarrhoea. In: Murray CJL, Lopez AD, eds. *The global epidemiology of infectious diseases.* Cambridge, Harvard University Press.

Bonita R et al. (1996) Cerebrovascular disease. In: Murray CJL, Lopez AD, eds. *Global perspectives on non-communicable diseases: the epidemiology of cancers, cardiovascular diseases, diabetes mellitus, respiratory disorders and other major conditions.* Cambridge, Harvard University Press.

Bundy D et al. (1996) Intestinal nematodes. In: Murray CJL, Lopez AD, eds. *The global epidemiology of infectious diseases.* Cambridge, Harvard University Press.

Clements CJ, Hussey GD (1996) Measles. In: Murray CJL, Lopez AD, eds. *The global epidemiology of infectious diseases.* Cambridge, Harvard University Press.

Cook C et al. (1996) Drowning. In: Murray CJL, Lopez AD, eds. *The global burden of injuries: mortality and disability from suicide, violence, war, and unintentional injuries.* Cambridge, Harvard University Press.

Daumerie DPJ (1996) Leprosy. In: Murray CJL, Lopez AD, eds. *The global epidemiology of infectious diseases.* Cambridge, Harvard University Press.

Desjeux PMP (1996) Leishmaniasis. In: Murray CJL, Lopez AD, eds. *The global epidemiology of infectious diseases.* Cambridge, Harvard University Press.

Donoghoe M et al. (1996) Drug use. In: *Neuro-psychiatric disorders and global health: the epidemiology of schizophrenia, dementia, substance abuse, epilepsy and affective, neurotic and stress-related disorders.* Cambridge, Harvard University Press.

Fullerton C et al. (1996) Falls. In: Murray CJL, Lopez AD, eds. *The global burden of injuries: mortality and disability from suicide, violence, war, and unintentional injuries.* Cambridge, Harvard University Press.

Gakidou E et al. (1996a) Cirrhosis. In: Murray CJL, Lopez AD, eds. *Global perspectives on non-communicable diseases: the epidemiology of cancers, cardiovascular diseases, diabetes mellitus, respiratory disorders and other major conditions.* Cambridge, Harvard University Press.

Gakidou E et al. (1996b) Chronic obstructive pulmonary disease. In: Murray CJL, Lopez AD, eds. *Global perspectives on non-communicable diseases: the epidemiology of cancers, cardiovascular diseases, diabetes mellitus, respiratory disorders and other major conditions.* Cambridge, Harvard University Press.

Galazka A (1996a) Diphtheria. In: Murray CJL, Lopez AD, eds. *The global epidemiology of infectious diseases.* Cambridge, Harvard University Press.

Galazka A (1996b) Pertussis. In: Murray CJL, Lopez AD, eds. *The global epidemiology of infectious diseases.* Cambridge, Harvard University Press.

Galazka A, Gasse FL, Torel CA (1996) Tetanus. In: Murray CJL, Lopez AD, eds. *The global epidemiology of infectious diseases.* Cambridge, Harvard University Press.

Goodreau S et al. (1996) Fires. In: Murray CJL, Lopez AD, eds. *The global burden of injuries: mortality and disability from suicide, violence, war, and un-intentional injuries.* Cambridge, Harvard University Press.

Government of India, Registrar-General (1992a) *Mortality statistics of causes of death.* New Delhi, Government of India.

Government of India, Registrar-General (1992b) *Survey of causes of death (rural). Annual report, 1990.* New Delhi, Government of India.

Greenwood M (1948) *Medical statistics from Graunt to Farr. The Fitzpatrick Lectures for the years 1941 and 1943.* Cambridge, Cambridge University Press.

Hakulinen T et al. (1986) Global and regional mortality patterns by cause of death in 1980. *International journal of epidemiology,* 15:226-233.

Hill K, Yazbeck A (1994) *Trends in child mortality, 1960-90: estimates for 84 developing countries.* (The World Bank World Development Report 1993: Investing in Health. Background Paper Series, No.6).

Hull TH et al. (1981) A framework for estimating causes of death in Indonesia. *Majalah demografi Indonesia,* 15:77-125.

Kane M, Schatz G, Hadler S (1996) Hepatitis B. In: Murray CJL, Lopez AD, eds. *The global epidemiology of infectious diseases.* Cambridge, Harvard University Press.

Kumaresan J et al. (1996) Tuberculosis. In: Murray CJL, Lopez AD, eds. *The global epidemiology of infectious diseases.* Cambridge, Harvard University Press.

LeDuc J, Esteves K, Glatz N (1996) Dengue haemorrhagic fever. In: Murray CJL, Lopez AD, eds. *The global epidemiology of infectious diseases.* Cambridge, Harvard University Press.

de L'Horne DJ (1996) Post-traumatic stress disorder. In: Murray CJL, Lopez AD, eds. *Neuro-psychiatric disorders and global health: the epidemiology of schizophrenia, dementia, substance abuse, epilepsy and affective, neurotic and stress-related disorders.* Cambridge, Harvard University Press.

Lob-Levyt J, Arthur P, Gove S (1996) Respiratory infections. In: Murray CJL, Lopez AD, eds. *The global epidemiology of infectious diseases.* Cambridge, Harvard University Press.

Lopez AD et al. (1996) Alcohol use. In: Murray CJL, Lopez AD, eds. *Neuro-psychiatric disorders and global health: the epidemiology of schizophrenia, dementia, substance abuse, epilepsy and affective, neurotic and stress-related disorders.* Cambridge, Harvard University Press.

Lopez AD, Hull TH (1983) A note on estimating the cause of death structure in high mortality populations. *Population bulletin of the United Nations,* 14:66-70.

Low-Beer D et al. (1996) HIV. In: Murray CJL, Lopez AD, eds. *Health dimensions of sex and reproduction: the global burden of sexually transmitted diseases, HIV, maternal conditions, perinatal disorders, and congenital anomalies.* Cambridge, Harvard University Press.

Lozano R (1996) Inflammatory heart disease. In: Murray CJL, Lopez AD, eds. *Global perspectives on non-communicable diseases: the epidemiology of cancers, cardiovascular diseases, diabetes mellitus, respiratory disorders and other major conditions.* Cambridge, Harvard University Press.

Mahapatra P et al. (1996a) Asthma. In: Murray CJL, Lopez AD, eds. *Global perspectives on non-communicable diseases: the epidemiology of cancers, cardiovascular diseases, diabetes mellitus, respiratory disorders and other major conditions.* Cambridge, Harvard University Press.

Mahapatra P et al. (1996b) Peptic ulcer disease. In: Murray CJL, Lopez AD, eds. *Global perspectives on non-communicable diseases: the epidemiology of cancers, cardiovascular diseases, diabetes mellitus, respiratory disorders and other major conditions.* Cambridge, Harvard University Press.

Mason JB et al. (1996) Undernutrition. In: Murray CJL, Lopez AD, eds. *Malnutrition and the burden of disease: the global epidemiology of protein-energy malnutrition, anaemias and vitamin deficiencies.* Cambridge, Harvard University Press.

McKeigue P, King H (1996) Diabetes mellitus. In: Murray CJL, Lopez AD, eds. *Global perspectives on non-communicable diseases: the epidemiology of cancers, cardiovascular diseases, diabetes mellitus, respiratory disorders and other major conditions.* Cambridge, Harvard University Press.

Michael E, Bundy D (1996) Lymphatic filariasis. In: Murray CJL, Lopez AD, eds. *The global epidemiology of infectious diseases.* Cambridge, Harvard University Press.

Michaud C (1996) Rheumatic heart disease. In: Murray CJL, Lopez AD, eds. *Global perspectives on non-communicable diseases: the epidemiology of cancers, cardiovascular diseases, diabetes mellitus, respiratory disorders and other major conditions.* Cambridge, Harvard University Press.

Miller AB (1996) Diet and cancer. In: Murray CJL, Lopez AD, eds. *Malnutrition and the burden of disease: the global epidemiology of protein-energy malnutrition, anaemias and vitamin deficiencies.* Cambridge, Harvard University Press.

Moncayo A, Myoshi C (1996) Chagas disease. In: Murray CJL, Lopez AD, eds. *The global epidemiology of infectious diseases.* Cambridge, Harvard University Press.

Mott KE (1996) Schistosomiasis. In: Murray CJL, Lopez AD, eds. *The global epidemiology of infectious diseases.* Cambridge, Harvard University Press.

Murray CJL (1994) Quantifying the burden of disease: the technical basis for disability adjusted life years. *Bulletin of the World Health Organization,* 72(3):429-445.

Murray CJL et al. (1996) Neoplasms. In: Murray CJL, Lopez AD, eds. *Global perspectives on non-communicable diseases: the epidemiology of cancers, cardiovascular diseases, diabetes mellitus, respiratory disorders and other major conditions.* Cambridge, Harvard University Press.

Murray CJL, Lopez AD (1994a) Global and regional cause-of-death patterns in 1990. *Bulletin of the World Health Organization,* 72(3):447-480.

Murray CJL, Lopez AD (1994b) Quantifying disability: data, methods and results. *Bulletin of the World Health Organization,* 72(3):481-494.

Murray CJL, Lopez AD eds. (1994c) *Global comparative assessments in the health sector disease burden, expenditures and intervention packages.* Geneva, World Health Organization.

Murray CJL, Lopez AD (1996a) Alternative visions of the future: projecting mortality and disability 1990-2010. In: Murray CJL, Lopez AD, eds. *The global burden of disease: a comprehensive assessment of mortality and disability from diseases, injuries and risk factors in 1990 and projected to 2020.* Cambridge, Harvard University Press.

Murray CJL, Lopez AD (1996b) Estimating causes of death: new methods with global and regional applications. In: Murray CJL, Lopez AD, eds. *The global burden of disease: a comprehensive assessment of mortality and disability from diseases, injuries and risk factors in 1990 and projected to 2020.* Cambridge, Harvard University Press.

Murray CJL, Lopez AD, Jamison DT (1994) The global burden of disease in 1990: summary results, sensitivity analysis and future directions. *Bulletin of the World Health Organization,* 72(3):495-509.

Murray CJL, Yang G, Qiao X (1992) Adult mortality: levels, patterns and causes. In: Feachem, RGS et al. *The health of adults in the developing world.* Oxford, Oxford University Press, pp. 23-111.

Najera JA et al. (1996) Malaria. In: Murray CJL, Lopez AD, eds. *The global epidemiology of infectious diseases.* Cambridge, Harvard University Press.

Negrel AD, Thylefors B, Pararajasegaram R (1996) Cataract. In: Murray CJL, Lopez AD, eds. *Global perspectives on non-communicable diseases: the epidemiology of cancers, cardiovascular diseases, diabetes mellitus, respiratory disorders and other major conditions.* Cambridge, Harvard University Press.

Orzeszyna M et al. (1996) Nephritis and nephrosis. In: Murray CJL, Lopez AD, eds. *Global perspectives on non-communicable diseases: the epidemiology of cancers, cardiovascular diseases, diabetes mellitus, respiratory disorders and other major conditions.* Cambridge, Harvard University Press.

Peto R et al. (1994) *Mortality from smoking in developed countries 1950-2000. Indirect estimates from national vital statistics.* New York, Oxford University Press.

Preston SH (1976) *Mortality patterns in national populations.* New York, Academic Press.

Pronczuk J, Hong CJ (1996) Poisonings. In: Murray CJL, Lopez AD, eds. *The global burden of injuries: mortality and disability from suicide, violence, war, and unintentional injuries.* Cambridge, Harvard University Press.

Regier DA (1996) Schizophrenia. In: Murray CJL, Lopez AD, eds. *Neuro-psychiatric disorders and global health: the epidemiology of schizophrenia, dementia, substance abuse, epilepsy and affective, neurotic and stress-related disorders.* Cambridge, Harvard University Press.

Remme H (1996) Onchocerciasis. In: Murray CJL, Lopez AD, eds. *The global epidemiology of infectious diseases.* Cambridge, Harvard University Press.

Reynolds EH et al. (1996) Epilepsy. In: Murray CJL, Lopez AD, eds. *Neuropsychiatric disorders and global health: the epidemiology of schizophrenia, dementia, substance abuse, epilepsy and affective, neurotic and stress-related disorders.* Cambridge, Harvard University Press.

Ritchie K et al. (1996) Dementia. In: Murray CJL, Lopez AD, eds. *Neuro-psychiatric disorders and global health: the epidemiology of schizophrenia, dementia, substance use, epilepsy and affective, neurotic and stress-related disorders.* Cambridge, Harvard University Press.

Ruzicka L, Gakidou E (1996) Suicide. In: Murray CJL, Lopez AD, eds. *The global burden of injuries: mortality and disability from suicide, violence, war, and unintentional injuries.* Cambridge, Harvard University Press.

Sandiford P (1996) Homicide and violence. In: Murray CJL, Lopez AD, eds. *The global burden of injuries: mortality and disability from suicide, violence, war, and unintentional injuries.* Cambridge, Harvard University Press.

Schillinger J, Wenger J, Perkins B (1996) Meningitis. In: Murray CJL, Lopez AD, eds. *The global epidemiology of infectious diseases.* Cambridge, Harvard University Press.

Shibuya K, Murray CJL (1996a) Perinatal disorders: low birth weight. In: Murray CJL, Lopez AD, eds. *Health dimensions of sex and reproduction: the global burden of sexually transmitted diseases, HIV, maternal conditions, perinatal disorders, and congenital anomalies.* Cambridge, Harvard University Press.

Shibuya K, Murray CJL (1996b) Perinatal disorders: birth trauma and asphyxia. In: Murray CJL, Lopez AD, eds. *Health dimensions of sex and reproduction: the global burden of sexually transmitted diseases, HIV, maternal conditions, perinatal disorders, and congenital anomalies.* Cambridge, Harvard University Press.

Shibuya K, Murray CJL (1996c) Congenital anomalies. In: Murray CJL, Lopez AD, eds. *Health dimensions of sex and reproduction: the global burden of sexually transmitted diseases, HIV, maternal conditions, perinatal disorders, and congenital anomalies.* Cambridge, Harvard University Press.

Shibuya K, Murray CJL (1996) Polio. In: Murray CJL, Lopez AD, eds. *The global epidemiology of infectious diseases.* Cambridge, Harvard University Press.

Symmons D (1996) Rheumatoid arthritis, osteoarthritis and lower back pain. In: Murray CJL, Lopez AD, eds. *Global perspectives on non-communicable diseases: the epidemiology of cancers, cardiovascular diseases, diabetes mellitus, respiratory disorders and other major conditions.* Cambridge, Harvard University Press.

Thylefors B (1996) Trachoma. In: Murray CJL, Lopez AD, eds. *The global epidemiology of infectious diseases.* Cambridge, Harvard University Press.

Timaeus IM (1991) Adult mortality: levels, trends and data sources. In: Feachem RG, Jamison DT, eds. *Disease and mortality in sub-Saharan Africa.* New York, Oxford University Press.

Tsai F (1996) Japanese encephalitis. In: Murray CJL, Lopez AD, eds. *The global epidemiology of infectious diseases.* Cambridge, Harvard University Press.

Underwood B (1996) Vitamin A deficiency. In: Murray CJL, Lopez AD, eds. *Malnutrition and the burden of disease: the global epidemiology of protein-energy malnutrition, anaemias and vitamin deficiencies.* Cambridge, Harvard University Press.

United Nations (1992) *Child mortality since the 1960s. A database for developing countries.* New York, United Nations.

United Nations (1995) *Terminology Bulletin No.347.* ST/CS/SER.F/347 New York, United Nations.

Ustün BT et al. (1996) Depressive disorders. In: Murray CJL, Lopez AD, eds. *Neuro-psychiatric disorders and global health: the epidemiology of schizophrenia, dementia, substance abuse, epilepsy and affective, neurotic and stress-related disorders.* Cambridge, Harvard University Press.

World Bank (1993) *World development report 1993. Investing in Health.* New York, Oxford University Press.

World Bank (1995) *The World Bank Atlas 1995.* Washington, D.C.

Zwi A (1996) War. In: Murray CJL, Lopez AD, eds. *The global burden of injuries: mortality and disability from suicide, violence, war, and unintentional injuries.* Cambridge, Harvard University Press.

Zwi A et al. (1996) Motor vehicle accidents. In: Murray CJL, Lopez AD, eds. *The global burden of injuries: mortality and disability from suicide, violence, war, and unintentional injuries.* Cambridge, Harvard University Press.

Alphabetical List of Tables